Transplant Infections

Transplant Infections

Editors

Raleigh A. Bowden, M.D.
Fred Hutchinson Cancer Research Center
Program in Infectious Diseases
Seattle, Washington

Per Ljungman, M.D., Ph.D.
Associate Professor
Department of Medicine
Huddinge Hospital
Huddinge
Sweden

Carlos V. Paya, M.D., Ph.D.
Department of Infectious Diseases
Immunology and Experimental Pathology
Mayo Clinic
Rochester, Minnesota

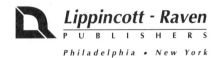
Lippincott - Raven
P U B L I S H E R S
Philadelphia • New York

Acquisitions Editor: Ruth W. Weinberg
Developmental Editor: Ellen DiFrancesco
Manufacturing Manager: Kevin Watt
Production Manager: Robert Pancotti
Production Editor: Jeff Somers
Indexer: Deana Reese Fowler
Compositor: Lippincott–Raven Desktop Division
Printer: Maple Press

Library of Congress Cataloging-in-Publication Data

Transplant infections / editors, Raleigh A. Bowden, Per Ljungman, Carlos V. Paya.
    p.   cm.
    Includes bibliographical references and index.
    ISBN 0-397-58776-7 (alk. paper)
    1. Communicable diseases.   2. Transplantation of organs, tissues, etc.—
Complications.   3. Nosocomial infections.   I. Bowen, Raleigh A.   II. Ljungman, Per.   III. Paya, Carlos V.
    [DNLM: 1. Transplants—adverse effects.   2. Virus Diseases—etiology.
3. Bacterial Infections—etiology.   4. Mycoses—etiology.   WO 660 T7691 1998]
RC112.T73   1998
617.9'5—dc21
DNLM/DLC
For Library of Congress   98-17118
                                                                        CIP

Contents

DIAGNOSTIC TOOLS

Carlos V. Paya, Section Editor

SPECIFIC SITES OF INFECTION

Catherine Cordonnier, Section Editor

BACTERIAL INFECTIONS

Dan Engelhard, Section Editor

VIRAL INFECTIONS

Per Ljungman, Section Editor

FUNGAL INFECTIONS

Raleigh A. Bowden, Section Editor

IMMUNE RECONSTITUTION STRATEGIES FOR PREVENTION AND TREATMENT OF INFECTIONS

John R. Wingard, Section Editor

Contributing Authors

Allen J. Aksamit, M.D.
Associate Professor of Neurology
Mayo Medical School
Department of Neurology
Mayo Clinic
200 First Street SW
Rochester, Minnesota 55905

Robert L. Atmar, M.D.
Department of Medicine
Baylor College of Medicine
Houston, Texas 77030

Michael J. Boeckh, M.D.
Associate in Clinical Research
Program in Infectious Diseases
Fred Hutchinson Cancer Research Center
1100 Fairview Avenue N
Seattle, Washington 98109

Raleigh A. Bowden, M.D.
Fred Hutchinson Cancer Research Center
Program in Infectious Diseases
1124 Columbia Street
Seattle, Washington 98104

Natalie H. Bzowej, M.D., Ph.D.
Gastroenterology Fellow
Department of Gastroenterology
University of California San Francisco
4150 Clement Street, 111B
San Francisco, California 94121

Stephen J. Chanock, M.D.
Senior Staff Fellow
Pediatric Oncology Branch
National Cancer Institute
Immunocompromised Host Section
Building 10
Room 13N-240
Bethesda, Maryland 20892

Gillian S. Clewley, B.Sc., FIMLS
Principal Virologist
Department of Virology
The Royal Free Hospital
Pond Street, Hampstead
London NW3 2QG
United Kingdom

Franklin R. Cockerill III, M.D.
Professor of Microbiology and Laboratory
  Medicine and Pathology and Medicine
Mayo Medical School
Chair, Division of Clinical Microbiology
Mayo Clinic and Foundation
200 First Street SW
Rochester, Minnesota 55905

Sandra M. Cockfield, B.Sc., M.D.
Associate Professor of Medicine
Division of Nephrology and Immunology
Department of Medicine
University of Alberta
11-107D Clinical Sciences Building
8440-112 Street
Edmonton, Alberta T6G 2B7
Canada

Catherine Cordonnier, M.D.
Professor of Hematology
Service D'Hématologie Clinique
Hopital Henri Mondor
51 Avenue du Maréchal de Lattre de Tassigny
94000 Créteil
France

Isabel Cunningham, M.D.
Associate Professor
Department of Medicine
Albert Einstein College of Medicine
1300 Morris Park Avenue
Bronx, New York 10461

David C. Dale, M.D.
Professor of Medicine
Department of Medicine
University of Washington
1959 NE Pacific
Seattle, Washington 98195-6422

Mazen S. Daoud, M.D.
Fellow, Dermatopathology
Department of Dermatology
Mayo Clinic
200 First Street SW
Rochester, Minnesota 55905

H. Joachim Deeg, M.D.
Professor of Medicine
University of Washington
Member
Fred Hutchinson Cancer Research Center
1100 Fairview Avenue North
Seattle, Washington 98109

Ben E. De Pauw, M.D., Ph.D.
Professor of Medicine
Department of Hematology
Blood Transfusion Service
St. Radboud University Hospital
Geert Grooteplein Z6
6525 GA Nijmegen
The Netherlands

J. Stephen Dummer, M.D.
Professor of Medicine
Associate Professor of Surgery
Department of Medicine
Division of Infectious Diseases
Vanderbilt University School of Medicine
911 Oxford House
Nashville, Tennesee 37232

David Emanuel, M.D.
Director, Stem Cell Transplantation Program
Riley Hospital for Children
Professor of Pediatrics
Indiana University School of Medicine
Riley Hospital
702 Barnhill Drive, Room 2600
Indianapolis, Indiana 46202

Vincent C. Emery, Ph.D.
Reader in Virology
Department of Virology
Royal Free Hospital
Rowland Hill Street
London NW3 2PF
United Kingdom

Dan Engelhard, M.D.
Professor
Pediatric Infectious Diseases
Department of Pediatrics
Hadassah University Hospital
Ein Kerem, POB 12000
Jerusalem, 91120
Israel

Janet A. Englund, M.D.
Associate Professor
Departments of Microbiology and Immunology
and Pediatrics
Baylor College of Medicine
One Baylor Plaza
Houston, Texas 77030

Nina Geller, Ph.D.
Investigator, Pediatric Infectious Diseases
Department of Pediatrics
Hadassah University Hospital
Ein Kerem, POB 12000
Jerusalem 91120
Israel

Lawrence E. Gibson, M.D.
Professor of Dermatology
Department of Dermatology
Mayo Clinic
200 First Street SW
Rochester, Minnesota 55905

John W. Gnann, Jr., M.D.
Associate Professor of Medicine
Division of Infectious Diseases
Department of Medicine
University of Alabama at Birmingham
845 19th Street South
Birmingham, Alabama 35294

Michael Green, M.D., M.P.H.
Associate Professor of Pediatrics and Surgery
Division of Allergy, Immunology and
Infectious Diseases
University of Pittsburgh School of Medicine
Children's Hospital of Pittsburgh
3705 Fifth Avenue
Pittsburgh, Pennsylvania 15213

Philip D. Greenberg, M.D.
Professor of Medicine and Immunology
University of Washington and Fred Hutchinson
Cancer Research Center
BB1325 Health Sciences Building
Box 356527
Seattle, Washington 98195-6527

Paul Griffiths, M.D., DSc, FRCPath
Department of Virology
Royal Free Hospital and School of Medicine
Rowland Hill Street
London NW3 2PF
United Kingdom

Barry D. Kahan, M.D., Ph.D.
Professor of Surgery and Director
Division of Immunology and Organ
*   Transplantation*
University of Texas Medical School-Houston
6431 Fannin, Suite 6.240
Houston, Texas 77030

Sharon Krystofiak, M.S.
Infection Control Practitioner
UPMC-Presbyterian
200 Lothrop Street
Pittsburgh, Pennsylvania 15213

Shimon Kusne, M.D.
Associate Professor of Medicine and Surgery
Division of Transplantation Medicine and
*   Division of Infectious Diseases*
University of Pittsburgh
Thomas E. Starzl Transplantation Institute
423 Lhormer Building
3515 Fifth Avenue
Pittsburgh, Pennsylvania 15213

Per Ljungman, M.D., Ph.D.
Head, Department of Hematology
Huddinge University Hospital
S-141 86 Huddinge
Sweden

Marian G. Michaels, M.D., M.P.H.
Associate Professor of Pediatrics and Surgery
Division of Allergy, Immunology and
*   Infectious Diseases*
University of Pittsburgh School of Medicine
Children's Hospital of Pittsburgh
3705 Fifth Avenue
Pittsburgh, Pennsylvania 15213

Robin Patel, M.D.
Assistant Professor of Medicine
Mayo Graduate School of Medicine
Senior Associate Consultant
Division of Infectious Diseases
Mayo Clinic
200 First Street SW
Rochester, Minnesota 55905

Carlos V. Paya, M.D., Ph.D.
Department of Infectious Diseases,
*   Immunology and Experimental Pathology*
Mayo Clinic
200 SW First Street
501 Guggenheim Bldg.
Rochester, Minnesota 55905

Jutta K. Preiksaitis, M.D.
Associate Professor of Medicine
Division of Infectious Diseases
WMC 2B1.03
8440 112th Street
University of Alberta
Edmonton, Alberta T6G 2B7
Canada

Stanley R. Riddell, M.D.
Immunology Program
Fred Hutchinson Cancer Research Center
1124 Columbia Street, M-758
Seattle, Washington 98104

Vivek Roy, M.D., MRCP, MRCPath
Assistant Professor of Medicine
Hematology-Oncology Section
Bone Marrow Transplantation Program
University of Oklahoma Health Science Center
WP 2010
920 SL Young Boulevard
Oklahoma City, OK 73104

Steven M. Standaert, M.D.
The Division of Infectious Diseases
*   Department of Medicine*
The Department of Surgery and
*   The Transplant Center*
Vanderbilt University School of Medicine
Nashville, Tennessee 37232

W.P. Daniel Su, M.D.
Professor of Dermatology
Department of Dermatology
Mayo Clinic
200 First Street SW
Rochester, Minnesota 55905

Jan G. Tollemar, M.D., Ph.D.
Associate Professor of Transplantation
*   Immunology*
Department of Transplantation Surgery
Karolinska Institute
Department of Clinical Immunology
Huddinge University Hospital
S-14186 Huddinge
Sweden

Pablo Troncoso, M.D.
Division of Immunology and
  Organ Transplantation
The University of Texas
  Medical School at Houston
6431 Fannin, Suite 6.240
Houston, Texas 77030

Randall C. Walker, M.D.
Assistant Professor of Medicine
Division of Infectious Diseases and
  Internal Medicine
Mayo Clinic
200 First Street SW
Rochester, Minnesota 55905

Thomas J. Walsh, M.D.
Medical Officer
Infectious Disease Section
Pediatric Branch
National Cancer Institute
National Institute of Health
Building 10, Room 13N240
Bethesda, Maryland 20892

Daniel Weisdorf, M.D.
Professor of Medicine
Division of Hematology
University of Minnesota
Box 480 Mayo
420 Delaware Street SE
Minneapolis, Minnesota 55455

Estella E. Whimbey, M.D.
Director of Clinical Virology
Department of Medical Specialties
The University of Texas
  M.D. Anderson Cancer Center
1515 Holcombe Boulevard, Box 47
Houston, Texas 77030

John R. Wingard, M.D.
Professor of Medicine
Department of Medicine
University of Florida College of Medicine
1600 SW Archer Road
Gainesville, Florida 32610

Teresa L. Wright, M.D.
Chief, Gastroenterology Section
Associate Professor of Medicine
Veterans Affairs Medical Center
Room 1A-13C, G.I. Unit
4150 Clement Street, Bldg. 203-111B
San Francisco, California 94121

Foreword

The last quarter of the twentieth century has witnessed a remarkable explosion in biomedical science, particularly in three important areas: a) the delineation of basic mechanisms of human disease, including quantitative physiology, molecular genetics, and signal transduction pathways; b) the discovery and development of new therapeutic molecules, many of them stemming directly from recombinant technology and the burgeoning of the new field of molecular pharmacology; and c) the deployment of new diagnostic technology, from flow cytometry to polymerase chain reaction to such new imaging modalities as computed tomography, magnetic resonance, and positron emission tomography. It can be effectively argued that the outstanding achievement in clinical application of these basic science advances is in transplantation, both bone marrow and solid organ. Over the last twenty-five years these two forms of treatment have evolved from interesting experiments in human immunobiology to the most practical means of rehabilitating individuals with end-stage kidney, heart, liver, and lung disease, aplastic anemia, certain leukemias and lymphomas, and certain tumors.

One measure of the progress in clinical transplantation is the constant effort to expand the spectrum of disease that can be successfully treated with either solid organ or bone marrow transplantation. Thus, such experimental efforts as small bowel and pancreatic islet transplantation are well launched, as are efforts to expand the range of indications for bone marrow transplantation. Indeed, the very success of transplantation has placed a particular emphasis on the shortage of donors, with long lists of individuals awaiting organs, national searches for histocompatibility matched bone marrow donors established, and an exponentially growing interest in xenotransplantation to assure an adequate supply of donor organs and tissues.

Despite the success being achieved, the two major hurdles to successful transplantation remain unchanged: allograft rejection and graft vs. host disease (GVHD) on the one hand, and infection, especially opportunistic infection, on the other. For many years we have known that these processes are inextricably linked, both modulated by the immunosuppressive therapy being administered. In the past few years this linkage has been shown to be even tighter than previously imagined, as cytokines released in the course of infection or GVHD or allograft rejection have been shown to be quite similar and capable of modulating each other; that is, there is a bidirectional signaling via cytokines that affects both the immunologic events and the infectious disease events. Thus, the long debated question, "Which comes first, infection or rejection?" has been clearly answered: either.

With this recognition, coupled with the frequency of infectious disease syndromes in these patients, the importance of transplantation infectious disease as a field integral to the success of clinical transplantation has been firmly established. This volume has been organized in response to these events, and is meant to serve the medical community at large—not just the transplant physicians and surgeons carrying out these procedures, but also the primary care physicians who increasingly are sharing the responsibility in managing these patients.

The infectious disease challenges facing the clinician charged with the care of these patients are formidable:

1. The range of organisms capable of causing life-threatening infections in these patients is broad, ranging from endogenous flora (including latent organisms that travel with the graft and then are reactivated, thus challenging a potentially naive transplant recipient), to commensal organisms ubiquitous in the environment, to the classic virulent microbes that affect anyone.

2. The impact of these infections is equally broad, including not only the **direct** production of clinical infectious disease syndromes, but also such **indirect** effects as immunomodulation, allograft injury and GVHD, and oncogenesis.

3. Because of the impaired inflammatory response present in many of these patients, signs and symptoms of infection may be greatly attenuated, resulting in delay in presentation, diagnosis, and therapy. Since success in treating virtually all clinically important infection in these patients is predicated on early diagnosis and treatment, the acumen of the physician in evaluating these patients is sorely tested, requiring an aggressive approach to the evaluation of subtle radiologic findings, skin lesions, and other early findings of invasive infection. This volume provides guidelines for accomplishing this task from experienced clinicians who are experts in their field.

4. Because of the linkage between infection and its indirect effects, particularly allograft rejection and GVHD, the goal of the clinician must be to prevent infection, not to treat it.

The editors and contributors to this volume have taken on the formidable task of answering these challenges. They have assembled a monograph that is scientifically rigorous and clinically useful. They have answered the inherent challenges in transplantation infectious disease in admirable fashion, adhering to the basic tenet: the risk of infection, particularly opportunistic infection, is largely determined by the interaction among three factors: the epidemiologic exposures the patient encounters; the technical skill with which such invasive procedures as surgery, vascular access, and intubation are accomplished; and the net state of immunosuppression. All of these subjects are covered, with particular attention to infection control. A unified approach that includes attention to the environment, targeted deployment of antimicrobial agents, and, in some instances, isolation techniques is appropriately emphasized. Transplant patients may be likened to "sentinel chickens" placed in the swamps of our hospitals and communities, such that any excess traffic in microbes will be seen first and foremost in these immunosuppressed hosts. These considerations apply not only to such community-acquired infections as influenza and other respiratory viruses, the endemic mycoses, and bacterial causes of gastroenteritis, but also to nosocomial infections due to such commensal organisms as *Aspergillus* species, and *Candida* species. Newly emerging pathogens such as methicillin-resistant *Staphylococcus aureus* and vancomycin-resistant enterococci have already been shown to have a particularly great impact on transplant patients, and the care and attention shown throughout this volume to issues of infection control are clearly warranted.

A second major tenet of transplantation infectious disease is that the therapeutic prescription for the transplant patient has two components: the immunosuppressive strategy required to prevent and treat GVHD and allograft rejection, and an antimicrobial strategy to make it safe. By its very nature, the antimicrobial strategy must be linked to the nature of the immunosuppressive therapy required. Throughout this book, a careful, balanced assessment of the advantages and disadvantages of a particular infection prevention strategy is presented, whether the author is discussing anti-cytomegalovirus options or antifungal prophylaxis. Clearly, the clinician is between a rock and a hard place—the need for preventing infection versus the possibility of selecting antimicrobial resistant infection. Among the greatest virtues of this volume is that it pilots the reader so well between these two dangers. The use of both prophylactic and preventive strategies is carefully and critically presented, and will be of great value for the clinician caring for transplant recipients.

One of the major trends in medical practice today is so-called evidence-based medicine, wherein recommendations are based on well-controlled and well-designed clinical studies. In a field evolving as rapidly as transplantation infectious disease, this is often difficult to do. What the editors and contributors together have accomplished in admirable fashion is a three-pronged approach to both diagnosis and management: present evidence-based recommendations when data to support such recommendations are clearly available; provide a logical approach with appropriate options when data for definite recommendations are not available; and delineate the research priorities in order to transform logical suggestions into evidence-based recommendations. Only a group of individuals with the broad expertise of the editors and the contributors could have accomplished these tasks so admirably. They have truly advanced the field by this effort, and merit our thanks and congratulations.

Robert H. Rubin, M.D., FACP, FCCP
Osborne Chair of Health Sciences and Technology
Chief of Surgical and Transplant Infectious Disease
Massachusetts General Hospital
Boston, Massachusetts 02114

Preface

This book is the first of its kind to bring together information specific to the management of infectious complications that occur specifically in immunocompromised patients undergoing transplantation. Although there are many texts with chapters on "Infection after Transplantation," and books that focus on infections in immunocompromised patients, immunocompromised patients differ from one another and many specialists now focus primarily on a single population. Further, we thought that the growing number of transplants being performed yearly around the world has provided more information about infectious diseases than can be well covered in a more general text on transplantation.

We also believe that it is of value to provide a single forum that not only summarizes the dramatic successes we have achieved in managing infections (such as the control of cytomegalovirus) but also reviews new strategies being developed (i.e., invasive aspergillosis) and discusses relatively rare problems that are encountered and for which there is little information in one place.

This book is intended to provide a comprehensive review of epidemiology, diagnosis, and management of opportunistic infections. The book focuses on the needs of the busy clinician at either a hematopoietic stem cell transplant (HCT) or solid organ transplant (SOT) center.

Infections continue to be one of the most important impediments to successful outcome after transplantation of both hematopoietic stem cells as well as solid organs. Although each transplant setting involves specific risks for opportunistic infections, the types of infections that occur are similar across the transplant setting. We believe that there is much to be learned from appreciating the similarities and differences in the patterns of infection and the resulting spectrum of morbidity and mortality among the various settings, thus justifying combining the fields of HCT and SOT into one text. We also acknowledge that significant differences exist with regard to the pathogenesis of infectious complications among the different SOT settings. However, for a clearer presentation of the specific infectious issues, the book has been structured according to infectious agents rather than types of SOT, and specific differences between SOT types have been highlighted within the chapter for each infectious agent.

Finally, we would like to consider this book as a launching pad for providing not only the basic and current knowledge of this topic in a comprehensive manner, but from which carefully conducted studies will be designed that will contribute to future developments and progress in the field of transplant infectious diseases.

R. B.
P. L.
C. P.

We would like to acknowledge the many patients we have cared for over the years. They have not only taught us the importance of examining and listening to each patient carefully, but have inspired us to ask the questions which have resulted in this book.

Transplant Infections

Transplant Infections edited by
Raleigh A. Bowden, Per Ljungman, and Carlos V. Paya.
Lippincott–Raven Publishers, Philadelphia © 1998

CHAPTER 1

Introduction to Marrow and Blood Stem Cell Transplantation

H. Joachim Deeg and Raleigh A. Bowden

Reports on the therapeutic use of marrow for the treatment of anemia associated with parasitic infections date back about a century (reviewed in ref. 1). However, it was not until the development of the atomic bomb and the observations in Hiroshima and Nagasaki that systematic research into the possibility of marrow transplantation got underway (2). Studies on total body irradiation (TBI) in rodents, dogs, and nonhuman primates revealed that a "marrow syndrome" (i.e., severe myelosuppression) developed at 500–700 cGy. Shielding of the spleen during TBI, implantation of autologous or syngeneic spleen, or infusion of syngeneic marrow following TBI resulted in rescue of the animals (1,3).

Initially, a humoral factor (growth factor?) released by the spleen or by other hematopoietic cells was thought to be responsible for marrow recovery. It was soon shown, however, that hematopoietic reconstitution originated from infused or implanted cells (4). Intravenous injection was the most effective way of transplanting hematopoietic cells that "homed" to the marrow cavity and other hematopoietic organs. In a rat model, lethally irradiated animals were rescued by parabiosis with a normal animal (5), suggesting the presence of stem cells circulating in peripheral blood. Although the infusion of autologous or syngeneic cells rescued animals without complications, animals given cells from a histoincompatible (allogeneic) donor developed "secondary disease," now known as graft-versus-host disease (GVHD) (3). Thus transplantation of spleen or marrow cells not only comprised a transfer of stem cells but also mediated immune effects (6,7).

The development of GVHD resulted in significant morbidity and mortality. At the same time, however, moderate GVHD was associated with improved survival in transplanted mice with leukemia due to a graft-versus-leukemia (GVL) effect (8).

Beginning in 1957, the first clinical transplant attempts of the modern era were undertaken (1,9,10). Overall results were discouraging: although patients transplanted from a syngeneic (monozygotic twin) donor did well immediately post transplant, they generally died from progressive leukemia; patients transplanted from an allogeneic donor generally died with severe GVHD. In most of these patients, however, the actual cause of death was infection, which has remained a major problem after transplantation until the present (11). Work by van Rood, Dausset, and others then showed that histocompatibility antigens (12) that differed between donor and recipient were responsible for the development of GVHD (13). In agreement with this concept infections appear to be less of a problem in patients given HLA-identical transplants (see later). Since then—driven by the pioneering work by Thomas, Good, Santos, and others—marrow and hematopoietic stem cell transplantation has evolved as the treatment of choice for diseases such as chronic myelogenous leukemia, severe aplastic anemia, myelodysplastic syndrome, and others. Although initially the main or only source of stem cells was marrow, peripheral blood stem cells (PBSC) harvested during recovery from chemotherapy induced marrow suppression or after growth factor stimulation have been used with rapidly increasing frequency in recent years (14,15). Since hematopoietic and immunologic recovery may be faster after PBSC than after marrow transplantation, this may also be reflected in a different pattern of infections.

Current indications for marrow transplantation are summarized in Table 1. These indications are continu-

From the Clinical Research Division, Fred Hutchinson Cancer Research Center, Seattle, WA. Supported by PHS grants CA18105, CA31787 and HL36444. HJD is also supported by a grant from the National Marrow Donor Program/Baxter Health Care Division.

TABLE 1. *Diseases treated by bone marrow transplantation*

Acquired		Congenital	
Malignant	Nonmalignant		
Acute nonlymphoblastic leukemia	Aplastic anemia	Immunodeficiencies Severe combined immunodeficiencies Combined immunodeficiencies Leukocyte adhesion defects Actin deficiency Chronic mucocutaneous candidiasis Others	Mucopolysaccharides Hurler syndrome Hunter syndrome Maroteaux-Lamy syndrome Others
Acute lymphoblastic leukemia	Pure red cell aplasia		
	Paroxysmal nocturnal hemoglobinuria		
Chronic myelogenous leukemia			Mucolipodises Metachromatic leukodystrophy Adrenoleukodystrophy Other lipidoses
Chronic lymphocytic leukemia	Acquired immunodeficiency syndrome		
Non-Hodgkin's lymphoma	Autoimmune disorders	Hematologic defects Wiscott-Aldrich syndrome Fanconi anemia Blackfan-Diamond anemia Thalassemia Sickle cell disease Glanzmann's thrombasthenia Gaucher's disease Chronic granulomatous disease Congenital neutropenia Chediak-Higashi syndrome Langerhans cell histiocytosis Dyskeratosis congenita Congenital amegakaryocytosis Thrombocytopenia-absent-radius (TAR) syndrome Familial erythrophagocytic lymphohistiocytosis (FEL) Others	Other lysosomal diseases Lesch-Nyhan syndrome Type IIa glycogen storage disease
Hodgkin's disease			
Multiple myeloma disease			
Myelodysplastic syndrome			
Hairy cell leukemia			
Neuroblastoma			
Hypereosinophilic syndrome			
Myelofibrosis			
Breast cancer			
Other selected solid tumors		Osteopetrosis	

ously under revision, because nontransplant modalities such as combination chemotherapy, hematopoietic growth factors, cytokines, immunotoxins, and antisense RNA continue to evolve, and improved results with nontransplant therapy may be observed. Even though the number of separate diseases amenable to this form of therapy is considerable, currently the large majority of transplants are performed to cure malignancy.

RATIONALE AND INDICATIONS FOR MARROW OR HEMATOPOIETIC STEM CELL TRANSPLANTATION

Myelosuppression is the most frequent dose-limiting toxicity of chemoradiotherapy used for treatment of malignancies. Myelosuppression and the risk of bleeding and infection can be overcome by the infusion of stem cells capable of hematopoietic reconstitution as a "rescue" procedure. This rescue then allows dose escalation of cytotoxic therapy to the point where toxicity in the next most sensitive organs such as the intestinal tract, liver, or lungs becomes dose limiting. Hematopoietic stem cells for transplantation can be obtained from various donor

sources (Table 2) (16). The use of cells from an allogeneic donor may increase the tumor cell kill above what is achieved with cytotoxic therapy by means of an allogeneic or GVL effect (17).

A second use of hematopoietic stem cells is as "replacement" therapy in patients with congenital or acquired marrow failure or immunodeficiencies. With these indications, there is generally no beneficial effect of GVHD.

Third, hematopoietic stem cells (or more mature precursors) may be effective "vehicles" for gene therapy (18). Objectives of such therapy include the replacement of defective or missing enzymes (e.g., adenosine deaminase; glucocerebrosidase) as well as the introduction of genes that may mediate antitumor activity (e.g., interleukin-2).

Finally, it was noted that some patients with aplastic anemia or leukemia who also suffered from an autoimmune disease (e.g., rheumatoid arthritis) when transplanted with allogeneic marrow not only were cured from their hematologic disease but also had sustained improvement or resolution of their autoimmune disease (reviewed in ref. 19).

TABLE 2. *Potential marrow or stem cell donors and risk of infections*

| | | Histocompatibility barrier | | |
		Minor	Major	Risk of infection
Autologous:	Patients are their own donors	−	−	+
Syngeneic:	Monozygotic (identical) twin	−	−	+
Allogeneic:	HLA genotypically identical donor	+	−	++
	HLA phenotypically identical donor			
	Related	+	−/+	++
	Unrelated	+++	−/+	+++
	HLA-nonidentical donor			
	Related	+	++	+++
	Unrelated	+++	++	++++
Xenogeneic:	Different species donor	+++	+++	?

SOURCES OF STEM CELLS AND DONOR SELECTION

Hematopoietic stem cells can be obtained from different donors (see Table 2) and different compartments (Table 3). The choice of a source of stem cells is dependent upon several factors. Although autologous marrow or PBSC should be available for every patient (except possibly patients with severe aplastic anemia), it would not be useful for genetically determined disorders or for acquired malignant disorders because of the concern about contamination with malignant cells. A haploidentical donor (parent, sibling, child) would be available for almost all patients, but significant HLA differences still represent major problems to transplantation because of GVHD, the risk of rejection, and an increased risk of infection with increasing degrees of histoincompatibility between donor and patient (see Table 2).

Approximately 25% to 30% of patients who have siblings can be expected to have an HLA genotypically identical donor. In addition, phenotypically matched donors can be identified among closely related family members in about 1% of patients, and somewhat less than 1% of patients will have an identical twin donor. These statistics (i.e., the lack of a matched related donor in approximately 70% of patients who could benefit from hematopoietic stem cell transplantation) have stimulated the development of transplantation in two directions: (a) the establishment of large data banks of volunteer unrelated donors, and (b) the development of techniques to "purge" autologous marrow.

Mostly thanks to the efforts of the National Marrow Donor Program (NMDP) in the United States, more than 2 million volunteer donors have been typed for HLA-A

TABLE 3. *Sources of stem cells*

Bone marrow
Peripheral blood
Cord blood
Fetal liver

and -B and many for HLA-DR (MHC class II) antigens (20). Similar registries have been established in Great Britain, France, Germany, and other countries. The probability of finding an HLA-A,-B,-DR match during the initial search currently is about 50% to 55%; an additional 10% to 15% of patients will find a match when available HLA-A- and B-matched donors are typed for DR, and 20% of patients have a 1-HLA-locus incompatible unrelated donor available (21).

Autologous marrow or PBSCs can be purged of contaminating malignant cells by chemical means (e.g., 4-hydroperoxycyclophosphamide) or with antibodies that recognize tumor cells (22). Limitations to this approach are slow engraftment of the treated marrow and residual tumor cells that resisted the purging regimen. A complementary approach, facilitated by the characterization of antigens expressed on putative stem cells (CD34), purifies stem cells with specific antibodies by a process of positive selection (23). It appears that at least in a proportion of patients these approaches allow for successful hematopoietic rescue.

Finally, cord blood and fetal liver are rich in hematopoietic stem cells that can be used for transplantation. As discussed below, the source of stem cells and the compartment from which they are derived are relevant to the tempo of hematopoietic recovery and immunologic reconstitution (24–26).

TRANSPLANT PROCEDURE

Preparation for Transplantation

In preparation for hematopoietic stem cell transplantation it is necessary for several reasons to "condition" the patient:

1. To eradicate the patient's disease or at least reduce the number of malignant or abnormal cells below detectable levels. (This applies for allogeneic, syngeneic, and autologous donors.)
2. To suppress the patient's immunity ("natural" or acquired through allosensitization) and prevent rejec-

tion of donor cells. (This applies to allogeneic but not to the autologous cells that constitute an "*auto*plantation" rather than a *trans*plantation.) Immunosuppression is also needed in preparation for some syngeneic transplants, apparently to eliminate autoimmune reactivity that may interfere with sustained hematopoietic reconstitution.

3. To create "space" so that donor cells can establish themselves in the recipient marrow, although this concept has recently been challenged (27).

Exceptions to the requirement of conditioning exist in children with severe combined immunodeficiency (SCID) because of the nature of the underlying disease, which does not allow them to reject transplanted donor cells, and in whom partial donor engraftment can completely correct the genetic defect (14,28).

Therapeutic modalities used to prepare patients for transplantation have been reviewed extensively elsewhere (16,29). In principle, they comprise the following:

1. Irradiation, either in the form of TBI, total lymphoid irradiation, or modifications thereof. Dose rate, fractionation, and total dose are still controversial, but most regimens deliver 1,200–1,400 cGy over 4–6 days. In addition, bone-seeking isotopes (e.g., holmium) and isotopes (e.g., ^{131}I) conjugated to monoclonal antibodies directed at lymphoid or myeloid antigens (e.g., anti-CD20, CD45) are being tested. It is of note that irradiation is a major risk factor for the development of interstitial pneumonia.

2. Chemotherapy (e.g., cyclophosphamide, 120–200 mg/kg over 2–4 days) is included in most regimens. Busulfan (16 mg/kg over 4 days) is frequently used instead of TBI. Other agents—including etoposide, melphalan, thiotepa, and cytarabine—may be used, sometimes without inclusion of irradiation where myeloablation is not required. Chemotherapy similar to TBI results in mucositis. Damage to the mucosal barrier increases the risk of infection.

3. Biological reagents (e.g., antithymocyte globulin [ATG]) or monoclonal antibodies (MAb) directed at T-cell antigens or adhesion molecules to suppress recipient immunity; or antibodies directed at antigens expressed on the recipient's malignant cells. In addition, cytokines or cytokine antagonists are being investigated for their therapeutic potential. Anti-T-cell therapy predisposes to viral infection, in particular cytomegalovirus (CMV) and the development of lymphoproliferative disorders related to Epstein-Barr virus (EBV) after transplantation (30).

4. Cellular therapy. Viable donor buffy coat cells have been used to facilitate engraftment in patients with severe aplastic anemia. The observation that broad T-lymphocyte depletion of donor marrow (see later) resulted in graft failures has led to protocols of selective T-cell addback to ensure engraftment. In addi-

tion, the use of buffy coat cells later is being explored for treatment and prevention of relapse in high-risk patients.

Additional procedures may involve plasmapheresis of the patient to remove isoagglutinins directed against the donor's ABO blood group or, vice versa, removal of plasma from the donor marrow to remove isoagglutinins directed at recipient cells. Alternatively, the donor red blood cells with which recipient antibodies may react can be removed, thus minimizing the transfusion reaction (13).

Stem Cell Harvest and Infusion

The donor receives anesthesia, and under sterile conditions, multiple aspirates of marrow are obtained from both posterior iliac crests (31). Additional potential aspiration sites are the anterior iliac crests and occasionally the sternum. Approximately 10–15 ml/kg donor weight are collected. If no ABO incompatibility exists and if the marrow is not to be subjected to any *in vitro* purging procedure, the resulting cell suspension is infused intravenously, generally via an indwelling intravenous (e.g., Hickman line) catheter, and hematopoietic stem cells and progenitor cells home to the marrow cavity.

If autologous marrow is used, many investigators apply in vitro purging with antibody and complement, with solid phase separation or chemicals prior to cryopreservation or reinfusion into the patient after conditioning. Other approaches at purging have involved, for example, short-term *in vitro* culture to select against clonogenic leukemic cells.

Alternative Stem Cell Sources

Hematopoietic stem cells are present at low concentrations outside of the bone marrow (32). One such alternative source, peripheral blood, contains dramatically increased frequencies of early hematopoietic precursors during the recovery phase following cytotoxic therapy or after administration of recombinant hematopoietic growth factors, such as G-CSF or c-kit ligand (Steel factor). A single leukapheresis may be sufficient to harvest the number of cells required for a transplant. For autologous procedures the goal is to harvest $2–5 \times 10^6$ CD34$^+$ cells/kg of recipient weight (15,33).

Umbilical cord blood, representing a segment of the "peripheral" circulation of the fetus, represents another rich and easily accessible source of hematopoietic stem cells (34,35). Also, cord blood cells may be less immunocompetent than adult cells and may carry a lower risk of inducing GVHD than adult marrow cells. The concentration of stem cells is high (frequency of long-term culture-initiating cells approximately 1:100 as compared with 1:500 in peripheral blood), but the small volume usually available (100–150 ml) may limit the use of these cells for transplantation.

In experimental models, fetal liver obtained at the optimum time of gestation can also provide a rich source of hematopoietic stem cells (35). However, because of unpredictable availability and ethical concerns, fetal liver cells do not currently play a major role in transplantation and are unlikely to do so in the future.

POST-TRANSPLANT CARE

Complications of hematopoietic stem cell transplantation, including infections, are related to the underlying disease, the preparative regimen (regimen-related toxicity [RRT]), and the interactions of donor cells with recipient tissue. The timing of complications is directly related to the immunodeficiency caused by the conditioning, GVHD, and its therapy or both (Fig. 1). All patients experience transient severe pancytopenia. This period may last 2–4 weeks with marrow cells, but possibly only 10–12 days with the use of mobilized PBSCs. The administration of "growth" factors such as G-CSF or c-kit ligand (or both) early after transplantation accelerates recovery of granulocytes. It is not clear that growth factors can further accelerate recovery with mobilized PBSCs; there

appears to be a minimum time interval that is required for cell replication and differentiation, although it may be possible to modify the function of cells (15,33).

Virtually all patients require transfusion support with platelets and red blood cells. The use of IL-11 or Oncostatin M and certainly the recently cloned thrombopoietin (36) may enhance platelet recovery. Erythropoietin administration post transplant has been shown to speed reticulocyte recovery and moderately reduce the red blood cell transfusion requirement in some patients (37).

However, it is predominantly the lack and functional deficiency of granulocytes and lymphocytes for various periods of time post transplant that are responsible for infectious complications. All patients receive prophylactic or empiric broad-spectrum antibiotics (11). Figure 2 shows the timing of infection with the rise of standard prophylactic regimens. Granulocyte transfusions are not given routinely. Treatment of patients in laminar air flow (LAF) rooms and with gastrointestinal decontamination may reduce the frequency of infections and the duration of febrile episodes, but neither are being used routinely now due to high cost of LAF and the availability of more effective broad-spectrum antibiotics (38).

With allogeneic transplantation some form of GVHD prophylaxis is required (39,40). The most widely used

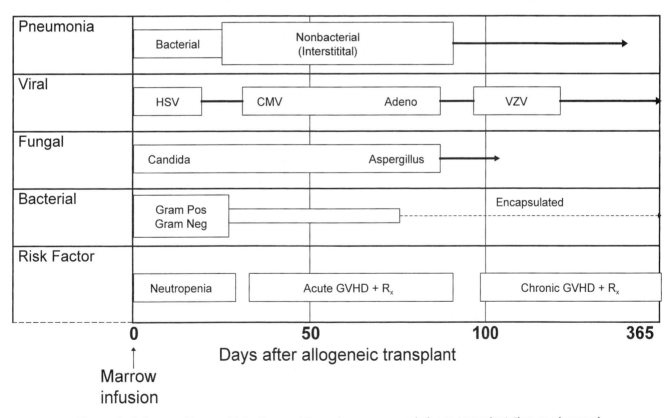

Figure 1. Scheme of types of infection and time of occurrence relative to transplantation as observed before the implementation of prophylaxis. HSV = Herpes simplex virus; CMV = cytomegalovirus; adeno = adenovirus; VZV = varicella zoster virus; GVHD = graft-vs-host disease; Rx = treatment.

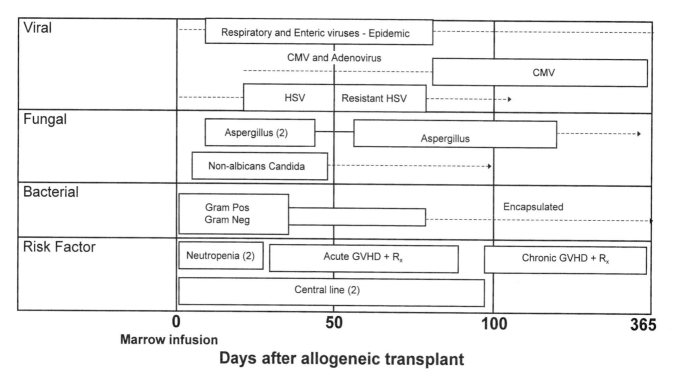

Figure 2. Risk periods for opportunistic infections with prophylaxis currently considered standard. Abbreviations as for Fig. 1.

modality involves *in vivo* administration of immunosuppressive agents such as methotrexate, cyclosporine, glucocorticoids, or FK506, either alone or in combination (41). The current standard at most institutions is a combination of methotrexate plus cyclosporine; some investigators add glucocorticoids (41). The role of FK506 is still incompletely defined. Because of the nonselectivity of these agents, patients are broadly immunosuppressed and susceptible to infections. T-lymphocyte depletion of donor marrow circumvents direct *in vivo* effects of immunosuppressive agents. However, the elimination of mature T cells is associated with a delay in immunologic reconstitution. Both immunodeficiency and therapeutic immunosuppression predispose the patient to infections, as discussed later and in other chapters.

HEMATOLOGIC RECOVERY

As indicated earlier, a severe risk period for infections is the time interval of granulocytopenia due to the decline in enodogenous marrow function and the lag time to proliferation of transplanted (donor) cell. With conventional marrow transplants granulocytes begin to recover at 12–14 days but occasionally not until 3 weeks post transplant. If at least 200 granulocytes/μl are not reached by day 21, patients generally are given G-CSF or GM-CSF. If the donor marrow is T-cell depleted, recovery may be even more protracted. After PBSC transplant engraftment as determined by >500 granulocytes/μl may occur as early as day 9 or 10, clearly shortening the length of gran-

ulocytopenia. Rather slow recovery, over several weeks, may be seen with cord blood transplants (34).

IMMUNOLOGIC RECOVERY

Virtually all components of the innate and of the adaptive immune systems are deficient after hematopoietic stem cell transplantation. Cell-mediated immunity, chemotaxis, and neutrophil function are severely impaired. Time post transplant, histocompatibility barriers, and GVHD and its treatment are also major factors (30).

Uncomplicated Recovery

Epithelial barriers are damaged by cytotoxic therapy, thereby facilitating the penetration of pathogenic bacterial or fungal organisms early post transplant. The risk may be reduced with intestinal decontamination and will resolve with healing. With time post transplant there will also be improvement in the volume and composition (IgA) of saliva. As discussed earlier, granulocyte counts may become normal by 1 month, but chemotaxis, phagocytosis, and superoxide production may still be impaired. Even in patients with uncomplicated recovery post transplant, both T-cell and B-cell-mediated immune responses against viral, bacterial, fungal, and other organisms are broadly suppressed because of the fact that the recipient's immune system has basically been eliminated. NK cells recover quickly. Complement abnormalities have not been reported post transplant (30). As discussed later, the pattern of immune recovery is to some extent dependent upon the immunity of the donor from whom the transplanted cells originated and is influenced by the patient's exposure.

B Cells

B-cell numbers are undetectable or very low early post transplant but rise to supranormal levels by 1–2 years (42,43). Recovery is faster with autologous than with allogeneic cells; memory B cells lag behind naive cells. Early (but not late) recovery for both populations is faster for allogeneic PBSC than for marrow recipients (44). With a successful transplant the B-cell compartment is generally replaced completely by donor-derived cells, except in patients with $T^+ B^-$ SCID in whom recipient B cells tend to reconstitute (45).

Following transplant, fewer B cells express CD25 and CD62L, and more express CD9c, CD38, IgM, and IgD, and the antigen density is increased (as in neonatal B cells). $CD5^+$ cells may be increased or not (43,46). Ig gene usage appears to be restricted early post transplant and skewed toward V-segments used frequently in neonatal B cells (e.g., V_H6). Concordantly, the antibody repertoire is restricted. IgG and IgA production may be abnormal for 1–2 years post transplant. Serum isotype levels after grafting recover in the same sequence in which they evolve in neonates; that is, IgM, IgG, and IgG_3 recover early, but IgG_2, IgG_4, and IgA may follow only much later. Many of the antibodies produced early following transplant are autoantibodies or have irrelevant specificities (47). Antibodies with relevant specificities recover only if the antigen is encountered and do so faster if both patient and donor are immune (48). IgG levels early post transplant may be lower with PBSCs. Antibodies to polysaccharide antigens tend to recover later than those directed at proteins. By 3 months post transplant, total IgG levels in recipients of allogeneic PBSCs tend to be lower than in the marrow recipients, but these areas require further study.

Antibody responses to vaccination after transplantation are almost universally lower than in normal controls, and repeated boosters are required to achieve good antibody levels (30). Responses are better in younger individuals and with T-cell-replete grafts, possibly related to CD4 recovery, which is faster in younger individuals. The policy has been to delay revaccination until 1–2 years post transplant to minimize the risk of potential side effects and to increase the probability of antibody responses.

Some antibodies of host origin (e.g., isoagglutinins), derived from long-lived plasma cells, may be detectable for months or even years after transplantation.

T Cells

CD4+ T Cells

$CD4^+$ cells are very low for 1–3 months after transplantation; they rise only slowly toward normal over several years, faster in children than in adults (30,49,50). The tempo appears to be similar after autologous and allogeneic transplants. The recovering cells are mostly composed of memory T cells; naive T cells follow very gradually, particularly in older patients, possibly related to diminished thymic function. After PBSC transplants, $CD4^+$ T cells, both naive and memory, are more abundant than after marrow transplants. Although early after transplant most $CD4^+$ T cells appear to be derived from transplanted T cells, later on they are stem cell derived, at least in pediatric patients.

After transplant, $CD4^+$T cells generally express CD11a, CD29, CD45RO, and HLA-DR, but they express less CD28, CD45RA, and CD62L, consistent with the prominence of memory cells (30,51). The responses to polyclonal stimuli (except possibly for Ca^{2+} flux) are low. Proliferative responses to antigens that are likely to be encountered (e.g., *Candida*) usually become normal late (i.e., years) after transplantation, whereas responses to unlikely antigens (e.g., tetanus) remain subnormal. *In vivo*, there are abnormally low responses to neoantigens (e.g., dinitrochlorobenzene) and recall antigens (e.g., mumps) for at least 2–3 years after transplant.

CD8+ Cells

Similar to $CD4^+$ cells, $CD8^+$ T cells are low for 2–3 months post transplant (49,50). However, subsequently $CD8^+$ cells rise quickly, resulting in an inversion of the typical CD4:CD8 ratio. The post-transplant CD8 cells are largely memory cells, expressing CD11a, CD11b, CD29, CD57, HLA-DR, and CD45RO but showing little CD28, CD45RA, and CD62L. The presence of a $CD11b^+$, $CD57^+$, $CD28^-$ phenotype suggests anergic or suppressive CD8 cells. $CD8^+$ cells appear to be derived from both T cells and stem cells; further studies are needed.

Nonspecific $CD8^+$ suppressor cells are found early post transplant and in patients with GVHD (52,53). Recent studies show that CMV- or EBV-specific $CD8^+$ cells can be transferred successfully and may persist for at least 18 months (54). The role of $CD4^- CD8^-$ or $CD4^+ CD8^+$ T cells post transplant is incompletely defined. $CD4^- CD8^-$ γ/δ T cells may exert an antileukemia effect (55).

Antigen-Presenting Cells

Monocytes reach normal levels within 1 month post transplant, although their function may remain impaired for 1 year (56). G-CSF-mobilized PBSCs contain large numbers of monocytes that may suppress allogeneic responses of T cells; however, they appear to settle in tissue rather early post transplant.

The reconstitution of various members of the dendritic cell family has been studied only incompletely. Langerhans cells are low early but return toward normal by 6 months. Follicular dendritic cells are reconstituted rather slowly, possibly accounting for the very delayed function of germinal centers and memory B cells (30,57).

GRAFT-VERSUS-HOST DISEASE (GVHD) AND GRAFT-VERSUS-LEUKEMIA (GVL) EFFECT

GVHD is a major complication of allogeneic marrow transplantation (39,40). Acute and chronic GVHD occur in 10% to 50% and 20% to 50%, respectively, of patients given an HLA-identical transplant, and in 50% to 90% and 30% to 70%, respectively, of patients transplanted from an alternative donor. Acute GVHD is the single most important risk factor for the development of chronic GVHD (58,59). Without prophylaxis, virtually all recipients of an allogeneic transplant develop GVHD (60). Acute GVHD may occur within days (e.g., among HLA-nonidentical transplant recipients) or 3–5 weeks post transplant. Main target organs are the immune system, skin, liver, and intestinal tract (61). Only skin, liver, and intestinal tract are generally considered in GVHD grading systems (62).

The immunopathophysiology of GVHD is complex, and detailed discussions have recently been presented elsewhere (39,40,63). Several lines of evidence suggest that inflammatory cytokines are critical mediators of GVHD, and in fact the pathophysiology of acute GVHD has been described as a "cytokine storm" (Fig. 3) (64). First, the conditioning regimen damages host tissues (intestinal mucosa, liver, etc.) that release inflammatory cytokines (e.g., TNFα and IL-1) (65). These cytokines increase the expression of human leukocyte antigen (HLA) and other molecules, such as LFA1 and CD44 (40). During autologous transplants this generation of cytokines is self-limited and resolves in 7–10 days. However, in allogeneic transplantation, mature donor T cells recognize alloantigens in the host and become activated. This recognition is facilitated by consequences of the first step, that is, cytokine-induced increases in host cell surface receptors. Both CD4+ cells, which recognize MHC class II antigens, and CD8+ cells, which react to MHC class I antigens and their associated peptides (in the case of GVHD minor antigen peptides), can be involved. Activated donor T cells then proliferate and secrete IL-2. When the principal T-cell response is a "Th1" or inflammatory response (mainly IL-2 and IFNγ), these cytokines activate additional donor (and residual host) mononuclear cells and macrophages to secrete IL-1 or TNFα. The resulting inflammatory response causes additional release of cytokines that amplifies local tissue injury, at least in part through active nitrogen intermediates such as nitric oxide. The overall result is the acute "suppressive" form of GVHD. When the principal T-cell response is a Th2 or "helper" response in which IL-4 and IL-10 predominate, the overall result is the chronic form or "stimulatory" form of GVHD with increased IgE synthesis and exaggerated lymphoproliferation (66–69).

The chronic GVHD syndrome has prominent features of autoreactivity (39,63), and T-lymphocytes with abnormal cytokine profiles (secreting, for example, IL-4 and interferon gamma) may be present (70). Experimental evidence suggests that thymic damage, inflicted by the conditioning regimen and preceding acute GVHD, results in a failure of intrathymic selection and an escape of autoreactive cells to the periphery (69). A similar mechanism appears to be responsible for syngeneic or autologous GVHD.

As stated before, a major target organ of GVHD is the immune system. As a result, immunodeficiency is a key feature of GVHD that is further amplified by immunosuppressive therapy of GVHD, rendering patients highly susceptible to infections. The risk is further accentuated by damage to various barrier structures, particularly skin and intestinal tract. It appears that all aspects of immune recovery after transplantation described earlier are impaired or delayed in patients with GVHD. In patients with chronic GVHD the immunoincompetence may extend over years.

Methods of GVHD prophylaxis are summarized in Table 4. Combination regimens of methotrexate and cyclosporine with or without the addition of intravenous immunoglobulins (see later) are the most effective currently available regimens (71,72). In a recent study the addition of prednisone to methotrexate and cyclosporine increased (rather than decreased) the incidence of acute GVHD, presumably as a result of interference with the antimetabolite effect of methotrexate (73). However, another study reported a highly significant beneficial effect with this triple combination if glucocorticoid administration was delayed (72). Results in ongoing trials with FK506 are encouraging and expected to be similar to those using cyclosporine, but it is too soon to draw definitive conclusions (74). *In vivo* administration of MAB (murine or the humanized form) against the interleukin-2 receptor or MAB neutralizing TNFα has only been of transient benefit (75–78). Soluble IL-1 receptor or IL-1 receptor antagonist has yielded encouraging results in prevention and treatment of GVHD (66,79). Although these agents are antigen-nonspecific and may not interfere with the initial steps of allogeneic activation, they may be able to prevent the manifestation of the graft-versus-host reaction (i.e., GVHD) and possibly interfere with other disease processes (e.g., septicemia or capillary leak syndrome) associated with diffuse tissue damage. Experiments are under way to determine whether such anti-inflammatory approaches will allow control of GVHD without interfering with a specific T-cell-mediated GVL effect.

T-cell depletion of donor marrow, clearly effective in reducing the incidence of GVHD, has increased the probability of graft failure (10% to 30% with HLA-identical, 30% to 60% with HLA-nonidentical bone marrow transplant [BMT]) and leukemia recurrence, particularly in

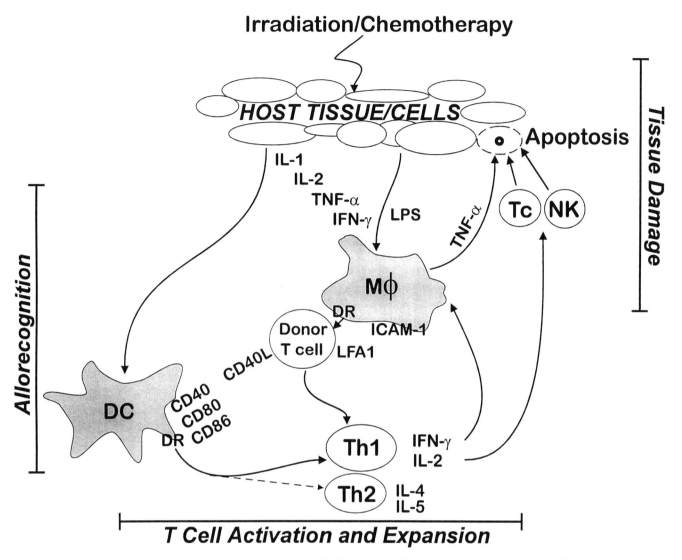

Figure 3. Schematic representation of the role of cells and cytokines in acute graft-versus-host disease. Initially, injury to host tissues, either directly by the conditioning regimen or indirectly through the production of cytokines, results in alterations of host tissues, including expression of HLA molecules, adhesion molecules, procoagulants, and nitric oxide production. Next, mature cells infused with the marrow or peripheral blood stem cells respond to these changes in the allogeneic host tissues. Responses include the autocrine production of "Th1" cytokines IL-2 and IFNγ, which in turn activate mononuclear cell effectors, primarily from among donor cells. Finally, additional production of inflammatory cytokines (e.g., IL-1) by donor mononuclear cells results in further direct tissue injury. Endotoxin (LPS) released by Gram-negative bacteria as well as production of other cytokines such as IL-6 and IL-8 may further amplify the injury and recruit additional effectors. If the development of Th2 cells and the corresponding cytokines (IL-4, IL-5) is favored, the reaction of the cells may be counterbalanced and tolerance may be more likely to develop. DC = dendritic cells; MO = macrophages; DR = HLA-DR (class II) antigens. Tc = cytotoxic T cells; NK = natural killer cells. ICAM-1 = intracellular adhesion molecule 1; LFA-1-lymphocyte function antigen 1. CD = cluster of differentiation; L = ligand.

patients with CML (80–82). These observations have led to the design of studies aimed at inducing GVHD or, more important, a GVL effect, by omitting or abbreviating prophylactic regimens or by adding viable donor buffy coat cells (83). Although this approach was generally successful in inducing GVHD, it has not been associated with a significant improvement in survival. Current trials are aimed at determining whether depletion of

subsets of T-lymphocytes (e.g., CD8+ cells) may provide GVHD prophylaxis without adversely affecting engraftment or eradication of leukemia (84,85). Experimental models suggest, on the other hand, that donor CD8+ cells have a graft-facilitating effect (86).

GVHD is an important risk factor for long-term survival in particular because GVHD and prolonged immunosuppression are associated with a high risk of

TABLE 4. *GVHD prophylaxis*

T-lymphocyte depletion of donor marrow *in vitro*
  Complete
  Selective (CD4, CD8)
  With partial addback
In vivo treatment of patient
  MTX, CSP, FK506, etc.
  Polyclonal anti-T-cell antibodies
  Monoclonal anti-T-cell antibodies
    Murine
    Humanized
Cytokine blockade
Gnotobiosis

TABLE 5. *Delayed complications*

Chronic GVHD
Infections
Airway and pulmonary disease
Autoimmune dysfunction
Impaired growth and development
Endocrine dysfunction
Sterility
Cataracts
Dental problems
Aseptic necrosis of the bone
New malignancies
Psychosocial dysfunction

potentially lethal infections. If GVHD develops despite prophylaxis, it requires aggressive therapy. This applies not only to acute, but also to chronic GVHD. Successful therapy of GVHD does not appear to interfere with an associated GVL effect (87). The GVL effect has recently been reviewed in detail elsewhere (88).

GRAFT FAILURE

With unmanipulated marrow grafts from an HLA-identical sibling, graft failure (either primary or secondary) is a minor problem. Graft failure does occur, however, in allosensitized patients conditioned with less intensive regimens (e.g., patients with aplastic anemia prepared with cyclophosphamide), in patients given transplants from alternative donors, and in patients given T-cell-depleted grafts. Preliminary results suggest that graft failure may be less frequent in patients transplanted with PBSCs.

Among patients with lymphohematopoietic malignancies given HLA-nonidentical transplants, 5% to 15% given unmanipulated bone marrow fail to engraft permanently, compared with 30% to 60% with T-cell-depleted bone marrow (80). Several host cell types participate in the rejection of bone marrow, particularly CD8$^+$ cytotoxic T-lymphocytes and natural killer cells (86). The depletion of T cells from the donor marrow removes an important element of GVHD that counteracts these host cells, thus making T-cell-depleted marrow more susceptible to rejection. The probability of rejection is further aggravated by recipient sensitization to HLA antigens, probably through blood transfusions, which results in a positive cross-match (89,90).

DELAYED COMPLICATIONS

Many patients have led normal lives for 20–25 years post transplant; others have developed delayed complications (Table 5). These complications are thought to be due either to the conditioning regimen (most important, irradiation) or to conditions relating to the transplant (e.g., chronic GVHD, immunodeficiency) (91,92). Life-threatening complications include infections and pulmonary dysfunction, particularly bronchiolitis obliterans, as a manifestation of chronic GVHD (93).

An interesting observation has been the development of autoimmune disorders, such as myasthenia gravis, post transplant. Autoimmune conditions may be due to adoptive transfer or to GVHD, or may occur in an idiopathic way. Vice versa, as discussed before, autoimmune diseases have improved in patients transplanted for other reasons. These observations provide another illustration of the effect of transplantation on immunity in general and autoimmunity in particular, an insight that may be applicable to the treatment of autoimmune disorders.

SUMMARY

Bone marrow transplantation is a successful therapy for many life-threatening diseases. The sequelae of this therapy include side effects mediated by immunologic mechanisms, such as GVHD. Recent work in basic immunology has brought significant advances in our understanding of the processes involved with T-cell responses to alloantigens (including the molecular mechanisms of immunosuppressive drugs) and the importance of inflammatory mediators (including cytokines) in the systemic pathophysiology initiated by these alloreactions. Novel reagents and approaches currently being tested in animal models will almost certainly modify some elements of current transplantation protocols. Although no single reagent or technique is likely to eliminate transplant-associated complications, potential synergy among several of these approaches is likely, and with it the possibility of more widespread application of this important therapeutic modality.

ACKNOWLEDGMENT

We thank B. Larson, H. Childs, and A. Owens for typing the manuscript.

REFERENCES

1. Santos GW. History of bone marrow transplantation. *Clin Haematol* 1983;12:611–639.
2. Committee for the Compilation of Materials on Damage Caused by the

Atomic Bombs in Hiroshima and Nagasaki. *Hiroshima and Nagasaki: the physical, medical, and social effects of the atomic bombings,* Ishikawa E, Swain D, trans. New York: Basic Books; 1981.

3. Van Bekkum DW, de Vries MJ. *Radiation chimaeras.* New York: Academic Press; 1967.

4. Ford CE, Hamerton JL, Barnes DWH, Loutit JF. Cytological identification of radiation-chimaeras. *Nature* 1956;177:452–454.

5. Brecher G, Cronkite EP. Post-radiation parabiosis and survival in rats. *Proc Soc Exp Biol Med* 1951;77:292.

6. Billingham RE. The biology of graft-versus-host reactions. In: *The Harvey lectures.* New York: Academic Press; 1966:21–78.

7. Grebe SC, Streilein JW. Graft-versus-host reactions: a review. *Adv Immunol* 1976;22:119–221.

8. Barnes DWH, Loutit JF. Treatment of murine leukaemia with x-rays and homologous bone marrow: II. *Br J Haematol* 1957;3:241–252.

9. Thomas ED, Lochte HL Jr, Lu WC, Ferrebee JW. Intravenous infusion of bone marrow in patients receiving radiation and chemotherapy. *N Engl J Med* 1957;257:491–496.

10. Mathe G, Amiel JL, Schwarzenberg L, et al. Bone marrow graft in man after conditioning by antilymphocytic serum. *Br Med J* 1970;2:131–136.

11. Bowden RA. Infections in patients with graft-vs.-host disease. In: Burakoff SJ, Deeg HJ, Ferrara J, Atkinson K, eds. *Graft-vs.-host disease: immunology, pathophysiology, and treatment.* New York: Marcel Dekker; 1990:525–538.

12. Dausset J. Iso-leuco-anticorps. *Acta Haematol* 1958;20:156–166.

13. Epstein RB, Storb R, Ragde H, Thomas ED. Cytotoxic typing antisera for marrow grafting in littermate dogs. *Transplantation* 1968;6:45–58.

14. Fischer A, Landais P, Friedrich W, et al. Bone marrow transplantation (BMT) in Europe for primary immunodeficiencies other than severe combined immunodeficiency: a report from the European Group for BMT and the European Group for Immunodeficiency. *Blood* 1994;83: 1149–1154.

15. Shpall DJ, Jones RB. Mobilization and collection of peripheral blood progenitor cells for support of high-dose cancer therapy. In: Forman SJ, Blume KG, Thomas ED, eds. *Bone marrow transplantation.* Boston: Blackwell Scientific Publications; 1994:913–918.

16. Deeg HJ, Klingemann HG, Phillips GL. *A guide to bone marrow transplantation,* 2nd ed. New York: Springer-Verlag; 1992.

17. Weiden PL, Flournoy N, Thomas ED, et al. Antileukemic effect of graft-versus-host disease in human recipients of allogeneic-marrow grafts. *N Engl J Med* 1979;300:1068–1073.

18. Miller AD. Genetic manipulation of hematopoietic stem cells. In: Forman SJ, Blume KG, Thomas ED, eds. *Bone marrow transplantation.* Boston: Blackwell Scientific Publications; 1994:72–78.

19. Marmont AM. Immune ablation followed by allogeneic or autologous bone marrow transplantation: a new treatment for severe autoimmune diseases? *Stem Cells* 1994;12:125–135.

20. Perkins HA, Hansen JA. The U.S. National Marrow Donor Program. *Am J Pediatr Hematol Oncol* 1994;16:30–34.

21. Anasetti C, Hansen JA. Bone marrow transplantation from HLA-partially matched related donors and unrelated volunteer donors. In: Forman SJ, Blume KG, Thomas ED, eds. *Bone marrow transplantation.* Boston: Blackwell Scientific Publications; 1994:665–680.

22. Rowley SD. Pharmacological purging of malignant cells. In: Forman SJ, Blume KG, Thomas ED, eds. *Bone marrow transplantation.* Boston: Blackwell Scientific Publications; 1994:164–178.

23. Andrews RG, Bryant EM, Bartelmez SH, et al. CD34+ marrow cells, devoid of T and B lymphocytes, reconstitute stable lymphopoiesis and myelopoiesis in lethally irradiated allogeneic baboons. *Blood* 1992;80:1693–1701.

24. Locatelli F, Maccario R, Comoli P, et al. Hematopoietic and immune recovery after transplantation of cord blood progenitor cells in children. *Bone Marrow Transplant* 1996;18:1095–1101.

25. Shpall EJ, Cagnoni PJ, Bearman SI, et al. Peripheral blood stem cells for autografting. *Ann Rev Med* 1997;48:241–251.

26. Mavroudis D, Read E, Cottler-Fox M, et al. CD34+ cell dose predicts survival, posttransplant morbidity, and rate of hematologic recovery after allogeneic marrow transplants for hematologic malignancies. *Blood* 1996;88:3223–3229.

27. Rao SS, Peters SO, Crittenden RB, et al. Stem cell transplantation in the normal nonmyeloablated host: relationship between cell dose, schedule, and engraftment. *Exp Hematol* 1997;25:114–121.

28. O'Reilly RJ, Friedrich W, Small TN. Transplantation approaches for severe combined immunodeficiency disease, Wiskott-Aldrich syn-drome, and other lethal genetic, combined immunodeficiency disorders. In: Forman SJ, Blume KG, Thomas ED, eds. *Bone marrow transplantation.* Boston: Blackwell Scientific Publications; 1994:849–873.

29. Petersen FB, Bearman SI. Preparative regimens and their toxicity. In: Forman SJ, Blume KG, Thomas ED, eds. *Bone marrow transplantation.* Boston: Blackwell Scientific Publications; 1994:79–95.

30. Storek J, Witherspoon RP. Immunological reconstitution after hemopoietic stem cell transplantation. In: Atkinson K, ed. *Clinical bone marrow and blood stem cell transplantation: a reference textbook,* 2nd ed. New York: Cambridge University Press (*in press*).

31. Thomas ED, Storb R. Technique for human marrow grafting. *Blood* 1970;36:507–515.

32. McCredie KB, Hersh EM, Freireich EJ. Cells capable of colony formation in the peripheral blood of man. *Science* 1971;171:293–294.

33. Bensinger WI. Peripheral blood stem cell transplantation. In: Buckner CD, ed. *Technical and biological components of marrow transplantation,* vol. 7. Boston: Kluwer Academic Publishing; 1995:169–193.

34. Wagner JE. Umbilical cord blood stem cell transplantation. In: Buckner CD, Clift R, eds. *Technical and biological components of marrow transplantation.* Boston: Kluwer Academic Publishers; 1995:195.

35. Touraine JL, Roncarolo MG, Bacchetta R, et al. Fetal liver transplantation: biology and clinical results. *[Rev] Bone Marrow Transplant* 1993; 11[Suppl 1]:119–122.

36. Kaushansky K, Lok S, Holly RD, et al. Promotion of megakaryocyte progenitor expansion and differentiation by the c-Mpl ligand thrombopoietin. *Nature* 1994;369:568–571.

37. Mitus AJ, Antin JH, Rutherford CJ, et al. Use of recombinant human erythropoietin in allogeneic bone marrow transplant donor/recipient pairs. *Blood* 1994;83:1952–1957.

38. Petersen FB, Buckner CD, Clift RA, et al. Infectious complications in patients undergoing marrow transplantation: a prospective randomized study of the additional effect of decontamination and laminar air flow isolation among patients receiving prophylactic systemic antibiotics. *Scand J Infect Dis* 1987;19:559–567.

39. Ferrara J, Deeg HJ, Burakoff SJ, 2nd ed. *Graft vs. host disease: immunology, pathophysiology, and treatment.* New York: Marcel Dekker; 1996.

40. Ringden O, Deeg HJ. Clinical spectrum of graft-versus-host disease. In: Ferrara JLM, Deeg HJ, Burakoff S, eds. *Graft vs. host disease,* revised and expanded, 2nd ed. New York: Marcel Dekker; 1997:525–559.

41. Chao NJ, Deeg HJ. *In vivo* prevention and treatment of GVHD. In: Ferrara JLM, Deeg HJ, Burakoff S, eds. *Graft vs. host disease,* 2nd ed. New York: Marcel Dekker; 1996:639–666.

42. Kook H, Goldman F, Padley D, et al. Reconstitution of the immune system after unrelated or partially matched T cell-depleted bone marrow transplantation in children: immunophenotypic analysis and factors affecting the speed of recovery. *Blood* 1996;88:1089–1097.

43. Storek J, Ferrara S, Ku N, et al. B cell reconstitution after human bone marrow transplantation: recapitulation of ontogeny? *Bone Marrow Transplant* 1993;12:387–398.

44. Ottinger HD, Beelen DW, Scheulen B, et al. Improved immune reconstitution after allotransplantation of peripheral blood stem cells instead of bone marrow. *Blood* 1996;88:2775–2779.

45. Stiehm ER, Roberts RL, Hanley-Lopez J, et al. Bone marrow transplantation in severe combined immunodeficiency from a sibling who had received a paternal bone marrow transplant. *N Engl J Med* 1996; 335:1811–1814.

46. Drexler HG, Brenner MK, Wimperis JZ, et al. CD5 positive B cells after T cell depleted bone marrow transplantation. *Clin Exp Immunol* 1987;68:662–668.

47. Gerritsen EJA, Van Tol MJD, Ballieux P, et al. Search for the antigen specificity of homogeneous IgG components (H-IgG) after allogeneic bone marrow transplantation. *Bone Marrow Transplant* 1996;17:825–833.

48. Lutz E, Ward KN, Szydlo R, et al. Cytomegalovirus antibody avidity in allogeneic bone marrow recipients: evidence for primary or secondary humoral responses depending on donor immune status. *J Med Virol* 1996;49:61–65.

49. Storek J, Witherspoon RP, Storb R. T cell reconstitution after bone marrow transplantation into adult patients does not resemble T cell development in early life. *Bone Marrow Transplant* 1995;16:413–425.

50. Ashihara E, Shimazaki C, Yamagata N, et al. Reconstitution of lymphocyte subsets after peripheral blood stem cell transplantation: two-color flow cytometric analysis. *Bone Marrow Transplant* 1994;13: 377–381.

51. Weinberg K, Annett G, Kashyap A, et al. The effect of thymic function on immunocompetence following bone marrow transplantation. *Biol Blood Marrow Transplant* 1995;1:18–23.

52. Autran B, Leblond V, Sadat-Sowti B, et al. A soluble factor released by CD8+CD57+ lymphocytes from bone marrow transplanted patients inhibits cell-mediated cytolysis. *Blood* 1991;77:2237–2241.

53. Tsoi MS, Storb R, Dobbs S, et al. Nonspecific suppresser cells in patients with chronic GVHD after marrow grafting. *J Immunol* 1981; 127:244–251.

54. Riddell SR, Watanabe KS, Goodrich JM, et al. Restoration of viral immunity in immunodeficient humans by the adoptive transfer of T cell clones. *Science* 1992;257:238–241.

55. Cela ME, Holladay MS, Rooney CM, Richardson S. Gamma/delta T lymphocyte regeneration after T lymphocyte-depleted bone marrow transplantation from mismatched family members or matched unrelated donors. *Bone Marrow Transplant* 1996;17:243–247.

56. Winston DJ, Territo MC, Ho WG, et al. Alveolar macrophage dysfunction in human BMT recipients. *Am J Med* 1982;73:859–865.

57. Walsh LJ, Athanasas-Platsis S, Savage NW. Reconstitution of cutaneous neural-immunological networks following bone marrow transplantation. *Transplantation* 1996;61:413–417.

58. Storb R, Prentice RL, Sullivan KM, et al. Predictive factors in chronic graft-versus-host disease in patients with aplastic anemia treated by marrow transplantation from HLA-identical siblings. *Ann Intern Med* 1983;98:461–466.

59. Atkinson K, Horowitz MM, Gale RP, et al. Risk factors for chronic graft-versus-host disease after HLA-identical sibling bone marrow transplantation. *Blood* 1990;75:2459–2464.

60. Sullivan KM, Deeg HJ, Sanders J, et al. Hyperacute GVHD in patients not given immunosuppression after allogeneic marrow transplantation. *Blood* 1986;67:1172–1175.

61. Deeg HJ, Cottler-Fox M. Clinical spectrum and pathophysiology of acute graft-vs.-host disease. In: Burakoff SJ, Deeg HJ, Ferrara J, Atkinson K, eds. *Graft-vs.-host disease: immunology, pathophysiology, and treatment.* New York: Marcel Dekker; 1990:311–335.

62. Thomas ED, Storb R, Clift RA, et al. Bone-marrow transplantation. *N Engl J Med* 1975;292:832–843, 895–902.

63. Shulman HM. Is graft-versus-host disease an alloimmune or autoimmune disorder? In: Tan EM, ed. *Clinical aspects of autoimmunity,* vol. 2. New York: Fones & Mann Projects Division; 1988:18–30.

64. Antin JH, Ferrara JLM. Cytokine dysregulation and acute graft-versus-host disease. *Blood* 1992;80:2964–2968.

65. Xun CQ, Thompson JS, Jennings CD, Brown SA, Widmer MB. Effect of total body irradiation, busulfan-cyclophosphamide, or cyclophosphamide conditioning on inflammatory cytokine release and development of acute and chronic graft-versus-host disease in H-2-incompatible transplanted SCID mice. *Blood* 1994;83:2360–2367.

66. Ferrara JL. Cytokine dysregulation as a mechanism of graft versus host disease. *[Rev] Curr Opin Immunol* 1993;5:794–799.

67. Sakamoto H, Michaelson J, Jones WK, et al. Lymphocytes with a CD4+CD8-CD3- phenotype are effectors of experimental cutaneous graft-versus-host disease. *Proc Nat Acad Sci USA* 1991;88: 10890–10894.

68. Deeg HJ, Storb R. Graft-versus-host disease: pathophysiological and clinical aspects. *Annu Rev Med* 1984;35:11–24.

69. Korngold R, Sprent J. T cell subsets in graft-vs.-host disease. In: Burakoff SJ, Deeg HJ, Ferrara J, Atkinson K, eds. *Graft-vs.-host disease: immunology, pathophysiology, and treatment.* New York: Marcel Dekker; 1990:31–50.

70. Allen RD, Staley TA, Sidman CL. Differential cytokine expression in acute and chronic murine graft-versus-host disease. *Eur J Immunol* 1993;23:333–337.

71. Storb R, Deeg HJ, Whitehead J, et al. Methotrexate and cyclosporine compared with cyclosporine alone for prophylaxis of acute graft versus host disease after marrow transplantation for leukemia. *N Engl J Med* 1986;314:729–735.

72. Chao NJ, Schmidt GM, Niland JC, et al. Cyclosporine, methotrexate, and prednisone compared with cyclosporine and prednisone for prophylaxis of acute graft-versus-host disease. *N Engl J Med* 1993;329:1225–1230.

73. Storb R, Pepe M, Anasetti C, et al. What role for prednisone in prevention of acute graft-versus-host disease in patients undergoing marrow transplants? *Blood* 1990;76:1037–1045.

74. Fay JW, Weisdorf DJ, Wingard JR, et al. FK506 monotherapy for prevention of graft versus host disease after histocompatible sibling marrow transplantation. *Blood* 1992;80(10, suppl. 1):135a. [Abstract]

75. Anasetti C, Hansen JA, Waldmann TA, et al. Treatment of acute graft-versus-host disease with humanized anti-Tac: an antibody that binds to the interleukin-2 receptor. *Blood* 1994;84:1320–1327.

76. Anasetti C, Martin PJ, Hansen JA, et al. A phase I-II study evaluating the murine anti-IL-2 receptor antibody 2A3 for treatment of acute graft-versus-host disease. *Transplantation* 1990;50:49–54.

77. Hervé P, Wijdenes J, Bergerat JP, et al. Treatment of corticosteroid resistant acute graft-versus-host disease by *in vivo* administration of anti-interleukin-2 receptor monoclonal antibody (B-B10). *Blood* 1990; 75:1017–1023.

78. Hervé P, Flesch M, Tiberghien J, et al. Phase I-II trial of a monoclonal anti-tumor necrosis factor a antibody for the treatment of refractory severe acute graft-versus-host disease. *Blood* 1992;79:3362–3368.

79. McCarthy PL Jr, Abhyankar S, Neben S, et al. Inhibition of interleukin-1 by an interleukin-1 receptor antagonist prevents graft-versus-host disease. *Blood* 1991;78:1915–1918.

80. Kernan NA. Graft failure following transplantation of T-cell-depleted marrow. In: Burakoff SJ, Ferrara J, Deeg HJ, Atkinson K, eds. *Graft-vs.-host disease.* New York: Marcel Dekker; 1990:557.

81. Apperley JF, Jones L, Hale G, et al. Bone marrow transplantation for patients with chronic myeloid leukaemia: T-cell depletion with Campath-1 reduces the incidence of graft-versus-host disease but may increase the risk of leukaemic relapse. *Bone Marrow Transplant* 1986; 1:53–66.

82. Mitsuyasu RT, Champlin RE, Gale RP, et al. Treatment of donor bone marrow with monoclonal anti-T-cell antibody and complement for the prevention of graft-versus-host disease. *Ann Intern Med* 1986;105: 20–26.

83. Sullivan KM, Storb R, Buckner CD, et al. Graft-versus-host disease as adoptive immunotherapy in patients with advanced hematologic neoplasms. *N Engl J Med* 1989;320:828–834.

84. Champlin R, Ho W, Gajewski J, et al. Selective depletion of CD8+ T lymphocytes for prevention of graft-versus-host disease after allogeneic bone marrow transplantation. *Blood* 1990;76:418–423.

85. Maraninchi D, Mawas C, Guyotat D, et al. Selective depletion of marrow-T cytotoxic lymphocytes (CD8) in the prevention of graft-versus-host disease after allogeneic bone-marrow transplantation. *Transplant Int* 1988;1:91–94.

86. Martin PJ. Donor CD8 cells prevent allogeneic marrow graft rejection in mice: potential implications for marrow transplantation in humans. *J Exp Med* 1993;178:703–712.

87. Weisdorf D, Haake R, Blazar B, et al. Treatment of moderate/severe acute graft-versus-host disease after allogeneic bone marrow transplantation: an analysis of clinical risk features and outcome. *Blood* 1990;75:1024–1030.

88. Truitt RL, Johnson BD, McCabe CM, et al. Graft versus leukemia. In: Ferrara JLM, Deeg HJ, Burakoff SJ, eds. *Graft vs. host disease,* 2nd ed. New York: Marcel Dekker; 1997:385–423.

89. Storb R, Deeg HJ. Failure of allogeneic canine marrow grafts after total body irradiation: Allogeneic "resistance" vs transfusion induced sensitization. *Transplantation* 1986;42:571–580.

90. Storb R, Epstein RB, Rudolph RH, Thomas ED. The effect of prior transfusion on marrow grafts between histocompatible canine siblings. *J Immunol* 1970;105:627–633.

91. Deeg HJ. Delayed complications after bone marrow transplantation. In: Forman SJ, Blume KG, Thomas ED, eds. *Bone marrow transplantation.* Boston: Blackwell Scientific Publications; 1994:538–544.

92. Kolb HJ, Bender-Götze C. Late complications after allogeneic bone marrow transplantation for leukemia. *Bone Marrow Transplant* 1990; 6:61–72.

93. Clark JG, Crawford SW, Madtes DK, Sullivan KM. The clinical presentation and course of obstructive lung disease after allogeneic marrow transplantation. *Ann Intern Med* 1989;111:368–376.

Transplant Infections edited by
Raleigh A. Bowden, Per Ljungman, and Carlos V. Paya.
Lippincott–Raven Publishers, Philadelphia © 1998

CHAPTER 2

Introduction to Solid Organ Transplantation

Barry D. Kahan and Pablo Troncoso

HISTORY OF TRANSPLANTATION

Mythology

For more than three millennia organ replacement has been the medicine of mythology. The mythic literature of several cultures alludes to organ transplantation both as a symbol of renewal and as a cure for disease. An Indian legend from the twelfth century B.C. recounts the powers of Shiva, the Hindu god who xenotransplanted an elephant head onto his child, creating Ganesha, the god of wisdom and vanquisher of obstacles (1). Eight centuries later, Pien Chi'ao (born 430 B.C.) exchanged the hearts of two patients afflicted with an unbalanced equilibrium of energies; he administered powerful herbs after the transplant to promote acceptance of the hearts (2). The classic *Leggenda Aurea* of Jacopo da Varagine (3) describes the "miracle of the black leg"—the limb of a deceased Ethiopian gladiator was retrieved by the Saints Cosmas and Damian and transplanted to the gangrenous leg of a Roman sacristan. Today, after decades of laboratory experiments and clinical trials, kidney, liver, and heart transplants are considered routine, and lung and pancreas replacements are becoming increasingly common. At the dawn of the next millennium, transplant technology has been successfully transferred from the realm of mythology to the arena of fact.

Surgical Advances

The modern era of transplant surgery began in the 1900s, owing in part to the discovery of new techniques for vascular anastomosis. In 1902 Ullman of Vienna performed the first successful experimental transplant in

dogs, and within 8 years he reported having performed more than 100 technically successful canine kidney transplants (4). In Lyon, Jaboulay and his assistant Carrell devised the modern techniques of vascular suture (5). By 1933 the first human kidney transplant had been performed, albeit unsuccessfully, by the Ukrainian surgeon Yu. Yu. Voronoy. His five subsequent attempts (6) also failed (7); consequently, the interest in organ transplantation diminished.

Hume (8), however, succeeded in performing an *ex vivo* human kidney transplant that transiently functioned in 1947. During the same time period, surgeons in Paris and Boston were developing surgical techniques for kidney transplantation. In Paris, Kuss (9), Servelle (10), and Dubost (11) reported having successfully transplanted kidney allografts in human patients using a heterotopic placement in the iliac fossa, and in Boston Hume (12) utilized a femoral approach in conjunction with the emerging practice of hemodialysis to prepare patients for transplantation. Although all the grafts in these pioneering studies eventually failed, in 1954 Murray (13,14) documented the permanent survival of identical twin donor kidney transplants. By the fall of 1963, approximately 30 isografts had been performed worldwide. Also in 1963, the first human liver transplant was performed (15). One year later, Barnard (16) performed the first successful human heart transplant.

Discoveries in Immunosuppression

Based upon Medawar's seminal experiments (17) with which he documented the immunologic basis of graft rejection, it was recognized that for organ transplantation to be successful immunosuppression was required. Among the 12 kidney transplant patients Murray (18) treated with total body irradiation in 1960, only one was a long-term survivor. Hamburger obtained similar results with his experiments in total body irradiation (19).

From the Division of Immunology and Organ Transplantation, The University of Texas Medical School at Houston, Houston, Texas 77030.

Schwartz and Dameshek (20) initiated the modern era of pharmacologic immunosuppression by documenting that the antiproliferative drug, 6-mercaptopurine (6-MP), dampened antibody production and prolonged skin allograft survival. Thereafter, Calne and Murray (21) introduced the imidazole derivative of 6-MP, azathioprine (AZA), for human use. Although corticoids had been added intermittently to therapy with immunosuppressive drugs, the regular use of both together became a standard regimen after reports by Starzl (22) and Goodwin (23).

The present era of organ transplantation began in 1980, when cyclosporine (CsA) was introduced into immunosuppressive regimens; CsA was the first drug that selectively inhibited specific adaptive immunity, sparing nonspecific host resistance.

CLINICAL IMMUNOSUPPRESSION

Initially, radiation and chemicals were used as nonselective immunosuppressive agents. The pharmacologic era of development began in 1914, when Murphy (24) documented the effects of the simple organic compounds benzene and toluene. In 1952 Baker (25) noted that the combination of nitrogen mustards, cortisone, and splenectomy prolonged the survival of canine allografts. Between 1959 and 1962, 6-MP, AZA, and glucocorticoids were developed as immunosuppressants for organ transplantation. In addition, antilymphocyte antibody therapy was tested in organ transplant protocols. Although polyclonal antisera showed a broad degree of T-cell inactivation, they also inhibited nonspecific host resistance elements. Monoclonal antibodies (MAb), produced by a technology that generates reagents selectively directed against cells bearing specific surface markers, were tested in the early 1980s. During the same era, OKT3, a murine IgG_{2a} monoclonal antibody directed against the CD3 component of the T-cell receptor (TcR)–CD3 complex, was rapidly accepted as an effective reagent for rejection reversal (26). However, the combination of glucocorticoids and AZA remained the conventional therapy for nearly 20 years, until CsA was introduced for clinical use (27).

In 1969 CsA was isolated from *Tolypocladium inflatum Gams*, representing the first of a group of agents that inhibit the cells regulating the maturation of alloreactive immune elements. Seven years later, CsA was rediscovered as a potent immunosuppressive agent for transplantation by Jean-François Borel (27). By the mid-1980s, two CsA/prednisone regimens, one with and one without AZA, were used as maintenance immunosuppressive protocols.

CsA affects lymphokine synthesis by inhibiting calcineurin phosphatase action, thereby preventing dephosphorylation of the nuclear factor of activated T cells (28,29). Patients receiving CsA maintain a degree of immunoresponsiveness that affords substantial host defenses, in contradistinction to radiation therapy, which paralyzes the entire immune system. However, the side effects of CsA prevent administration of sufficient doses to exploit its full potential (30). Neither CsA analogs (CsA G and SDZ IMM-125) (31,32) nor tacrolimus (FK506), an actinomycete macrolide product that also inhibits calcineurin activity (33–35), has improved the modest therapeutic window of CsA.

In an effort to discover an agent with a broader therapeutic window than AZA or CsA, several more selective inhibitors of *de novo* nucleoside synthesis—such as mizorbine (MZB) (36), mycophenolate mofetil (MMF) (37), and brequinar (BQR) (38)—were evaluated. Although clinical experience suggests that BQR offers little advantage over other nucleoside synthesis inhibitors and the distribution of MZB has been restricted to Japan, the FDA recently approved MMF for maintenance therapy based upon multicenter phase III trials that showed that in conjunction with CsA and steroids, MMF reduced the rate of allograft rejection episodes to 30%, compared with 50% with Aza (39,40).

An alternate approach to improving outcomes is the use of CsA-based synergistic drug combination regimens. Rapamycin (SRL) (41,42), an agent that blocks lymphokine signal transduction, is currently being evaluated in several clinical trials for its efficacy when combined with CsA. The synergistic interaction between SRL and CsA may be related to their sequential molecular mechanisms of action. Studies have shown that a combination of immunosuppressive agents that act during two sequential phases of the cell cycle—namely, the G_0 to G_1 transformation (CsA) and the G_1 buildup (SRL)—display a greater degree of immunosuppressive synergism than two agents that both act on the G_0 to G_1 transformation (CsA and anti-TcR MAb), or two agents that interrupt the nonsequential G_0 to G_1 and S phases (CsA and BQR) of the cell cycle.

Other agents that are under clinical development are deoxyspergualin (43,44), which apparently disrupts lymphocyte differentiation; leflunomide (45), the mechanism of action of which is unclear; antisense oligonucleotides (46); and products of recombinant DNA technology, including molecular mimics of cytokine receptors (47).

Although several drugs are available for use in clinical transplantation, present immunosuppressive protocols are very often transplant center-specific and are based upon empirical rather than scientific foundations. Moreover, transplant centers tend to use uniform regimens despite the fact that all patients do not have an equal propensity for rejection or degree of risk with regard to the hazards of immunosuppression.

Induction Therapy

The purpose of induction regimens is to promptly establish an adequate level of immunosuppression during the immediate post-transplant period. Many clinicians initiate CsA therapy before or immediately after the transplant procedure, according to a concentration-controlled (48) or a fixed-dose strategy (49). Others prefer to administer sequential immunosuppression with an anti-lymphocyte antibody preparation as induction therapy, followed by delayed administration of CsA, based on the belief that achieving therapeutic concentrations of CsA not only can be difficult but also can carry a risk of allograft damage. Little evidence suggests that such antilymphocyte induction protocols are beneficial (50). Moreover, any benefit must be considered alongside the increased risks of infection and malignancy, as well the greater expense of therapy (51,52). Although some transplant centers continue to employ sequential therapy for all cadaveric organ recipients, its use is increasingly being reserved for immunologically high-risk recipients or for patients with delayed renal graft function.

Several randomized studies show similar rates of graft survival and eventual levels of transplant function among patients treated with various induction protocols. Polyclonal antilymphocyte sera (equine anti-human thymocyte globulin, ATGAM) provide rapid T-lymphocyte depletion accompanied by variable but significant effects on granulocytes and platelets. OKT3, a murine MAb, offers a greater degree of selectivity against T cells; however, its administration may be associated with a severe first-dose lymphokine release syndrome and the risk of developing human anti-mouse antibodies. These effects may preclude its subsequent use in induction regimens.

Maintenance Therapy

Short-Term Regimens

The risk of acute rejection is highest during the first 3 months after transplant. The goal of short-term maintenance therapy is to avert early acute rejection episodes, the occurrence of which appears to increase the risk of eventual graft loss (53). Many short-term maintenance immunosuppressive regimens involve the administration of excessive quantities of drugs, even though high levels of toxic drug exposure may compromise long-term renal function.

CsA, administered alone, in combination with steroids, or in a triple-drug combination with AZA, has become the most popular form of long-term maintenance immunosuppression for organ transplants. Most protocols begin with a twice-a-day regimen of oral CsA (a divided dose of 8–10 mg/kg), the new microemulsion of which more rapidly achieves the steady-state concentration than the previous formulation (54). Doses of CsA are adjusted based on measured trough levels, and most workers consider the therapeutic target to be whole blood concentrations between 175 and 350 ng/ml, as measured with ^{3}H or ^{125}I tracer in a specific MAb-based fluores-

cence polarization immunoassay or by high-performance liquid chromatography. By 3 months following transplant, most patients receive 4–7 mg/kg CsA daily.

A major obstacle to monitoring CsA trough levels to assess the tremendous intra- and interpatient pharmacokinetic variability is the poor correlation between trough levels and CsA exposure, as estimated by the area under the concentration–time curve (AUC) (48,55). Because many studies have documented that adequate early exposure to CsA reduces the incidence of acute rejection episodes, a pharmacokinetic strategy in which parameters are measured pretransplant after intravenous and oral doses of CsA are administered can aid physicians in rapidly determining a suitable concentration (48). In addition, a pharmacokinetic approach is rewarded by early hospital discharge, avoidance of concomitant AZA therapy, and reduced incidence of acute rejection episodes, as compared with empirical dose-seeking strategies.

Corticosteroids are valuable adjuncts to the basic immunosuppressive protocols. Experimental and clinical data suggest a modestly synergistic effect between CsA and corticosteroids. Also, evidence suggests that the use of a high dose of steroids in the early post-transplant period may reduce the injury secondary to graft reperfusion. Consequently, most regimens include a massive (250–1,000 mg) intraoperative dose of methylprednisolone. Thereafter, the doses are reduced to 200 mg, then to 30 mg, and then to 20 mg per day, followed by a more gradual taper to 15 mg between 30 and 90 days following transplant.

The roles of AZA and MMF in current short-term maintenance immunosuppressive therapy remain controversial. Some physicians add these agents in an attempt to increase immunosuppression, thereby allowing for a reduction in CsA dose, which will presumably decrease drug-induced toxicity. Because both AZA and MMF only act additively with CsA, the level of immunosuppression results from cumulative effects; administration of suboptimal amounts of CsA may lead to an increased incidence of rejection (55,56). Furthermore, addition of nucleoside synthesis inhibitors to the regimen is likely to increase the frequency of cytomegalovirus infection, malignant disease, and papillomatosis, as well as introducing side effects inherent to the drug itself, such as hepatotoxicity for AZA, diarrhea for MMF, and bone marrow depression for both AZA and MMF.

Long-Term Regimens

Nearly all long-term maintenance immunosuppression regimens are CsA based and include corticosteroids, with or without AZA. Although CsA has reduced the incidence and severity of acute rejection episodes, it has had less impact on reducing the incidence of chronic rejection observed with AZA/prednisone therapy (range of 6% to 10%) (57). Although this failure of CsA may result from the resistance of B cells to CsA, some evidence suggests that patients who have been inconsistently exposed to CsA are at a greater risk for chronic rejection. It has been documented that the new microemulsion formulation of CsA improves drug exposure, and our clinical trial is presently exploring its impact on the incidence of chronic rejection (58).

Although it is generally believed that CsA and steroid doses can be reduced over time, immunosuppression is required for the functional life of the graft. The discontinuation of immunosuppression, even many years after transplantation, may lead to late acute rejection or accelerated chronic rejection episodes.

Antirejection Therapy

Rejection remains the most frequent cause of transplant failure. Because of the significant risks associated with excessive immunosuppression, one of the most important issues in the treatment of rejection is the certainty of the diagnosis. Although some physicians empirically initiate treatment, most centers prefer to rely on histopathological confirmation.

For mild to moderate episodes of rejection corticosteroids continue to be the most important, cost-effective first line of treatment. Steroid regimens consist of large intravenous doses of methylprednisolone with an oral taper to maintenance prednisone doses within a few weeks. A favorable response to treatment is characterized by a rapid reversal of symptoms and of abnormal laboratory tests. The risks of corticosteroid therapy include exacerbating or inducing diabetes mellitus, producing gastrointestinal irritation/perforation, and triggering psychoses. High doses of pulse steroids reverse approximately 80% of first acute cellular rejection episodes.

The definition of steroid-resistant rejection remains ambiguous. Usually, after 2–5 days of treatment, physicians at most centers assess the success of steroid therapy based upon remission of symptoms and graft dysfunction. If the response is deemed unsatisfactory, antilymphocyte antibody preparations are employed. Steroid-resistant rejection is reversed in 80% to 90% of cases with either OKT3 or polyclonal sera (59–61). At most centers OKT3 is used because it may be administered by peripheral vein, whereas polyclonal sera demands central venous delivery. Immunologic monitoring by FACS analysis is used to assess patient response and guide dose adjustments. $CD3^+$ peripheral blood T cells usually fall to less than 10% following the first dose of OKT3; with ATGAM, absolute $CD2^+$ T-cell counts should remain between 50 and 150 per milliliter within a few days of administration. OKT3 may be a better first-line option for severe, particularly vascular, rejection episodes. Unfortunately, no secure algorithms exist to determine the proper duration of OKT3 therapy, because the therapeutic effects of the agent may be delayed by 7–10 days and the long-term toxic effects may be delayed by 14–30 days.

In patients who experience acute rejection refractory to corticosteroid and antilymphocyte antibody treatments, grafts are almost destined to fail. In these cases, physicians have used either FK506 or MMF as immunosuppressive salvage regimens with variable results (39,40,62). Some promising data have also been shown with SRL rescue treatment (63).

CURRENT RESULTS IN SOLID ORGAN TRANSPLANTATION

The number of organs transplanted in the United States increases each year. It is currently reported that more than 20,000 transplants are performed yearly; this is 57% more than in 1988 (64). The increase in transplant operations may be related to an increase in donors. Unfortunately, this increase in the donor pool has been achieved primarily through the use of organs from living donors and from cadaveric donors who are older than 50 years of age. Thus the shortage of suitable donor organs continues to be a limiting factor for organ transplants, a particular tragedy because overall graft and patient survival rates are improving every year and for every organ (64).

Kidney Transplantation

The United Network for Organ Sharing (UNOS) Scientific Transplant Registry reported that from 1988 through 1994 more than 80,000 renal transplants were performed in 251 U.S. transplant centers (64). The overall 1- and 5-year graft survival rates are 81% and 59%, respectively, for recipients of cadaveric donor transplants and 91% and 75% for recipients of living donor kidneys. The patient survival rate is higher among recipients of living donor transplants: 97% and 90% at 1 and 5 years, compared with 93% and 80%, respectively, for recipients of cadaveric transplants. According to UNOS data, the predicted 10-year survival rates are 79% for HLA-identical sibling transplants, 52% for parent-to-child transplants, and 44% for cadaveric transplants (65). Although many factors influence transplant outcome, the UNOS analysis identifies the following as key factors: HLA matching, race, center, original disease, early renal function, and early rejection episodes (65).

Liver Transplantation

UNOS data show that more than 23,000 liver transplants were performed in U.S. centers between 1988 and 1995 (64). Current 1- and 5-year graft survivals are 75% and 57%, respectively. Retransplantation, severity of the patient's conditions, diagnosis for the primary liver disease (survival is worst for recipients transplanted for malignancies and best for patients with metabolic diseases), and donor/recipient ABO match seem to be the most important factors affecting survival (66). In the UNOS analysis 1- and 5-year patient survivals are 80% and 68% respectively.

However, it is reported that rehabilitation rates are greater than 80%, with most liver transplant recipients claiming that their quality of life is good or excellent.

Thoracic Transplantation

From January 1988 though December 1995, 20,803 thoracic transplants were reported to the UNOS Registry (64). All thoracic organs have shown steady increases in survival rates over time. For most thoracic organs patient survival rates are equivalent to graft survival rates. The 1-year survival rate for a heart transplant recipient increased from 80% in 1988 to 84% in 1994, and for lung transplants recipients from 42% to 74%, respectively. Similarly, heart-lung composite graft survival rate has increased from 51% to 74% in the same period. Current 5-year graft survival rates are 65%, 39%, and 39% for heart, lung, and heart/lung transplants, respectively.

Pancreas Transplantation

The first pancreas transplant was performed in 1966 at the University of Minnesota (67). The current UNOS report shows 1- and 5-year survival rates of 79% and 56% for grafts and 90% and 79% for patients, respectively. Recipients of simultaneous kidney transplants have higher survival rates than those who did not receive a kidney transplant or received the kidney prior to the pancreas transplant.

FUTURE PROSPECTS

Xenografting

Although xenotransplants have been attempted in humans, few have been successful (68–70). There are major immunologic and ethical obstacles to successful clinical xenografting. The most important mechanism of xenograft rejection is the presence of natural anti-species antibodies that bind to the endothelial cells of the graft, activate the complement cascade, and trigger hyperacute rejection. This type of rejection is not controlled with current immunosuppressive regimens. In addition, complement regulatory proteins such as CD59, DAF, and MCP show strict species specificity, so that the complement regulatory proteins on xenogenic endothelial cells do not protect them from attack by human xenoantibodies and complement. In an attempt to solve this problem studies are being conducted with transgenic animals with inhibitors of the human complement on their vascular endothelium (71). An alternate approach seeks to immunoisolate the xenogeneic tissue in capsules or membranes. Early trials on pancreatic islet transplantation show promising results (72,73).

Induction of Donor-Specific Tolerance

The ultimate goal for transplantation therapy is to achieve selective tolerance toward donor antigens without the need for permanent immunosuppression. In animal models special circumstances are associated with an increased likelihood of tolerance induction, including transplantation in the neonatal (or prenatal) period, across weak histocompatibility barriers, or to privileged sites (74,75). Neonatal tolerance depends primarily upon a central thymic process of selective depletion of antidonor immunoreactive cells (76). However, production of this deletional tolerance status in adult animals with cellular chimerism requires abolition of the intrinsic immune system by total-body or total-lymphoid irradiation or intense antibody and chemical immunosuppressants that presently seem to preclude the safe clinical application of these modalities (77–80).

A less hazardous approach seeks to cajole mature lymphocytes to develop tolerance peripherally. Mechanisms that may explain post-thymic peripheral unresponsiveness include T-cell anergy, immune deviation or blocking antibodies, and/or negative regulatory cell induction (81,82). Anergy emerges when antigenic stimulation occurs in the absence of an appropriate second activation signal. It has been reported that anergy is induced after treatment with anti-CD4, CTLA4-Ig, or MAb such as anti-CD2, anti-intercellular adhesion molecule-1, and anti-lymphocyte function antigen (LFA), which block costimulatory signal induction (83–86). Immune deviation is associated with the predominance of the T-helper-2 (Th2) phenotype of CD4$^+$ T cells and the presence of cytokines IL-4, IL-5, and IL-10 (87).

The induction of negative regulatory cells is associated with the infusion of donor-specific cells, such as those from blood or bone marrow, in combination with CsA, ATG, and SRL (88). The use of donor cells to induce transplantation tolerance has been a subject of intense interest. Several donor cell treatment protocols, including bone marrow and peripheral blood transfusions, may contain veto cells that act to promote clonal deletion or anergy (89). Most of these treatment regimens are also related to the development of blocking antibodies and/or to the deletion of specific effector cells, which generates an unresponsive state in the host toward the donor.

Another area of interest has been the development of peptides derived from polymorphic regions of donor major histocompatibility complex (MHC) molecules; these peptides induce tolerance via the indirect route of antigen presentation (90). The utility of this approach in humans has yet to be determined.

Unfortunately, clinical trials of tolerance induction demand that the manipulation be performed within the context of some conventional immunosuppression, such as CsA. This requirement may prevent lymphocyte differentiation along a tolerogenic pathway. In addition, because no assays exist to document the tolerant status, extreme caution must be exercised when baseline immunosuppression is withdrawn.

SUMMARY

Organ transplantation has evolved from an experimental practice to a therapeutic modality. Technical advances have improved the safety of the surgical procedures, and the major thrust of research efforts is focused on improving the efficacy and safety of immunosuppressive therapy. Unfortunately, present clinical protocols more often include empirically rather than scientifically selected combinations of immunosuppressive drugs. However, with the advent of more rigorous trial designs for testing new immunosuppressive regimens, it is likely that the overall success of organ transplantation will be achieved by an incisive cost/benefit analysis of the short- and long-term advantages of emerging clinical strategies. Rejection still represents a major barrier to transplant success, and its prevention and treatment demand regimens that display a more narrow spectrum of iatrogenic side effects. The ultimate goal of achieving transplant tolerance is now being attempted in clinical studies and remains the major challenge for the coming years.

REFERENCES

1. Kahan BD. Ganesha: the primeval Hindu xenograft. *Transplant Proc* 1989;21[Suppl 1]:1–8.
2. Kahan BD. Pien Ch'iao, the legendary exchange of hearts, traditional Chinese medicine, and the modern era of cyclosporine. *Transplant Proc* 1988;20[Suppl 2]:2–12.
3. Kahan BD. Cosmas and Damian revisited. *Transplant Proc* 1983;15 [Suppl 1]:2211–2216.
4. Ullman E. Experimentalle nierentransplantation. *Wie Klin Wochenschr* 1902;15:281.
5. Carrel A. La technique opératoire des anastomoses vasculairs et la transplantation des viscères. *Lyon Med* 1902;98:859.
6. Voronoy Y. Sobre el bloqueo del aparato reticuloendotelial del hombre en algunas formas de intoxicacion por el sublimado y sobre la tranplantacion del rinon cadaverico como metodo de tratamiento de la anuria consecutiva a aquella intoxicacion. *El Siglo Med* 1936;97:296.
7. Hamilton DN, Reid WA. Yu Yu Voronoy and the first human kidney allograft. *Surg Gynecol Obstet* 1984;159:289–294.
8. Moore FD. *Transplantation: the give and take of tissue transplantation.* New York: Simon & Schuster, 1972.
9. Kuss R, Teinturier J, Milliez P. Quelques essais de greffe de rein chez l'homme. *Mem Acad Chir* 1951;77:155.
10. Servelle M, Soulie P, Rougeulle J. La Greffe rénale. *Rev Chir* 1951;70: 186.
11. Dubost C. Resultants d'une tentative de greffe rénale. *Bull Soc Med Hosp Paris* 1951;67:1732.
12. Hume DM, Merrill JP, Miller BF, Thorn GW. Experiences with renal homotransplantation in man in modified recipients. *Ann Surg* 1963; 158:608.
13. Merrill JP, Murray JE, Harrison JH, Guild WR. Successful homotransplantation of the human kidney between identical twins. *JAMA* 1956;160:277.
14. Murray JE, Merrill JP, Harrison JH. Kidney transplantation between seven pairs of identical twins. *Ann Surg* 1958;148:343.
15. Starzl RE, Marchioro TL, Von Kaulla KN. Homotransplantation of the liver in humans. *Surg Gynecol Obstet* 1963;117:659–676.
16. Barnard CN. A human cardiac transplant. The operation: an interim report of a successful operation performed at Groote Schuur Hospital, Cape Town. *S Afr Med J* 1967;41:1271–1274.
17. Medawar PB. The behavior and fate of skin autografts and skin homografts in rabbits. *J Anat* 1945;79:157.
18. Murray JE, Merrill JP, Dammin GJ, et al. Study of transplantation immunity after total body irradiation: clinical and experimental investigation. *Surgery* 1960;48:272.
19. Hamburger J, Vaysse J, Crosnier J, et al. Transplantation of a kidney

between non-monozygotic twins after irradiation of the recipient: good function at the fourth month. *Presse Med* 1959;67:1771.
20. Schwartz RS, Dameshek W. Drug induced immunological tolerance. *Nature* 1959;65:702.
21. Calne RY, Alexandre GP, Murray JE. A study of the effects of drugs in prolonged survival of homologous renal transplants in dogs. *Ann NY Acad Sci* 1962;99:743.
22. Starzl TE, Marchioro TL, Waddell WR. The reversal of rejection in human renal homografts with subsequent development of homograft tolerance. *Surg Gynecol Obstet* 1963;117:385.
23. Goodwin WE, Mims MM, Kaufman JJ. Human renal transplant III. Technical problems encountered in six cases of kidney homotransplantation. *Trans Am Assoc Genitourin Surg* 1963;54:116.
24. Murphy JB. Heteroplastic tissue grafting effected through roentgen ray lymphoid destruction. *JAMA* 1914;62:1459.
25. Baker R, Gordon R, Huffer J, Miller GH. Experimental renal transplantation: I. Effect of nitrogen mustard, cortisone and splenectomy. *Arch Surg* 1952;65:702.
26. Cosimi AB, Colvin RB, Goldstein G, et al. Treatment of acute allograft rejection with OKT3 monoclonal antibody. *Transplantation* 1981;32: 535–539.
27. Borel JF, Feurer C, Gubler HU, Stähelin H. Biological effects of cyclosporine A: a new antilymphocyte agent. *Agents Actions* 1976;6: 468–475.
28. Granelli-Piperno A, Andrus L, Steinman RM. Lymphokine and non-lymphokine mRNA levels in stimulated human T cells: kinetics, mitogen requirements and effects of cyclosporine A. *J Exp Med* 1986; 163:922–937.
29. Orosz CG, Adams PW, Ferguson RM. Frequency of human alloantigen-reactive T lymphocytes: III. Evidence that cyclosporine has an inhibitory effect on human CTL and CTL precursors, independent of CsA mediated helper T cell dysfunction. *Transplantation* 1988;46 [Suppl 2]:735–795.
30. Kahan BD. Cyclosporine. *N Engl J Med* 1989;321:1725–1738.
31. Heistand PC, Gunn HC, Gale JM, Ryffel B, Borel JF. Comparison of the pharmacological profiles of cyclosporine (Nva-2)-cyclosporine and (Val2) dihydro-cyclosporine. *Immunology* 1985;55:249–255.
32. Donatsch P, Mason N, Richardson BP, Ryffel B. Toxicologic evaluation of the new cyclosporine derivate, SDZ IMM 125, in a comparative, subchronic toxicity in rats. *Transplant Proc* 1992;24:39–42.
33. Ochiai T, Nakajima K, Nagata M, Hori S, Asano T, Isono K. Studies of the induction and maintenance of long-term graft acceptance by treatment with FK506 in heterotopic cardiac allotransplantation in rats. *Transplantation* 1987;44:734–738.
34. Ochiai T, Nagata M, Nakajima K, et al. Studies of the effects of FK506 on renal allografting in the beagle dog. *Transplantation* 1987;44: 729–733.
35. Shapiro R, Jordan M, Scantlebury V, et al. FK506 in clinical kidney transplantation. *Transplant Proc* 1991;23:3065–3067.
36. Turka LA, Dayton J, Sinclair G, Thompson CB, Mitchell BS. Guanine ribonucleotide depletion inhibits T cell activation: mechanism of activation of the immunosuppressive drug mizoribine. *J Clin Invest* 1991;87:940–948.
37. Sollinger SW, Deierhoi MH, Belzer FO, Diethelm AG, Kauffman RS. RS-61443: a phase I clinical trial and pilot rescue study. *Transplantation* 1992;53:428–432.
38. Kahan BD, Tejpal N, Gibbons-Stubbers S, et al. The synergistic interactions *in vitro* and *in vivo* of brequinar sodium with cyclosporine or rapamycin alone and in triple combination. *Transplantation* 1993;55: 894–900.
39. Sollinger HW for the U.S. Renal Transplant Mycophenolate Mofetil Study Group. Mycophenolate mofetil for prevention of acute rejection in primary cadaveric renal allograft recipients. *Transplantation* 1995; 60:225–232.
40. The European Mycophenolate Mofetil Cooperative Study Group. Placebo controlled study of mycophenolate mofetil combined with cyclosporine and corticosteroids for prevention of acute rejection. *Lancet* 1995;345:1321–1325.
41. Eng CP, Sehgal SN, Vezina C. Activity of rapamycin (AY-22,989) against transplanted tumors. *J Antibiot (Tokyo)* 1984;37:1231–1237.
42. Calne RY, Collier DS, Lim S, et al. Rapamycin for immunosuppression in organ allografting. *Lancet* 1989;2:227.
43. Ochiai T, Hori S, Nakajima K, et al. Prolongation of rat heart allograft survival by 15-deoxyspergualin. *J Antibiot (Tokyo)* 1987;40:249–250.
44. Dickneite G, Schorlemmer HU, Sedlacek HH, Falk W, Urlich SK,

Muller-Rucholtz W. Suppression of macrophage function and prolongation of graft survival by the new guanidinic-like structure, 15 deoxyspergualin. *Transplant Proc* 1987;19:1301–1304.

45. Bartlett RR, Dimitrijevic M, Mattar T, et al. Leflunamide (HWA 486), a novel immunomodulating compound for the treatment of autoimmune disorders and reactions leading to transplantation rejection. *Agents Actions* 1991;32:10–21.

46. Stepkowski SM, Tu Y, Condon T, Bennet FC. Blocking of heart allograft rejection by ICAM-1 antisense oligonucleotides alone or in combination with other immunosuppressive modalities. *J Immunol* 1994;153:5336–5346.

47. Fanslow WC, Sims JE, Sasenfeld H, et al. Regulation of alloreactivity *in vivo* by a soluble form of the interleukin-1 receptor. *Science* 1990;248:739–742.

48. Kahan BD, Welsh M, Rutzky L, et al. The ability of pretransplant test-dose pharmacokinetic profiles to reduce early adverse events after renal transplantation. *Transplantation* 1992;53:345–351.

49. Belitsky P, MacDonald AS, Cohen AD, et al. Comparison of antilymphocyte globulin and continuous i.v. cyclosporine A as induction immunosuppression for cadaver kidney transplants. A prospective randomized study. *Transplant Proc* 1991;23:999–1000.

50. Shield CF. Effective induction immunosuppression for cadaver renal transplantation at the St. Francis Regional Medical Center. Clin Transplant 1990;265–274.

51. Slakey DP, Johnson CP, Callaluce RD, et al. A prospective randomized comparison of quadruple versus triple therapy for first cadaver transplants with immediate function. *Transplantation* 1993;56:827–831.

52. Hanto DW, Jendrisak MD, So SK. Induction immunosuppression with antilymphocyte globulin or OKT3 in cadaver kidney transplantation: results of a single institution prospective randomized trial. *Transplantation* 1994;57:377–381.

53. Montandon A, Wegmueller E, Hodler J. Early rejection crises and prognosis of the renal graft. *Nephrologie* 1985;6:59–63.

54. Amante AJ, Kahan BD. Abbreviated AUC strategy for monitoring cyclosporine microemulsion therapy in the immediate post-transplant period. *Transplant Proc* 1996;28:2162–2163.

55. Kahan BD, Grevel J. Overview: Optimization of cyclosporine therapy in renal transplantation by a pharmacokinetic strategy. *Transplantation* 1988;46:631–644.

56. Lindholm A, Kahan BD. Influence of cyclosporine pharmacokinetics, trough concentrations, and AUC monitoring on outcome after kidney transplantation. *Clin Pharmacol Ther* 1993;54:205–218.

57. Knight RJ, Kerman RH, Welsh M, et al. Chronic rejection in primary renal allograft recipients under cyclosporine-prednisone immunosuppressive therapy. *Transplantation* 1991;51:355–359.

58. Kahan BD, Welsh M, Schoenberg L, et al. Variable oral absorption of cyclosporine: a biopharmaceutical risk factor for chronic renal allograft rejection. *Transplantation* 1996;62:599–606.

59. Mochon M, Kraiser B, Palmer JA, et al. Evaluation of OKT3 monoclonal antibody and anti-thymocyte globulin in the treatment of steroid resistant acute allograft rejection in pediatric renal transplants. *Pediatr Neprhol* 1993;7:259–262.

60. Norman DJ, Barry JM, Bennett WM, et al. The use of OKT3 in cadaveric renal transplantation for rejection that is unresponsive to conventional anti-rejection therapy. *Am J Kid Dis* 1988;1:90–93.

61. Ortho Multicenter Transplant Study Group. A randomized clinical trial of OKT3 monoclonal antibody for acute rejection of cadaveric renal transplants. *N Engl J Med* 1985;313:337–342.

62. Woodle ES, Thistlethwaite JR, Gordon JH, et al. A multicenter trial of FK506 (tacrolimus) therapy in refractory acute renal allograft rejection. A report of the Tacrolimus Kidney Transplantation Rescue Study Group. *Transplantation* 1996;62:594–599.

63. Slaton JW, Kahan BD. Case report-sirolimus rescue therapy for refractory renal allograft rejection. *Transplantation* 1996;61:977–979.

64. UNOS, Richmond Virginia and the Division of Transplantation, Bureau of Health Resources Development, Health Resources and Services Administration, U.S. Department of Health and Human Services 1996 Annual Report of the U.S. Scientific Registry for Transplant Recipients and the Organ Procurement and Transplantation Network: Transplant Data: 1988–1995. Rockville, MD.

65. Terasaki PI, Cecka JM, Gjertson DW, Cho Y, Takemoto S, Cohn M. A ten year prediction for kidney transplant survival. In: Terasaki PI, Cecka JM, eds. *Clinical transplants 1992*. Los Angeles: UCLA Tissue Typing Laboratory, 1993:501–512.

66. Belle SH, Berlinger KC, Detre KM. An update on liver transplantation in the United States: recipient characteristics and outcome. In: Cecka JM, Terasaki PI, eds. *Clinical transplants 1995*. Los Angeles: UCLA Tissue Typing Laboratory, 1996:19–33.

67. Kelly WD, Lillehei RC, Merkel FK, Idezuki Y, Goetz FC. Allotransplantation of the pancreas and duodenum along with the kidney in diabetic nephropathy. *Surgery* 1967;61:827–837.

68. Starzl TE, Fung J, Tzakis A, et al. Baboon to human liver transplantation. *Lancet* 1993;341:65–71.

69. Starzl TI, Tzakis A, Fung J. Prospects of clinical xenotransplantation. *Transplant Proc* 1994;26:1082–1088.

70. Smith JA, Rosengard BR, Wallwork J. Cardiopulmonary xenotransplantation: the past, present, and future prospects. *J Thorac Cardiovasc Surg* 1995;4:8–16.

71. Dunning JJ, White DJ, Wallwork J. Xenografts. Its current status and the future prospects. *Rev Esp Cardiol* 1995;48:145–148.

72. Tibbell A, Groth CG, Moller E, Korsgren O, Andersson A, Hellerstrom C. Pig to human islet transplantation in eight patients. *Transplant Proc* 1994;26:762–763.

73. Robertson RP. Pancreatic and islet transplantation for diabetes: cures or curiosities? *N Engl J Med* 1992;327:1861–1868.

74. Wood K. Alternative approaches for the induction of transplantation tolerance. *Immunol Lett* 1991;29:133–137.

75. Streilein JW, Klein J. Neonatal tolerance induction across regions of H-2 complex. *J Immunol* 1977;119:2147–50.

76. Kappler JW, Roehm N, Marrack P. T cell tolerance by clonal elimination in the thymus. *Cell* 1987;49:273–280.

77. Chavin KD, Qin L, Lin J, Yasita H, Bromberg JS. Combined anti-CD2 and anti-CD3 receptor monoclonal antibodies induce donor-specific tolerance in a cardiac transplant model. *J Immunol* 1993;151:7249–7259.

78. Matsura A, Katsuno M, Suzuki Y, et al. Cyclophosphamide-induced tolerance in fully allogeneic heart transplantation in mice. *Cell Immunol* 1994;155:501–507.

79. Perico N, Rossini M, Imberti O, Remuzzi G. Thymus mediated immune tolerance to renal allograft is donor but not tissue specific. *J Am Soc Nephrol* 1991;2:1063–1071.

80. Moller F, Hoyt G, Farfan F, Starnes VA, Clayberger C. Cellular mechanisms underlying differential rejection of sequential heart and lung allografts in rats. *Transplantation* 1993;55:650–655.

81. Wood KJ. New concepts in tolerance. *Clin Transplant* 1996;10:93–99.

82. Shoskes DA. Immunologic tolerance in renal transplantation. *World J Urol* 1996;14:218–224.

83. Alters S, Song H, Fathman C. Evidence that clonal anergy is induced in thymic migrant cells after anti-CD4-mediated transplantation tolerance. *Transplantation* 1993;56:633–638.

84. Van Gool S, de Boer M, Ceuppens J. The combination of anti-B-7 monoclonal antibody and cyclosporine A induces alloantigen-specific anergy during a primary mixed lymphocyte reaction. *J Exp Med* 1994;179:715–720.

85. Wolf H, Wang J, Salmen S. Induction of anergy in resting human T lymphocytes by immobilized anti-CD3 antibodies. *Eur J Immunol* 1994;24:1410–1417.

86. Ma J, Wang J, Guo Y, Sy MS, Bigby M. *In vivo* treatment with anti-ICAM-1 and anti-LFA-1 antibodies inhibits contact sensitization-induced migration of epidermal Langerhans cells to regional lymph nodes. *Cell Immunol* 1994;158:389–399.

87. Onodera K, Hancock WW, Graser E, et al. Type 2 helper T cell-type cytokines and the development of "infectious" tolerance in rat cardiac allograft recipients. *J Immunol* 1997;158:1572–1581.

88. Mottram PL, Mirisklavos A, Dumble LJ, Clunie GJ. T suppressor cells induced by transfusions and cyclosporine. Studies in the murine cardiac allograft model. *Transplantation* 1990;50:1033–1037.

89. Hiruma K, Nakamura H, Henkart P, Gress RE. Clonal deletion of post-thymic T cells: veto cells kill precursor T lymphocytes. *J Exp Med* 1992;175:863–868.

90. Sayegh MH, Krensky MH. Novel immunotherapeutic strategies using MHC derived peptides. *Kidney Int* 1996;49:S13–S20.

Transplant Infections edited by
Raleigh A. Bowden, Per Ljungman, and Carlos V. Paya.
Lippincott–Raven Publishers, Philadelphia © 1998

CHAPTER 3

Infection Control Issues After Bone Marrow and Solid Organ Transplantation

Shimon Kusne and Sharon Krystofiak

Over the last decade, transplantation has been accepted as a treatment modality for terminal illnesses. Therapies used to prevent rejection suppress the immune system; as a result, the transplant recipient is often at high risk for infection. The indiscriminate use of multiple antibiotics may predispose the individual to colonization or infection with drug-resistant organisms. Good infection control practices are very important in the care of transplant recipients because nosocomial infections result in increased morbidity and mortality.

This chapter reviews selected infection control issues that impact transplant recipients. In general, both bone marrow transplantation (BMT) and solid organ transplantation (SOT) recipients have similar risks for infection. Because of their cytoablative therapy, compromised anatomic barriers, and long-term immunodeficiency, BMT recipients may have additional infection risks. The Centers for Disease Control and Prevention (CDC) has issued various guidelines for the prevention of infection, resulting in similar patient management practices in most institutions. As practices are evaluated, new guidelines are developed to direct clinicians and infection control practitioners. CDC guidelines for the prevention of infection after BMT are to be published in 1998. As managed care changes the delivery of health services, multiple patient care options may exist. We describe some of the practices in our institution, acknowledging that there may be several valid approaches to the same problem.

PRETRANSPLANT EVALUATION

History of Past Infection

As part of the pretransplant evaluation, past infection history should be explored. If a history of recurrent infection is identified, it may be very useful to use previous information to prevent infections. For example, cystic fibrosis patients evaluated for lung transplantation could have respiratory tract and sinus colonization with very resistant Gram-negative rods like *Burkholderia cepacia* and *Stenotrophomonas maltophilia*. To select adequate antibiotics for empiric treatment and prophylaxis, it is useful to be familiar with previous bacterial isolates and their antibiotic sensitivity patterns. A history of infection or colonization with *Aspergillus* species is important to note for antifungal prophylaxis after transplantation.

Serologic Screening

Serologic screening prior to transplantation is important in order to evaluate infection risks. In general, seronegative recipients are considered at risk for infections transmitted from the donor transplant organ or from blood transfusions. Titers that are routinely obtained at pretransplant evaluation include Cytomegalovirus (CMV), Epstein-Barr virus (EBV), Herpes simplex virus (HSV), Varicella zoster virus (VZV), and *Toxoplasma gondii*. Seronegative recipients should be screened again at time of transplant. Comparison of donor and recipient results will identify patients who may require prophylaxis or preemptive therapy regimens after receiving seropositive donor organs.

Certain transplant populations are particularly susceptible to specific infections. For example, although there are cases of toxoplasmosis reported after BMT and solid organ transplantation, most cases are seen in heart transplant recipients, as cysts are transmitted within the donor

From the Division of Transplantation Medicine and Division of Infectious Diseases, University of Pittsburgh, Pittsburgh, PA 15213 and Infection Control Department, UPMC-Presbyterian, Pittsburgh, PA 15213.

heart muscle. Seronegative heart transplant recipients who receive an organ from a positive donor are usually given pyrimethamine for prophylaxis (1).

Vaccination

Pretransplant evaluation provides an opportunity to review the vaccination history of the candidate and to update vaccines if necessary. Special attention is usually given to three vaccines: influenza, pneumococcus, and hepatitis B (2). Flu vaccine is usually administered yearly to transplant recipients. Most authors now believe that reimmunization with pneumococcus vaccine might be indicated if more than 5–6 years have elapsed since vaccination. In general, the ability to respond to vaccination with protective titers is significantly reduced after transplantation. We have unsuccessfully attempted to vaccinate liver transplant recipients with the yeast-derived hepatitis B vaccine. Therefore an effort is now made in our institution to vaccinate these patients before transplantation; if necessary, we give a booster during candidacy. Poor response to influenza, pneumococcus, and hepatitis B vaccine has been documented in both solid organ and BMT recipients (3–5). In allogeneic BMT recipients poor antibody production is associated with chronic graft-versus-host disease (GVHD), the use of antithymocyte globulin, and the first 6 months after transplant (6). In the absence of GVHD, patients who are about 1 year after BMT are able to develop protective titers after vaccination. For more details on various types of vaccines in transplant recipients, the reader is referred to chapter 25.

Dental/Ear-Nose-Throat Evaluation

Dental infection or sinusitis may cause fever in the transplant recipient. BMT recipients may develop bacteremia after transplantation as a result of mucositis. It is therefore important to evaluate the patient prior to transplantation for such foci of infection. Ideally, the patient should see the dentist before transplantation occurs, so any necessary dental extractions or fillings can be completed during transplant evaluation process. For example, we have cared for a liver transplant patient who had been treated for *Aspergillus* sinusitis 1 year prior to transplant and had reexacerbation of severe sinusitis in the immediate postoperative period.

TB Exposure

All candidates for transplantation should be evaluated by tuberculin skin testing [purified protein derivative (PPD)] for previous exposure to tuberculosis. An anergy panel should also be placed. Antigens used to test for delayed cutaneous hypersensitivity usually include candida, mumps, trichophyton, or tetanus. This background information may be very useful if a contact investigation must be undertaken once a transplant recipient is exposed to an active case of TB. A previous administration of bacille Calmette-Guérin (BCG) does not represent a con-

traindication for PPD testing unless there is a history of severe skin reaction to TB testing. At our institution, PPD-positive solid organ transplant candidates are placed on INH prophylaxis at candidacy or in the immediate postoperative period. Anergic candidates from areas with endemic TB are also considered for prophylaxis, especially if there are any radiologic changes consistent with previous granulomatous disease in the lungs. The decision whether to give additional INH prophylaxis to a transplant candidate who had previously completed treatment for active TB is a particular dilemma. We have elected to give prophylaxis to such individuals, because theoretically some inactive mycobacteria could still be present and cause active infection after the institution of immunosuppressive therapy after transplantation (7). After transplantation, INH is given only to patients who are PPD positive at the pre-transplantation evaluation.

Special Risks

Travel or residency in areas known to have particular endemic pathogens should be ascertained as part of the pretransplant evaluation. Fungal infections caused by dimorphic fungi—including histoplasmosis, blastomycosis, and coccidioidomycosis—may be remotely acquired by the patient and then be reactivated, causing active infection after transplantation (8). *Strongyloides stercoralis* is an endemic parasite in certain areas of the world that may be silently carried in the GI tract for many years. Larval migration may cause pulmonary infiltrates, bacteremia, or even Gram-negative meningitis after transplantation. If a prolonged febrile illness of unclear etiology occurs, it is helpful to have travel data and consider any unusual infections in the differential diagnosis. Although these infectious complications are uncommon, prompt diagnosis and early institution of treatment may lead to decreased mortality from life-threatening pathogens.

Active Infection

If the candidate appears to be actively infected, transplantation is usually withheld because infection may progress and be life-threatening after immunosuppression is initiated. Therefore most infections should be adequately treated before a candidate may be placed on the active transplant list. It is very difficult to determine when the candidate can be safely transplanted. Colonization with potential pathogens should also be evaluated. *Aspergillus* colonization of the upper airways or sinuses may become invasive after BMT or SOT. Therefore an attempt is made to eradicate the colonizing fungus before transplantation takes place. Each case should be carefully assessed with the pros and cons evaluated. In light of the shortage of solid organs available, a decision not to perform transplant surgery may take away the patient's only chance for survival. The infectious disease consultant often encounters complex questions concerning the duration of therapy and potential risks from chronic infections such as osteomyelitis. The answer to these questions is complex and requires individual evaluation.

Prevention and Isolation Practices

It is essential that caregivers maintain good infection control practices to minimize the transmission of nosocomial infections. The use of invasive devices such as central lines, indwelling urinary catheters, and ventilators exposes the patient to additional risks of infection. Careful attention should be given to good hand-washing practices, central line care, and practices to decrease the risk of pneumonia. Patients may also be isolated as a precaution against the transmission of infectious disease.

Whereas the 1991 OSHA Bloodborne Pathogens Standard focused primarily on employee protection, in 1996 the CDC and the Hospital Infection Control Practices Advisory Committee (HICPAC) published a patient-focused isolation guideline that mandates the use of Standard Precautions for all patients (9). Combining Universal Precautions and Body Substance Isolation precautions, contact with human blood, body fluids, secretions, excretions except sweat, nonintact skin, mucous membranes, and contaminated items requires personal protective equipment. Additional Transmission-Based Precautions are used to prevent infections spread by the airborne, droplet, and direct-contact routes. Certain infections that required disease-specific isolation precautions are now included under Standard Precautions.

Airborne Precautions are used if a patient has a known or suspected infection with an agent that can be transmitted by evaporated droplets (droplet nuclei <5 μm) that remain suspended in the air and may be carried away from the infected patient. Measles, varicella, and tuberculosis are the primary infections included in this category and all require rooms with controlled ventilation. Specialized air filters and negative pressure in the room prevent the infectious droplets from entering the general air supply and infecting others.

Droplets larger than 5 μm are generated in certain diseases, such as influenza and adenovirus. These larger-sized particles do not remain suspended in the air, and no special ventilation is required. Close contact with respiratory tract secretions is required for transmission, so masks should be worn when working within 3 feet of an infected patient to prevent inhalation of infectious droplets.

Contact Precautions are used to prevent the transmission of certain microorganisms that may be found on the patient's skin or on inanimate objects in the patient's environment. Epidemiologically, significant organisms such as vancomycin-resistant enterococci, *Clostridium difficile*, and respiratory syncytial virus (RSV) are included in this category. Private rooms are recommended, but patients infected with the same organism may be cohorted together. If neither of these options is achievable, the immunosuppressed state of potential roommates should be considered.

A Protective Isolation category was defined in the 1975 CDC isolation techniques manual to protect neutropenic or immunosuppressed patients. Whereas other isolation categories were designed to prevent the transmission of disease from an infected patient to others, Protective or "Reverse" Isolation is used to protect the neutropenic patient. The term *neutropenic precautions* refers to practices designed to reduce microbial contamination in the immunosuppressed patient's environment. Because many infections in neutropenic patients have been attributed to the patient's own flora, the use of special environmental precautions is controversial. To reduce the risk of infection, nursing care often focuses on skin integrity, indwelling IV devices, and good oral hygiene (10).

Table 1 presents a summary of the CDC Isolation Precautions Guideline, listing some of the more common infections in the transplant recipient and the type of precautions necessary (9).

Intravascular Catheter-Related Infections

There has been a general increase in the incidence of infections secondary to Gram-positive bacteria, particularly *Staphylococcus* species, attributed to the increased use of various indwelling central lines. The use of antimicrobial prophylaxis may select for fungal species, particularly *Candida albicans*; immunosuppressive agents such as methylprednisolone may also increase the risk of bacteremia (11). Line-related bacteremia is one of the primary infections seen in the immunosuppressed patient, because normal skin flora may colonize long-term access devices. In 1995 the CDC published *Guidelines for the Prevention of Intravascular Device–Related Infections* to address this problem (12). Good hand-washing procedures, barrier precautions, and effective skin decontamination techniques must be used. Antimicrobial ointments for catheter insertion sites are no longer recommended. Catheters should not be routinely replaced, but the site should be diligently monitored for evidence of infection. Guidewires should not be used for catheter exchange if there is any redness, tenderness, or purulent material at the insertion site. The vascular device should be removed as soon as it is no longer needed for therapy.

The incidence of infection and other risk factors varies with the type and intended use of intravascular devices. The two basic types of devices include short-term or temporary devices and those used for long-term access. Every device involves some advantages and some risks. Special attention should be focused on prevention of site infections, and education of the patient is an important part of the process.

Prevention of Exposure from Health Care Workers and Visitors

Employees and visitors may transmit infections to the transplant patient. Health care workers (HCW) should be

TABLE 1. *CDC isolation precautions for selected infections*

Infection	Precautions	Comments
Abscess, draining, minor	Standard	Contact for major draining abscesses
Adenovirus	Droplet, contact	
Aspergillosis	Standard	
Blastomycosis	Standard	
Candidiasis	Standard	
Cellulitis	Standard	
Clostridium difficile	Contact	Isolate incontinent patients, increase environmental cleaning
Coccidioidomycosis	Standard	
Cryptococcosis	Standard	
Cytomegalovirus	Standard	
Epstein-Barr virus	Standard	
Hepatitis, viral (HBV, HCV)	Standard	
Herpes simplex	Standard	Recurrent-skin, oral, genital
	Contact	Mucocutaneous, disseminated or severe cases
Histoplasmosis	Standard	
Influenza	Droplet	Private room preferred
Legionnaire's disease	Standard	
Listeriosis	Standard	
Multidrug-resistant organisms	Contact	Private room preferred
Mycobacteria, nontuberculous	Standard	
Nocardiosis	Standard	
Parvovirus B19	Droplet	
RSV	Contact	BMT—add droplet precautions
Rotavirus	Contact	Diapered or incontinent patients
Tuberculosis, pulmonary	Airborne	
Varicella	Airborne	
Zygomycosis (*Mucor, Rhizopus*)	Standard	

evaluated for health history and immunization status at the beginning of employment (13). Varicella vaccine is recommended for seronegative health care workers, as is hepatitis B vaccine and annual influenza vaccination. Facilities should have well-defined policies to define when potentially infectious personnel may not have patient contact. These policies should encourage the HCW to report any potential exposures or illnesses, and permit temporary reassignment or furlough from duty options to prevent the exposure of transplant patients to potentially deadly infections. Visitors should also be screened for communicable diseases by clinical personnel.

Nutrition and Flowers

Diets that restrict certain foods associated with higher bacterial counts or fungal spores and drinking sterile water have been used by many centers performing BMT (14,15). The value of this practice is unclear, because most authors believe that the source of infection in this population is the patient's own flora colonizing the gastrointestinal tract. Consumption of fresh fruit and vegetables that cannot be effectively washed or peeled may be restricted during periods of neutropenia. Sterile plates and utensils are no longer considered necessary; however, appropriate dish-washing practices should be used. Fresh flowers and plants may increase the number of fungal spores in the environment, and vase water may contain increased quantities of *Pseudomonas* species. Dried flower arrangements may also have large quantities of fungal spores, particularly if dried moss is used.

NOSOCOMIAL INFECTIONS

Aspergillosis

Definition of Nosocomial Infection

Although definition criteria have been established, nosocomial pneumonia is one of the most difficult infections for the infection control practitioner to ascertain. In the case of fungal isolates, there is no defined incubation period, so the "onset of infection 48 hours after admission" standard that separates community-acquired from hospital-acquired infections is not valid. The isolation of fungal species from expectorated sputum may not be diagnostic, but the clinician will often start antifungal therapy. Such isolates may represent transient colonization, a lab contaminant or invasive disease (16). Because of the ubiquitous nature of fungal spores and the significantly higher concentrations found outdoors, if a discharged patient is readmitted with invasive fungal pneumonia, we may be unable to determine if the infection was due to sources within the hospital. Comparative data on the incidence of nosocomial fungal pneumonia is unavailable, and many institutions have attempted to develop their own definition of nosocomial aspergillosis. Our Infection Control Department is

TABLE 2. *Case definitions*

Nosocomial infection	(a) The patient has one or more positive cultures with the same pathogenic fungal species and clinical signs of infection, histopathology, or radiologic evidence of invasive fungal disease. *Or* (b) Histopathology or radiographic evidence of invasive disease with no microbiological culture confirmation may be considered an infection if the patient is treated with an antifungal agent. Date of onset should be more than the seventh day after admission with no evidence of active or incubating infection at the time of admission.
Colonization	Significant isolate(s) that cannot be classified as disseminated or locally invasive; or if no systemic antifungal therapy if given.
Not significant	One isolate of a fungal species from a nonsterile site, no systemic antifungal therapy or no correlation of routine microbiological and fungal cultures.
Community-acquired infection	Signs or symptoms of infection are present at the time of admission and there was no hospitalization within the prior 2 weeks.

currently using the case definitions shown in Table 2, using an arbitrary 7-day stay to define an incubation period for fungal infections in the SOT setting.

Environmental Concerns

Nosocomial aspergillosis is associated with three main mechanisms: airborne acquisition, which is typically secondary to contaminated ventilation systems; direct contact, through contaminated objects such as wound dressings; and airborne/contact, where possibly both mechanisms are implicated, as seen in sternal fungal osteomyelitis after sternotomy (17). There are no recognized "safe levels" for bioaerosols, or standards for frequency of air sampling. Rural outdoor air concentrations of fungi may be as high as 10,000 colony-forming units of air per cubic meter (CFU/m^3) and not cause pulmonary infections in the general population. It is difficult to establish a safe threshold limit in the indoor environment. However, studies have established a positive correlation between increased airborne spore counts and the incidence of invasive aspergillosis (17–19).

Many authors have collected air samples to quantify the number of airborne spores. Open petri dishes, commonly referred to as "settle plates," may be used to estimate airborne concentration of fungal spores. The number of spores that settle on the agar due to effects of gravity are assumed to be proportional to the airborne concentration. Results are expressed as colonies per unit time of exposure. This method does not provide comparative information, because there is no quantifiable volume of air sampled. Air-sampling methods that use calibrated sieve impactors or centrifugal samplers provide standardized counts, and results are expressed as colony-forming units per cubic meter of air (CFU/m^3).

Routine air sampling for fungi is not generally recommended. During construction/renovation or when isolates of *Aspergillus* or other fungi are identified in patient cultures, air sampling may be performed to assess the relative level of spores in the environment. Outdoor samples may be collected as appropriate controls. Fungal colony

types found in the indoor samples should be the same as those from outdoor samples, with a 10-fold (1 log) reduction in indoor counts due to air handler filtration (20). Indoor samples that have a predominance of a particular fungus which is not in proportion to outdoor samples may reflect contamination of the indoor environment (21).

Environmental Controls

Specially designed isolation rooms that utilize laminar air flow (LAF) and/or high-efficiency particulate air (HEPA) filtration may be used to provide the cleanest air possible. HEPA filtration, which provides a minimum of 10 air changes per hour, is often used to reduce fungal spore counts. HEPA filters remove 99.97% of particles larger than 0.3 µm. HEPA filters may be installed in the ventilation system to provide a highly filtered, positively pressurized room, or portable units may be placed in any patient room for additional air filtration. Patient rooms should be tightly sealed to prevent contamination from outdoor sources, and doors should remain closed to ensure positive pressurization. It has been proposed that areas that utilize HEPA filtration and positive pressurization of patient rooms (Fungal Spore Control Ventilation [FSCV]) have total spore counts of less that 15 CFU/m^3, with *Aspergillus* counts less than 0.1 CFU/m^3 (20).

Laminar air flow (LAF) rooms provide the most effective air filtration, increasing air exchanges and utilizing large banks of HEPA filters on the head wall of the patient room (15,22). This combination significantly reduces the spore count, with the number of fungal spores present inversely proportional to the air change rate (14). Room design is similar to glove boxes used in laboratories, with sleeved gloves used on a plastic barrier to allow patient care without entering the controlled environment (15,22). LAF units are expensive, and their use has been limited primarily to BMT units. The routine use of these systems is controversial. In one study from Seattle, allogeneic BMT patients who received prophylaxis and LAF room isolation had the lowest infection rate, but their survival rate was not different from that of patients who had no prophylaxis and were placed in conventional rooms without laminar flow (22). Most institutions that are routinely performing BMT rely on HEPA filtration and not on LAF, because significant differences in nosocomial infection rates between the two have not been observed.

Room design should be focused on easy-to-clean surfaces. Walls and horizontal surfaces should be smooth and nonporous to prevent trapping bacteria and spores and to facilitate cleaning. Porous ceiling tiles and carpeting should also be avoided. Window shades and curtains may attract dust particles. New designs are available that house either curtains or shades within two glass panels to minimize dust collection while providing privacy and controlling light. Vinyl or plastic blinds can be used safely if they are frequently cleaned. Hospitalized BMT and SOT patients should avoid construction areas. If the patient must be transported out of the protective environment, a mask should be worn to prevent the inhalation of particulates. Transplant recipients should also avoid dusty, construction, or excavation/landscaping sites after discharge. The use of other Protective Isolation strategies, such as restriction of fresh fruit and flowers, has been associated with a decrease in the incidence of infection in some studies. It is now assumed that extreme isolation measures such as the sterilization of all objects in the room is unnecessary.

Length of stay in the hospital is being reduced dramatically, and the benefits of a protective environment are being reevaluated. Some authors have shown that BMT can be done without protective isolation, with the patients allowed in some cases to spend time at home even before engraftment (23,24). The most important risk factor for invasive aspergillosis remains the patient's underlying immunosuppressive condition. High-risk patients may develop invasive aspergillosis even with low fungal spore counts (19).

Construction Guidelines

Construction and renovation in the hospital are often associated with an increase in the number of cases of aspergillus. At the beginning of renovation, airborne particulates and fungal spore counts may be exceptionally high because spores are dispersed into the environment during the demolition process. When construction or renovation activities are to be performed in or near facilities that handle high-risk transplant patients, guidelines and monitoring requirements should be established during the planning process (17). Such guidelines help to define the appropriate barriers and techniques to prevent the spread of dust and debris into other areas of the facility. Construction and housekeeping personnel should be trained about the dangers of aspergillosis with emphasis on control measures. Strategies for prevention of nosocomial aspergillosis will also control any other fungi that can be transmitted by dust, such as the zygomycetes (e.g., *Mucor*

and *Rhizopus*). Infection control interventions to prevent nosocomial aspergillosis were well illustrated during one construction-associated outbreak, where the incidence of invasive aspergillosis rose from 3.18 to 9.88 cases per 1,000 patient days at risk during construction (25). Control measures used included portable HEPA filtration units, the installation of sealed windows, easy-to-clean tiles and shades, and increased maintenance of the ventilation system. The introduction of portable HEPA filters units was identified as the most important step in this undertaking. After the institution of control measures, the infection rate decreased to 2.91 per cases per 1,000 patient days.

When construction activities are outdoors, air intakes for the ventilation system may also become heavily loaded with construction dust, potentially leading to increased contamination of the indoor environment. Increased focus on filter maintenance is important, and successful containment may be possible, as reported during the construction of a BMT unit (21). Maintaining the construction area at negative pressure, establishing plastic sheet barriers, and establishing controlled access to construction zones prevented dust from contaminating patient areas.

Aspergillus flavus has frequently been identified in reports of construction-related contamination of the indoor environment (26). Arnow and colleagues reported an increase in spore counts of *Aspergillus fumigatus* and *Aspergillus flavus* with a mean of >1 CFU/m³ associated with the opening of a new hospital (27). Environmental assessment identified fungal contamination of the carpet, fireproofing material, and ventilation filters. Damp areas, discolored ceiling tiles, and peeling wallpaper may be contaminated with fungi. Most studies document decreased indoor spore counts after the institution of appropriate control measures (21,26). Air sampling is frequently recommended to assess air contamination after construction or HEPA filter changes and as part of an outbreak investigation if nosocomial aspergillosis is suspected. Repeat air samples may be collected after an identified source is decontaminated or removed. Periodic sampling may also be performed as part of an environment audit.

Aspergillus are certainly not the only significant fungal pathogen found in the environment. *Fusarium* and *Trichosporon* species, dematiaceous molds, zygomycetes, and normally innocuous soil and plant fungi may cause infections in the immunocompromised patient (28). Good housekeeping practices are vital in high-risk patient areas. These areas should be visually monitored to ensure that any dust is contained and removed from the patient environment. If nosocomial infections occur within an institution, renovation of ventilation systems to provide highly filtered air in high-risk patient areas may be considered. Although antifungal prophylaxis of patients may be useful, cases may still occur, necessitating the temporary closure of contaminated patient units or suspension of transplant activities during hospital construction projects.

Legionellosis

Transplant recipients are considered to be at increased risk of developing *Legionella* pneumonia, commonly known as Legionnaires' disease. Even after water treatment plant processing, small quantities of this aquatic bacteria may enter homes and buildings, and live in the biofilm that lines the pipes. *Legionella* multiply in warm water, with the temperature range of 35–46°C considered ideal (29,30). Regulations concerning maximum water temperature designed to prevent scalding accidents often fall into this range, which increases the possibility that a facility will become contaminated with *Legionella* and several other species of nontuberculous mycobacteria, including *Mycobacterium xenopi* (31,32). Inhalation of contaminated aerosols generated by humidifiers, air-conditioning units, cooling towers, and showers was traditionally considered to be the primary route of transmission of this bacteria into the lungs. Aspiration of contaminated water is now considered an additional transmission mechanism (33,34). Although there are different opinions on the need for control measures, common sources, and methods of transmission, it is becoming more common for health care facilities to identify *Legionella* contamination and assess the levels in their potable water supplies. *Legionella pneumophila* strains may be more virulent than non-*pneumophila* strains. Of 10 culture-proven cases of legionellosis found in BMT patients over a 6-year period, five of the seven patients with non-*pneumophila* isolates recovered. None of the three patients with *L. pneumophila* pneumonia survived (35). Advances in molecular fingerprinting techniques have been instrumental in associating patient isolates with *Legionella* species cultured from a facility's potable water supply. Lawsuits have successfully linked nosocomial infection to perceived facility negligence (30).

Environmental Monitoring

Culturing plumbing fixtures such as sink spouts, showerheads, ice makers, and drinking fountains for *Legionella* will identify potential sources of the bacteria in high-risk patient areas. The degree of contamination (percent of positive fixtures and quantity of bacteria present) varies significantly from building to building. The type of hot water system, water temperature, location, and building age all play a role in the colonization of pipes within a facility (36). The monitoring and control of *Legionella* in a health care facility requires a team effort, with microbiology laboratory, Infection Control, and maintenance departments working together to provide a safe environment for high-risk patients. There are no guidelines regarding culturing frequency or acceptable levels of positivity. Generally, each facility will establish a policy on environmental monitoring, depending on the patient population. Hospital areas with transplant patients may require more stringent monitoring and control programs than the general hospital population would require.

Control Measures in the Hospital

As a general rule, if significant quantities of *Legionella* are isolated in a facility, control measures to reduce the level of colonization should be instituted. Systems that use holding tanks or heaters that allow water to stagnate in the bottom of the tank provide a reservoir for the multiplication of *Legionella*. The newest approach to eradicate *Legionella* from the plumbing system involves the use of copper/silver ionization systems, which release low concentrations of metal ions into the water distribution system (37). Hyperchlorination of the hot water supply, thermal eradication (heat and flush method), UV light sterilization, and elevation of the water temperature may also successfully decrease contamination of the water distribution system (30,38,39).

Even when control mechanisms are in place, nosocomial legionellosis may occur. Disruptions in the water distribution system—such as water main breaks, use of fire hydrants, floods, and internal maintenance disruptions—may cause changes in water pressure that disrupt the biofilm within the potable water system (30). When pieces of the biofilm break free and enter the water supply, water may appear cloudy or dirty. Local water authorities may issue water restrictions in the event of major contamination of the drinking water supply. It is helpful to establish water service disruption policies to protect immunosuppressed patients. Substitution of appropriate bottled water is encouraged for drinking and mouth care. Ice machine filters may become contaminated and should be changed after water service is restored (40). Showering may be suspended until the water is determined to be safe. When service is restored, all fixtures should be flushed until the water appears clear. Tub bathing may be acceptable because there is little aerosolization of the water during the bathing process. Bed baths or other systems that do not generate aerosols are recommended.

Recommendations for the Discharged Patient

In areas where *Legionella* has been identified in the water supply, patients who rely on well or spring water may be encouraged to have their own water supply checked (36). It is often mistakenly assumed that all bottled water is safer or more healthy than tapwater, but many water products are not processed to reduce bacterial contamination. Products such as spring water that emphasize natural properties may contain more bacteria than other water products.

Antibiotic Resistant Organisms: Enterococci and Vancomycin Resistance

Nosocomial infections caused by resistant organisms have emerged as a serious problem in hospitals all over the world. This is due in part to an increase in nonselective use of broad-spectrum antibiotic agents. In an effort to prevent infection, patients are often placed on various prophylactic antimicrobial agents after SOT and before BMT engraftment (41). Although this practice decreases the incidence of infection, pathogens may develop resistance to the agents being used. The emergence of *Streptococcus viridans* which is highly resistant to penicillin, has been associated with the use of beta-lactam antibiotics in neutropenic cancer patients (42). Centers that are routinely using quinolones for neutropenic patient prophylaxis have reported coagulase negative *Staphylococcus* and Gram-negative blood culture isolates that are resistant to these agents (43,44). Infections caused by non-*albicans Candida* species, particularly *Candida krusei* and *Candida glabrata*, have been reported in centers using fluconazole as a prophylactic agent in neutropenic BMT patients (45,46). Nosocomial infections with resistant Gram-negative organisms (*Klebsiella, Stenotrophomonas maltophilia, Burkholderia cepacia*) are increasing and are believed to be related to the use of broad-spectrum antibiotics (47–49). Gram-negative bacteria that produce extended-spectrum beta lactamase are becoming more prevalent. Vancomycin-resistant enterococci (VRE) are used in this chapter as a model to describe control rationale and strategies to prevent the transmission of antibiotic-resistant organisms.

Enterococci have become a significant infection control problem, as evidenced by a twenty-fold increase in nosocomial infections reported to the CDC National Nosocomial Infections Surveillance (NNIS) System from 1989 through 1993 (50). Enterococci differ from other streptococci in their relative resistance to penicillins and cephalosporins and their intrinsic low-level resistance to aminoglycosides and lincosamide antibiotics (51). They are also resistant to bile, are considered normal enteric flora in adults, and generally exhibit low virulence. They may be isolated from the mouth, vagina, groin, and anterior urethra. Using molecular typing techniques, VRE strains have been identified as three resistance phenotypes—van A, van B, and van C (51). The van A phenotype is plasmid mediated and is by definition resistant to high levels of vancomycin and teicoplanin. Van B strains exhibit high-level resistance to vancomycin but are susceptible to teicoplanin. Class C is a constitutive low-level resistance to vancomycin and is found in *Enterococcus gallinarum* and *Enterococcus casseliflavus.*

Risk Factors for Infection

Epidemiological analysis has shown that often enterococcal infection has originated from the patient's colonizing flora. Intra-abdominal and cardiothoracic surgery and manipulation of the urinary tract have been previously identified as risk factors for enterococcal infection. Severity of illness has been identified as one of the main risk factors for development of VRE bacteremia (52–55). Critically ill ICU patients or those with underlying medical conditions, including immunocompromised patients on oncology and transplant units, are also at increased risk of colonization and infection with VRE strains. Increased length of hospitalization and antibiotic use contribute to the patient's risk (56). Although vancomycin use has been identified as a predisposing factor for acquisition of the organism, any antimicrobial agent that alters the normal Gram-positive and anaerobic gut flora may allow VRE to flourish (54,55). Recent reports have shown contact spread of the bacteria directly from patient to patient and indirectly on the hands of health care workers (57,58). Contaminated equipment and environmental surfaces have also been identified as sources for disease transmission (59). Liver transplant patients who developed VRE bacteremia were retrospectively compared with transplant recipients who developed bacteremia with vancomycin-sensitive enterococci (VSE) (60). VRE was associated with increased episodes of recurrent bacteremia and persistent isolation of this bacteria from the original site of infection. Whether VRE strains are more virulent than sensitive enterococci is still a controversial issue, but in this study there were few cases of endovascular infection among VRE patients and none among the VSE control patients.

Fecal carriage of VRE was studied in an outbreak on a renal unit. The authors used restriction enzyme analysis and ribotyping and were able to show that the outbreak isolate was clonally related (56). VRE was isolated from the stool of 15% of renal patients, 5% of other patients in the hospital, and 2% of sampled patients in the community with no history of hospitalization or antibiotic use (56). Many studies have shown by DNA analysis that nosocomial transmission is the primary route for VRE colonization among patients.

Infection Control Measures

The CDC Hospital Infection Control Practices Advisory Committee (HICPAC) developed guidelines for preventing the spread of VRE (61). Four main points were identified as crucial for prevention: prudent vancomycin use, an education program, an effective microbiology laboratory, and a multidisciplinary effort to control the organism.

The microbiology laboratory initiates the process of VRE control by promptly and accurately identifying the organism. When antibiotic susceptibility testing identifies a vancomycin-resistant strain, Infection Control, the patient's physician, and unit personnel should be notified. Patients colonized or infected should be placed in single rooms or cohorted with other VRE-positive patients. Because this bacteria may colonize the intestinal tract, patients with poor personal hygiene or fecal incontinence may contaminate the environment with the bacteria. Gloves are therefore recommended when entering the room of colonized patients. Gowns should also be worn if substantial contact with environmental surfaces is expected.

Various reports have documented the isolation of VRE strains from environmental surfaces (57,58,62). Noncritical items such as stethoscopes or thermometers should not be used on other patients unless they are thoroughly disinfected after use on a VRE patient. Dedicated equipment is preferred but may be shared among cohorted patients. Patients may be screened for VRE carriage by collecting rectal or stool cultures to identify additional cases. This information is useful to determine transmission between roommates or others on a unit where infected patients have been identified. Despite the institution of Contact Precautions for carriers, the incidence of carriage may remain about the same (53). VRE colonization may persist for long periods of time (63), and therefore colonized or infected patients may require continuous isolation until discharge. If a patient is to be transferred to another facility, it is imperative to notify the receiving institution about the patient's VRE status, so that appropriate precautions are taken. Readmitted VRE-positive patients may be placed in Contact Isolation until surveillance cultures are completed.

There are concerns that a plasmid that carries the vancomycin resistance gene could transmit this resistance to other Gram-positive bacteria, particularly *Staphylococcus aureus*. Because of the multiple virulence factors associated with this pathogen, infections would be very serious if the organism is already resistant to all antimicrobial agents.

Clostridium difficile infection

Numerous factors may cause diarrhea in transplant recipients: antibiotics, enteral nutrition, and other agents that affect bowel motility. Extended use of antimicrobials reduces the bacterial flora of the gut, providing a niche for the multiplication of *Clostridium difficile*, an anaerobic, spore-forming Gram-positive rod that is resistant to many antimicrobic agents. Although the organism may be found as normal enteric flora in approximately 4% of adults, it may also cause severe gastroenteritis manifested with either diarrhea or colitis. *C. difficile* is known to produce two toxins: toxin A, or enterotoxin, and toxin B, or cytotoxin. These toxins act synergistically, resulting in cellular damage, hemorrhage, and accumulation of fluid in the colon. In most patients, there is a history of antibiotic usage before the onset of diarrhea. *C. difficile* is recognized as the most common cause of nosocomial diarrhea, with higher rates of carriage reported in hospitalized patients, ranging from 15% to 30% (64).

Risk Factors

Although any antibiotic agent can affect the normal balance of the intestinal flora, clindamycin, penicillins, and third-generation cephalosporins have been particularly associated with the development of infection (65). Other factors that alter the gut flora also increase the risks of both carriage of the organism and disease. One study noted that the use of stool softeners and antacids was associated with increased carriage (66). Diarrhea has also been associated with older age, underlying disease, and enemas. Symptomatic patients usually have more risk factors, and certain intrinsic patient factors influence the relative risk of developing symptomatic infection (67).

Nosocomial Transmission

Documented clusters of cases due to nosocomial transmission have frequently been associated with environmental contamination with bacterial spores. In one study, 21% of culture-negative patients admitted to a general ward acquired *C. difficile* while in the hospital; of these, 37% developed diarrhea (68). The authors were able to prove transmission between patients by using an immunoblot technique, and documented clustering in patient rooms with two occupants. Other authors have suggested other patterns of acquisition, with no evidence of transmission to roommates (69). One nosocomial cluster investigation identified two case strains of bacteria by restriction endonuclease testing, associating most of the strains with abdominal surgery performed by one particular surgical team (70).

Because of spore production, the organism can survive well in the environment. *C. difficile* has been cultured from inanimate objects such as medical instruments, toilets, bathroom floors, and furniture (71). Bacteria have been cultured from the hands of medical personnel, with confirmation that strains isolated from medical staff caring for patients with *C. difficile* were the same as patient isolates (68).

Patients may become colonized with *C. difficile* transmitted by contact with other patients, contaminated rooms or equipment, or medical personnel carrying these bacteria on their hands. More environmental contamination with spores occurs if a patient has *C. difficile*–associated diarrhea than if carriage is asymptomatic. Nosocomial attack rates vary from facility to facility, with an approximate linear rate of 8% per week reported in high-risk hospitals (72). Clinicians taking care of transplant recipients should therefore be aware that nosocomial transmission of *C. difficile* is a real possibility, and early implementation of infection control measures may prevent other cases from occurring. Patients should be placed in private rooms or cohorted with other infected patients. Symptomatic patients should be placed in Contact Precautions. Health care personnel should wear gloves when entering the patient room. Gowns should be worn if significant contact with the environment is anticipated. Patient transport outside the unit should be minimized if the patient has diarrhea, to avoid contaminating other areas with the bacterial spores. Good hand washing is essential. Staff members must observe proper procedures; visitors also should be encouraged to wash their hands thoroughly before leaving the patient's room. If multiple cases of *C. difficile* colitis are noted on a patient unit, horizontal surfaces may be disinfected with a 1% hypochlorite solution (73). During outbreaks, environmental decontamination, isolation or cohorting of patients, and limitation of clindamycin were able to significantly reduce *C. difficile*–associated disease (74). Use of dedicated patient equipment or disposables such as rectal thermometers may significantly reduce the incidence of *C. difficile* diarrhea in both acute care and chronic facilities (75).

Antimicrobial Therapy Issues

Although the initial step in the treatment of *C. difficile* is to discontinue the antibiotic agent(s) to allow recolonization of the gut with normal flora, oral metronidazole or oral vancomycin is often used to treat the infection. Vancomycin use has been identified as a risk factor for colonization and infection with vancomycin-resistant enterococci (VRE), and its use for *C. difficile* is now recommended only in cases in which the patient fails to respond to metronidazole or if the infection is severe or life-threatening (61). Because antimicrobial agents associated with *C. difficile* infection also increase the risk of VRE colonization, many institutions are now attempting to use these agents more prudently.

COMMUNITY-ACQUIRED INFECTIONS

Tuberculosis

Increased disease prevalence in the community increases the possibility that an immunosuppressed individual will be exposed to a case of active TB. Transplant recipients are susceptible to infection with *Mycobacterium* species, and progression to active disease can be quite rapid, similar to the experiences of HIV-infected patients (76). Although stem cell transplant recipients have severe cell-mediated immunodeficiency, the incidence of MTB infection is relatively low. In a review of 2,241 BMT recipients at the University of Minnesota performed over a 20-year period, there were 11 cases of mycobacterial infection. These cases were comprised of nine atypical *Mycobacterium* species infections and only two MTB infections (31). MTB appears to be more of a problem after SOT than HCT.

Isolation

In the transplant unit it is essential that appropriate isolation be instituted as quickly as possible if TB is considered as a possible diagnosis. Some institutions require that any patient who has a respiratory tract culture submitted to the microbiology lab for TB culture automatically be placed in an appropriate isolation room until the diagnosis of TB is excluded. At our institution, three sputum cultures for TB collected on separate days must have negative smear results before isolation can be discontinued. Between 1983 and 1994, we treated 14 liver transplant recipients (0.5%) for active TB. We found that the most important risk factor was birth in a foreign country with endemic tuberculosis (77). Those patients who have increased potential for TB should be placed in isolation rooms if active disease is even remotely possible. In a 1990 nosocomial outbreak of TB that occurred among renal transplant recipients, disease was transmitted from the source patient to five other patients on the same unit. The institution of isolation was delayed because the TB infection had an atypical early presentation (78). Strain confirmation was performed by Restriction Fragment Length Polymorphism (RFLP) analysis. Mortality in this patient group was 50%, with the shortest incubation time between exposure and active infection approximately 5 weeks.

Ventilation system criteria for TB isolation rooms are described in the 1994 CDC TB Guidelines (79). Engineering controls are designed to contain any droplet nuclei, preventing the contamination of the patient units(s) and other public areas. The room must be at negative pressure to the corridor, with exhaust air vented to the outside of the building or filtered through high-efficiency particulate air filters (HEPA) before recirculation. Air changes per hour and other system parameters will vary, depending on the ventilation system design. Facilities may have to replace or retrofit their ventilation system to fulfill safety criteria. The 1996 CDC Guideline for Isolation Precautions in Hospitals uses the term *Airborne Precautions* to identify these room requirements for TB isolation (9). Although this ventilation design is also required for varicella isolation, requirements for respiratory protection differ between these two types of airborne infections. Approved particulate filter respirators are used by employees when entering the isolation room of patients with active or suspected TB.

Diagnosis

Active infection in the transplant patient may not present with the traditional symptoms found in the general population (80). Pulmonary infiltrates or pleural effusion may represent TB infection without other typical symptoms. After transplantation, most recipients remain or become anergic secondary to immunosuppressive agents that are administered to prevent organ rejection. Therefore PPD testing rarely provides useful information for monitoring transplant recipients. Important information is provided when conversion from negative to positive tuberculin skin testing (TST) occurs, but negative results do not rule out infection.

Tuberculin testing of close family members may provide additional information on the patient's potential to spread this infection. Disseminated TB is found more frequently in transplant recipients, because the major host defense against tuberculosis is cell-mediated immunity (80). After allogeneic BMT, patients are usually anergic for the first 3 months, but GVHD is associated with longer intervals of depressed delayed cutaneous hypersensitivity (81).

Many microbiology laboratories now use rapid testing methods to detect and confirm tuberculosis. Fluorescent microscopy for the evaluation of AFB smears and radiometric culture methods provide important diagnostic information, which may lead to earlier initiation or discontinuation of patient isolation.

Postexposure Follow-up

If transplant recipients are exposed to a person with active tuberculosis, a contact investigation should be initiated. Recent tuberculin skin test results and chest radiographs taken before the exposure may be used for baseline data. Additional PPD testing should be performed 12 weeks after the exposure to evaluate skin test conversion. Prophylactic INH therapy should be considered for the prevention of disease if the exposure is considered significant. If the source patient has a documented or suspected drug-resistant strain of TB, alternative prophylactic regimens should be considered (76).

Varicella-zoster Virus

Isolation

The infection control management of varicella-zoster virus (VZV) in the immunosuppressed population involves some difficult issues. It has long been recognized that varicella is transmitted by the airborne route during the primary infection (chickenpox) as virus particles are released from the airways of the patient into the environment. Transmission may also occur after direct contact with moist vesicles. Eighty-four percent of cases in adult BMT recipients are reactivations of the patient's latent virus, presenting as herpes zoster (28). Most cases occur after discharge; however, the patient may be readmitted to the hospital for treatment. CDC Guidelines require the use of Airborne Precautions and Contact Precautions for patients infected with varicella, and disseminated zoster (9). In dermatomal zoster, transmission occurs primarily through direct contact with the skin lesions. One of the most difficult tasks for infection control is to define "disseminated" zoster, to institute isolation room use.

In the immunosuppressed host, even small numbers of moist lesions and possibly respiratory secretions may contain enough viral particles to transmit the infection to other susceptible individuals through airborne routes or through shedding of viral particles from skin lesions into the surrounding air. An adult cadaveric renal transplant recipient that occupied a private room adjacent to a patient with zoster developed fatal hepatitis after nosocomial transmission of primary varicella infection (82). Sawyer and colleagues were able to demonstrate by PCR technique VZV DNA in 82% of air samples collected in varicella patient rooms and in 70% of air samples collected in zoster patient rooms (83). In a few samples, virus was detected outside the door of negatively pressurized isolation rooms. Although this may represent a failure of the ventilation system to maintain negative pressurization of the room or staff members leaving the door to the room open, obvious aerosolization of virus particles does occur. Virus was also detectable up to 6 days after the onset of rash using the same technique (83).

Patient Screening

Varicella infection in susceptible immunosuppressed patients may result in visceral disease and is associated with high mortality. We have reported a series of three adult liver transplant patients who developed varicella hepatitis; one patient died after developing adult respiratory distress syndrome (ARDS) and disseminated intravascular coagulation (DIC) (84). Varicella vaccine is contraindicated in the transplant recipient, because it is made from a live attenuated virus. After vaccination there is some risk of inducing visceral disease in patients who are taking immunosuppression that affects T cells (85). The risk of healthy individuals developing a rash after vaccination and transmitting it to an immunosuppressed patient is very low, and therefore there is no contraindication to vaccinate susceptible individuals (including health care workers) living in the same household with transplant recipients (86). It is recommended by the manufacturer that health care workers who develop vesicles not care for susceptible individuals, although it is hypothesized that this vaccine strain of virus may not be capable of causing secondary infections (87).

VZV susceptibility may last for years after BMT and is related to the severe immunologic deficiencies of these patients. Both allogeneic and autologous transplant recipients are susceptible to infection, and acyclovir prophylaxis may be efficacious in prevention (28,88,89).

Postexposure Management

Transplant coordinators must frequently evaluate an exposure of a transplant recipient to an individual with "possible" chickenpox. Most commonly, the exposure occurs after contact with a family member, usually a child. Defining the nature of the exposure as duration, proximity, and disease progression is an important step in the assessment process. Direct exposure is traditionally defined as one that occurred face to face for more than an hour; however, a significant exposure may be much shorter in this population.

It is essential that documentation concerning each patient's immune status be easily accessible. On a few occasions after an exposure occurred on the transplant ward, minor panic ensued because some patients did not remember if they had had chickenpox. Most adult patients are seropositive for VZV even if they do not recall their status. Varicella-zoster immune globulin (VZIG) prophylaxis after an exposure of seronegative patients to a case of VZV should be considered. An IM injection should be given within 96 hours after an exposure. When titers were unavailable, VZIG prophylaxis was given, because serologies would not have been readily available within the 96-hour time frame for treatment. The usual dosage is 125 units for each 10 kg of weight, up to a maximum of 625 units. If another exposure occurs more than 3 weeks after the VZIG dose was given, an additional dose of VZIG should be given to provide continued passive immunity (86). Acyclovir taken after VZV exposure may prevent or attenuate infection and may be a valid alternative after exposure.

Staff Considerations

Not all susceptible health care workers who report exposure to VZV actually develop chickenpox; in one report the incidence of varicella after exposure approached 10% (90). Traditionally, susceptible health care workers who report such exposure have been furloughed from work from the tenth to the twenty-first day after the exposure. This is based on the average incubation period of 14 days and the knowledge that transmission may occur up to 5 days before and 6 days after the onset of rash (91). Health care workers who receive acyclovir prophylaxis may exhibit a longer incubation period before the development of a rash. It is important to have accurate employee data concerning vaccination or previous history of chickenpox. Susceptible employees should be actively encouraged to receive the varicella vaccine.

RSV and Other Respiratory Viruses

Most of the respiratory tract viral infections are seasonal, are more prevalent in children than in adults, and are transmitted by droplets rather than aerosols. Coughing, sneezing, or talking may generate droplets, which are not usually projected farther than 3 feet from the source patient. Special ventilation is not required for inpatient isolation. In the hospital setting, suctioning respiratory secretions and performing bronchoscopy may also generate droplets. The most common respiratory viral infections include respiratory syncytial virus (RSV), influenza, parainfluenza, and adenovirus. The infection control aspects of respiratory viral infections are similar, and RSV is used as an example of infection control in the transplant population.

RSV is an RNA virus that causes upper and lower respiratory tract infections, usually before 3 years of age. Reinfection is common, but in the normal host is self-limited and generally mild. Outbreaks in the community usually occur seasonally, with peaks in the late spring and autumn, lasting until winter (92). The virus may be spread in nurseries, causing severe respiratory infection in infants which have underlying medical conditions, such as bronchopulmonary dysplasia, congenital heart disease or prematurity (93). Viral shedding usually lasts for a week, but may be longer in infants that are less than 1 month old or those with pneumonia (94). Nosocomial infections often parallel outbreaks in the community.

RSV can survive drying and can stay viable for about 6 hours on surfaces and fomites, including gloves (95). Transmission occurs by direct contact with a person who sheds the virus in the form of droplets or from contact with contaminated hands, handkerchiefs, eating utensils, or other articles. Viral particles may be inoculated into the eyes and nasal mucosa by touching these areas with contaminated hands (95). Therefore nosocomial outbreaks may occur not only from patient to patient, but also from caregivers or visitors who may think they have a cold (96,97).

Immunocompromised patients may develop lower tract lung infection with pneumonia. Most of the cases reported in the literature with severe infection and fatal outcomes occurred in patients after BMT, in adults as well as children. BMT patients are extremely vulnerable to infection in the aplastic phase after marrow grafting, and RSV acquired at this time may be fatal (10,98,99). In one outbreak in a BMT center, 14 of 18 (78%) who developed pneumonia died (100). Solid organ transplant recipients may also become infected with RSV (99,101). Two liver transplant recipients, who were less than 15 months old and were intubated when symptoms began soon after transplantation, died from RSV pneumonia (101). This may suggest direct inoculation of the virus in the lower respiratory tract, by-passing the upper airways. Ribavirin used orally or intravenously may reduce the morbidity and mortality due to RSV, influenza B, and parainfluenza (102). A study of intravenous ribavirin treatment of 10 BMT patients with significant RSV pneumonia performed at the Fred Hutchinson Cancer Research Center found no significant improvement in mortality rates when compared with historical controls treated with the aerosolized drug (103).

Infection Control Measures

Infection control measures should be promptly instituted to prevent nosocomial transmission. Contact Precautions should be used for infants, young children, and immunosuppressed individuals. In outbreaks, cohorting of symptomatic patients, with emphasis on hand washing, may reduce transmission to others. It is crucial for successful cohorting that early diagnosis of RSV be made when an epidemic is starting in the community. The use of shell vial cultures and rapid antigen detection by IFA or ELISA have greatly accelerated diagnosis compared with viral isolation techniques (104,105). The University of Texas M. D. Anderson Cancer Center found that contact isolation measures practiced on its BMT ward were inadequate to prevent the nosocomial transmission of RSV (106). An infection control intervention was instituted that included multiple strategies. Symptomatic BMT recipients were screened with DFA, ELISA, and culture of respiratory specimens. Infected patients were transferred to another unit where they were isolated, cohorted, and treated with aerosolized ribavirin. Masks and gloves were required for room entry. Visitors with symptoms of infection and children under 12 years were not permitted to visit. Symptomatic staff members were restricted from the unit. Using this multifaceted approach, nosocomial RSV infections were significantly decreased (106).

Other Respiratory Viruses

Other respiratory viral infections that usually manifest as self-limited upper respiratory tract illness may result in potentially life-threatening lower respiratory infections in immunocompromised patients, particularly after BMT. During an influenza A epidemic in Houston, eight of 28 BMT recipients were diagnosed with influenza. Five of these cases were nosocomially acquired (107). Six of the eight patients developed pneumonia, with a 17% mortality rate. None of the patients had received influenza vaccination or amantadine, illustrating the importance of yearly influenza vaccine for immunocompromised patients. It is also important for health care providers and the families of immunosuppressed patients to receive annual influenza vaccine, to further reduce the risk of disease transmission. Parainfluenza and adenoviruses may also cause life-threatening infection and be spread nosocomially (108,109). Rapid identification of the respiratory viruses, especially in pediatric wards, will help in cohorting staff and patients when an epidemic is recognized in the community (110).

Rotavirus and Viral Gastroenteritis

Viral gastroenteritis is usually a self-limited syndrome in the normal host. Several viruses are associated with gastroenteritis, including rotavirus, Norwalk and Norwalklike viruses, enteric adenovirus, caliciviruses, enteric coronavirus, and astrovirus (111). Rotaviruses and the Norwalk virus group have been considered the most epidemiologically significant agents of the gastroenteritis viruses, causing endemic and epidemic dis-

ease throughout the world. The rotaviruses have particularly been associated with outbreaks in children and in developing countries where they have been associated with high mortality rates (112). Symptoms often include vomiting, diarrhea, and dehydration. Fever may be present. Dehydration may be severe enough to require hospitalization for intravenous fluid replacement. The incubation period ranges from 1 to 3 days, with symptoms usually lasting for less than 1 week. Transmission of rotavirus occurs through the fecal/oral route, with maximum viral shedding in the stool 2–5 days after the onset of diarrhea. Nosocomial infections have been associated with insufficient use of appropriate infection control measures. Rotavirus infections represent between 20% and 40% of nosocomial diarrhea in children (113–115).

In the United States most infections occur in children between the ages of 6 and 24 months, after maternal antibody protection wanes (116). Infections are more frequent between October and April. Usually the virus gives a self-limited diarrhea; however, premature infants and transplant recipients may get severe disease (111). Although rotaviruses do not generally cause bloody stool, fecal occult blood loss has been reported in pediatric liver transplant recipients (117). It has also been found that viral gastroenteritis in BMT recipients was associated with higher mortality rates (114).

Nosocomial Transmission

Rotaviruses are relatively resistant to chemical disinfectants, with 95% alcohol (ethanol) considered more effective than formalin or phenolics. Sodium hypochlorite is also generally considered to be an effective disinfectant for environmental surfaces (111). The virus can remain viable in water and on dry inanimate objects and hands for many days. Rotavirus may be transmitted by aerosols, with inanimate objects contaminated not only by feces, but also by aerosols generated by cleaning bedpans (112). Patient-to-patient transmission may result in mini-epidemics within the hospital (111). Adult contacts of patients with rotavirus may exhibit subclinical illness (115). As a general rule, infection control measures should be instituted promptly whenever patients are incontinent or develop diarrhea. Standard Precautions are adequate unless the patient is incontinent or diapered, in which case Direct Contact Precautions should be added. Good hand washing is essential, with glove and gown usage for patient contact if fecal contamination is likely.

SUMMARY

Good infection control practices are essential to protect highly susceptible transplant recipients. Some management issues are still unresolved and are being handled according to internal policies in various medical centers. Cost-effectiveness is also becoming a very important issue in the practice of infection control. Although some preventive measures (like laminar flow) are very effective, they may be too costly for routine use if no additional benefit is provided to the patient. Until the use of new strategies can be validated, a common sense approach to patient care issues, such as focusing on appropriate hand washing, is essential.

REFERENCES

1. Hakim M, Esmore D, Wallwork J, English TAH. Toxoplasmosis in cardiac transplantation. *Br Med J* 1986;292:1108.
2. Centers for Disease Control and Prevention. Recommendations of the Advisory Committee on Immunization Practices (ACIP): Use of Vaccines and Immune Globulins for Persons with Altered Immunocompetence. *MMWR* 1993;42 (No. RR-14):1–18.
3. Winston DJ, Ho WG, Schiffman G, Champlin RE, Feig SA, Gale RP. Pneumococcal vaccination of recipients of Bone Marrow Transplants. *Arch Intern Med* 1983;143:1735–1737.
4. Versluis DJ, Beyer WEP, Masurel N, Wenting GJ, Weimar W. Impairment of the immune response to influenza vaccination in renal transplant recipients by cyclosporine, but not azathioprine. *Transplantation* 1986;42:376–379.
5. Jacobson IM, Jaffers G, Dienstage JL, et al. Immunogenicity of hepatitis B vaccine in renal transplant recipients. *Transplantation* 1985;39:393–395.
6. Witherspoon RP, Strob R, Ochs HD, et al. Recovery of antibody production in human allogeneic marrow graft recipients: influence of time posttransplantation, the presence or absence of chronic graft-versus-host disease, and antithymocyte globulin treatment. *Blood* 1981;58:360–368.
7. Higgins RM, Cahn AP, Porter D, Richardson AJ, Mitchell RG, Hopkin JM, Morris PJ. Mycobacterial infections after renal transplantation. *Q J Med* 1991;78:145–153.
8. Tolkoff-Rubin NE, Rubin RH. Clinical approach to viral and fungal infections in the renal transplant patient. *Semin Nephrol* 1992;12: 364–375.
9. Garner JS. Hospital Infection Control Practices Advisory Committee. Guideline for isolation precautions in hospitals. *Infect Control Hosp Epidemiol* 1996;17:53–80.
10. Sable CA, Donowitz GR. Infections in bone marrow transplant recipients. *Clin Infect Dis* 1994;18:273–284.
11. Sayer HG, Longton G, Bowden R, Pepe M, Storb R. Increased risk of infection in marrow transplant patients receiving methylprednisolone for graft-versus-host disease Prevention. *Blood* 1994;84(4): 1328–1332.
12. Centers for Disease Control and Prevention. Intravascular Device-Related Infections Prevention. *Federal Register*, vol. 60, no. 187, 9/27/95:49978–50003.
13. Centers for Disease Control and Prevention. Draft guideline for infection control in health care personnel, 1997. *Federal Register,* vol. 62, no. 173, 9/8/97:47276–47327.
14. Fenelon LE. Protective isolation: who needs it? *J Hosp Infect* 1995;30: 218–222.
15. Mooney BR, Reeves SA, Larson E. Infection control and bone marrow transplantation. *Am J Infect Control* 1993;21(3):131–138.
16. Wald A, Leisenring W, van Burik JA, Bowden RA. Epidemiology of Aspergillus infections in a large cohort of patients undergoing bone marrow transplantation. *J Infect Dis* 1997;175(6):1459–1466.
17. Walsh TJ, Dixon DM. Nosocomial aspergillosis: environmental microbiology, hospital epidemiology, diagnosis and treatment. *Eur J Epidemiol* 1989;5(2):131–142.
18. Iwen PC, Davis JC, Reed EC, Winfield BA, Hinrichs SH. Airborne fungal spore monitoring in a protective environment during hospital construction, and correlation with an outbreak of invasive aspergillosis. *Infect Control Hosp Epidemiol* 1994;15(5):303–306.
19. Hay RJ, Clayton YM, Goodley JM. Fungal aerobiology: how, when and where? *J Hosp Infect* 1995;30:352–357.
20. Streifel AJ. Air cultures for fungi. In: *Clinical microbiology procedures handbook.* Minneapolis: Department of Environmental Health and Safety, University of Minnesota, 1994.

21. Overberger PA, Wadowsky RM, Schaper MM. Evaluation of airborne particulates and fungi during hospital renovation. *Am Ind Hyg Assoc J* 1995;56:706–712.
22. Schuler U, Ehninger G. New approaches to the prophylaxis and treatment of bacterial and fungal infections in allogeneic marrow transplant recipients. *Bone Marrow Transplant* 1994;14(4):S61–S65.
23. Serody JS, Shea TC. Prevention of infections in bone marrow transplant recipients. *Infect Dis Clin N Am* 1997;11:459–477.
24. Russell JA, Poon M, Jones AR, Woodman, Ruether BA. Allogeneic bone-marrow transplantation without protective isolation in adults with malignant disease. *Lancet* 1992;339:38–40.
25. Loo VG, Bertrand C, Dizon C, et al. Control of construction-associated nosocomial aspergillosis in an antiquated hematology unit. *Infect Control Hosp Epidemiol* 1996;17(6):360–364.
26. Sarubbi FA, Kopf HB, Wilson MB, McGinnis MR, Rutala WA. Increased recovery of *Aspergillus flavus* from respiratory specimens during hospital construction. *Am Rev Respir Dis* 1982;125:33–38.
27. Arnow PM, Sadigh M, Costas C, Weil D, Chudy R. Endemic and epidemic aspergillosis associated with in-hospital replication of *Aspergillus* organisms. *J Infect Dis* 1991;164(Nov):998–1002.
28. Walter EA, Bowden RA. Infection in the bone marrow transplant recipient. *Infect Dis Clin North Am* 1995;9:823–847.
29. Brundrett GW. *Legionella and building services.* Oxford, UK: Butterworth-Heinmann; 1992:7.
30. Freije MR. *Legionella control in health care facilities: a guide for minimizing risk.* Indianapolis: HC Information Resources; 1996:15, 18–25, 65–77.
31. Roy V, Weisdorf D. Mycobacterial infections following bone marrow transplantation—a 20 year review. *Bone Marrow Transplant* 1997;19: 467–470.
32. Mandel AS, Sprauer MA, Sniadack DH, Ostroff SM. State regulation of hospital water temperature. *Infect Control Hosp Epidemiol* 1993; 14:642–645.
33. Yu VL. Could aspiration be the major mode of transmission for *Legionella*? *Am J Med* 1993;95:13–15.
34. Blatt SP, Parkinson MD, Pace E, et al. Nosocomial legionnaires' disease: aspiration as a primary mode of disease acquisition. *Am J Med* 1993;95:16–22.
35. Harrington RD, Woolfrey AE, Bowden RA, McDowell MG, Hackman RC. Legionellosis in a bone marrow transplant center. *Bone Marow Transplant* 1996;18(2):361–368.
36. Stout JE, Yu VL, Muraca PW, Joly J, Troup N, Tompkins LS. Portable water as a cause of sporadic cases of community acquired Legionnaires' disease. *N Engl J Med* 1992;326:151–155.
37. Liu Z, Stout JE, Tedesco L, et al. Controlled evaluation of copper-silver ionization in eradicating *Legionella pneumophila* from a hospital water distribution system. *J Infect Dis* 1994;169:919–922.
38. Muraca PW, Yu VL, Goetz A. Disinfection of water distribution systems for *Legionella*: a review of application procedures and methodologies. *Infect Control Hosp Epidemiol* 1990;11(2) :79–88.
39. Matulonnis U, Rosenfeld CS, Shadduck RK. Prevention of *Legionella* infections in a bone marrow transplant unit: multifaceted approach to decontamination of a water system. *Infect Control Hosp Epidemiol* 1993;14:571–575.
40. Stout JE, Yu VL, Muraca PW. Isolation of *Legionella pneumophila* from the cold water of hospital ice machines: implications for origin and transmission of the organism. *Infect Control* 1985;7786(4): 141–146.
41. Karp JE, Merz WG, Dick JD, Saral R. Strategies to prevent or control infections after bone marrow transplants. *Bone Marrow Transplant* 1991;8:1–6.
42. Carratala J, Alcaide F, Fernandez-Sevilla A, Corbella X, Linares J, Gudiol F. Bacteremia due to viridans streptococci that are highly resistant to penicillin: increase among neutropenic patients with cancer. *Clin Infect Dis* 1995;20:1169–1173.
43. Kotilainen P, Nikoskelainen J, Huovinen P. Emergence of Ciprofloxacin-resistant coagulase-negative *Staphylococcus* skin flora in immunocompromised patients receiving Ciprofloxacin. *J Infect Dis* 1990;161:41–44.
44. Carratala J, Fernandez-Sevilla A, Tubau F, Callis M, Gudiol F. Emergence of quinolone-resistant *Escherichia coli* bacteremia in neutropenic patients with cancer who have received prophylactic norfloxacin. *Clin Infect Dis* 1995;20:557–560.
45. Wingard JR, Merz WG, Rinaldi MG, Milleer CB, Karp JE, Saral R.

Association of *Torulopsis glabrata* infections with *Fluconazole prophylaxis* in neutropenic bone marrow transplant patients. *Antimicrob Agents Chemo* 1993;37(9):1847–1849.

46. Wingard JR, Merz WG, Rinaldi MG, Johnson TR, Karp JE, Saral R. Increase in *Candida krusei* infection among patients with bone marrow transplantation and neutropenia treated prophylactically with *Fluconazole*. *N Engl J Med* 1991;325(18):1274–1277.

47. Meyer KS, Urban C, Eagan JA, Bberger BJ, Rahal JJ. Nosocomial outbreak of *Klebsiella* infection resistant to late-generation cephalosporins. *Ann Intern Med* 1993;119:353–358.

48. Maningo E, Watanakunakorn C. *Xanthomonas maltophilia* and *Pseudomonas cepacia* in lower respiratory tracts of patients in critical care units. *J Infect* 1995;31:89–92.

49. Khardori N, Etting L, Wong E, Schable B, Body GP. Nosocomial infections to *Xanthomonas maltophilia* in patients with cancer. *Rev Infect Dis* 1990;12:997–1003.

50. Roper WL, Peterson HB, Curran JW. Nosocomial enterococci resistant to vancomycin—United States, 1989–1993. *MMWR* 1993;42:597–599.

51. Moellering RC Jr. Emergence of *Enterococcus:* a significant pathogen. Clin Infect Dis 1992;14:1173–1178.

52. Shay DK, Maloney SA, Montecalvo M, et al. Epidemiology and mortality risk of vancomycin-resistant enterococcal bloodstream infections. *J Infect Dis* 1995;172(4):993–1000.

53. Wells CL, Juni BA, Cameron SB, et al. Stool carriage, clinical isolation, and mortality during an outbreak of vancomycin-resistant enterococci in hospitalized medical and/or surgical patients. *Clin Infect Dis* 1995;21:45–50.

54. Edmond MB, Ober JF, Weinbaum DL, et al. Vancomycin-resistant *Enterococcus faecium* bacteremia: risk factors for infection. *Clin Infect Dis* 1995;20:1126–1133.

55. Murray BE. Editorial response: what can we do about vancomycin-resistant enterococci? *Clin Infect Dis* 1995;20:1134–1136.

56. Jordens JZ, Bates J, Griffiths DT. Faecal carriage and nosocomial spread of vancomycin-resistant *Enterococcus faecium*. *J Antimicrob Chemother* 1994;34:512–528.

57. Boyce JM, Opal SM, Chow JW, et. al. Outbreak of multi-drug resistant *Enterococcus faecium* with transferable vanB class vancomycin resistance. *J Clin Microbiol* 1994;32:1148–1153.

58. Rhinehart E, Smith N, Wennerstern C, et al. Rapid dissemination of beta-lactamase producing aminoglycoside-resistant *Enterococcus faecium*. *N Engl J Med* 1990;323:1814–1818.

59. Livornese LL Jr, Dias S, Samel C, et al. Hospital-acquired infection with vancomycin-resistant *Enterococcus faecium* transmitted by electronic thermometers. *Ann Intern Med* 1992;117:112–116.

60. Linden PK, Pasculle AW, Manez R, et al. Differences in outcomes for patients with bacteremia due to vancomycin-resistant *Enterococcus faecium* or vancomycin-susceptible *E. faecium*. *Clin Infect Dis* 1996;22:663–670.

61. Centers for Disease Control and Prevention. Recommendations for preventing the spread of vancomycin resistance. *MMWR* 1994;59:25758–25763.

62. Karanfil LV, Murphy M, Josephson A, et al. A cluster of vancomycin-resistant *Enterococcus faecium* in an intensive care unit. *Infect Control Hosp Epidemiol* 1992;13:195–200.

63. Morris JG, Shay DK, Hebden JN, et al. Enterococci resistant to multiple antimicrobial agents, including vancomycin. *Ann Intern Med* 1995;123:250–259.

64. Samore MH. Epidemiology of nosocomial *Clostridium difficile* infection. *Compr Ther* 1993;19(4):151–6.

65. Brown E, Talbot GH, Axelrod P, Provencher M, Hoegg C. Risk factors for *Clostridium difficile* toxin-associated diarrhea. *Infect Control Hosp Epidemiol* 1990;11(6):283–290.

66. McFarland LV, Surawicz CM, Stamm WE. Risk factors for *Clostridium difficile* carriage and *C. difficile*-associated diarrhea in a cohort of hospitalized patients. *J Infect Dis* 1990;162:689–684.

67. McFarland LV, Elmer GW, Stamm WE, Mulligan ME. Correlation of Immunoblot type, enterotoxin production, and cytotoxin production with clinical manifestations of *Clostridium difficile* infection in a cohort of hospitalized patients. *Infect Immun* 1991;59(7):2456–2462.

68. McFarland LV, Mulligan ME, Kwok RYY, Stamm WE. Nosocomial acquisition of *Clostridium difficile* infection. *New Engl J Med* 1989;320(4):204–210.

69. Clabots CR, Johnson S, Olson MM, Peterson LR, Gerding DN. Acqui-

sition of *Clostridium difficile* by hospitalized patients: evidence for colonized new admissions as a source of infection. *J Infect Dis* 1992;166:561–567.

70. Johnson S, Clabots CR, Linn FV, Olson MM, Peterson LR, Gerding DN. Nosocomial *Clostridium difficile* colonization and disease. *Lancet* 1990;336:97–100.

71. Fekety R, Kim K, Brown D, Batts DH, Cudmore M, Silva J Jr. Epidemiology of antibiotic-associated colitis. *Am J Med* 1981;70:906–908.

72. Gerding DN. *Clostridium difficile*. In: *APIC infection control and applied epidemiology: principles and practice.* St. Louis: Mosby; 1996:54-1–54-3.

73. Kaatz GW, Gitlin SD, Scheberg DR, et al. Acquisition of *Clostridium difficile* from the hospital environment. *Am J Epidemiol* 1988;127:1289–1294.

74. Struelens MJ, Maas A, Nonhoff C, et al. Control of nosocomial transmission of *Clostridium difficile* based on sporadic case surveillance. *Am J Med* 1991;91(3B):138S–144S.

75. Brooks SE, Veal RO, Kramer M, Dore L, Schupf N, Adachi M. Reduction in the incidence of *Clostridium difficile*-associated diarrhea in an acute care hospital and a skilled nursing facility following replacement of electronic thermometers with singe-use disposables. *Infect Cont Hosp Epidemiol* 1992;13(2):98–103.

76. Centers for Disease Control and Prevention. Management of persons exposed to multidrug-resistant tuberculosis. *MMWR* 41(RR-11):61–69.

77. Wada S, Kusne S, Fung J, Rakela J. Foreign born is the most important risk factor for tuberculosis in adult liver transplant recipients. The 36th ICAAC, New Orleans, 1996. [Abstract]

78. Jereb JA, Burwen DR, Dooley SW, et al. Nosocomial outbreak of tuberculosis in a renal transplant unit: application of a new technique for restriction fragment length polymorphism analysis of *Mycobacterium* tuberculosis isolates. *J Infect Dis* 1993;168:1219–1224.

79. Centers for Disease Control and Prevention. Guidelines for preventing the transmission of *Mycobacterium* tuberculosis in health-care facilities 1994. *MMWR* 1994;43(No. RR-13):60.

80. Lichtenstein I, MacGregor R. Mycobacterial infections in renal transplant recipients: report of five cases and review of the literature. *Rev Infect Dis* 1983;5:216–226.

81. Kurzrock R, Zander A, Vellekoop L, Kanojia M, Luna M, Dicke K. Mycobacterial pulmonary infections after allogeneic bone marrow transplantation. *Am J Med* 1984;77:35–40.

82. Patti ME, Selvaggi KJ, Kroboth FJ. Varicella hepatitis in the immuno-compromised adult: a case report and review of the literature. *Am J Med* 1990;88:77–80.

83. Sawyer MH, Chamberlin CJ, Wu YN, Aintablian N, Wallace MR. Detection of varicella-zoster virus DNA in air samples from hospital rooms. *J Infect Dis* 1994;169:91–94.

84. Kusne S, Pappo O, Manez R, et al. Varicella-zoster virus hepatitis and a suggested management plan for prevention of VZV infection in adult liver transplant recipients. *Transplantation* 1995;60(6):619–621.

85. Takahashi M. The varicella vaccine: vaccine development. *Infect Dis Clin N Am* 1996;10(3):469–488.

86. Centers for Disease Control and Prevention. Prevention of varicella: recommendations of the advisory committee on immunization practices. *MMWR* 1996;45(RR-11):1–36.

87. Merck & Co., West Point, PA. Varivax package insert 1995.

88. Ljungman P, Lonqvist B, Gahrton G. Clinical and subclinical reactivation of varicella-zoster virus in immunocompromised patients. *J Infect Dis* 1986;153:840–847.

89. Han CS, Miller W, Haake R, Weisdorf D. Varicella zoster infection after bone marrow transplantation: incidence, risk factors and complications. *Bone Marrow Transplant* 1994;13:277–283.

90. Haiduven D, Stevens DA, Hench C. Postexposure varicella management: further comments. *Infect Control Hosp Epidemiol* 1994;15(12):740–741.

91. Lund J. Varicella zoster virus in the health care setting: risk and management. *AAOHN J* 1993;4(8):369–373.

92. McIntosh K, Halonen P, Ruuskanen O. Report of a workshop on respiratory viral infections: epidemiology, diagnosis, treatment, and prevention. *Clin Infect Dis* 1993;16:151–164.

93. Hall CB, Douglas RD Jr. Nosocomial respiratory syncytial viral infections: should gowns and masks be used? *Am J Dis Child* 1981;135:512–515.

94. Hall CB, Douglas RB Jr, Geiman JM. Respiratory syncytial virus infections in infants: Quantitation and duration of shedding. *J Pediatr* 1976;89:11–15.

95. Wright SA, Bieluch VM. Selected nosocomial viral infections. *Heart Lung* 1993;22(2):183–187.

96. Madeley CR. Viral infections in children's wards—how well do we manage them? *J Hosp Infect* 1995;30:163–171.

97. Leclair JM, Freeman J, Sullivan BF, Crowley CM, Goldmann DA. Prevention of nosocomial respiratory syncytial virus infections through compliance with glove and gown isolation precautions. *N Engl J Med* 1987;317:329–334.

98. Fouillard L, Mouthon L, Laporte JPH, et al. Severe respiratory syncytial virus pneumonia after autologous bone marrow transplantation: a report of three cases and review. *Bone Marrow Transplant* 1992;9:97–100.

99. Englund JA, Sullivan CJ, Jordan MC, Dehner LP, Vercellotti GM, Balfour HH Jr. Respiratory syncytial virus infection in immunocompromised adults. *Ann Intern Med* 1988;109:203–8.

100. Harrington RD, Hooton RD, Hackman RC, et al. An outbreak of respiratory syncytial virus in a bone marrow transplant center. *J Infect Dis* 1992;165:987–993.

101. Rohl C, Green M, Wald ER, Ledesma-Medina J. Respiratory syncytial virus infections in pediatric liver transplant recipients. *J Infect Dis* 1992;165:166–169.

102. Sparrelid E, Ljungman P, Ekelof-Andstrom E, et al. Ribavirin therapy in bone marrow transplant recipients with viral respiratory tract infections. *Bone Marrow Transplant* 1997;19(9):905–908.

103. Lewinsohn DM, Bowden RA, Mattson D, Crawford SW. Phase I study of intravenous ribavirin treatment of respiratory syncytial virus pneumonia after marrow transplantation. *Antimicrob Agents Chemother* 1996;40(11):2555–2557.

104. Matthey S, Nicholson D, Ruhs S, et al. Rapid detection of respiratory viruses by shell vial culture and direct staining by using pooled and individual monoclonal antibodies. *J Clin Microbiol* 1992;30:540–544.

105. Rabalais G, Stout G, Ladd K, Clost K. Rapid diagnosis of respiratory viral infections by using a shell vial assay and monoclonal antibody pool. *J Clin Microbiol* 1992;30:1505–1508.

106. Garcia R, Raad I, Abi-Said D, et al. Nosocomial respiratory syncytial virus infections: prevention and control in bone marrow transplant patients. *Infect Control Hosp Epidemiol* 1997;18:412–416.

107. Whimbey E, Elting LS, Couch RB, et al. Influenza A virus infections among hospitalized adult bone marrow transplant recipients. *Bone Marrow Transplant* 1994;13:437–440.

108. Wendt CH, Weisdorf DJ, Jordan MC, Balfour HH, Hertz MI. Parainfluenza virus respiratory infection after bone marrow transplantation. *N Engl J Med* 1992;326:921–926.

109. Brummitt CF, Cherrington JM, Katzenstein DA, et al. Nosocomial adenovirus infections: molecular epidemiology of an outbreak due to adenovirus 3a. *J Infect Dis* 1988;158:423–431.

110. Ruuskanen O. Respiratory syncytial virus—is it preventable? *J Hosp Infect* 1995;30:494–497.

111. Rao GG. Control of outbreaks of viral diarrhoea in hospitals—a practical approach. *J Hosp Infect* 1995;30(1):1–6.

112. Ansari SA, Springthorpe S, Sattar SA. Survival and vehicular spread of human rotaviruses: possible relation to seasonality of outbreaks. *Rev Infect Dis* 1991;12:448–461.

113. Pacini DL, Brady MT, Budde CT, Connell MJ, Hamparian VV, Hughes JH. Nosocomial rotaviral diarrhea: pattern of spread on ward in a children's hospital. *J Med Virol* 1987;23:359–366.

114. Yoken RH, Bishop CA, Townsend TR, et al. Infectious gastroenteritis in bone-marrow-transplant recipients. *New Engl J Med* 1982;306(17):1009–1012.

115. Evans AS, ed. *Viral infections of humans, epidemiology and control*, 3rd ed. New York: Plenum; 1991:104.

116. Centers for Disease Control and Prevention. Viral agents of gastroenteritis: public health importance and outbreak management. *MMWR* 1990;39(RR-5):1–24.

117. Fitts SW, Green M, Reyes J, Nour B, Tzakis AG, Kocoshis SA. Clinical features of nosocomial rotavirus infection in pediatric liver transplant recipients. *Clin Transplant* 1995;9(3Pt1):201–204.

Transplant Infections edited by
Raleigh A. Bowden, Per Ljungman, and Carlos V. Paya.
Lippincott–Raven Publishers, Philadelphia © 1998

CHAPTER 4

Diagnosis of Bacterial and Parasitic Infection

Franklin R. Cockerill III

BACTERIA

Introduction

Bacteria are among the most commonly encountered microbial pathogens in patients who have undergone solid organ or bone marrow transplantation (1–7). Transplant recipients are susceptible to common bacterial pathogens that cause disease in normal hosts and, in addition, are susceptible to unusual bacterial pathogens that infrequently cause disease in normal hosts. These latter organisms—which include *Legionella* spp., *Nocardia* spp., *Rhodococcus* spp., *Listeria monocytogenes,* and *Mycobacteria* spp.—are opportunists, and by virtue of humoral or cell-mediated immune dysfunction within the host, produce life-threatening disease. Another bacterial pathogen, *Bartonella henselae,* has been recently determined to be the etiologic agent for cat scratch disease, an infection that can occur in all hosts. This organism also appears to be an opportunist and has been demonstrated to cause disseminated disease in immunocompromised hosts.

Other bacteria may cause disease in these patients as the result of anatomic barrier disruption. For example, endotracheal intubation results in a conduit between the upper airway that is normally colonized with bacteria and the lower respiratory tract, which is normally sterile. Bacteria that may be introduced through this artificial conduit to the lower respiratory tract and that may cause disease in the bronchial tubes or lung parenchyma include *Streptococcus pneumoniae, Haemophilus influenzae, Neisseria meningitidis,* group A streptococci, and *Klebsiella pneumoniae* (8). In hospital settings, the oropharynx may become colonized with nosocomial pathogens. These

include Gram-negative facultatively anaerobic bacteria, especially members of the family Enterobacteriaceae (*Escherichia coli, Klebsiella* spp., *Enterobacter* spp., *Proteus* spp., *Serratia* spp.); Gram-negative obligately aerobic bacteria, notably *Pseudomonas* spp., *Stenotrophomonas maltophilia,* or *Burkholderia cepacia*; or Gram-positive facultatively anaerobic bacteria, especially methicillin-resistant staphylococci (methicillin-resistant *S. aureus* [MRSA] and methicillin-resistant coagulase-negative staphylococci) and vancomycin-resistant *Enterococcus* spp. (VRE). Any of these nosocomial bacteria may colonize the upper respiratory tract and spread to the lower respiratory tract secondary to endotracheal intubation (8). Mucositis, as the result of total body irradiation and chemotherapy, may be associated with bacteremia as a result of oral flora, especially *Streptococcus* spp., viridans group (2,6). Intravascular catheters may become infected with cutaneous flora or nosocomial pathogens. These organisms include *Staphylococcus* spp., coagulase-negative; *Streptococcus* spp., viridans group; and *Corynebacterium* spp., including *Corynebacterium jeikeium* and the same nosocomial Gram-positive and Gram-negative bacteria described earlier. All these organisms may be introduced into the bloodstream directly if intravenous fluids or medications are injected through an infected catheter port. Alternatively, these organisms may first colonize a proximal port and then over time ascend to catheter tip (9,10).

Neutropenia following bone marrow transplantation is frequently associated with bacteremia. Enteric Gram-negative bacteria, notably members of the family Enterobacteriaceae, *Pseudomonas* spp., and the Gram-positive organisms *Staphylococcus* spp., or *Enterococcus* spp. account for most of these bacteremias (2).

The mechanics of solid organ transplantation may predispose to bacterial infections. Hepatic transplantation requires choledocojejunostomy (commonly a Roux-en Y procedure), which results in direct contact of the trans-

Chair, Division of Clinical Microbiology, Mayo Clinic, Professor of Microbiology, Laboratory Medicine and Pathology and Medicine, Mayo Medical School, Mayo Clinic, Division of Clinical Microbiology, 200 First Street SW, Hilton 470, Rochester, MN 55905.

planted liver with fecal flora (4,7). Before broad-spectrum antimicrobial prophylaxis programs targeted against enteric flora (e.g., selective decontamination of the digestive tract [SDD]) were used, serious bacterial infections occurred frequently with liver transplantation. However, selective decontamination protocols like SDD may further predispose the transplant recipient to infections with other bacteria such as VRE, MRSA, methicillin-resistant coagulase-negative staphylococci, and other unusual Gram-positive bacteria such as *Lactobacillus* spp. or *Leuconostoc* spp, and multidrug-resistant Gram-negative bacteria such as *Stenotrophomonas maltophilia* (11–15).

Because of the wide variety of bacteria that can cause infections in these patients, in some instances, test-ordering protocols may be useful to ensure that appropriate specimen processing and analyses are performed. This is especially important for specimens that are obtained using relatively invasive procedures. For example, at the Mayo Clinic, a standard battery of microbiology tests is performed on all specimens obtained by bronchoalveolar lavage, transbronchoscopic, transthorascopic, or open lung biopsies from immunocompromised patients. Clinicians simply indicate on a written form or by an electronic order that the patients are immunocompromised.

Table 1 summarizes the more commonly encountered bacterial pathogens in transplant patients. A review of the patient's clinical history and a comprehensive physical exam may disclose a source for infection or limit the differential diagnosis for bacterial etiologies. Communication with the clinical microbiology personnel is important so that appropriate cost-effective testing can be performed quickly and proficiently. Identification of the responsible bacteria and the provision of appropriate antimicrobial therapy according to susceptibility test results may impact significantly on the outcome of the transplant patient. Development of disease management strategies for infections in transplant patients may also facilitate these efforts.

Tables 2 through 4 summarize currently available recommended test methods for the detection of bacterial pathogens from human specimens. For completeness, the tables include pathogens common to both normal hosts and transplant patients, as well as pathogens that occur primarily in transplant patients. Not shown are specimen collection procedures. However, this important step in the diagnostic testing process cannot be overstated. An adequate amount of specimen (using sterile technique when appropriate) should be placed in the appropriate transport device, and the specimen should be transported under appropriate environmental conditions within a reasonable time period to the laboratory. As a large number of transport devices are available, consultation with the laboratory personnel is important, especially when unusual bacteria are considered. Comprehensive reviews of the specifics of specimen collection, transport, and storage are described elsewhere (16,17). As a general point, spec-

TABLE 1. *Bacteria that commonly cause disease in solid organ transplant or bone marrow transplant recipients*

Bone marrow transplant (neutropenia-associated infection)
  Gram-positive aerobic or facultatively anaerobic cocci
    Staphylococcus aureus (including MRSA[a])
    Staphylococcus spp., coagulase-negative
    Streptococcus spp., viridans group
    Enterococcus spp. (including VRE[b])
  Gram-negative aerobic or facultatively anaerobic bacilli
    Enterobacteriaceae
    Pseudomonas spp.
    Stenotrophomonas maltophilia

Solid organ transplant (postoperative infection)
  Heart/lung transplant
    Encapsulated bacteria[c]
      Streptococcus pneumoniae
      Haemophilus influenzae
      Neisseria meningitidis
      Klebsiella pneumoniae
    Other
      Group A streptococci (*Streptococcus pyogenes*)
      Burkholderia cepacia[d]
  Hepatic transplant
    Enterobacteriaceae[e]
    Staphylococcus spp.[f] (including MRSA[a])
    Enterococcus spp.[f] (including VRE[b])
    Leuconostoc spp.[f]
    Lactobacillis spp.[f]
    Obligately anaerobic bacteria
  Renal transplant
    Enterobacteriaceae
    Enterococcus spp.

Cell-mediated immune deficiency-associated and/or intracellular infections
  Gram-negative bacilli
    Legionella spp.
    Bartonella spp.
  Gram-positive bacilli
    Listeria monocytogenes
  Gram-positive, partially acid-fast bacilli
    Rhodococcus spp.
    Nocardia spp.
    Mycobacteria spp.

Postsplenectomy-associated infection
  Encapsulated bacteria
    S. pneumoniae
    H. influenzae
    N. meningitis
    K. pneumonia

Intravenous catheter-associated infection
  Staphylococcus aureus (including MRSA[c])
  Staphyloccous spp., coagulase-negative
  Enterococcus spp. (including VRE[d])
  Streptococcus spp., viridans group
  Leuconostoc spp.
  Lactobacillus spp.
  Stomatococcus spp.
  Corynebacterium jeikeium
  Enterobacteriaceae
  Pseudomonas spp. and other nonfermenting gram-negative bacilli

[a]MRSA refers to methicillin-resistant *Staphyloccus aureus*.
[b]VRE refers to vancomycin-resistant *Enterococcus* spp.
[c]May also occur with humoral immune deficiency.
[d]Especially prevalent in patients with cystic fibrosis.
[e]Common Enterobacteriaceae include *Escherichia coli*, *Klebsiella* spp., *Enterobacter* spp., *Proteus* sp., and *Serratia* spp.
[f]Especially prevalent if selective decontamination of the digestive tract (SDD) prophylaxis is used.

imens requiring strictly anaerobic conditions for viability must be sent in appropriate anaerobic transport devices (16,18). Depending on the volume, most other specimens can be sent in either a swab transport device (swab is immersed in nutrient broth) or a sterile container (16,19). Some studies have demonstrated the utility of blood culture bottles for transporting as well as culturing sterile body fluids, especially peritoneal fluid (20).

In general, rapid diagnostic test methods if available should be used in addition to conventional culturing techniques for diagnosing infection in transplant patients. These patients, because of significant immunoincompetence, may have rapidly progressive fatal infection if not diagnosed early.

Blood

Tables 2 and 3 summarize rapid detection and culture methods that may be useful for identifying both common and uncommon bacterial pathogens in blood. Some of the specialized testing methods shown are generally only available at reference laboratories. Therefore if the clinician feels strongly that one of these tests is useful, an aliquot of the specimen should be sent to a reference laboratory. Rapid test methods for the detection of bacterial pathogens in blood are limited in the number of different bacteria they can detect and are less sensitive than culture methods. Bacterial antigen tests for commonly encountered encapsulated organisms (*H. influenza, N. meningitidis,* or *S. pneumoniae*) are easy to perform and available in most laboratories (21).

Blood cultures should be obtained from all transplant patients in whom sepsis is considered. The standard blood culture set for adults consists of 20–30 ml of blood equally distributed between two or among three culture receptacles. When 20 ml of blood are drawn, the standard practice is to culture 10 ml in an aerobic atmosphere and 10 ml in an anaerobic atmosphere. If 30 ml of blood are drawn, the same practice is followed except the additional 10 ml is cultured under aerobic conditions. In patients with suspected endocarditis or endovascular infection, conditions in which bacteremia is continuous, two or three separate blood cultures collected at varying time intervals over a 24-hour period are nearly always sufficient. For other types of bacteremia, 99% will be detected by three separate blood cultures collected at varying time intervals over a 24-hour period (22).

Recently, some authorities have questioned whether anaerobic blood cultures should be performed routinely in all patients, especially those in whom anaerobic bacteremia is unlikely (23). We have recently demonstrated that anaerobic blood cultures may recover some facultatively anaerobic bacteria (e.g., *Enterococcus* spp., some viridans streptococci) more efficiently than aerobic blood cultures (24). Anaerobic blood cultures should be obtained in patients who have undergone liver trans-

plants and have signs and symptoms of sepsis (4). In this group, bacteremias caused by obligately anaerobic bacteria may occur because of the contiguity of the transplanted liver with the gastrointestinal tract. The lysis centrifugation method is a specialized blood culture method that is useful for recovering both common and many unusual bacterial pathogens and fungi (25–28). In this system, blood is inoculated into a test tube containing saponin, a chemical that lyses red and white blood cells, thereby releasing intracellular bacteria. The tube is centrifuged and the sediment is inoculated onto solid agar plates or into broth. *Mycobacteria* spp., especially *Mycobacterium avium-intracellulare,* occasionally produce bacteremias in severely immunocompromised patients. The inoculation of the sediment from a lysis centrifugation blood culture tube onto specialized mycobacteria agar or into BACTEC 13A broth bottles is useful for recovering mycobacteria (29). Controversy exists as to whether blood cultures can be obtained from intravascular lines (30–34). It has been shown by several investigators that such a practice results in the isolation of more contaminating microorganisms than if blood is obtained from peripheral veins (30–32). Contaminant blood cultures are associated with the increased length of hospital stay, and unnecessary use of antimicrobics and additional testing (35,36). These factors may result in more than 50% additional hospital charges (36). It is therefore advised that, whenever possible, blood for culturing be obtained from peripheral veins. This recommendation must be taken in the context of the clinical situation of the patients. For example, phlebotomy using peripheral veins may be risky in severely thrombocytopenic bone marrow transplant patients.

Other Sterile Body Fluids or Tissues

Bacterial antigen testing for *H. influenzae, N. meningitidis,* and *S. pneumoniae* can also be performed on cerebrospinal fluid (CSF) or urine. Bacterial antigen testing for *L. pneumophila* can be performed on urine. For staining and culturing methods, CSF, joint, peritoneal, or pleural fluids should be concentrated by filtering or centrifugation. In contrast, Gram stains of urine should be performed on unconcentrated specimens. The presence of ≥ 2 bacteria per oil immersion field ($\times 1,000$) in a Gram-stained smear of a drop of unconcentrated urine should represent $\sim 10^5$ colony forming units of bacteria per milliliter of urine. Bone marrow specimens may be particularly valuable for diagnosing *Salmonella typhi* (agent of typhoid fever) (37), *Brucella* spp. (38), or disseminated mycobacteria infections (*M. avium-intracellulare*) (17) and can be processed using the lysis centrifugation method (17). Granulomas surrounding small vessels in a bone marrow biopsy (ring granulomas) are associated with *Coxiella burnetti* (agent of Q fever) infection (39).

TABLE 2. Recommended rapid diagnostic tests for detecting bacteria in human specimens

Specimen	Stains	Immunologic tests[a]	Other	Bacteria detected
Blood	Acridine orange	LA, CIE, COA, FA		Haemophilus influenzae, Neisseria meningitidis, Streptococcus agalactiae (group B streptococcus), Streptococcus pneumoniae
				Generally, all bacteria but may be especially useful for detecting organisms present <10^4 colony-forming units (CFU)/ml or organisms that do not stain well with the Gram stain method, such as Bartonella henselae (agent of cat scratch disease, bacillary angiomatosis, and peliosis hepatis)
	Wright's, Giemsa, or Darkfield examination			
	Giemsa or Diff-Quik (buffy coat)			Borrelia recurrentis (agent of relapsing fever) or other spirochetes
	Dark field			Ehrlichia spp.
				Leptospira spp.
	Acid-fast or auramine-rhodamine			Mycobacteria species (occasionally positive when the quantity of organisms is high, as may occur with severe immunodeficiency)
Cerebrospinal fluid	Gram	LA, CIE, COA, FA		Generally all bacteria, although typical morphologies may not be present in cerebrospinal fluid
				H. influenzae, N. meningitidis, S. agalactiae, S. pneumoniae
	Acid-fast or auramine-rhodamine			Mycobacteria spp.
	Modified acid-fast			Nocardia spp., Rhodococcus spp.[b]
Brain tissue	Gram			Generally all bacteria
	Acid-fast or auramine-rhodamine			Mycobacteria spp.
	Modified acid-fast			Nocardia spp.
				Rhodococcus spp.[b]
Bone marrow	Gram			Brucella spp.
				Salmonella typhi
	Acid fast or auramine rhodamine			Mycobacteria spp.
	H&E			Coxiella burnettii[c] (agent of Q fever) (Organisms are not visualized but perivascular or ring granulomas may be seen which are characteristic.)
Sterile body fluids other than blood, CSF, or urine; sterile tissues; exudates or pus	Gram			Generally all bacteria
	Acid-fast or auramine-rhodamine			Mycobacteria spp.
	Modified acid-fast			Nocardia spp., Rhodococcus spp.[b]
	Warthin-Starry			Bartonella spp., Borrelia spp.
	FA			Borrelia burgdorferi, Rickettsia spp.
Eye fluid, tissue	Gram			Generally all bacteria
	Acid-fast or auramine-rhodamine			Mycobacteria spp.
	Modified acid-fast			Rhodococcus spp.[b]
				Nocardia spp.

TABLE 2. (Continued)

Specimen	Stains	Immunologic tests[a]	Other	Bacteria detected
Upper respiratory tract secretions	Gram	FA COA, LA, FA		*Bordetella pertussis* *Streptococcus pyogenes* (group A streptococcus)
Lower respiratory tract secretions including bronchial alveolar lavage [BAL], transtracheal or transbronchoscopic aspirates) and lung tissue (transbronchoscopic biopsy or open lung biopsy)	Gram Acid-fast or auramine-rhodamine Modified acid-fast	FA		Generally all bacteria *Mycobacteria* spp. *Nocardia* spp., *Rhodococcus* spp.[b] *Legionella* spp. (see also urine, below) for *Legionella pneumophila*
Urethral exudate (male)	Gram	EIA		*Neisseria gonorrhoeae*
Cervical or vaginal exudate		EIA		*Neisseria gonorrhoeae*
Stomach	Gram; Warthin–Starry or Giemsa (tissue)		Rapid urease test (biopsy) Urea breath test	*Helicobacter pylori*
Small bowel or colon tissue	PAS (periodic acid Schiff) Acid-fast or auramine-rhodamine			*Tropheryma whippelii* (agent of Whipple's disease) *Mycobacterium* spp.
Feces	Wet mount Methylene blue	EIA (O157 antigen and/or Shiga-like toxin [verocytotoxin]) EIA, LA		*Campylobacter jejuni* Evaluation for white blood cells associated with invasive bacterial diarrhea *Escherichia coli* O157:H7 *Clostridium difficile*
Genital chancer or chancroid lesion (male or female)	Gram Darkfield examination			Donovan bodies (associated with *Calymmatobabacterium granulomatis*, agent of granuloma inguinale) *Treponema pallidum* (agent of syphilis)
Urine	Gram Acid-fast or auramine rhodamine Dark field	EIA, RIA		Generally all bacteria (observation of ≥2 bacteria per oil immersion field ($\times$1000) in a Gram-stained smear of a drop of unconcentrated urine indicates ~10^5 bacteria/ml) *Mycobacteria* spp. Limited to *Legionella pneumophila* *Leptospira* spp.

[a]*LA* refers to "latex agglutination," *CIE* to "counterimmunoelectrophoresis," *COA* to "coagglutination," *FA* to "fluorescent antibody," *RIA* to "radioimmunoassay," *H&E* to "hematoxylin and eosin."

[b]*Rhodococcus* spp. may not stain by the modified acid-fast method.

[c]*Coxiella burnettii* is a Rickettsia-like bacterium.

41

TABLE 3. *Recommended culture methods for detecting bacteria in human specimens*

Specimen	Media[a]	Incubation	Bacteria
Blood	*Broth-based systems (manual or automated)* Effective broths that are most commonly used include tryptic or trypticase soy broth with ~0.025% SPS. One bottle is vented (aerobic) and the second is unvented (anaerobic). Manual or automated systems are incubated 5–7 d, or longer if fastidious organisms are anticipated. *Lysis centrifugation* Blood is added to a test tube containing saponin, a chemical that lyses white and red blood cells. The contents are centrifuged and the sediment is cultured to:	Incubation conditions: 35°C/room air.	Generally all commonly encountered aerobic, facultatively anaerobic and obligately anaerobic bacteria can be isolated with broth-based blood culture systems. Some fastidious organisms may require prolonged incubation (e.g., HACEK bacteria, which most frequently cause endocarditis).
	BA and CBA	35°C/5–10% CO_2/3 d	Most aerobic and facultatively anaerobic bacteria (including *Rhodococcus* spp.)
	MB7H10, MB7H11, and a BACTEC bottle containing 13A media	35°C/5–10% CO_2/60d[c]	*Mycobacteria* spp. *Nocardia* spp.
	CBA and TSB-TS	35°C/5–10% CO_2/6–8 wk	*Bartonella* spp.
	BRA	35°C/5–10% CO_2 28 d	*Brucella* spp. *Legionella* spp. *Francisella* spp. *Nocardia* spp.
	BCYE	35°C/2–5% CO_2/1–2 wk	*Brucella* spp.
	Other		
	FL, EH	20°C/Room air/4–6 wk	*Leptospira* spp.
	BSK-H	30°C/Room air/4 wk (tubes examined by Darkfield microscopy twice weekly)	*Borrelia burgdorferi*
Cerebrospinal fluid	BA, CBA, TGB(A) (specimen should be concentrated)	35°C/5–10% CO_2/2 d	Most aerobic and facultatively anaerobic bacteria
	BSK-H	30°C/Room air/4 wk (tubes examined by Darkfield microscopy twice weekly)	*Borrelia burgdorferi*
Bone marrow	LJ, MB7H10, MB7H11, BACTEC 13A	35°C/5–10% CO_2/60 d[c]	*Mycobacterium* spp., *Nocardia* spp.
	BCYE	35°C/5–10% CO_2/2 wk	*Nocardia* spp.
	BRA	35°C/5–10% CO_2/28 d	*Brucella* spp.
	BRA	35°C/5–10% CO_2/28 d	*Brucella* spp.
	BA, CBA, TGB(A)	35°C/5–10% CO_2/2 d	*Salmonella* spp.
	LJ, MB710, MB7H11, BACTEC 13A	35°C/5–10% CO_2/60 d	*Mycobacteria* spp., *Nocardia* spp.
	BCYE	35°C/5–10% CO_2/2 wk	*Nocardia* spp.
Brain tissue	BA, CBA, TGB	35°C/5–10% CO_2/2 d	Most aerobic and facultative anaerobic bacteria
	Abscess, aerobic media: BA, CBA, TGB(A) and EMB or MAC	35°C/5–10% CO_2/2 d	Aerobic and facultatively anaerobic
	Abscess, anaerobic media: TGB(An)	Anaerobic atmosphere/7 d	Obligately anaerobic bacteria

continued

42

TABLE 3. *(Continued)*

Specimen	Media[a]	Incubation	Bacteria
Sterile body fluids other than blood, CSF or urine; sterile tissues	BA, CBA	35°C/5–10% CO_2/2 d	Most aerobic and facultatively anaerobic bacteria
	CBA or TSB-RS	35°C/5–10% CO_2/6–8 wks	*Bartonella* spp.
	LJ, MB7H10, MB7H11, BACTEC 13A	35°C/5–10% CO_2/60 d[c]	*Mycobacteria* spp.
			Nocardia spp.
	BCYE	35°C/5–10% CO_2/2 wk	*Nocardia* spp.
	BSK-H, skin, or rarely blood and CSF		*Borrelia burgdorferi*
Exudate or pus	BA; CBA; EMB or MAC; CNA; TGB(A)	35°C/5–10% CO_2/2d	Most aerobic and facultatively anaerobic bacteria.
	CBA or TSB-RS	35°C/5–10%/ CO_2/6–8 wk	*Bartonella* spp.
	LJ, MB7H10, MB7H11, BACTEC 13A	35°C/5–10% CO_2/60 d[c]	*Mycobacteria* spp.
			Nocardia spp.
			Nocardia spp.
Eye fluid, tissue	BCYE	35°C/5–10% CO_2/2 wk	Most aerobic and facultatively anaerobic bacteria
	BA; CBA; EMB or MAC; CNA; TGB(A)	35°C/5–10% CO_2/2 d	*Mycobacteria* spp.
	LJ, MB7H10, MB7H11, BACTEC 13A	35°C/5–10% CO_2/60[c]	*Nocardia* spp.
			Nocardia spp.
Upper respiratory	BCYE	35°C/5–10% CO_2/2 wk	*Bordetella pertussis*
	BG or RL	35°C/room air/7–10 d	*S. pyogenes*
	BA	35°C/5–10% CO_2 or room air/2 d	
	BA and TA or CTA and LA	35°C/5–10% of CO_2 or room air/2–3 d	*Corynebacterium diphtheria*
Lower respiratory tract secretions (including BAL, transtracheal or transbronchoscopic aspirates) and lung tissue (trans-bronchoscopic biopsy or open lung biopsy)	BA; CBA; EMB or MAC; CNA; consider BC for cystic fibrosis patients	35°C/5–10% CO_2/2 d	Most aerobic and facultatively anaerobic bacteria
	BCYE	35°C/2–5% CO_2/5 d	*Legionella* spp.
		35°C/5–10% CO_2/2 wk	*Nocardia* spp.
	LJ, MB7H10, MB7H11 BACTEC 13A	35°C/5–10% CO_2/6–8 wk[b]	*Mycobacteria* spp., *Nocardia* spp.
Urethral exudate, cervical or vaginal exudate	CBA, TM	35°C/5–10% CO_2/3 d	*N. gonorrhoeae*
Urine	BA and EMB or MAC	35°C/5–10% CO_2/2 d	Most aerobic and facultatively anaerobic bacteria
	FL, EH	20°C/Room air/4–6 wk	*Leptospira* spp.
	LJ, MB7H10, MB7H11, BACTEC 13A	35°C/5–10% CO_2/60 d[a]	*Mycobacteria* spp., *Nocardia* spp.
	BCYE	35°C/5–10% CO_2/2 wk	*Nocardia* spp.
Gastric tissue	HP	35–37°C/5–7% O_2, 5–10% CO_2/7 d	*Helicobacter pylori*
	MB7H11, BACTEC 13A	35°C/5–10% CO_2/60 d[c]	*Mycobacterium* spp.
Small or large bowel tissue	B4; EMB or MAC; HE, XLD and/or SS; SB or 6NB	35°C/Room air/3 d	*Salmonella* spp.
Feces			*Shigella* spp.
	TCBS	35°C/Room air/3 d	*Vibrio cholera*
	CIN	30°C/Room air/2 d	*Yersinia entercolitica*

continued

43

TABLE 3. *(Continued)*

Specimen	Media[a]	Incubation	Bacteria
Feces *(contd.)*	SMAC CA	35°C/room air/3 d 42°C/5% O_2, 10% CO_2/85% N/3 d	*E. coli* O157:H7 *Campylobacter jejuni*
intracellulare	MB7H11	35°C/5–10% CO_2/60 d[c]	*Mycobacteria* spp., especially *M. tuberculosis* and *M. avium-intracellulare* (should only be performed on acid-fast positive specimens)
Intravascular catheters			
Ports (swabs)	Plate and incubate as per exudate or pus described earlier		Most aerobic and facultatively anaerobic bacteria
Blood cultures	See blood cultures earlier; simultaneous peripheral blood cultures should be obtained.		Most aerobic and facultatively anaerobic bacteria
Catheter tip cultures	CBA	35°C/5–10% CO_2/2 d and then room temp/room air/5 d	Most aerobic and faculatative anaerobic bacteria; ≥15 CFU colony forming units considered significant, Maki criteria, (ref. 38)
Surveillance cultures			
Upper respiratory tract (throat swabs or sputum) and *gastro-intestinal tract* (rectal swab)	BA; EMB or MAC; BHIB	35°C/room air/1 d	Most aerobic and facultatively anaerobic bacteria
Vancomycin-resistant enterococci (VRE) screen (rectal swab or feces)	ES	35°C/room air/2 d	Vancomycin-resistant *Enterococcus* spp.
Urine	BA; EMB or MAC	35°C/room air/1 d	Most aerobic and facultatively anaerobic bacteria.

[a]BA, blood agar; BC, *Burkholderia cepacia* agar; BCYE, buffered charcoal yeast extract agar; BG, Bordet-Gengou agar; BHIB, brain heart infusion broth; BRA, Brucella agar; BSK-H, Barbour-Stoenner-Kelly agar; CA, Campylobacter agar [types Skirrow, CVA, (Campylobacter-cefoperazone-vancomycin-amphotericin), CCDA (blood-free charcoal cefoperazone deoxycholate agar) or CSM (charcoal-based selective medium)]; CBA, chocolate blood agar; CIN, cefsulodin-irgasan-novobiocin agar; CNA, colistin nalidixic acid agar; CTA, cysteine tellurite agar; EH, Ellinghausen's agar; EMB, eosin methylene blue agar; ES, Enterococcosel agar; FL, Fletcher's agar; GNB, Gram-negative broth; HA, *Helicobacter pylori* agar; HE, Hektoen enteric agar; LA, Loefflers agar; LJ, Lowenstein Jensen agar; MAC, MacConkey agar; MB7H10, Middlebrook 7H10 agar; MB7H11, Middlebrook 7H11 agar; RA, Regan-Lowe agar; SMAC, sorbitol MacConkey agar; SPS, sodium polyanethol sulfonate; SB, Sellenite broth; SS, *Salmonella shigella* agar; TA, Tindale's agar; TCBS, thiosulfate-citrate-bile salts-sucrose agar; TGB, thioglycollate broth; TGB(A), thioglycollate broth used for aerobic isolation, containing rabbit serum; TGB(An), thioglycollate broth with vitamin K, hemin, and rabbit serum used for anaerobic isolation; TM, Thayer-Martin agar; TSB-RS, tryptic soy agar with defibrinated rabbit serum; XLD, xylose-lysine-deoxycholate agar

[b]The HACEK group includes the following bacteria: *Haemophilus aphrophilus/paraphrophilus, Actinobacillus actinomycetemcomitans, Cardiobacterium hominis, Eikenella corrodens,* and *Kingella* spp.

[c]Also incubate separate plates at 30°C if *M. marinum, M. ulcerans, M. chelonae,* or *M. haemophilum* is possible.

TABLE 4. *Molecular test methods currently available for direct detection of bacteria in human specimens*

Organism	Test method	Commercial kits
Streptococcus pyogenes	Specific ribosomal RNA (rRNA) sequences unique to *S. pyogenes* are detected using a single-stranded DNA probe.	Gen-Probe Group A Streptococcus Direct Test (Gen-Probe, Inc., San Diego, CA)
Mycobacterium tuberculosis	Transcription mediated replication and hybridization protection assay to detect rRNA	Amplified MTB Direct Test (Gen-Probe)
	DNA probing of a conserved region of the 16S rRNA gene amplified by the polymerase chain reaction (PCR)	Roche Amplicor MTB PCR Test (Roche Molecular Systems, Branchburg, NJ)
	DNA probing of an insertion sequence unique to *M. tuberculosis* (IS6110) amplified by PCR	
Neisseria gonorrhoeae	DNA probing of the *opa* gene amplified by the ligase chain reaction (LCR)	Abbott LCx Probe System (Abbott Laboratories, Abbott Park, IL)
Borellia burgdorferi (agent of Lyme disease)	DNA probing of the outer surface protein A gene—*ospA* amplified by PCR	
Bordetella pertussis	DNA probing of an insertion sequence amplified by PCR	
Bartonella henselae (agent of cat scratch disease, bacillary angiomatosis, and peliosis hepatis)	DNA probing of a conserved region of the 16S rRNA gene, or the citrate synthase gene (*gltA*) amplifeid by PCR	
Bartonella quintana (agent of trench fever)		
Tropheryma whippelii (agent of Whipple's disease)	DNA probing of a conserved region of the 16S rRNA gene amplified by PCR	
Ehrlichia spp. (agent of human granulocytic ehrlichiosis [HGE])	DNA probing of a conserved region of the 16S rRNA genes of *E. equi* and *E. phagocytophila* (which are closely related to the agent for HGE) amplified by PCR	

In addition, bone marrow specimens are frequently positive by stain or culture in patients infected with the fungus *Histoplasma capsulatum* (28).

Respiratory Tract Specimens

Legionella spp., *Mycobacteria* spp., and *Nocardia* spp. frequently cause pulmonary disease in transplant recipients (1–7). Using a direct fluorescent antibody technique, *Legionella* spp. can be diagnosed by direct examination of pulmonary secretions or alveolar tissue. Alternatively, acute infection with the most frequently encountered *Legionella* spp., *L. pneumophila,* can be diagnosed by screening for antigen in the urine (40). *Legionella* antigenuria can persist for months following acute infection, a factor that may limit the usefulness of this direct test for diagnosing subsequent *L. pneumophila* infections (41). Microorganisms that stain poorly by the Gram stain method and that appear to branch or are beaded in appearance, should be suspect for *Nocardia* spp. These organisms frequently stain acid-fast by a modified acid-fast staining method. This method uses less intense decolorizing agents than those used for conventional acid-fast staining of mycobacteria. *Nocardia* spp. grow more slowly than other bacteria but can be recovered on standard bacteriologic media. *Nocardia* spp. also grow well on media used for isolating fungi and mycobacteria and on media used to isolate *Legionella* spp. (buffered charcoal yeast extract, BCYE) (42). A recently described

opportunist Gram-positive bacillus, *Rhodococcus equi,* also may cause pulmonary infection in immunocompromised patients, including transplant recipients, and like *Nocardia* spp., may branch and stain acid-fast using a modified acid-fast staining method (43).

Feces

Occasionally, in severely immunocompromised patients, acid-fast staining and culture may be useful for diagnosing enteric infection caused by *Mycobacterium tuberculosis* or *M. avium-intracellulare.* It is advised, however, that cultures for mycobacteria be performed only on stools with positive acid-fast strains (44). If mycobacteria are recovered from feces, disseminated disease is frequently present.

Intravascular Catheters

Transplant patients may have indwelling central intravascular catheters for prolonged time periods. If other sources for infection are ruled out, then infection related to the intravascular catheter must be considered. Diagnosing intravascular catheter-associated infection can be challenging for the clinician considering the fact that a definitive diagnosis cannot be achieved unless the catheter is removed and a culture of the tip yields potentially pathogenic bacterium in sufficient quantity (i.e., ≥15 colony forming units of bacteria) (45). Some recent studies suggest that determining the ratio of colony counts of the bacteria isolated from blood drawn from the catheter and peripheral veins may be used for diagnosing catheter-related infection (46,47). However, further studies are necessary to confirm these findings. As previously emphasized, routine blood cultures should be obtained from peripheral veins and not intravascular catheters whenever possible. Bacteria growing from these cultures may simply represent flora colonizing the port. If there is evidence for a catheter tunnel infection (subcutaneous infection around the catheter), swabs of the affected area or pus if present should be stained and cultured for bacteria, mycobacteria, and fungi.

Surveillance Cultures

Surveillance cultures for bacteria (and fungi) may be useful, especially in settings where broad-spectrum antimicrobial prophylaxis is provided to transplant patients. As mentioned previously, one example of this is selective decontamination of the digestive tract (SDD) whereby the digestive tract is decontaminated of most Gram-negative and Gram positive aerobic or facultatively anaerobic bacteria (14,15).

Surveillance cultures of the oropharynx and the feces in patients receiving SDD or other forms of antimicrobial prophylaxis grow sparse amounts of Gram-positive facultatively anaerobic bacteria, notably *Staphylococcus* spp., *Enterococcus* spp., *Lactobacillus* spp., and *Leuconostoc* spp. In addition, yeasts may be recovered. If patients develop signs of sepsis while on SDD, it is usually the result of infection with one of these organisms. Based on the susceptibility patterns of the bacteria recovered by surveillance cultures, antimicrobic strategies may be developed for these septic patients. The true value of these cultures, including their cost-effectiveness, remains controversial.

Molecular Test Methods

Molecular test methods, including nucleic acid probing and sequencing techniques, allow for the detection of bacterial pathogens directly from human specimens. Currently available molecular test methods and nucleic acid amplification techniques are shown in Table 4. These methods are particularly useful for fastidious or slow-growing bacteria like *Legionella* spp., *Bartonella* spp., *Mycobacterium* spp., or *Borrelia burgdorferi*. The bacterial agent of Whipple's disease, *Tropheryma whippelii,* has never been recovered by conventional culture methodsd and presently can only be diagnosed by nucleic acid testing methods. It must be emphasized that some studies, particularly those that have evaluated molecular identification methods for group A streptococci and mycobacteria, have demonstrated that these methods, including those that use nucleic acid amplification techniques, are less sensitive than culture (48,489). Therefore if the results for molecular test methods such as these are negative, other diagnostic test methods, including culture techniques, should be considered.

Serological Test Methods

Indirect serological methods may be useful for diagnosing infections caused by certain bacteria and in some cases may be the only means by which a diagnosis is achieved. For *Rickettsia* spp., where alternative diagnostic test methods are limited (attempts at culturing these organisms should be avoided due to their high infectivity), these tests may be the only means by which a diagnosis is established. Table 5 shows the serological test methods currently available for bacteria at most reference laboratories. Of note, these methods detect IgG and/or IgM antibody to specific bacteria pathogens and for the most part require that the infection have existed in a

TABLE 5. *Serologic methods currently available for detecting antibodies to bacterial pathogens*

Organism	Technique[a]
Brucella spp.[b]	TA
Francisella tularensis	EIA, TA
Helicobacter pylori	EIA
Legionella spp.	IFA, EIA
Leptospira spp.	IHA
Bartonella henselae (agent of cat scratch disease, bacillary angiomatosis, and peliosis hepatis)	IFA, EIA
Borrelia burgdorferi (agent of Lyme disease)	EIA, WB
Treponema pallidum (agent of syphilis)	Nonspecific treponemal tests: RPR, VDRL
	Specific treponemal tests: IFA: FTA-ABS, IgG, IgM; MH: MHA-TP
	EIA
Ehrlichia spp. (agent of human granulocytic ehrlichiosis [HGE])	EIA
Rickettsia spp. (*R. rickettsia, R. typhi*)	IFA, CF, EIA
Coxiella burnetii	IFA, CF

[a]CF, complement fixation; EIA, enzyme immunoassay; FL, fluoculation; IFA, indirect fluorescent antibody; IHA, indirect hemagglutination; MH, microhemagglutination; SA, slide agglutination; TA, tube agglutination; WB, Western blot.
[b]Not all test profiles may include *Brucella canis*.

patient for a finite period so that detectable levels of antibody exist. For IgG analyses, a fourfold increase between baseline and convalescent antibody titers may be required to confirm infection. Because the demonstration of a fourfold rise in antibodies may require ≥4 weeks, the diagnostic utility of IgG analyses may be limited, especially in the acute disease phase. However, in some situations, baseline IgG antibody levels may exceed a critical threshold that is considered diagnostic for infection. Except for the last example, indirect serological methods cannot be considered as rapid diagnostic tests, and therefore may be of limited utility. These tests may also be of limited value in patients who lack a humoral response, especially bone marrow transplant recipients.

Susceptibility Testing of Bacterial Isolates to Antimicrobial Agents

The National Committee for Clinical Laboratory Standards (NCCLS) provides published guidelines for conventional susceptibility test methods for commonly encountered organisms that grow aerobically or anaerobically (50,51). These methods include disk diffusion, broth dilution, and agar dilution. For disk diffusion, the inhibition of growth of an organism on solid media is assessed around a paper disk from which antimicrobic diffuses.

The greater the zone of inhibition of bacterial growth, the more effective the antimicrobic. In the broth dilution procedure, the effect of a known concentration of antimicrobic dispersed along with the organism in liquid media is assessed. No growth of the organism (the broth remains clear) indicates that the organism is inhibited at the concentration of antimicrobic tested. For agar dilution, a known amount of antimicrobic is dispersed in solid media and the effect on growth of spot inocula of organism onto the surface of the media is assessed. No visible growth of the organism means that it is inhibited by the specific concentration of antimicrobic present in the solid media.

Interpretation of the results for each of these methods may differ as to the antimicrobic and organism tested, and guidelines for such are provided by the NCCLS. These interpretations are provided as the following categories: resistant, susceptible, or intermediately susceptible. If an organism is identified as resistant to a particular antimicrobic, it should not be used in the clinical setting. For some fastidious or slow-growing bacteria like *Nocardia* spp. or mycobacteria, no standard test methods are available. The automated BACTEC method, however, appears to be the preferred method for antimicrobial susceptibility testing of both *Nocardia* spp. (52) and *Mycobacteria* spp. (53). For other bacteria, which are not culturable or

TABLE 6. *Recommended testing methods for detecting parasites in human specimens*

Specimen	Stains	Immunologic tests	Parasite detected
Tissue Cerebrospinal fluid Bronchial alveolar lavage fluid Localized disease	Giemsa[a]	EIA, FA (IgG, IgM[b])	*Toxoplasma gondii*
Feces	Wet mount (direct or concentrated)		*Strongyloides stercoralis*
Disseminated disease			
Sputum	Wet mount (direct or concentrated)		
Tissue	H&E[c]		
Feces	Wet mount (direct or concentrated) and acid-fast		*Isospora* spp., *Sarcocystis* spp., *Cryptosporidium* spp.,[d] *Cyclospora* spp.[d,e,f] and genera of *Microsporidia*
	PAS, modified trichrome[g]		Genera of *Microsporidia*
	Electron microscopy		*Cyclospora* spp., and genera of *Microsporidia*
		EIA, FA	*Cryptosporidium parvum*
Tissue			
Fixed or embedded	H&E, electron microscopy		Genera of *Coccidia* and *Microsporidia*
	PAS, silver		Genera of *Microsporidia*
Touch prep	Giemsa (touch prep)		Genera of *Microsporidia*

[a]Identification of tachyzoites in tissue or fluid is required; identification of cysts does not imply active disease because many individuals may have cysts related to prior infection.
[b]The detection of IgM antibodies provides a more accurate indication of infection in the newborn.
[c]H&E refers to hematoxylin and eosin, PAS to periodic acid-schiff.
[d]Confirm oocyst size: *Cryptosporidium* oocysts measure from 4 to 6 μm and *Cyclospora* oocysts measure from 8 to 10 μm.
[e]Modified acid-fast staining may be required for *Cyclospora* spp.
[f]Cyclospora species will autofluoresce (strong green or intense blue) under UV epifluorescence (57).
[g]See ref. 52.

are poorly so (e.g., *Bartonella* spp., *Ehrlichia* spp., or *Tropheryma whippeli*), antimicrobial susceptibility testing is currently impossible.

PARASITES

Parasitic infections, in contrast to bacterial infections, are much less common in patients who have undergone solid organ or bone marrow transplantation (1–3,54). *Pneumocystis carinii,* originally classified as a protozoan, is now classified as a fungus and is not discussed here.

As mentioned for bacterial infections, transplant recipients are susceptible to a large number of common parasitic pathogens that cause disease in normal hosts. However, the current discussion will be limited to parasites that are opportunists in immunocompromised patients. These include *Toxoplasma gondii,* species of four genera of *Coccidia* (*Isospora, Sarcocystis, Cryptosporidium,* and *Cyclospora*), and species of five genera of *Microsporidia* (*Enterocytozoon, Septata, Nosema, Encephalitozoon,* and *Pleistophora*). *Toxoplasma gondii* infections have long been documented in transplant patients (1,2,54). Infections caused by the *Coccidia* or *Microsporidia* have recently been reported in immunosuppressed patients, notably those patients coinfected with human immunodeficiency virus (55–59). Isolated cases of these infections have been documented in transplant recipients (55,56). Intestinal disease has been demonstrated to occur with all *Coccidia* genera, *Enterocytozoon* spp., and *Septata* spp. Extraintestinal disease has been reported with *Sarcocystis* spp., *Cryptosporidium* spp., *Septata* spp., *Encephalitozoon* spp., *Nosema* spp., and *Pleistophora* spp. One helminth, *Strongyloides stercoralis,* can cause severe disseminated disease in the immunocompromised hosts and should therefore also be considered in the differentiated diagnosis of parasitic disease in transplant recipients.

Table 6 shows recommended test methods. Of note, it is advised that all patients who are candidates for transplantation undergo screening tests for these pathogens. In the case of *T. gondii,* a baseline serology should be performed. For the other organisms, stool exams should be done. Although DNA amplification tests have been developed for the detection of *T. gondii* in human specimens, no standardized procedures or commercial procedure kits are available.

REFERENCES

1. Miller LW, Naftel DC, Bourge RC, et al. Infection after heart transplantation. *J Heart Lung Transplant* 1994;13:381–393.
2. Walter EA, Bowden RA. Infection in the bone marrow transplant recipient. *Infect Transplant* 1995;9:823–847.
3. Kontoyiannis DP, Rubin RH. Infection in the organ transplant recipient. *Infect Transplant* 1995;9:811–822.
4. Paya CV, Hermans PE, Washington II JA, Smith TF, Anhalt JP. Incidence, distribution, and outcome of episodes of infection in 100 orthotopic liver transplants. *Mayo Clin Proc* 1989;64:555–564.
5. George DL, Arnow PM, Fox AS, et al. Bacterial infection as a compli-

6. Donnelly JP. Bacterial complications of transplantation: diagnosis and treatment. *J Antimicrob Chemother* 1995;36[Suppl B]:59–72.
7. Paya CV, Hermans PE. Bacterial infections after liver transplantation. *Eur J Clin Microbiol Infect Dis* 1989;8:499–504.
8. Deutsch E, End AE, Grimm M, Graninger W, Klepetko W, Wölner E. Early bacterial infections in lung transplant recipients. *Chest* 1993;104:1412.
9. Groeger JS, Lucas AB, Thaler HT, et al. Infectious morbidity associated with long-term use of venous access devices in patients with cancer. *Ann Int Med* 1993;119:1168–1174.
10. Raad II, Bodey GP. Infectious complications of indwelling vascular catheters. *Clin Infect Dis* 1992;15:197–210.
11. Patel R, Badley AD, Larson-Keller J, et al. Relevance and risk factors of enterococcal bacteremia following liver transplantation. *Transplantation* 1996;61:1192–1197.
12. Patel R, Cockerill FR, Porayko MK, Osmon DR, Ilstrup DM, Keating MR. Lactobacillemia in liver transplant patients. *Clin Infect Dis* 1994;18:207–212.
13. Steffen R, Reinhartz, Blumhardt G, et al. Bacterial and fungal colonization and infections using oral selective bowel decontamination in orthotopic liver transplantations. *Transplant Int* 1994;7:101–108.
14. Cockerill III FR, Muller SR, Anhalt JP, et al. Prevention of infection in critically ill patients by selective decontamination of the digest tract. *Ann Intern Med* 1992;117:545–553.
15. Cockerill III FR. Indications for selective decontamination of the digestive tract. *Semin Resp Med* 1994;8:300–307.
16. Miller JM, Holmes HT. Specimen collection, transport and storage. In: Murray P, Baron EJ, Pfaller MA, Tenover FC, Yolken RH, eds. *Manual of clinical microbiology.* Washington, DC: ASM Press; 1995:19–48.
17. Introduction to Microbiology Part II: Guidelines for the collection, transport, processing, analysis, and reporting of cultures from specific specimen types. In: Koneman EW, Allen SD, Janda WM, Schreckenberger PC, Winn WC, eds. *Color atlas and textbook of diagnostic microbiology.* Philadelphia: JB Lippincott; 1992:61–104.
18. Holden J. Collection and transport of clinical specimens for anaerobic culture. In: Isenberg H, ed. *Clinical microbiology procedures handbook,* vol. 1. Washington, DC: ASM Press; 1992:2.2.1–2.2.6.
19. Shea YR. Specimen collection and transport. In: Isenberg H, ed. *Clinical microbiology procedures handbook,* vol. 1. Washington, DC: ASM Press 1992:1.1.1–1.1.30.
20. Hay JE, Cockerill III FR, Kaese D, et al. Clinical comparison of Isolator, Septi-Chek, nonvented tryptic soy broth, and direct agar plating combined with thioglycollate broth for diagnosing spontaneous bacterial peritonitis. *J Clin Microbiol* 1996;34:34–37.
21. Cuevas LE, Hart CA, Muchogho G. Latex particle agglutination tests as an adjunct to the diagnosis of bacterial meningitis: a study from Malowi. *Ann Trop Med Parasitol* 1989;83:375–379.
22. Washington II JA. Blood cultures: principles and techniques. *Mayo Clin Proc* 1975;50:91–95.
23. Sharp SE. Routine anaerobic blood cultures: still appropriate today? *Clin Microbiol Newslett* 1991;13:179–181.
24. Cockerill III FR, Hughes JG, Vetter EA, et al. Analysis of 281,797 consecutive blood cultures over an eight-year period: trends in microorganisms isolated and the value of anaerobic culture of blood. *Clin Infect Dis* 197;24:403–418.
25. Hellinger WC, Cawley JJ, Harmsen WS, Ilstrup DM, Cockerill III FR. Clinical comparison of the Isolator and BacT/Alert aerobic blood culture systems. *J Clin Microbiol* 1995;33:1787–1790.
26. Cockerill III FR, Torgerson CA, Reed GS, et al. Clinical comparison of DIFCO ESP, Wampole Isolator, and Becton Dickinson Septi-Chek aerobic blood culturing systems. *J Clin Microbiol* 1996;34:20–24.
27. Cockerill III FR, Reed GS, Hughes JG, et al. Clinical comparison of the BACTEC 9240 PLUS Aerobic/F Resin bottle and aerobic culture of the Isolator for detection of bloodstream infection. *J Clin Microbiol* 1997;35:1469–1472.
28. Paya CV, Roberts GD, Cockerill III FR. Laboratory diagnosis of disseminated histoplasmosis—clinical importance of the lysis-centrifugation blood culture technique. *Mayo Clin Proc* 1987;62:480–485.
29. Kiehn TE, Commarato R. Comparative recoveries of *Mycobacterium avium*–*M. intracellulare* from Isolator lysis-centrifugation and BACTEC 13A blood culture systems. *J Clin Microbiol* 1988;26:760–761.

cation of liver transplantation: epidemiology and risk factors. *Rev Infect Dis* 1996;13:387–396.

30. Washington JA. Collection, transport, and processing of blood cultures. *Clin Lab Med* 1994;14:59–68.
31. Felices FJ, Hernandez JL, Ruiz J, Meseguer J, Gomez JA, Molina E. Use of the central venous pressure catheter to obtain blood cultures. *Crit Care Med* 1979;7:78–79.
32. Reller LR, Murray PR, MacLowry JD. Cumitech 1A, blood cultures II. In: Washington JA II, ed. Washington, DC: American Society for Microbiology; 1982.
33. Bryant JK, Strand CL. Reliability of blood cultures collected from intravascular catheter versus venipuncture. *Am J Clin Pathol* 1987;88:113–116.
34. Tonnesen A, Peuler M, Lockwood WR. Cultures of blood drawn by catheters vs venipunctures. *JAMA* 235:1877.
35. Dunagan WC, Woodward RS, Medoff G, et al. Antimicrobial misuse in patients with positive blood cultures. *Am J Med* 1989;87:253–259.
36. Bates DW, Goldman L, Lee TH. Contaminant blood cultures and resource utilization: the true consequences of false-positive results. *JAMA* 1991;265:365–369.
37. Vallenas C, Hernandez H, Kay B, et al. Efficacy of bone marrow, blood, stool, and duodenal content cultures for bacteriologic confirmation of typhoid fever in children. *Pediatr Infect Dis* 1985;4:496.
38. Entemadi HA, Raissadat A, Pickett MJ, Zafari Y, Vahedifar P. Isolation of *Brucella* spp. from clinical specimens. *J Clin Microbiol* 1984;20:586.
39. Voigtz J, Delsol G, Fabre J. Liver and bone marrow granulomas in Q fever. *Gastroenterology* 1983;84:887–888.
40. Sathapatayavongs B, Kohler RB, Wheat LJ, White A, Winn Jr WC. Rapid diagnosis of Legionnaires' disease by latex agglutination. *Am Rev Resp Dis* 1983;127:559–562.
41. Kohler RB, Winn Jr WC, Wheat LJ. Onset and duration of urinary antigen excretion in Legionnaires' disease. *J Clin Microbiol* 1984;20:605–607.
42. Vickers RM, Rihs JD, Yu VL. Clinical demonstration of isolation of *Nocardia asteroides* on buffered charcoal-yeast extract media. *J Clin Microbiol* 1992;30:227–228.
43. Prescott JF. *Rhodococcus equi: an animal and human pathogen.* Clin Microbiol Rev 1991;4:20–24.
44. Havlik JA, Metchock B, Thompson III SE, Barett K, Rimland D, Horsburgh CR Jr. A prospective evaluation of *Mycobacterium avium-complex* colonization of the respiratory and gastrointestinal tracts of persons with human immunodeficiency virus infection. *J Infect Dis* 1993;168:1045–1048.
45. Maki DG, Weiss CE, Sarafin HW. A semiquantitative culture method for identifying intravenous catheter-related infection. *N Engl J Med* 1977;296:1305–1309.
46. Douard MC, Arlet G, Leverger G, et al. Quantitative blood cultures for diagnosis and management of catheter-related sepsis in pediatric hematology and oncology patients. *Intensive Care Med* 1991;17:30–35.
47. Mosca R, Curtas S, Forbes B, Meguid M. The benefits of Isolator cultures in the management of suspected catheter sepsis. *Surgery* 1987:718–722.
48. Pokorski SJ, Vetter EA, Wollan PC, Cockerill III FR. Comparison of Gen-Probe Group A *Streptococcus* Direct Test with culture for diagnosing streptococcal pharyngitis. *J Clin Microbiol* 1994;32:1440–1443.
49. Dalovisio JR, Montenegro-James S, Kemmerly SA, et al. Comparison of the amplified *Mycobacterium tuberculosis* (MTB) direct test, Amplicor MTB PCR, and IS6110-PCR for detection of MTB in respiratory specimens. *Clin Infect Dis* 1996;23:1099–1106.
50. National Committee for Clinical Laboratory Standards. *Performance Standards for Antimicrobial Susceptibility Testing*, Eighth Informational Supplement. NCCLS Publication No. M100-S8. Villanova, PA: National Committee for Clinical Laboratory Standards; 1998.
51. National Committee for Clinical Laboratory Standards. Methods for Antimicrobial Susceptibility Testing of Anabolic Bacteria, approved standard—fourth edition. NCCLS Publication No. M11-A4. Villanova, PA: National Committee for Chemical Laboratory Standards, 1997.
52. Ambaye A, Kohner PC, Wollan PC, Roberts KL, Roberts GD, Cockerill III FR. Comparison of agar dilution, broth microdilution, disk diffusion, E-test, and BACTEC radiometric methods for antimicrobial susceptibility testing of clinical isolates of the Nocardia asteroides complex. *J Clin Microbiol* 1997;35:847–852.
53. Inderlied CB, Salfinger M. Antimicrobial agents and susceptibility tests: mycobacteria. In: Murray P, Baron EJ, Pfaller MA, Tenover FC, Yolken RH, eds. *Manual of clinical microbiology.* Washington, DC: ASM Press; 1995:1385–1404.
54. Renoult E, Georges E, Biava M-F, et al. Toxoplasmosis in kidney transplant recipients: report of six cases and review. *Clin Infect Dis* 1997;24:625–634.
55. Weber R, Bryan RT, Schwartz ↓, Owen RL. Human microsporidial infections. *Clin Microbiol Rev* 1994;7:426–461.
56. Current WL, Garcia LS. Cryptosporidiosis. *Clin Microbiol Rev* 1991;4:325–358.
57. Ortega Y, Sterling CR, Gilman RH, Cama VA, Diaz F. Cyclospora species: a new protozoan pathogen of humans. *N Engl J Med* 1993;328:1308–1312.
58. Long EG, White E, Carmichael WE, et al. Morphologic and staining characteristics of a *Cyanobacterium*-like organism associated with diarrhea. *J Infect Dis* 1991;164:199–202.
59. Weber R, Bryan RT, Owen RL, Wilcox CM, Gorelkin L, Visvesvara GS. Improved light-microscopical detection of microsporidia spores in stool and duodenal aspirates. *N Engl J Med* 1992;362:161–166.

Transplant Infections edited by
Raleigh A. Bowden, Per Ljungman, and Carlos V. Paya.
Lippincott–Raven Publishers, Philadelphia © 1998

CHAPTER 5

Diagnosis of CMV and Other Herpesviruses

Gillian S. Clewley, Vincent C. Emery, and Paul Griffiths

INTRODUCTION

Eight herpesviruses are now known to infect humans. We will discuss these in order, according to their significance for transplant patients and finally summarize cost-effective approaches to diagnosis.

Objectives of Laboratory Testing

The objective of laboratory testing and the techniques used cannot be considered in isolation. Furthermore, laboratory techniques must be chosen with knowledge of how the results may affect patient management. There must be clear, two-way communication between the laboratory staff and the clinicians who care for the various transplant patient groups. The laboratory techniques must be constantly audited to ensure that they still provide useful information when clinical protocols change (e.g., with the introduction of prophylactic antiviral drugs or changes in immunosuppressive medication). Routine use of old assays should be discarded as new treatments are developed that significantly decrease the incidence of infection (e.g., antiviral prophylaxis for herpes simplex virus [HSV] has eliminated the need to screen routinely for this virus). Likewise, new assays must be designed and introduced when new clinical challenges appear (e.g., strains of virus clinically resistant to antiviral chemotherapy).

These principles can be illustrated by describing the ideal assay for cytomegalovirus (CMV) infection. As described earlier, clinicians wish to treat CMV infection promptly, before it can trigger secondary pathological consequences. Clinical samples must therefore be collected prospectively and tested with assays that are sensitive enough to be predictive of disease but not so sensitive as to commit all patients, including those who never

would have developed disease, to treatment (Table 1). Clearly, not all these objectives can be achieved currently, but they provide a framework for assessing the laboratory services required for these complex patients. A summary of the attributes of various diagnostic tests for herpesvirus infections in the transplant recipient is shown in Table 2. Aspects of this table are expanded in the following sections, which describe each herpesvirus infection in detail.

Herpes Simplex Viruses

Serology

The presence of IgG antibodies against HSV indicates a previous infection with either HSV-1 or HSV-2 or both. In the transplant patient, it is usually only necessary to determine past infection with HSV, and there is no need to differentiate between HSV-1 and HSV-2 type specific antibodies. A positive antibody result indicates the possibility of reactivation post transplant, and marrow transplant patients and some solid organ transplant patients are treated prophylactically with antiviral drugs. Patients most at risk are those with high antibody titers pretransplant (1), so prophylaxis could be limited to these. The most commonly used assay to detect HSV IgG antibodies is enzyme immunoassay.

Collection of Clinical Specimens

Vesicular fluid and cells from the base of the ulcer from a fresh lesion are most suitable for electron microscopy, direct antigen detection, and virus isolation. Once lesions have crusted over, viruses can rarely be isolated. For viral culture, vesicular fluid, and throat swabs, swabs from the base of ulcers, saliva, and biopsy material should all be collected into viral transport medium. The specimens should be sent directly to the laboratory, but if there is a delay they should be refrigerated. For

From the Department of Virology, Royal Free Hampstead NHS Trust, London, UK NW3 2QG.

TABLE 1. *Objectives of laboratory testing for CMV*

Pretransplant
  Test donor and recipient for IgG antibodies to detect patients at risk for reactivation of infection.
Posttransplant
  Receive regular surveillance samples from the recipient.
  Process these samples by methods that:
  - Give rapid results.
  - Are sensitive and specific.
  - Provide prognostic information regarding risk for disease.
  Receive other samples from patients with conditions where CMV is in the differential diagnosis; for example,
  - Bronchial washings in cases of pneumonitis
  - Biopsies of affected organs
  - CSF
  Receive samples from patients with suspected resistance to anti-CMV drugs:
  - Rapid identification or exclusion of resistance
  - Advice on alternative drugs to be used

---

electron microscopy or direct antigen detection, the vesicular fluid and cells should be smeared onto a clean glass slide, placed in a slide box, and immediately transported to the laboratory for examination. Cerebrospinal fluid (CSF) specimens should be collected aseptically into a sterile container without any preservatives because these may inhibit PCR tests.

Methods for Rapid Diagnosis

Electron Microscopy Electron microscopy is probably the most rapid method to identify herpesviruses in vesicular fluid. The vesicular fluid is mixed with a small drop of phosphotungstic acid (3% in distilled water), a drop of the mixture placed on a carbon and formvar-coated copper grid, and excess fluid removed using a small piece of filter paper. On examination by electron microscopy, herpesvirus particles may be seen, but the type of herpesvirus cannot be distinguished because all types look the same. Although electron microscopy is quick to perform, it is an insensitive method, and a high titer of virus, at least 10^6 viral particles per milliliter, is required. The cost per test is low if the capital cost of the equipment is ignored. Thus electron microscopy is used only by laboratories that already have this equipment for other reasons.

Immunofluorescence An alternative method, which is more sensitive and specific than electron microscopy, is immunofluorescence examination using cells collected from the base of vesicular lesions. The cells are scraped from the lesion and smeared onto a glass slide. After the slide is dried and fixed in acetone, the cells can be stained with antibodies to HSV that are directly conjugated to fluorescein isothiocynate (FITC). Monoclonal antibodies to HSV-1 and HSV-2 are also available should serotyping of the virus be necessary.

Enzyme Immunoassay Commercially available enzyme immunoassays, or EIAs, for the detection of HSV antigen are also available. These procedures are rapid but tend to be less sensitive and less specific than immunofluorescence and can give false-positive results due to nonspecific binding of the conjugate. Any positive samples should be reassayed after being neutralized with HSV-specific antibody to confirm a true positive.

Cell Culture HSV can be isolated and propagated easily in many different primary and continuous cell lines. Cell cultures inoculated with 0.2 ml of clinical specimen will develop a typical cytopathic effect (CPE) of ballooning, degenerating cells, and occasionally multinucleated giant cells, within 1–7 days. Depending upon the cell line used and the titer of virus in the specimen, many of the cultures show a CPE within 24 hours.

Although the CPE produced by HSV replication is usually characteristic, the changes seen may be similar to those produced by other viruses. Therefore CPE should be confirmed by HSV-specific assays (e.g., neutralization

---

TABLE 2. *Choice of diagnostic test for the detection of herpesvirus infections in the transplant recipient*

Virus	\multicolumn{5}{c}{Diagnostic technique}
	EM	Direct immunofluorescence	PCR	DEAFF/Shell vial	Cell culture
HSV	++	+++	++ (for CSF samples)	–	+
VZV	++	+++	++ (for CSF samples)	–	+
CMV	–	+++ (antigenemia test)	+++	+	+
EBV	–	–	+++	–	–
HHV-6	–	–	+++	–	+
HHV-7	–	–	+++	–	+
HHV-8	–	–	++	–	+/–

with specific antibody or immunofluorescence using monoclonal antibodies to HSV-1 and HSV-2). Immunofluorescence is a quicker assay to perform, and the availability of commercially produced conjugated monoclonal antibodies has made subtyping of HSV isolates routine in many laboratories.

The amount of virus present in a clinical specimen can be semiquantitated using a tissue culture infectious dose 50% ($TCID_{50}$) end-point assay. This is the highest dilution of clinical specimen that produces CPE in 50% of the cell cultures inoculated. These assays are only rarely performed but are becoming increasingly important in the identification of drug-resistant strains of virus. After the virus has been quantitated using a $TCID_{50}$ assay, a known amount of virus can be cultured with varying concentrations of antiviral drug and 50% inhibitory concentration can be determined. This will identify drug-resistant strains of virus, and alternative antivirals can be assayed in this way to identify one for clinical use.

Cell culture is an extremely sensitive method of viral detection, providing the clinical material is collected, transported, and stored correctly, but cell culture facilities are needed and the procedure is very labor intensive and, hence, expensive. It should be part of routine clinical laboratory procedure because it provides a virus substrate for sensitivity testing.

PCR With suspected cases of herpes simplex encephalitis, HSV DNA can be looked for in the CSF by a PCR assay. Because of the low level of viral nucleic acid in the CSF, a nested PCR assay should be used. PCR has been shown to be a sensitive and specific method for the diagnosis of acute herpes simplex encephalitis (2). However, HSV is widespread in the environment, especially in a diagnostic virology laboratory, so great care must be taken not to contaminate any samples that are to be processed by PCR. Amplified product from previous HSV PCR reactions can also be a source of contamination, so as with other PCR assays, there is a stringent need to physically separate the individual processes of the PCR technique and incorporate negative controls into each assay to test for contamination.

Varicella-zoster

Serology

The presence of IgG antibodies against varicella-zoster virus (VZV) indicates a past infection with the virus and hence the possibility of reactivation after transplant. All transplant patients should have their VZV antibody status determined pretransplant. They can be monitored clinically for reactivation (if seropositive) or to ensure they do not come into contact with anyone with chickenpox or zoster (if seronegative). Many different methods are available for the detection of VZV IgG antibodies, the most sensitive being radioimmunoassay (RIA) and

enzyme immunoassay. Many are commercially available EIAs, and for practical reasons EIA tends to be the assay of choice rather than RIA. Latex agglutination tests are also commercially available and are particularly useful when a rapid antibody test is required. These assays are sensitive but prozones may occur with high titer serum samples, giving a false-negative result, so for this reason all negative samples should also be tested diluted to overcome this problem.

Collection of Clinical Specimens

As for HSV infections, the best specimen for the detection of VZV is vesicular fluid plus cells collected from a fresh lesion onto a glass slide for electron microscopy or direct antigen detection, and on a cotton swab in viral transport medium for viral culture. VZV is rarely isolated from any other site, although in the cases of disseminated infection it may be grown from multiple dermatomes and, if fatal, from various tissues collected at autopsy. VZV DNA is also rarely detected in CSF specimens from patients with encephalitis following acute or reactivated infection with VZV. The CSF specimen should be collected into a sterile container and sent to the laboratory for PCR.

Methods for Rapid Diagnosis

Electron Microscopy Exactly the same procedure is carried out as for HSV detection, and as with HSV, a positive specimen will show herpesvirus particles by electron microscopy, but the type of herpesvirus present cannot be determined.

Immunofluorescence The cells obtained from the base of a VZV vesicular lesion can also be stained with FITC-conjugated VZV monoclonal antibodies. As with HSV detection this is a more sensitive and specific method of rapid VZV diagnosis than electron microscopy and is the preferred assay. Cells are scraped from the lesion and smeared on to a glass slide. After the slide is dried and fixed in acetone, the cells can be stained with FITC-conjugated VZV monoclonal antibodies. This will give a differential diagnosis between VZV and HSV, whereas electron microscopy will not.

Cell Culture VZV will replicate in a wide variety of human, and in several simian, cell lines. Probably the best cells to use are human fibroblasts, which are very sensitive and can be maintained without passage for long periods to allow for the development of VZV CPE, which can take from 3 days to more than 2 weeks to appear. The CPE is focal, and virus spreads from cell to cell, so that the focal sites gradually enlarge. The CPE of VZV in fibroblasts is very characteristic and further identification is usually not required. The focal lesions are oval in shape and enlarge as the CPE develops, with many of the cells being multinucleated and on staining showing intranuclear inclusions. VZV remains strongly cell associated and can only be passaged into fresh cells by inoculation with infected cells and not with cell-free media.

PCR VZV DNA can be detected in CSF in patients with VZV encephalitis by PCR (3). As with the HSV PCR, a nested assay is required to increase the sensitivity because of the probable low level of DNA in the CSF.

Cytomegalovirus

Pretransplant

Detection of IgG antibodies

The presence of IgG antibodies against CMV is a clear indication of past infection. Although the seropositive individual is immune in the immunologic sense, the individual is latently infected with virus that is capable of reactivation, especially when the immune system is ablated as part of conditioning, and may become reinfected with a different strain of CMV (e.g., from a donated organ). Many different types of assays have been described for the detection of IgG and IgM antibodies against CMV, including neutralization, complement fixation, indirect hemagglutination, indirect immunofluorescence, latex agglutination, radioimmunoassay, and enzyme immunoassay. Many of these have been useful for epidemiological studies and for the diagnostic purposes. The AD169 strain of CMV is recommended for routine diagnostic work because of its broad spectrum of reactivity. However, wild-type viruses contain an additional 22 genes (4) that have presumably been lost from Ad169 during passage *in vitro*.

For the detection of IgG antibodies against CMV in the immunocompromised patient, a more sensitive assay, such as an EIA, should be used. If an immunofluorescence assay is to be used, it should be the anticomplementary immunofluorescence test because it is not affected by IgG binding to Fc receptors induced by CMV infection. There is no indication for IgM testing at present.

Post Transplant

Collection of Clinical Specimens

The mainstay of diagnosis is the collection of regular blood samples. Blood for PCR can be either an ethylenediaminetetraacetic acid (EDTA) or citrated sample, but blood for CMV culture should be collected into 500 units of preservative-free heparin per 10 ml of blood. Historically, blood, urine, and saliva have been the clinical specimens collected for the routine surveillance of CMV infection. Urine must be fresh and sent to the laboratory without additives because CMV is stable in urine. Saliva should be collected with a plain cotton-tipped swab and sent to the laboratory in viral transport medium.

Tissue biopsies in viral transport medium, bronchoalveolar lavage, or CSF samples collected in sterile containers can also be processed for CMV. All specimens should be sent directly to the laboratory. If there is a delay in transporting the specimens, they should be refrigerated, but under no circumstances should they be frozen.

Cell Culture Human fibroblasts are the only cells fully permissive for CMV replication *in vitro*, whereas *in vivo* CMV infects mainly tissues of epithelial origin as well as endothelial cells. Although CMV can infect and replicate in other cells, such as human thyroid endothelial cells and rabbit fibroblasts, only a low level of virus is produced.

Semicontinuous fibroblast cells grown from foreskin or embryo lungs can be used for CMV culture but must be used at a low passage (<20). To detect wild strains of CMV great care must be taken in the propagation of the cells, ensuring that they are free from other microorganisms such as mycoplasmas. The culture medium should be removed from the cells, 0.2 ml of clinical specimen inoculated and the cultures incubated at 37°C for 1 hour to allow virus adsorption. The cultures should then be washed and refed to help prevent the toxic effect of the specimen. The cell culture should be observed every other day for the development of the typical CPE produced by CMV. The CPE of CMV usually develops slowly and the cultures must be maintained for a minimum of 21 days.

Detection of Early Antigen Fluorescent Foci Test/Shell Vial Culture The detection of early antigen fluorescent foci (DEAFF) test and the shell vial culture are methods that allow the sensitivity and specificity of cell culture to be retained, but by the detection of immediate-early or early gene products of CMV replication, there is no need to wait for full productive viral replication before a diagnostic result is obtained.

For the DEAFF test, clinical specimens are inoculated onto cell cultures and grown, as described earlier, on chamber slides or shell vials. The cultures are incubated for 18–24 hours before being fixed and stained with monoclonal antibodies directed against immediate-early and/or early CMV gene products that will have accumulated within the nuclei of the infected cells. After the cells are stained with a secondary FITC labeled antibody, a positive culture will show fluorescent nuclei when viewed under a UV microscope (5).

For the shell vial assay, fibroblasts are grown on round coverslips placed in the bottom of shell vials. These are inoculated with clinical samples and centrifuged at room temperature for 1 hour at 700 *g*. The cultures are incubated for 18–24 hours and the coverslips are fixed and stained, as in the DEAFF test. The low-speed centrifugation of the cultures enhances the sensitivity of the test (6).

Antigenemia Assay Circulating polymorphonuclear leukocytes (PMNL) are separated from whole blood, fixed, and stained with monoclonal antibodies directed against pp65, an early matrix protein of CMV, followed by immunoperoxidase staining (7). This will detect the presence of pp65 in the PMNL, and the number of positive PMNLs provides a semiquantitative estimate of viral load (8,9). The source of pp65 within the PMNLs remains ill defined but may represent phagocytosed virion protein, the major component of dense bodies, an aberrant form of CMV, rather than active viral replication in the cells (10).

The detection of pp65 antigen in PMNs using specific monoclonal antibodies provides a relatively rapid and semiquantitative method for the identification of active CMV infection. The original antigenemia methods have been substantially modified and improved by the laboratories of Professors Thé (7) and Gerna (11). The results of antigenemia testing in immunocompromised hosts have been shown in a limited series of publications to provide both diagnostic and prognostic information that can be used in patient management and to direct antiviral chemotherapy (12–15). However, the assay is most accurate when the blood sample is processed relatively rapidly after being obtained. In addition, in patients who are neutropenic, such as bone marrow transplant recipients and patients undergoing ganciclovir therapy, obtaining sufficient cells for meaningful results is one of the limitations of the test.

Notwithstanding these practical difficulties, the utility of the antigenemia assay has been aptly demonstrated in the identification of HIV-positive patients and bone marrow transplant patients at risk of CMV disease (15–17).

The study by Bacigalupo and colleagues (16) of 134 consecutive bone marrow transplant patients showed that 43% of patients developed antigenemia at a median of 40 days post transplant, with a median number of positive cells of $4/2.5 \times 10^5$ PBMCs. Both T-cell depletion and acute graft-versus-host disease were predictive of CMV antigenemia. In the antigenemic patients, risk of CMV interstitial pneumonitis was significantly higher ($p = 0.0005$). In addition, transplant-related mortality was significantly higher in patients with antigenemia, even when stratified according to numbers of antigenemia-positive cells.

The use of antigenemia to guide ganciclovir therapy has been investigated by Boeckh and colleagues (17). Compared with patients receiving ganciclovir prophylaxis, more patients managed by antigenemia-guided ganciclovir therapy developed disease (14% versus 2.7%; $p = 0.02$). However, there was no difference in hazard of CMV disease by day 180. In this study, the majority (82.3%) of patients presenting with low-grade antigenemia (less than three positive cells in two slides) progressed to high-grade antigenemia (more than three positive cells in two slides) within a median of 8 days.

A caveat remains concerning the comparison of antigenemia results among different laboratories: What is the threshold at which patients are at increased risk of disease? A survey of the literature reveals that some authors will act upon a single antigenemia-positive cell in 50,000 PBMCs, whereas others may use 5, 10, or even 100 cells per 50,000 PBMCs to direct therapeutic intervention. Standardization procedures to allow more uniform thresholds to be obtained are currently being planned within multicenter collaborations (18).

PCR Multiple PCR primers and conditions have been described for the detection of CMV in biologically relevant fluids from immunocompromised hosts. Both nested and nonnested procedures are utilized in laboratories along with a broad range of samples, including urine, semen, whole blood, serum or plasma, CSF (for the diagnosis of encephalitis), and vitreous fluid (for the diagnosis of CMV ocular disease). The choice of sample and method depends upon the quantity of DNA used in the PCR itself and the requirement that latent DNA should not be detected with high frequency if blood (whole or fractionated) is the sample of choice.

Numerous prospective studies have shown that plasma, serum, and blood (whole or fractionated) provide prognostic information that enables more efficient patient management through preemptive therapy. For example, the study by Kidd and colleagues (19) demonstrated that PCR was superior to conventional cell culture and DEAFF methods in identifying renal transplant, bone marrow transplant, and liver transplant patients at risk of future CMV disease.

The advantages of PCR-directed preemptive therapy over conventional cell culture directed to therapy have been aptly demonstrated by Einsele and colleagues (20). In this study, bone marrow transplant patients who were prescribed preemptive therapy with ganciclovir on the basis of two consecutive PCR-positive results 1 week apart were less likely to have CMV disease than patients treated on the basis of detection of CMV by conventional cell culture. In addition, patients managed using the PCR approach had an overall decrease in the duration of ganciclovir prescribed. The latter reduction would be expected to reduce the duration of neutropenia and hence reduce the probability of problems associated with bacterial or fungal infections.

Many cross-sectional and a small number of longitudinal studies have shown that CMV load is elevated in patients with symptomatic CMV infection (21–23). The possibility that further quantitative PCR methods may allow thresholds to be designated above which a patient is at high risk of CMV disease has been demonstrated by our group (24). In this study of renal transplant recipients, viral loads in the urine between 10^5 and 10^6 were associated with a rapid increase in the probability of disease from <10% to approximately 80%. Thus the prospect of analyzing temporal increases in viral load and using thresholds to initiated preemptive therapy before the attainment of high viral loads, is likely to be a future development in the diagnostic setting.

Resistance of CMV Strains to Antiviral Chemotherapy
Since the advent of more widespread use of anti-CMV

drugs, the appearance of CMV strains resistant to these compounds has become clinically apparent. *In vitro* isolates of ganciclovir-resistant virus were obtained some years prior to the molecular basis of the resistance to ganciclovir being identified. As a consequence of the work described by Littler (25) and Sullivan (26), we know that the UL97 gene product of CMV is able to phosphorylate both ganciclovir (GCV) and acyclovir to their monophosphate forms. Subsequent phosphorylation to the triphosphate form is via cellular kinases, and the active triphosphate is then a potent inhibitor of the CMV DNA polymerase. Perhaps not surprisingly, a range of mutants has been identified *ex vivo* that fail to phosphorylate GCV due to amino acid alterations within the UL97 gene (27).

In addition to the appearance of UL97 mutants, mutations within the DNA polymerase can give rise to viruses that are resistant to GCV or, if therapy is with foscarnet or cidofovir, to these agents. In some instances, cross-resistance to these compounds via DNA polymerase mutations can occur.

At present, most antiviral susceptibility testing of CMV strains is performed using conventional cell culture methods or rapid culture methods and, in the majority of centers, is not routinely undertaken. Because the greatest frequency of mutations in resistant strains appears to reside in UL97 (at least with respect to GCV), the possibility of using molecular methods to identify resistant strains more rapidly is manifest (28).

Histology The histologic findings associated with CMV rely on the presence of classic changes of cytomegaly and nuclear and cytoplasmic inclusions. The distinct features include large cells 20–30 μm in diameter, with a large nucleus containing round, oval, or reniform inclusions. These large inclusions are separated from the nuclear membrane by a clear zone that gives the inclusions the owl's eye appearance, by which name they are typically known.

Immunocytochemical staining using CMV-specific monoclonal antibodies, and *in situ* DNA hybridization techniques, can be used to show CMV-specific proteins and nucleic acid within tissue biopsies. These methods have been shown to be of value in the diagnosis of CMV hepatitis in liver allografts, especially in tissue sections with a histologic appearance of disseminated focal hepatitis where inclusion bodies are sparsely distributed or absent (29,30). However, *in situ* hybridization is often not as sensitive as immunohistochemistry/classical hemotoxylin and eosin histology, whereas nested PCR for CMV DNA in biopsies frequently identifies CMV DNA in liver from patients without liver disease. It is possible that quantitative PCR methods may be of value in this setting.

CMV DNA or antigens can also be detected in lung biopsies from patients following transplantation (31,32). Both procedures are more sensitive than the detection of CMV by standard histologic methods. However, the significance of these observations remains to be assessed formally with regard to risk of CMV pneumonia.

Human Herpesvirus 6

Human herpesvirus type-6 (HHV-6) was discovered in 1986 (33), and the first viral isolates were derived from cultured leukocytes of immunocompromised patients with lymphoproliferative disorders.

HHV-6 is subdivided into two strains: HHV-6A and HHV-6B; the complete sequence of the HHV-6B strain U1102 has been completed recently (34). HHV-6 is acquired almost universally within the first 2 years of life (reviewed in Lusso, ref. 35), with salivary transmission being the most likely route. Indeed, HHV-6 can be frequently detected by PCR in the saliva of seropositive individuals.

Serology

The majority of the serological assays reported to date rely on infected cell culture material to provide a source of antigen, and the detection of positive reactions using immunofluorescent techniques. Whereas these methods are inherently confounded by false-positive reactions, the data show that seroprevalence of HHV-6 in the adult population is in excess of 95% and are therefore consistent with the results of saliva PCR data. Thus it is unlikely that after transplant many patients will suffer from primary HHV-6 infection; rather, they are more like to suffer from reactivation or reinfection. Comparison with CMV indicates that both of these situations are less likely to produce pathogenic consequences. Most studies indicating high seroprevalence use human sera at low dilution (usually 1:10 or 1:20). If higher dilutions of sera are used, then the frequency of apparent seropositivity in the population also decreases (cf. PCR positivity versus total input DNA in the previous section) (36). Because of the cross-reactivity between HHV-6 antigens and their CMV and HHV-7 homologs, the most rigorous results are obtained when the sera are preabsorbed against HHV-7-infected cells or HCMV-infected cells (37,38). In our experience, the major problem arises from cross-reaction with HHV-7. Commercial assays for HHV-6 antibodies are available but await formal evaluation and application.

Collection of Viral Specimens

PBMCs isolated for Ficoll-Hypaque separation of heparinized blood can be used as a source of virus for cell culture. PCR can also be performed on these samples following DNA extraction. Saliva samples can also be used for PCR and culture analysis. Saliva can be diluted with RPMI1640 and inoculated onto PHA-stimulated adult PBL or CBL as indicated.

HHV-6 can be propagated in cord blood lymphocytes and in established cell lines such as HSB2. Virus isolation methods have been used to demonstrate the presence of HHV-6 in samples from individuals, sometimes in association with clinical syndromes (39,40). Nevertheless, virus isolation methods do not distinguish between active and latent infection and often require the cells to be activated artificially prior to supporting replication.

Methods of Diagnosis

PCR To a large extent, PCR has become the mainstay for the identification of HHV-6A and HHV-6B strains. Both qualitative and, more recently, quantitative methods have been described for the detection of HHV-6 DNA in blood and other body fluids (41–45). The frequency of PCR positivity in blood cell DNA extracts increases as the quantity of input DNA (i.e., the number of cell equivalents) is increased, reaching some 50% at 1 μg (1.5×10^5 cell equivalents; unpublished data), whereas in otherwise healthy individuals virus is not detected in the plasma or serum phase. Nevertheless, in immunocompromised hosts following transplantation and in children suffering primary infection, viral DNA can be detected in both blood and plasma/serum phases (46).

The aim of PCR in the context of HHV-6 should be the identification of the agent to confirm a diagnosis of primary infection yielding Exanthem Subitum-like symptoms or in the identification of post-transplant reactivation, allowing the differential contributions of CMV and HHV-6 to be evaluated. At present, most laboratories do not routinely test for HHV-6 in either of these contexts, and it is unlikely that there will be widespread testing for these agents until sufficiently persuasive data are published indicating the full pathogenic potential of HHV-6 in the immunocompromised host. In addition, the availability of compounds that inhibit HHV-6 replication are also required to manage the infection once diagnosed.

Human Herpesvirus 7

Since the discovery of HHV-7 in 1990 (47), a variety of PCR-based and serological methods have shown that this virus is highly prevalent in the human population, with comparable seroprevalence rates to HHV-6 ie >95%. Primary infection with HHV-7 in the absence of HHV-6 infection has been associated with *Exanthem subitum,* but there is *in vitro* evidence that HHV-7 can also reactivate HHV-6 (48,49). As a consequence, this reactivation may lead to *Exanthem subitum*–like symptoms due to the reactivation of HHV-6 rather than to HHV-7 primary infection per se.

Serology

To date, most serological investigations of HHV-7 have relied upon immunofluorescence using cells infected with HHV-7 and relatively low dilutions of human sera (i.e., 1:10; cf. HHV-6 serology). Similar to the situation described for HHV-6, the apparent seroprevalence of HHV-7 decreases as the serum is diluted. Nevertheless, in most studies, HHV-7 seroprevalence in the adult population is in excess of 95%.

Collection of Viral Specimens

The collection of viral specimens for HHV-7 analysis parallels that described for HHV-6 (*vide supra*).

Methods of Diagnosis

Cell Culture HHV-7 can be propagated in cord blood lymphocytes following activation. In addition, and somewhat more conveniently, it can be cultured in Sup T1 cells. Given the nature of HHV-7 infection, the use of cell culture to differentiate active from latent infection is questionable, and most studies to date have not used cell culture to provide information on the association between HHV-7 and disease.

PCR A limited number of primer pairs (predominantly nested) and conditions have been described for the detection of HHV-7 in whole blood, plasma, serum, and saliva (38,50,51). In general, data from whole blood indicate that increasing quantities of input DNA (i.e., cell equivalents) results in increasing frequency of detection of HHV-7 by PCR such that at 1 μg DNA, 83% of the healthy human population is positive for HHV-7 DNA (50).

Quantitative PCR methods for HHV-7 have been described and used to show that the viral burden in saliva of healthy individuals is approximately 10^6 genomes/ml, whereas in PBMC DNA the viral burden is relatively low (approximately 40 genomes/μg cellular DNA) and remains relatively constant over time (50). However, in children with primary HHV-7 infection, viral loads can be substantially elevated and may reach in excess of 10^7 genomes/ml (46).

Epstein-Barr Virus

Serology

All patients should be screened pretransplant for the presence of IgG antibodies against Epstein-Barr virus viral cupsid antigens (EBV VCA). This indicates past infection with the virus, and hence reactivation may occur after transplant, depending on the level of immunosuppression and the type of transplant. Patients most at risk of lymphoma are EBV seronegative recipients of seropositive organs (52). Serology for EBV is of little use after transplant to monitor reactivation, although antibodies to the lytic antigens of EBV, VCA, and Early antigens (EA), may show a rising titer. Primary infection with EBV post transplant may produce a heterophile antibody response but EBV-specific antibodies may be slow to develop.

Collection of Clinical Specimens

CSF and tissue samples from biopsies or post mortem should be collected into sterile containers and stored at −70°C if they are not to be processed immediately. DNA must be extracted from the tissue samples prior to EBV PCR testing.

Methods of Diagnosis

PCR PCR has not been routinely used in the diagnosis of EBV infection post transplantation except to define EBV-related lymphoproliferation in tissue. This is partly reflective of the ability of PCR methods to frequently detect EBV DNA in patients following transplant who never develop EBV-related diseases. However, PCR amplification of repetitive genomic sequences has been used for research purposes to distinguish between EBV isolates directly from clinical samples (52). This study showed that EBV transmission in cadaveric organs from a donor to two recipients resulted in both recipients developing post-transplant lymphoproliferative disease (PTLD). These tumors were directly related to the donor EBV isolate as RFLP and PCR amplification of EBNA-1 repeat regions were identical between donor and recipient tissues.

A more extensive study by Haque and colleagues (53) using PCR amplification of an EBNA-6 repeat region in heart/heart-lung transplant recipients showed that the seropositive recipients did not acquire reinfection from donor virus, whereas a high proportion of the seronegative recipients seroconverted within the first year through exposure to the donor virus. Thus the acquisition of donor EBV strains is a risk factor for PTLD in previously seronegative transplant recipients.

PCR for EBV in the CSF of patients with primary central nervous system lymphoma has been shown to detect most individuals with disease (3) and can therefore an adjunct in the diagnosis of primary CNS lymphoma.

The relative utility of *in situ* hybridization and PCR in the diagnosis of oral hairy leukoplakia (OHL) has been investigated by Mabruk and colleagues (54). PCR for EBV was positive in 10 biopsy specimens, with a definitive diagnosis of OHL by *in situ* hybridization. However, exfoliated cytology samples from the lateral border of the tongue also produced positive results in one-third of healthy controls due to the presence of EBV in saliva at the time of sampling. Thus the highly sensitive nature of the PCR assay may not be sufficiently specific for routine identification of patients with OHL.

The relationships between EBV infection following liver transplantation and occurrence of hepatitis/graft failure and benign and malignant lymphoproliferative disorders has been investigated by Alshak and colleagues (55). Sixty-one liver biopsy samples from 37 patients were analyzed by histopathology and PCR for EBV. Interestingly, only three biopsies suggestive of EBV lymphoma were also positive for EBV DNA, and the authors concluded that identification of EBV infection in liver biopsies is satisfactorily performed using histopathological criteria without the requirement for PCR.

Whereas data suggest that PCR has the potential for the early identification of patients at risk of EBV lymphomas, there are insufficient data in the literature to warrant recommending routine surveillance of biopsy samples from solid organ recipients. Nevertheless, results from larger, prospective studies may modify this situation.

Human Herpesvirus 8

Human herpesvirus type-8 (HHV-8) or Kaposi's sarcoma herpesvirus (KSHV) is the most recent addition to the Herpesviridae family. The virus was first identified in Kaposi's sarcoma (KS) tissue in 1994 and has been demonstrated to be associated with all forms of KS, together with body cavity lymphomas and Castleman's disease (56–58). The virus is most closely related to the gamma herpesviruses and, in particular, the gamma-2 herpesvirus group.

The complete sequence of HHV-8 has been published (59) and the virus encodes numerous genes important in the manipulation of the cellular environment and the host immune system. Because of the relative difficulty of culturing HHV-8 to high titer (60), most studies to date have used PCR or, more recently, serological methods.

Serology

Initial attempts at producing serological assays for the detection of HHV-8 antibodies were hampered by the cell lines available, because they were co-infected with HHV-8 and EBV (57,61). More recently, cell lines solely infected with HHV-8 have been characterized (e.g., BCBL-1), and these form the basis for the serological methods described later (62).

As expected, there is a high consistency between the results of many studies with respect to patients with KS exhibiting very high, if not universal seropositivity to HHV-8 (63–65). However, more discrepancies have arisen in the seropositivity among the healthy population in different countries. Seroprevalence rates to HHV-8 are higher in endemic areas (e.g., southern Europe, Africa), but in northern Europe and the United States seroprevalence rates range from 3% to approximately 20%, depending on the methodology used.

It should be noted that, at high dilutions of serum, the seroprevalence of the human population to HHV-6 and HHV-7 is substantially lower than the true seroprevalence; hence the dilution of serum used in assays of these types is important, as is the inherent sensitivity of the immunofluorescent procedure. Nevertheless, data suggest that patients with HIV infection who are destined to develop KS show a rise in antibody against HHV-8 substantially before the clinical appearance of KS (66). This phenomenon has been described as seroconversion but more likely represents reactivation of virus, or reinfection boosting humoral immune responses.

In the context of transplant recipients, the expected seroprevalence of HHV-8 is likely to be akin to the normal population, which itself will depend upon the country of origin of the transplanted individual. To date, there have been no prospective studies using either serology or PCR to identify alterations in antibody levels against HHV-8 and the risk associated with this increase for the future development of KS or the appearance of HHV-8 in the blood following transplantation. Historically, it has been noted that renal transplant recipients are at a substantially increased risk of KS (67). It will be interesting to ascertain whether these patients can be identified through transplant screening via the presence of antibodies to HHV-8. It should be remembered that the mere presence of antibodies against HHV-8 will reflect patients at risk of KS but does not necessarily mean that all patients with antibodies to KS HHV-8 will ultimately develop KS. Hence identification of other risk factors that contribute to the appearance of KS is required.

Collection of Viral Samples

DNA can be isolated from whole blood using commercially available methods or further separation of PBMCs in Ficoll-Hypaque. In addition, for the detection of KS in the lung, sputum samples can also be used.

Methods of Diagnosis

PCR Most PCR-based studies for HHV-8 DNA detection have used either nested or nonnested procedures based upon the original sequence described by Chang and colleagues in 1994 (68). These methods have allowed the identification of HHV-8 DNA in samples from organs with KS lesions and also in the blood of patients with KS.

A study by Whitby and colleagues (69) reported that HIV-infected patients with HHV-8 in their blood constituted a high-risk population for the future development of KS. However, in this study, many patients who went on to develop KS did not appear to have HHV-8 detected in their blood prior to KS development. These data may be explained by the frequency of sampling, but it should be borne in mind that viral loads for HHV-8 in the blood may not represent the local tissue burden of HHV-8 and, hence, because of the infrequent detection of HHV-8 in the blood prior to the onset of KS, PCR of this body fluid may not be useful diagnostically.

One quantitative PCR methodology for HHV-8 has been described recently (70) and has shown that, in a renal transplant patient with KS, viral load in the blood

rapidly declined when immunosuppressive therapy was reduced. Resolution of the KS lesion occurred over the ensuing months. These data imply that the quality of the immune system is important in controlling HHV-8 replication. However, the KS lesions take substantially longer to heal, presumably due to the cellular events that have already occurred in the cells exhibiting the KS phenotype.

Histology A formal diagnosis of KS can be performed histopathologically on tissue biopsy samples. In the case of cutaneous KS, biopsies are frequently not performed because of the obvious nature of the lesion. In contrast, lesions within other organs, such as the lung, are frequently diagnosed histopathologically. Most of these biopsies would be expected on the basis of the data currently published to contain HHV-8. Whether the detection of HHV-8 itself in tissues without evidence of KS histopathologically will be substantially related to the future development of KS in these organs has not yet been determined.

REFERENCES

1. Berry NJ, Grundy JE, Griffiths PD. Radioimmunoassay for the detection of IgG antibodies to herpes simplex virus and its use as a prognostic indicator of HSV excretion in transplant recipients. *J Med Virol* 1987;21:147–154.
2. Aurelius E, Johansson B, Skoldenberg B, Staland A, Forsgren M. Rapid diagnosis of herpes simplex encephalitis by nested polymerase chain reaction assay of cerebrospinal fluid. *Lancet* 1991;337:189–192.
3. Cinque P, Vago L, Dahl H, et al. Polymerase chain reaction on cerebrospinal fluid for diagnosis of virus-associated opportunistic diseases of the central nervous system in HIV-infected patients. *AIDS* 1996;10:951–958.
4. Cha T-A, Tom E, Kemble GW, Duke GM, Mocarski ES, Spaete RR. Human cytomegalovirus clinical isolates carry at least 19 genes not found in laboratory strains. *J Virol* 1996;70:78–83.
5. Griffiths PD, Panjwani DD, Stirk PR, et al. Rapid diagnosis of cytomegalovirus infection in immunocompromised patients by detection of early antigen fluorescent foci. *Lancet* 1984;2:1242–1245.
6. Gleaves CA, Smith TF, Shuster EA, Pearson GR. Rapid detection of cytomegalovirus in MRC-5 cells inoculated with urine specimens by using low-speed centrifugation and monoclonal antibody to an early antigen. *J Clin Microbiol* 1984; 19:917–919.
7. Thé TH, van der Bij W, van den Berg AP, et al. Cytomegalovirus antigenemia. *Rev Infect Dis* 1990;12[Suppl 7]:S734–S744.
8. Grefte A, Blom N, van der Giessen M, van Son W, The TH. Ultrastructural analysis of circulating cytomegalic cells in patients with active cytomegalovirus infection: evidence for virus production and endothelial origin. *J Infect Dis* 1993;168:1110–1118.
9. Grefte JM, van der Gun BT, Schmolke S, et al. The lower matrix protein pp65 is the principal viral antigen present in peripheral blood leukocytes during an active cytomegalovirus infection. *J Gen Virol* 1992;73:2923–2932.
10. Grefte A, Harmsen MC, van der Giessen M, Knollema S, van Son WJ, Thé TH. Presence of human cytomegalovirus (HCMV) immediate early mRNA but not ppUL83 (lower matrix protein pp65) mRNA in polymorphonuclear and mononuclear leukocytes during active HCMV infection. *J Gen Virol* 1994;75:1989–1998.
11. Gerna G, Revello MG, Percivalle E, Morini F. Comparison of different immunostaining techniques and monoclonal antibodies to the lower matrix phosphoprotein (pp65) for optimal quantitation of human cytomegalovirus antigenemia. *J Clin Microbiol* 1992;30:1232–1237.
12. Van den Berg AP, Klompmaker IJ, Haagsma EB, et al. Antigenemia in the diagnosis and monitoring of active cytomegalovirus infection after liver transplantation. *J Infect Dis* 1991;164:265–270.
13. Van den Berg AP, Tegzess AM, Scholten-Sampson A, et al. Monitoring

antigenemia is useful in guiding treatment of severe cytomegalovirus disease after organ transplantation. *Transplant Int* 1992;5:101–106.

14. Mazzulli T, Rubin RH, Ferraro MJ, et al. Cytomegalovirus antigenemia: clinical correlations in transplant recipients and in persons with AIDS. *J Clin Microbiol* 1993;31:2824–2827.

15. Dodt KK, Jacobsen PH, Hofmann B, et al. Development of cytomegalovirus (CMV) disease may be predicted in HIV-infected patients by CMV polymerase chain reaction and the antigenaemia test. *AIDS* 1997;11:F21–F28.

16. Bacigalupo A, Tedone E, Isaza A, et al. CMV-antigenemia after allogeneic bone marrow transplantation: correlation of CMV-antigen positive cell numbers with transplant-related mortality. *Bone Marrow Transplant* 1995;16:155–161.

17. Boeckh M, Gooley TA, Myerson D, Cunningham T, Schoch G, Bowden RA. Cytomegalovirus pp65 antigenemia-guided early treatment with ganciclovir versus ganciclovir at engraftment after allogeneic marrow transplantation: a randomized double-blind study. *Blood* 1996;88: 4063–4071.

18. Thé TH, van den Berg AP, Harmsen MC, van der Bij W, van Son WJ. The cytomegalovirus antigenemia assay: a plea for standardization. *Scand J Infect Dis* 1995;99[Suppl]:25–29.

19. Kidd IM, Fox JC, Pillay D, Charman H, Griffiths PD, Emery VC. Provision of prognostic information in immunocompromised patients by routine application of the polymerase chain reaction for cytomegalovirus. *Transplantation* 1993;56:867–871.

20. Einsele H, Ehninger G, Hebart H, et al. Polymerase chain reaction monitoring reduces the incidence of cytomegalovirus disease and the duration and side effects of antiviral therapy after bone marrow transplantation. *Blood* 1995;86:2815–2820.

21. Saltzman RL, Quirk MR, Jordan MC. High levels of circulating cytomegalovirus DNA reflect visceral organ disease in viremic immunosuppressed patients other than marrow recipients. *J Clin Invest* 1992;90:1832–1838.

22. Fox JC, Kidd IM, Griffiths PD, Sweny P, Emery VC. Longitudinal analysis of cytomegalovirus load in renal transplant recipients using a quantitative polymerase chain reaction: correlation with disease. *J Gen Virol* 1995;76:309–319.

23. Kuhn JE, Wendland T, Schafer P, et al. Monitoring of renal allograft recipients by quantitation of human cytomegalovirus genomes in peripheral blood leukocytes. *J Med Virol* 1994;44:398–405.

24. Cope AV, Sweny P, Sabin C, Rees L, Griffiths PD, Emery VC. Quantity of cytomegalovirus viruria is a major risk factor for cytomegalovirus disease after renal transplantation. *J Med Virol* 1997;52:200–205.

25. Littler E, Stuart AD, Chee MS. Human cytomegalovirus UL97 open reading frame encodes a protein that phosphorylates the antiviral nucleoside analogue ganciclovir. *Nature* 1992;358:160–162.

26. Sullivan V, Talarico CL, Stanat SC, Davis M, Coen DM, Biron KK. A protein kinase homologue controls phosphorylation of ganciclovir in human cytomegalovirus-infected cells. *Nature* 1992;358:162–164.

27. Chou SW, Erice A, Jordan MC, et al. Analysis of the UL97 phosphotransferase coding sequence in clinical cytomegalovirus isolates and identification of mutations conferring ganciclovir resistance. *J Infect Dis* 1995;171:576–583.

28. Bowen EF, Johnson MA, Griffiths PD, Emery VC. Development of a point mutation assay for the detection of human cytomegalovirus UL97 mutations associated with ganciclovir resistance. *J Virol Meth* 1997;68: 225–234.

29. Colina F, Juca NT, Ballestin C, et al. Histological diagnosis of cytomegalovirus hepatitis in liver allografts. *J Clin Pathol* 1995;48: 351–357.

30. Brainard JA, Greenson JK, Vesy CJ, et al. Detection of cytomegalovirus in liver transplant biopsies: a comparison of light microscopy, immunohistochemistry, duplex PCR, and nested PCR. *Transplantation* 1994; 57:1753–1757.

31. Solans EP, Garrity ER Jr, Mccabe M, Martinez R, Husain AN. Early diagnosis of cytomegalovirus pneumonitis in lung transplant patients. *Arch Pathol Lab Med* 1995:119:33–35.

32. Arbustini E, Morbini P, Grasso M, et al. Human cytomegalovirus early infection, acute rejection and major histocompatibility class II expression in transplanted lung. Molecular, immunocytochemical, and histopathologic investigations. *Transplantation* 1996;61:418–427.

33. Salahuddin SZ, Ablashi DV, Markham PD, et al. Isolation of a new virus, HBLV, in patients with lymphoproliferative disorders. *Science* 1986;234:596–601.

34. Gompels UA, Nicholas J, Lawrence G, et al. The DNA sequence of human herpesvirus-6: structure, coding content, and genome evolution. *Virology* 1995;209:29–51.

35. Lusso P. Human herpesvirus 6 (HHV-6). *Antiviral Res* 1996;31:1–21.

36. Clark DA, Alexander FE, McKinney PA, et al. The seroepidemiology of human herpesvirus-6 (HHV-6) from a case-control study of leukaemia and lymphoma. *Int J Cancer* 1990;45:829–833.

37. Adler SP, McVoy M, Chou S, Hempfling S, Yamanishi K, Britt W. Antibodies induced by a primary cytomegalovirus infection react with human herpesvirus 6 proteins. *J Infect Dis* 1993;168:1119–1126.

38. Berneman ZN, Ablashi DV, Li G, et al. Human herpesvirus 7 is a T-lymphotropic virus and is related to, but significantly different from, human herpesvirus 6 and human cytomegalovirus. *Proc Natl Acad Sci USA* 1992;89:10552–10556.

39. Carrigan DR, Knox KK. Human herpesvirus 6 (HHV-6) isolation from bone marrow: HHV-6-associated bone marrow suppression in bone marrow transplant patients. *Blood* 1994;84:3307–3310.

40. Drobyski WR, Knox KK, Majewski D, Carrigan DR. Brief report: fatal encephalitis due to variant B human herpesvirus-6 infection in a bone marrow-transplant recipient. *N Engl J Med* 1994;330: 1356–1360.

41. Cone RW, Hackman RC, Huang ML, et al. Human herpesvirus 6 in lung tissue from patients with pneumonitis after bone marrow transplantation. *N Engl J Med* 1993;329:156–161.

42. Cone RW, Huang ML, Ashley R, Corey L. Human herpesvirus 6 DNA in peripheral blood cells and saliva from immunocompetent individuals. *J Clin Microbiol* 1993;31:1262–1267.

43. Gopal MR, Thomson BJ, Fox J, Tedder RS, Honess RW. Detection by PCR of HHV-6 and EBV DNA in blood and oropharynx of healthy adults and HIV-seropositives. *Lancet* 1990;335:1598–1599.

44. Clark DA, Ait-Khaled M, Wheeler AC, et al. Quantification of human herpesvirus 6 in immunocompetent persons and post-mortem tissues from AIDS patients by PCR. *J Gen Virol* 1996;77:2271–2275.

45. Secchiero P, Zella D, Crowley RW, Gallo RC, Lusso P. Quantitative PCR for human herpesviruses 6 and 7. *J Clin Microbiol* 1995;33: 2124–2130.

46. Clark DA, Kidd IM, Collingham KE, et al. Primary human herpesvirus-6 and -7 infections in febrile infants. *Arch Dis Child* 1997;77: 42–45.

47. Frenkel N, Schirmer EC, Wyatt LS, et al. Isolation of a new herpesvirus from human CD4+ T cells. *Proc Natl Acad Sci USA* 1990;87: 748–752.

48. Tanaka K, Kondo T, Torigoe S, Okada S, Mukai T, Yamanishi K. Human herpesvirus 7: another causal agent for roseola (exanthem subitum). *J Pediatr* 1994;125:1–5.

49. Katsafanas GC, Schirmer EC, Wyatt LS, Frenkel N. *In vitro* activation of human herpesviruses 6 and 7 from latency. *Proc Natl Acad Sci USA* 1996;93:9788–9792.

50. Kidd IM, Clark DA, Ait-Khaled M, Griffiths PD, Emery VC. Measurement of human herpesvirus 7 load in peripheral blood and saliva of healthy subjects by quantitative polymerase chain reaction. *J Infect Dis* 1996;174:396–401.

51. Wilborn F, Schmidt CA, Lorenz F, et al. Human herpesvirus type 7 in blood donors: detection by the polymerase chain reaction. *J Med Virol* 1995;47:65–69.

52. Cen H, Breinig MC, Atchison RW, Ho M, McKnight JL. Epstein-Barr virus transmission via the donor organs in solid organ transplantation: polymerase chain reaction and restriction fragment length polymorphism analysis of IR2, IR3, and IR4. *J Virol* 1991;65:976–980.

53. Haque T, Thomas JA, Falk KI, et al. Transmission of donor Epstein-Barr virus (EBV) in transplanted organs causes lymphoproliferative disease in EBV-seronegative recipients. *J Gen Virol* 1996;77: 1169–1172.

54. Mabruk MJ, Flint SR, Toner M, et al. *In situ* hybridization and the polymerase chain reaction (PCR) in the analysis of biopsies and exfoliative cytology specimens for definitive diagnosis of oral hair leukoplakia (OHL). *J Oral Pathol* 1994;23:302–308.

55. Alshak NS, Jiminez Am, Gedebou M, et al. Epstein-Barr virus infections in liver transplantation patients: correlation of histopathology and semiquantitative Epstein-Barr virus-DNA recovery using polymerase chain reaction. *Human Pathol* 1993;24:1306–1312.

56. Moore PS, Chang Y. Detection of herpesvirus-like DNA sequences in Kaposi's sarcoma in patients with and without HIV infection. *N Engl J Med* 1995;332:1181–1185.

57. Ambroziak JA, Blackbourn DJ, Herndier BG, et al. Herpes-like sequences in HIV-infected and uninfected Kaposi's sarcoma patients. *Science* 1995;268:582–583.
58. Cesarman E, Chang Y, Moore PS, Said JW, Knowles DM. Kaposi's-sarcoma-associated herpesvirus-like DNA sequences in AIDS-related body-cavity-based lymphomas. *N Engl J Med* 1995;332:1186–1191.
59. Russo JJ, Bohenzky RA, Chien MC, et al. Nucleotide sequence of the Kaposi sarcoma-associated herpesvirus (HHV8). *Proc Natl Acad Sci USA* 1996;93:14862–14867.
60. Foreman KE, Friborg J Jr, Kong WP, et al. Propagation of a human herpesvirus from AIDS-associated Kaposi's sarcoma. *N Engl J Med* 1997;336:163–171.
61. Miller G, Rigsby MO, Heston L, et al. Antibodies to butyrate-inducible antigens of Kaposi's sarcoma-associated herpesvirus in patients with HIV-1 infection. *N Engl J Med* 1996;334:1292–1297.
62. Renne R, Zhong W, Herndier B, et al. Lytic growth of Kaposi's sarcoma-associated herpesvirus (human herpesvirus 8) in culture. *Nature Med* 1996;2:342–346.
63. Gao SJ, Kingsley L, Li M, et al. KSHV antibodies among Americans, Italians and Ugandans with and without Kaposi's sarcoma. *Nature Med* 1996;2:925–928.
64. Kedes DH, Operskalski E, Busch M, Kohn R, Flood J, Ganem D. The seroepidemiology of human herpesvirus 8 (Kaposi's sarcoma–associated herpesvirus): distribution of infection in KS risk groups and evidence for sexual transmission. *Nature Med* 1996;2:918–924.
65. Lennette ET, Blackbourn DJ, Levy JA. Antibodies to human herpesvirus type 8 in the general population and in Kaposi's sarcoma patients. *Lancet* 1996;348:858–861.
66. Gao S-J, Kingsley L, Hoover DR, et al. Seroconversion to antibodies against Kaposi's sarcoma-associated herpesvirus-related latent nuclear antigens before the development of Kaposi's sarcoma. *N Engl J Med* 1996;335:233–241.
67. Myers BD, Kessler E, Levi J, et al. Kaposi sarcoma in kidney transplant recipients. *Arch Intern Med* 1974;133:307–311.
68. Chang Y, Cesarman E, Pessin MS, et al. Identification of herpesvirus-like DNA sequences in AIDS-associated Kaposi's sarcoma. *Science* 1994;266:1865–1869.
69. Whitby D, Howard MR, Tenant-Flowers M, et al. Detection of Kaposi's sarcoma associated herpesvirus in peripheral blood of HIV-infected individuals and progression to Kaposi's sarcoma. *Lancet* 1995;346:799–802.
70. Lock MJ, Griffiths PD, Emery VC. Development of a quantitative competitive polymerase chain reaction for human herpesvirus 8. *J Virol Meth* 1997;64:19–26.

Transplant Infections edited by
Raleigh A. Bowden, Per Ljungman, and Carlos V. Paya.
Lippincott–Raven Publishers, Philadelphia © 1998

CHAPTER 6

Laboratory Methods for the Diagnosis of Respiratory Viral Diseases

Janet A. Englund, Estella Whimbey, and Robert L. Atmar

The importance of common respiratory viruses in immunocompromised patients is increasingly appreciated, in part because of the improved ability of the virology laboratory to document infection with these viral agents. The diagnosis of respiratory virus infection requires the active search for these agents using appropriate clinical specimens and laboratory techniques. Seroprevalence studies, based on detecting changes in antibody concentrations, have been important in determining the epidemiology of respiratory viruses, but these methods have not been useful in studies of the severely immunocompromised patient. By contrast, the use of relatively simple and rapid diagnostic techniques has assisted greatly in the identification of respiratory viral infections in these patients (1). Advances in molecular biotechnology also have revolutionized the ability to detect viral agents. The ability to trace the spread of viruses by "fingerprinting" or by partial sequencing viral genomes has resulted in important new clinical and epidemiological observations. Commercially available monoclonal antibodies and other reagents, the availability of antiviral therapy, and the recognition of antiviral resistance have created new opportunities for the clinician and increased demands on viral laboratories to provide rapid, sensitive, and specific diagnostic tests. An understanding of various detection methods is important in the interpretation of results obtained from the virology laboratory.

Respiratory viruses differ from the common herpes group of viruses in that the isolation of a respiratory virus is generally significant and usually establishes the etiology of a disease. Furthermore, with the exception of aden-oviruses and measles virus, respiratory viruses are not generally considered to produce latent infections. A positive culture for a respiratory virus is usually associated with symptomatic disease, particularly in otherwise healthy subjects. The isolation of viruses such as influenza or rhinoviruses from patients with respiratory symptoms is diagnostic because an asymptomatic carrier state has not been recognized. Although prolonged shedding of respiratory viruses, particularly respiratory syncytial virus (RSV) and parainfluenza viruses, is common in immunocompromised patients, it is generally associated with continued or at least intermittent respiratory symptoms. Conversely, failure to detect a virus does not necessarily mean that a virus was not present previously or did not cause disease. Failure to detect a virus may be a result of inappropriate or inadequate specimen collection and handling, or may be a function of the time course of the disease, the age or antibody status of the patient, and the technical resources available to detect or cultivate the virus.

SPECIMEN COLLECTION

The appropriate collection of specimens is critical for the successful identification of viruses in clinical samples (2). The source of the specimen, the timing of collection in relation to onset of symptoms, the rapidity and method of delivery to the laboratory, and the clinical and epidemiological data provided to the laboratory are important factors that directly affect the likelihood of successful isolation and/or identification of a viral pathogen.

Sample Site

The clinical syndrome caused by a virus and its pathogenesis determine the specimen(s) most appropriate for virus identification. Viruses that cause respiratory tract disease, such as influenza viruses, RSV, and rhinoviruses,

JAE, RLA: From the Departments of Microbiology and Immunology, Pediatrics, and Medicine of the Baylor College of Medicine, Houston, TX 77030. EW: From the section of Infectious Diseases, University of Texas M.D. Anderson Cancer Center, Houston, TX 77030.

are most frequently identified in respiratory secretions. Viruses associated with localized and systemic disease, such as enteroviruses, may be identified in throat swabs as well as cerebrospinal fluid or fecal specimens; viruses that cause generalized disease, such as measles and mumps, may be identified from multiple sources, including respiratory secretions, urine, and blood.

The upper respiratory tract may be sampled by nasopharyngeal aspirates, nasal wash, nasopharyngeal swab, throat wash, pharyngeal swab, or a combination of these methods. Limited data are available comparing the optimal specimen for the identification of respiratory viruses in immunocompromised patients. However, nasal wash methods have been shown to be superior for the isolation of RSV in infants and children (3) and for the isolation of rhinoviruses in healthy adults (4). The nasal wash method is the preferred method for obtaining upper respiratory tract specimens in both children and adults in our center (1), whereas a nasopharyngeal swab has been advocated at other centers (5).

Nasal aspiration or wash is most easily performed in children using a bulb syringe or suction catheter with the child sitting and being held firmly in a parent's lap. In cooperative adults, a nasal wash specimen is also best obtained with the patient sitting. The subject is coached to not swallow while up to 5 ml normal saline is instilled in a nostril using a needle-less syringe. The saline is allowed to run out the nose into a clean receptacle by the subject, leans his/her head forward and gently blows out the nose. The contralateral nostril can be pinched to ensure good expulsion of the saline. The procedure can then be repeated on the contralateral nostril. The saline is immediately added to sterile viral transport media containing selective antibiotics and placed on ice.

The selection of a sampling method may be influenced by the virus(es) targeted for identification and the identification method (6). RSV is more likely to be identified in a nasopharyngeal specimen than from a pharyngeal swab, whereas adenoviruses are more likely to be identified from a pharyngeal swab (7). A combination of sampling methods, such as nasopharyngeal aspirate or wash with a pharyngeal swab, provides the greatest likelihood of detecting the broadest range of the more common respiratory viruses by culture. When swabs are used for sample collection, calcium alginate swabs should be avoided because they may be responsible for decreased rates of viral recovery (2,8–11). Cotton or Dacron swabs are generally felt to be comparable for recovery of viruses (9).

The lower respiratory tract is sampled using sputum specimens, endotracheal tube aspirates, or bronchoalveolar lavage (BAL) fluid, with the latter being particularly useful in immunocompromised hosts (11–13). In general, BAL should be considered for the diagnosis of viral respiratory infections in immunocompromised patients prior to more invasive procedures such as open lung biopsy. Tissue biopsy specimens may be helpful when BAL results are inconclusive for the diagnosis of certain diseases such as measles pneumonia. Cerebrospinal fluid can be useful in establishing a viral etiology for aseptic meningitis. Urine and blood specimens are used to identify systemic viral infections. Table 1 lists the different clinical specimens from which respiratory viruses may be identified.

Clinical specimens optimally are obtained early in the course of respiratory illness. Viral shedding frequently begins shortly before the onset of symptoms, peaks during the illness, and disappears when symptoms resolve. There are some notable exceptions—for example, enteroviruses may be shed in the feces for weeks to months, and RSV may be shed for months in some immunocompromised patients such as HIV-infected children (14). Factors that influence the likelihood of successful virus identification include the type of virus, the site from which the sample was obtained, the test being used, the age of the patient being sampled (e.g., younger children shed influenza viruses longer than adults), and the immune competence of the patient.

Transport to the Laboratory

Once a clinical specimen has been collected, it should be transported to the virus laboratory for inoculation as soon as possible. Increased diagnostic yields are associated with shorter times to collaborative inoculation because virus viability decreases with time. This is par-

TABLE 1. *Specimen source for identification of common respiratory viruses by culture or other laboratory techniques*

	NW	NP SWAB	Throat	BAL	Blood	Urine	CSF	Stool
RSV	+++	+++	+	+++	−	−	−	−
Influenza A, B	+++	+++	++	+++	−	−	−	−
Parainfluenza 1–3	+++	+++	++	+++	−	−	+	−
Rhinovirus	+++	+++	++	++	−	−	−	−
Enterovirus	++	++	+++	++	−	−	+++	+++
Adenovirus	+++	+++	+++	+++	+++	++	+	+++
Coronavirus	++	?	?	?	−	−	−	−
Measles virus	+	+	++	+++	++	+++	++	−

Keys: +++ = excellent; ++ = good; + = satisfactory/sometimes useful; − = rare/never.
Abbreviations: NW, Nasal wash; NP, nasopharyngeal swab; BAL, bronchoalveolar lavage; CSF, cerebrospinal fluid.

ticularly true with labile viruses such as RSV. Several steps also can be taken to enhance the likelihood of preserving viruses during the transportation of a specimen. First, the specimen should be transported on wet ice or placed in a refrigerator at 4°C. A decline in infectivity for most viruses has been demonstrated to be temperature dependent, and cooling of the specimen (without freezing) improves virus stability (15). Second, a good viral transport medium should be used. A suitable transport medium generally contains protein, antibiotics to prevent bacterial growth, and a buffer to control the pH (16). Several different viral transport media have been described and used successfully. However, charcoal-containing media have repeatedly been shown to reduce virus recovery (16–18). Some clinical specimens, such as CSF and urine, can be transported without the use of a viral transport medium (16). Third, avoid freezing the specimen unless the specimen will not be examined within 2–5 days of collection (18–20). Couch and colleagues (21) showed no loss of influenza virus or parainfluenza virus infectivity after storage of specimens for up to 5 days at 4°C. The freeze/thaw cycle is harmful to many viruses, particularly enveloped viruses. If specimens must be frozen, storage at <−70°C is usually advised, as warmer temperatures (e.g., −20°C) may lead to the rapid loss of infectivity (16). Quick-freezing a specimen in a dry ice/ethanol bath may enhance recovery of labile viruses such as RSV.

Storage of Specimens

Virus recovery from stored specimens can be optimized by using appropriate storage temperatures and cryoprotectants. As noted earlier, −70°C is a better storage temperature for many viruses than is −20°C, although the latter is adequate for the recovery of enteroviruses from stool specimens (18). Cryoprotectants used to enhance virus recovery after freezing of a specimen include dimethyl sulfoxide (DMSO), serum, skim milk, other proteins, sucrose, glycerol, and sorbitol (16).

RESPIRATORY SYNCYTIAL VIRUS (RSV)

RSV, a member of the paramyxoviridae, is an enveloped virus that has a negative-sense single-strand RNA genome. Many different laboratory methods and procedures are available to document infection with RSV (Tables 2 and 3). The choice of method(s) used to document infection is dependent on the patient population, epidemiological factors, and available resources. The following sections will review important factors related to the laboratory identification of RSV.

Direct Visualization

Viral diagnosis by electron microscopy relies on the identification of virus based on typical morphological characteristics. Major advantages for the use of electron microscopy include the ability to visualize a virus quickly without the need for replication. Because identification is based on morphology alone, there is no need to maintain viral or host cell viability. Specific identification of RSV may be problematic because of its morphologic similarity of various paramyxoviruses. Further limitations of electron microscopy include the need to have a relatively high concentration of viral particles, with a titer of approximately 10^6–10^7 particles/ml generally required (7). Although such concentrations of RSV are seen in respiratory secretions of infected infants and immunocompromised children, they are uncommon in immunocompromised adults (22). Electron microscopy is not generally utilized to diagnose RSV infections.

Cytology and Histopathology

Cytologic examination can be extremely useful in the hands of experienced laboratory personnel because, with appropriate specimens, prompt and clinically useful information may be obtained. Histopathological diagnosis, commonly applied to lung biopsy samples, also may prove diagnostic of RSV infection (Fig. 1). Other samples

TABLE 2. *Laboratory methods used to detect selected viruses*

Virus	Direct visualization or histology	Culture	Ag detection (EIA,IF,RIA)	Nucleic acid detection
Adenoviruses	++	+++	+	+
Coronaviruses		+	+	+
Enteroviruses*		+++	+	+
Influenza		+++	++	+
Measles		++	+	+
Parainfluenza		+++	++	+
RSV	+++	+++	+++	+
Rhinoviruses		+++	+	+

*Adapted from Atmar and Englund, Laboratory methods. In: Evans AS, Kaslow RA, eds. *Viral infections in humans: epidemiology and control.* New York: Plenum, 1997, p. 64.

Key: +=method mainly used in research setting; ++=method available in specialized reference laboratories; +++=method readily available and frequently used in many laboratories.

TABLE 3. *Comparison of laboratory methods used in the diagnosis of respiratory viruses**

Method	Sensitivity	Specificity	Cost	Time to Dx	Availability
Electron Microscopy	+	+	Moderate	Hours	Research Setting
Direct Cytology	+	+	Least	Hours	Clinical Lab.
Tissue Culture	++/+++	+++	Expensive	>3 days	Clinical Lab.
Immunofluorescence	++	++	Moderate	Hours	Clinical Lab.
Antigen Detection	++	+++	Least	Hours	Clinical Lab.
Radioimmunoassay	++	++	Moderate	1–3 days	Research Setting
Elisa Assays	++	++	Least	Hours	Clinical Lab.
In situ Hybridization	++	++	Expensive	1–3 days	Reference Lab.
Polymerase Chain Reaction	+++	++/+++	Moderate/Expensive	Hours to days	Reference Lab.

*Adapted from Evans AS, Kaslow RA, eds. *Viral infections in humans,* New York: Plenum, 1997, p. 65.

commonly evaluated include smears of respiratory secretions and bronchoalveolar lavage specimens that have undergone cytocentrifugation. Infection with RSV is identified by the relatively virus-specific intracytoplasmic inclusions in multinucleated cells during RSV infection; however, immunologic techniques are generally used to confirm the diagnosis. The advent of rapid antigen detection techniques applied to respiratory specimens has decreased the need for biopsy procedures for the diagnosis of RSV.

Viral Isolation

Detection of viral replication in cell culture remains the gold standard for much of clinical virology and currently, for the diagnosis of RSV infection (Fig. 2). Isolation of RSV by culture confirms the presence of a complete infectious unit capable of further multiplication. Positive results may be obtained with as little as a single infectious virion, which is well below the threshold of detection for most other detection methods. In addition, several viruses may be identified in a single specimen. The major limitations of viral isolation include the dependence on biological systems that can vary in quality and availability, and the time, expense, and expertise required for virus isolation and identification.

The presence of viral replication in cell cultures is traditionally detected by the observation of typical morphological changes, generally referred to as "cytopathic effect" (CPE), in the cell culture line. Either semicontinuous (diploid) cell lines, with the capacity for 20–50 passages, or continuous (heteroploid) cell lines, with the capacity for indefinite passaging, may be used for the isolation of RSV. Continuous cell lines derived from an epithelial malignancy source (e.g., laryngeal [HEp-2 cells], lung [A549 cells], and cervical [HeLa] carcinoma) are frequently used to detect RSV. Advantages of continuous cell lines include ease and cost of preparation, general availability, and the ability to detect viruses or contaminants endogenous to the cell line prior to its use. However, the sensitivity of some continuous cell lines, such as HEp-2 and Vero cells, to RSV may change after serial passages so that careful quality control is required.

Isolation of RSV Using Physical Refinements

Methods that enhance virus isolation or speed the detection of an agent are highly desirable for the virology laboratory. A variety of physical and chemical techniques may increase the speed and sensitivity of a viral diagnosis (23). Roller culture methods, first introduced by Gey in 1933 (24), are known to increase rates of propagation of eukaryotic cells. This method also has been shown to increase both cellular RNA and viral RNA synthesis (23). Low-speed rolling, high-speed rolling, rocking, and orbital motion have all been found to be advantageous in certain culture conditions. Centrifugation of a clinical specimen or viral isolate onto a cell culture monolayer also can enhance viral detection. The improved detection is probably not due to enhanced pen-

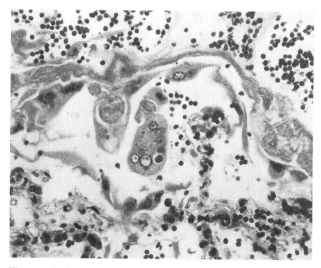

Figure 1. Autopsy lung specimen showing characteristic histopathology of infection with respiratory syncytial virus. A multinucleated giant cell is seen in the middle of the photomicrograph, with inflammatory cells in the periphery. Early hyaline membranes and macrophages are also present.

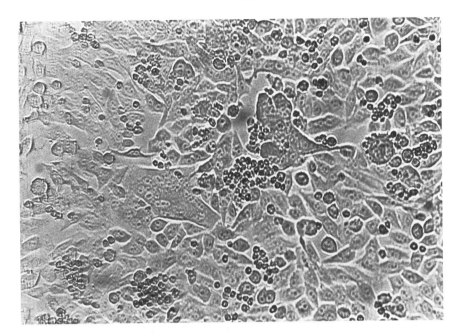

Figure 2. Cytopathic effect (CPE) of respiratory syncytial virus in culture of Hep-2, a human-derived continuous epithelial cell line. Two syncytial characteristics of RSV, a result of the fusion of infected cells, are seen in the middle of the photomicrograph.

etration of the virus into the cell but to stimulation of cell proliferation and activation of gene expression (23,25). Methods utilizing centrifugation of clinical samples are used routinely in many clinical virology laboratories, frequently in conjunction with viral antigen detection to provide rapid diagnosis (26,27). The use of short-term centrifugation of 10 minutes to 2 hours at 500–1,500 *g* has been reported to increase detection of a variety of viruses, including RSV (23). The centrifugation of viruses onto tissue culture monolayers has been shown to reduce the time to viral detection and to increase plaque or foci formation by two- to 100-fold (23). Culture vessels commonly used in this method are either shell vials (cylindrical, flat-bottomed vials that may contain a removable round coverslip at the bottom on which tissue culture cells are attached), or multiwell plastic plates containing either 24, 48, or 96 wells.

Detection of Viral Antigens

Immunofluorescence (IF) assays are widely used for the rapid detection of RSV in clinical samples and for the definitive identification of RSV in tissue culture (28–30) (Tables 2–4). IF assays allow viral antigens to be detected whether or not visible changes in cell culture are evident, but the specimen examined must contain cellular material to be evaluated. In the direct IF test, specific antibody labeled with a fluorescent dye such as fluorescein isothiocyanate is allowed to react with cells obtained from a clinical specimen or from an inoculated cell culture. After allowing time for an antigen/antibody reaction to occur, the slides are washed and examined microscopically for direct visualization of fluorescence of the infected cells in the specimen. In the indirect IF test, two different antisera are used: an unlabeled virus-specific antibody is used

TABLE 4. *Examples of rapid diagnostic test kits approved for laboratory use and marketed in the United States*

Antigen Detection Kitrs	Company	Location
Respiratory syncytial virus		
Directigen	BectonDickinson Microbiology Systems	Cockeysville, MD
Testpak	Abbott Laboratories	North Chicago, IL
Influenza:		
Directigen	BectonDickinson Microbiology Systems	Cockeysville, MD
ZstatFlu	ZymeTx, Inc.	Oklahoma City, OK
Immunofluorescence Kits		
Prima System EIA:; (RSV, influenza, parainfluenza, adenovirus)	Bartels Inc.; Intracel Corporation	Issaquah, WA
Chemicon Direct and Indirect IF Assay for RSV, influenza, parainfluenza, adenovirus	Chemicon International, Inc.	Temecula, CA
Imagen (RSV, influenza, parainfluenza, adenovirus)	DAKO Diagnostics, Ltd.	Cambridgeshire, UK

Note: Other approaches and testing methods are being rapidly developed by other manufacturers, and this table is only an example of the variety of tests available.

first and is followed by a fluorescein-labeled, species-specific antibody directed against the species in which the first antiserum was made. If a reaction occurs between the first antiserum and the clinical specimen, the second antibody will bind to the antigen/antibody complex and fluorescence of the virus-infected cells can be detected.

The use of IF for the direct detection of RSV antigens in clinical samples and the confirmation of viral growth in cell cultures have increased with the widespread commercial availability of relatively inexpensive RSV-specific antibody. The IF method has the advantage of both allowing rapid viral diagnosis and confirming that the specimen has been properly obtained (31–36). When working with large numbers of clinical specimens, the time required for sample collection, processing, and interpretation of the stained slide becomes substantial. The enthusiasm for this technique in clinical specimens has varied because of the time and degree of technical competence required to read such samples; the availability of other, less labor-intensive antigen detection methods; and the possibility of false-negative results. Nevertheless, reliable and sensitive rapid diagnoses may be made quickly from clinical samples using this method. IF techniques in pediatric patients, when performed by an experienced laboratory, can detect up to 95% of the samples positive by culture (35,37), although many clinical laboratories report rates of 70% to 80% (34).

The combination of IF techniques with cell culture has increased the sensitivity of cell culture while providing a positive result in a shorter time period. With the use of centrifugation or other methods of enhancement of viral replication, and pools of virus-specific antibodies, cell cultures can be incubated between 1 and 3 days and then stained for a variety of virus antigens using indirect or direct IF methods (23). Disadvantages of IF techniques include the need for fluorescent microscopes, the requirement for expertise in the interpretation of results, difficulty in the interpretation of clinical specimens that have a high level of nonspecific background fluorescence, and instability of prepared slides over periods longer than 1 month (32).

Enzyme-Linked Immunoassays

Enzyme-based immunoassays, or EIAs, have gained widespread acceptance in virology laboratories (2) and are commonly utilized in many pediatric hospitals and medical centers. The assays rely on antibodies directed against a specific viral antigen, generally the fusion protein of RSV, which are adsorbed or directly linked to polystyrene wells in microtiter plates, plastic beads, or membrane-bound material. When viral antigen is present in a specimen, it binds to the immobilized antibody and a second "detecting" antibody conjugated to an enzyme such as horseradish peroxidase or alkaline phosphatase

then attaches to the antigen. This forms a three-layer "sandwich" consisting of the immobilized antibody, antigen, and detecting antibody with enzyme attached. A substrate specific for the enzyme is added and a color reaction occurs that can be monitored by spectrophotometry or by direct visualization. The test is quite simple to run, requiring only standardization of reagents and techniques such as dilution, incubation, and washing. The principles in EIA are similar to those in immunofluorescence, but the EIA test has the advantage of being simple to perform, utilizing reagents that have long shelf-lives and are inexpensive, and requiring less expertise in the interpretation of test results. Advantages of the EIA technique include sensitivity, specificity, rapidity, safety, automation potential, and low cost, particularly when many specimens require evaluation. Disadvantages of the test include the inability to evaluate the quality of the clinical specimen and the fact that test results may remain positive in the face of antiviral therapy, such as ribavirin, when cultures are negative.

Variations in the methodology for EIA testing include the materials used, the procedures for incubation and detection, and the interpretation of results. Many different test kits are commercially available and in widespread clinical use for the detection of RSV in immunocompetent and immunocompromised children (34,38). A drawback of EIA testing in immunocompromised adults has been the lack of sensitivity, particularly when applied to specimens from the upper respiratory tract. The decreased sensitivity of antigen detection test in adults is associated with low levels of infectious virus in upper respiratory secretions (22).

The availability of semi-invasive procedures to obtain clinical specimens, such as bronchoalveolar lavage, has led to more demands for the rapid detection of viral infections from these specimens. The diagnosis of RSV using enzyme-linked immunosorbent assays or commercial antigen detection kits has been more sensitive and specific in lower respiratory tract samples than in upper respiratory specimens of nasal washes combined with throat swabs. However, most commercially available RSV-antigen detection test kits are not currently licensed for use in BAL samples.

Reverse Transcription Polymerase Chain Reaction (RT-PCR)

The detection of viral nucleic acids is another strategy for the identification of SV in clinical samples. The detection of viral RNA may provide information that otherwise cannot be obtained (39). In some instances, the virus cannot be isolated in tissue culture because of virus inactivation during collection, transport, or storage; contamination with other microbes, particularly other viruses; lack of an available *in vitro* culture system; or slow growth of the virus. Nucleic acid detection (*in situ*) can be used to identify cells containing viral nucleic acids within a tissue sample.

The polymerase chain reaction (PCR) has revolutionized the detection of small quantities of nucleic acid. First described in 1985, PCR became more practical with the development of a thermostable DNA polymerase, Taq (from *Thermus aquaticus*) polymerase, and an automated thermocycler apparatus (40,41). The use of a reverse transcription step to make a complimentary DNA from RNA has allowed the detection of small quantities of RNA (42,43). PCR products, or amplicons, are detected by visualization of silver- or ethidium bromide–stained gels after electrophoresis or by detection of a hybridization signal (e.g., dot-blot, Southern, or liquid hybridization). Because nonspecifically amplified DNA may occasionally be the same length as the desired amplicon, an additional test of specificity, such as by probe hybridization or restriction enzyme digestion of the amplicon, should be performed (2). The extreme sensitivity of the PCR reaction has led to the recognition of problems of false-positives due to carry-over contamination. Several precautions have been used to overcome this problem, including physical separation of pre- and post-PCR areas, the use of positive displacement pipettes, the use of disposable gloves, and premixing and aliquotting of reagents (44).

When PCR methods have been applied to the diagnosis of RSV infections, they have generally identified more infections than either antigen detection methods or cell culture (45–48). The clinical samples in these studies have come from young children and infants, and the utility of these techniques in immunocompromised hosts remains to be determined.

Multiplex PCR may be used to detect RSV in addition to other viruses or virus types in a single PCR assay. Several different primers or primer sets are utilized in the reaction mix. The virus type is identified by the size of the amplicon detected after amplification. This method has been used successfully and relatively rapidly in respiratory specimens obtained from children (49) with good sensitivity and specificity reported. However, the utility of this method for immunocompromised children and adults has not yet been demonstrated. A potential disadvantage of multiplex PCR is that several different primer sets may adversely affect the efficiency of the nucleic acid amplification.

Laboratory Methods for Viral Identification and Characterization

Further characterization of RSV or other viruses obtained from a clinical specimen is frequently desirable once an agent has been isolated. Immunofluorescence, radioimmunoassay, and enzyme immunoassay formats may be used as described for direct virus detection. Other methods for virus identification and characterization include virus neutralization assays and epitope-blocking enzyme-linked assays. Antigenic differences or similarities among virus strains that have been isolated from different geographic locations or at different times may be examined in a number of ways. The availability of pools of monoclonal antibodies permits the examination of these relationships and has been used in the analysis of RSV strains in nosocomial outbreaks (50,51). RNA fingerprinting is another method that has been utilized to examine RSV isolate variability in an outbreak (52,53).

RSV subgroup determination has been performed using either subgroup-specific PCR reactions (54,55) or subgroup-specific probes (56). RSV strains have been characterized further by restriction of endonuclease digestion of PCR products. Such virus characterization also has been used in the evaluation of nosocomial transmission of virus (51–53).

Antiviral Susceptibility

The development of clinical resistance to antiviral agents has been documented in a variety of viruses, but resistance of RSV to ribavirin, the only licensed antiviral against RSV, has not yet been documented in clinical practice. Methods used to determine antiviral susceptibility to RSV generally include bioassays that evaluate RSV replication in cell culture during or after exposure to an effective antiviral and EIA methods that evaluate antigen production after drug exposure (57).

Serology

The detection of virus-specific antibody or the detection of an increase in titer of preexisting antibody has been an important element of viral diagnosis and epidemiological studies because most primary infections or reinfections result in the production of specific antibodies. However, the utility of antibody detection for the diagnosis of infection in the immunocompromised patient is problematic because of the likelihood of a suppressed or delayed appearance of antibody, the time lag between infection and when a diagnosis can be made, and the frequency with which blood products that contain antibodies are administered to many immunocompromised patients, such as bone marrow transplant recipients. Although the detection of specific IgM antibody may be used to suggest a recent infection in a single serum specimen, this method is not generally rapidly available in clinical settings and may not be present in a timely fashion in an immunocompromised patient. Because a timely diagnosis of RSV is important, the diagnosis of RSV should not rely on serological parameters. Such methods may be useful in less seriously immunocompromised patients or in studies of family members or health care workers associated with these patients.

Many different serological techniques have been used in the diagnosis of RSV and other viral infections. Factors involved in the selection of a specific antibody assay include specificity, sensitivity, speed, technical complexity, cost, and availability of reagents. All antibody assays rely on the proper collection and storage of sera and, ideally, the comparison of acute and convalescent specimens collected at an interval of at least 2 weeks.

Serum specimens may be assayed for neutralizing antibody against RSV by testing serial dilutions of the serum against a standard dose of the virus. The antibody titer is expressed as the highest serum dilution that neutralizes the test dose of virus. As a bioassay, neutralization assays are highly specific and quite sensitive. The neutralizing antibody level is directly correlated with immunity, an important clinical and epidemiological end point (58). Similar assays have been used to assay effective RSV antibody in commercially available immunoglobulin preparations, including the licensed immunoglobulin containing high levels of RSV-specific antibody, Respigam (MedImmune, Inc., Gaithersburg, MD). Disadvantages of the assay include the time required to obtain a result and the relatively high cost resulting from the labor intensity and requirement for cell culture and titered viral stocks. Neutralization assays can be carried out in a variety of systems and the end point can be measured by a number of different procedures.

Although neutralization tests are rather expensive and technically difficult, they should be considered for use in place of less sensitive tests such as complement fixation (CF). The CF test was of great use in demonstrating an increase in antibody level in convalescent compared with acute sera, but newer, more sensitive assays have replaced this test in recent studies (59).

Enzyme-based immunoassays (EIA) are also widely used for the detection of RSV-specific antibody. This method has gained widespread use because of its sensitivity, specificity, safety, simplicity, low cost, and ability to be automated. The system lends itself to automation because of readily available microtiter diagnostic systems. Difficulties inherent in immunoassay techniques include those associated with obtaining and standardizing purified, sensitive, and specific IgG and IgM reagents. Specific antibody subclasses can be purified directly from serum samples using techniques such as column chromatography, sucrose gradient ultracentrifugation, ion-exchange chromatography, or absorption with material such as staphylococcal protein, which causes insoluble matrices to form between the reagent and specific IgG subclasses (60). In general, results from different laboratories using different reagents are not directly comparable.

Another commonly used immunohistochemical technique to detect RSV-specific antibody is the immunofluorescence technique (IF). Whereas direct techniques are used commonly to detect antigen in infected tissue or cells, indirect immunohistochemical techniques are used to detect antibody in sera or other bodily fluids. Variations on the indirect IF test, such as amplification immunoassay systems utilizing various sandwich techniques (double indirect IF or anticomplement IF) or chemical amplification systems utilizing biotin/avidin complexes are used in some research settings (2).

Western blot (WB) has been used for the detection of antibody to specific viral antigens of RSV (61). WB methods are useful for determining the viral subtype from which an immunocompetent patient has been infected or to differentiate infection from vaccination. This technique relies on the incubation of patient serum with partially purified whole virus from which the viral proteins have been separated by electrophoresis in a polyacrylamide gel and transferred onto nitrocellulose paper. The assay has the advantage of identifying antibodies specific for several antigens of the same virus simultaneously. Difficulties of WB include the expense and time required for the test, the technical requirements for performing and interpreting the test, and the problems encountered with preparing reagents.

INFLUENZA

Influenza viruses are members of the orthomyxoviridae and have a single standard negative-sense, segmented RNA genome. The diagnosis of infection by characteristic cytology or histopathology is not applicable for influenza viruses. Influenza virus infection in immunocompromised patients generally results in relatively nonspecific histopathological changes (62,63), although intracytoplasmic inclusions and syncytial cells may be seen in infected tissue. However, immunologic or other virus-specific techniques may be used to directly confirm the clinical diagnosis on various specimens, including tissue and respiratory secretions.

Virus Isolation

Detection of influenza virus in cell culture remains the gold standard for viral diagnosis. Commonly used cell lines for the detection of influenza virus include primary cell cultures—including cell lines derived from monkey, chicken, or bovine kidney cells—as well as continuous cell lines such as the Madin-Darby canine kidney cell line. The addition of trypsin to culture medium is helpful in the isolation of certain influenza viruses, particularly in nonprimary cell lines, because the proteolytic cleavage of viral hemagglutinin is required for efficient viral replication, and many nonprimary cell lines lack the protease needed for this cleavage. Trypsin therefore enhances the initiation and spread of virus within the cell culture (64).

Influenza viruses, as well as parainfluenza viruses, measles, arboviruses, and some rhinoviruses, bind to the erythrocytes of certain animal species (e.g., guinea pigs, goats, or chickens). This property permits the use of hemadsorption assays in the laboratory as a rapid and economical method of detecting virus infection in cell culture. In the laboratory, a suspension of fresh erythrocytes (from a suitable animal species, such as chicken) is added at varying time points following inoculation of the clinical specimen into cell culture and adherence of erythrocytes to the cell membrane is evaluated, generally using light microscopy. When hemadsorption is documented, the supernatant fluid may be subcultured onto fresh tissue or tested using specific antigen detection methods to determine virus identity. Hemadsorption can be detected prior to, or in some instances in the absence of, detectable CPE, and is frequently used in the laboratory for identification of cell cultures infected with influenza viruses.

Low-speed rolling and centrifugation of a clinical specimen onto a cell culture monolayer can be used to enhance viral detection and is frequently used in conjunction with viral antigen detection to provide a rapid diagnosis (23,65). Shell vials or multiwelled plastic plates also may be used for this method, as has been reported for RSV (31).

Detection of Viral Antigen

Both direct and indirect immunofluorescence (IF) assays have been used for the rapid detection of influenza A and B viruses in clinical samples and for definitive identification of these viruses in cell culture. The use of IF assays similar to those described for RSV allows detection of viral antigens even before viral CPE or hemadsorption is evident (30). The combination of IF and cell culture has increased the sensitivity of detecting influenza viruses in some studies, and the combined use of centrifugation with antigen detection methods or hemadsorption has been shown to result in earlier and sometimes more sensitive diagnoses of influenza (23,66).

Laboratory-specific EIAs are utilized in research laboratories, but results from a single laboratory cannot be generalized to other settings. Commercially available test kits, such as the Flu A Directigen kit (Becton Dickinson Diagnostics, Cockeysville, MD), are utilized in many clinical laboratories for the rapid detection of influenza A virus in patients. This test appears to have a specificity approaching 100% and a sensitivity of 75% in pediatric patients in one study (34). Of note is the increased sensitivity of the assay in children below the age of 6 months. Although specificity remains high, the sensitivity is considerably lower in immunocompromised adults (approximately 50%) (67). However, the sensitivity of the influenza A Directigen kit for influenza is substantially greater than that of the RSV Directigen kit utilized in the same patient population (22).

RT-PCR

RT-PCR detection is another method used for the viral identification of influenza virus in clinical samples. This method has been shown to be consistently more sensitive than antigen detection methods for the diagnosis of

influenza virus infection (68,69), although its superiority over culture methods has been less consistent (70,71). PCR methods may be particularly useful in settings where culture is not readily available or if specific genetic information about a virus is desired. For example, RT-PRC was recently used for rapid identification of a swine influenza virus causing an infection in humans (72).

Laboratory Methods for Viral Identification and Characterization

Further characterization of hemadsorbing viruses obtained from clinical specimens is important because of the potential for specific antiviral therapy, depending on the virus identified. The method traditionally used for identification of influenza viruses has been the virus hemagglutination-inhibition assay performed with type-specific antisera. Immunofluorescence (34), enzyme immunoassays (64), and PCR (69) are more frequently used today, based on methods described for the direct detection of viruses in clinical specimens.

PCR techniques have been used to further characterize influenza virus isolates. In addition to typing or subtyping influenza virus isolates (73–75), PCR has been used to obtain virus sequence genomes to identify drug-resistant isolates (76), identifying reassortant viruses, and even to characterize the 1918 influenza virus responsible for the pandemic "Spanish flu" from archived autopsy specimens (77).

Antiviral Susceptibility

The development of resistance of influenza A viruses to amantadine and rimantadine has been well documented in treated healthy and immunocompromised patients (78,79). As antiviral therapy becomes more widely utilized, laboratory documentation of antiviral susceptibility becomes increasingly important. Methods used to determine antiviral susceptibility to influenza viruses from clinical specimens or cultured viruses include bioassays, which evaluate viral replication in cell culture during or after exposure to an effective antiviral, enzyme-linked immunoassays, which can quantitate specific influenza-related antigens, and sequence analysis of RNA. However, sensitivity testing systems for influenza viruses are not standardized, and results may depend on the assay system, cell line used, viral inoculum, and number of viral passages prior to testing (80).

The detection of amantadine/rimantadine resistance based on RNA sequence changes takes advantage of the fact that amino acid changes in the M2 region of the influenza virus are associated with drug resistance. Using RT-PCR techniques followed by digestion with specific restriction enzymes, rapid detection of resistance may be made without requiring viral isolation or passages of the virus in cell culture. RT-PCR of a portion of the M2 gene

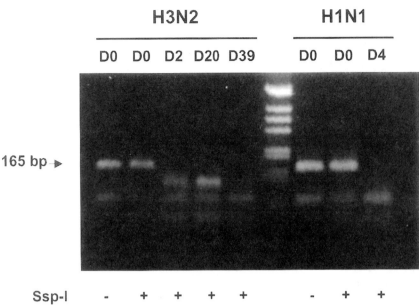

Figure 3. Detection of rimantadine resistance using RT-PCR techniques. Mutations caused by changes at amino acid 31 of the M2 gene of type A influenza viruses result in resistance to both amantadine and rimantadine, both in vitro and in vivo. Serial isolates of influenza A/H3N2 and A/H1N1 from two immunocompromised patients were collected prior to, during, and/or after rimantadine therapy. The M2 gene was amplified by PCR and amplicons were digested with Ssp-1. Day of isolation after initial viral isolate is indicated above the gel. Rimantadine-resistant isolates were digested by Ssp-1, as indicated by loss of the 165 base pair-sized band (arrow). Isolates collected after Day 0 show this resistance pattern.

of influenza A strains followed by direct sequencing or restriction endonuclease restriction analysis has proven useful in detecting the development of viral resistance in immunocompromised patients (Fig. 3) (79).

Serology

The detection of changes in influenza-specific antibody has been important historically for studying the epidemiology of influenza but has not been proven practical in severely immunocompromised patients. The time lag between infection and time of diagnosis, the frequent administration of blood products, and immunosuppressive regimens that block or delay antibody production are important reasons for this.

Serological methods may be useful, however, for determining the epidemiology of outbreaks in the community, for determining the potential protection of various vaccines in health care workers or immunocompromised patients (64), or in diagnosing infections retrospectively. Different assays that may be utilized include neutralization and microneutralization assays, hemagglutination-inhibition assays (HAI), EIA, immunofluorescence, and complement fixation. HAI is commonly used to determine antibody to specific influenza viruses, and its advantages include simplicity, the low cost for reagents and equipment, and speed of the assay. Disadvantages of this assay include the fact that nonviral-specific serum components may also inhibit hemagglutination, thereby making the test results uninterpretable.

PARAINFLUENZA VIRUSES

The laboratory detection of parainfluenza viruses relies on similar parameters required for the detection of RSV and influenza viruses, namely, the quality of the clinical specimen, the handling of the specimen prior to arriving at the laboratory, and the knowledge in the laboratory that a respiratory pathogen may be suspected. Identification of parainfluenza virus infections by direct electron microscopy or histologic examination is possible. In one report of bone marrow transplant recipients with culture-confirmed parainfluenza virus infection, six of seven lung tissue specimens (six autopsy specimens and one open lung biopsy) had evidence of intracytoplasmic viral inclusions consistent with invasive parainfluenza virus infection when the specimens were evaluated histopathologically (Fig. 4) (81).

Culture Methods

Cell culture methods remain the mainstay of the diagnosis of parainfluenza viruses in the laboratory. Parainfluenza viruses have been collected from primary monkey kidney cells in many clinical studies, but continuous monkey kidney cell lines such as LLC-MK2, with trypsin added in the medium, are equally sensitive and less expensive than primary cell lines (82). Infection of cell cultures with parainfluenza viruses may be detected by the addition of animal (guinea pig, chicken) erythrocytes, which will adsorb to the infected cells 5–14 days following inoculation. In many laboratories, routine hemadsorption is performed at regular intervals and virus is commonly detected within 10 days of inoculation. Hemadsorbing viruses can then be further characterized using HI or IF (83). Parainfluenza virus type 3 produces a recognizable cytopathic effect in continuous cell lines. However, cytopathic effect in cell culture is usually not seen with other types of parainfluenza viruses.

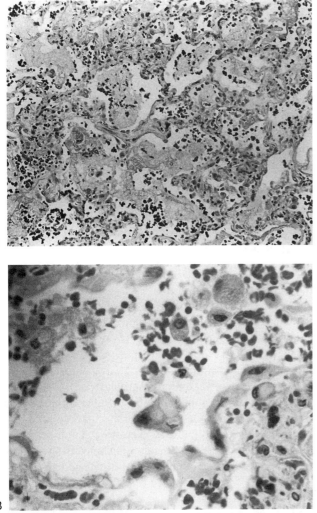

Figures 4a and 4b. Lung tissue taken at autopsy from 27-year-old male bone marrow transplant recipient infected with parainfluenza type 3 virus. Figure 4a demonstrates diffuse pneumonitis and alveolar damage, with obliteration of normal architecture, chronic inflammatory infiltrate, and interstitial fibrosis. Eosinophilic granular cytoplasmic inclusions are seen in Figure 4b.

Antigen Detection

Fluorescein-labeled antibodies have been utilized in the study of parainfluenza viruses for many years. Rapid antigen tests are currently commercially available only for parainfluenza type 3. Originally, such reagents were used to confirm virologic identity of tissue culture isolates, but now they are being increasingly used to detect the presence of parainfluenza viruses directly in respiratory secretions and in cell cultures that have been incubated for 48 hours or less. Variations of this technique—including simultaneous rapid culture using differential multicolored fluorescent confirmatory stains (84), respiratory virus panels containing a pool of monoclonal antibodies (65), and short-term centrifugation of shell vials at 700 *g* with subsequent immunofluorescent stain-

ing (85)—have been reported to be effective for the diagnosis of parainfluenza virus infections in pediatric specimens. Little information is available on the relative ease of detection or viral loads in immunocompromised patients, although prolonged shedding of virus in pediatric patients with severe combined immunodeficiency is well established (86–88). High morbidity and mortality rates associated with infection in bone marrow transplant recipients early post transplantation (81) and lung transplant recipients (89) have been associated with positive cultures or antigen deletion of parainfluenza viruses.

RT-PCR

The length of time required to grow some parainfluenza viruses and the relatively poor sensitivity of tissue culture for parainfluenza virus type 1 probably result in the underdiagnosis of these viruses in the clinical laboratory (90). The use of RT-PCR detection of viral nucleic acid may provide enhanced detection of these viruses. However, RT-PCR assays to detect parainfluenza virus have not been widely used directly in respiratory secretions, in part because of the success of antigen detection methods (para 3 only) in respiratory secretions and shell vial amplification of respiratory viruses in culture (91). Furthermore, the relative complexity, time, and cost of PCR reactions compared with antigen detection methods may favor the latter in some clinical laboratories. The sensitivity of various detection methods in immunocompromised patients is not known. The use of multiple PCR probes to attempt to define the etiology of respiratory infections has been approached using primers to parainfluenza types 1, 2, and 3 simultaneously with primers to RSV and influenza viruses in a single test, the Hexaplex assay (Prodesse, Inc, Madison, WI). This assay, performed in freshly collected nasal washes or nasopharyngeal swabs from 69 children, demonstrated good sensitivity and specificity, with results available more quickly than standard virus isolation with results equivalent or superior to culture (49). Sequencing of PCR products has also been useful in molecular epidemiological studies of parainfluenza virus type 3 (92).

Serology

Serological methods have been frequently used to determine the epidemiology of parainfluenza virus infections in otherwise healthy adults and children. However, the usefulness of antibody determinations against parainfluenza viruses in the immunocompromised host is unlikely to provide rapid diagnosis or to be a sensitive measure of infection. Antibody in serum and nasal secretions can be measured by neutralization, HAI, EIAs, and CF tests (82,93,94).

RHINOVIRUSES

Rhinoviruses belong to the Picornaviridae and are positive-sense single-stranded RNA viruses. Unlike the other Paramyxoviruses, rhinovirus infection cannot be suspected based on characteristic histopathological changes or changes in cell morphology. Because the amount of virus present on respiratory secretions is low, it also is not diagnosed by electron microscopy. In most clinical laboratories, cell culture is used to diagnose rhinovirus infection. Several different cell lines may be used, including diploid strains of human embryonic lung cells (WI-38 or MRC-5), primary cell lines such as rhesus monkey kidney cells, and a strain of HeLa cells that has enhanced sensitivity to rhinoviruses (95). Temperatures of 33° to 34°C with rolling of tubes is useful for virus isolation. In general, cytopathic effect due to infection of rhinovirus in sensitive cells is apparent in 5–14 days. Continuous cell lines require monitoring for continued sensitivity to rhinoviruses because these cells may vary in their detection sensitivity to these viruses for unknown reasons (96). Other sensitive culture methods have included the use of organ cultures of fetal human trachea. The cell lines utilized for the detection of rhinoviruses may detect enteroviruses; rhinovirus isolates may be distinguished from enteroviruses by their lability in acid (loss in viral titer following exposure to a pH of 5).

Antigen Detection

Assays for the detection of rhinovirus antigen have been developed using immunofluorescence and enzyme immunoassays. However, these assays are serotype-specific, and because there are more than 100 serotypes of rhinovirus, these methods are not useful in the clinical laboratory. In addition, because the concentration of rhinovirus in respiratory secretions is low, the sensitivity of these assays is problematic. Thus there are no commercially available antigen-detection assays for rhinovirus (96).

RNA Detection

The use of RT-PCR has improved the ability to both detect and characterize rhinoviruses. RT-PCR assays have been two to three times more sensitive than conventional culture methods in some clonal studies (97). Some assays do not distinguish rhinovirus from enteroviruses, but others can distinguish viruses in these two genera (98,99). RT-PCR also has been used to distinguish rhinovirus isolates from enteroviruses instead of using the conventional acid lability assays. *In situ* hybridization studies have been used in human challenge studies (100) but have not been used for routine clinical diagnosis of rhinovirus infection. Typing of rhinoviruses based on PCR amplification sequence variations in 5' noncoding region has also been

described (101). The utility of these methods in immunocompromised patients requires further evaluation.

Serology

The standard serological method for documenting rhinovirus infection is the virus neutralization assay (102). This assay has been used to measure antibody in serum and nasal secretions. The utility of serology for the diagnosis of rhinovirus infection is limited because of the large number of viral serotypes and requires that the patient be able to mount an appropriate immune response. Thus serological methods are not generally applicable to the diagnosis of these infections.

CORONAVIRUSES

The reliable and sensitive identification of coronaviruses in the laboratory remains a major hurdle in their study (103). The coronaviruses were first isolated in organ cultures of human embryonic trachea by Tyrrell and Bynoe (104), and the morphology was determined using negative staining of the specimen under electron microscopy. The two main types of coronavirus are 229E and OC43. Sensitive diploid fibroblast cell lines have been used in some laboratories for the detection of 229E viruses in humans, but OC43 strains have only been detected using organ cultures. Newer detection methods utilizing nucleic acid hybridization techniques have been developed for the detection of 229E strains and are sensitive and specific, but no more sensitive than cell culture (105,106). RT-PCR assays also have been developed and used in a limited number of clinical studies and may facilitate further studies of these viruses.

Many epidemiological studies of these viruses have relied on serological techniques such as CF, EIAs, and HAI tests (OC43 strain only) for the detection of these viruses. The application of serological methods for immunocompromised hosts has not generally been useful. Thus little is known about the incidence of disease or presentation of clinical disease associated with coronaviruses in immunocompromised hosts.

FUTURE DIRECTIONS

Advances in viral diagnoses and the development of new modes of antiviral therapy are likely to result in the desire to detect viral respiratory infections accurately and as early as possible in the severely immunocompromised patient. Increased demand for rapid and cost-effective measures for determining the etiology of viral infections, in conjunction with improved methods of detection based on advances in molecular biotechnology, will likely lead to better methods to diagnose respiratory viral infections in the future. Of some concern, however, is the ability of the clinician to effectively culture patients for viruses, because of cost containment issues and because of regionalization and consolidation of clinical virology laboratories.

REFERENCES

1. Couch RB, Englund JA, Whimbey E. Respiratory viral infections in immunocompetent and immunocompromised persons. *Am J Med* 1997;102:2–8.
2. Atmar RL, Englund JA. Laboratory methods for the diagnosis of viral diseases. In: Evans AS, Kaslow RA, eds. *Viral infections of humans*, 4th ed. New York: Plenum; 1997:59–88.
3. Hall CB, Douglas RG Jr. Clinically useful methods for the isolation of respiratory syncytial virus. *J Infect Dis* 1975;131:1–5.
4. Cate TR, Couch RB, Johnson KM. Studies with rhinoviruses in volunteers; production of illness effect of naturally acquired antibody, and demonstration of a protective effect not associated with serum antibody. *J Clin Invest* 1964;43(1):56–60.
5. Bowden RA. Respiratory virus infections after marrow transplant; the Fred Hutchinson Cancer Research Center experience. *Am J Med* 1996;102(3A):27–30.
6. Smith TF. Specimen requirements: selection, collection, transport and processing. In: Specter S, Lancz G, eds. *Clinical virology manual*. New York: Elsevier Publishing; 1992:19–41.
7. Menegus MA, Douglas RG Jr. Viruses, rickettsiae, chlamydiae and mycoplasmas. In: Mandell GL, Douglas RG Jr, Bennett JE, eds. *Principles and practice of infectious diseases*. New York: Churchill Livingstone; 1990:193–205.
8. Ahluwalia G, Embree J, McNicol P, Law B, Hammond GW. Comparison of nasopharyngeal aspirate and nasopharyngeal swab specimens for respiratory syncytial virus diagnosis by cell culture, indirect immunofluorescence assay, and enzyme-linked immunosorbent assay. *J Clin Microbiol* 1987;25:763–767.
9. Crane LR, Gutterman PA, Chapel T, Lerner AM. Incubation of swab materials with herpes simplex virus. *J Infect Dis* 1990;141:531.
10. Frayha H, Castrucuabi S, Mahoney J, Chernesky MA. Nasopharyngeal swabs and nasopharyngeal aspirates equally effective for the diagnosis of viral respiratory disease in hospitalized children. *J Clin Microbiol* 1989;27:1387–1389.
11. Greenberg SB, Krilov LV. Laboratory diagnosis of viral respiratory disease. In: Drew WL, Rubin SJ, eds. *Cumulative techniques and procedures in clinical microbiology*. Washington, DC: American Society of Microbiology; 1986:1–21.
12. Hertz MI, Englund JA, Bitterman PB, McGlave PB. Respiratory syncytial virus-induced acute lung injury in adult patients with bone marrow transplants: a clinical approach and review of the literature. *Medicine* 1989;68:269–281.
13. Baselski VS, Wunderink RG. Bronchoscopic diagnosis of pneumonia. *Clin Microbiol Rev* 1994;533–558.
14. King JC, Burke AR, Clemens JD, et al. Respiratory syncytial virus illnesses in human immunodeficiency, virus-infected and noninfected children. *Pediatr Infect Dis J* 1993;12:733–739.
15. Hambling MH. Survival of respiratory syncytial virus during storage under various conditions. *Br J Exp Pathol* 1964;45:647–655.
16. Johnson FB. Transport of viral specimens. *Clin Microbiol Rev* 1990;3:120–131.
17. Huntoon CJ, House RF, Smith TF. Recovery of viruses from three transport media incorporated into culturettes. *Arch Pathol Lab Med* 1981;105:436–437.
18. Schmidt NJ, Emmons RW. General principles of laboratory diagnostic methods for viral, rickettsial and chlamydial infections. In: Schmidt NJ, Emmons RW, eds. *Diagnostic procedures for viral rickettsial and chlamydial infections*. Washington, DC: American Public Health Association; 1989:1–35.
19. Chernesky MA, Ray CG, Smith TF. Laboratory diagnosis of viral infections. In: Drew WL, ed. *Cumulative techniques and procedures in clinical microbiology*. Washington, DC: American Society for Microbiology; 1982:1–17.
20. Baxter BD, Couch RB, Greenberg SB, Kasel JA. Rapid methods for the diagnosis of viral infections. *Lab Med* 1987;18:16–20.
21. Couch RB, Greenberg SB, Kasel JA. Maintenance of viability and comparison of identification methods for influenza and other respiratory viruses of humans. *J Clin Microbiol* 1977;6:19–22.
22. Englund JA, Piedra PA, Jewell A. Rapid diagnosis of respiratory syncytial virus infection in immunocompromised adults. *J Clin Microbiol* 1996;34:1649.
23. Hughes JH. Physical and chemical methods for enhancing rapid detection of viruses and other agents. *Clin Microbiol Rev* 1993;6:150–175.
24. Gey GO. An improved technique for massive tissue cultures. *Am J Cancer* 1995;17:752–756.
25. Hudson JB, Misra V, Mosmann TR. Cytomegalovirus infectivity: analysis of the phenomenon of centrifugal enhancement of infectivity. *Virology* 1976;72:235–243.
26. Espy MJ, Hierholzer JC, Smith TF. The effect of centrifugation on the rapid detection of adenovirus in shell vials. *Am J Clin Pathol* 1987;88:358–360.
27. Matthey S, Nicholson D, Ruhs S, et al. Rapid detection of respiratory viruses by shell vial culture and direct staining by using pooled and individual monoclonal antibodies. *J Clin Microbiol* 1992;30(3):540.
28. Kisch AL, Chanock KM, Johnson KM. Immunofluorescence with respiratory syncytial virus. *Virology* 1974;26:177–182.
29. Parrott RH, Kim H, Brandt CD. Respiratory syncytial virus. In: Lennette EH, ed. *Diagnostic procedures for viral, rickettsial and chlamydial infections*, 5th ed.. Washington, DC: American Public Health Association; 1979:695.
30. Minnich LL, Ray CG. Immunofluorescence. In: Lancz G, Specter S, eds. *Clinical virology manual,* 2nd ed. New York: Elsevier Publishing; 1995:117–128.
31. Espy MJ, Smith TF, Harmon MW, Kendal AP. Rapid detection of influenza virus by shell vial assay with monoclonal antibodies. *J Clin Microbiol* 1986;24:677–679.
32. Ray CG, Minnich LL. Efficiency of immunofluorescence for rapid detection of common respiratory viruses. *J Clin Microbiol* 1997;25(2):355–357.
33. Todd S, Minnich LL, Warner JL. Comparison of rapid immunofluorescence procedure with TestPack RSV and directigen FLU-A for diagnosis of respiratory syncytial virus and influenza A virus. *J Clin Microbiol* 1995;33:1650.
34. Dominguez EA, Taber LH, Couch RB. Comparison of rapid diagnostic techniques for respiratory syncytial and influenza A virus respiratory infections in young children. *J Clin Microbiol* 1993;31:2286–2290.
35. Halstead DC, Todd S, Fritch G. Evaluation of five methods for respiratory syncytial virus detection. *J Clin Microbiol* 1990;28:1021–1025.
36. Waner JL, Whitehurst NJ, Todd S. Comparison of Directigen RSV with viral isolation and direct immunofluorescence for the identification of respiratory syncytial virus. *J Clin Microbiol* 1990;28:480.
37. Kim H, Wyatt RG, Fernie BF, et al. Respiratory syncytial virus detection by immunofluorescence in nasal secretions with monoclonal antibodies against selected surface and internal proteins. *J Clin Microbiol* 1983;18:1399–1404.
38. Swierkosz EM, Flanders R, Melvin L, Miller JD, Kline MW. Evaluation of the Abbott TESTPACK RSV enzyme immunoassay for detection of respiratory syncytial virus in nasopharyngeal swab specimens. *J Clin Microbiol* 1989;27:1151–1154.
39. Norval M, Bingham RW. Advances in the use of nucleic acid probes in diagnosis of viral diseases of man. *Arch Virol* 1987;97:151–165.
40. Saiki RK, Scharf S, Faloona F, et al. Enzymatic amplification of beta-globin genomic sequences and restriction site analysis for diagnosis of sickle cell anemia. *Science* 1985;230:1350–1354.
41. Saiki RK, Gelfand DH, Stoffel S, et al. Primer-directed enzymatic amplification of DNA with a thermostable DNA polymerase. *Science* 1988;239:487–491.
42. Atmar RL, Metcalf TG, Neill FH, Ester MK. Detection of enteric viruses in oysters using the polymerase chain reaction. *Appl Environ Microbiol* 1993;59:631–635.
43. Gama RE, Horsnell PR, Hughes PJ, North C, Bruce CB, Al-Nakib W. Amplification of rhinovirus specific nucleic acids from clinical samples using the polymerase chain reaction. *J Med Virol* 1989;28:73–77.
44. Kwok S, Higuchi R. Avoiding false positives with PCR. *Nature* 1989;339:237–238.
45. Yoshio H, Yamada M, Nii S. Reverse transcription-polymerase chain reaction amplification of respiratory syncytial virus genome from

neonatal nasal swab samples. *Acta Paediatrica Japonica* 1996;38 (5):429–433.

46. Gilbert LL, Dakhama A, Bone BM, Thomas EE, Hegele RG. Diagnosis of viral respiratory tract infections in children by using a reverse transcription-PCR panel. *J Clin Microbiol* 1996;34(1):140–143.

47. Freymuth F, Eugene G, Vabret A, et al. Detection of respiratory syncytial virus by reverse transcription-PCR and hybridization with a DNA enzyme immunoassay. *J Clin Microbiol* 1995;33(12):3352–3355.

48. Paton AW, Paton JC, Lawrence AJ, Goldwater PN, Harris RJ. Rapid detection of respiratory syncytial virus in nasopharyngeal aspirates by reverse transcription and polymerase chain reaction amplification. *J Clin Microbiol* 1992;30(4):901–904.

49. Fan J, Henrickson KJ, Savatski LL. Rapid simultaneous diagnosis of RSVA,B, influenza A B, Human parainfluenza virus types 1,2, and 3 infection by multiplex quantitative RP-PCR hybridization (Hexaplex™) assay. Clin Infect Dis 1998;26:1397–1402

50. Yewdell JW, Gerhard W. Antigenic characterization of viruses by monoclonal antibodies. *Ann Rev Microbiol* 1981;35:185–206.

51. Englund JA, Anderson LJ, Rhame FS. Nosocomial transmission of respiratory syncytial virus in immunocompromised adults. *J Clin Microbiol* 1991;29:115.

52. Harrington RD, Hooton TM, Hackman RC, et al. An outbreak of respiratory syncytial virus in a bone marrow transplantation center. *J Infect Dis* 1992;165:987.

53. Storch GA, Hall CB, Anderson LJ, Park CS, Dohner DE. Antigenic and nucleic acid analysis of nosocomial isolates of respiratory syncytial virus. *J Infect Dis* 1993;167:562–566.

54. Gottschalk J, Zbiden R, Kaempf L, Heinzer I. Discrimination of respiratory syncytial virus subgroups A and B by reverse transcription-PCR. *J Clin Microbiol* 1996;34(1):41–43.

55. Sullender WM, Sun L, Anderson LJ. Analysis of respiratory syncytial virus genetic variability with amplified cDNAs. *J Clin Microbiol* 1993;31:1224–1231.

56. Van Milaan AJ, Sprenger MJW, Rothbarth PH, Brandenburg AH, Masurel N, Claas ECJ. Detection of respiratory syncytial virus by RNA-polymerase chain reaction and differentiation of subgroups with oligonucleotide probes. *J Med Virol* 1994;44:80–87.

57. Englund JA, Piedra PA, Ahn Y. High-dose, short duration ribavirin aerosol therapy compared with standard ribavirin therapy in children with suspected respiratory syncytial virus infection. *J Pediatr* 1994; 125:635.

58. Siber GR, Leszczynski J, Pena-Cruz V, et al. Protective activity of a human respiratory syncytial virus immune globulin prepared from donors screened by microneutralization assay. *J Infect Dis* 1992;165: 456.

59. Dowell SF, Anderson LJ, Gary HE Jr, et al. Respiratory syncytial virus is an important cause of community-acquired lower respiratory infection among hospitalized adults. *J Infect Dis* 1`996;174:456–62.

60. James K. Immunoserology of infectious diseases. *Clin Microbiol Rev* 1990;3:132–152.

61. Piedra PA, Glezen WP, Kasel JA. Safety and immunogenicity of the PFP vaccine against RSV: the Western blot assay aids in distinguishing immune responses of the PFP vaccine from RSV infection. *Vaccine* 1995;13:1095.

62. Yousef HM, Englund JA, Couch RB, et al. Influenza among hospitalized adults with leukemia. *Clin Infect Dis* 1997;24:1095–1099.

63. Whimbey E, Champlin RE, Couch RB, et al. Community respiratory virus infections among hospitalized adult bone marrow transplant recipients. *Clin Infect Dis* 1996;22:778–782.

64. Glezen WP, Couch RB. Influenza virus. In: Evans AS, Kaslow RA, eds. *Viral infections in humans*. New York: Plenum; 1997:473–505.

65. Engler HD, Preuss J. Laboratory diagnosis of respiratory virus infections in 24 hours by utilizing shell vial cultures. *J Clin Microbiol* 1997;35(8):2165–2167.

66. Waner JL, Todd S, Hamed S, Murphy P, Wall LV. Comparison of directigen FLU-A with viral isolation and direct immunofluorescence for the rapid detection and identification of influenza A virus. *J Clin Microbiol* 1991;29(3):479–482.

67. Atmar RL, Englund JA, Whimbey E, Mirza N, Lewis V, Baxter BD. Use of the Directigen Flu A kit to diagnose influenza A virus infection in immunocompromised adults. Ann Mtg of Pan Am Group for Rapid Viral Diagnosis 1994. [Abstract]

68. Claas ECJ, van Milaan AJ, Sprenger MJW, et al. Prospective application of reverse transcriptase polymerase chain reaction for diagnosing influenza infections in respiratory samples from a children's hospital. *J Clin Microbiol* 1993;31(8):2218–2221.

69. Atmar RL, Baxter BD, Dominguez EA, Taber LH. Comparison of reverse transcription-PCR with tissue culture and other rapid diagnostic assays for detection of type A influenza virus. *J Clin Microbiol* 1996;34(10):2604–2606.

70. Ellis JS, Fleming DM, Zambon MC. Multiplex reverse transcription-PCR for surveillance of influenza A and B viruses in England and Wales in 1995 and 1996. *J Clin Microbiol* 1997;35(8):2076–2082.

71. Cherian T, Bobo L, Steinhoff MC, Karron RA, Yolken RH. Use of PCR-enzyme immunoassay for identification of influenza A virus matrix RNA in clinical samples negative for cultivable virus. *J Clin Microbiol* 1994;32(3):623–628.

72. Wentworth DE, McGregor MW, Macklin MD, Neumann V, Hinshaw VS. Transmission of swine influenza to humans after exposure to experimentally infected pigs. *J Infect Dis* 1997;175(1):7–15.

73. Schweiger B, Lange I, Heckler R, Willers H, Schreier E. Rapid detection of influenza A neuraminidase subtypes by cDNA amplification coupled to a simple DNA enzyme immunoassay. *Arch Virol* 1994;139:439–444.

74. Wright KE, Wilson GAR, Novosad D, Dimock C, Tan D, Weber JM. Typing and subtyping of influenza viruses in clinical samples by PCR. *J Clin Microbiol* 1995;33(5):1180–1184.

75. Atmar RL, Baxter BD. Typing and subtyping clinical isolates of influenza virus using reverse transcription-polymerase chain reaction. *Clin Diagn Virol* 1996;7:77–84.

76. Klimov AI, Rocha E, Hayden FG, Shult PA, Floretta-Roumillat L, Cox NJ. Prolonged shedding of amanatadine-resistant influenza A viruses by immunodeficient patients: detection by polymerase chain reaction-restriction analysis. *J Infect Dis* 1995;172:1352–1355.

77. Taubenberger JK, Reid AH, Krafft AE, Bijwaard KE, Fanning TG. Initial genetic characterization of the 1918 "Spanish" influenza virus. *Science* 1997;275:1793.

78. Hayden FG. Prevention and treatment of influenza in immunocompromised patients. *Am J Med* 1997;102(3A):55–60.

79. Englund JA, Champlin RE, Wyde PR, et al. Commonemergence of amantadine- and rimantadine-resistant influenza A viruses in symptomiatic immunocompromised adults. *Clin Infect Dis* 1998;26: 1418–1424.

80. Decker C, Ellis MN, McLaren C, Hunter G, Rogers J, Barry DW. Virus resistance in clinical practice. *J Antimicrob Chemother* 1983; 12:137–152.

81. Lewis V, Champlin R, Englund JA, et al. Respiratory disease due to parainfluenza virus in adult bone marrow transplant recipients. *Clin Infect Dis* 1996;23:1033–1037.

82. Glezen WP, Denney FW. Parainfluenza Viruses. In: Evans AS, Kaslow RA, eds. *Viral infections in humans*, 4th ed. New York: Plenum; 1997:551–562.

83. Mufson MA. Parainfluenza viruses, mumps virus, and New Castle disease virus. In: Lennette EH, Schmidt NJ, eds. *Diagnostic procedures for viral, rickettsial and chlamydial infections*, 6th ed. Washington, DC: American Public Health Association; 1989:669.

84. Brumback BG, Wade CD. Simultaneous rapid culture for four respiratory viruses in the same cell monolayer using a differential multicolored fluorescent confirmatory stain. *J Clin Microbiol* 1996;34 (4):798–801.

85. McDonald JC, Quennec P. Utility of a respiratory virus panel containing a monoclonal antibody pool for screening of respiratory specimens in nonpeak respiratory syncytial virus season. *J Clin Microbiol* 1993;31(10):2809–2811.

86. Jarvis WR, Middleton PJ, Gelfand EW. Parainfluenza pneumonia in severe combined immunodeficiency disease. *J Pediatr* 1979;94:423.

87. DeLage G, Brochu P, Pelletier M. Giant-cell pneumonia caused by parainfluenza virus. *J Pediatr* 1979;94:426.

88. Frank JA Jr, Warren RW, Tucker JA, et al. Disseminated parainfluenza infection in a child with severe combined immunodeficiency. *Am J Dis Child* 1983;137:1172.

89. Wendt CH, Fox JMK, Hertz MI. Paramyxovirus infection in lung transplant recipients. *J Heart Lung Transp* 1995;14:479–485.

90. Fan J, Henrickson KJ. Rapid diagnosis of human parainfluenza virus type 1 infection by quantitative reverse transcription-PCR-enzyme hybridization assay. *J Clin Microbiol* 1996;34(8):1914–1917.

91. Piedra PA, Englund JA, Glezen WP. Respiratory syncytial virus and parainfluenza viruses. In: Richman DD, Whitley RJ, Hayden FG, eds. *Clinical virology.* New York: Churchill Livingstone; 1997: 787–819.

92. Karron RA, O'Brien KL, Froehlich JL, Brown VA. Molecular epidemiology of a parainfluenza type 3 virus outbreak on a pediatric ward. *J Infect Dis* 1993;167:1441.

93. Chanock RM, Parrott RH, Johnson KM, Kapikian AZ, Bell JA. Myxoviruses: parainfluenza. *Am Rev Resp Dis* 1963;88:152–166.

94. Julkunen I. Serological diagnosis of parainfluenza virus infections by enzyme immunoassay with special emphasis on purity of viral antigens. *J Med Virol* 1984;14:177–187.

95. Conant RM, Somerson NL, Hamparian VV. Rhinovirus: basis for a numbering system. 1. HeLa cell for propagation and serologic procedures. *J Immunol* 1968;100:107.

96. Gwaltney JM, Rueckert RR. Rhinovirus. In: Richman DD, Whitley RJ, Hayden FG, eds. *Clinical virology.* New York: Churchill Livingstone; 1997:1025–1047.

97. Johnson SL, Sanderson G, Pattemore PK, et al. Use of polymerase chain reaction for diagnosis of picornavirus infection in subjects with and without respiratory symptoms. *J Clin Microbiol* 1993;31(1): 111–117.

98. Atmar RL, Georghiou PR. Classification of respiratory tract picornavirus isolates as enteroviruses or rhinoviruses by using reverse transcription-polymerase chain reaction. *J Clin Microbiol* 1993;31(9): 2544–2546.

99. Olive DM, Siham AM, Wahiba AM, et al. Detection and differentiation of picornaviruses in clinical samples following genomic amplification. *J Gen Virol* 1990;71:2141–2147.

100. Bruce CB, Chadwick P, Widad AN. Detection of rhinovirus RNA in nasal epithelial cells by *in situ* hybridization. *J Virol Meth* 1990;30: 115–126.

101. Torgersen H, Skern T, Blaas D. Typing of human rhinoviruses based on sequence variations in the 5′ non-coding region. *J Gen Virol* 1989; 70:3111–3116.

102. Douglas RG, Jr, Fleet WF, Cate TR, Couch RB. Antibody to rhinovirus in human sera. I. standardization of a neutralization test. *Proc Soc Exper Biol Med* 1968;127:497–502.

103. Monto AS. Coronavirus. In: Evans As, Kaslow RA, eds. *Viral infections of humans: epidemiology and control,* 4th ed. New York: Plenum; 1997:211–228.

104. Tyrrell DAJ, Bynoe ML. Cultivation of a novel type of common-cold virus in organ cultures. *BMJ* 1965;1:1467.

105. Myint S, Harmsen D, Raabe R. Characterization of nucleic acid probe for the diagnosis of human coronavirus 229E infections. *J Med Virol* 1990;31:165–172.

106. Myint S, Siddell S, Tyrrell DAJ. Detection of human coronavirus. *J Med Virol* 1989;29:70–73.

Transplant Infections edited by
Raleigh A. Bowden, Per Ljungman, and Carlos V. Paya.
Published by Lippincott–Raven Publishers, Philadelphia, 1998

CHAPTER 7

Diagnosis of Invasive Fungal Infections in Transplant Recipients

Thomas J. Walsh and Stephen J. Chanock

Invasive fungal infections have emerged as one of the most challenging complications of marrow and solid organ transplantation (1,2). Over the past two decades, there has been an increase in the number of cancer and transplant (both solid and marrow) recipients with fungal infections, which is explained by two major trends: (a) more patients are undergoing transplantation or intensive chemotherapy regimens and (b) intensive cytotoxic and antirejection regimens are being used more aggressively. The latter two approaches are associated with more profound defects in host defense systems (3). Invasive fungal infections are also a significant complication in the expanded population of individuals infected with HIV. In addition, selective pressures increase the likelihood of colonization with pathogenic fungi; these include prolonged hospitalization and widespread use of antimicrobial therapy (especially antibacterial agents).

In all immunocompromised groups, the consequences of developing a deep fungal infection are associated with significant morbidity and mortality. Although the expanding repertoire of available antifungal agents may be encouraging, use of these therapies has been plagued by difficulties in early detection of fungal infection. For years we have appreciated that clinical resolution has been associated with early detection and recovery of host defects. Because clinical manifestations of fungal infections are unfortunately often nonspecific, indications for starting antifungal therapy are frequently based upon clinical suspicion in a high-risk patient.

The diagnosis of an invasive fungal infection is not always straightforward. A fungal pathogen in clinical specimens can be detected by many different methods. Direct microscopic examination and isolation of a spe-cific pathogen by standard culture techniques have been the gold standards for diagnosis until recently. Nonculture methods, many of which are still under active investigation, offer the promise of a quicker turnaround while preserving a high level of sensitivity. These new methods include detection of pathogen-specific antigens (i.e., cell wall mannan, enolase, HSP-90-related *Candida* antigen, D-arabinitol, and 1,3-beta-D-glucans). An excellent example of a rapid detection system is the agglutination technique for the polysaccharide capsule of *Cryptococcus neoformans*. The high level of sensitivity and specificity established for this test system is an excellent prototype for development of comparable systems for detection of *Candida* and *Aspergillus* spp. Laboratory identification of *Candida* and *Aspergillus* isolates at the level of different species carries important implications for both prognosis and therapeutic choices (4,5). The ability to detect specific diagnostic antibodies to circulating fragments of the organism has a restricted role in the initial management of patients with a suspected fungal infection. Recently, the explosion in recombinant DNA technology has led to amplification of nucleic acid sequences unique to species or genera of fungal pathogens. In many circumstances, diagnosis is confirmed by testing biopsy specimens with one or more of these tests. The use of polymerase chain reaction (PCR) technologies for detection of *Candida* and *Aspergillus* spp. has generated great interest but remains an unfulfilled promise. Although the sensitivity and specificity of PCR-based technologies may be high, clinical applications will have to be validated in prospective clinical trials.

The chapter will be divided into sections based upon detection of specific fungal pathogens. Within each section, standard methodologies and research approaches will be reviewed. In the process of reviewing diagnostic modalities, we will discuss the available techniques and

From the Infectious Disease Section, Pediatric Branch, National Cancer Institute, Bethesda, MD 90892.

highlight the problems associated with conventional approaches of relying upon microscopic examination of specimens or culture-based techniques. On the basis of reviewing the current approach to the more common and not so common fungal pathogens, it is easier to appreciate the limitations and pitfalls of diagnostic mycology. In turn, one can understand the need to develop new, more accurate detection systems. The latter may improve sensitivity and at the same time be performed in a shorter period of time.

MEDICALLY IMPORTANT YEAST PATHOGENS

Invasive Candidiasis

Clinical Manifestations of Invasive Candidiasis

Invasive candidiasis is a major cause of morbidity and mortality in hospitalized patients (6–12). In transplant recipients, candidiasis is the most commonly encountered fungal infection. The most frequently isolated species of *Candida* is *C. albicans*, but recent trends indicate that non-*albicans* species are increasingly prevalent. However, the clinical signs and symptoms of invasive candidiasis are rarely specific enough to establish a definitive diagnosis of candidiasis without laboratory confirmation. Instead, the clinician must rely upon recognition of cardinal features for deciding whether to initiate antifungal therapy. Important clues in the history and physical examination may indicate a high likelihood for invasive candidiasis (13–19). These include persistent or recurrent fever despite antibacterial therapy in a neutropenic patient; vitreal opacities, a hallmark of *Candida* endophthalmitis in the nonneutropenic host; erythematous maculopapular cutaneous lesions and myalgias indicative of acute disseminated candidiasis; and tenderness in the right or left upper quadrants consistent with hepatic or splenic candidiasis in chronic disseminated candidiasis. Still, it is incumbent upon the care providers to confirm the presence of invasive candidiasis by one of several different methodologies. Until recently, most laboratories relied upon direct examination of clinical specimens or detection of growth in media favorable for growth of *Candida*.

Direct Examination

Direct examination of a specimen can provide a number of important insights into a fungal infection. One can discriminate between different fungal pathogens on the basis of morphological features of an organism, such as the presence of blastoconidia (budding yeast forms), pseudohyphae, and hyphae (20–22). One can also estimate the burden of a pathogen present, using this as a rough marker for discriminating between infection and colonization. It is also possible to recognize other organisms, such as bacteria, that may be important pathogens

in a mixed infection. The cellular composition of the inflammatory reaction is also critical. For example, in hepatosplenic candidiasis, there may be a paucity of the organism seen but a characteristic pattern of incomplete granuloma formation. Inspection of homogenized liver biopsy tissue for fungal elements may rapidly establish a diagnosis of hepatic candidiasis, particularly because culture detection systems used for processing biopsy specimens are associated with a low diagnostic yield (19).

Invasive infection due to *Candida* spp. is characterized by the presence of pseudohyphae and blastoconidia in deep-tissue specimens; however, the presence of pseudohyphae or hyphae does not necessarily establish a diagnosis of mucosal invasion in oropharyngeal and vaginal candidiasis (23–25). Pure blastoconidia seen in a mucosal specimen could also suggest *Candida glabrata* causing oropharyngeal or esophageal lesions (e.g., from mucosal scrapings), *Cryptococcus neoformans* causing pneumonia (e.g., observed in bronchoalveolar lavage fluid), or *Histoplasma capsulatum* var. *capsulatum* causing oropharyngeal lesions (e.g., from mucosal scrapings) or pneumonia (e.g., observed in bronchoalveolar lavage fluid).

Because *Candida albicans* is a normal commensal organism of the oropharyngeal and vaginal flora, isolation from either oropharyngeal or vaginal secretions is not specific. However, in the context of a patient at risk, direct examination does provide a semiquantitative estimate of the amount of *Candida* spp. that can be useful for monitoring therapy as well as for starting a new antifungal agent. Most experts still agree that direct examination should be performed in concert with standard culture techniques. The rapid identification of *Candida* will frequently prompt initiation of systemic antifungal therapy (especially if the patient is immunocompromised) or topical therapy (if detected early) in the transplant recipient, particularly if there are any compatible signs or symptoms. Typically, one uses direct inspection of material from mucosal infections (e.g., scrapings from an oropharyngeal lesion, brushings from an esophageal plaque, swab from a vaginal discharge, or aliquot of urine) at the earliest suspicion of infection. However, the success of this approach is predicated upon the clinician's recognition of the signs and symptoms of infection. It is also difficult to discriminate between infection and colonization.

Examination of urine sediment is useful for the diagnosis of *Candida* spp. as the cause of a urinary tract infection. However, the significance of candiduria depends upon the immune status of the host and the presence or absence of specific risk factors for disseminated candidiasis (26). In addition, specimen collection must be factored into the analysis. It is important to emphasize that candiduria per se cannot establish a diagnosis of renal candidiasis. On the other hand, the absence of candiduria does not exclude the diagnosis. However, the identification of *Candida* casts in the urine specimen is highly suggestive of renal candidiasis (26). Renal *Candida* casts are detected by cytology with either Papanicolaou stain or direct inspection with a polarizing microscope. In experimental renal candidiasis in immunocompetent rabbits, the authors found no lower limit for the detection of *Candida albicans* in the urine below which the diagnosis of upper urinary tract infection can be excluded (27). Serial quantitative urine cultures capable of detecting 10 CFU/ml may not necessarily be diagnostic despite the renal candidiasis at a measured concentration of ε10⁵ CFU/ml.

Direct examination of a specimen for detection of *Candida* spp. can be performed using a number of different techniques (28). These include a wet-mount of unstained fluid (e.g., urine), Gram stain, calcofluor white potassium hydroxide (KOH), Wright-Giemsa stain, methylene blue, Papanicolaou stain (for cytopathological specimens), methenamine silver stain, and periodic acid-Schiff (PAS) stain (29). The last two stains are generally reserved for examining formalin-fixed and paraffin-embedded sections of tissue. Tissue specimens for suspected *Candida* infection and other mycoses should be subjected to homogenization before plating on conventional media. Most labs are equipped to use one or more of the following techniques: mortar and pestle, a glass homogenizer, or a sterile plastic bag (29).

Candida spp. are best recognized in tissue by PAS stain or by Gomori-Grocott methenamine silver (GMS) (20,21). Although *Candida* spp. can be seen after staining with hematoxylin-eosin, it is often faint and frequently overlooked. A brisk inflammatory response can obscure the recognition of Candida, whereas PAS or GMS may be more sensitive. The advantage of PAS stain is that it preserves the surrounding cellular architecture, whereas GMS highlights only silver-positive structures, particularly fungal elements.

Typically, *Candida* spp. in tissue as blastoconidia, pseudohyphae, and hyphae are seen in *Candida* spp. infection. There is one notable exception in which morphology is helpful for identifying at the level of species, *C. glabrata*. This is classically seen only in the blastoconidia form, but even this requires confirmation by culture or a PCR technique.

Microbiological Identification of Candida Species

Determination of *Candida* at the level of species should be made on all isolates from normally sterile body fluids (i.e., peritoneal fluid), and most cultures take from mucosal surfaces. The choice of antifungal agents is driven by knowledge of the species (i.e., fluconazole would not be given for *C. krusei* or *C. glabrata*), and in some instances, the decision to initiate therapy or remove a catheter may depend upon knowledge of the species (7,8,30–35). On the other hand, identification of yeast forms in respiratory secretions is controversial (36) and

should be fully evaluated, especially in the transplant recipient, because of the possibility of *Cryptococcus neoformans* infection.

There are many ways to differentiate *Candida* species in the laboratory, but most laboratories generally use a combination of the following: colonial morphology, germ tube test, cornmeal agar morphology, and biochemical analysis by carbohydrate assimilation and fermentation (37–39). The advent of PCR technology offers the promise of differentiating *Candida* species based upon known, single-base differences in nucleic acid sequences of selected genes.

Candida spp. are easily isolated on standard mycological and bacteriologic media, including Sabouraud glucose agar, sheep blood agar, and horse blood agar (22). *Candida albicans*, the most common isolate in diagnostic laboratories, may grow in the presence of cycloheximide or Mycosel (BBL Microbiology Systems, Cockeysville, MD). Colonies of *Candida* species grown at temperatures between 25° and 37°C have a characteristic white or beige color and smooth to wrinkled textured colony morphology. *Candida* species, especially *C. albicans*, demonstrate a fine stellate or fringed border of the colonies, which is due to the presence of pseudohyphae and hyphae at the advancing edge of the colony. Variations in colonial morphology, also known as phenotypic switching, occur with high frequency when *Candida* spp. are incubated at 25°C (38). *Candida* species in a mixed specimen may be distinguished on media containing tetrazolium dyes (40,41). Special media with colorimetric differences between species, based upon enzymatic reactions, have been developed and used in many laboratories (40,41). Still, the 2-hour germ tube test is used by most laboratories to distinguish between *C. albicans* (germ tube positive) and non-*albicans Candida* species (germ tube negative). Excess inoculation of the test broth may lead to suppression of germination and a false-negative result in detection of *C. albicans*. The germ tube of *C. albicans* has a recognizable morphology that can be easily differentiated from blastoconidial germination seen with *C. tropicalis*.

Candida albicans may also be identified by terminal chlamydospore formation on cornmeal agar with Tween-80 (22–24). The arrangement of blastoconidia and the morphological features of pseudohyphae and hyphae are useful for discriminating between non-*albicans* species. Since *Cryptococcus neoformans* and *Candida glabrata* produce only yeast forms, this test is also useful for confirmation. In general, *C. neoformans* is typically spherical, but significant variation in diameter and the capsule may not be well developed during early stages. *Trichosporon* species differ from *Candida* spp. because of the characteristic mixture of arthroconidia, blastoconidia, and hyphae, whereas *Geotrichum* spp. have yeastlike colonial morphological features, comprising only hyphae and arthroconidia.

Few laboratories use biochemical assays to identify a *Candida* species. A labor-intensive yet well-established assay is the carbohydrate assimilation test of Wickerham. The principle of the test is to measure specific carbohydrate assimilation or carbohydrate fermentation patterns in response to a sole source of energy in the presence or absence of oxygen, respectively. The API-20C carbohydrate assimilation test (Analytab Products, Plainview, NY) is a widely utilized rapid yeast identification system (42–46). Other rapid yeast identification systems include the Uni-Yeast-tek System (Remel Laboratories, Lenexa, KS) and the automated systems, such as the MicroScan (Baxter Healthcare Corp., West Sacramento, CA), AMS-YCB (Vitek Systems, Hazelwood, MO), and Quantum II (Abbott Laboratories, Dallas, TX) (47–49). Less commonly encountered yeasts are occasionally misidentified with these systems.

Differential Diagnosis of Other Yeast Isolates

The presence of a capsule around a yeast form suggests *Cryptococcus neoformans*, which can be further identified by its ability to grow selectively on birdseed agar (for detection of phenol oxidase), or use of positive urease reaction Caffeic-acid-containing medium or pigment tests (49–51). Still, one has to be careful because capsule formation may be incomplete, depending upon growth conditions. *Candida* species, with the exception of *C. lipolytica* and some *C. krusei*, are seldom urease positive. *Trichosporon beigelii* are urease positive but can be recognized by the presence of arthroconidia. *Rhodotorula* species are urease positive but have a distinct pink to orange-red color (52). Rapid nitrate utilization is also helpful for distinguishing *Candida* spp. from *Cryptococcus* spp., *Rhodotorula* spp., and *Trichosporon* spp. (53). Some of the rarer clinical isolates can be identified by morphological signatures observed in clinical isolates grown on different media. These include the asci- and ascospores of *Saccharomyces cerevisiae* or the internal spores (sporangiospores) of *Prototheca wickerhamii*, which can appear to be yeastlike under certain conditions (54). *Malassezia furfur* is grown optimally with supplementation of blood agar plate with a long-chain carbon source (e.g., olive oil) (55). However, *Malassezia furfur* may be directly isolated from a lysis centrifugation blood culture. *Malassezia furfur* and *Malassezia pachydermatis* are yeasts that appear to be flask shaped, often with a collarette detectable on wet mount (56,57).

Significance of Fungemia

Currently, isolation of *Candida* spp. from the bloodstream remains the most important tool for diagnosing invasive candidiasis (Table 1). In the past, *Candida* spp. isolated from routine blood cultures has generated controversy, but during the recent decade, an appreciation of the clinical implications of candidemia has emerged. The dismissal of *Candida* spp. in a single positive blood culture as a skin contaminant has fallen in disfavor, partly because of the significant implications of delaying therapy (58). Because of a better appreciation of the serious morbidity and mortality associated with candidemia and improved detection systems (see later), it is no longer necessary to wait for a second, confirmatory culture. Therefore a blood culture positive for *Candida* spp. in an immunocompromised host requires immediate consideration for therapeutic intervention (10,59,60). This is particularly critical in patients with an indwelling catheter, because vascular catheters may be the target of fungemia from a distal site or the portal of entry of *Candida* spp. Most experts recommend treatment with an antifungal agent and when possible, removal of the catheter (8,10,62,63). Negative peripheral blood cultures do not reliably exclude the diagnosis of disseminated candidiasis.

Methods for Detection of Fungemia

Detection of *Candida* spp. from blood cultures represents one of the major advances in diagnostic mycology. Previously, blood culture detection systems had a poor track record in identifying *Candida* spp. (Table 2). One of the consequences of this was a marked disparity between postmortem tissue findings of invasive candidiasis and the paucity of antemortem positive blood cultures. New methodologies have improved the rate of recovery as well as the time to detection of *Candida* spp. in blood cultures.

Overall, detection of *Candida* spp. in blood culture systems depends upon several variables: the volume of blood (greater volumes provide greater yield); the conditions of medium and atmosphere; the concentrations of *Candida* spp. within the bloodstream (e.g., 10^4 cells/ml will be detected more rapidly in most systems than will 101 cells/ml); and the particular species of *Candida*. For example, *C. albicans*, *C. tropicalis*, and *C. parapsilosis* are detected sooner (1–3 days) in conventional broth systems than *C. krusei* and *C. glabrata*. The latter may require a longer period of time for growth (4–9 days).

TABLE 1. *Significance of fungemia in transplant recipient*

All blood cultures positive for a fungal isolate should be considered clinically significant until proven otherwise.
It may not be possible to isolate a clinically significant isolate from a second culture.
Fungal pathogens isolated from the bloodstream of a transplant recipient with an indwelling catheter should be treated until proven otherwise.
Indwelling catheters may be the target of fungemia from a distal site or portal of entry.

TABLE 2. *Isolation of fungal pathogens by blood culture*

High yield
    Candida spp.
    Cryptococcus spp.
    Histoplasma spp.
    Fusarium spp.
    Trichosporon spp.
    Malassezia spp. (olive oil overlay)
Low yield
    Aspergillus spp.
    Zygomycetes
    Coccidioides immitis

Candida spp. grows poorly under anaerobic conditions and so venting of bottle has led to an enhancement in the rate of growth and the efficiency of recovery of *Candida* from blood (64–66). For example, in one study, *Candida* spp. grew in 16 of 16 vented broth cultures in comparison with two of 16 nonvented broth cultures (65). *Candida* spp. and other pathogenic yeasts can be isolated from media suitable for isolation of mycobacteria (66). Several techniques have been used to detect *Candida* in broth, including turbidity, radiometric signal of CO_2 generation, and infrared detection (67–69). A recently developed broth system known commercially as BacT/Alert Microbial Detection System (Organon Teknika Corp.) improves detection of *Candida* and bacteria by monitoring the rate of change of the infrared signal, unlike the previous systems designed to recognize growth when an absolute-threshold infrared signal was surpassed (70). This system may be more sensitive than lysis centrifugation for detection of *Candida* spp. but awaits larger studies for confirmation.

Biphasic media is employed by many diagnostic laboratories to improve recovery of *Candida* from blood cultures (66,69–71). An individual colony, which may be detected on the agar surface, allegedly correlates with a single *Candida* organism in the volume of the broth. The Roche Septi-Check (Roche Diagnostics) is designed to detect both bacteria and fungi. A brain/heart infusion (BHI) biphasic system has been reported to improve the efficiency for detection of fungemia in comparison with that of conventional broth systems (72). A biphasic system (GIBCO Laboratories) can accelerate the time to

detection of fungemia from a mean of 3.0 days to 2.3 days in broth (70).

Recent advances in blood culture systems are summarized in Table 3. Following the introduction of radiometric blood culture detection systems, particularly the BACTEC 225 and 460 (Johnson Laboratories, Cockeysville, MD), clinical laboratories demonstrated the utility of this method for detection of fungemia (67,69). Among 30 blood cultures growing yeasts, the mean time to detection was 2.4 days by the radiometric system versus 8.3 days by a BHI biphasic system. Using three different blood culture detection methods for analysis of 193 cultures, 141 (73%) were first detected radiometrically, versus 42 (22%) by subculture and 10 (5%) by Gram stain (68). The radiometric blood culture system has yielded to an infrared detection system (BACTEC 660), which is comparable in detection of fungemia but easier to operate (73).

The next major development in detection of fungemia was the introduction of the lysis centrifugation blood culture system (formerly Isolator by du Pont & Nemours, Delaware, and now manufactured as the Isostat by Wampole Laboratories, Cranbury, NJ). Recovery of *Candida* from a blood specimen is enhanced when the sample is lysed with a detergent (74). The net effect of the proprietary lytic mixture in the Isolator is to lyse cells and, at the same time, inactivate complement and selected antimicrobial agents prior to culturing the pellet in a semiquantitative manner. The semiquantitative measure of colony counts has been shown to correspond to the number of circulating colonies of *Candida* or other yeasts. Like other blood culture detection systems, for deep fungal infections, particularly in neutropenic hosts, the concordance with fungal burden is poor.

The superiority of lysis centrifugation technique has been demonstrated compared with other systems with respect to accelerating the efficiency and the time of recovery from the bloodstream (75–80). Studies comparing the lysis centrifugation system with the radiometric resin system (BACTEC 16B-17D) or infrared nonradiometric resin system (BACTEC 660) demonstrate these systems to have comparable abilities for detection of fungi (81,82). The addition of an antibiotic removal resin has contributed to this improved sensitivity. Culture of blood for 5 days using the BACTEC 660 was found to be

TABLE 3. *Blood culture methods for detection of* Candida *spp.*

Method	Principle of Detection
Lysis centrifugation Wampole Laboratories, Cranbury, NJ	Recovery of *Candida* is enhanced by inactivation of complement, inactivation of some antimicrobial agents, and lysis of host cells with a proprietary mixture.
BacT/Alert System Organon Teknika Corporation, Durham, NC	Broth culture is serially monitored for CO_2 production. Early detection is indicated by increasing signal consistent with growth curve.
Bactec with Infrared Detection Johnson Laboratories, Cockeysville, MD	Broth culture serially monitored for change in infrared signal.

sufficient to recover *Candida* spp. from all 22 positive blood cultures (83). At the same time, lysis centrifugation has permitted earlier and more accurate isolation of other yeastlike fungi—including *Histoplasma capsulatum* var. *capsulatum* and, in some studies, *Cryptococcus neoformans*—from the bloodstream (84,85). On occasion, filamentous fungi have been isolated by the lysis centrifugation technique.

The BacT/Alert Microbial Detection System (Organon Teknika Corporation, Durham, NC) rapidly detects fungi in blood and is used by many laboratories (86,87). It is based upon colorimetric detection using a semipermeable membrane of CO_2 generated in liquid culture media. The colorimetric changes are read by a photodiode every 10 minutes and analyzed by a microprocessor; detection is based upon a sustained increase in CO_2 production within the system. An acceleration in recovery time for detection of bacteremia and probably fungemia makes this an attractive system for routine blood cultures in the transplant setting. A modified bottle for fungal blood cultures has been developed for use in the BACTEC System, and it integrates the BACTEC of nonradiometric signal emission with a method of cell lysis but without centrifugation (Mirrett). The BACTEC selective fungal medium was equivalent to lysis centrifugation in detection of candidemia, whereas the Isolator lysis centrifugation performed better than the BACTEC selective fungal medium for detection of fungemia due to *H. capsulatum* var. *capsulatum*.

Berenguer and colleagues (88) demonstrated a significant relationship between the number of deep-tissue sites and the sensitivity of lysis centrifugation blood cultures in detection of candidemia. Patients with more than three deep-tissue sites infected had the highest level of fungemia, whereas those with only one deep-tissue site had the lowest level of detection of fungemia. Blood cultures were positive in seven (78%) of nine patients with more than three organs infected by *Candida* in comparison with five (28%) of 18 patients with one organ infected ($p = 0.024$). The mean recovery time for *Candida* in positive blood cultures was 2.6 days in disseminated candidiasis and 3.2 days in single organ candidiasis ($p = 0.017$). There may be a direct relation between the tissue burden of *Candida* and the frequency of detection of fungemia by lysis centrifugation.

Because intravascular catheters are an important source of fungemia, catheter tips are routinely removed and sent to the laboratory for evaluation. Typically, a 5-cm portion of the distal segment is sent and rolled on a sheep blood agar plate four times before the tip is placed in a tube of broth media (89,90). The plate is incubated for 48 hours and colonies are counted. Although the presence of ≥15 CFU has been suggested as an indicator for catheter associates of bacteremia, the interpretation of a certain number of colonies of *Candida* spp. as representing a "significant" recovery has not been established. The

recovery of one of more *Candida* spp. colonies from a vascular catheter tip should prompt a thorough clinical reevaluation for invasive candidiasis.

A recent study of fungemia in HIV-infected children identified the central venous catheter as the apparent portal of entry (91). Fungemia presented most frequently in these patients as a community-acquired process with new onset of fever. Blood cultures drawn from the central silastic venous catheters were positive in all cases. whereas fungemia was rarely isolated from peripheral blood cultures. Interestingly, in this study, half of the isolates were non-*albicans Candida* spp. or distinctly unusual isolates, such as *Bipolaris* and *Rhodotorula*.

Investigational Methods of Nonculture Diagnosis of Invasive Candidiasis

Because the standard tools for evaluating *Candida* infection, blood cultures, diagnostic imaging, and biopsies (as a source for histopathology and culture of tissue) lack sensitivity in early recognition of infection and are imprecise as markers of complete eradication of infection. Similarly, many techniques intended to establish a diagnosis by nonculture methods have lacked sensitivity for invasive candidiasis. Still, the promise of diagnosing candidemia within hours of harvesting the sample continues to generate interest in developing these lines of research. At present, there is great interest in antigen purification, monoclonal antibody production, epitope mapping, recombinant DNA techniques, and polymerase chain reaction methodology, but it is unlikely that any single system will supplant the standard diagnostic tools until careful, large prospective studies validate the sensitivity and specificity of the modalities (Table 4). Instead, one could imagine that data derived from a panel of diagnostic systems will likely prove most useful in early diagnosis and monitoring therapeutic response of invasive candidiasis.

A number of different systems have been evaluated for direct measurement of *Candida*-specific antigens in clinical specimens. To date, there have been a number of studies looking at *Candida* cell wall antigens, such as mannans (92,93), *Candida* metabolites (particularly d-arabinitol [94,95]), and *Candida* cytoplasmic antigens (96–106). The purpose of this line of study has been to develop a marker of invasive disease that will not only provide the initial diagnostic information but also permit monitoring of the burden of *Candida*. One of these cytoplasmic antigens is an immunodominant *Candida* enolase (107); another immunodominant antigen is a breakdown product of a *Candida* heat shock protein (HSP 90) (101,102).

Detection of Candida Antigens by Immunoassay

Since the development of the highly sensitive latex *Cryptococcus* antigen agglutination tests (LCAT) for

TABLE 4. *Investigational nonculture methods for detection of invasive candidiasis*

Target	Method of Detection
Cell wall components	
Mannan	RIA, ELISA
1,3-b-glucans	Amebocyte lysate assay
Chitin	Spectrophotometric assay
Cytoplasmic antigens	
Enolase	ELISA, Immunoblot
Anti-enolase antibody	ELISA
47 kD Breakdown product of HSP-90	Enzyme-linked dot immunobinding assay
Metabolite	
d-arabinitol	Rapid enzymatic detection (by spectrophotometer or fluorimetry), GLC/FID, Mass spectroscopy/GLC
Genomic DNA Sequences	
C-14-lanosterol demethylase	PCR
Ribosomal RNA genes Chitin synthase	
Intergenic DNA spacer region	

Abbreviations: RIA, radioimmunoassay; ELISA, enzyme-linked immunosorbent assay; GLC, gas-liquid chromatography; FID, flame ionization detector; PCR, polymerase chain reaction.

detection of circulating cryptococcal polysaccharide antigen, a comparable system with similar sensitivity for detection of invasive candidiasis has been sought. Unfortunately, detection of circulating *Candida* antigens has been elusive. Thus far, most immunodiagnostic studies for antigen detection have been targeted at identifying either *Candida* cell wall mannans or cytoplasmic antigens.

Great effort has been expended on reliable systems for detection of cell wall mannan and mannoproteins. A number of different systems have been studied, including the following techniques, radioimmunoassay (RIA), enzyme-linked immunoassay (ELISA), and latex agglutination (LA) (100,108–110) to identify circulating cell mannans and mannoproteins. Anti–cell wall mannan antibodies and other nonspecific binding proteins interfere with detection of cell wall mannan antigen. Consequently, heat and hydrolysis are necessary to liberate the detectable mannan antigen, but cell wall mannan antigen is cleared rapidly from serum, resulting in low serum levels (usually ≤100 ng/ml). Repeat serum sampling may be necessary to improve sensitivity for detection of cell wall mannan antigen. Based upon this, one would predict that immunocompromised patients, such as patients with acute leukemia, would be less likely to produce neutralizing antibody and thus the system would be more favorably employed for detection. This has been demonstrated but also highlights the pitfall of such a technique.

Biochemically defined cytoplasmic antigens have been studied as suitable markers for detection of invasive candidiasis. For example, *Candida* enolase and a breakdown product of a 90-kd heat shock protein (HSP-90) are two immunodominant cytoplasmic antigens that are detected during invasive candidiasis. Initially, the elucidation of *Candida* enolase as an antigenic marker for invasive candidiasis by Strockbine and colleagues identified an immunodominant cytoplasmic 48-kd antigen purified from *Candida* (103,104). Antibody production to this antigen was strongly associated with deep candidiasis in nonimmunocompromised patients (103), but the 48-kd immunodominant cytoplasmic antigen of *Candida albicans* was subsequently determined to be *Candida* enolase (103,111). Studies in experimental disseminated candidiasis in mice and rabbits demonstrated that *Candida* enolase antigenemia detected by ELISA was detectable in the absence of fungemia but still correlated with deep-tissue infection. Specifically, it distinguished gastrointestinal involvement from deep-tissue involvement, and declined in response to antifungal therapy. Initially, clinical investigation of the enolase antigen in immunocompromised cancer patients was based upon compelling animal data. *In vivo* studies showed that mice infected intraperitoneally or intravenously with *C. albicans* had deep visceral infection and enolase antigenemia but minimal to absent fungemia.

A multicenter 2-year prospective study of the expression of this *Candida* cytoplasmic antigen in the serum of high-risk cancer patients with deeply invasive candidiasis was conducted using a double-sandwich liposomal immunoassay (112). In 24 cases of invasive candidiasis in cancer patients, the detection sensitivity for *Candida* enolase antigenemia per serum sample was 54%. However, multiple serum sampling improved detection of antigenemia to 75% (18/24); 11 (85%) of 13 known cases of deep-tissue-proven infection and 7 (64%) of 11 known cases of fungemia were antigen positive. Specificity was 96% in comparison with control groups, which included patients with mucosal colonization, bacteremia, and other deep mycoses. Antigenemia was detected in the absence of fungemia in five cases of tissue-proven invasive candidiasis but was not detected in six cases of fungemia alone. The multicenter *Candida* enolase study was not specifically designed to determine whether detectable enolase antigenemia preceded positive blood cultures as the first indicator of invasive candidiasis. Among the 24 patients with invasive candidiasis, only six patients had simultaneous blood cultures and antigen determinations to permit comparison of time of detection. In comparing the time to early diagnosis of antigenemia with that of blood cultures, among six evaluable patients with comparably obtained positive samples for antigenemia and fungemia, all had antigenemia (1–8 days) before fungemia. With improvement of the assay's single-sample sensitivity, it may be a useful indicator of deep infection in neutropenic cancer patients and may complement the diagnostic utility of blood cultures.

The findings from this study were subsequently confirmed in two more prospective trials (113,114). The specificities and sensitivities of four tests used for the serodiagnosis of candidemia in 39 patients with candidemia were performed by Mitsutake and colleagues. The dot immunoblotting assay that detects the enolase antigen (48 kd) was compared directly with other assay systems, which detect mannan antigen, heat-labile antigen (a threshold titer of four times), or beta-glucan (≥60 pg/ml) (115). Enolase antigen was detected in 28 (71.8%) patients with candidemia, whereas 30 (76.9%), 10 (25.6%), and 27 (84.4%) patients were positive for the heat-labile antigen by the Cand-Tec assay, the mannan antigen by the Pastorex *Candida* assay, and beta-glucan by the Limulus test, respectively. Ten patients with *Candida* colonization, five patients with invasive pulmonary aspergillosis, five patients with cryptococcosis, and 20 healthy subjects had no circulating, detectable enolase antigen or mannan antigen. The specificity of enolase antigen in the serodiagnosis of candidemia was 100%, but the sensitivity was 71.8%. The specificity and sensitivity of Cand-Tec, the assay for mannan antigen, and the assay for beta-glucan were 76.9% and 87.5%, 25.6% and 100%, and 84.4% and 87.5%, respectively. Thus the enolase antigen in this study was sensitive and specific but not sufficiently so to detect all cases of candidemia. No cases of deeply invasive candidiasis without fungemia were included in this study.

The immunodominant *Candida* cytoplasmic antigen is a 47-kd antigen breakdown product of a 90-kd heat shock protein (HSP-90) of *C. albicans* (102,115). Since western blot analysis with polyclonal sera insufficiently resolves antigen bands between 47 and 52 kd, the success of the approach was achieved by development of monoclonal antibodies to the 48-kd *Candida* enolase Ag and the 47-kd antigen. Antibodies reactive to the 47-kd antigen or a synthetic peptide epitope derived from the antigen react with a band at 92 kd (101). An enzyme-linked dot immunobinding assay has been developed for detection of immunodominant 47-kd antigen in patients with invasive candidiasis (102) but its usefulness awaits further study.

The target of a commercially available latex agglutination assay (CAND-TEC, Ramco Laboratories, Inc.,

Houston, TX) is still not well characterized. Results with this test have been controversial, partly because of the differences in study design, patient populations, definitions, classification, and sampling frequency (116–120).

D-arabinitol, the cyclopentol metabolite of *C. albicans*, is a suitable target that can be detected in serum by gas-liquid chromatography or by mass spectroscopy with selected ion monitoring (121–126). The accuracy of the test depends upon proper extraction and derivitization of the sample (95,127). The high cost of the technology and quality assurance required to verify results have discouraged widespread use of this modality. Furthermore, the processing of specimens is labor intensive, permitting only a small number of samples to be processed daily. D-arabinitol is cleared by glomerular filtration, and therefore d-arabinitol levels may be elevated in the presence of impaired renal function. The final value of a d-arabinitol level is determined on the basis of the d-arabinitol-to-creatinine ratio. Elevated levels of d-arabinitol are detectable in cases of invasive candidiasis, but serum d-arabinitol is not elevated in infections because of two *Candida* species, *C. glabrata* and *Candida krusei*.

The demands of the d-arabinitol assay by older published methods precluded adequate clinical studies in large series that include serial samples (127). Consequently, the pattern of serum d-arabinitol detection in serum has not been well characterized for invasive candidiasis, limiting our understanding of its usefulness in monitoring therapeutic response. However, a rapid enzymatic system for detection of serum d-arabinitol concentration now affords an opportunity for this marker to be utilized in clinical practice (128–133). Moreover, automated systems permit measurement of serum d-arabinitol and creatinine concentrations for determination of d-arabinitol/creatinine ratio in large numbers of samples.

A large prospective study was performed using a rapid enzymatic assay for detection of invasive candidiasis and for monitoring therapeutic response in patients from two large oncology centers (140). A total of 3,223 serum samples were analyzed from 274 oncology patients. Serum d-arabinitol concentrations by rapid enzymatic assay and creatinine levels were measured in coded serum samples to determine a serum d-arabinitol and creatinine ratio (DA/Cr) (134). In patients with fungemia, the mean of the maximum serum DA/Cr was 11 times greater than the measured levels in normal blood bank donors and four times greater than all controls. An elevated DA/Cr (≥4.0 M mg^{-1} dl^{-1}) was detected in 31 (74%) of all 42 cases of fungemia and 25 (83%) of 30 cases in the subset of persistent fungemia. Elevated DA/Cr was detected in 42 (62%) of all 68 cases of invasive candidiasis. In patients with persistent fungemia, the highest DA/Cr values were consistently measured. In 26 evaluable cases of fungemia, elevated DA/Cr values were detected in 14 (54%) before, 10 (38%) after, and 2 (8%) simultaneously with the first microbiological report of fungemia. The trends of serial DA/Cr values correlated with therapeutic response in 29 (85%) of 34 patients with evaluable cases of fungemia. Mortality in fungemic patients was significantly related to the trend of serial DA/Cr values over time. Thus rapid enzymatic detection of DA in serially collected serum samples from high-risk cancer patients permitted detection of invasive candidiasis, early recognition of fungemia, and therapeutic monitoring in DA-positive cases.

D-arabinitol/L-arabinitol ratios (D/L-arabinitol ratios) in urine were evaluated in a prospective study that included 100 children with cancer. The technique used was gas chromatography and the intent was to determine if urine samples could be used for diagnosis of invasive candidiasis (135,136). Positive D/L-arabinitol ratios were found in 10 (100%) of 10 children with invasive candidiasis, 12 (52%) of 23 patients undergoing empiric antifungal chemotherapy, but 4 (6%) of 67 children not receiving antifungal treatment. The authors reported that the D/L-arabinitol ratio could be detected in urine well before either a positive blood culture or the start of empirical antifungal therapy; the median was 12 days. That urine can be utilized for rapid detection is encouraging, but further studies are needed to validate its utility, especially now that hematopoietic growth factors have significantly decreased the duration of neutropenia in transplant recipients.

The detection of circulating 1,3-b-D-glucan, a component of Candida cell wall, is another investigative strategy for diagnosis of invasive candidiasis. An amebocyte lysate assay for diagnosis of fungal infection has been developed from the Japanese horseshoe crab, *Tachypleus tridentatus*. The *Tachypleus* clotting cascade has two pathways that are differentially activated by fungal cell wall products and by endotoxin of which the gelation reaction of the amebocyte lysate assay is classically known to be initiated by bacterial endotoxin (137,138). The gelation reaction may also be activated by the complementary coagulation pathway by the synthetic carbohydrate, carboxymethyl-1,3-b-D-glucan in concentrations of ≥ 1 ng/ml (85). Removal of factor G from the lysate permitted activation only by endotoxin, whereas retaining factor G and removing factors B and C results in a 1,3-b-D-glucan-activated system.

The measured plasma concentration of 1,3-beta glucan at the time of routine blood cultures in febrile episodes has been studied (138). Using a cutoff value of 20 pg/ml, 37 of 41 episodes of proven fungal infections (confirmed at necropsy or by microbiology) were confirmed by the assay. In 59 episodes of fever due to infection caused by a pathogen other than a fungus, a tumor, or collagen-vascular disease, the measured value was below the cutoff value, giving a specificity of 100%. Of 102 episodes of fever of unknown origin, 26 had plasma glucan concentrations of more than 20 pg/ml. Based upon these data, the test has a positive predictive value estimated as 59%

(37/63), negative predictive value estimated as 97% (135/139), and efficiency estimated as 85% (172/202). These encouraging findings warrant further investigation in well-defined prospectively monitored patient populations.

Detection of Anti-Candida Antibodies

The detection of specific antibodies against *Candida spp.* has been studied extensively. Unfortunately, as a diagnostic tool, this method has not gained widespread use in the clinical venue (105,139–142). Initially, different groups reported the development of precipitins tests and passive hemagglutination tests, both of which have suffered from low sensitivity and specificity, partly because the tests were based upon crude preparations of cell wall or cytoplasmic constituents. Variations in the preparations between laboratories also plagued this approach and led to conflicting results among investigators. For example, cytoplasmic antigen preparations containing cell wall mannan have been used by different labs (100,142). Anti–cell wall mannan antibodies were found in most human sera, and patients with invasive candidiasis were not clearly distinguished from those who were not actively infected with *Candida*.

Antibodies detecting *Candida*-specific components of cytoplasmic extracts with mannan removed have also been developed (98,99,101,103). Detection of antibodies that recognize a range in proteins between 40 to 60 kd has been reported, but again this approach has not been validated in large studies. The expanding number of patients at risk, who also have significant defects in host defense due to transplant conditioning or post-transplant complications, is less likely to mount measurable antibody responses.

Amplification of Candida DNA by Polymerase Chain Reaction

The development of polymerase chain reaction (PCR) technology has had pleotropic effects in clinical microbiology (Table 5). The ability to detect small, unique fragments of DNA specific to an organism, such as *Candida*, and in some circumstances, even at the level of species, represents a major advance in nonculture methods (143). PCR technology is based upon the amplification of a unique stretch of DNA (known as an amplicon) from material collected from a patient. Confirmation of the identifying amplicon is determined by one of many different techniques designed to discriminate a difference as small as one base pair. The choice of amplicon permits speciation and possibly drug susceptibility profile. The latter is predicated upon the identification of unique mutations that confer a resistant phenotype. This has already been developed for rifampin sensitivity for isolates of *Mycobacterium tuberculosis* (144). Already,

TABLE 5. *Polymerase chain reaction techniques in the diagnosis of fungal infections in transplant recipients*

Rapid identification of a pathogen
    Rapid determination of genera and possibly species
    Direct detection in
        Biopsy specimen
        Blood culture
        Bronchoalveolar lavage fluid
Epidemiological tool
    Trace epidemiology/outbreak
Determine antifungal susceptibility of isolate
    Based upon known mutations correlating with resistance

PCR-based studies have been published that can differentiate between *Candida* species, such as *C. albicans*, *C. krusei*, *C. tropicalis*, and *T. glabrata* (145,146). Generally, one or more different techniques is required to identify an organism such as *Candida* and at the same time discriminate it from other genera of fungi.

Within hours of specimen collection, detection of fungal pathogens can be determined, well before an organism is detected by isolation from either liquid or solid media. In theory, clinical information may be available sooner on which to base therapeutic decisions (147). If a fungal infection can be accurately detected by PCR technology, clinicians will not have to wait for culture results, nor will they be left to rely upon starting therapy in response to clinical indications. Based upon an accurate system for rapid and sensitive turnaround, it may be possible to initiate antifungal therapy, frequently complicated by significant toxicity, on stronger evidence for a specific fungal pathogen. It may also be possible to select therapy according to the specific isolate detected by PCR.

In principle, PCR technology may yet overcome the classic problem of low sensitivity and specificity that has perennially plagued diagnostic mycology (100). However, the detection of very small amounts of DNA presents a complex set of problems.

PCR-based assays will have to be studied carefully, taking into account the clinical status of the patient. Specifically, the source of the material will need to be factored into interpretation, partly because of the power of detecting small fragments of DNA in clinical specimens. It should be stressed that PCR-based techniques cannot distinguish between viable and dead organisms. In this regard, nonquantitative PCR techniques are incapable of clearly delineating a site of colonization from one of true infection. Accordingly, detection of *Candida* amplicons must be interpreted in the context of the source and clinical profile of the collected material (i.e., the site from which the specimen was harvested).

The specific choice of unique oligonucleotide primers is a critical step in developing a PCR assay. Several groups have shown that *Candida* amplicons can easily be detected in clinical and laboratory samples (148,149). The usefulness of the assay is dependent upon whether the choice of the amplified region is common to all *Candida* spp., a specific *Candida* species, or common fungal pathogens. By choosing a region, known to be conserved in all *Candida* species, one can quickly establish the presence of *Candida* (see Table 1) (148,149). In some instances, a single base pair difference can distinguish between species, as has been widely used in the molecular detection of inherited human diseases. A number of techniques have been developed that permit single base discrimination as well as small differences (see Table 2). These techniques include endonuclease restriction digestion of the amplicon, allele-specific oligonucleotide hybridization, single-stranded conformational polymorphism, or heteroduplex analysis (150).

Prior to widespread use of PCR methods in diagnosis of *Candida* infection, high-throughput technology will have to be validated in a manner that will guarantee acceptable levels of sensitivity and specificity. Large prospective studies that correlate isolation techniques with PCR-based studies are required to establish the diagnostic usefulness of PCR. Another factor influencing the clinical usefulness of PCR is specimen processing. Material from a previously sterile site (such as CSF or blood) must be handled carefully prior to PCR amplification. Contamination of reagents or specimens will undermine the usefulness of the technique because of the potential amplification from picomolar amounts of a unique DNA sequence. To optimize conditions, protein debris and other extraneous materials must be eliminated prior to amplification. A number of variations on DNA extraction have been reported, but all have in common the importance of exposing or releasing fungal DNA from viable or killed organisms. Body fluids such as saliva or oral washings present technical problems. On a practical level, thickened secretions are more difficult to amplify and therefore require modification of the sample prior to analysis.

Similar to the basic principle of PCR, several other approaches have been studied; each of these is based upon the principle of amplification of a small quantity of unique genetic material. Branched DNA technology offers the potential for amplification (and quantitation) of target RNA prior to detection; it utilizes a unique detection system of hybridizing complex, branched DNA carrying indicator compounds (151,152). The hybrid capture assay has been targeted for high-throughput analysis of clinical specimens but as of yet has not been developed for fungal pathogens (153).

PCR technology has been successfully used to validate the usefulness of this approach for fungal pathogens. Detection of DNA amplicons from laboratory isolates was shown using the lanosterol C14-demethylase gene. Buchman detected amplicons from prepared clinical specimens from which *C. albicans* had previously been isolated by standard laboratory techniques (8). Other groups have utilized selected candidate genes for detection of *Candida* species that include ribosomal DNA subunits, actin, and chitin synthase (149,154–158).

Once an amplicon is generated by PCR, it is possible to perform further analysis to distinguish between species of *Candida* (see Table 2). For example, several groups have used primers that amplify a subunit of ribosomal DNA common to *C. albicans*, *C. glabrata*, *C. parapsilosis*, and *C. krusei* (145,146,159). Another approach has utilized restriction fragment length polymorphism analysis of intergenic spacer regions of ribosomal DNA (160,161) or hybridization of PCR amplicons derived from ribosomal DNA internal spacers (158,160). Primer pairs were designed to differentiate between four species of *Candida*. (162). A nested PCR-technique, which requires a second amplification of the first product, has been used for discriminating between *C. albicans* and *C. glabrata* on the basis of small differences in the cytochrome P450 lanosterol-alpha-demethylase (L1A1) gene (156).

Detection of *Candida* nucleic acid sequences in the bloodstream is particularly challenging. As the detection systems improve the level of detection, corresponding to the number of CFUs in circulation, it will be difficult to distinguish pathogenic fungemia from incidental fungemia. Quantitative tests linked to high-performance technologies will need validation prior to conducting large, prospective studies. This same problem applies to colonization of mucosal surfaces. Because fungal infection is often restricted to deep-tissue compartments and the absence of circulating fungal pathogens, the detection of *Candida* DNA by PCR results from blood may be of limited benefit. In these circumstances, when there is high suspicion for disseminated infection, PCR analysis of tissue material may be needed to confirm the diagnosis.

Preclinical studies have shown that *C. albicans* can be amplified by PCR in blood drawn from neutropenic mice with candidiasis (163). Buchman's original paper used specimens isolated from (148). Other groups have shown that *C. albicans* can be detected by PCR in blood or in serum (154,155,159). Another approach has been to develop a microtitration plate system for detecting PCR-amplified products derived from *Candida* species isolated from blood specimens (164). A semiquantitative PCR system for detection of *Candida* has been published and is a first step toward developing assays that may be of use for therapeutic monitoring, as well as detection (165).

The detection of small differences in either the sequence of known genes or polymorphisms apparent in spacer regions represents a potent tool for epidemiological analysis (145, 166–169). Some groups have applied PCR technology to study the spread of *Candida* infection in a burn or bone marrow transplant unit (161,167,168). This methodology can be applied to studies directed at transmission of *Candida* species (161,167).

PCR-based methods also permit study of variations in gene sequences that can be used for phylogenetic analysis as well as epidemiological studies (169). Sequence analysis of a conserved region can establish a phylogenetic relationship and in the process determine whether an organism is highly related to known fungi. For example, sequence analysis of ribosomal DNA of *Pneumocystis carinii*, previously believed to be a protozoa, indicates that it shares greater homology to fungus than protozoa (170). In addition, sequence homology between conserved genes may provide insights into possible pathogenesis factors that could be targets for drug development efforts or novel therapeutic interventions. Because only a few antifungal agents are commercially available and there is an emerging problem with resistant isolates, distinguishing between strains or species could be an important tool for therapeutic and epidemiological purposes (171–173).

Antifungal Susceptibility Testing of Yeasts

A standardized reference method for antifungal susceptibility of yeasts has been developed by the Antifungal Subcommittee of National Committee for Clinical Laboratory Standards (NCCLS) (174). This reference provides a basis for assessing the minimum inhibitory concentration (MIC) of an antifungal agent. Based upon this approach, newer methods can be evaluated against a standard methodology to further refine and improve antifungal susceptibility testing.

The availability of reproducible antifungal susceptibility testing methods for fluconazole and itraconazole against *Candida* spp. forms the basis for clinical studies (62). Breakpoints for MICs of fluconazole against *Candida* spp., as determined by the National Committee for Clinical Laboratory Standards' M27-T broth macrodilution methodology, have been established for *Candida* isolates from cases of fungemia and mucosal candidiasis. Isolates for which MICs are ≤8 µg/ml are susceptible to fluconazole, whereas those for which MICs are ≥64 µg/ml are resistant. Isolates for which the MIC of fluconazole is 16–32 µg/ml are considered susceptible, depending (S-DD) upon the dose on the basis of data indicating clinical response in adults when >100 mg of fluconazole per day is given. *Candida krusei* is excepted because it is intrinsically resistant to fluconazole. The MIC breakpoints for itraconazole that apply only to mucosal candidiasis are as follows: susceptible ≤0.125 µg/ml; S-DD, 0.25–0.5 µg/ml; and resistant, ≥1.0 µg/ml.

Cryptococcosis

Cryptococcal infection develops in patients with suppression or loss of cell-mediated immunity. The classical catalog of patients at risk includes those with Hodgkin's lymphoma, adult T-cell leukemia, lymphoma, chronic lymphocytic leukemia, HIV infection, chronic graft-versus-host disease, corticosteroid therapy, and deoxy-coformicin. The degree of immunosuppression is highly associated with the risk for cryptococcal infection and the propensity for dissemination. Cryptococcosis in immunocompromised patients may be present as pneumonia, meningitis, or disseminated infection. Interestingly, cryptococcosis seldom develops in neutropenic patients unless there is a concomitant loss of cellular immunity.

Disseminated cryptococcosis is frequently isolated from blood cultures, CSF culture, or biopsy specimens from cutaneous lesions.

Cryptococcus grows in blood cultures as an encapsulated yeast, which appears as a Gram-positive organism with stippling (20–26). It can be isolated from the different blood culture techniques discussed earlier with near comparable efficiency.

The detection of cryptococcal capsular polysaccharide by latex agglutination and, more recently, by EIA, has become the established modality for detection. Of the many antigen detection systems developed in clinical microbiology, the cryptococcal antigen detection test, which has a remarkably high degree of sensitivity and specificity, ranks as one of the most successful. Indeed, the success of the cryptococcal capsular polysaccharide antigen system serves as an example for further development of nonculture, surrogate marker systems for rapid and accurate detection of other medically important fungal pathogens (174).

In performing the LCAT, digestion with pronase is recommended to eliminate false-positive agglutination with rheumatoid factor. False-positive results may be observed in patients with disseminated trichosporonosis. The comparative procedures and results for performing LCAT and EIA for detection of cryptococcal antigen are well established (175).

Diagnosis of cryptococcal meningitis can be established by a combination of direct examination of CSF on a wet mount, including India ink preparations, CSF culture, and cryptococcal capsular polysaccharide antigen detection in CSF, serum, and other normally sterile body fluids. The capsule is routinely observed, but in rare circumstances some strains may appear to be "capsule-deficient," particularly in isolates from patients with HIV infection. These strains may be misdiagnosed upon direct exam as other yeasts or as contaminating particles (176). The CSF cell count, glucose, and protein in immunosuppressed patients may be normal, probably due to an ineffective inflammatory response.

Several features are distinctive in cryptococcal meningitis in HIV patients compared with other immunocompromised hosts, such as those with cancer or organ transplants. The CSF antigen in HIV-infected patients with meningeal involvement is substantially higher, frequently exceeding 1:1,024 (174). India ink preparation is usually positive in patients with HIV infection and cryptococcal meningitis. Culture and cryptococcal antigen titers by latex agglutination (LCAT) should be used to confirm the diagnosis even when a positive India ink test is determined. Although not always positive, cultures and LCAT should be performed on peripheral blood and CSF. Monitoring of serum and CSF levels are useful for guiding therapy and, in particular, the determination of when to shift from induction therapy to maintenance therapy. The sensitivity of serum and CSF titers in cryptococcal meningitis is routinely greater than 90%. Although a CT scan is usually nonspecific in most cases of CNS cryptococcosis, the presence of hydrocephalus or cryptococcomas can be useful.

Serial monitoring of serum samples from patients with disseminated cryptococcosis is recommended for therapeutic monitoring, especially in the HIV-infected host. In the transplant recipient, monitoring of cryptococcal antigen levels can be helpful for confirming eradication of infection, but cessation of treatment has to be based upon expected recovery of immune function. Generally, non-HIV-infected patients, whose antigen titers are usually <1:1,024, may demonstrate a therapeutic response resulting in resolution of titers to zero during therapy. HIV-infected patients with highly elevated titers (often >1,0124) may not demonstrate a complete resolution and the persistent antigen titers may reflect the residual burden of organisms kept in check by antifungal therapy. Although we have observed resolution of antigen titers to an undetectable level during chronic anticryptococcal therapy in HIV-infected children, we continue chronic suppressive antifungal therapy (177). A rise in serum antigen levels during chronic suppressive antifungal therapy in patients with disseminated cryptococcosis may indicate recurrence of infection, because of either waning cellular immunity or emergence of resistance.

Periodic acid-Schiff (PAS) staining of biopsy specimens of suspicious skin lesions is the best method to see encapsulated budding yeast cells. In addition, Mucicarmine or Alcian blue stains specifically stain the mucopolysaccharide capsule.

Trichosporonosis

Trichosporon infection in the neutropenic host and those receiving high-dose corticosteroids can be very difficult to manage (177). Although uncommon, infection due to *Trichosporon* is characterized by refractory fungemia, funguria, renal dysfunction, cutaneous lesions, chorioretinitis, and pneumonia. Persistent cultures of blood, urine, and sputum are seen despite the use of high-dose amphotericin B (177).

Trichosporon beigelii grows as a rugose or powdery yeast; morphology reveals a combination of blastoconidia, arthroconidia, hyphae, and occasionally pseudohyphae. Current knowledge indicates that *T. beigelii* is a heterogeneous group of organisms that includes more than one species (178,179). A classification for *T. beigelii* has been proposed that divides isolates into five different species. Although the taxonomic classification of *Trichosporon* may be complex, the taxon *T. beigelii* is most likely a group (180). Because conventional rapid yeast speciation kits still code for *T. beigelii*, *T. beigelii* is conveniently used for reporting isolates.

Trichosporon spp. germinates under the same conditions used for detection of *C. albicans* (181). Direct microscopic examination of biopsied cutaneous lesions displays arthroconidia, blastoconidia, pseudohyphae, true hyphae, and vascular invasion. The serum latex agglutination cryptococcal test may be positive because of shared antigens and resultant cross-reactivity between *T. beigelii* and *Cryptococcus neoformans* (182). Accordingly, the serum LCAT may occasionally call attention to the early detection of disseminated trichosporonosis (181–183), but once on antifungal therapy the serum LCAT may be negative (184). Reversion from a positive to a negative LCAT in patients with disseminated trichosporonosis cannot be reliably interpreted as suggesting a therapeutic response (185). The cross-reacting antigen in *T. beigelii* is a component of the cell wall (186) and appears to confer resistance to host response (187) in a manner analogous to the capsular polysaccharide of *C. neoformans* (188). *Trichosporon* antigen-mediated immunosuppression can be reversible by GM-CSF (187). Isolates of *T. beigelii* recovered from the bloodstream contain more cross-reactive antigen than those isolates derived from superficial infections (189).

Endemic Mycoses: Histoplasmosis, Coccidioidomycosis, Blastomycosis, and Penicilliosis

Histoplasma capsulatum var. *capsulatum*, *Coccidioides immitis*, *Blastomyces dermatitidis*, and *Penicillium marneffei* are endemic dimorphic fungi frequently encountered in patients with impaired cell-mediated immunity, similar to cryptococcosis. In most cases, the natural history of systemic dimorphic mycoses begins with inhalation of conidia that land in the lower respiratory tract (190). Initial containment is achieved by alveolar macrophages, which are modulated by T cells, resulting in a localized granulomatous inflammatory response for *H. capsulatum*, *P. brasiliensis*, and *P. marneffei*. A combined acute (pyogenic) and chronic (mononuclear/macrophage) inflammatory response is often observed with *C. immitis* and *B. dermatitidis*. Eventually, calcifications develop at the site of the resolving granulomatous foci of *H. capsulatum* and are often seen on chest radiographs of infected patients.

In most cases of infection in immunocompetent patients, the only evidence of infection is acquisition of immune response; this is manifested by positive delayed-type skin test and the production of specific antibodies, which are detected as precipitins or complement-fixing

antibodies (191). In a small percentage of the time, for reasons still not well understood, progressive pulmonary infection or clinically overt disseminated infection ensues, most often in patients with HIV infection or on corticosteroid therapy. The more clinically significant dimorphic fungi are identified by a combination of direct microscopic examination of specimens, isolation and characterization of the fungus in cultures, DNA probing of isolates, or demonstration of specific exoantigens produced in culture (191).

The mycelial forms *H. capsulatum*, *B. dermatitidis*, *C. immitis*, or *P. brasiliensis* can be confirmed by an exoantigen technique that detects the presence of cell-free antigens (192). A specific exoantigen detected in the aqueous extract of a mycelial culture indicates a systemic dimorphic fungi. The procedure can be performed rapidly and is readily applicable to nonsporulating cultures. Exoantigens are demonstrated by immunodiffusion of specific antigens in either a concentrated aqueous extract of the colony on solid medium or the supernatant fluid of a broth culture of the isolate. Reference antisera are used to identify specific antigens in the isolate and the control antigen.

A recent advancement in the identification of dimorphic fungi from cultures is the development of nucleic acid probes. Probes for the identification of *H. capsulatum*, *B. dermatitidis*, and *C. immitis* are commercially available in a nonisotopic kit format (193–195). A lysate from the organism is incubated with labeled DNA probe, using acridinium ester. The probe recognizes target rRNA, forming a stable double-stranded hybrid. Although the probe method is more expensive than exoantigen testing, probe technology offers the advantages of early testing on very young cultures, rapid processing, easy interpretation of results, and a high level of accuracy for the identification of *H. capsulatum*, *B. dermatitidis*, and *C. immitis*.

Histoplasma capsulatum

Most cases of asymptomatic infection due to the *H. capsulatum* var. *capsulatum* have a clinically asymptomatic fungemia, as evidenced by pulmonary and splenic calcifications. This "cryptic dissemination" to multiple organs permits subsequent reactivation at pulmonary and extrapulmonary sites if the host becomes immunocompromised or similarly stressed. This situation resembles the pathogenesis of tuberculosis.

Clinically overt acute disseminated histoplasmosis may develop in immunocompromised patients with cellular immunodeficiencies. However, disseminated histoplasmosis of infancy may develop in otherwise apparently healthy infants less than 2 years of age. Specimens for culture include blood, urine, bone marrow, and sputum. HIV-infected patients with disseminated histoplasmosis may have multiple necrotizing cutaneous lesions. Biopsy and culture of these cutaneous lesions may reveal poorly formed granulomas containing an abundant amount of small budding yeast forms due to *H. capsulatum.*

Special stains should be used for the direct examination of specimens with possible *H. capsulatum.* The budding yeast cells of *H. capsulatum* (2–4 μm) appear very small on a Calcofluor white or KOH preparation of sputum and may be confused with *Candida glabrata.* (20–26). A useful clue is the presence of small yeast cells of *H. capsulatum* within macrophages. In contrast, the yeast cells of *T. glabrata* are seldom found within macrophages. Giemsa or hematoxylin and eosin (H&E) stains highlight intracellular yeasts of *H. capsulatum* more readily, particularly in sputum, blood smears, bone aspirates, and biopsy specimens (191). The GMS stain yeast cells while not staining the cellular detail of the host inflammatory cells.

Histopathological examination of paraffin-embedded specimens with either H&E or PAS stains reveals a granulomatous inflammatory response to *H. capsulatum.* Collections of small yeast forms are abundant in the cytoplasm of macrophages in acute pulmonary or disseminated histoplasmosis. The yeast cells of *H. capsulatum* can be distinguished from other intracellular parasites *Leishmania donovani* and *Toxoplasma gondii.* For example, *L. donovani* have a characteristic a kinetoplast, which is not present in the yeast cells of *H. capsulatum.* The tachyzoites of *T. gondii* are not stained by GMS. As a lesion fibroses with calcification, the number of yeast forms decreases, and in this circumstance the GMS stain is preferable.

Plated culture specimens with presumed *H. capsulatum* should be incubated at 25–30°C, but growth is slow and often exhibits aerial mycelium that varies in color from white to buff to brown (1). During early growth of the mycelial culture, spherical or pyriform microconidia (2–5 μm in diameter) are seen. With further incubation, the mould develops slender conidiophores and characteristic globose and pyriform, tuberculate and nontuberculate macroconidia measuring 8–16 μm in diameter are apparent. Because these macroconidia resemble the saprophytic genus *Sepedonium,* the isolate should be converted to the yeast form. Additional tests should demonstrate production of the h or m exoantigen, or detection with a specific nucleic acid probe for *H. capsulatum. H. capsulatum* grows on media with cycloheximide, unlike the monomorphic *Sepedonium* spp., which are inhibited under this selective pressure.

The lysis-centrifugation technique (Isolator; Wampole Laboratories, Cranbury, NJ) is a highly sensitive method for rapid recovery of *H. capsulatum* and other dimorphic fungi (76,77,191). The time to detection is highly dependent upon the inoculum cultured.

Detection in serum and urine of a polysaccharide antigen of *H. capsulatum* is a valuable tool for both the diagnosis and therapeutic monitoring of disseminated histo-plasmosis (196). These detection systems are especially useful for patients with a high burden of the pathogen (e.g., in patients with advanced HIV infection). Antigen detection in serum and urine for non-HIV-infected patients with localized pulmonary disease is less sensitive. To ensure adequate quality control practices, urine and other specimens have been routinely submitted to a reference laboratory at Indiana University.

A new EIA method has been developed as an acceptable alternative for detection of carbohydrate antigen of *H. capsulatum* in urine (197). A comparison of the conventional radioimmunoassay and the enzyme-linked immunoassay for the measurement of *Histoplasma* antigen in banked urine specimens showed no significant difference. Both the EIA and RIA detected measurable antigen levels in urine from 50 of 56 patients (89%) with disseminated disease and 11 of 30 patients (37%) with self-limiting disease. Control specimens from healthy adults, patients with other fungal infections, urinary tract infections, or nonfungal pneumonia were also tested. One of 96 control specimens, from a patient with paracoccidioidomycosis, was positive with both systems.

Gomez and colleagues also recently reported the development of a novel ELISA system for detection of a 69–70-kd antigen of *H. capsulatum* that is distinct from the carbohydrate antigen measured in conventional assays (196–198). The new system performed comparably with an overall sensitivity for all cases of histoplasmosis at 71%; specificity was 98% measured in normal human sera from areas of endemicity and 85% in sera of patients with other chronic fungal or bacterial infections.

The cross-reactivity of the antigen assay developed at Indiana University was evaluated in patients with disseminated fungal infections (199). Cross-reacting antigen was detected in 12 of 19 patients with blastomycosis, eight of nine with paracoccidioidomycosis, 17 of 18 with *P. marneffei* infection, and one with disseminated *H. capsulatum* var. *duboisii* infection. Cross-reaction was not observed in six patients with disseminated coccidioidomycosis. Hence cross-reactivity between other endemic mycoses and *H. capsulatum* var. *capsulatum* remains an important consideration. Again the usefulness of the system must take into account both the risk for specific endemic infections and particularly the history of exposure.

Coccidioidomycosis

The incidence of pulmonary coccidioidomycosis continues to increase in endemic areas in the United States. Although primary infection in normal hosts rarely requires antifungal therapy, this paradigm has undergone modification because of the large number of immunocompromised hosts (especially those with HIV infection or a recent transplantation) who live in endemic areas. Dissemination to extrapulmonary sites may result in cutaneous and soft-tissue infection, osteomyelitis, arthritis, and meningitis.

Cerebrospinal fluid, other body fluids, and biopsies of tissues infected by *C. immitis* should be submitted to the clinical microbiology laboratory for microscopic examination and culture with ample warning for the staff. The mould form of *C. immitis* is highly contagious and thus requires adequate precautions in the laboratory. For this reason it is preferable to perform direct examinations of sputum, exudates, and tissue for pathognomonic spherules. Mature spherules are thick-walled, usually 20–60 μm in diameter, and easily recognized on wet mounts with either KOH or Calcofluor white. Endospores (2–4 μm) are seen in intact or recently disrupted spherules. In some circumstances, hyphae may develop in chronic cavitary and granulomatous lesions of pulmonary coccidioidomycosis or in a pleural space having low CO_2 content.

A wide spectrum of tissue inflammation can be observed in response to coccidioidomycosis, ranging from an acute pyogenic to a chronic granulomatous reaction (20–22). A granulomatous reaction is observed in response to intact spherules, which can be sparse in patients with resolving infection but are numerous during progressive disease. Spherules of *C. immitis* are identified easily in tissue by routine H&E, GMS, and PAS stains, particularly the latter.

The preparation of slide cultures from isolates that may contain viable *C. immitis* is strongly discouraged. When spherules of *C. immitis* cannot be identified on wet mounts, specimens should be cultured on slants instead of plates. *C. immitis* grows readily on conventional media at 25–30°C usually within 1 week as a floccose buff to yellow to tan colony composed of hyaline, septate hyphae with arthroconidia. The arthroconidia of *C. immitis* develop in the lateral hyphal branches and are generally thick-walled, barrel-shaped cells, 2–4 by 3–6 μm. One can appreciate an alternation of these forms with empty, thin-walled disjunctor cells. Conversion of the mould form of *C. immitis* to the tissue form is not recommended except under special circumstances.

Serum IgM precipitins, which may be demonstrated by a tube precipitin test, can be measured 1–3 weeks after the onset of symptoms due to primary infection in approximately 70% to 80% of patients but are no longer measurable after approximately 3–4 months (200). Complement-fixing serum IgG antibodies (CFA) emerge later and often persist for 6–9 months. An elevated CFA titer is characteristically observed in disseminated coccidioidomycosis. Falls in titers are followed for surrogate monitoring of response to therapy.

Blastomycosis

At 25–30°C, *B. dermatitidis* grows as a mould with conidia and septate hyphae. The mould form of *B. dermatitidis* is characterized by abundant conidia associated with both aerial hyphae and lateral conidiophores. These can be spherical, ovoid, or pyriform in shape; are 2–10 μm in diameter, similar to macroconidia of *H. capsulatum* but unlike the macroconidia of *H. capsulatum*; and are smooth. It is also possible to see thick-walled chlamydospores that are 7–18 μm in diameter. There is variation in the growth, colony appearance, and degree and type of conidiation, but colonies generally require 2 or more weeks before classic features are apparent. Plated on enriched media at 37°C, *B. dermatitidis* grows as a yeast that has characteristic morphology of folded, pasty, and moist colonies. The yeast forms are thick walled and spherical, and produce single buds with a broad base of attachment between the bud and parent cell.

Immunodiffusion tests for serum antibodies in patients with blastomycosis are preferred over complement fixation tests, but neither system is sufficiently sensitive or specific for detection of blastomycosis.

WI-1 is a 120-kd protein of the outer cell wall of *B. dermatitidis* that has been used to develop a serological test for the diagnosis of blastomycosis (201). One hundred thirty-two serum samples were assayed from 107 patients with possible blastomycosis. At least one sample was positive in 83% of the 23 patients with confirmed blastomycosis, but in only 5% of the 84 patients without confirmation of blastomycosis. The validity of this test awaits further study.

Penicilliosis

Recently, *P. marneffei* has been recognized as an endemic pathogen, particularly in immunocompromised patients from Southeast Asia (202,203). The diagnosis is made by direct smear and culture of clinical material. It is best to harvest material from umbilicated centrally necrotic lesions, bone marrow aspirate, or peripheral lymph node. *P. marneffei* is a dimorphic organism, but the yeastlike phase has a characteristic central transverse septum. It is routinely cultured from blood, bone marrow, skin, and lymph nodes as a hyaline mould with the typical phialide structure of *Penicillium* spp. The conidial chains are connected by an isthmus and the terminal conidia appear larger than the ones beneath them. During colony maturation, a diffusible, rose-red pigment is observed that is reminiscent of *Trichophyton rubrum*. The pigment alone is not diagnostic of the species because other *Penicillium* spp. produce a comparable, diffusible red pigment.

MEDICALLY IMPORTANT FILAMENTOUS FUNGI

Invasive Aspergillosis

Clinical and Radiographic Manifestations

Infection with *Aspergillus* spp. is a major complication of transplantation. It is difficult to recognize until an advanced stage is diagnosed, when the prognosis is guarded. Infection due to *Aspergillus* species can involve the pulmonary tree, including the sinuses but also skin or wound sites. It is rarely identified in the bloodstream, though the pattern of extension in some immunocompromised hosts clearly suggests a hematogenous route (see Table 2).

The most common site of involvement is pulmonary aspergillosis, which can be variable in its clinical course (5,204,205). Unfortunately, morbidity and mortality are high in the transplant setting. Patients who are neutropenic are at high risk for pulmonary aspergillosis, which may not be recognized until late in development because of the blunted inflammatory response. Fever and a nonproductive cough, especially during bouts of neutropenia, should prompt immediate evaluation for aspergillosis. Over time, patients develop pleuritic pain, nonproductive cough, hemoptysis, pleural rub, and occasionally adventitious breath sounds (206).

Radiographic manifestations of invasive pulmonary aspergillosis develop late and include bronchopneumonia, lobar consolidation, segmental pneumonia, multiple nodular lesions resembling septic emboli, and cavitary lesions (207,208). A classic "halo sign" is seen in neutropenic patients when recovery of peripheral counts is imminent (209,210). Radiographic detection, particularly by CT scan, has evolved as an important diagnostic strategy for prompt diagnosis of pulmonary aspergillosis (210). Computerized tomographic (CT) scans of the chest reveal more extensive involvement than the corresponding chest radiograph. Early lesions visible on CT scan are often peripheral or subpleural nodules contiguous to the pulmonary vascular tree. Cavitary lesions are also seen in more advanced cases. Early radiographic recognition of pulmonary lesions contributes to more prompt initiation of antifungal therapy appropriate for pulmonary aspergillosis (209,211,213). High-resolution rapid chest CT scanning (Imatron C-100) is more sensitive in bone marrow transplant recipients (212). A CT scan in neutropenic patients undergoing cancer chemotherapy permitted earlier recognition of invasive aspergillosis with improvement in time to detection from the onset of infiltrates from 7 to 1.9 days.

Microbiology and Direct Examination

There are more than 600 species of the genus *Aspergillus* but only a handful cause disease in humans (214). The two most common species are *Aspergillus fumigatus* and *Aspergillus flavus*, whereas the less commonly encountered species include *Aspergillus terreus*, *Aspergillus ustus*, and *Aspergillus nidulans*. *Aspergillus niger* can be isolated from patients with chronic obstructive pulmonary disease that is probably related to the saprophytic conditions amenable to growth. However, the clinical significance of these isolates is debated.

In culture, the genus *Aspergillus* is characterized by hyaline hyphae and conidiophores. The latter bear terminal vesicles, phialides, and spores that are termed *conidia*. *Aspergillus* conidia are spherical in shape, measuring 2.5–3.5 μm in diameter and have a remarkable tendency to form phialoconidia. Speciation of the genus *Aspergillus* is based upon the morphology of the phialides, conidia, and conidiophores. Conidia are probably the principal means for nosocomial transmission of *Aspergillus* (204). *Aspergillus* spp. in tissue form angular, dichotomously septate branching hyphae, a hallmark of infection. The invasive tissue form lacks conidiophores, vesicles, phialides, or conidia, but these structures may occasionally be seen in cavitary, pulmonary lesions. When *Aspergillus* hyphae in tissue are sectioned in cross-section they may resemble nonbudding yeast forms (214). The histopathological pattern of angular, dichotomously branching septate hyphae may also be observed in invasive mycoses due to *Aspergillus* spp., *Pseudallescheria boydii*, *Fusarium* spp., and several less common fungi. It is necessary to discriminate *Aspergillus* from the others on the basis of culture techniques.

Biopsy and culture of tissue is the definitive means for establishing a diagnosis of invasive aspergillosis. *Aspergillus* spp. grow on standard plate media without special conditions (20–26). On the other hand, growth in liquid media is very difficult and not recommended. Biopsy specimens should be processed immediately. However, because many patients at risk for invasive aspergillosis also have bleeding diatheses, alternative, less invasive approaches are usually pursued.

The use of surveillance cultures continues to generate controversy in the care of transplant recipients. Positive nasal surveillance cultures of *A. flavus* harvested during an outbreak of nosocomial aspergillosis in granulocytopenic patients correlated with invasive pulmonary aspergillosis (200,215). However, these findings have not been corroborated in general usage, prompting many to reserve this approach for containment of local outbreaks, associated with construction work in the hospital environment (216,217). Isolation of *Aspergillus* spp. from respiratory secretions from febrile granulocytopenic patients with pulmonary infiltrates is strongly associated with invasive pulmonary aspergillosis (215). Isolation of *Aspergillus* spp. from respiratory secretions of high-risk patients was highly predictive for invasive pulmonary aspergillosis in high-risk patients (216). Invasive aspergillosis was not present in nonimmunosuppressed patients or in nongranulocytopenic patients with solid tumors. The study also demonstrated a low predictive value for invasive disease, when *Aspergillus* spp. was recovered from respiratory secretions of nongranulocytopenic smokers with chronic lung disease. Still, granulocytopenia and absence of smoking were the most significant predictors of invasive aspergillosis in patients with positive respiratory tract cultures for *Aspergillus* spp. Because the consequences of delayed therapy are detrimental to outcome, most experts agree that isolation of *Aspergillus* spp. from respiratory tract cultures in a febrile granulocytopenic patients with pulmonary infiltrates should be considered a priori evidence of pulmonary aspergillosis.

Mucosal eschars along the nasal septum are an important clue for diagnosing *Aspergillus* sinusitis. Biopsy and culture of the lesion are indicated prior to prompt initiation of antifungal therapy. In some circumstances, if nasal septal lesions are not observed, a sinus aspirate may preclude the need for bronchoscopy. Although *Aspergillus* is the most common fungus isolated from the sinuses of immunocompromised patients, other fungi—including *Zygomycetes*, *Fusarium*, *P. boydii*, *Curvularia*, and *Alternaria*—should be excluded.

Bronchoalveolar lavage (BAL) is the standard approach for evaluating a transplant patient with pulmonary lesions who are at high risk for aspergillosis. However, the data are supportive of this approach, indicating that about half the patients with biopsy-proven aspergillosis have demonstrable *Aspergillus* after culture of washings (218,219). The absence of hyphal elements in a BAL specimen does exclude the diagnosis (220).

Open lung biopsy should be reserved for patients after a negative BAL but are at high risk for aspergillosis. It is recommended that the surgeon biopsy both the periphery and the central areas of abnormal lung, because the distribution of organism may vary. An early study failed to demonstrate a significant change in therapy following OLB, but since the completion of this study, data have been emerging to indicate that high doses of amphotericin B (1.0–1.5 mg/kg/day) may be more active against pulmonary aspergillosis than dosages used for empirical amphotericin B (0.5–0.6 mg/kg/day) (221). The administration of a lipid formulation of amphotericin B may be justified if a definitive diagnosis of invasive aspergillosis is established, though more data are needed to validate the administration of higher doses (in the range of 3–6 mg/kg/day).

Immunodiagnostic Methods for the Diagnosis of Aspergillosis

Immunodiagnostic methods for diagnosis of invasive aspergillosis have been developed using either antibody and antigenic detection methods (109,222). Table 6 summarizes the recent antigenic, metabolic, and molecular approaches for detection of invasive aspergillosis. Because nearly all immunocompromised patients have impaired antibody response, this approach has been unsuccessful for aspergillosis.

Galactomannan has been investigated as a target molecule for detection of aspergillosis. The presence of galactomannan antigenemia can be measured by counter immunoelectrophoresis, radioimmunoassay, or an enzyme-

TABLE 6. *Investigational nonculture methods for detection of invasive aspergillosis*

Antigenic, biochemical, or molecular target	Method of detection
Cell wall components	
Galactomannan	• Latex agglutination
	• ELISA
	• RIA
1,3-b-glucans	• Amebocyte lysate assay
Chitin	• Spectrophotometry
Metabolites	
d-mannitol	• GLC/FID
	• Mass spectroscopy/GLC
Genomic DNA sequences	
C-14-lanosterol demethylase	PCR
Ribosomal RNA genes	
Alkaline protease	

Abbreviations: RIA, radioimmunoassay; ELISA, enzyme-linked immunosorbent assay; GLC, gas-liquid chromatography; FID, flame ionization detector; PCR, polymerase chain reaction.

linked immunoassay on serum and urine samples (223,224). The detection of galactomannan in urine is more sensitive than serum for diagnostic purposes.

A latex agglutination assay using an antigalactomannan monoclonal antibody (EB-A2) is commercially available (225). Its usefulness is limited by several factors, a discrepancy between the first clinical signs of infection and a positive test result and a high rate of false-negative test results. The antigalactomannan monoclonal antibodies used in the latex agglutination assay cross-reacts with the laboratory contaminants such as *Penicillium chrysogenum*, *Cladosporium herbarum*, *Acremonium* species, and *Alternaria alternata*, as well as established pathogens, including *Fusarium oxysporum*, *Wangiella dermatitidis*, and *Rhodotorula rubra* (226). *Penicillium marneffei*, the dimorphic endemic fungal pathogen of Southeast Asia, also has been reported to cross-react with the EB-A2 monoclonal antibody.

A double-sandwich ELISA using a monoclonal antibody is more sensitive than the latex agglutination system and is reported to be useful in patients with proven or probable aspergillosis (227). Verweij and colleagues compared results of the direct sandwich ELISA for detecting *Aspergillus* galactomannan with that of the Pastorex *Aspergillus* antigen latex agglutination (LA) test. The authors analyzed 532 serum samples from 61 patients at risk for invasive aspergillosis and the ELISA test results, when positive, were apparent earlier than the LA test. The sensitivity and specificity were 90% and 84% for the ELISA versus 70% and 86% for the LA test.

A heat-stable carbohydrate antigen has been reported and studied in both an animal model and on collected patient samples. The active moiety is most likely a galactomannan-like antigen that can be measured by ELISA. It may be used for both diagnostic and monitoring of aspergillosis (228–230). Antigen levels were higher in disseminated infection than in invasive pulmonary aspergillosis (median levels, 500 and 121 ng/ml, respectively). Higher antigen levels were useful in predicting disseminated disease, and the course of antigenemia correlated with clinical outcome, including survival. This nonculture strategy coupled with early CT scanning has been reported to permit an earlier diagnosis and subsequent improvement in outcome (210).

PCR-Based Technology

Polymerase chain reaction (PCR)–based methods have been developed for early detection of invasive aspergillosis (231,232). Proof-of-principle was first established in a small study designed to detect *A. fumigatus* and *A. flavus* by PCR from BAL. Six (13%) of 46 BAL specimens from control patients had a positive PCR signal (231). Another group has reported a PCR assay for the detection and identification of *Candida* and *Aspergillus* species (233). The oligonucleotide primer pair consisted of a consensus sequence for a variety of fungal pathogens and the species-specific probes used for species identification were derived from a comparison of the sequences of the 18S rRNA genes of *Candida* spp. and *Aspergillus* spp.

An interesting approach has been to evaluate the double-sandwich ELISA for *Aspergillus* galactomannan and a PCR-based system in BAL fluid samples from 19 patients with probable or established pulmonary aspergillosis (234). *Aspergillus* species were detected by PCR or ELISA from BAL fluid samples from five of seven patients. Serum results for all patients were ELISA positive in BAL fluid. Interestingly, in four patients, the serum ELISA was positive before the BAL fluid was obtained. This preliminary investigation further found that GM may be detected by ELISA in BAL fluid samples from patients at risk of invasive pulmonary aspergillosis but that monitoring of serum GM levels may allow for the earlier diagnosis of invasive pulmonary aspergillosis.

Using a nested PCR method, one group evaluated a PCR strategy that uses serum instead of the more commonly whole blood or respiratory secretions (235). Two sets of oligonucleotide primers derived from the sequence of the variable regions V7 to V9 of the 18S rRNA genes of *Aspergillus fumigatus* were chosen. The single-strand conformational polymorphism (SSCP) technique has been reported to detect a spectrum of fungal pathogens and/or genera (150). In particular, *Aspergillus* spp. were readily amplified from known clinical samples using primers that target the 18S rRNA gene. The SSCP pattern could distinguish between species of *Aspergillus* as well as for other medically important opportunistic fungi, such as *Cryptococcus neoformans*, *Pseudallescheria boydii*, and *Rhizopus arrhizus*.

Zygomycosis

The class Zygomycetes is composed of two important orders: the Mucorales and the Entomophthorales (20–24). Respiratory infections are generally caused by fungi of the order Mucorales, of which *Rhizopus oryzae* is the most commonly isolated. Among the order Mucorales, other species, such as *Cunninghamella bertholettiae* and *Absidia corymbifera*, have been reported to be respiratory pathogens (236). Members of the Entomophthorales, typically cause tropical subcutaneous zygomycosis (lobomycosis) and another form of zygomycosis affecting the nasal submucosa (rhinoentomophthoromycosis); they rarely cause pulmonary and disseminated zygomycosis (237). Because organisms from both the Mucorales and the Entomophthorales can cause life-threatening infections and are grouped together in immunocompromised patients, the term *zygomycosis* is used throughout this text.

The spectrum of zygomycosis in patients undergoing transplantation includes rhinocerebral infections (as is seen in patients with diabetes mellitus), pulmonary infections emerging during granulocytopenia or corticosteroids, and disseminated infection observed in patients receiving chronic desferroxamine therapy. Most of the zygomycetes causing respiratory infections in transplant recipients are complicated by thrombotic invasion of blood vessels and clinically significant bleeding. The diagnosis of pulmonary zygomycosis requires a high degree of suspicion and a biopsy specimen. (238).

In tissue specimens, broad (15–20), irregular, usually sparsely septate (coenocytic) hyphae with nondichotomous side-branching are observed (239). The formation of chlamydoconidia in tissue has been reported in cases of zygomycosis due to either *Absidia* or *Rhizopus* spp. (240). Tissue specimens should be stained with Gomorri's methenamine silver nitrate and with hematoxylin and eosin. In addition, a portion should be examined on a slide with 20% aqueous potassium hydroxide with Calcofluor under a fluorescent microscope. Examination by Calcofluor staining or by KOH-digested sputum and cultures of respiratory tract secretions are frequently negative in patients with a pulmonary infarct syndrome. Biopsy of a skin lesion is required to definitely diagnose cutaneous infection.

When culturing biopsied tissue, specimens should be inoculated onto standard media, such as Sabouraud dextrose agar and potato dextrose agar (containing no added cycloheximide) and incubated at room temperature and at 37°C (241). Zygomycetes may not grow well if infected tissue is ground or homogenized in preparation for plating on culture media. Therefore the recovery rate may be enhanced if the tissue specimen is sliced into small pieces without grinding or homogenization. Zygomycetes can be inhibited by residual amphotericin B in tissue. Recent studies using PCR-SSCP have been useful for identifying zygomycetes.

The importance of a definitive diagnosis is important because antifungal azoles are not active and amphotericin B has been associated with treatment failure. Surgery is still the cornerstone of therapy; hence the importance of making a tissue diagnosis must be stressed. Definitive diagnosis of rhinocerebral or pulmonary zygomycosis requires a biopsy to demonstrate of tissue invasion. Examination of the wet mount on sputum or other liquid cultures from the respiratory tract are frequently negative. Recovery of a zygomycete from bronchoalveolar lavage specimen in an immunocompromised patient with fever and pulmonary infiltrate is considered to be indicative of infection, requiring immediate consideration for therapeutic intervention (242).

Fusariosis

Disseminated infection due to *Fusarium* spp. in granulocytopenic patients undergoing intensive antileukemic chemotherapy or bone marrow transplantation has emerged as a new problem (243–246). Four different species of *Fusarium—F. solani, F. oxysporum, F. moniliforme* and *F. chlamydosporum*—have been reported to cause disseminated infection in immunosuppressed patients. Manifestations of infection include pulmonary infiltrates, cutaneous lesions, positive blood cultures, and sinusitis (247). Biopsy specimens of cutaneous lesions reveal fine, dichotomously branching, acutely angular, septate hyphae that are not easily distinguishable from those of other hyaline moulds.

Fusarium species can be detected with a lysis centrifugation system. *Fusarium* spp. grow on solid media with hyphae with phialides and microconidia, and typical plantain-shaped macroconidia (phragmospores) develop as the culture matures. This leads to an initial erroneous report of a similar organism, such as *Acremonium* spp. Further evaluation will confirm the presence of *Fusarium* spp, based upon the recognition of phragmospores. Even though early detection is generally desirable, isolates of *Fusarium* spp. are resistant to amphotericin B and triazoles, resulting in infection with high morbidity and mortality.

Current diagnostic approaches depend upon bedside evaluation, diagnostic imaging, biopsy, and culture, but PCR methods also are being developed for improved detection. Using primer pairs common to several different medically important pathogens, a PCR assay has been developed that requires discrimination at the level of probe or gel separation technology (150,248–250).

Pseudallescheriasis

Pseudallescheria boydii is rarely seen in transplant patients, but the consequences of missing the diagnosis can be devastating. It is also known to cause mycetoma in immunocompetent patients. Examination by Calcofluor staining or by KOH-digested sputum and cultures of respiratory tract secretions is frequently negative in patients with a pulmonary infarct syndrome. Biopsy of a skin lesion is required to definitely diagnose cutaneous infection. Overall, pneumonia due to *P. boydii* is clinically indistinguishable from *Aspergillus* spp. and carries a similar poor prognosis; it also has a propensity for dissemination to the central nervous system (251–256). The diagnostic approach parallels that for *Aspergillus* spp. but appears to be angular with septate, dichotomously branching hyphae. Terminal annelloconidia are seen histologically. The definitive microbiological diagnosis is established by culture, in which the organism may grow as the synanamorph *Scedosporium apiospermum* or as the teleomorph *P. boydii* with cleistothecia (259).

Infections due to *P. boydii* are refractory to antifungal therapy, including amphotericin B. Immunocompromised patients with pneumonia, cerebral abscesses, endophthalmitis, osteomyelitis, or disseminated infections due to *P. boydii* often fail to respond to single agent azole therapy. In one study, seven (32%) of the 22 clinical isolates of *P. boydii* were resistant *in vitro* to concentrations of amphotericin B ≥2.0 μg/ml and eight (36%) consistently had MICs ≤0.5 μg/ml. This has led some to recommend amphotericin B in combination with antifungal azoles. The study found enhanced *in vitro* antifungal activity when amphotericin B was combined with itraconazole or fluconazole (257).

Universal primers and specific probes detection of the less common but emerging pathogenic fungi have been investigated (258). A section of the 28S rRNA gene from approximately 100 fungi, representing approximately 50 species of fungal pathogens and commonly encountered saprophytes, was sequenced to develop universal PCR primers and species-specific oligonucleotide probes. Twenty-one separate nucleic acid probes that target the large subunit rRNA genes were developed. These recognized eight *Candida* spp., five *Aspergillus* spp., *Pseudallescheria boydii, Blastomyces dermatitidis, Coccidioides immitis, Histoplasma capsulatum, Sporothrix schenckii, Cryptococcus neoformans* var. *gattii, Cryptococcus neoformans* var. *neoformans, Filobasidiella neoformans* var. *bacillispora,* and *Filobasidiella neoformans* var. *neoformans.* Each step in the process was designed for detection under universal conditions, thus simplifying the technique and at the same time permitting identification of a wide range of pathogens.

CONCLUSION

An expanding population of transplant candidates (both solid and marrow recipients) will result in more cases of invasive fungal infections unless we develop strategies to use prophylaxis effectively during periods of high risk. The success of fluconazole in preventing *Candida* infection in the marrow recipient population may be short-lived because of the emergence of fluconazole-resistant isolates and a shift in colonization patterns. Heavy antibiotic usage of both antibacterial and antifungal compounds will continue to shift the patterns of infecting fungal pathogens. At the same time, it is incumbent upon the medical community to improve diagnostic modalities, not only because of the need to contain economic costs but also to limit the use of empirical antifungal therapy. However, the utility of applying these new molecular, antigenic, and analytical diagnostic tools in an era of cost containment depends greatly upon the patient population. Advances in new blood culture systems, as well as diagnostic biochemical, antigenic, and molecular markers will permit earlier detection and therapeutic monitoring. Continued development of standardized antifungal susceptibility systems with clinical and *in vivo* correlations is crucial for rational use of antifungal compounds. In the long run, it will be necessary to link new diagnostic modalities with outcome.

REFERENCES

1. Meyers J. Fungal infections in bone marrow transplant patients *Semin Oncol* 1990;17:S10–S17.
2. Walter E, Bowden R. Infection in the bone marrow transplant recipient. *Infect Dis Clin North Am* 1995;9:823–847.
3. Lehrnbecher TL, Foster C, Vazquez N, Mackall CL, Chanock SJ. Therapy-induced alterations in host defense in children receiving therapy for cancer. *Am J Pediatr Hematol/Oncol* 1997;19:399–417.
4. Wey SB, Motomi M, Pfaller MA, Woolson RF, Wenzel RP. Hospital acquired candidemia: the attributable mortality and excess length of stay. *Arch Intern Med* 1988;148:2642–2645.
5. Pannuti CS, Gingrich RD, Pfaller MA, Wenzel RP. Nosocomial pneumonia in adult patients undergoing bone marrow transplantation: a 9-year study. *J Clin Oncol* 1991;77–84.
6. Armstrong D. Problems in management of opportunistic fungal diseases. *Rev* Infect Dis 1989;2 [Suppl.7]:S1591–S1599.
7. Bodey GP. Candidiasis in cancer patients. *Am J Med* 1984;77[Suppl]:13–19.
8. Horn R, Wong B, Kiehn TE, Armstrong D. Fungemia in a cancer hospital: changing frequency, earlier onset, and results of therapy. *Rev Infect Dis* 1985;7:646–655.
9. Komshian SV, Uwaydah AK, Sobel JD, Croue LR. Fungemia caused by *Candida* species and *Torulopsis glabrata* in the hospitalized patient: frequency, characteristics, and evaluation of factors influencing outcome. *Rev Infect Dis* 1989;11:379–390.
10. Leccciones JA, Lee JW, Navarro E, Witebsky FG, Marshall DJ, Steinberg SM, Pizzo PA, Walsh TJ. Vascular catheter-associated fungemia in cancer patients: analysis of 155 episodes. *Rev Infect Dis* 1992;14:875–883.
11. Maksymiuk AW, Thongprasert S, Hopfer R, et al. Systemic candidiasis in cancer patients. *Am J Med* 1984;77[Suppl]:20–27.
12. Walsh TJ, Pizzo PA. Nosocomial fungal infections. *Annual Rev Microbiol* 1988;42:517–546.
13. Arena FP, Perlin M, Brahman H, Weiser B, Armstrong D. Fever, rash and myalgias of disseminated candidiasis during antifungal therapy. *Arch Int Med* 1981;141:1233–1237.
14. Bodey GP, Luna M. Skin lesions associated with disseminated candidiasis. *JAMA* 1974;229:1466–1468.
15. Edwards JE. *Candida* endophthalmitis. In: Bodey GP, Fainstein V, eds. *Candidiasis.* New York: Raven Press; 1985:211–225.
16. Jarowski CI, Fialk MA, Murray HW, Gottlieb GJ, Coleman M, Steinberg CR, Silver RT. Fever, rash and muscle tenderness. *Arch Int Med* 1978;138:544–546.
17. Pizzo PA, Robichaud KJ, Wesley R, Commers J. Fever in the pediatric and young adult patient with cancer: a prospective study of 1,001 episodes. *Medicine* 1982;61:153–165.
18. Solomon SL, Khabbaz RF, Parker RH, et al. An outbreak of *Candida parapsilosis* bloodstream infections in patients receiving parenteral nutrition. *J Infect Dis* 1984;149:98–102.
19. Thaler M, Pastakia B, Shawker TH, O'Leary T, Pizzo PA. Hepatic candidiasis in cancer patients: the evolving picture of the syndrome *Ann Int Med* 1988;108:88–100.
20. Kwon-Chung J, Bennett JE. *Medical mycology.* Melvern, PA: Lea & Febiger; 1994.
22. Larone DH. *Medically important fungi: a guide to identification,* 2nd ed. New York: Elsevier; 1987.
21. Kreger-van Rij NJW. *The yeasts: a taxonomic study,* 3rd ed. Amsterdam: Elsevier Science Publishers; 1984.
23. McGinnis MR. *Yeast identification. Laboratory handbook of medical mycology.* New York: Academic Press; 1980:337–410.
24. Rippon JW. *Medical mycology: the pathogenic fungi and the pathogenic actinomycetes,* 3rd ed. Philadelphia: WB Saunders; 1988.
25. Warren NG, Shadomy HJ. Yeasts of medical importance. *Manual of clinical microbiology,* 5th ed. Washington, DC: American Society for Microbiology; 1991:617–629.
26. Navarro EE, Almario JS, King C, Bacher J, Pizzo PA, Walsh TJ. Candida casts in experimental renal candidiasis in rabbits: implications for diagnosis and pathogenesis of upper urinary tract infection. *J Med Vet Mycol* 319942;415–426.
27. Navarro E, Almario JS, Schaufele RL, Bacher J, Walsh TJ. Quantitative urine cultures do not reliably detect renal candidiasis. *J Clin Microbiol* 1997 (*in press*).
28. Merz WG, Roberts GD. Detection and recovery of fungi from clinical specimens. *Manual of clinical microbiology.* In: Murray P, Baron EJ, Pfaller MA, Tenover FC, Yolken RH, eds. *Manual of clinical microbiology,* 6th. ed. Washington, DC: American Society for Microbiology 1995;709–722.
29. Walsh TJ, McEntee C, Dixon DM. Tissue homogenization for quantitative cultures of *Candida albicans* using sterile reinforced polyethylene bags. *J Clin Microbiol* 1987;25:931–932.
30. Hadfield TL, Smith MB, Winn RE, Rinaldi MG, Guerra C. Mycoses caused by *Candida lusitaniae. Rev Infect Dis* 1987;9:1006–1012.
31. Walsh TJ, Salkin IF, Dixon DM, Hurd NJ. Clinical microbiological and experimental animal studies of *Candida lipolytica. J Clin Microbiol* 1989;27:927–931.
32. Merz WG, Khazan U, Jabra-Rizk MA, Wu LC, Osterhout GJ, Lehmann PF. Strain delineation and epidemiology of *Candida (Clavispora) lusitaniae. J Clin Microbiol* 1992;30:449–454.
33. Wingard JR, Merz WG, Saral R. *Candida tropicalis*: a major pathogen in immunocompromised patients. Ann Int Med 1979;91:539–543.
34. Wingard JR, Merz WG, Rinaldi MG, Johnson TR, Karp JE, Saral R. Increase in *Candida krusei* infection among patients with bone marrow transplantation and neutropenia treated prophylactically with fluconazole. *N Engl J Med* 1991;325:12740–1277.
35. Wingard JR, Merz WG, Rinaldi MG, Miller CB, Karp JE, Saral R. Association of *Torulopsis glabrata* infections with fluconazole prophylaxis in neutropenic bone marrow transplant patients. *Antimicrob Agents Chemother* 1993;37:1847–1849.
36. Murray PR, Van Scoy RE, Roberts GD. Should yeasts in respiratory secretions be identified? *Mayo Clin Proc* 1977;52:42–45.
37. Slutsky B, Buffo J, Soll DR. High frequency switching of colony morphology in *Candida albicans. Science* 1985;230:666–669.
38. Yamane N, Saitoh Y. Isolation and detection of multiple yeasts from a single clinical sample by use of Pagano-Levin agar medium. *J Clin Microbiol* 1985;21:276–277.
39. Allison, RT. An evaluation of Pagano-Levin medium in a quantitative study of *Candida albicans*: preliminary communication. *J Med Lab Technol* 1967;24:199–202.
40. Odds FC, Bernaerts R. CHROMagar Candida, a new differential isolation medium for presumptive identification of clinically important *Candida* species. *J Clin Microbiol* 1994;32:1923–1929.
41. Pfaller MA, Houston A, Coffmann S. Application of CHROMagar Candida for rapid screening of clinical specimens for *Candida albicans, Candida tropicalis, Candida krusei,* and *Candida (Torulopsis) glabrata. J Clin Microbiol* 1996;34:58–61.
42. Land GA, Harrison BA, Hulme KL, Cooper BH, Byrd JC. Evaluation of a new API 20C strip for yeasts identification against a conventional method. *J Clin Microbiol* 1979;10:357–364.
43. Bowman PI, Ahearn DG. Evaluation of commercial systems for identification of clinical yeast isolates. *J Clin Microbiol* 1976;4:49–53.

44. Buesching WJ, Kurek K, Roberts GD. Evaluation of the modified API 20C system for identification of clinically important yeasts. *J Clin Microbiol* 1979;9:565–569.

45. Kiehn TE, Edwards FF, Tom D, Lieberman G, Bernard EM, Armstrong D. Evaluation of the Quantum II yeast identification system. *J Clin Microbiol* 1985;22:216–219.

46. Pfaller MA, Preston T, Bale M, Foontz FP, Body BA. Comparison of the Quantum II, API Yeast Ident, and AutoMicrobic systems for identification of clinical yeast isolates. *J Clin Microbiol* 1988;26: 2054–2058.

47. Cooper BH, Johnson JB, Thaxton ES. Clinical evaluation of the Uni-Yeast-Tek system for rapid presumptive identification of medically important yeasts. *J Clin Microbiol* 1978;7:349–355.

48. Oblack DL, Rhodes JC, Martin WJ. Clinical evaluation of the AutoMicrobic System Yeast Biochemical Card for rapid identification of medically important yeasts. *J Clin Microbiol* 1981.13:351–355.

49. Sekhon AS, Padhye AA, Gorg AK, Pruitt WR. Evaluation of the Abbott Quantum II yeast identification system. *Mykosen* 1986;30: 408–411.

50. Hopfer RL, Blan F. Caffeic-acid containing medium for identification of *Cryptococcus neoformans*. *J Clin Microbiol* 1975;2:115–120.

51. Kaufmann CS, Merz WG. Two rapid pigmentation tests for identification of *Cryptococcus neoformans*. *J Clin Microbiol* 1982;15: 329–331.

52. Pien FD, Thompson RL, Deye D, Roberts GD. *Rhodotorula septicemia*: two cases and a review of the literature. *Mayo Clin Proc* 1980;55:258–260.

53. Hopkins JM, Land GA. Rapid methods for determining nitrate utilization by yeasts. *J Clin Microbiol* 1977;5:497–500.

54. Pore RS. Prototheca taxonomy. *Mycopathologia* 1985;90:129–139.

55. Danker WM, Spector SA, Fierer J, Davis CE. *Malassezia fungemia* in neonates and adults: complication of hyperalimentation. *Rev Infect Dis* 1987;9:743–753.

56. Gueho E, Simmons RB, Pruitt WR, Meyer SA, Ahearn DG. Association of *Malassezia pachydermatis* with systemic infections of humans. *J Clin Microbiol* 1987;25:1789–1790.

57. Richet HM, McNeil MM, Edwards MC, Jarvis WR. Cluster of *Malassezia furfur* pulmonary infections in infants in a neonatal intensive-care unit. *J Clin Microbiol* 1989;27:1197–1200.

58. Odds FC. *Candida and candidosis*. Philadelphia: Bailliere Tindall; 1988:206–234.

59. Brooks RG. Prospective study of *Candida endophthalmitis* in hospitalized patients with candidemia. *Arch intern Med* 1989;149: 2226–2228.

60. Edwards JE Jr, Bodey GP, Bowden RA, et al. International Conference for the Development of a Consensus on the Management and Clin Infect Dis 1997;25:43–59.

61. Rex JH, Bennett JE, Sugar AM, et al. Intravascular catheter exchange and duration of candidemia. *Clin Infect Dis* 1995;21:994–996.

62. Rex JH, Pfaller MA, Galgiani JN, et al. Development of interpretive breakpoints for antifungal susceptibility testing: conceptual framework and analysis of *in vitro–in vivo* correlation data for fluconazole, itraconazole, and *Candida* infections. *Clin Infect Dis* 1997;24: 235–247.

63. Walsh TJ, Bustamante C, Vlahov D, Standiford HC. *Candida* suppurative peripheral thrombophlebitis: prevention, recognition and management. *Infect Control* 1986;7:16–22.

64. Braunstein H, Tomaasulo M. A quantitative study of the growth of *Candida albicans* in vented and unvented blood-culture bottles. *Am J Clin Pathol* 1976;66:87–90.

65. Gantz NM, Medeiros AA, Swain JL, O'Brien TF. Vacuum blood-culture bottles inhibiting growth of *Candida* and fostering growth of Bacteroides. *Lancet* 1974;2:1174–1176.

66. Roberts GD, Horstmeier C, Hall M, Washington JA II. Recovery of yeast from vented blood culture bottles. *J Clin Microbiol* 1975;2: 18–20.

67. Hopfer RL, Orengo A, Chesnut S, Wenglar M. Radiometric detection of yeasts in blood cultures of cancer patients. *J Clin Microbiol* 1980; 12:329–331.

68. Kiehn TE, Capitolo C, Mayo JB, Armstrong D. Comparative recovery of fungi from biphasic and conventional blood culture media. *J Clin Microbiol* 1981;14:681–683.

69. Prevost E, Bannister E. Detection of yeast septicemia by biphasic and radiometric methods. *J Clin Microbiol* 1981;13:655–660.

70. Weckbach LS, Stasneck JL. Performance characteristics of a commercially prepared biphasic blood culture bottle. *J Clin Microbiol* 1986;23:700–703.

71. Murray PR. Comparisons of lysis centrifugation and agitated biphasic blood culture systems for detection of fungemia. *J Clin Microbiol* 1991;29:96–98.

72. Roberts GD, Washington JA. Detection of fungi in blood cultures. *J Clin Microbiol* 1975;1:309–310.

73. Jungkind D, Millan J, Allen S, Dyke J, Hill E. Clinical comparison of a new automated infrared blood culture system with the BACTEC 460 system. *J Clin Microbiol* 1986;23:262–266.

74. Komorowski RA, Farmer SG. Rapid detection of candidemia. *Am J Clin Pathol* 1973;59:56–61.

75. Henry NK, McLimans CA, Wright AJ, Thompson RL, Wilson WR, Washington JA II. Microbiological and clinical evaluation of the isolator lysis centrifugation blood culture tube. *J Clin Microbiol* 1983;17: 864–869.

76. Bille J, Edson R, Roberts G. Clinical evaluation of the lysis centrifugation blood culture system for the detection of fungemia and comparison with a conventional biphasic broth blood culture system. *J Clin Microbiol* 1984;19:126–128.

77. Bille J, Stockman L, Roberts GD, Horstmeier CD, Ilstrup DM. Evaluation of a lysis-centrifugation system for recovery of yeasts and filamentous fungi from blood. *J Clin Microbiol* 1983;18:469–471.

78. Buck GE, Hanes V, Kelly MT, Alexander JA. Clinical comparison of the Roche Septi-Chek and Dupont Isolator blood culture systems. *Am J Clin Pathol* 1987;87:396–398.

79. Guerra-Romero L, Edson RS, Cockerill FR III, Horstmeier CD, Roberts GD. Comparison of DuPont Isolator and Roche Septi-chek for detection of fungemia. *J Clin Microbiol* 1987;25:1623–1625.

80. Kiehn TE, Wong B, Edward FF, Armstrong D. Comparative recovery of bacteria and yeasts from lysis-centrifugation and a conventional blood culture system. *J Clin Microbiol* 1983;18:300–304.

81. Brannon P, Kiehn TE. Large scale clinical comparison of lysis centrifugation and radiometric systems for blood culture. *J Clin Microbiol* 1986;24:886–887.

82. Kelly MT, Roberts FJ, Henry D, Geere I, Smith JA. Clinical comparison of isolator and BACTEC 660 resin media for blood culture. *J Clin Microbiol* 1990;28:1925–1927.

83. Masterson KC, McGowan JE. Detection of positive blood cultures by the BACTEC NR660. The clinical importance of five versus seven days of testing. *Am J Clin Pathol* 1988;90:91–94.

84. Mirrett S, Davis T, Wilson M, et al. Controlled evaluation of BACTEC selective fungal medium for detection of fungemia. *Abstr Am Soc Microbiol* 400; (abst C-351).

85. Morita T, Tanaka S, Nakamura T, Iwanaga S. A new 1,3-b-D-glucan-mediated coagulation pathway found in *Limulus* amebocyte. *FEBS Lett* 1981;129:318–321.

86. Alpert NL. Microbial detection system. *Clin Instr Systems* 1990;11: 1–5.

87. Wilson ML, Weinstein MP, Reimer LG, Mirrett S, Reller LB. Controlled comparison of the BacT/Alert and BACTEC 660/730 nonradiometric blood culture systems. *J Clin Microbiol* 1992;30:323–329.

88. Berenguer J, Buck M, Witebsky F, Stock F, Pizzo PA, Walsh TJ. Lysis-centrifugation blood cultures in the detection of tissue-proven invasive candidiasis: disseminated versus single organ infection. *Diagnost Microbiol Infect Dis* 1993;17:103–109.

89. Haslett TM, Isenberg HD, Tucci V, Kay BG, Vellozzi EM. Microbiology of in-dwelling central intravascular catheters. *J Clin Microbiol* 1988;26:696–701.

90. Linares J, Stiges-Serra A, Garan J, Perez JL, Martin R. Pathogenesis of catheter sepsis: a prospective study with qualitative and semiquantitative cultures of catheter hub and segments. *J Clin Microbiol* 1985; 21:357–360.

91. Walsh TJ, Gonzalez C, Roilides E, et al. Fungemia in HIV-infected children: new epidemiologic patterns, emerging pathogens, and improved antifungal outcome. *Clin Infect Dis* 1995;20:900–906.

92. Bousgnoux ME, Hill C, Moissenet D, et al. Comparison of antibody, antigen, and metabolite assays for hospitalized patients with disseminated or peripheral candidiasis. *J Clin Microbiol* 1990;28:905–909.

93. Lemieux C, St. Germain G, Vincelette J, Kaufman L, DeRepentigny L. Collaborative evaluation of antigen detection by a commercial latex agglutination test and enzyme immunoassay in the diagnosis of invasive candidiasis. *J Clin Microbiol* 1990;28:249–253.

94. Gold JWM, Wong B, Bernard EM, Kiehn TE, Armstrong D. Serum arabinitol concentrations and arabinitol/creatinine ratios in invasive candidiasis. *J Infect Dis* 1983;147:504–513.

95. Wong B, Bernard EM, Armstrong D, Roboz J, Suzuki R, Holland JF. [Letter]. *J Clin Microbiol* 1985;21:478–479.

96. Araj GF, Hopfer RL, Chesnut S, Fainstein V, Bodey GP. Diagnostic value of the enzyme-linked immunosorbent assay for detection of *Candida albicans* cytoplasmic antigen in sera of cancer patients. *J Clin Microbiol* 1982;16:46–52.

97. Greenfield RA, Jones JM. Purification and characterization of a major cytoplasmic antigen of *Candida albicans*. *Infect Immun* 1981;34:469–477.

98. Greenfield RA, Bussey MJ, Stephens JL, Jones JM. Serial enzyme-linked immunosorbent assays for antibody to *Candida* antigens during induction chemotherapy for acute leukemia. *J Infect Dis* 1983;148:275–283.

99. Jones JM. Kinetics of antibody responses to cell wall mannan and a major cytoplasmic antigen of *Candida albicans* in rabbits and humans. *J Lab Clin Med* 1980;96:845–860.

100. Jones JM. Laboratory diagnosis of invasive candidiasis. *Clin Microbiol Rev* 1990;3:32–45.

101. Matthews RC, Burnie JP, Tabaqchali S. Isolation of immunodominant antigens from sera of patients with systemic candidiasis and characterization of serological response to *Candida albicans*. *J Clin Microbiol* 1987;25:230–237.

102. Matthews R C, Burnie J P. Diagnosis of systemic candidiasis by an enzyme-linked immunodot immunobinding assay for a circulating immunodominant 47 kD antigen. *J Clin Microbiol* 1988;26:459–463.

103. Strockbine NA, Largen MT, Buckley HR. Production and characterization of three monoclonal antibodies to *Candida albicans* proteins. *Infect Immun* 1984;43:1012–1018.

104. Strockbine NA, Largen MT, Zweibel SM, Buckley HR. Identification and molecular weight characterization of antigens from *Candida albicans* that are recognized by human sera. *Infect Immun* 1984;43:715–721.

105. Taschdjian CL, Kozinn PJ, Cuesta MV, Toni EF. Serodiagnosis of candidal infections. *Am J Clin Pathol* 1971;57:195–205.

106. Taschdjian CL, Seelig MS, Koznin PJ. Serological diagnosis of candidal infections. *CRC Crit Rev Lab Sci* 1973;4:19–59.

107. Mason AB, Brandt ME, Buckley HR. Enolase activity associated with a *Candida albicans* cytoplasmic antigen. *Yeast* 1988;5:S231–S240.

108. Bennett JE. Rapid diagnosis of candidiasis and aspergillosis. *Rev Infect Dis* 1987;9:398–401.

109. De Repentigny L. Serodiagnosis of candidiasis, aspergillosis, and cryptococcosis. *Clin Infect Dis* 1992;14[Suppl 1]:S11–S22.

110. Reiss E, Morrison CJ. Nonculture methods for diagnosis of disseminated candidiasis. *Clin Microbiol Rev* 1993;6:311–323.

111. Franklyn KM, Warmington JR, Ott AK, Ashman R. An immunodominant antigen of *Candida albicans* shows homology to the enzyme enolase. *Immunol Cell Biol* 1990;68:173–178.

112. Walsh TJ, Hathorn JW, Sobel JD, et al. Detection of circulating *Candida* enolase by immunoassay in patients with cancer and invasive candidiasis. *N Engl J Med* 1991;324:1026–1031.

113. Mitsutake K, Takasshige M, Takayoshi T, et al. Enolase antigen, mannan antigen, Cand-Tec antigen, and b-glucan in patients with candidemia. *J Clin Microbiol* 1996;34:1918–1921.

114. Gutierrez J, Maroto C, Piedrola G, Martin E, Perez JA. Circulating *Candida* antigens and antibodies: useful markers of candidemia. *J Clin Microbiol* 1993;31:2550–2552.

115. Matthews RC, Burnie JP, Tabaqchali S. Immunoblot analysis of the serological response in systemic candidosis. *Lancet* 1984;ii:1415–1418.

116. De Bernardis F, Girmenia C, Boccanera M, Adriani D, Martino P, Cassone A. Use of a monoclonal antibody in a dot immunobinding assay for detection of a circulating mannoprotein of *Candida* spp. in neutropenic patients with invasive candidiasis. *J Clin Microbiol* 1993;31:3142–3146.

116. Bailey JW, Sada E, Brass C, Bennett JE. Diagnosis of systemic candidiasis by latex agglutination for serum antigen. *J Clin Microbiol* 1985;21:749–752.

117. Fung JC, Donta ST, Tilton RC. *Candida* detection system [CAND-TEC] to differentiate between *Candida albicans* colonization and disease. *J Clin Microbiol* 1986;24:542–547.

118. Gentry LO, Wilkinson ID, Lea AS, Price MF. Latex agglutination test for detection of *Candida* antigen in patients with disseminated disease. *Eur J Clin Microbiol* 1983;2:122–128.

119. Kahn FW, Jones JM. Latex agglutination tests for detection of *Candida* antigens in sera of patients with invasive candidiasis. *J Infect Dis* 1986;153:579–585.

120. Ness JJ, Vaugh WP, Woods GL. *Candida* antigen latex test for detection of invasive candidiasis in immunocompromised patients. *J Infect Dis* 1989;159:495–501.

121. Bernard EM, Christiansen KJ, Tsang SF, Kiehn TE, Armstrong D. Rate of arabinitol production by pathogenic yeast species. *J Clin Microbiol* 1981;189–194.

122. Bernard EM, Wong B. Armstrong D. Stereoisomeric configuration of arabinitol in invasive candidiasis. *J Infect Dis* 1985;151:711–715.

123. Roboz J, Suzuki R, Holland JF. Quantification of arabinitol in serum by selected ion monitoring as a diagnostic technique in invasive candidiasis. *J Clin Microbiol* 1980;12:594–602.

124. Wong B, Bernard EM, Gold JWM, Fong D, Armstrong D. The arabinitol appearance rate in laboratory animals and humans: estimation from the arabinitol/creatinine ratio and relevance to the diagnosis of candidiasis. *J Infect Dis* 1982;146:353–359.

125. Wong B, Bernard EM, Gold JWM, Fong D, Silber A, Armstrong D. Increased arabinitol levels in experimental candidiasis in rats: arabinitol appearance rates, arabinitol/creatinine ratios, and severity of infection. *J Infect Dis* 1982;146:346–352.

126. Wong B, Castellanos M. Enantioselective measurement of the *Candida* metabolite D-arabinitol in human serum using multidimensional gas chromatography and a new chiral phase. *J Chromatography* 1989;495:21–30.

127. de Repentigny L, Marr LD, Keller JW, Carter AW, Kuykendall RJ, Kaufman L, Reiss E. Comparison of enzyme immunoassay and gas-liquid chromatography for the rapid diagnosis of invasive candidiasis in cancer patients. *J Clin Microbiol* 1985;21:972–979.

128. Quong M, Miyada CG, Switchenko AC, Goodman TC. Identification, purification, and characterization of a D-arabinitol-specific dehydrogenase from Candida tropicalis. *Biochem Biophys Res Com* 1994;196:1323–1329.

129. Switchenko AC, Miyada CG, Goodman TC, Walsh TJ, Wong B, Becker MJ, Ullman EF. An automated enzymatic method for the measurement of D-arabinitol in human serum. *J Clin Microbiol* 1994;32:92–97.

130. Walsh TJ, Lee JW, Sien T, et al. Serum D-arabinitol measured by automated enzymatic assay for detection and therapeutic monitoring of experimental disseminated candidiasis: correlation with tissue concentrations of *Candida albicans*. *J Med Vet Mycol* 1994;32:205–215.

131. Soyama K, Ono E. Enzymatic fluorometric method for the determination of serum D-arabinitol in serum by initial rate analysis. *Clin Chim Acta* 1985;149:149–154.

132. Soyama K, Ono E. Improved procedure for determination of serum D-arabinitol by resazurin-coupled method. *Clin Chim Acta* 1987;168:259–260.

133. Soyama K, Ono E. Enzymatic and gas-liquid chromatographic measurement of D-arabinitol compared. *Clin Chem* 1988;3:432.

134. Walsh TJ, Merz WG, Lee JW, et al. Diagnosis and therapeutic monitoring of invasive candidiasis by rapid enzymatic detection of serum D-arabinitol. *Am J Med* 1995;99:164–172.

135. Christensson B, Wiebe T, Pehrson C, Larsson L. Diagnosis of invasive candidiasis in neutropenic children with cancer by determination of D-arabinitol/L-arabinitol ratios in urine. *J Clin Microbiol* 1997;35:636–640.

136. Lehtonen L, Anttila VJ, Ruutu T, et al. Diagnosis of disseminated candidiasis by measurement of urine D-arabinitol/L-arabinitol ratio. *J Clin Microbiol* 1996;34:2175–2179.

137. Obayashi T, Tamura H, Tanaka S, et al. A new chromogenic endotoxin-specific assay using recombined *Limulus* coagulation enzyme and its clinical applications. *Clin Chem Acta* 1985;149:55–65.

138. Obayashi T, Yoshida M, Mori T, et al. Plasma (1→3)-beta-D-glucan measurement in diagnosis of invasive deep mycosis and fungal febrile episodes. *Lancet* 1995;345:17–20.

139. Harding SA, Sanford GR, Merz WG. Three serologic tests for candidiasis: diagnostic value in distinguishing deep or disseminated infection from superficial infection or colonization. *Am J Clin Pathol* 1976;65:1001–1009.

140. Kozinn PJ, Taschdjian CL, Goldberg PK, et al. Efficiency of serologic

tests in the diagnosis of systemic candidiasis. *Am* J Clin Pathol 1978; 70:893–898.

141. Kozinn PJ, Taschdjian CL, Goldberg PK, Wise GJ, Toni EF, Seelig MS. Advances in the diagnosis of renal candidiasis. *J Urol* 1978;119: 184–187.

142. Meckstroth KL, Reiss E, Keller JW, Kaufman L. Detection of antibodies and antigenemia in leukemic patients with candidiasis by enzyme-linked immunosorbent assay. *J Infect Dis* 1981;144:24–32.

143. Mitchell TG, Sandin RL, Bowman BH, Meyer W, Merz WG. Molecular mycology: DNA probes and applications of PCR technology. *J Med Vet Mycol* 1994;32:3351–3366.

144. Heym B, Honore N, Truffot-Pernot C, et al. Implications of multidrug resistance for the future of short-course chemotherapy of tuberculosis: a molecular study. *Lancet* 1994;344:293–298.

145. Pfaller MA. The use of molecular techniques for epidemiologic typing of *Candida* species. *Curr Top Med Mycol* 1992;4:43–63.

146. Sullivan DJ, Henman MC, Moran GP, et al. Molecular genetic approaches to identification, epidemiology and taxonomy of non-*albicans Candida* species. *J Med Microbiol* 1996;44:399–408.

147. Walsh TJ, Hiemenz J, Anaissie E. Recent progress and current problems in treatment of invasive fungal infections in neutropenic patients. *Hematol/Oncol Clin North Am* 1996;10:365–400.

148. Buchman TG, Rossier M, Merz WG, Charache P. Detection of surgical pathogens by *in vitro* DNA amplification. Part I. Rapid identification of *Candida albicans* by *in vitro* amplification of a fungus specific gene. *Surgery* 1990;108:338–346.

149. Kan VL. Polymerase chain reaction for the diagnosis of candidemia. *J Infect Dis* 1993;168:779–783.

150. Walsh TJ, Francesconi A, Kasai M, Chanock SJ. PCR and single-strand conformational polymorphism for recognition of medically important fungi. *J Clin Microbiol* 1995;33:3216–3220.

151. Hendricks DA, Stowe BJ, Hoo BS, et al. Quantitation of HBV DNA in human serum using a branched DNA (bDNA) signal amplification assay. *Am* J Clin Pathol 1995;104:537–546.

152. Wolcott M. Advances in nucleic acid-based detection methods. *Clin Microbiol Rev* 1992;5:370–382.

153. Ferenczy A, Franco E, Arseneau J, Wright TC, Richart RM. Diagnostic performance of hybrid capture human papillomavirus deoxyribonucleic acid assay combined with liquid-based cytologic study. *Am J Obstet Gynecol* 1996;175:651–656.

154. Holmes AR, Cannon RD, Shepherd MG, Jenkinson HF. Detection of *Candida albicans* and other yeast in blood by PCR. *J Clin Microbiol* 1994;32:228–231.

155. Miyakawa Y, Mabuchi T, Fukazawa Y. New method for detection of *Candida albicans* in human blood by polymerase chain reaction. *J Clin Microbiol* 1993;31:3344–3347.

156. Burgener-Kairuz P, Zuber JP, Jaunin P, Buchman TG, Bille J, Rossier M. Rapid detection and identification of *Candida albicans* and *Torulopsis (Candida) glabrata* in clinical specimens by species- specific nested PCR amplification of a cytochrome P-450 lanosterol-alpha-demethylase (L1A1) gene fragment. *J Clin Microbiol* 1994;32: 1902–1907.

157. Chryssanthou E, Andersson B, Petrini B, Lofdahl S, Tollemar J. Detection of *Candida albicans* DNA in serum by polymerase chain reaction. *Scand J Infect Dis* 1994;26:479–485.

158. Botelho AR, Planta RJ. Specific identification of *Candida albicans* by hybridization with oligonucleotides derived from ribosomal DNA internal spacers. *Yeast* 1994;10:709–717.

159. Haynes KA, Westerneng TJ. Rapid identification of *Candida albicans*, *C. glabrata*, *C. parapsilosis* and *C. krusei* by species specific PCR of large subunit ribosomal DNA. *J Med Microbiol* 1996;44:390–396.

160. Williams DW, Wilson MJ, Lewis, Potts AJ. Identification of *Candida* species by PCR and restriction fragment length polymorphism analysis of intergenic spacer regions of ribosomal DNA. *J Clin Microbiol* 1995;33:2476–2479.

161. Robert F, Lebreton F, Bougnoux ME, et al. Use of random amplified polymorphic DNA as a typing method for *Candida albicans* in epidemiological surveillance of a burn unit. *J Clin Microbiol* 1995;33: 2366–2371.

162. Jordan JA. PCR identification of four medically important *Candida* species by using a single primer pair. *J Clin Microbiol* 1994;32: 2962–2967.

163. Van Deenter AJ, Goessens WH, van Belkum A, van Vliet HJ, van Etten EW, Verbrugh HA. Improved detection of *Candida albicans* by

164. Fujita SI, Lasker B, Lott TJ, Reiss E, Morrison CJ. Microtitration plate enzyme immunoassay to detect PCR-amplified DNA from *Candida* species in blood. *J Clin Microbiol* 1995;33:962–967.

165. Burnie JP, Golbang N, Matthews RC. Semiquantitative polymerase chain reaction enzyme immunoassay for diagnosis of disseminated candidiasis. *Eur* J Clin Microbiol Infect Dis 1997;16:346–350.

166. Lischewski A, Ruhnke M, Tennagen I, Schonian G, Morschlauser J, Hacker J. Molecular epidemiology of *Candida* isolates from AIDS patients showing different fluconazole resistance profiles. *J Clin Microbiol* 1995;33:769–771.

167. Van Belkum A, Mol W, van Saene R, Ball LM, van Velzen D, Quint W. PCR-mediated genotyping of *Candida albicans* strains from bone marrow transplant patients. *Bone Marrow Transplant* 1994;13:811–815.

168. Van Belkum A, Melchers W, de Pauw BE, Scherer S, Quint W, Meis JF. Genotypic characterization of sequential *Candida albicans* isolates from fluconazole treated neutropenic patients. *J Infect Dis* 1994;169: 1062–1070.

169. White TJ, Burns T, Lee S, Taylor J. Amplification and direct sequencing of fungal ribosomal RNA genes for phylogenetics. In: Innis M, et al, *PCR Protocols*. San Diego: Academic Press; 1990:315–324.

170. Stringer JR. The identity of *Pneumocystis carinii*: not a single protozoan, but a diverse group of exotic fungi. *Infect Agents Dis* 1993;2: 109–117.

171. Schonian G, Meusel O, Tietz HJ, et al. Identification of clinical strains of *Candida albicans* by DNA fingerprinting with the polymerase chain reaction. *Mycoses* 1993;36:171–179.

172. Lin D, Lehmann PF. Random amplified polymorphic DNA for strain delineation with *Candida tropicalis*. *J Med Vet Mycol* 1995;33: 241–246.

173. Bostock A, Khattak MN, Matthews R, Burnie J. Comparison of PCR fingerprinting, by random amplification of polymorphic DNA, with other molecular typing methods for *Candida albicans*. *J Gen Microbiol* 1993;139:2179–2184.

174. National Committee for Clinical Laboratory Standards. Reference method for broth dilution antifungal susceptibility testing of yeasts. Proposed Standard. NCCLS document M27-P. NCCLS, Villanova, PA 1992.

174. Powderly WG, Cloud GA, Dismukes WE, Saag MS. Measurement of cryptococcal antigen in serum and cerebrospinal fluid: value in the management of AIDS-associated cryptococcal meningitis. *Clin Infect Dis* 1994;18:789–792.

175. Tanner DC, Weinstein MP, Fedorciw B, Joho KL, Thorpe JJ, Reller L. Comparison of commercial kits for detection of cryptococcal antigen. *J Clin Microbiol* 1994;32:1680–1684.

176. Bottone E, Wormser G. Capsule-deficient cryptococci in AIDS. *Lancet* 1985;2:553.

177. Gonzalez C, Shetty D, Lewis L, Mueller B, Pizzo PA, Walsh TJ. Cryptococcosis in HIV-infected children. *Pediatr Infect Dis J* 1996;15: 796–800.

177. Walsh TJ, Melcher GP, Lee JW, Pizzo PA. Infections due to *Trichosporon* species: new concepts in mycology, pathogenesis, diagnosis, and treatment. *Curr Top Med Mycol* 1993;5:79–113.

178. Gueho E, Smith MT, de Hoog GS, Billon-Grand G, Christen R, Batenburg-van der Vegte WH. Contributions to a revision of the genus Trichosporon. *Antonie Van Leeuwenhoek* 1992;61:289–316.

179. Lee JW, Melcher GA, Rinaldi MG, Andrews J, Pizzo PA, Walsh TJ. Patterns of morphologic variation in strains of *Trichosporon beigelii*. *J Clin Microbiol* 1990;28:2823–2827.

180. Seeliger HPR, Schroter R. A serological study on the antigenic relationship of the form genus Trichosporon. *Sabouraudia* 1963;2: 248–263.

181. Walsh TJ, Kelly P, Peebles R, Lee JW, Lecciones J, Pizzo PA. Biochemical and physiological variables regulating germination of Trichosporon beigelii. *J Med Vet Mycol* 1994;32:123–132.

182. McManus EJ, Jones JM. Detection of a *Trichosporon beigelii* antigen cross-reactive with *Cryptococcus neoformans* capsular polysaccharide in serum from a patient with disseminated Trichosporon infection. *J Clin Microbiol* 1985;21:681–685.

183. McManus EJ, Bozdech MJ, Jones JM. Role of the latex agglutination test for cryptococcal antigen in diagnosing disseminated infections with *Trichosporon beigelii*. *J Infect Dis* 1985;151:1167–1169.

184. Walsh TJ, Newman KA, Moody M, Wharton R, Wade JC. Tri-

chosporonosis in patients with neoplastic disease. *Medicine (Baltimore)* 1986;65:268–279.

185. Walsh TJ, Lee JW, Melcher GP, et al. Experimental *Trichosporon* infection in persistently granulocytopenic rabbits: implications for pathogenesis, diagnosis, and treatment of an emerging opportunistic mycosis. *J Infect Dis* 1992;166:121–133.

186. Melcher GP, Reed KD, Rinaldi MG, Lee JW, Pizzo PA, Walsh TJ. Demonstration of a cell wall antigen cross-reacting with cryptococcal polysaccharide in experimental disseminated trichosporonosis. *J Clin Microbiol* 1991;29:192–196.

187. Lyman CA, Garrett KF, Pizzo PA, Walsh TJ. Response of human polymorphonuclear leukocytes and monocytes to *Trichosporon beigelii*: host defense against an emerging pathogen. *J Infect Dis* 199470: 1557–1565.

188. Kozel TR, Mastroianni RP. Inhibition of phagocytosis by cryptococcal polysaccharide: dissociation of the attachment and ingestion phases of phagocytosis. *Infect Immun* 1976;14:62–67.

189. Lyman CA, Devi S, Nathanson J, Frasch CE, Pizzo PA, Walsh TJ. Detection and quantification of the glucuronoxylomannan-like polysaccharide antigen from clinical and non-clinical isolates of *Trichosporon beigelii*: implications for pathogenecity. *J Clin Microbiol* 1994;33:126–130.

190. Walsh TJ, Mitchell T, Larone DH. Histoplasma, Blastomyces, Coccidioides, and other dimorphic fungi causing systemic mycoses. In: Murray P, Baron EJ, Pfaller MA, Tenover FC, Yolken RH, eds. *Manual of clinical microbiology*, 6th ed. Washington, DC: American Society for Microbiology; 1995;749–764.

191. Paya CV, Roberts GD, Cockerill FR III. Laboratory methods for the diagnosis of disseminated histoplasmosis: clinical importance of the lysis-centrifugation blood culture technique. *Mayo Clin Proc* 1987;62: 480–485.

192. Kaufman L, Standard PG. Specific and rapid identification of medically important fungi by exoantigen detection. *Ann Rev Microbiol* 1987;41:209–225.

193. Hall GS, Pratt-Rippin K, Washington JA. Evaluation of a chemiluminescent probe assay for identification of *Histoplasma capsulatum* isolates. *J Clin Microbiol* 1992;30:3003–3004.

194. Huffnagle KE, Gander RM. Evaluation of Gen-Probe's *Histoplasma capsulatum* and *Cryptococcus neoformans* AccuProbes. *J Clin Microbiol* 1993;31:419–421.

195. Padhye AAG, Smith D, McLaughlin PG, Standard, Kaufman L. Comparative evaluation of a chemiluminescent DNA probe and an exoantigen test for rapid identification of Histoplasma capsulatum. *J Clin Microbiol* 1992;30:3108–3111.

196. Wheat LJ, Kohler RB, Tewari RP. Diagnosis of disseminated histoplasmosis by detection of Histoplasma capsulatum in serum and urine specimens. *N Engl J Med* 1986;314:83–88.

197. Durkin MM, Connolly PA, Wheat LJ. Comparison of radioimmunoassay and enzyme-linked immunoassay methods for detection of *Histoplasma capsulatum* var. *capsulatum* antigen. *J Clin Microbiol* 1997;35:2252–2255.

198. Gomez B, Figueroa, Hamilton AJ, Oritz BL, Robeldo MA, Restrepo A, Hay RJ. Development of a novel antigen detection test for histoplasmosis. *J Clin Microbiol* 1997;2618–2622.

199. Wheat J, Wheat H, Connolly P, et al. Cross-reactivity in *Histoplasma capsulatum* variety capsulatum antigen assays of urine samples from patients with endemic mycoses. *Clin Infect Dis* 1997;24:1169–1171.

200. Pappagianis D, Zimmer BL. Serology of coccidioidomycosis. *Clin Microbiol Rev* 1990;3:247–268.

201. Soufleris AJ, Klein BS, Courtney BT, Proctor ME, Jones JM. Utility of anti-WI-1 serological testing in the diagnosis of blastomycosis in Wisconsin residents. *Clin Infect Dis* 1994;19:87–92.

202. Supparatpinyo K, Khamwan C, Baosoung V, Nelson KE, Sirisanthana T. Disseminated *Penicillium marneffei* infection in southeast Asia. *Lancet* 1994;344 [8915]:110–113.

203. Sirisanthana V, Sirisanthana T. *Penicillium marneffei* infection in children infected with human immunodeficiency virus. *Pediatr Infect Dis J* 1993;12:1021–1025.

204. Walsh TJ, Dixon DM. Nosocomial aspergillosis: environmental microbiology, hospital epidemiology, diagnosis, and treatment. *Eur J Epidemiol* 1989;5:131–142.

205. Denning DW, Stevens DA. Antifungal and surgical treatment of invasive aspergillosis: review of 2,121 cases. *Rev Infect Dis* 1990;12: 1147–1201.

206. Panos R, Barr L, Walsh TJ, et al. Factors associated with fatal hemoptysis in cancer patients. *Chest* 1988;94:1008–1013.

207. Orr DP, Myerowitz RL, Dubois PJ. Patho-radiologic correlation of invasive pulmonary aspergillosis in the compromised host. *Cancer* 1978;41:2028.

208. Slavin ML, Knowles GK, Phillips MJ, et al. The air crescent sign of invasive pulmonary aspergillosis in acute leukemia. *Thorax* 1982;37: 554.

209. Kuhlman JE, Fishman EK, Burch PA, Karp JE, Zerhouni EA, Siegelman SS. Invasive pulmonary aspergillosis in acute leukemia. The contribution of CT to early diagnosis and aggressive management. *Chest* 1987.92:95–99.

210. Caillot D, Casasnovas O, Bernard A, et al. Improved management of invasive pulmonary aspergillosis in neutropenic patients using early thoracic computed tomographic scan and surgery. *J Clin Oncol* 1997; 15:139–147.

211. Aisner J, Schimpff SC, Wiernik PH. Treatment of invasive aspergillosis: relationship of early diagnosis and treatment to response. *Ann Intern Med* 1977;86:539.

212. Barloon TJ, Galvin JR, Mori M, Stanford W, Gingrich RD. Ultrafast chest CT in the clinical management of febrile bone marrow transplant patients with normal or nonspecific chest roentgenograms. *Chest* 1991;99:928–933.

213. Walsh TJ, Garrett K, Feuerstein E, et al. *Therapeutic* monitoring of experimental invasive pulmonary aspergillosis by ultrafast computerized tomography: a novel non-invasive method for measuring responses of organism-mediated tissue injury. *Antimicrob Agents Chemother* 1995;39:1065–1069.

214. Rinaldi MG. Invasive aspergillosis. *Rev Infect Dis* 1983;5:1061–1069.

215. Aisner J, Murillo J, Schimpff SC, et al. Invasive aspergillosis in acute leukemia: correlation with nose cultures and antibiotic use. *Ann Intern Med* 1979;90:4–10.

216. Yu VL, Muder RR, Poorsattar A. Significance of isolation of *Aspergillus* from the respiratory tract in diagnosis of invasive pulmonary aspergillosis. Results of a three-year prospective study. *Am J Med* 1986;81:249–56.

217. Treger TR, Visscher DW, Bartlett MS, et al. Diagnosis of pulmonary infection caused by *Aspergillus*: usefulness of respiratory cultures. *J Infect Dis* 1985;152:572–578.

218. Albelda SM, Talbot GH, Gerson SL, et al. Role of fiberoptic bronchoscopy in the diagnosis of invasive pulmonary aspergillosis in patients with acute leukemia. *Am J Med* 1984;76:1027.

219. Kahn FW, Jones JM, England DM. The role of bronchoalveolar lavage in the diagnosis of invasive pulmonary aspergillosis. *Am J Clin Pathol* 1986;86:518–24.

220. Saito H, Anaissie EJ, Morice RC, Dekmezian R, Bodey GP. Bronchoalveolar lavage in the diagnosis of pulmonary infiltrates in patients with acute leukemia. *Chest* 1988;94:745–749.

221. Burch PA, Karp JE, Merz WG. et al. Favorable outcome of invasive aspergillosis in patients with acute leukemia. *J Clin Oncol* 1987;5: 1985–1993.

222. Lehmann PF, Reiss E. Invasive aspergillosis: antiserum for circulating antigen produced after immunization with serum from infected rabbits. *Infect Immun* 1978;20:570–572.

223. Reiss E, Lehmann PF. *Galactomannan antigenemia* in invasive aspergillosis. *Infect Immun* 1979;25:357–365.

224. Dupont B, Huber M, Kim SJ, et al. *Galactomannan antigenemia* and antigenuria in aspergillosis: studies in patients with experimentally infected rabbits. *J Infect Dis* 1987;155:1–9.

225. Verweij PE, Rijs AJ, De Pauw BE, Horrevorts AM, Hoogkamp-Korstanje JA, Meis JF. Clinical evaluation and reproducibility of the Pastorex *Aspergillus* antigen latex agglutination test for diagnosing. *J Clin Pathol* 1995;48:474–476.

226. Kappe R, Schulze-Berge A. New cause for false-positive results with the Pastorex *Aspergillus* antigen latex agglutination test. *J Clin Microbiol* 1993;31:2489–2490.

227. Verweij PE, Stynen D, Rijs AJ, de Pauw BE, Hoogkamp-Korstanje JA, Meis JF. Sandwich enzyme-linked immunosorbent assay compared with Pastorex latex agglutination test for diagnosing invasive aspergillosis in immunocompromised patients. *J Clin Microbiol* 1995; 33:1912–1914.

228. Patterson TF, George D, Miniter P, Andriole VT. Saperconazole therapy in a rabbit model of invasive aspergillosis. *Antimicrob Agents Chemother* 1992;36:2681–2685.

229. Patterson TF, Miniter P, Patterson JE, Rappeport JM, Andriole VT. *Aspergillus* antigen detection in the diagnosis of invasive aspergillosis. *J Infect Dis* 1995;171:1553–1558.

230. Patterson TF, Miniter P, Ryan JL, Andriole VT. Effect of immunosuppression and amphotericin B on *Aspergillus* antigenemia in an experimental model. *J Infect Dis* 1988;158:415–422.

231. Tang CM, Holden DW, Aufauvre-Brown A, Cohen J. The detection of *Aspergillus* spp. by the polymerase chain reaction and its evaluation in bronchoalveolar lavage fluid. *Am Rev Respir Dis* 1993;148:1313–1317.

232. Hopfer RL, Walden P, Setterquist S, Highsmith WE. Detection and differentiation of fungi in clinical specimens using polymerase chain reaction [PCR] amplification and restriction enzyme analysis. *J Med Vet Mycol* 1993;31:65–75.

233. Einsele H, Hebart H, Roller G, et al. Detection and identification of fungal pathogens in blood by using molecular probes. *J Clin Microbiol* 1997;35:1353–1360.

234. Verweij PE, Latge JP, Rijs AJ, et al. Comparison of antigen detection and PCR assay using bronchoalveolar lavage fluid for diagnosing invasive pulmonary aspergillosis in patients receiving treatment for hematological malignancies. *J Clin Microbiol* 1995;33:3150–3153.

235. Yamakami Y, Hashimoto A, Tokimatsu I, Nasu M. PCR detection of DNA specific for *Aspergillus* species in serum of patients with invasive aspergillosis. *J Clin Microbiol* 1996;34:2464–2468.

236. Sugar AM. Mucormycosis. *Clin Infect Dis* 1992;14[Suppl 1]:S126–S129.

237. Walsh TJ, Renshaw G, Andrews J, et al. Invasive zygomycosis due to *Conidiobolus incongruus*. *Clin Infect Dis* 1994;19:423–430.

238. Agger WA, Maki DG. Mucormycosis: a complication of critical care. *Arch Intern Med* 1978;138:925–931.

239. Chandler FW, Kaplan W, Ajello L. *Color atlas and text of the histopathology of mycotic diseases.* Chicago: Year Book; 1980:122–127, 294–301.

240. Chandler FW, Watts JC, Kaplan W, et al. Zygomycosis. Report of four cases with formation of chlamydoconidia in tissue. *Am J Clin Pathol* 1985;84:9–14.

241. Goodman NL, Rinaldi MG. Agents of zygomycosis. In: Balows A, Hausler WJ, Herrmann K, Isenberg HD, Shadomy HJ, eds. *Manual of clinical microbiology,* 5th ed. Washington, DC: American Society of Microbiology 1991;674–692.

242. Rozich J, Oxendine D, Heffner J, Brzezinski W. Pulmonary zygomycosis. A cause of positive lung scan diagnosed by bronchoalveolar lavage. *Chest* 1989;95:238–240.

243. Anaissie E, Bodey GP, Kantarjian H, Ro J, Vartivarian SE, Hopfer R, Hoy J, Rolston K. New spectrum of fungal infections in patients with cancer. *Rev Infect Dis* 1989;11:369–378.

244. Anaissie E, Kantarjian H, Jones P, et al. Fusarium: a newly recognized fungal pathogen in immunosuppressed patients. *Cancer* 1986;57:2141–2145.

245. Martino P, Gastaldi R, Raccah R, Girmenia C. Clinical patterns of *Fusarium* infections in immunocompromised patients. *J Infect* 1994;[Suppl 1]:7–15.

246. Merz W, Karp J, Hoagland M, et al. Diagnosis and successful treatment of fusariosis in the compromised host. *J Infect Dis* 1988;158:1046–1055.

247. Anaissie E, Kantarjian H, Ro J, et al. The emerging role of *Fusarium* infections in patients with cancer. *Medicine* 1988;67:77–83.

248. Kappe R, Fauser C, Okeke CN, Maiwald M. Universal fungus-specific primer systems and group-specific hybridization oligonucleotides for 18S rDNA. *Mycoses* 1996;39:25–30.

249. Appel DJ, Gordon TR. Intraspecific variation within populations of *Fusarium oxysporum* based on RFLP analysis of the intergenic spacer region of the rDNA. *Exp Mycol* 1995;19:120–128.

250. Appel DJ, Gordon TR. Relationships among pathogenic and nonpathogenic isolates of *Fusarium oxysporum* based on the partial sequence of the intergenic spacer region of the ribosomal DNA. *Mol Plant Microbe Interact* 1996;9:125–138.

251. Alsip SG, Cobbs CG. *Pseudallescheria boydii* infection of the central system in a cardiac transplant recipient. *South Med J* 1986;79:383–384.

252. Armin AR, Reddy VB, Orfei E. Fungal endocarditis caused by *Pseudallescheria [Petriellidium] boydii* in an intravenous drug user, *Tex Heart Inst J* 1987;14:321–324.

253. Berenguer J, Diaz-Mediavilla J, Urra D, Munoz P. Central nervous system infection caused by *Pseudallescheria boydii*: case report and review. *Rev Infect Dis* 1990;11:890–896.

254. Galgiani JN, Stevens DA, Graybill JR, Stevens DL, Tillinghest AJ, Levine HB. *Pseudallescheria boydii* infections treated with ketoconazole. Clinical evaluations of seven patients and *in vitro* susceptibility results. *Chest* 1984;86:219–224.

255. Travis LB, Roberts GD, Wilson WR. Clinical significance of *Pseudallescheria boydii*: a review of 10 years' experience. *Mayo Clin Proc* 1985;60:531–537.

256. Welty FK, McLeod GX, Ezratty C, Healy RW, Karchmer AW. *Pseudallescheria boydii* endocarditis of the pulmonic valve in a liver transplant recipient. *Clin Infect Dis* 1992;15:858–860.

257. Walsh TJ, Peter J, McGough DA, Fothergill AW, Rinaldi MG, Pizzo PA. Activity of amphotericin B and antifungal azoles alone and in combination against *Pseudallescheria boydii*. *Antimicrob Agents Chemother* 1995;39:1361–1364.

258. Sandhu GS, Kline BC, Stockman L, Roberts GD. Molecular probes for diagnosis of fungal infections. *J Clin Microbiol* 1995;33:2913–2919.

259. Wood GM, McCormack JG, Muir DB, Ellis DH, et al. Clinical features of human infection with *Scedosporium inflatum*. *Clin Infect Dis* 1992;14:1027–1033.

Transplant Infections edited by
Raleigh A. Bowden, Per Ljungman, and Carlos V. Paya.
Lippincott–Raven Publishers, Philadelphia © 1998

CHAPTER 8

Pneumonia

Catherine Cordonnier and Isabel Cunningham

Pneumonia is the most common infection after transplant of any organ and is the infection with the highest mortality. Improvement in overall results in all transplants has resulted from improvements in recognizing and treating post-transplant pneumonias. Features common to all transplant patients are immunocompromise, interventions with surgery and/or diagnostic procedures, and treatment with antibiotics, all of which affect the risk for pneumonia. The underlying disease and prior treatment and complications may increase the risk for certain patients. Because individual infections are discussed in detail in other parts of this book, this chapter will focus on the factors that make the lungs particularly susceptible to infections after transplant, the time after transplant when they most commonly occur, and principles of diagnosis and management in the most commonly performed transplants.

ALTERED PULMONARY DEFENSE AFTER TRANSPLANT

The normally sterile lung has surveillance mechanisms that attempt to prevent colonization of airways with air-borne pathogens and to paralyze or kill those that pass the first barriers (1). In transplantation, normal surveillance may be altered. Marrow transplant candidates usually have had multiple chemotherapeutic agents, many of which may affect the lung prior to initiation of specific therapy for transplant. Surgery, ventilatory support, immunosuppressive therapy (including radiation), and infection itself may impair both immunologic and nonimmunologic lung defenses in any transplant patient. The presence of both donor and recipient cells in the lung, particularly in marrow and lung transplants, may cause local immunologic reactions and the release of a variety of cytokines, which can additionally impair native defenses and increase the risk of pulmonary infection.

Alterations in the mucosa, particularly the mucociliary apparatus, and the alveolar cell populations, particularly the macrophages, are especially important after transplant. The ciliated and squamous epithelium, from nasopharynx to distal bronchioles, is the first line of defense against pathogens in the airways. Surgical resection in lung or heart–lung transplants impairs the integrity of the mucosal surface. Mucociliary transport changes and mucosal damage may also be due to a patient's underlying disease, as in cystic fibrosis or primary immunodeficiency, or to prior infection with virus or mycoplasma. These conditions are at least transiently ciliolytic (1,2). The loss of cough reflex for several years after lung transplant may worsen this damage. Damage has been documented to persist long after transplant, particularly that due to bronchial clearance in lung transplants (3) and impairment of ciliated epithelium after lung and marrow transplant (4,5). Among other factors, irradiation in bone marrow transplant (BMT) conditioning protocols may be responsible for the latter.

Alveolar macrophages are important in lung defense, both as phagocytes and as immune effector cells. Immunosuppressive agents have been reported to affect the number and function of alveolar macrophages after transplant. Studies after BMT and lung transplant have shown impaired chemotaxis, phagocytosis, and killing of bacteria and fungi (6,7). In heart transplant patients, pulmonary edema has been associated with decreased antibacterial defenses by alveolar macrophages. Viral infections may also modify the phagocytic and killing properties of these cells. This effect may partially explain the observation that transplant patients who develop cytomegalovirus (CMV) infection have an increased incidence of co-morbid infection and an increase in other opportunistic infections. Prolonged neutropenia, as after BMT, may also be associated with a decreased number of alveolar macrophages (8).

The existence of two different cell populations may pose other problems in the lung (9–13). After lung trans-

CC: From Hopital Henri Mondor, 51 Av. du Maréchal de Lattre de Tassigny, 94000 Créteil, France. IC: Albert Einstein College of Medicine, 1300 Morris Park Avenue, Bronx, New York 10461.

plant, macrophages in the allografted lung come from recipient monocytes and dendritic cells of the donor are replaced by those of the recipient as well. The opposite occurs after allogeneic marrow transplant where donor monocyte precursors enter the lung. Post-transplant immune reactions—including graft rejection, bronchiolitis obliterans, and pulmonary fibrosis, related directly or indirectly to graft-versus-host disease (GvHD) after allogeneic BMT—may result from this mixed chimerism. Such immune reactions and the increased immunosuppression needed to treat them prolong the risk period for infectious complications past the first few months, and sometimes indefinitely. After lung transplant, local and systemic alterations of cytokine production have been found (13). Alveolar macrophages obtained from heart–lung transplant recipients have been shown to have a decreased production of TNFα. Moreover, when acute lung rejection occurs, many additional alterations are observed, including CD4 and CD8 lymphocyte activation; increased production of IL2; interferon-γ; TNFα; stimulation of the production of IL1, TNF, IL6, and IL8; and changes in the surfactant composition (13). Some of these events may alter the epithelial barrier and favor infection.

There are three main ways by which infectious pneumonia may occur after transplant: as a result of the surgical procedure and postoperative ventilation; as a consequence of environmental exposure, either nosocomial or in the community; and finally, by transplantation of an infected organ or by reactivation of latent infection in an immunosuppressed recipient.

MAGNITUDE OF THE PROBLEM

Recipients of all types of transplant are at risk for infectious pneumonia, and the causative infectious agents are the same in all transplants. However, the morbidity and mortality of these infections vary. In general, they are highest in transplants of lung and of stem cells and lowest in renal transplants. The occurrence of pneumonia in any recipient depends on the interrelationship of infectious exposure or reactivation, the condition of the lungs, and the degree of immunosuppression. Bacterial pneumonia is a risk for all transplanted patients early after transplant, which is the peri-operative period for solid organs and the period of conditioning-related neutropenia for bone marrow transplants.

Opportunistic pneumonias generally occur subsequent to the early risk period, and correlate with the degree and duration of immunosuppression. Immunosuppressive agents are given to all solid organ recipients, to prevent or treat rejection, from the time of transplant, and are usually continued indefinitely at the lowest possible levels. Almost all recipients of allogeneic stem cell transplants receive continuous immunosuppression for months to years, not to prevent rejection but to control graft-versus-

host reaction. The only recipients who require no post-transplant immunosuppression are recipients of syngeneic (identical twin) cells or of allogeneic cells from which most T cells have been removed. Likewise, most recipients of autologous grafts do not receive immunosuppression, unless they receive cyclosporine in an effort to induce a graft-versus-tumor effect. Patients in whom immunosuppression is required at the higher levels are at highest risk for mortality from pneumonia. These include allogeneic BMT recipients with GvHD and solid organ recipients needing increased immunosuppression to control rejection.

Since 1980, key pharmacological advances, including cyclosporine, trimethoprim-sulfamethoxazole, and ganciclovir, have decreased early morbidity and mortality in all types of transplants, so that the 1-year survival for heart, lung, liver, and pancreas transplants is now at least 75% to 95% in the worldwide registry (14). In solid organ transplants, the introduction of cyclosporine was associated with a decreased incidence in all types of pneumonias, related to its effect on reducing organ rejection, which lessened the requirement for heightened immunosuppression. The incidence of early bacterial pneumonia, which occurred in more than half of organ and marrow transplant patients, has steadily decreased, so that it is now reported in 10% to 15% of patients or less (15,16).

The pneumonias with the greatest potential for morbidity and mortality for all transplant patients are still those caused by cytomegalovirus and aspergillus, although the incidence of both infections was reported to decrease in solid organ transplant after the introduction of cyclosporine. Evidence of CMV infection was reported in most transplant patients before effective antiviral prophylaxis. CMV pneumonia was seen in up to 20% of all transplants but was observed in up to 40% of lung transplant patients. This pneumonia was associated with mortality of 50% to 90% in solid organ and invariably closer to 100% in allogeneic stem cell transplants, prior to the availability of ganciclovir, which has decreased the mortality to 15% or less in most types of transplants. Fungal pneumonia, and aspergillus in particular, is the infection whose mortality has changed little over this time. Its incidence is generally reported from 9% to 27% in both solid organ and stem cell transplants, and the mortality remains high, from 60% to 100%. It is highest in stem cell and liver transplants and in those in whom immunosuppression is profound and protracted.

PRINCIPLES OF MANAGEMENT

Management of pulmonary infections after transplant requires a high degree of suspicion and early use of diagnostic procedures (17,18). In the last 20 years bronchoscopy and endobronchial sampling using bronchoalveolar lavage (BAL) have become the established primary technique for investigating pulmonary infection.

Its use in routine surveillance, which is standard practice after pulmonary and heart transplants, allows for earlier initiation of therapy, and contributes to the improved survival after pneumonia. Invasive diagnostic procedures, mainly used secondarily, need to be selected in situations where BAL is noncontributory, weighing the risk of increased morbidity.

Clinical Approach to Pneumonia

A systematic approach to pneumonia in any transplant patient should include consideration of the following:

History

Knowledge of a patient's exposure, travel, environmental risks, and previous infection, the hospital epidemiology, and the pretransplant serology of both recipient and donor, particularly for CMV and toxoplasmosis, is essential in evaluating a transplant patient with evidence of pneumonia. Exposure to tuberculosis should be evaluated in all candidates for organ transplantation by PPD testing during screening. Donor infectious history may be unavailable, and Gram stain of the donor trachea before lung transplant has been used in individualizing perioperative antibiotics for certain transplant patients. A history of recurrent bacterial infection, which may occur in cystic fibrosis, may require special consideration in choosing antibiotics.

Clinical Presentation

Symptoms and signs of pneumonia may or may not be typical of a known infectious cause. As in all immunosuppressed patients, there may be scarce findings, so any symptoms must be carefully and quickly evaluated, considering that any infection can progress rapidly in the immunosuppressed patient. Fever or cough or sputum production may be absent. Hypoxemia may be the sole finding, and even if the x-ray is normal, bronchoscopic evaluation should be considered. The presence of any such symptom may, however, reflect a noninfectious etiology, such as idiopathic fibrosis or alveolar hemorrhage. For example, dyspnea is characteristic of interstitial processes but is not pathognomonic for any one cause, and an inactive patient may not manifest hypoxemia, even in the setting of a widespread process. Acute thoracic pain, with or without hemoptysis, may indicate embolic disease (Fig. 1), but may also indicate aspergillus. Pneumothorax may be seen in *P. carinii* pneumonia, particularly in patients who receive aerosolized pentamidine, but may also occur in mycobacterial or aspergillus infection, or fibrosis (Fig. 2). The rapid onset of pneumonia is consistent with bacterial pneumonia and pulmonary edema with thromboembolism but may also occur in viral infections in immunosuppressed patients. A subacute or chronic onset can suggest fungal or parasitic infection, although either may present abruptly.

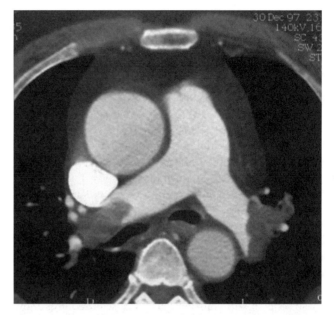

Figure 1. Pulmonary embolism (Helical CT-scan). Bilateral proximal obliteration of both pulmonary arteries due to massive embolism occurring 3 weeks after a liver transplant in a 55-year-old man, revealed by fever and dyspnea. No infection was found at autopsy.

Imaging

Post-transplant pneumonia may be focal, multifocal, or diffuse; interstitial, alveolar, or mixed. Evaluation requires a chest x-ray of good quality. When patients are housed in intensive care or laminar airflow rooms, or are

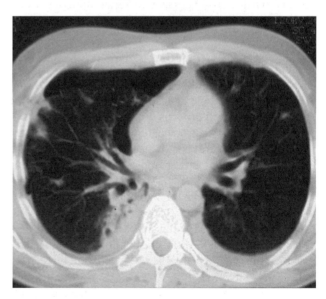

Figure 2. Pneumothorax revealing idiopathic fibrosis after allogeneic SCT (high-resolution CT scan). Patchy alveolar lesions with hydropneumothorax in a 35-year-old man 6 months after allogeneic SCT for acute lymphoid leukemia. The lung lesions were found on biopsy to be due to idiopathic fibrosis.

on mechanical ventilation, good-quality x-rays may be impossible. Every effort must be made to obtain optimal studies, and ones that can be compared with others, with consideration of moving to bronchoscopy quickly. Most x-ray patterns are nonspecific. Where an x-ray appears negative in a symptomatic patient, chest CT scan may reveal abnormalities (19,20). CT may additionally provide localization of lesions and proximity to pulmonary vessels, important if lung biopsy is contemplated, and may detect small pleural effusions. Certain CT findings may suggest particular infections (19,20). For example, the halo sign, a zone of lower attenuation surrounding a pulmonary mass, has been associated with aspergillus infection. This may be present early in a neutropenic patient after BMT, whereas the presence of an air crescent sign on x-ray requires neutrophils. However, even with improved definition of pneumonia, CT scan does not replace the isolation of the pathogen for diagnosis. Also, one should consider that a CT scan requires moving a patient from a protected room, which may provide an opportunity for exposure to infection such as aspergillus. Thoracic imaging with ^{67}Ga-citrate or indium-labeled IgG may be useful in transplant patients, especially in the setting of an apparently negative chest x-ray. Although diffuse gallium uptake has had more than 90% sensitivity for *P. carinii* in AIDS (21), in transplant there are other etiologies for positive gallium, which include infectious and noninfectious pneumonia (22), so that a positive result should be interpreted cautiously.

Any work-up using radiologic procedures should be done expeditiously to avoid delay in obtaining the pathogen. They should be completed rapidly and lead quickly to a diagnostic procedure. Serial follow-up x-rays are essential in evaluating treatment.

Diagnostic Investigation

Blood cultures should be done routinely but are of limited value in diagnosing pneumonia except where the pathogen has a high propensity for the blood, such as *S. pneumoniae*, or in neutropenia. Special culture media are required when nocardia or atypical mycobacteria are suspected. Other specimens should be obtained, depending on the clinical setting, such as skin biopsy, CSF, serologies where likely to be reliable (unlikely early after BMT), and antigenemia (of documented usefulness in cryptococcus and CMV, currently being studied in candida and aspergillus). At the present time, no noninvasive examinations can replace the specificity of direct pulmonary investigation.

Sputum analysis should be reviewed, considering that it may yield only organisms colonizing the oropharynx. The results may be difficult to interpret, especially in the transplant patient who receives multiple antibiotics. A positive culture may be valuable when agents are isolated that do not normally inhabit the oropharynx, especially

Legionella, mycobacteria, and certain fungi. The importance of finding aspergillus in the sputum depends on the degree of immunosuppression of the patient and the risk of withholding antifungal therapy until further documentation. In BMT patients with pneumonia, a positive sputum culture may be highly suspicious for pulmonary aspergillosis. In the same way, the presence of *Mycobacterium tuberculosis* in the sputum of a transplant patient may be considered as the cause of the pneumonia when clinical and radiologic signs support this etiology. Induced sputum has not been shown to be useful in transplant patients for diagnosing *P. carinii* pneumonia, unlike in AIDS patients.

The standard for diagnosing pulmonary infection is bronchoscopic sampling with lavage (23–25) (Table 1). The yield of protected brushing and transbronchial biopsy in the same procedure may be additive but increases the potential for complications. Lavage is safe, minimally invasive, and reproducible. Lavage, usually with biopsy, is performed routinely in lung transplant patients in the first month after lung transplant in most large centers, to monitor rejection and to seek occult infection. In the transplant of other organs and stem cells, BAL is the first investigative procedure performed for pulmonary symptoms. The clinician who seeks consultation from a pulmonary specialist for BAL should address the likely thrombocytopenia with transfusion and alert the microbiology laboratories to ensure that all potential organisms are sought. Close follow-up after the procedure is mandatory, with knowledge that fever may be expected in up to half of patients, and chest x-rays may be transiently worse the day following the procedure (26). A routine BAL protocol should include at least total and differential cell counts on cytocentrifuge preparations using May-Grünwald-Giemsa (MGG) stains, and cytologic examination on cell pellets obtained by centrifugation and cytocentrifugation stained with MGG and Papanicolaou for virus and the Gomori-Grocott method for *P. carinii* and fungi. Other stains are necessary to identify alveolar proteinosis (periodic acid-Schiff), mycobacteria (Zielh), and siderophages (Prussian Blue) (27) (see Table 1).

A sample of fluid should be sent for bacteriologic, viral, and fungal cultures. Aspiration and BAL fluids should be examined for *Legionella pneumophilia* by direct immunofluorescence and cultures, and for nocardia and mycobacteria. Immunofluorescent assays using specific monoclonal antibodies for detecting *P. carinii* have been recently reported as more sensitive than stains (24). The viruses to be detected on alveolar fluid by culture, immunologic assay, or polymerase chain reaction (PCR) should be determined with the laboratory according to the clinical setting. Because the principal viral infections documented after transplants are herpes simplex virus and mainly CMV, they should be routinely searched, even if prophylactic and preemptive antiviral treatments have

TABLE 1. *Investigations on bronchoscopic samples in transplant patients*

Sample	Laboratory investigations	
	Essential	Optional
Protected bacteriologic sample (brush or catheter)	Gram stain	Search for bacteria in neutrophils
	Quantitative culture	
Aspiration	Legionella (IFA/DFA stains, culture on BCYE[a] medium)	India ink
	Mycobacteria and nocardia (AFB stain, culture)	
	Fungi (wet mount, culture)	
Lavage fluid	Cytologic exam of lavage fluid on smear and after cytocentrifugation: direct examination, differential count, viral inclusions, pathogens	Stains: Papanicolaou Periodic Acid Schiff Perls' Prussian Blue (hemosiderin-laden macrophages)
	Stains: May Grunwald Giemsa Gomori methamine silver (or alternative stain for *P. carinii*)	Immunodetermination of CD4/CD8 alveolar lymphocytes
	Microbiologic processing: Gram stain, culture Legionella (IFA/DFA, culture on BCYE medium) Mycobacteria Fungi (Wet mount stain, culture)	Toxoplasmosis: IFA Aspergillus antigen
	Virus: All possible viruses, particularly the herpes family: centrifugation culture, antigen detection	Adeno- and respiratory viruses: IFA/DFA, culture
Transbronchial biopsy[b]	Histology	

[a]BCYE, buffered charcoal yeast extract; IFA, indirect immunofluorescence; DFA, direct immunofluorescence.
[b]Transbronchial biopsy is essential for noninfectious processes and less contributive than BAL for infectious pneumonia.

dramatically decreased their incidence as causes of pneumonia after transplant. Some teams look at the same time for HHV6. Adenovirus and other respiratory viruses (including respiratory syncytial virus, influenza, parainfluenza) should be considered, particularly in the setting of known exposures and during seasonal outbreaks (28–30).

In one-half to two-thirds of cases, BAL yields a diagnosis in transplant patients similar to that of other immunocompromised patients, and the diagnosis is most often infectious. The yield may vary with the type of pneumonia, being more than 90% in *P. carinii* pneumonia and CMV, and much lower in mycobacteria or aspergillus, where up to 50% of infections may be missed or misdiagnosed (24).

A protected bacteriologic sample should be considered with BAL, in the patient not on broad-spectrum antibiotics and where the clinical pattern is consistent with a bacterial pneumonia. This can be done by protected brush specimen or by plugged telescoping catheter, and processed by quantitative culture techniques. The minimal threshold bacterial concentration required to consider the isolated pathogen as the cause of the pneumonia with both techniques is $\geq 10^3$ CFU (colony-forming units) per milliliter. Otherwise, the commonly accepted criteria for bacterial pneumonia on culture of BAL fluid is $\geq 10^4$–10^5 CFU/ml (31,32). If the patient is ventilated, these samples may be obtained through the endotracheal

tube, provided that the positive expiratory pressure is less than 10 cm and inspired oxygen is greater than 60%. However, many feel that cytologic examination of alveolar fluid recovered in this setting is more difficult to interpret, as the quality may be suboptimal.

Transbronchial biopsy is routine in surveillance and evaluation of symptoms in patients with lung transplants, but it is not routine in BMT patients because of the risks of bleeding and the fact that it does not add significantly to BAL in identifying pathogens. It is particularly important in differentiating infectious from immunologic processes such as graft rejection in lung transplants or bronchiolitis obliterans in both BMT and lung transplants (33). The investigative procedures to be performed on lavage samples are listed in Table 1 and should be discussed according to the transplant setting, seasonal considerations, and hospital epidemiology. This list is not exhaustive, and new sensitive and specific laboratory tests are currently being investigated and could be added in the near future if relevant (24).

In cases where bronchoscopy does not yield a pathogen, one may consider a second BAL, and/or a transbronchial biopsy, or transthoracic needle aspiration under CT scan when a lesion is considered accessible. The final decision between lung biopsy (through open or video-assisted thoracoscopy) or empiric treatment to cover the most likely organisms should be made by the transplant physician and the lung specialist after weighing the risks of surgery, empiric treatment, and failure to reach a diagnosis. After BMT, focal lesions that develop or persist despite antibiotics are mostly of fungal origin. Successful fine-needle aspiration has been reported, with a 15% rate of complications (34). Lung biopsy is more helpful in prolonged clinical course, and in nodular or cavitary patterns, than in acute and/or nonnodular diseases (35).

Consideration of Noninfectious Processes

The lung is also the site of numerous noninfectious injuries (Table 2). These need to be considered, as they may require specific treatments such as diuresis or anticoagulation. The probability may vary by time after transplant and by type of transplant. Alveolar hemorrhage may complicate any transplant, and should be differentiated from infections that may cause hemorrhage, such as aspergillus or pseudomonas. It has been found in 11% to 26% of autologous stem cell transplants, and an incidence of 41% of allogeneic BMT recipients with acute GvHD was reported in one study where autopsies were available (27,36). Alveolar proteinosis may rarely occur in the setting of BMT in hematologic diseases, especially during the first 3 months. Its diagnosis requires special stains (37). The lung may also be the site of a neoplastic process.

Acute respiratory distress syndrome may complicate pulmonary infection and may occur in the setting of a nonpulmonary infection, such as in some cases of alfa-streptococcal bacteremia occurring in neutropenic patients (see the section entitled "Stem Cell Transplant") or of a noninfectious process. It may also occur in the first 2 weeks following liver transplantation, and especially after retransplantation (38), or within 48 hours of cardiopulmonary bypass (39). After lung transplant, lesional pulmonary edema may be observed during the first days, as a result of several factors, including ischemia, denervation, and graft rejection (40,41). The occurrence of mediastinitis should always be suspected after any thoracic surgery.

The lung may be the site of immunologic conflict when the immune system of one of the donor–recipient pair develops cytotoxicity against the lung structures of the other (10). This is observed after lung or heart–lung transplant, where graft rejection may mimic infection, especially viral infection, and is often associated with it.

Idiopathic interstitial pneumonia is a complication reported in most allogeneic SCT studies, with more than 70% in-hospital mortality rate (42). It has been associated with acute and chronic GvHD, high-dose total-body irradiation, and older age (42–44). The responsibility of some pathogens may be underestimated in this syndrome, either because they are not systematically searched (i.e., respiratory viruses or HHV6) or because they are still unidentified.

Finally, bronchiolitis obliterans (or obliterative bronchiolitis) is an important factor contributing to death after 6 months in lung and stem cell transplants. Its incidence varies from 7% to 54% after lung transplant with a mortality rate of 30% to 40% (45). After allogeneic SCT, the overall incidence of bronchiolitis obliterans has been reported to be 2% (46), and it has not been reported after syngeneic or autologous transplant. The condition has been related to decreased serum IgG and chronic GvHD, with a frequency varying between 6% and 10% of patients with chronic GvHD who survive 120 days (46,47). As in most obstructive lung diseases, it is associated with sinusitis in half the cases and is often complicated by infections, especially due to *Haemophilus influenzae* (Fig. 3), *S. pneumoniae*, *Aspergillus* spp., and respiratory viruses. Alveolar or nodular infiltrates may be seen in the setting of allogeneic marrow transplant, as a result of bronchiolitis obliterans organizing pneumonia (48).

TABLE 2. *Main noninfectious causes of pneumonia in transplant patients*

Clinical setting	Cause
Any transplant	Fluid overload/pulmonary edema
	Alveolar hemorrhage
	Pulmonary embolism
	Leukoagglutin reaction
	Acute respiratory distress syndrome
	Hypersensitivity drug reaction
	Tumor
	EBV-associated lymphoma
	Pulmonary calcinosis
Lung and Heart-lung transplants	Intrathoracic bleeding postprocedure
	Graft rejection
	Bronchiolitis obliterans
Bone marrow transplant	Alveolar proteinosis
	Pulmonary veno-occlusive disease
	Radiation pneumonitis
	Idiopathic interstitial pneumonia
	Bronchiolitis obliterans

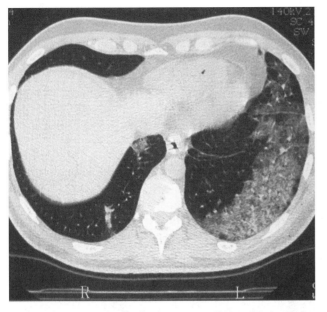

Figure 3. Haemophilus influenzae pneumonia (high-resolution CT scan). Alveolo-interstitial infiltrate of left lower lobe in acute lymphoid leukemia patient 5 months after receiving pheno-identical SCT while on steroids and cyclosporine for GvHD, found to be H. influenzae. The slight peribronchial vascular thickening developed into bronchiolitis obliterans several weeks thereafter.

Starting Treatment and Reevaluation of Efficacy

Because any pneumonia occurring in the setting of transplant may be life-threatening, empiric antibiotics against the likely organisms must be started without delay. Consideration should be given to the likelihood of fungus in patients with prolonged neutropenia and those on steroid therapy. Some empiric treatments can negate subsequent results, especially for bacteria and viruses, but may be warranted. It is essential to investigate these patients as early as possible in the course of the pneumonia and to be sure the laboratories look for all possible pathogens so that no time will be lost making the diagnosis. Some empirical treatments will not change the chance of isolating the pathogen for at least several days so that investigation may be delayed while empiric treatment is begun (as in Cotrimoxazole for *P. carinii*, antifungals for aspergillosis). Decreasing immunosuppression may be beneficial as part of the treatment of pneumonia, especially when the occurrence of the infection is clearly related to the depth of immunosuppression, as for post-transplant lymphoma associated with Epstein-Barr virus (EBV).

Clinical and etiologic reevaluation should be done at regular intervals, especially when no diagnosis was initially established. New investigations should be undertaken rapidly when the pneumonia does not respond to empirical treatment. Even when the cause of the pneumonia has been established, the occurrence of new signs or new infiltrates should be regarded as suspicious for new infections, keeping in mind that the association of several pathogens or the successive occurrence of different causes of pneumonia is usual in this setting.

Place of Intensive Care and of Ventilatory Support

The treatment of pneumonia may require intensive care and ventilatory support. The decision to transfer a patient to an intensive care unit (ICU) is particularly difficult in terms of physical and emotional burden for the patient, his family, and the caregivers. Data on survival after ICU admission are available for BMT patients, compiled mainly in the 1980s. Survival was low (0 to 11%) and best for nonrespiratory primary problems, such as neurological or surgical complications, and worst when multiple organs were failing in addition to the lung (49–52). Even when patients survived the ICU episode, there was high mortality from other events within 6 months. Guidelines for decision making have been published (52). It should be remembered that since the 1980s there have been improvements in the diagnosis and treatment of viral and fungal infections, the infections with the highest mortality after transplant of any organ. Together with greater ICU experience with such patients, these factors may result in improved survival statistics in the future (52a).

ICU transfer may be addressed very differently from one country to another, because of differences in culture, and in consideration of financial and emotional implications of the decisions. The prognosis of ventilated transplant patients may well continue to improve in the future. Guidelines should be adaptable to new data on the prognosis for ventilated patients, but in general, one should consider the chance of survival and return to acceptable life for the individual patient before transfer to an ICU. The patient and family should be provided with reasonable estimations of prognosis prior to transfer; in addition, the likelihood of continuing life support should be considered regularly during the course of treatment. In all series, the duration of ventilation was correlated with survival.

SPECIAL CONSIDERATIONS ACCORDING TO THE TYPE OF TRANSPLANT

Solid Organ Transplants

Heart

Heart transplants have been performed successfully for almost 30 years. The heart is the second most commonly transplanted organ after the kidney. Progressive improvements in surgical technique, immunosuppression protocols, and methods of diagnosing and treating infections have resulted in 1-year survival that is now greater than 85%, approaching that of renal transplants (14,16). Pneumonia is the most common infectious complication. Bacterial pneumonia is most common in the first month after cardiac transplant, and the risk is increased in older patients and those with chronic pulmonary edema, prolonged ventilator time, and CMV infection (15). In early reports, bacterial pneumonia occurred in more than two-thirds of patients, most frequently due to Gram-negative enteric organisms, but legionella and nocardia were also reported. The reported incidence of bacterial pneumonia has since declined to less than 5% (15,16) with the use of perioperative antibiotics, surveillance x-rays, and bronchoscopy, and the widespread use of cyclosporine and prophylactic trimethoprim-sulfamethoxazole. Since the introduction of this prophylaxis, cases of nocardia, legionella, and *P. carinii* are rarely seen (53,54). Prior to the general use of prophylaxis, pneumocystis pneumonia was seen in 9% to 11% of patients, an incidence similar to that of liver and kidney transplants, and mortality was 11% to 38% (54). The most common fungal pneumonia, due to aspergillus, has been reported in 14% at medians of 1–2 months after transplant (55). A decrease in aspergillus was noted after the introduction of cyclosporine, but the high mortality persists, variously reported between 60% and 75%, and is felt to be lower than those of marrow or liver transplant patients (16,55).

Prior to ganciclovir, almost all patients seropositive for cytomegalovirus prior to transplant developed evidence of CMV infection (16,53), dangerous for its morbidity but also both for its association with increased risk of cardiac graft rejection and for its immunomodulating effects that lead to other opportunistic infections. Pneumonia due to CMV was reported in 11% to 25% of cardiac transplant patients, at a mean of 3 months, and was rarely seen after 7 months (56). The mortality of CMV pneumonia was at least 75% before ganciclovir was used (53,56). More recently, prophylactic ganciclovir in seropositive patients has been demonstrated to decrease the incidence of pneumonia from 13% to 2% (57). For seronegative patients who receive seronegative hearts and are transfused with filtered and/or CMV-negative blood products, the risk of pneumonia is very low. Primary CMV infection, occurring in the seronegative recipient of a seropositive heart, continues to be a risk, even with prophylaxis (57).

The incidence of other viral pneumonias is rarely reported, and the true incidence may vary with the availability of specific diagnostic methods and the incidence of autopsies in a particular center. Pulmonary involvement by post-transplant EBV-associated lymphoproliferative disorder is more common in thoracic organ transplants than in renal transplants, and the risk in cardiac transplant persists for years after transplant, unlike in renal transplant patients in whom the risk decreases after the first year (58). This is presumably related to the need for prolonged use of high levels of immunosuppression in cardiac transplants, which lengthens the period at risk for opportunistic infections, which have been reported late after transplant (59). Pulmonary infiltrates are usually

nodular and associated with unremitting fever and high LDH levels. Generally, a biopsy specimen is required to make the diagnosis. This is one example where, in the appropriate setting, a negative BAL should be quickly followed by biopsy so that the treatment can be urgently initiated. Toxoplasmosis pneumonia has been rarely reported but can be rapidly fatal in the early post-transplant period in patients who are seronegative prior to transplant, even when myocardial biopsy is negative (53,60). The incidence of *Mycobacterium tuberculosis* pneumonia has decreased with universal PPD screening and prophylaxis where necessary, and since the use of cyclosporine, but may be increased in settings where history of exposure is high. Atypical mycobacterial infections involving the lungs may occur as late as 3 years after transplant (53).

Lungs

Since 1980 the most commonly performed lung transplant procedure has evolved from heart–lung and double-lung to single-lung transplants, for which the most common indication is chronic obstructive pulmonary disease (61). The incidence of most types of pneumonia has been higher in lung than in the other solid organ transplants, and the site of most pneumonias is the transplanted lung. Surgical denervation and lymphatic disruption impair the cough reflex and innate clearance mechanisms that greatly increase the risk in these patients (61).

Bacterial pneumonia is a risk throughout the post-transplant period, both early and late, with significant mortality. With improved protocols the incidence of early bacterial pneumonia has decreased from 35–66% to 10–13%, and mortality has dropped from 27–50% to 2% (53,62). Most large groups report the routine use of perioperative antibiotics that include an antipseudomonas agent and clindamycin, to cover anaerobes and staphylococci, for 3–5 days unless there is a positive culture, or underlying cystic fibrosis, where two antipseudomonas agents may be given for 10–14 days (63,64). Patients with cystic fibrosis, formerly felt to be at prohibitive risk from chronic and resistant pseudomonas and *Burkholderia cepacia* (formerly *P. cepacia*) infection, have not been found to have an increased risk of post-transplant pneumonia, if careful monitoring is instituted (63).

A significant percentage of lung transplant patients (24% to 50%) will develop obstructive bronchiolitis as a consequence of chronic rejection, and the resultant bronchiectasis puts them at risk for recurrent bacterial pneumonias, with a high incidence of pseudomonas and acinetobacter in most reports (61,63,65). Increased immunosuppression is usually undertaken to treat obstructive bronchiolitis, and in this set of patients, long-term survival is substantially lower than in those without bronchiolitis (30% vs. 60%) (64). Fungal infections also occur more frequently in lung transplants, mainly in the first month, but may also be seen as late as 2 years or more in patients still immunosuppressed (65). Although candida may be isolated from 50% to 100% of patients and may be considered colonization, pneumonia due to candida may occur early after transplant (66).

Aspergillus lung disease has been documented in 11% to 40% of heart–lung and lung transplants, varying in presentation from localized airway disease to nodular, cavitary, and interstitial infiltrates, and occurs frequently in association with CMV or other infection (61,66,67). *Aspergillus* tracheobronchitis has been responsive to itraconazole or aerosolized amphotericin (61), but aspergillus pneumonia treated with intravenous amphotericin has been difficult to eradicate, with mortality of more than 80% (61,62,66). Other fungi—including fusarium, cryptococcus, and histoplasma—should be considered and sought in the lung transplant patient. The risk of *P. carinii* pneumonia, between the third and sixth month, was reported to be 26% to 88% prior to the use of prophylaxis, higher in lung transplant than any other organ transplant (53,54,62,68). Prophylaxis with trimethoprim-sulfamethoxazole for 1 year is currently considered adequate unless immunosuppression is increased, when it is advised that prophylaxis should be resumed and continued indefinitely (68).

CMV infection is an important cause of morbidity and may be associated with an increased risk of rejection, the development of obliterative bronchiolitis, and other infections (61,69,70). Prior to ganciclovir, it was noted in 60% to 80% of those at risk for primary infection, and in 37% to 100% of patients overall (53,61). Pneumonia was the most common form of CMV infection, occurring in up to 50% of patients with CMV infection, with mortality variously reported at 27% to 67%. It must be differentiated from allograft rejection pathologically, as correct treatment is crucial. CMV pneumonia usually occurs within the first 3 months and may appear only in the transplanted lung (61,71). Treatment with ganciclovir reduced mortality to 1% in one report (62), with failures seen among seronegative recipients of positive organs. Results of prophylaxis and preemptive trials showed decrease in CMV infection similar to studies in cardiac transplants, except in those seronegative patients receiving lungs from positive donors, where the incidence remained 67% to 80%.

Herpes simplex pneumonia had been a significant risk, particularly in the setting of increased immunosuppression, but it has generally been prevented since the introduction of prophylactic acyclovir for seropositive patients. The potential for recurrence should be considered. Pneumonia with respiratory viruses—including influenza, parainfluenza, and RSV—may be associated with long-lasting decreased pulmonary function and bronchiolitis obliterans after lung transplant (61,72). Annual flu vaccination has been advocated for lung transplant patients (61). EBV-associated lymphoproliferative disease has been reported to occur twice as often in lung

transplants as in others (6.2% to 9.4%) with at least 40% mortality (62,73). Most cases involve the allografted lung. Reduction in immunosuppression and the use of acyclovir or ganciclovir resulted in resolution in a significant number of cases. Adenovirus pneumonia was reported in four of 308 transplants at Pittsburgh, three of which occurred in children, at 20–43 days after transplant. These pneumonias were severe and rapidly fatal (74). Pneumonias due to mycobacteria have been reported rarely but are noteworthy for their heterogeneous presentations, and their reported responsiveness to aggressive long-term therapy (61,62,75).

Kidney

Experience with renal transplants is longer and larger than with other transplants, with approximately 500,000 recorded in the worldwide registry through 1996 (14). Survival is highest in these transplants, with only 5% to 8% 1-year mortality reported to the registry for at least the last 10 years (14). The incidence of pneumonia is the lowest of all transplants (8% to 16%) (53). Bacterial pneumonia is reported in less than 5% in recent reviews (15), and most occur later in the first year, unlike bacterial pneumonia in other organ transplants (15,76). An increased risk has been correlated with the use of ALG or OKT3, with CMV infection, azotemia, and hypogammaglobulinemia (15). Pneumococcal pneumonia, which had been reported in more than 6%, has been generally preventable with pretransplant immunization. *Nocardia asteroides,* which had been reported in up to 20% of patients has, along with pneumocystis (Fig. 4), been effectively prevented with trimethoprim-sulfamethoxazole (77).

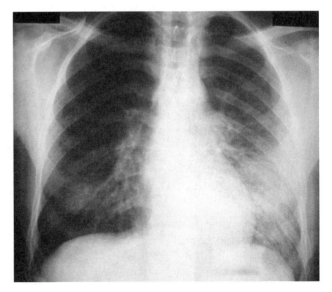

Figure 4. Pneumocystis carinii pneumonia. Diffuse interstitial pneumonia related to P. carinii diagnosed on BAL 5 months after kidney transplant.

As in other organ transplants, CMV pneumonia in renal transplants is no longer associated with 50% to 90% mortality, since the availability of ganciclovir, which is successful treatment in up to 90% of patients. Pneumonia due to respiratory viruses and adenovirus may also occur in these patients and should be considered in the appropriate setting (72,76,78). Aspergillus pneumonia has been reported in up to 10% of patients (67,76,79) with extremely high mortality and may occur later in renal than in transplants of other organs (79). Histoplasmosis, where pulmonary involvement is usual, has been reported in both endemic and nonendemic areas, up to 14 years after transplant, and often in the setting of increased immunosuppression (80).

Blastomycosis dermatiditis pneumonia was reported in five cases with both early and late presentations. Diagnosis may be difficult but serology may be useful, and surgical removal may be required (81). Toxoplasmosis pneumonia is a rare but important infection and should be considered, particularly in the first 3 months after transplant. In one report, both recipients of kidneys from a single donor developed toxoplasmosis pneumonia on days 39 and 41 following transplant, and the diagnosis was made at autopsy in both. With early recognition, treatment is generally successful (82). The incidence of *Mycobacterium tuberculosis* infection has been reported to be 0.65% to 2.3%, and up to 9.5% in endemic areas, occurring from 1 to 78 months after transplant, and most commonly involving the lung (53,75). A literature review of nontuberculous mycobacterial infections in solid organ tranpslants noted that most of the reported patients had had renal transplants. Twenty-eight percent of patients with nontuberculous infection had pulmonary involvement (83). The problems of drug interactions and the potential for graft rejection make treating these infections challenging, but the majority of mycobacterial infections may be successfully treated.

Liver

The incidence of bacterial pneumonia in liver transplants was 16% to 25%, second only to that of lung transplants in the 1980s, and associated with more than 40% mortality (15,53). Prolonged intubation and atelectasis, and impaired neutrophil chemotaxis have been suggested as predisposing factors (15,53). Prophylactic measures to decrease infection with enteric organisms have included perioperative antibiotics, antibiotics before and after cholangiograms, and selective bowel decontamination protocols used before and/or after transplant (84). The latter has been associated with a decrease in early Gram-negative pneumonia, but opinions vary as to its benefit in the absence of large trials (15,53,84).

Legionella has been a source of bacterial pneumonias in reports in the past 10 years, which emphasizes the importance of continuous monitoring of the water supply in transplant areas (84). Fungal infection occurs in up to 42% of liver transplant patients, in whom surgical disruption of the biliary tract and small bowel increases the risk of dissemination of gastrointestinal fungal organisms (84). Pneumonia due to fungi has the highest mortality of any infection after liver transplant. Aspergillus pneumonia has been reported in approximately 15% of liver transplant patients, with almost universal mortality (67,84) (Fig. 5).

Other fungal pneumonias, particularly from coccidiomycosis or cryptococcus, are occasionally reported (84,85). CMV infection occurs in 25% to 85% of patients within the first 3 months. Pneumonia is the second most frequent disease, after disease of the allografted liver, and has been reported in 13% to 30% of patients, with more than 75% survival after treatment with ganciclovir (84,86). EBV-associated lymphoproliferative disease involving the lungs may occur early after transplant, but the mean time in one study was 1.6 years.

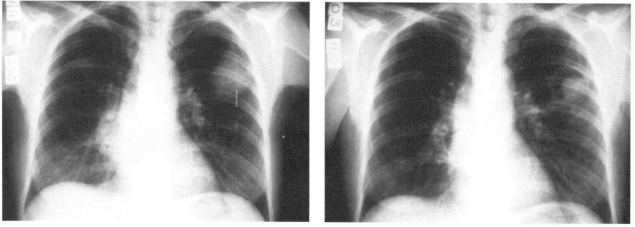

A   B

Figure 5. Fungus ball. Aspergillus may appear as a round lesion (**A**) that evolves into a fungus ball (**B**), as in this 22-year-old patient 45 days after liver transplant, which resolved after 6 months treatment and surgery.

These infections are important because their x-ray presentations are variable and because successful treatment depends on early diagnosis. In the past, the correct diagnosis has been made only at autopsy in more than 50% of cases (87). Other viral pneumonias, particularly due to adenovirus or respiratory syncytial virus, occur in 3% to 10% of patients, usually in the first month after transplant, and frequently in association with other infections (84,88). In one study of 17 cases of RSV, two deaths occurred in infants (88).

Pneumocystis pneumonia has been effectively prevented by the routine use of trimethoprim-sulfamethoxazole. Toxoplasmosis pneumonia, though rare, has been reported early after liver transplant and may be rapidly fatal (85,89). *M. tuberculosis* pneumonia, also rare, is important for its high mortality and the problems its treatment poses for drug interactions, particularly with cyclosporine. Because it has been reported early in the post-transplant period in patients in whom PPD testing was not done prior to transplant, testing is part of pre-transplant evaluation in most centers (90).

Stem Cell Transplant

Immunosuppression is profound from the time of allogeneic stem cell transplant, and the recovery time for immune reconstitution lasts at least several months, and may be years, or indefinitely, in those who have GvHD and require continued immunosuppressive therapy. In allogeneic transplant patients, infections occur in predictable risk periods. Gram-negative bacterial infections usually complicate the early transplant course, followed by opportunistic fungal and viral infections. The risk for opportunistic infection decreases after the first 6 months, except in patients with severe chronic GvHD. GvHD is the major factor influencing the incidence and severity of pneumonia. In situations where the donor cells are from an unrelated or mismatched donor, the risk of GvHD is significantly greater, as is the use of high-dose immunosuppressive therapy, and prolongation of immune recovery. In such cases, the risk for opportunistic infection continues indefinitely, such that the predictability of certain infections is no longer applicable for these patients. However, where the transplanted cells are autologous and there is generally no GvHD or continued immunosuppression, the incidence and mortality of pneumonia are significantly lower (42,91).

Bacterial pneumonias occurring during the initial neutropenia after stem cell transplant, either allogeneic or autologous, are caused by pathogens common to all neutropenic patients or those with comparable mucositis. Data on such infections are sparse, as empiric antibiotics are traditionally begun quickly without bronchoscopic evaluation, but the most common pathogens are Gram-negative (92).

One should also consider the possibility of streptococcal pneumonia or of acute respiratory distress syndrome related to streptococcal sepsis, in light of the observed increase in Gram-positive infections in neutropenic patients. These infections are particularly due to *S. viridans,* with a reported incidence of up to 22% and a mortality rate of 10% to 15%. These streptococcal infections have been correlated with the presence of mucositis, the use of prophylactic quinolones, and the use of high-dose arabinosylcytosine (93,94). The approach to bacterial pneumonias in transplant is similar to that in other neutropenic hosts and should include coverage for pseudomonas species. The recovery of neutrophils may increase the size of pulmonary infiltrates, which may evolve to abscess formation, particularly in *St. aureus* or Gram-negative pneumonias. The period of neutropenia has been shortened with the use of growth factors and peripheral blood stem cells, so it is hoped that a decrease in bacterial infections reported during this period should follow.

Pneumonias from intracellular pathogens such as mycobacteria are rarely reported after transplant but may recur in previously exposed patients. Most patients maintain indwelling intravenous catheters throughout this time, and seeding of the lungs from a bacteremia continues to be a risk. After recovery from neutropenia, allogeneic transplant recipients continue to be at risk for Gram-negative and other nosocomial infections. Microbiological documentation may be more feasible through bronchoscopy during this time, and such evaluation is important, as the patient will have already received antibiotics, so that resistant bacteria, mixed infections, or co-infection with a nonbacterial organism may be identified. Bacterial infections occurring in the late post-transplant period, usually considered to be after 6 months, may be related to persistent immunoglobulin deficiency, which increases the risk for pneumonia due to encapsulated bacteria. A specific deficiency in anti-*Streptococcus pneumoniae* antibodies has been noted, which may predispose the patient to pneumococcal infection, which is often of abrupt onset and rapidly fatal.

Pneumococcal infection was found historically in 27% of 7-month survivors followed to 36 months (95) and was the most commonly documented bacterial infection in a large recent British study, where mortality was 33% (96). This risk is increased fourfold where there is functional asplenia with GvHD, as in splenectomized patients. Severe chronic GvHD may prolong the risk indefinitely. The risk in autologous patients is less, except in those with a history of Hodgkin's disease and/or splenectomy. There is no consensus on prophylaxis for this problem. The use of oral penicillin or amoxicillin may not be justified in view of the reported increased incidence of penicillin resistance (97). Immunization with a polysaccharide vaccine is of limited efficacy, particularly in view of the prolonged immunosuppression of these patients (6).

Similarly, *Haemophilus influenzae* may cause pneumonia and sinus infection, usually after the third month following transplant. Its incidence has been a significant problem in European centers (98) and could vary with the immunization policies of the normal population. Immunization against type b, the most frequent type found in human infection, with a conjugated vaccine, has been recommended in Europe after the fourth month in allogeneic patients, particularly those with chronic GvHD and obstructive pulmonary disease (97).

Pneumonia due to *Legionella* species, both pneumophila and nonpneumophila species, has been occasionally reported, most often as a nosocomial infection in patients with prolonged hospitalization, in the setting of outbreaks (99,100). Radiologic findings may be variable, may mimic fungal nodules, and may not be apparent at the onset of high fever and pleuritic pain. Seroconversion may not be seen or may be delayed. Invasive nocardiosis has been reported in 0.3% to 1.7% of allogeneic patients and must be differentiated from fungal infections (101,102).

Mycobacterial infections, due to *M. tuberculosis, M. avium intracellulare,* or other species, have been reported rarely but should be considered in the appropriate setting. They have generally been diagnosed between 2 and 18 months after transplant but may occur early where there has been prior infection (103). The Minneapolis team reported an incidence of 0.4%, which is approximately 10 times the annual U.S. incidence (104). In this study, the lung was involved in only 1 out of 11 patients (104).

Aspergillus is the most worrisome fungal infection after marrow transplant. It has been reported in from 0% to 20% of transplants; the most common site is the lung (105–107). A first peak of incidence occurs during the neutropenic period, particularly in leukemic patients who had been previously colonized. Early recurrence may also occur in patients with a previous aspergillus infection. It may also occur at any time after transplant, particularly where corticosteroids have been used for prolonged periods. The second peak incidence is generally between the second and third months. Some centers feel that the use of laminar flow isolation in the early transplant course decreases the chance of early aspergillus, but opinions vary.

The mortality of aspergillus pneumonia approaches 100% in most studies, and it is generally acknowledged that delay in initiation of antiaspergillus treatment may be partly responsible for this outcome. The optimal approach is the earliest possible diagnosis and treatment initiation, so that this infection must be considered in any case of fever, particularly in the patient on broad-spectrum antibiotics, or in any pneumonia, either of new onset or of one previously diagnosed that does not resolve on appropriate therapy. A negative bronchoscopy result should not diminish the suspicion for this pathogen, as the false-negative rate is at least 50%, and repeat or further diagnostic procedures must be considered. In retrospective studies, the risk of relapse of prior aspergillus infection has been estimated to be 15% to 33% (108,109).

In such cases, efforts should be made prior to beginning transplant, to eliminate the potential for relapse, with surgery where possible, and to initiate antiaspergillus prophylaxis early. Efforts to find the best prophylaxis regimen and to find methods to differentiate colonization from infection are being studied, as is the use of PCR and antigenemia before and early after transplant, as a means of improving the detection of infection (110).

Besides the lung parenchyma, aspergillus may be found isolated to the tracheo-bronchial tree, where it may be responsible for significant airway obstruction and symptoms. White, adherent plaques may be seen at bronchoscopy, particularly in the setting of chronic GvHD and steroid use. This infection must be differentiated from a worsening of bronchiolitis, so that inappropriate and dangerous increases in immunosuppression may be avoided and antifungal treatment may be initiated.

Pneumonia due to *Candida* species is reported rarely, partly because there are no firm criteria for differentiating invasive infection from colonization on the basis of bronchoscopy without biopsy. The lungs may be involved in any systemic *albicans* or non-*albicans Candida* infection.

The diagnosis of fungal pneumonia relies on pathological specimens and in large numbers of cases is made only at autopsy. For this reason the true incidence in transplants is unknown. Pneumonias due to endemic fungi in North America, such as histoplasmosis or coccidioidomycosis, must be considered in these patients, as well as in the emerging fungi, including trichosporon, alternaria, fusarium, and the mucorales (Fig. 6). Any of these fungi can cause pneumonia in transplant patients, as in similarly immunocompromised hosts.

The incidence of *P. carinii* pneumonia had been historically found to be 5% to 30% of the cases of interstitial pneumonia, which was seen in 20% to 50% of allogeneic BMT recipients (43,111). This incidence has dramatically decreased with the widespread use of prophylaxis with trimethoprim-sulfamethoxazole for 6–12 months after allogeneic transplant, especially for patients receiving steroids. Late occurrence of *P. carinii* pneumonia may be observed more than 6 months after transplant in patients with chronic GvHD and receiving prolonged immunosuppression, emphasizing the necessity for continued prophylaxis beyond 1 year in some patients (112). *P. carinii* may be initially minimally symptomatic, and manifest only by prolonged fever and slight dyspnea. Around 15% of patients may have no or minimal x-ray findings (113), but BAL should be done rapidly where there is no other obvious explanation for fever, because mortality of *P. carinii* pneumonia approaches 60%, and seems worst in patients developing it within 6 months of BMT (96,113). There are no data specifically in BMT patients to compare the respective prophylactic efficacy of trimethoprim-sulfamethoxazole and aerosolized pentamidine, although this latter is generally considered a possible alternative (114,115).

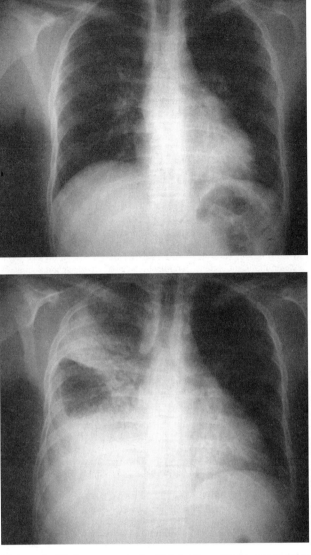

Figure 6. Trichosporon beigelii infection. Right upper lobe infiltrate occurring in aplastic anemia patient 10 days prior to SCT (**A**). Bronchoscopy was noncontributory. Despite amphotericin therapy, the patient died 7 days after SCT, 4 days after endotracheal sample (**B**) and blood cultures demonstrated *T. beigelii.*

During the neutropenic phase after both autologous and allogeneic transplant, and partly because of the mucosal damage due to chemo- and radiotherapy, there is a high incidence of HSV reactivation. HSV pneumonia has been reported rarely and may be rapidly fatal in this setting (116). With the wide use of acyclovir, either as systematic prophylaxis or at the first sign of mucositis, the incidence of extramucosal disease has been greatly reduced.

Cytomegalovirus was, until recently, the most significant pathogen for pneumonia in allogeneic BMT, responsible for 40% to 50% of interstitial pneumonias occurring in allogeneic BMT recipients, or 15% of these patients

(43,44). CMV pneumonia is usually a febrile disease, with possible different radiologic patterns, primarily interstitial, but there may be also alveolar or micronodular infiltrates. CMV pneumonia is often associated with other lung infections, such as bacterial, fungal, or *P. carinii* pneumonia. The occurrence of CMV pneumonia has been correlated with the serological status of donor and host, and with allogeneic reaction, as it is unusual in syngeneic transplants (117) and has been reported in only 1% to 6% of autologous transplants, despite an incidence of reactivation comparable to that of allogeneic BMT (118).

In allogeneic transplant, patients in whom the presence of CMV was found in surveillance BAL at the end of the first month had a higher risk of pneumonia (119). As surveillance for virus by culture, antigenemia, or PCR has become routine after allogeneic transplants, surveillance BAL is not routinely used. Pre-emptive therapy has greatly decreased the incidence of CMV pneumonia, particularly in genoidentical transplants, but the best approach for recipients of mismatched or unrelated transplants, who may be indefinitely immunosuppressed is not yet known. In the setting of pneumonia, the optimal approach to identifying the virus is to combine indirect immunofluorescence and rapid culture of BAL fluid. It has been shown that the identification of CMV through PCR on BAL fluid does not correlate with CMV pneumonia (120). Identification of characteristic inclusions is a sign of advanced infection.

Other herpesviruses—including varicella-zoster, EBV, and HHV6—have been reported in BMT patients. HHV6 is frequently found together with CMV or other pathogens, and its clinical significance and pathogenicity are unclear. High levels of HHV6-DNA have been found in lung tissue of patients with idiopathic, or CMV interstitial pneumonitis. Because of higher concentrations of HHV6 genome in lung tissue from marrow recipients when compared with controls, it has been suggested that HHV6 infection could be associated with idiopathic pneumonia in this setting, but this remains to be confirmed (121). As HHV6 is sensitive to ganciclovir and foscarnet, preemptive therapy to prevent CMV should also decrease the risk of HHV6 infection during that time.

The incidence of respiratory virus infections is estimated to be 1% to 3% of patients after BMT (72). They include respiratory syncytial virus, followed by parainfluenza virus, rhinovirus, and influenza virus. The incidence of pneumonia due to RSV varies greatly in the literature, from 0 to 16% during outbreaks (122). The mortality of these infections also varies among series, and with the time after transplant and the degree of immunosuppression, but it may be significant (29). There is much to be learned about differentiating infection from disease, and about the best means of identifying these viruses in routine practice. It should be possible to arrive at a consensus policy on the place of culture, immunofluorescence, and PCR, as has been done in the case of CMV.

Measles pneumonia has been rarely reported after BMT and has a 65% mortality rate, because it may occur without rash (123). Adenovirus infection occurs with different rates in the literature. Adenovirus pneumonia occurred in 3% of 201 consecutive BMT recipients in the experience of Carrigan and colleagues (124), more often in children than in adults, and more often in unrelated transplants, but seems to be less frequent in other centers (30).

Pulmonary toxoplasmosis has been reported rarely, usually in the setting of disseminated infection resulting from reactivation, usually during the first year after transplant (125). The pattern is usually a diffuse interstitial disease, and neurological symptoms may be absent, which makes the diagnosis difficult. Toxoplasmosis may be identified in BAL fluid through immunofluorescence or in blood through PCR (126).

CONCLUSION

As pneumonia is a principal determinant of post-transplant survival, it is essential that the mechanisms and timing of infections after transplant be understood. Because of the predictable timing of certain infections, some prophylactic regimens have been instituted with far-reaching benefit. The increasing use of transplantation and the introduction of different immunosuppressive regimens may alter the timing or types of pneumonias in the future. Although solid organ transplantation has been limited by a finite number of donor organs, the accessibility of donors of stem cells will expand as results using mismatched and unrelated donors improve. Additionally, new pathogens are emerging and familiar pathogens are becoming more resistant. A high level of suspicion when pneumonia occurs in a transplant patient, and vigilance in diagnosing and treating, will continue to be required to prevent an increase in mortality from pneumonia.

REFERENCES

1. Reynolds HY. Normal and defective respiratory defenses. In: Remington JE, ed. *Respiratory infections: diagnosis and management,* 2nd ed. New York: Raven Press; 1988:1–33.
2. Wilson R, Alton E, Rutman A, et al. Upper respiratory tract viral infection and mucociliary clearance. *Eur J Respir Dis* 1987;70:272–279.
3. Hervé P, Silbert D, Cerrina J, Simonneau G, Dartevelle P. Impairment of bronchial mucociliary clearance in long-term survivors of heart/lung and double-lung transplantation. *Chest* 1993;103:59–63.
4. Read RC, Shankar S, Rutman A, Yacoub M, Cole PJ, Wilson R. Ciliary beat frequency and structure of recipient and donor epithelia following lung transplantation. *Eur Respir J* 1991;4:796–801.
5. Cordonnier C, Gilain L, Ricolfi F, et al. Acquired ciliary abnormalities of nasal mucosa in marrow recipients. *Bone Marrow Transplant* 1996;17:611–616.
6. Winston DJ, Territo MC, Ho WG, Miller MJ, Gale RP, Golde DW. Alveolar macrophage dysfunction in human bone marrow transplant recipients. *Am J Med* 1983;73:859–866.
7. Paradis I, Rabinowich H, Zeevi A, et al. Life in the allogeneic environment after lung transplantation. *Lung* 1990;168[Suppl.]:1172–1181.
8. Cordonnier C, Escudier E, Verra F, Brochard L, Bernaudin JF, Fleury-Feith J. Bronchoalveolar lavage during neutropenic episodes: diagnostic, yield and cellular pattern. *Eur Respir J* 1994;7:114–120.
9. Starzl TE, Demetris AJ, Murase N, Ildstad S, Ricordi C, Trocco M. Cell migration, chimerism, and graft acceptance. *Lancet* 1992;339:1579–1582.
10. Fung JJ, Kaufman C, Paradis IL, et al. Interactions between bronchoalveolar lymphocytes and macrophages in heart-lung transplant recipient. *Hum Immunol* 1985;14:287–294.
11. Kubit V, Sonmez-Alpan E, Zeevi A, et al. Mixed allogeneic chimerism in lung allograft recipients. *Hum Pathol* 1994;25(4):408–412.
12. Springmeyer SC, Altman LC, Kopecky KJ, Deeg HJ, Storb R. Alveolar macrophage kinetics and function after interruption of canine marrow function. *Am Rev Respir Dis* 1982;125:347–351.
13. Etienne B, Morneix JF. Aspects immunologiques de la greffe pulmonaire. *Rev Mal Respir* 1996;13:S15–S22.
14. Data Highlights from the 1996 United Network of Organ Sharing Annual Report 1996.
15. Mermel LA, Maki DG. Bacterial pneumonia in solid organ transplantation. *Semin Respir Infect* 1990;5(1):10–29.
16. Hofflin JM, Potasman I, Baldwin JC, Oyer PE, Stinson EB, Remington JS. Infectious complications in heart transplant recipients receiving cyclosporine and corticosteroids. Ann Int Med 1987;106:209–216.
17. White DA. Pulmonary infection in the immunocompromised patient. *Semin Thor Cardiovasc Surg* 1995;7(2):78–87.
18. Dichter JR, Levine SJ, Shelhamer JH. Approach to the immunocompromised host with pulmonary symptoms. *Hematol Oncol Clin North Am* 1993;7(4):887–912.
19. Caillot D, Casasnovas O, Bernard A, et al. Improved management of invasive pulmonary aspergillosis in neutropenic patients using early thoracic computed tomographic scan and surgery. *J Clin Oncol* 1997;15:139–147.
20. Blum U, Windfuhr M, Buitrago-Tellez C, et al. Invasive pulmonary aspergillosis: MRI, CT, and plain radiographic findings and their contribution for early diagnosis. *Chest* 1994;106:1156–1161.
21. Bitran J, Bekerman C, Weinstein R, Bennet C, Ryo U, Pinsky S. Patterns of Gallium-67 scintigraphy in patients with acquired immunodeficiency syndrome and the AIDS related complex. *J Nucl Med* 1987;28:1103–1106.
22. Mazzoni G, Lee S, Tomer A, Gittes RF. Indium-labeled presensitized T cells for diagnosis of graft rejection. *J Surg Res* 1992;52(1):85–88.
23. Stover DE, Zaman MB, Hadju SI, Lange M, Gold J. Bronchoalveolar lavage in the diagnosis of diffuse pulmonary infiltrates in the immunosuppressed host. *Ann Intern Med* 1984;101:1–7.
24. Shelhamer J, Gill V, Quinn T, et al. The laboratory evaluation of opportunistic pulmonary infections. *Ann Intern Med* 1996;124(6):585–599.
25. Sternberg RI, Baughman RP, Dohn MN, First MR. Utility of bronchoalveolar lavage in assessing pneumonia in immunosuppressed renal transplant recipients. *Am J Med* 1993;95:358–364.
26. Verra F, Hmouda H, Rauss A, et al. Bronchoalveolar lavage in immunocompromised patients: clinical and functional consequences. *Chest* 1992;101:1215–1220.
27. De Lassence A, Fleury-Feith J, Escudier E, Beaune J, Bernaudin JF, Cordonnier C. Alveolar hemorrhage: diagnostic criteria and results in 194 immunocompromised hosts. *Am J Respir Crit Care Med* 1995;151:157–163.
28. Cough RB, Englund JA, Whimbey E. Respiratory viral infections in immunocompetent and immunocompromised persons. *Am J Med* 1997;102(3A):2–9.
29. Bowden RA. Respiratory virus infections after marrow transplant: The Fred Hutchinson Cancer Research Center experience. *Am J Med* 1997;102(3A):27–30.
30. Ljungman P. Respiratory virus infections in bone marrow transplant recipients: the European perspective. *Am J Med* 1997;102(3A):44–47.
31. Griffin JJ, Meduri GU. New approaches in the diagnosis of nosocomial pneumonia. *Med Clin North Am* 1994;78:1091–1122.
32. American Thoracic Society. Hospital-acquired pneumonia in adults: diagnosis, assessment of severity, initial antimicrobial therapy, and preventive strategies. A consensus statement. *Am J Respir Crit Care Med* 1996;153:1711–1725.
33. Scott JP, Fradet G, Smyth RL, et al. Prospective study of trans-

bronchial biopsies in the management of heart-lung and single lung transplant patients. *J Heart Lung Transplant* 1991;10:626–637.

34. Crawford SW, Hackman RC, Clark JG. Biopsy diagnosis and clinical outcome of persistent focal pulmonary lesions after marrow transplantation. *Transplantation* 1989;48:266–271.

35. Travis WD, Roth DB. Histopathologic evaluation of lung biopsy specimens. In: Shelhamer J, Parrillo JE, ed. *Respiratory disease in the immunosuppressed host.* Philadelphia: Lippincott 1991;182–217.

36. Jules-Elysee K, Stover D, Yalahom J, White DA, Gulati SC. Pulmonary complications in lymphoma patients treated with high dose therapy and autologous bone marrow transplantation. *Am Rev Respir Dis* 1992;146:485–491.

37. Cordonnier C, Fleury-Feith J, Escudier E, Atassi K, Bernaudin JF. Secondary alveolar proteinosis is a reversible cause of respiratory failure in leukemic patients. *Am J Respir Crit Care Med* 1994;149(3):788–794.

38. Takaoka F, Brown MM, Paulsen AW, Ramsay MAE, Klintman GB. Adult respiratory distress syndrome following orthotopic liver transplantation. *Clin Transplant* 1989;3:294–299.

39. Royston D, Minty BD, Biol MI, Hingenbottam TW, Wallwork J, Jones GJ. The effect of surgery with cardiopulmonary bypass on alveolar-capillary barrier function in human beings. *Ann Thorac Surg* 1985;40:139–143.

40. Bergin CJ, Castellino RA, Blank N, Sibley RK, Starnes VA. Acute lung rejection after heart-lung transplantation: correlation of findings on chest radiographs with lung biopsy results. *Am J Radiol* 1990;155:23–27.

41. Bonser RS, Jamieson SW. Heart-lung transplantation. *Clin Chest Med* 1990;11:235–246.

42. Clark JG, Hansen JA, Marshall I, Parkman R, Jensen L, Peavy HH. Idiopathic pneumonia syndrome after bone marrow transplantation. *Am Rev Respir Dis* 1993;147:1601–1606.

43. Winston DJ, Ho WG, Champlin RE. Cytomegalovirus infection and interstitial pneumonia after bone marrow transplantation. In: Champlin R, ed. *Bone marrow transplantation.* Boston: Kluwer 1990;113–128.

44. Wingard JR, Mellits ED, Sostrin MB, et al. Interstitial pneumonia after allogeneic marrow transplantation. *Medicine (Baltimore)* 1988;67:175–186.

45. Spector NM, Connoly MA, Garrity ER. Lung transplant rejection: obliterative bronchiolitis. *Am J Crit Care* 1996;5(5):366–372.

46. Holland HK, Wingard JR, Beschorner WE, Saral R, Santos GW. Bronchiolitis obliterans in bone-marrow transplantation and its relationship to chronic graft-versus-host diseases and low serum IgG. *Blood* 1988;72(2):621–627.

47. Clark JG, Crawford SW, Madtes DK, Sullivan KM. Obstructive lung diseases after allogeneic marrow transplantation. *Ann Intern Med* 1989;111:368–376.

48. Matthew P, Bozeman P, Krance R, Brenner M, Heslop H. Bronchiolitis obliterans organizing pneumonia in children after allogeneic bone marrow transplantation. *Bone Marrow Transplant* 1994;13:221–223.

49. Crawford SC, Schwartz DA, Petersen FB, Clark JG. Mechanical ventilation after marrow tansplantation. *Am Rev Respir Dis* 1988;137:682–687.

50. Denardo SJ, Oye RK, Bellamy PE. Efficacy of intensive care for bone marrow transplant patients with respiratory failure. *Crit Care Med* 1989;17:4–6.

51. Todd K, Wiley F, Landaw E, et al. Survival outcome among 54 intubated pediatric bone marrow transplant patients. *Crit Care Med* 1994;22:171–176.

52. Rubenfeld GD, Crawford SC. Withdrawing life support from mechanical ventilated recipients of bone marrow transplants: a case for evidence-based guidelines. *Ann Intern Med* 1996;125:625–633.

52a. Jackson SR, Tweeddale MG, Barnett MJ, et al. Admission of bone marrow transplant recipients to the intensive care unit: outcome, survival and prognostic factos. *Bone Marrow Transplant* 1998;21:697–704.

53. Ettinger NA. Solid organ and bone marrow transplantation: clinical approach to upper and lower respiratory infections. In: Neiderman MS, Sarosi GA, Glassroth J, eds. *Respiratory infections: a scientific basis for management.* Philadelphia: WB Saunders; 1994.

54. Dummer SJ. Pneumocystis carinii infections in transplant recipients. *Semin Respir Infect* 1990;5(1):50–57.

55. Denning DW, Stevens DA. Antifungal and surgical treatment of invasive aspergillosis: review of 2121 published cases. *Rev Infect Dis* 1990;12:1147–1201.

56. Dummer JS, White LT, Ho M, Griffith BP, Hardesty RL, Bahnson HT. Morbidity of cytomegalovirus infection in recipients of heart or heart-lung transplants who received cyclosporine. *J Infect Dis* 1985;152(6):1182–1191.

57. Merigan TC, Renlund DG, Keay S, Bristow MR, et al. A controlled trial of ganciclovir to prevent cytomegalovirus disease after heart transplantation. *N Engl J Med* 1992;326:1182–1186.

58. Opelz G, Henderson R, for the Collaborative Transplant Study: Incidence of non-Hodgkin lymphoma in kidney and heart transplant recipients. *Lancet* 1993;342:1514–1516.

59. Hosenpud JD, Hershberger RE, Pantely GA, et al. Late infection in cardiac allograft recipients: profiles, incidence, and outcome. *J Heart Lung Transplant* 1991;10:380–386.

60. Gordon SM, Gal AA, Hertzle RGL, Bryan JA, Perlino C, Kanter KR. Diagnosis of pulmonary toxoplasmosis by bronchoalveolar lavage in cardiac transplant recipients. *Diagn Cytopathol* 1993;9(6):650–654.

61. Trulock EP. Lung transplantation. *Am J Respir Crit Care Med* 1997;155:789–818.

62. Paradis IL, Williams P. Infection after lung transplantation. *Semin Respir Infect* 1993;8(3):207–215.

63. Flume PA, Egan TM, Paradowski LJ, Detterbeck FC, Thompson JT, Yankaskas JR. Infectious complications of lung transplantation: impact of cystic fibrosis. *Am J Respir Crit Care Med* 1994;149:1601–1607.

64. Kawai A, Paradis IL, Keenan RJ, et al. Lung transplantation at the University of Pittsburgh: 1982 to 1994. In: Terasaki PI, Cecka JM, eds. *Clinical Transplants 1994.* Los Angeles: UCLA Tissue Typing Laboratory; 1994:111–120.

65. Kramer MR, Marshall SE, Starnes VA, Gamberg P, Amitai Z, Theodore J. Infectious complications in heart-lung transplantation. *Arch Intern Med* 1993;153:2010–2016.

66. Kanj SS, Welty-Wolf K, Madden J, et al. Fungal infections in lung and heart-lung transplant recipients. *Medicine* 1996;75(3):142–156.

67. Paya CV. Fungal infections in solid-organ transplantation. *Clin Infect Dis* 1993;16:677–688.

68. Kramer MR, Stoehr C, Lewiston NJ, Starnes VA, Theodore J. Trimethoprim-sulfamethoxazole prophylaxis for *Pneumocystis carinii* infections in heart-lung and lung transplantation: how effective and for how long? *Transplantation* 1992;53(3):586–589.

69. Keenan RJ, Lega ME, Dummer JS, et al. Cytomegalovirus serologic status and postoperative infection correlated with risk of developing chronic rejection after pulmonary transplantation. *Transplantation* 1991;51:433–438.

70. Paradis I, Yousem S, Griffith B. Airway obstruction and *Bronchiolitis obliterans* after lung transplantation. *Clin Chest Med* 1993;14(4):751–762.

71. Horvath J, Dummer S, Loyd J, Walker B, Merrill WH, Frist WH. Infection in the transplanted and native lung after single lung transplantation. *Chest* 1993;104:681–685.

72. Sable CA, Hayden FG. Orthomyxoviral and paramyxoviral infections in transplant patients. *Infect Dis Clin North America* 1995;9(4):987–1003.

73. Aris RM, Maia DM, Neuringer IP, Gott K, Kiley GK, Handy J. Post-transplantation lymphoproliferative disorder in the Epstein-Barr virus-naive lung transplant recipient. *Am J Respir Crit Care Med* 1996;154:1712–1717.

74. Ohori NP, Michaels MG, Jaffe R, Williams P, Yousem SA. Adenovirus pneumonia in lung transplant recipients. *Hum Pathol* 1995;26(10):1073–1079.

75. Dromer C, Nashef SAM, Velly J-F, Martigne C, Couraud L. Tuberculosis in transplanted lungs. *J Heart Lung Transplant* 1993;12:924–927.

76. Ramsey PG. The renal transplant patient with fever and pulmonary infiltrates: etiology, clinical manifestations, and management. *Medicine* 1980;59(3):206–222.

77. Ruiz LM, Montejo M, Benito JR, et al. Simultaneous pulmonary infection by *Nocardia asteroides* and *Pneumocystis carinii* in a renal transplant patient. *Nephrol Dial Transplant* 1996;11:711–714.

78. Miller R, Chavers BM. Respiratory syncytial virus infections in pediatric renal transplant recipients. *Pediatr Nephrol* 1996;10:213–215.

79. Guillemain R, Lavarde V, Amrein C, Chevalier P, Guivarch A, Glotz D. Invasive aspergillosis after transplantation. *Transplant Proc* 1995;27:1307–1309.

80. Peddi VR, Hariharan S, First MR. Disseminated histoplasmosis in renal allograft recipients. *Clin Transplant* 1996;10(2):160–165.

81. Winkler S, Stanek G, Hubsch P, et al. Pneumonia due to *Blastomyces dermatitidis* in a European renal transplant recipient. *Nephrol Dial Transplant* 1996;11:1376–1379.

82. Renoult E, Georges E, Biava M-F, et al. Toxoplasmosis in kidney transplant recipients: report of six cases and review. *Clin Infect Dis* 1997;24:625–634.

83. Patel E, Roberts GD, Keating MR, Paya C. Infections due to nontuberculous mycobacteria in kidney, heart, and liver transplant recipients. *Clin Infect Dis* 1994;19:263–273.

84. Winston DJ, Emmanouilides C, Busuttil RW. Infections in liver transplant recipients. *Clin Infect Dis* 1995;21:1077–1091.

85. Singh N, Gayowski T, Wagener M, Marino IR, Yu VL. Pulmonary infections in liver transplant recipients receiving tacrolimus. *Transplantation* 1996;61(3):396–401.

86. Kanj SS, Sharara AI, Clavien P-A, Hamilton JD. Cytomegalovirus infection following liver transplantation: review of the literature. *Clin Infect Dis* 1996;22:537–549.

87. Dodd GDI, Ledesma-Medina J, Baron RL, Fuhrman CR. Posttransplant lymphoproliferative disorder: intrathoracic manifestations. *Radiology* 1992;184:65–69.

88. Pohl C, Green M, Wald ER, Ledesma-Medina J. Respiratory syncytial virus infections in pediatric liver transplant recipients. *J Infect Dis* 1992;165:166–169.

89. Mayes JT, O'Connor BJ, Avery R, Castellani W, Carey W. Transmission of *Toxoplasma gondii* infection by liver transplantation. *Clin Infect Dis* 1995;21:511–515.

90. Higgins RSD, Kusne S, Reyes J, et al. *Mycobacterium tuberculosis* after liver transplantation: management and guidelines for prevention. *Clin Transplant* 1992;6:81–90.

91. Gentile G, Micozzi A, Girmenia C, et al. Pneumonia in allogeneic and autologous bone marrow recipients. *Chest* 1993;104(2):371–375.

92. Pannuti C, Gingrich R, Pfaller M, et al. Nosocomial pneumonia in adult patients undergoing bone marrow transplantation. *J Clin Oncol* 1991;9:77–84.

93. Bochud PY, Calandra T, Francioli P. Bacteremia due to viridans streptococci in neutropenic patients: a review. *Am J Med* 1994;97:256–64.

94. Elting LS, Bodey GP, Keefe BH. Septicemia and shock syndrome due to *viridans* streptococci: a case-control study of predisposing factors. *Clin Infect Dis* 1992;14(6):1201–1207.

95. Winston DJ, Schiffman G, Wang DC, Feig SA, Lin CH, Marso EL. Pneumococcal infections after bone marrow transplantation. *Ann Intern Med* 1979;91:835–841.

96. Hoyle C, Goldman JM. Life-threatening infections occurring more than 3 months after BMT. *Bone Marrow Transplant* 1994;14:247–252.

97. Ljungman P, Cordonnier C, de Bock R, et al. Immunisations after bone marrow transplantation: results of a European survey and recommendations from the Infectious Diseases Working Party of the European Group for Blood and Marrow Transplantation. *Bone Marrow Transplant* 1995;15:455–460.

98. Cordonnier C, Bernaudin JF, Bierling P, et al. Pulmonary complications occurring after allogeneic bone marrow transplantation. *Cancer* 1986;58:1047–1054.

99. Kugler JW, Armitage JO, Helms CM, et al. Nosocomial Legionnaires' disease: occurrence in recipients of bone marrow transplants. *Am J Med* 1983;74:281–288.

100. Harrington RD, Woolfrey AE, Bowden R, McDowell MG, Hackman RC. Legionellosis in a bone marrow transplant center. *Bone Marrow Transplant* 1996;18(2):361–368.

101. Choucino C, Goodman SA, Greer JP, Stein RS, Wolff SN, Dummer JS. Nocardial infections in bone marrow transplant recipients. *Clin Infect Dis* 1996;23(5):1012–1019.

102. Van Burik JA, Hackman RC, Nadeem SO, et al. Nocardiosis after bone marrow transplantation: a retrospective study. *Clin Infect Dis* 1997;24(6):1154–1160.

103. Kurzrock R, Zander A, Vellekop L, Kanojia M, Luna M, Dicke K. Mycobacterial pulmonary infections after allogeneic bone marrow transplantation. *Am J Med* 1984;77:35–40.

104. Roy V, Weisdorf D. Mycobacterial infections following bone marrow transplantation: a 20 year retrospective review. *Bone Marrow Transplant* 1997;19:467–470.

105. Meyers JD. Infection in bone marrow transplant recipients. *Am J Med* 1986;81[Suppl. 1A]:27–38.

106. Sheretz RJ, Belani A, Kramer BS, et al. Impact of air filtration on nosocomial *Aspergillus* infections. *Am J Med* 1987;83:709–718.

107. Cunningham I. Pulmonary infections after bone marrow transplant. *Semin Respir Infect* 1992;7(2):132–138.

108. Offner F, Cordonnier C, Ljungman P, et al. Impact of previous aspergillosis on the outcome of bone marrow transplantation. *Clin Infect Dis* (in press).

109. Martino R, Lopez R, Sureda A, Brunet S, Domingo-Albos A. Risk of reactivation of a recent invasive fungal infection in patients with hematological malignancies undergoing further intensive chemoradiotherapy. A single center experience and review of the literature. *Haematologica* 1997;82:297–304.

110. Einsele H, Hebart H, Roller G, et al. Detection and identification of fungal pathogens in blood by using molecular probes. *J Clin Microbiol* 1997;35(6):1353–1360.

111. Krowka MJ, Rosenow EC, Hoagland JC. Pulmonary complications of bone marrow transplantation. *Chest* 1985;87:237–246.

112. Lyytikäinen O, Ruutu T, Volin L, et al. Late onset *Pneumocystis carinii* pneumonia following allogeneic bone marrow transplantation. *Bone Marrow Transplant* 1996;17(6):1057–1059.

113. Tuan IZ, Dennison D, Weisdorf DJ. *Pneumocystis carinii* following bone marrow transplantation. *Bone Marrow Transplant* 1992;10(3):267–272.

114. Momin F, Chandrasekar PH. Antimicrobial prophylaxis in bone marrow transplantation. *Ann Intern Med* 1995;123:205–215.

115. Link H, Vöhringer HF, Wingen F, Brägas B, Schwardt A, Ehninger G. Pentamidine aerosol for prophylaxis of *Pneumocystis carinii* pneumonia after BMT. *Bone Marrow Transplant* 1993;11(5):403–406.

116. Ramsay PG, Fife KH, Hackman RC, Meyers JD, Corey L. Herpes simplex virus pneumonia: clinical, virological, and pathological features in 20 patients. *Ann Intern Med* 1982;97:813–820.

117. Appelbaum FR, Meyers JD, Fefer A, et al. Nonbacterial nonfungal pneumonia following marrow transplantation: comparison to infection after allogeneic bone marrow transplantation. *Transplantation* 1982;33:265–268.

118. Wingard JR, Chen DY, Burns WH, et al. Cytomegalovirus infection after autologous bone marrow transplantation with comparison to infection after allogeneic bone marrow transplantation. *Blood* 1988;71:1432–1437.

119. Schmidt GM, Horak DA, Niland JC, et al. A randomized, controlled trial of prophylactic ganciclovir for cytomegalovirus pulmonary infection in recipients of allogeneic bone marrow transplants. *N Engl J Med* 1991;324:1005–1011.

120. Cathomas G, Morris P, Oekle K, Cunningham I, Emanuel D. Rapid diagnosis of cytomegalovirus pneumonia in marrow transplant recipients by bronchoalveolar lavage using the polymerase chain reaction, virus culture, and the direct immunostaining of alveolar cells. *Blood* 1993;81:1909–1914.

121. Cone R, Hackman R, Huang M, et al. Human Herpesvirus 6 in lung tissue from patients with pneumonitis after bone marrow transplantation. *N Engl J Med* 1993;329:156–161.

122. Sable CA, Donowitz GR. Infections in bone marrow transplant recipients. *Clin Infect Dis* 1994;18:273–284.

123. Kaplan LJ, Daum RS, Smaron M, McCarthy CA. Severe measles in immunocompromised patients. *JAMA* 1992;267:1237–1241.

124. Carrigan DR. Adenovirus infections in immunocompromised patients. *Am J Med* 1997;102(3A):71–74.

125. Derouin F, Devergie A, Auber P, et al. Toxoplasmosis in bone-marrow transplant recipients: report of seven cases and review. *Clin Infect Dis* 1992;15:267–276.

126. Bretagne S, Costa J, Kuentz M, et al. Late toxoplasmosis evidenced by PCR in a marrow transplant recipient. *Bone Marrow Transplant* 1995;15(5):809–11.

Transplant Infections edited by
Raleigh A. Bowden, Per Ljungman, and Carlos V. Paya.
Lippincott–Raven Publishers, Philadelphia © 1998

CHAPTER 9

Skin Infections

Mazen S. Daoud, Lawrence E. Gibson, W. P. Daniel Su

Dermatologic diseases are increasingly recognized as a significant complication of immunosuppression. The increasing availability of organ transplantation and immunosuppressive medications has resulted in a large population of patients with a variety of skin diseases. Neoplasms, infections, graft-versus-host disease, and drug-related dermatoses such as xerosis, hirsutism, and steroid acne are among the most common diseases encountered in transplant patients. Infections are a common immediate cause of death in the transplant patients. Morphology of infectious skin lesions in the transplant patients is of limited diagnostic value because of the altered inflammatory response to microbial invasion. Routine dermatologic screening is a crucial step in early detection and successful treatment. A thorough evaluation including skin biopsy for routine examination and culture is essential in any transplant patient with an unexplained rash or skin lesion.

The risk of infection is determined by the net state of immunosuppression and the epidemiological exposure to the infective agent. A trivial exposure to a usually "harmless" organism can result in a life-threatening disease in this patient population. Epidemiological exposure is very important in developing countries and may explain the increased incidence of infections in transplant patients in these countries over developed counterparts, since immunosuppressive protocols are similar worldwide (1).

Certain circumstances may predispose transplant patients to primary dermatologic infections such as destruction of keratinized layer of the skin by trauma from intravenous lines, alteration of normal flora of the skin leading to infections with opportunistic organisms, thinning of skin, and inhibition of fibroblast proliferation secondary to chronic corticosteroid use (2). Skin lesions may be the only accessible site for culture in few patients with disseminated bacterial or fungal infections.

Infectious complications occur in about 75% of transplant recipients (3). The inflammatory response to infections in immunocompromised patients is usually altered from that encountered in immunocompetent host, which gives an atypical presentation in the majority of skin infections. Unusual pathogens should always be considered even in what appears to be a usual skin infection. For example, cryptococcal cellulitis appears very similar to cellulitis caused by staphylococcal or streptococcal bacteria. The combination of atypical clinical presentation of infections and the broad spectrum of potential pathogens that can cause infections in transplant patients makes the clinical diagnosis very difficult. Definitive diagnosis often relies on skin biopsy for routine tissue examination, special stains, and tissue culture. The likelihood of an infectious complication is more common with prolonged time after transplantation. Certain pathogens tend to occur more frequently at certain intervals after transplantation. Herpes simplex infection, for example, tends to occur in the first 12 months, while warts are more common many years later. Herein we will review the various skin infections encountered in the post-transplant era. A brief description of the skin biopsy procedure in the diagnosis of skin infections is also presented.

BACTERIAL INFECTIONS

Bacterial infections are common in solid organ transplant (SOT) recipients. Bacteria may cause surgical wound infections or infections related to indwelling catheters and intravenous lines early in the course of transplant. The more serious complications of erysipelas and cellulitis may appear many years later. The incidence of wound infections in solid organ transplant patients varies between 2% and 56% (4). Folliculitis, cellulitis, and abscesses are the most common bacterial infections in the skin, tending to occur early in the first few months after surgery (5,6). The causative bacteria include streptococcus, staphylococcus, and less commonly, Gram-negative

From the Department of Dermatology, Mayo Clinic, Rochester, MN 55905.

bacilli. Cellulitis and folliculitis may take an unfamiliar presentation with mild infiltration and erythema; however, they may become more aggressive and involve extensive areas of the skin, leading to necrosis and gangrene. Cellulitis can be caused by *Cryptococcus neoformans, Candida* spp., and occasionally atypical mycobacteria. These organisms should be kept in mind in differential diagnosis of cellulitis, especially if the response to antibiotic is inadequate (2). Recurrent cellulitis of the elbow in SOT patients, a condition called *transplant elbow*, is caused by thinning of the skin secondary to chronic corticosteroid use and frequent trauma to the area (7). The most common causative agent is *Staphylococcus aureus.* Pseudomonas folliculitis is usually a self-limited process obtained from hot tub use. Rarely, this process may progress to destructive ulcerative lesions, termed *ecthyma gangrenosum*, that are difficult to heal (Fig. 1).

Unlike in SOT recipients, patients with stem cell transplant (SCT) are more susceptible to infections with Gram-positive cocci. Prophylactic oral antibiotics and use of central intravenous catheters increase the likelihood of bacterial infections. The prolonged deficiency of IgG from high doses of immunosuppressants renders these patients unable to opsonize the encapsulated bacteria such as *Streptococcus pneumoniae* and *Haemophilus influenzae* (8). Unlike in patients with SOT, recipients of BMT are much less likely to develop bacterial infections once the engraftment has occurred and the immunosuppressant medications are discontinued or decreased. Finally, rare cases of necrotizing fasciitis were reported in children with BMT (9). Pseudomonas and enteric Gram-negative organisms were the most common cause and should be considered in selecting the appropriate antibiotics.

Mycobacterial Infections

Mycobacterial infections are rare complications of SOT and BMT recipients. The incidence is estimated at around 0.5% of BMT recipients (10). The manifestations include unexplained fever, pulmonary infiltrate, osteomyelitis, and central venous catheter tunnel inflammation. Primary extrapulmonary localization (in skin and joint) account for almost half of the cases (11). In BMT patients, most cases of mycobacterial infections are related to central venous catheters (10). In contrast to infections in SOT, Acid-fast bacilli (AFB) staining of draining material is often positive. Rapid-growing mycobacteria are the most common cause (10). The infection usually occurs early in the course of the transplantation.

Cutaneous lesions in SOT patients typically start as erythematous and indurated nodules with central necrosis, and occasionally as granulomatous plaques after an average of 2–4 years following transplant. The most common locations are the lower legs and arms. The lesions are not associated with lymphadenopathy, fever, or leukocytosis. A history of penetrating localized trauma is occasionally present. Infection of surgical wounds or sites of medical injections is seen (11). A sporotrichoid spread is unusual in contrast to the immunocompetent host. Associated osteomyelitis is not uncommon and needs to be ruled out. Lesions are occasionally more inflammatory with pus production. AFB stain of draining material is usually negative. The most common pathogens are *Mycobacterium kansasii, M. fortuitum,* or *M. chelonae* (11).

Histologically, acute inflammation with preponderance of neutrophils is seen in early lesions. Chronic inflammation with many histiocytes forming dermal and subcutaneous granulomas with or without giant cells usually follows. The AFB stain rarely demonstrates the organism on tissue examination. A mixed acute and chronic inflammation is often seen in the same biopsy specimen. Multiple biopsies are often necessary to confirm the diagnosis, and tissue culture is always recommended. The laboratory should be notified that atypical mycobacterium is a potential pathogen to ascertain proper culture technique. Chest x-ray and intradermal tuberculin testing are usually not helpful. Dissemination from a primary cutaneous lesion can occur in SOT patients (12). *In vitro* antimicrobial sensitivity is not a standard procedure because the correlation between *in vitro* and *in vivo* susceptibilities is unclear. However, susceptibility data may still be used to guide selection of antimicrobials. Combination treatment with isoniazid and ethambutol or rifampin, or all three, is usually successful. Prolonged treatment is necessary (11,13). Amikacin, with or without cefoxitin or erythromycin, was advocated as an empirical therapy until susceptibility results are known. Other agents such as tetracyclines, erythromycin, minocycline, ciprofloxacin, sulfonamides, and clarithromycin were used singly or in combination with variable results (11). Debridement of catheter tunnel tract in addition to appropriate antimycobacterial agents is often essential for complete resolution of infection.

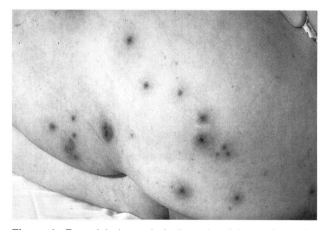

Figure 1. Round, indurated, dusky red nodules and papules with central necrotic black eschar and surrounding erythema characteristic of ecthyma gangrenosum.

Leprosy may develop or become activated after transplantation (14). The disease is seen more often in endemic areas. It usually occurs 3–4 years after the transplantation.

Nocardiosis

Nocardia is an infection caused by the aerobic actinomycete. The infection usually occurs after inhalation of the organism; however, direct cutaneous inoculation may occur in immunocompromised patients. The disease is very rare in the United States. The incidence of nocardiosis among alogeneic BMT recipients is 0.3% (15). None of 1,284 solid organ transplant recipients from multiple studies developed nocardiosis (3,16–21). The cardiac transplant service at Stanford University has described cutaneous nocardiosis in four (2.5%) of their 160 patients in 1975 (22), but in none of 107 patients in 1986 (16). An incidence of 2% to 15% as reported in the literature is probably an overestimation but may reflect epidemiological differences in exposure based on country of residence (23). The median time to the diagnosis of nocardiosis after BMT is 7 months. Cutaneous involvement occurs in one of four patterns:

Mycetoma with draining sinus tracts;
Localized cutaneous disease, such as cutaneous and subcutaneous nodule;
Abscess or cellulitis-like lymphocutaneous disease with the characteristic sporotrichoid pattern;
Disseminated disease with skin involvement.

Dissemination to the central nervous system may occur in one-third of the primary cutaneous cases and lead to high mortality. Trimethoprim/sulfamethoxazole (TMP/SMX) given as prophylaxis for *Pneumocystis carinii* may prevent nocardiosis in BMT patients, which explains the low prevalence of nocardiosis in BMT patients. However, patients may acquire the disease despite TMP/SMX prophylaxis (15,24). TMP/SMX is considered the treatment of choice for nocardiosis. Other therapeutic alternatives include amikacin, ceftriaxone, imipenem, and cefotaxime. The combination of low-dose TMP/SMX and minocycline is preferred in BMT recipients to reduce the risk of bone marrow suppression (24,25). Long-term therapy has been recommended because premature termination of therapy may activate a quiescent focus of the disease.

Malakoplakia

Malakoplakia is an uncommon granulomatous disease seen in immunocompromised patients and results from impaired macrophagic phagocytic activity of bacteria. Partially digested bacterial fragments accumulate in the cytoplasm. Transplant patients are at risk. Twenty-seven percent of patients with malakoplakia have had renal

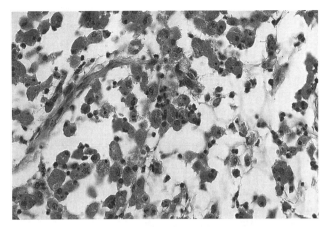

Figure 2. A predominantly histiocytic infiltrate in the dermis with scattered lymphocytes. The histiocytes have a large, finely granular eosinophilic cytoplasm with round to oval intracytoplasmic inclusions (center of photograph) characteristic of malakoplakia. (PAS stain.)

transplantation (26). The disease is most commonly seen in the urinary tract but may rarely affect the skin. The lesions are hard nodules and plaques that may ulcerate. The perianal and inguinal areas are commonly affected. Histologic examination reveals a predominantly histiocytic infiltrate in the dermis with scattered lymphocytes and plasma cells. The histiocytes have a large, finely granular eosinophilic cytoplasm with round to oval intracytoplasmic inclusions that stain with PAS, Von Kossa, and Giemsa stains (Fig. 2). The skin biopsy is often needed for diagnosis of systemic malakoplakia. Tissue culture usually reveals Gram-negative rods such as *Escherichia coli*, *Klebsiella* spp., and *Enterobacter* spp. (26,27). Gram-positive cocci like *Staphylococcus aureus*, *Streptococcus*, and *Enterococcus* are cultured occasionally. Systemic and topical antibiotics give variable results despite selection based on culture and sensitivity. Few lesions developed in some patients while on chronic antibiotic treatment (26). Surgical excision of skin nodules is often curative. Spontaneous resolution has been reported.

VIRAL INFECTIONS

Viral infections are common in transplant patients. It is estimated that 55% of heart transplant patients (16) and 22% to 35% of kidney transplant patients (3,5) develop at least one episode of cutaneous viral infection in the first year following the transplant. The annual incidence of certain viral infections varies with the time from the transplant. First-year infections are almost exclusively due to herpes virus; warts tend to appear many years later (3). In one study, up to 92% of renal transplant recipients of more than 5 years developed warts (28). The more severe viral infections tend to occur in the first year after transplant.

Herpesvirus Infections

Herpes Simplex Virus

Reactivation of herpes simplex virus (HSV) I and II is common in organ transplantation. In renal transplant patients, 4% to 47% are expected to develop at least one episode of HSV infection (16,29,30). Furthermore, It is estimated that HSV develops in 10% to 30% of heart transplant patients (12,25,26). In BMT recipients the incidence is much less common because of the use of prophylactic acyclovir. Only one BMT patient out of 83 on prophylactic acyclovir developed oral herpetic lesions after transplant (31). The lesions are usually localized and commonly affect the perioral skin, oral and nasal mucosa, or the genital area. The eruptions tend to occur in the first 1–3 months after solid organ transplantation but may occur later (19). The lesions result in shallow, grouped, painful ulcers. They are occasionally multifocal, extensive, hemorrhagic, and persistent. Severe mucosal ulcerations could also result. Half the cases reported in one study were asymptomatic and diagnosis was made by culture (32). Medical personnel who follow transplant patients should question and examine patients for new mucosal and genital lesions. The disease is rarely associated with dissemination. Usually the lesions respond well to oral or intravenous acyclovir (30). The oral dose is 200 mg five times a day for 10 days, and the intravenous dose is 5 mg/kg every 8 hours for 7 days. Untreated cases may persist for many weeks (30). The role of prophylactic antiviral therapy in SOT patients is not certain yet. Patients with frequent recurrences of HSV preoperatively or patients with positive antibody titer may become good candidates for prophylactic antiviral treatment. Saral and colleagues (33) demonstrated that intravenous acyclovir in BMT patients eliminate HSV infection during the first weeks following the transplant. Viral shedding and clinical infection are also reduced in BMT patients on standard acyclovir prophylaxis (31).

Cytomegalovirus

Cytomegalovirus (CMV) infection is a significant complication among recipients of bone marrow, renal, and liver transplants. Cutaneous eruptions develop in about 10% to 25% of patients with CMV infection (34). Skin involvement is far more common in SOT than in BMT patients. Specific cutaneous lesions in CMV infection manifest as localized cutaneous ulcers, or widespread, exanthematous, maculopapular eruptions. The localized ulcerations are purulent, are sharply demarcated, and tend to occur in the perianal, genital, and less likely perioral skin (35). CMV infections tend to occur between 1 and 6 months after SOT (6). The median interval after BMT is 2 months. Histologically, the ulcerative lesions show a perivascular infiltrate with lymphocytes, histiocytes, and neutrophils in middle and upper dermis that occasionally resemble leukocytoclastic vasculitis. Many large, irregularly shaped endothelial cells are usually present (Fig. 3). The most characteristic finding in cutaneous CMV infection is the formation of large intracytoplasmic and intranuclear inclusion bodies. These inclusions may be sparse and difficult to detect. Immunoperoxidase staining for CMV viral antigens is available and helpful in establishing the diagnosis before tissue culture results are available (36). DNA hybridization technology can be used on formalin-fixed, paraffin-embedded tissues and may help to establish the diagnosis earlier (36). Mixture of CMV and other infections such as herpes simplex, candida, and atypical mycobacterium is not uncommon (34). These subtle clinical and pathological findings and the frequent association of other infections may explain the occasional underdiagnosis of cutaneous CMV. Cutaneous CMV infection appears to be associated with grave prognosis; most patients die within 6 months from diagnosis. The cause of death is either from CMV dissemination or from concurrent systemic or cutaneous mixed infection (34). Disseminated purpuric maculopapular lesions have a worse prognosis than localized ulcerated lesions.

Varicella-Zoster Virus

Varicella-zoster virus (VZV) infection is an uncommon complication seen in about 5% of SOT recipients (16,32,37) and up to 23% to 28% of BMT patients (38,39). One-third of adults and children with BMT develop herpes zoster (38–40).

The disease occurs after an average of 1–2 years from the initial surgery in SOT (1). In BMT patients, VZV occurs within the first 6 months (38,39). The median onset of infection was day 96, with 89% of cases occurring within 1 year (40). The incidence of VZV was slightly more common in allogeneic than in autologous transplantation. Reactivation of VZV infection is more

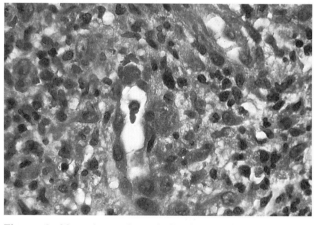

Figure 3. Many large, irregularly shaped endothelial cells with the formation of large intracytoplasmic inclusion bodies in a transplant patient with CMV infection.

common than primary VZV. A history of varicella infection is often present (17). Reactivation of VZV manifests as grouped vesicular eruptions on an erythematous base that involve two or three neighboring dermatomes. The thoracic and abdominal dermatomes are often affected. The lesions are occasionally gangrenous and hemorrhagic. Dissemination and multifocal involvement are not common in SOT; however, cutaneous dissemination and visceral dissemination occur in 15% and 5%, respectively, of patients with BMT (38). Postherpetic neuralgia occurs in half of the patients (30). Furthermore, if untreated, primary cutaneous VZV could be fatal. Intravenous acyclovir is the treatment of choice, and healing occurs in 3–5 weeks with therapy. VZV is more common in patients with hematologic malignancies for which BMT was performed than in patients with solid tumors requiring BMT (38,40). Total body irradiation may be responsible for the difference (40).

Human Herpesvirus-6

Human Herpesvirus-6 (HHV-6) is a virus that causes exanthem subitum (roseola infantum), usually in the first year of life. HHV-6 remains latent in the body after the primary infection and reactivates in the immunosuppressed state. A skin rash has been described between the sixth and fortieth days following BMT in children (41). The rash is associated with fever. HHV-6 was isolated from the blood and bone marrow around the time of the illness. Further data are needed to confirm and characterize this phenomenon.

Papillomavirus Infections

Warts are the most commonly encountered cutaneous virus infection in SOT recipients (16,29). Common warts (verruca vulgaris) are the most common type; however, plane, plantar, and perianal warts are also seen. The frequency and number of warts increase with the degree of immune suppression and with increased time after transplantation (37). The prevalence of common warts in transplant patients is related to the length of followup on these patients and hence varies in different studies. The prevalence of common warts in renal transplant patients is about 11% in the first year and increases to as high as 92% in those surviving more than 5 years (28,37,42). Among heart transplant patients, 43% acquire common warts within 5 years of the surgery (29). The prevalence of warts does not seem to increase by short-term immunosuppression in BMT recipients (43). The warts usually develop on sun-exposed areas of the extremities (3,42). In renal transplant patients, HPV2 and HPV4 are the most common types. Dysplastic changes are common in warts in transplant patients. Changes range from focal intraepidermal atypia of keratinocytes to frank squamous cell carcinoma. The latter occur more frequently than

expected in SOT patients, especially renal transplant patients. Clinically, the appearance of all warts with or without dysplasia is similar, which stresses the need for frequent histologic examination of these lesions. HPV types 2, 4, 5, and 8 were identified from squamous cell carcinoma lesions. Cryotherapy remains the simplest and most effective form of treatment for warts. Recurrence is common. Squamous cell carcinomas are best treated surgically.

Molluscum Contagiosum

Molluscum contagiosum is a rare infectious complication of SOT and BMT recipients (16,20). The disease is characterized by small, firm, umbilicated papules, far more common in children than in adults. The lesions spread by close contact or autoinoculation. The disease is more common in HIV-infected patients than in transplant recipients.

FUNGAL INFECTIONS

Fungal infections are the most common cutaneous infections encountered in transplant patients (3). The prevalence of cutaneous fungal diseases varies among studies, geographic areas, country of origin, duration of transplantation, and degree of immune suppression. Low socioeconomic status, hot climate, high humidity, and lack of personal hygiene are likely to increase the prevalence of fungal diseases (17). The average prevalence of cutaneous fungal infections in SOT is about 50%, and the vast majority of these are of the superficial type (3,17,18). Cutaneous fungal infections are far less common in BMT than in SOT recipients. Invasive fungal infections occur in about 2.3% of BMT patients within the first month of transplant (44). A strong association was noted between the occurrence of these invasive infections and the degree of neutropenia. The use of growth factors and primed peripheral blood progenitor cells was associated with shorter duration of neutropenia and a decrease in the overall incidence of fungal infections (44). Cutaneous fungal infections occur in one of three situations:

1. Primary skin infections with fungi that usually cause limited or localized disease in immunocompetent host. These superficial infections can result in widespread disease but remain limited to skin. Examples include tinea corporis and tinea versicolor.
2. Primary skin infections caused by opportunistic pathogens. These infections may remain localized or disseminate to systemic disease.
3. Secondary skin fungal infections caused by dissemination from systemic foci. Infections in groups 2 and 3, being invasive, are important causes of morbidity and mortality in transplant patients. Their incidence

has increased over the last three decades coincident with the use of immunosuppressive and cytotoxic agents.

Superficial Mycoses

Various superficial fungal diseases have been seen in SOT and to a lesser degree in BMT patients. The prevalence of superficial mycoses in renal transplant patients varies between 7% and 76% in different studies from different countries around the world (18,29,45). The incidence was reported around 20% in patients with heart transplant (16). Superficial fungal infections are more common in tropical areas (17) and are more likely to develop in patients receiving cyclosporine (45).

Tinea versicolor is a common infection seen in as many as 77% of kidney transplant patients from Puerto Rico (37) and as few as 4% in patients with heart transplant from Norway (29). The disease is caused by a saprophytic fungus called *Malassezia furfur.* The clinical features are similar to those in immunocompetent patients; however, the lesions are more likely to be nonpruritic and less inflammatory, and tend to involve larger areas of the body. Flexural distribution can also be seen. Occasionally, multiple papulonodular and pustular eruptions caused by *Pityrosporum* organisms are called *Pityrosporum* folliculitis.

Tinea corporis and tinea pedis have been reported to occur in 25% to 50% in one series (37) and are usually caused by *Trichophyton rubrum.* These figures are much higher than what we see in our practice. The lesions are usually nonpruritic and noninflammatory, and tend to involve extensive areas. A common misdiagnosis is dermatitis, and topical corticosteroids are often prescribed. A simple scraping of the scales to a slide followed by the application of 20% potassium hydroxide (KOH) preparation often yields diagnostic hyphae on microscopic examination. Dermal and subcutaneous abscesses caused by *T. rubrum* are occasionally seen and result from invasion of dermis through the hair follicles. Topical agents often fail to clear the infection; however, they respond dramatically to oral ketoconazole.

Onychomycosis is seen in 43% of patients with kidney transplant. The most common cause is *Trichophyton rubrum*; however, few cases have been reported with *Candida albicans* (37,45). The disease is characterized by subungual hyperkeratosis with onycholysis (separation of nail plate from nail bed) and discoloration of nail plate. Candidal and bacterial paronychia with red, tender, edematous proximal nail folds are also seen. The prevalence and severity of onychomycosis and other dermatophytosis are increased with the duration of transplantation (16,37,45).

Mucocutaneous candidiasis is seen in about 8% of patients with kidney transplant (37). The disease is caused by *Candida albicans,* a ubiquitous and common skin yeast that can cause extensive disease in transplant patients. Oral thrush, balanitis, vaginitis, and cutaneous flexural involvement are common. Renal transplant patients are predisposed to candidal onychomycosis (45). Clinical features of candidal infections are similar to those in immunocompetent host, but distribution is more extensive.

Invasive Opportunistic Mycoses

Fungal infections cause significant morbidity and mortality in transplant patients. The incidence of invasive fungal infections in renal transplant patients was 3% in one study from the tropics (1). Most of these infections were caused by *Candida, Aspergillus, Cryptococcus,* and *Mycoraceae* spp. Infections tend to occur 20–30 months after surgery (1) and have been reported as early as 2 months after transplantation (5). In contrast to SOT, BMT recipients are more likely to develop invasive fungal infections in the first few weeks after surgery. This seems to correlate with the transient neutropenia often following BMT. In a study of 290 patients with autologous BMT with a median duration of neutropenia of 12 days, seven patients (2.3%) developed invasive fungal infections in the first 30 days after surgery (56).

The type of fungal infection seen in transplant patients depends on the underlying immune defect. Generally, defects in neutrophil function or number (early after BMT) predispose patients to infections with *Candida* and *Aspergillus* spp. Defects in T-lymphocytes or mononuclear phagocytic function—as in patients on long-term corticosteroids, cyclosporine, azathioprine, or other cytotoxic agents—predispose patients to infections with more virulent fungal pathogens.

Candidiasis

Candidal infections are common opportunistic fungal infections in BMT and SOT patients. Skin lesions appear as maculopapular and erythematous with necrotic centers (Figs. 4 and 5). Lesions may resemble drug eruptions occasionally. Common predisposing factors include neutropenia, chronic immunosuppressant therapy, long-term broad-spectrum antibiotic use, and intravenous catheterization. Skin biopsy usually shows microabscesses in upper dermis centered around blood vessels (Fig. 6). Inflammation is usually minimal and nonspecific. A few budding yeasts with pseudohyphae may be found in the dermis using PAS or GMS stains. Tissue and blood cultures often yield positive results. Candidal cellulitis is indistinguishable from that caused by Gram-positive bacteria. It has a propensity to disseminate and cause systemic disease.

Candidiasis may affect the skin as part of systemic infection. The portal of entry is usually the gastrointestinal tract or intravascular devices. Oral colonization with

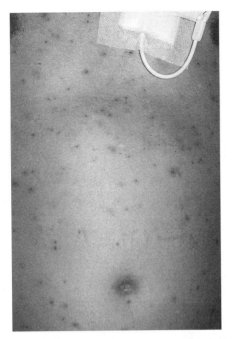

Figure 4. Small erythematous maculopapular lesions with necrotic center on the abdomen of a liver transplant patient with fever and disseminated *C. tropicalis* infection.

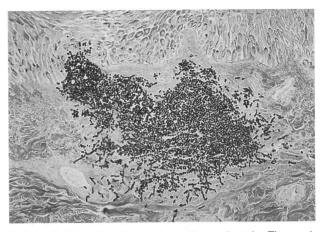

Figure 6. The skin biopsy from the patient in Figure 4. Microabscesses in upper dermis centered around blood vessels is evident. Inflammation is minimal and budding yeasts with pseudohyphae are seen (Gomori's methenamine silver).

Candida spp. is a common problem in BMT patients (46). The problem is reduced using prophylaxis with fluconazole (47). *C. albicans* is the predominant species isolated; however, others—such as *C. tropicalis* and *C. glabrata*—are also seen. The latter is found in high numbers in the gastrointestinal tract in pediatric BMT patients receiving prophylactic fluconazole. Because *C. glabrata* have variable sensitivity to fluconazole, infections with this pathogen may occur in transplant patients receiving prophylactic fluconazole. BMT patients are also susceptible to infection by *C. krusei*, which is resistant to fluconazole and rarely to *C. lusitaniae* (48).

Aspergillosis

Aspergillus spp. can involve the skin of immunocompromised patients as a primary or secondary process (49). *Aspergillus fumigatus* and *Aspergillus flavus* are the most common organisms. The former causes most of the disseminated cases; the latter causes most of the primary cutaneous cases. In a few SOT and BMT patients, primary infection may occur in association with contaminated intravenous catheters or extensive trauma or burns. Primary infections ultimately spread to distant sites, causing death. Clinically, skin lesions appear as erythematous edematous papules and plaques that resemble cellulitis and become necrotic and purpuric with a hemorrhagic eschar.

Secondary cutaneous disease results either from direct invasion from underlying infectious foci or as hematogenous spread from distant infectious sites, usually the lungs. This is the typical presentation of cutaneous aspergillosis in BMT patients and most SOT recipients. The disease almost invariably results in death. The skin lesions of disseminated aspergillosis include subcutaneous abscesses, pustules, nodules, hemorrhagic blisters, cellulitis-like patch, or ulcerations. Examination of surface exudate or scales with potassium hydroxide (KOH) may provide an immediate presumptive diagnosis by showing septate hyphae. Skin biopsy shows involvement of blood vessels by the organism, often leading to thrombosis, infarction, and necrosis. In tissue, *Aspergillus* spp. produce the characteristic 45-° dichotomous branching. The hyphae are septate and measure 3–4 mm on average. The recovery of *Aspergillus* spp. on culture is of little value unless the organism can be demonstrated in skin tissue. In primary cutaneous disease, extensive surgical debridement with intravenous amphotericin B is often needed. In secondary cutaneous disease, the mortality rate approximates 98%, despite antifungal treatment.

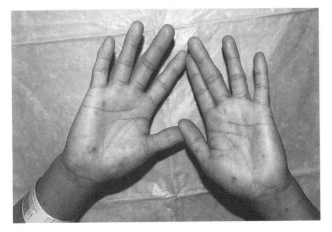

Figure 5. Multiple erythematous purpuric lesions on dorsal hands in the patient in Figure 4. Note the resemblance to drug eruptions and vasculitis.

Cryptococcosis

Cryptococcus neoformans can cause primary or secondary cutaneous infection in SOT patients. Skin involvement by a hematogenous spread, from the pulmonary foci usually, occurs in 10% to 15%. Primary cryptococcosis is uncommon in transplant patients and results from disruption of skin barrier. Dissemination to systemic involvement is common. Cryptococcosis usually occurs 3–10 years after transplant. No accurate estimate of the risk of cryptococcosis in organ transplant patients is available, and numbers vary with the different geographic areas and risks of exposure (16,17,20,30). Cutaneous lesions may present as subcutaneous abscess, dermal plaque or nodule, ecchymosis, purpura, or ulcers (50). Other presentations include cellulitis (Fig. 7) with tender warm erythema that later develop blisters and vesicles. The cellulitis does not respond to antibiotics and raises suspicion of a nonbacterial cause. Molluscum contagiosum–like lesions, described in patients with acquired immunodeficiency syndrome, may occur in transplant patients. Multiple lesions with different morphologies can be seen. The most reliable diagnostic test is skin biopsy for routine examination and culture. The presence of 5–10 mm ovoid to oval bodies surrounded by a clear halo with narrow-based budding is suggestive of the diagnosis. Numerous organisms are often seen in transplant patients with minimal inflammation (Figs. 8 and 9). Confirmation is by tissue culture. The prognosis is poor despite antifungal treatment, and death occurs in 50% to 60% of patients with cutaneous infection. Intravenous amphotericin B efficacy can be enhanced by 5-flucytosine and is considered the treatment of choice. Ketoconazole 400 mg a day is a good alternative in non-meningeal cryptococcosis. Ketoconazole treatment is difficult to manage in transplant patients, especially because of interference with cyclosporine. A decrease in immunosuppressant medications is also helpful. Fluconazole

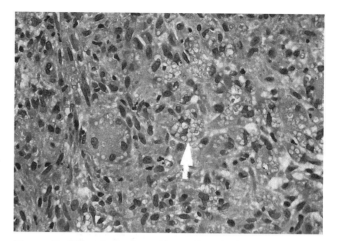

Figure 8. Skin biopsy from the patient in Figure 7 showing numerous ovoid to oval bodies in groups (*arrow*) and individually between the collagen bundles and in giant cells. Note the minimal inflammatory reaction typical of gelatinous reaction.

should be considered as an alternative treatment to amphotericin B.

Mucormycosis

Mucormycosis could be a life-threatening invasive infection caused by fungi of the family Mucoraceae. The most important of these are *Rhizopus, Mucor,* and *Absidia* spp. Infections occur almost exclusively in diabetic patients, including diabetic transplant patients. Less commonly, mucormycosis can occur in other SOT and BMT recipients (51,52). Catheters and external stents and tubes may serve as a portal of entry. Most often necrotic eschars develop that rapidly enlarge (Fig. 10). These infections are often fatal if disseminated and not treated. Secondary mucormycosis is seen after dissemination from a pulmonary foci. The diagnosis of cutaneous mucormycosis is made by biopsy as well as tissue culture.

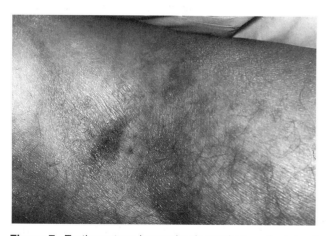

Figure 7. Erythematous hemorrhagic patches on the lateral arm of a renal transplant patient with disseminated cryptococcosis. Note the resemblance to bacterial cellulitis.

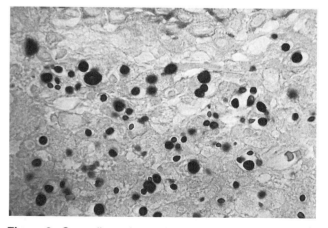

Figure 9. Gomori's methenamine silver showing the characteristic *Cryptococcus neoformans* organism with variable-sized yeast cells.

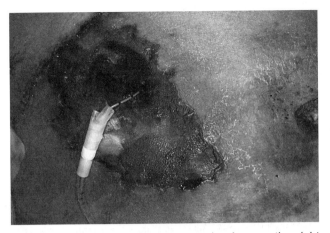

Figure 10. A rapidly enlarging necrotic ulcer on the right side of the abdomen of this liver transplant patient. Note the necrotic bullae formation (below), and surrounding erythema and ecchymosis.

In tissue, broad, nonseptated 90° branching hyphal elements are seen usually invading blood vessels (Fig. 11). Surgical debridement and liposomal amphotericin B for 6 months were reported to be effective (52).

Histoplasmosis

Histoplasmosis is a rare infectious complication of SOT patients caused by *Histoplasma capsulatum* (21). The disease is very rare in BMT patients and is often a manifestation of a disseminated disease. A warm, tender, indurated plaque resembling cellulitis could be the first sign of systemic histoplasmosis (53). Tender, erythematous, subcutaneous nodules that resemble erythema nodosum in a transplant patient should alert the physician to a possible diagnosis of histoplasmosis. Rapid diagnosis with introduction of normal saline into the lesion fol-

lowed by the aspiration of fluid, slide preparation, and appropriate staining may show the organism. Skin biopsy for routine examination and tissue culture is always recommended. Prognosis for secondary histoplasmosis is poor.

Others

Coccidioidomycosis and North American blastomycosis have rarely been diagnosed in BMT and SOT patients (20,54). Skin lesions are usually seen as part of systemic disease.

Protothecosis is a rare complication of organ transplantation. The lesions start as papulonodular lesions that ulcerate and drain a sanguinopurulent discharge. Culture of the draining material usually reveals a yeastlike organism with characteristic cleavage planes (55). The morula forms are best shown in tissue using PAS or methenamine silver stains.

PARASITIC INFECTIONS

Parasitic infections in general are rare complications of organ transplant patients. Overall, these infections are more common in SOT than in BMT patients. There are rare reports of *Pneumocystis carinii* and *Toxoplasma gondii* causing skin disease in organ transplant patients (56,57), although systemic infections are encountered.

Leishmaniasis is a rare protozoal disease in the United States. Cutaneous leishmaniasis encountered in the United States is most likely caused by *Leishmania braziliensis* or *L. Mexicana*. The lesions start as a papulonodule that ulcerates. Skin biopsy often reveals an intracellular organism that is best visualized by Giemsa stain. The diagnosis is often confirmed by tissue culture. There is no evidence that the incidence of leishmaniasis is increased in organ transplant patients or that visceral involvement can result from cutaneous leishmaniasis.

Strongyloidiasis is a disease caused by *Strongyloides stercoralis,* an intestinal nematode endemic to tropical and subtropical areas. Cutaneous signs could be the presenting complaints characterized by maculopapular or urticarial eruptions on the buttocks, trunk, and lower extremities. In transplant patients, eosinophilia may be absent. Most infections are diagnosed 1–3 months after transplant (58).

Norwegian scabies represents a heavy infestation with *Sarcoptes scabiei.* Immunocompromised patients are susceptible to this infection. Extensive hyperkeratotic crusts of the palms and soles are usually seen (Fig. 12). Treatment consists of repeated topical application of lindane.

Skin Biopsy

Skin biopsy is a very important tool in the diagnosis of skin infections in transplant patients. The procedure is

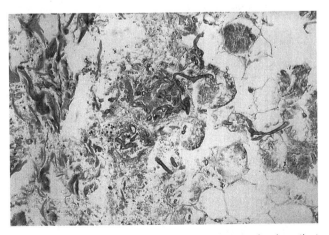

Figure 11. A mass of large, broad, nonseptate hyphae that occlude the deep dermal and subcutaneous fat blood vessels. Note the tissue necrosis and the lack of inflammatory tissue reaction (hematoxylin and eosin).

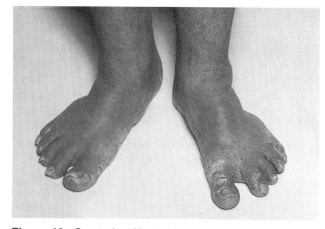

Figure 12. Crusted or Norwegian scabies with the characteristic hyperkeratosis and excessive scaling. The condition is extremely contagious and many thousands of mites are present.

easy to perform and results could be obtained within 24–48 hours in well-established laboratory.

The skin is usually cleansed with alcohol at the site of biopsy. Preservative-free, epinephrine-free lidocaine is recommended as local anesthetic. Methylparaben is often used as preservative in lidocaine and has some antimicrobial properties that may interfere with tissue culture. Furthermore, bicarbonate and epinephrine should be avoided for their antibacterial and antifungal effect (59). A ring-block at the lowest possible concentration of lidocaine is recommended, because lidocaine may have a growth-inhibiting effect on certain fungi (59).

A 5- or 6-mm punch biopsy is recommended. After removal, the specimen is divided into two equal parts—one for routine histology, the other for tissue culture. Multiple biopsies are often performed. The first part of the sliced specimen is then placed in formalin and submitted for routine histology. We recommend that a panel of special stains such as GMS or PAS (for fungus), Fite stain (for mycobacterium), and Gram stain (for bacteria)—in addition to hematoxylin and eosin—be ordered initially when submitting the tissue because valuable time could be saved. Immunoperoxidase stains and *in situ* hybridization are also available for some viral antigens and could be performed on paraffin-embedded tissue upon request. Multiple sections are often necessary to detect an infectious process with sparse organisms.

The second part of the sliced tissue is placed in a sterile physiologic saline and sent for bacterial, viral, fungal, and mycobacterial cultures. The laboratory should be notified about the possibility of infectious etiology in transplant patients. The skin defect is often closed with cutaneous nylon sutures. Wound care consists of twice-daily cleansing with alcohol or hydrogen peroxide, followed by application of topical antibiotic ointment.

REFERENCES

1. John GT, Date A, Mathew CM, Jeyaseelan L, Jacob CK, Shastry JC. A time table for infections after renal transplantation in the tropics. *Transplant* 1996;61:970–972.
2. Gorensek MJ. The immunocompromised host. *Dermatol Clin* 1989;7: 353–367.
3. Bencini PL, Montagnino G, De Vecchi A, Tarantino A, Crosti C, Caputo R, Ponticelli C. Cutaneous manifestations in renal transplant recipients. *Nephron* 1983;34:79–83.
4. Hibberd PL, Rubin RH. Renal transplantation and related infections. *Semin Respir Infect* 1993;8:216–224.
5. Martinez-Marcos F, Cisneros J, Gentil M, et al. Prospective study of renal transplant infections in 50 consecutive patients. *Eur J Clin Microbiol Infect Dis* 1994;13:1023–1028.
6. Granger DK, Burd RS, Schmidt WJ, Dunn DL, Matas AJ. Incidence and timing of infections in pediatric renal transplant recipients in the cyclosporine era. *Transp Proc* 1994;26:64.
7. Wolfson JS, Sober AJ, Rubin RH. Dermatologic manifestation of infections in imunocompromised patients. *Medicine (Baltimore)* 1985;64: 115.
8. Donnelly JP. Bacterial complications of transplantation: diagnosis and treatment. *J Antimicrob Chemother* 1995;36(Suppl):59–72.
9. Murphy JJ, Granger R, Blair GK, Miller GG, Fraser GC, Magee JF. Necrotizing faciitis in childhood. *J Pediatr Surg* 1995;30:1131–1132.
10. Roy V, Weisdorf D. Mycobacterial infections following bone marrow transplantation: a 20 year retrospective review. *Bone Marrow Transplant* 1997;19:467–470.
11. Lloveras J, Peterson PK, Simmons RL, Najarian JS. Mycobacterial infections in renal transplant recipients. Seven cases and a review of the literature. *Arch Intern Med* 1982;142:888–892.
12. Gombert ME, Goldstein EJC, Corrado ML, Stein AJ, Butt KMH. Disseminated mycobacterium marinum infection after renal transplantation. *Ann Intern Med* 1981;94:486–487.
13. Neeley SP, Denning DW. Cutaneous mycobacterium thermoresistible infection in a heart transplant recipient. *Rev Infect Dis* 1989;11: 608–611.
14. Adu D, Evans DB, Millard PR, et al. Renal transplantation in leprosy. *Br Med J* 1973;2:280–281.
15. van Burik JA, Hackman RC, Nadeem SQ, Hiemenz JW, White MH, Flowers ME, Bowden RA. Nocardiosis after bone marrow transplantation: a retrospective study. *Clin Infect Dis* 1997;24:1154–1160.
16. O'Connell BM, Abel EA, Nickoloff BJ, et al. Dermatologic complications following heart transplantation. *J Heart Transplant* 1986;5: 430–436.
17. Chugh KS, Sharma SC, Singh V, Sakhuja V, Jha V, Gupta KL. Spectrum of dermatological lesions in renal allograft recipients in a tropical environment. *Dermatologica* 1994;188:108–112.
18. Strumia R, Perini L, Tarroni G, Fiocchi O, Gili P. Skin lesions in kidney transplant recipients. *Nephron* 1992;62:137–141.
19. Bencini PL, Montagnino G, Sala F, De Vecchi A, Crosti C, Tarantino A. Cutaneous lesions in 67 cyclosporine-treated renal transplant recipients. *Dermatologica* 1986;172:24–30.
20. Cohen EB, Komorowski RA, Clowry LJ. Cutaneous complications in renal transplant recipients. *Am J Clin Pathol* 1987;88:32–37.
21. Bergfeld WF, Roenigk HH. Cutaneous complications of immunosuppressive therapy. A review of 215 renal transplant patients. *Cutis* 1978; 22:169.
22. Krick JA, Stinson EB, Remington JS. Nocardia infection in heart transplant patients. *Ann Intern Med* 1975;82:18–26.
23. Wilson JP, Turner HR, Kirchner KA, Chapman SW. Nocardia infections in renal transplant recipients. *Medicine* 1989;68:38–57.
24. Freites V, Sumoza A, Bisotti R, et al. Subcutaneous *Nocardia asteroides* abscess in a bone marrow transplant recipient. *Bone Marrow Transplant* 1995;15:135–136.
25. Hodohara K, Fujiyama Y, Hiramitu Y, et al. Disseminated subcutaneous nocardia asteroides abscesses in a patient after bone marrow transplantation. *Bone Marrow Transplant* 1993;11:341–343.
26. Lowitt MH, Kariniemi AL, Niemi KM, Kao GF. Cutaneous malakoplakia: a report of two cases and review of the literature. *J Am Acad Dermatol* 1996;34:325–332.
27. Palou J, Torras H, Baradad M, Bombi JA, Matin E, Mascaro JM. Cutaneous malakoplakia. Report of a case. *Dermatologica* 1988;176: 288–292.

28. Dyall-Smith D, Trowell H, Dyall-Smith ML. Benign human papillomavirus infection in renal transplant recipients. *Intern J Dermatol* 1991;30:785–789.

29. Jensen P, Clausen OP, Geiran O, et al. Cutaneous complications in heart transplant recipients in Norway 1983–1993. *Acta Dermatol Venereol* 1995;75:400–403.

30. Goldstein GD, Gollub S, Gill B. Cutaneous complications of heart transplantation. *J Heart Transp* 1986;5:143–147.

31. Epstein JB, Ransier A, Sherlock CH, Spinelli JJ, Reece D. Acyclovir prophylaxis of oral herpes virus during bone marrow transplantation. *Eur J Cancer. Part B, Oral Oncology* 1996;32B:158–162.

32. Dummer JS, Hardy A, Poorsattar A, Ho M. Early infections in kidney, heart, and liver transplant recipients on cyclosporine. *Transp* 1983;36:259–267.

33. Saral R, Burns WH, Laskin OL, Santos GW, Lietman PS. Acyclovir prophylaxis of herpes-simplex-virus infections. *N Eng J Med* 1981;305:63–67.

34. Lee JYY. Cytomegalovirus infection involving the skin in immunocompromised. hosts. A clinicopathologic study. *Am J Clin Pathol* 1989;92:96–100.

35. Pariser RJ. Histologically specific skin lesions in disseminated cytomegalovirus infection. *J Am Acad Dermatol* 1983;9:937–946.

36. Patterson JW, Broecker AH, Kornstein MJ, Mills AS. Cutaneous cytomegalovirus infection in a liver transplant patient. Diagnosis by *in situ* DNA hybridization. *Am J Dermatopathol* 1988;10:524–530.

37. Lugo-Janger G, Sanchez JL, Santiago-Delpin E. Prevalence and clinical spectrum of skin diseases in kidney transplant recipients. *J Am Acad Dermatol* 1991;24:410–414.

38. Schuchter LM, Wingard JR, Piantadosi S, Burns WH, Santos GW, Saral R. Herpes zoster infection after autologous bone marrow transplantation. *Blood* 1989;74:1424–1427.

39. Wacker P, Hartmann O, Benhamau E, Salloum E, Lemerle J. Varicella-zoster virus infection after autologous bone marrow transplantation in children. *Bone Marrow Transplant* 1989;4:191–194.

40. Kawasaki H, Takayama J, Ohira M. Herpes zoster infection after bone marrow transplantation in children. *J Pediatr* 1996;128:353–356.

41. Yoshikawa T, Suga S, Asano Y, et al. Human herpesvirus-6 infection in bone marrow transplantation. *Blood* 1991;78:1381–1384.

42. Barba A, Tessari G, Boschiero L, Chieregato GC. Renal transplantation and skin diseases: review of the literature and results of a 5-year follow up of 285 patients. *Nephron* 1996;73:131–136.

43. Kirchner H. Immunobiology of human papillomavirus infection. *Prog Med Virol* 1986;33:1–41.

44. Mossad SB, Longworth DL, Goormastic M, Serkey JM, Keys TF, Bolwell BJ. Early infectious complications in autologous bone marrow transplantation: a review of 219 patients. *Bone Marrow Transplant* 1996;18:265–271.

45. Lugo-Janger GJ, Pedraza R, Morales Otero LA, et al. Superficial mycosis in renal transplant recipients. *Transplant Proc* 1991;23:1787–1788.

46. Hoppe JE, Klingebiel T, Niethammer D. Orointestinal yeast colonization of pediatric bone marrow transplant recipients: surveillance by quantitative culture. *Mycoses* 1995;38:51–57.

47. Goodman JL, Winston DJ, Greenfield RA, Chandrasekar PH. A controlled trial of fluconazole to prevent fungal infections in patients undergoing bone marrow transplantation. *N Engl J Med* 1992;326:845–851.

48. Wingard JR. Importance of *Candida* species other than *C. albicans* as pathogens in oncology patients. *Clin Infect Dis* 1995;20:115–125.

49. Watsky KL, Eisen RN, Bolognia JL. Unilateral cutaneous emboli of *Aspergillus. Arch Dermatol* 1990;126:1214–1217.

50. Mayers DL, Martone WJ, Mandell GL. Cutaneous cryptococcosis mimicking Gram-positive cellulitis in a renal transplant patient. *South Med J* 1981;74:1032–1033.

51. Leong KW, Crowley B, White B, et al. Cutaneous mucormycosis due to *Absidia corymbifera* occurring after bone marrow transplantation. *Bone Marrow Transplant* 1997;19:513–515.

52. Jantunen E, Kolho E, Ruutu P, et al. Invasive cutaneous mucormycosis caused by *Absidia corymbifera* after allogenic bone marrow transplantation. *Bone Marrow Transplant* 1996;18:229–230.

53. Cooper PH, Walker AW, Beachman BE. Cellulitis caused by histoplasma organisms in a renal transplant patient [letter]. *Arch Dermatol* 1982;118:3–4.

54. Serody JS, Mill MR, Detterbeck FC, Harris DT, Cohen MS. Blastomycosis in transplant recipients: report of a case and review. *Clin Infect Dis* 1993;16:54–58.

55. Dagher FJ, Smith AG, Pankoski D, Ollodart RM. Skin protothecosis in a patient with renal allograft. *South Med J* 1978;71:222–224.

56. Gentry LO, Zeluff B, Kielhofner MA. Dermatologic manifestations of infectious diseases in cardiac transplant patients. *Infect Dis Clin North Am* 1994;8:637–654.

57. Leyva WH, Santa Cruz DJ. Cutaneous toxoplasmosis *J Am Acad Dermatol* 1986;14:600–605.

58. Morgan JS, Schaffner W, Stone WJ. Opportunistic strongyloidiasis in renal transplant recipients. *Transplantation* 1986;42:518–523.

59. Williams BJ, Hanke CW, Bartlett M. Antimicrobial effects of lidocaine, bicarbonate, and epinephrine. *J Am Acad Dermatol* 1997;37:662–664..

Transplant Infections edited by
Raleigh A. Bowden, Per Ljungman, and Carlos V. Paya.
Lippincott–Raven Publishers, Philadelphia © 1998

CHAPTER 10

Central Nervous System

Allen J. Aksamit

NEUROLOGICAL SYNDROMES

Organ transplantation recipients are challenging patients when considering possible central nervous system (CNS) infection complicating transplantation. The two major questions that are important to ask to devise a differential diagnosis are (a) "What is the neurological syndrome?" and (b) "What is the temporal profile of disease?" The neurological syndromes can be simply broken down into three major categories. They are seizures, focal brain parenchymal disease, and diffuse meningoencephalitis.

Seizures

Seizures are a common presentation of neurological infection (1). However, they do not distinguish whether the offending infection is a diffuse or focal process. Both focal parenchymal involvement of the cerebral hemisphere and diffuse meningoencephalitis can be associated with irritability of the cerebral cortex, leading to seizures. Generalized tonic/clonic seizures are not difficult to recognize clinically. However, the generalized nature of the seizure does not specifically identify whether the origin of the seizure discharge was focal, arising from localized parenchymal disease, or cortical irritability from a diffuse meningoencephalitic process. Therefore an isolated seizure should prompt an evaluation for both focal and diffuse disease. Focal seizures causing clonic movements of a limb or transient sensory symptoms of a positive quality (e.g., tingling, marching paresthesias) suggest focal cortical involvement. This is a common manifestation of cerebritis from a variety of opportunistic infections. However, diffuse meningoencephalitis with focal cortical infiltration of the organism through the perivascular Virchow-Robin space can also lead to seizures without frank neuroimaging focal cortical abnormalities.

Assessment of seizures should include a neuroimaging technique of at least a CT (computed tomography) scan, though a MRI (magnetic resonance imaging) scan of the head is more sensitive. If imaging excludes the possibility of cerebral mass effect, then spinal fluid should be analyzed, if safe from a coagulation standpoint. In patients with bone marrow transplant with thrombocytopenia or patients with liver transplantation with qualitative platelet defects, thrombocytopenia, and synthetic defects of coagulation factors, bleeding diasthesis may prohibit spinal fluid analysis.

An unusual but underrecognized cause for change in mental status due to CNS infection is nonconvulsive status epilepticus. In this circumstance, there is a fluctuating level of mental alertness without frank convulsive activity observable. The usual clue is the variability of responsiveness of the patient. This is a potentially treatable condition and is a neurological emergency. It can only be satisfactorily diagnosed with urgent EEG evaluation.

Focal Brain Parenchymal Infection

Focal cerebral cortical syndromes are common with focal parenchymal brain disease related to infection complicating transplantation. Most commonly, the infection is hematogenously born to the brain from systemic sources. Therefore the cerebral gray/white matter junction is the initial site of infection. However, there are exceptions to this rule, as different pathogens have different mechanisms of pathogenetic spread to the brain. The predilection for the gray/white matter junction is also present with metastatic disease such as metastatic tumors. Therefore the neuroimaging differential diagnostic possibilities of focal brain parenchymal disease usually include infection versus metastases. Deep-seated lesions affecting the basal ganglia structures or white matter structures in the area of the internal capsule of the cerebral hemispheres may suggest specific kinds of infectious organisms. Toxoplasmosis has a predilection for the

From the Department of Neurology, Mayo Medical School, Mayo Clinic, Rochester, MN 55905.

periventricular locations in the brain, as does CNS lymphoma, and either can occur in transplant patients.

Focal parenchymal CNS infection can be manifest clinically as multiple syndromes. The most easily recognized is hemiparesis. However, there is no specific predilection for the motor system to be selectively involved, and indeed any area of the cerebral cortex can be equally likely affected. Therefore a variety of syndromes—including aphasia, hemisensory syndrome, cortical syndromes (e.g., hemineglect), cortical sensory loss (i.e., loss of discriminative function such as stereognosis or graphesthesia with preserved pin and light-touch sensation), or visual deficits (e.g., homonymous hemianopsia, alexia, or alexia without agraphia) or cortical blindness—may occur. When the cerebellar hemisphere is affected by parenchymal disease, the most common presentation is either hemiataxia, when the lateral hemisphere is affected, or nystagmus, truncal ataxia, dysarthria, nausea, and vomiting, when the midline structures of the cerebellum are affected. Brain stem involvement by a parenchymal mass is usually cued clinically by the presence of cranial nerve deficits often in conjunction with long-tract signs such as corticospinal tract or sensory tract deficits.

Diffuse Meningoencephalitis

Meningoencephalitis due to neurological infection complicating transplantation classically presents with headache and stiff neck. The absence of these clinical signs in transplant patients, however, does not exclude meningitis. That is, patients with meningoencephalitis may not have headache or stiff neck because of altered state of consciousness from metabolic or drug effect. Likewise, stiff neck, which is dependent on spinal fluid inflammation with leukocytes and cytokines being released into the CSF space, may not occur because immunosuppression or lack of bone marrow reserves may limit the patient's CSF (cerebrospinal fluid) cellular response. Also, practical factors may interfere with the ability to determine these clinical signs. Specifically, paralytic agents used for neuromuscular blockade and intubation make reliability of nuchal signs low.

Unexplained altered state of consciousness should always trigger a search for possible CNS infection. Change in sensorium from infection is difficult to distinguish from toxic and metabolic effects. Still, disorientation, somnolence, stupor, and coma are all signs that are consistent with a diffuse meningoencephalitic infection. Also, focal parenchymal disease from frontal lobe disease or multiple, particularly small disseminated foci infection in the brain can produce a diffuse encephalopathy without gross focal clinical signs.

The involvement of the subarachnoid space by infections that cause meningoencephalitis can also commonly affect cranial nerves with focal or multifocal syndromes produced. The sixth cranial nerve is most likely to be affected because of its long course external to the brain stem originating at the level of the pontomedullary junction running along the base of the pons and laterally through the cavernous sinus and eventually through the superior orbital fissure. This long exposure to the subarachnoid space makes it potentially vulnerable to pressure effects, infiltrative processes, or focal suppuration. However, any cranial nerve can be affected, and other common syndromes include syndromes of the cerebellopontine angle, including deafness, facial paralysis, and vertigo. The third cranial nerve is also commonly affected, causing oculomotor paresis. The early involvement of the pupil may mimic signs of increased intracranial pressure. This is because of the external orientation of the pupillomotor fibers in the third nerve, which make it vulnerable to infiltration by an external infectious, purulent process.

TEMPORAL PROFILE

Relationship to Transplantation

There are two important aspects regarding the temporal profile of potential infection in deciding about potential etiologic agents in the circumstance of transplantation (2,3). First, the temporal relationship of the neurological syndrome to the date of transplant will help establish potential organisms (Table 1). Specifically, bacterial infections and infections such as cytomegalovirus occur frequently in the first month following transplantation. This is because of a combination of the intensity of the immunosuppression that is administered and the systemic operative potential sources of infection present around the time of organ transplantation. In the circumstance of bone marrow transplantation, cytopenias may be most severe during this time period and may predispose to reactivation of rapidly replicating viral infections. On the other hand, other indolent, relatively weak pathogens require long-term immunosuppression for systemic reactivation and eventual spread to the CNS. Progressive multifocal leukoencephalopathy or cryptococcal meningitis are typical examples (see Table 1). Some organisms, however, may occur early or late. Aspergillosis, for example, can occur early because of colonization of the endotracheal tube and respiratory equipment (in the intensive care unit) during the early post-transplantation period or can occur as a consequence of colonization of the tracheobronchial tree leading to hematogenous dissemination of organism to the CNS late after transplantation.

Evolution of the Clinical Syndrome

The second important aspect of the temporal profile is the evolution of the clinical neurological syndrome. Rapid, acute, focal evolution of a neurological syndrome suggests either a vascular invasive organism, such as

TABLE 1. *Temporal relationship of the neurological syndrome to the date of transplant*

	Focal parenchymal disease	Diffuse meningoencephalitis

Early (≤1 month post-transplant)	Bacterial brain abscess
	  Staphylococcus abscess
	  Gram-negative abscess
	  Anaerobe abscess
	Aspergillosis brain abscess
	Candida brain abscess
		Candida meningitis
		Bacterial meningitis
		  Gram-positive meningitis (Strep or Staph)
		  Gram-negative meningitis
		Herpes simplex meningoencephalitis

Late (>1 month post-transplant)	Progressive multifocal
	  leukoencephalopathy (PML)
	
	Aspergillosis brain abscess
	Toxoplasmosis brain abscess
	Nocardia brain abscess
	Mucor/Rhizopus encephalitis
		Listeria meningitis
		
		Cryptococcal meningitis
		Varicella-zoster meningoencephalitis
		Human herpesvirus 6 (HHV6)
		  meningoencephalitis
		CMV encephalitis

Aspergillus, or rapid replication of the organism, as is associated with bacterial abscess. If the evolution is more subacute but focal and causes evolving neurological deficit over days to weeks, then an indolent opportunistic infection should be suspected, such as progressive multifocal leukoencephalopathy. Nonfocal neurological syndromes that are acute include bacterial meningoencephalitis, *Candida* meningoencephalitis, and aspergillosis with multiple disseminated brain abscesses. Subacute nonfocal meningoencephalitis suggests *Cryptococcus.* These guidelines, however, are approximations, and it is certainly possible for organisms such as *Cryptococcus* to present acutely and occasionally for bacterial infections (e.g., those resulting from *Listeria*) to present more chronically. More specific discussions of individual organisms, their temporal profile, and relationship to the timing and type of transplantation will follow for each of the individual organisms.

OPPORTUNISTIC INFECTIONS

Bacterial Infections

Gram-Negative and Gram-Positive Infections

Gram-positive and Gram-negative bacterial infections of the CNS are relatively rare in the circumstance of solid organ transplantation. The strongest predilection occurs in patients who have bone marrow transplantation and who have more severe and prolonged granulocytopenia following immunosuppression (4). Bacterial infection usually corresponds to systemic infection and occurs as a consequence of seeding of the nervous system with either bacteremia or other systemic source.

The incidence of bacterial infections involving the CNS following solid organ transplantation has been estimated at between 1% and 4%.

Bacterial infections can present as a frank meningitis. Altered sensorium is common and may be the most common manifestation. More than 50% of patients will pre-

sent with high fever and commonly will have accompanying complaints of headache. Stiff neck may be variably present. Because of the accompanying granulocytopenia, particularly in bone marrow transplant patients, a meningeal reaction with pleocytosis may be mild, and profound fever and stiff neck may not be present.

Alternatively, seizures can occur as a consequence of meningitis, and meningitis should be suspected if there is headache, stiff neck, and fever without evidence of abnormality on neuroimaging studies.

Brain abscess, on the other hand, or early development of cerebritis secondary to bacterial seeding of the CNS often presents with obtundation and focal neurological deficit. Headache is somewhat less common, and fever is present in only 50%. The focal neurological deficits include hemiparesis, which sometimes leads to the mistaken diagnosis of "stroke" because of rapid evolution.

Bacterial abscesses are hematogenously disseminated to the CNS and tend to occur at the gray/white matter junction. Therefore seizures are a common presenting manifestation. It is estimated that in the first month after transplantation, seizures associated with fever and focal neurological deficit are due to a bacterial abscess and cerebritis formation in approximately 70% (1).

Solid organ transplantation can be associated with bacterial infection of the CNS. However, the bacterial source is usually systemically evident, either occurring at the site of the surgical procedure or associated with contaminated intravenous lines with secondary hematogenous seeding. In bone marrow transplantation, the source of septicemia is often less clear. Therefore the bacterial spectrum of organisms is much broader.

The timing of dissemination of bacterial infection to the nervous system is usually simultaneous with systemic bacterial infection. Infection therefore occurs any time in the first month after transplantation. The role of immunosuppressive agents is not as large. In bone marrow transplantation, it is the granulocytopenia that mainly correlates with bacterial infection.

Fever is common and occurs in most patients, but it is not inevitably present. This is true for both meningitis and brain abscess formation. Again, coincident signs of systemic infection are often present and may be associated with hypotension, disseminated intravascular coagulation, and cutaneous lesions. Meningitis is most commonly associated with no focal abnormalities. Focal parenchymal involvement secondary to arterial involvement of meningeal blood vessels with associated petechial hemorrhage or infarction is commonly seen pathologically, however. Focal accentuation of meningeal infections can be associated with both focal neurological deficits, seizures, or profound obtundation usually ascribed to parenchymal encephalitic processes.

Brain abscess is characteristically associated with a rapidly evolving focal neurological deficit. Because of the predilection for the gray/white matter junction, hyporeflexia rather than hyperreflexia may be present early associated with weakness. A Babinski sign is typically present. Later, a spasticity may develop associated with hyperreflexia in the affected limbs. Sensory focal deficits, visual field deficits, and language difficulty all can be seen but are much more difficult to detect in the obtunded patient.

Focal spinal cord involvement can also occur with paraparesis or quadriparesis. This typically occurs associated with back pain because the infection has caused an epidural abscess or disk space infection.

The bacteria involved with meningitis or early abscess formation after transplantation usually reflect the bacterial pathogens common following procedures or invasive interventions performed as part of the postoperative care of surgical patients. Bacterial infections include *Streptococcus pneumoniae*, *Klebsiella pneumoniae*, *Escherichia coli*, and alpha hemolytic *Streptococcus*. Paranasal or sinus origin can also be another source of bacterial spread to the nervous system. *Staphylococcus aureus* or *Staphylococcus epidermidis* can occur commonly from cutaneous or intravenous-line-associated infection. Mixed flora can occur when oral dentition is poor, including anaerobic bacterial infection or microaerophilic bacteria. Bacterial abscess or parameningeal infection can be polymicrobial. Meningitis is usually associated with septicemia by a single organism.

It is always important to remember that in the circumstance of suspected meningitis or cerebritis, even in the absence of obvious systemic sepsis, blood cultures should be performed to identify a hematogenous source of bacterial infection. Also, other suspected sites such as intravenous lines, purulent material from nasal or sinus passages, and cutaneous abscesses provide culturable material that may give important microbiological information as to the etiologic agent causing nervous system infection. The urinary tract, lungs, and surgical wounds are also easily culturable sites that should not be neglected in the course of evaluating possible neurological infection. Ultimately, early stereotactic brain biopsy for microbiology may be necessary.

The imaging of CNS and infection is important to distinguish meningitis from focal brain involvement where headache, fever, and obtundation may be the only signs and symptoms of neurological involvement. Likewise, seizures may be generalized from onset, not giving a clue as to the focal nature of parenchymal involvement. Because there is urgency in performing spinal fluid examination, a prior urgency for imaging the brain to exclude serious mass effect is important.

CT scanning of the head is less sensitive than MRI scan in detecting focal parenchymal involvement by bacterial infection. However, it excludes serious mass effect in the circumstance of bacterial infection. Typically, in association with meningitis, CT scanning is normal. In the circumstance of cerebritis or early brain abscess formation, CT scan shows hypodensity and focal mass effect. With contrast, CT scan of a brain abscess will show ring enhancement.

Transporting an ill patient with systemic sepsis and unstable hemodynamic status for head scanning is always problematic. The clinician must weigh the potential risks of moving the patient for scanning procedure versus the risk of herniation from spinal tap. Unfortunately, clinical signs of mass effect, such as papilledema or focal abnormalities on neurological examination, may not be obvious early in the comatose patient with large mass effect. However, because of the risk of cerebral herniation, if these signs are present, spinal fluid analysis should not be performed.

MRI scan of the head, particularly performed with gadolinium enhancement, is a very sensitive indicator of focal parenchymal infection. MRI scan T2-weighted images are extremely sensitive to increased water content in the brain and are always abnormal with bacterial brain abscess. Gadolinium enhancement is a sensitive indicator of leaking blood/brain barrier and is seen as a ring or solid enhancement in cerebritis and early abscess formation. More variable degrees of gadolinium enhancement occur in the meningeal coverings of patients with meningitis, but focal or diffuse meningeal enhancement can be seen with higher sensitivity on MRI scan than on CT. The purulence tends to be more common in the basal cisterns of the brain, and therefore gadolinium enhancement may be more prominent in these locations. Secondary vascular injury to brain with infarction due to arterial or venous occlusion is more likely to be seen on MRI scan than on CT of the head.

Although the gray/white matter junction of the cerebral hemispheres is the most common location for brain abscess, deep white matter structures, basal ganglia, cerebellum, and brain stem are all potential sites for hematogenous seeding by bacteria. Multiple abscesses are detected by MRI much more often and reliably than by CT.

Cerebrospinal fluid examination may be dangerous in the transplant patient who has suspected meningitis because of abscess mimicking the clinical features or because of epidural bleeding. The urgency of diagnosing meningitis does require urgent CSF if it can be practically obtained. Imaging is discussed earlier. The risk of epidural hematoma is from bleeding diasthesis. Absolute contraindications for spinal fluid examination include platelet counts <20,000, prothrombin time with International Normalized Ratio (INR) >1.5, or activated partial thromboplastin time (APTT) longer than 80 seconds. The risk of epidural hematoma at the site of lumbar puncture is still significant with platelet counts <50,000, particularly if there are associated qualitative platelet defects. This is often the case in association with liver transplantation. Other parameters, such as bleeding time or thromboelastogram, may provide additional information about the safety of doing lumbar puncture if time is available.

The microbiology of the spinal fluid is helpful in defining the cause of bacterial meningitis. Rapid identification of bacterial pathogens by Gram stain and counterimmunoelectrophoresis should be performed. Bacterial culture is definitive. Brain abscess or early cerebritis is usually associated with sterile spinal fluid. Low CSF glucose (<40% of the coincident blood glucose) is more likely to be associated with meningitis than with brain abscess or cerebritis. Gram stain in meningitis is positive in only 50% to 60% of patients.

The diagnosis of brain abscess or early cerebritis formation may only be definitively confirmed microbiologically by brain biopsy. Modern stereotactic neurosurgical techniques provide a relatively less invasive means of obtaining culturable material directly from brain with precise localization afforded by stereotactic methods. The reason for neurosurgical intervention is the absence of a likely bacterial pathogen, progressing neurological deficit associated with suspected brain abscess or cerebritis, or absence of a systemic source of infection.

Listeria monocytogenes

Listeria monocytogenes is a Gram-positive bacillus and is probably the most common cause of CNS bacterial infection in immunosuppressed hosts, including those with organ transplantation (5–7). Its most common clinical manifestations are associated with acute purulent meningitis. Why *Listeria* has a strong predilection for CNS seeding with meningitis is poorly understood (8). Parenchymal brain stem involvement can rarely occur associated with meningitis. Specifically, brain stem invasion with microabscess formation is most common (9,10).

Listeria meningitis typically presents with the nonspecific findings of fever and headache typical for acute meningitis. The temporal profile of the evolution of these symptoms may be somewhat more subacute, often occurring over 2–10 days rather than being as fulminant as

other forms of bacterial meningitis. Nuchal signs are frequent but are not an inevitable accompaniment of the meningitis, particularly in severely immunosuppressed patients. The degree of meningeal signs usually correlates with the degree of inflammatory response the patient can mount in the spinal fluid. In severely suppressed individuals, the signs may be absent.

Obtundation and focal signs, particularly cranial nerve palsies, can occur with parenchymal invasion by *Listeria*. Seizures are a rare manifestation of this infection. Corticospinal signs such as Babinski signs or hyperreflexia on physical examination may also give a clue to the parenchymal invasion of this organism affecting the pyramidal tracts.

Bone marrow transplantation is the most common associated condition (8). Incidence has been calculated to be 0.39 per 100 transplants. *Listeria* has also been observed to be associated with renal, liver, or heart transplantation (11). *Listeria* complicating transplantation almost always occurs more than 1 month after transplant. *Listeria* infection usually follows gastrointestinal ingestion of the organism, penetration, and subsequent bacteremia. These invasive mechanisms by *Listeria* are much less likely to occur in immunopreserved individuals. A correlation between the use of corticosteroids and *Listeria* has also been observed. Cell-mediated immunity defects pose the greatest risk (8).

The usual signs of meningitis, such as fever, stiff neck, and obtundation, are the most common signs associated with *Listeria* meningitis. Seizures occur frequently in up to 40% of patients (8). Increased intracranial pressure may occur rarely. Nuchal rigidity signs with Kernig's and Brudzinski's signs are frequent.

Brain stem encephalitis (rhombencephalitis) and microabscess formation are relatively unique to *Listeria* meningitis. When this occurs, the clinical manifestations include cranial nerve palsies, nystagmus, ataxia, and dysarthria. Likewise, long tract signs of hemiparesis, hyperreflexia, and Babinski signs may be present.

Listeria monocytogenes invasion with meningitis is almost always associated with bacteremia. Therefore blood cultures and examination of the spinal fluid are important in establishing the organism. This is particularly important in *Listeria* meningitis, where CSF culture may not be uniformly positive for the organism. However, if the CSF formula shows an acute purulent meningitis, and blood cultures are positive, *Listeria* is the likely cause of the meningitis even if CSF cultures are negative.

CT scan of the head is usually unremarkable with *Listeria* infection. It is helpful as a screening test in the acute setting to establish the safety of lumbar puncture in a patient who has suspected meningitis. CT scan in the circumstance of acute meningitis is sometimes practically difficult. Some patients with brain stem encephalitis and abscess formation may show contrast enhancement and mass effect, emphasizing the need for imaging if possible (9).

Imaging of *Listeria* meningitis and the associated focal brain stem encephalitis by MRI scanning has been described (12). As with most forms of bacterial acute meningitis, MRI imaging even with gadolinium enhancement may be negative, particularly in the early stages of disease.

With brain stem invasion by *Listeria* in association with meningitis, MRI scans may show increased T2 signal within the brain parenchyma in a multifocal or irregular pattern. Gadolinium enhancement can be seen in the basilar cisterns. If brain stem involvement is present, it may enhance with gadolinium.

Listeria meningitis is typically associated with an acute purulent reaction of CSF. The cell count usually ranges from 100 to 1,000 nucleated cells. The degree of neutrophilia versus lymphocytosis comprising the CSF cellular reaction is related to the acuteness of evolution of the meningitic syndrome. If the meningitis is more acutely evolving, CSF pleocytosis is typically neutrophilic. A more subacute evolving meningitis over days to a week or more is associated with a predominance of lymphocytes.

Typically, there is elevation of CSF protein in the range of 50–500 mg%. CSF glucose is frequently normal but may be depressed and more commonly occurs when the neutrophilic CSF cellular reaction is present.

The Gram stain on the spinal fluid for this Gram-positive rod is usually negative in *Listeria monocytogenes* meningitis. When it is positive, it may be mistaken for a Gram-positive coccus, most commonly confused with *Streptococcus*. Cultures are positive in the spinal fluid in 70% to 90% of patients with *Listeria* meningitis. However, as mentioned earlier, blood cultures are important supporting evidence for *Listeria* infection.

Pathology of acute purulent meningitis is a leptomeningeal infiltration by polymorphonuclear and lymphocytic cells. Particularly with *Listeria*, there can be dissection of this lymphocytic infiltrate down the Virchow-Robin spaces into the brain parenchyma with formation of small microabscesses (9,10). Presumably the predilection for the brain stem ventral surface comes from an invasiveness of this organism along these perivascular spaces and subsequent expansion into the substance of the brain. The pyramidal tracts of the pons and medulla are particularly prone to this invasion, accounting for the frequent accompaniment of long tract signs with hyperreflexia and extensor toe signs. Also, cerebellar folia or the cerebellar peduncles may be involved, accounting for unifocal or bilateral cerebellar signs on the physical examination. Again, microscopically, microabscesses with parenchymal invasion can be found, with focal neuronal destruction occurring at the sites of the lymphocytic infiltration.

Nocardia

Nocardia species is a weakly acid-fast, Gram-positive, branching filamentous bacterium that causes brain abscess in immunocompromised patients. The infection usually occurs as a consequence of hematogenous dissemination from primary pulmonary infection.

The presenting manifestations of *Nocardia* brain abscess are similar to other brain abscesses. Headache, confusion or obtundation, fever, and seizures are the most common symptoms. Focal neurological symptoms can also occur, depending on the location of the abscess. It has been estimated that seizures occur as the presenting manifestation of nocardia brain abscess in 30% of all nocardial nervous system infections (13).

Nocardia is thought to be an opportunistic infection requiring an impairment of cell-mediated immunity. Therefore *Nocardia* brain abscesses occur more than 1 month after transplantation and often later after transplantation. The most common associated transplantation is renal transplantation. One study estimated that the incidence of *Nocardia* brain abscess in renal transplantation was 0.7% (14).

As noted earlier, headache is the most common presenting symptom, but obtundation is the most common sign found associated with nocardia brain abscess. The temporal profile of the evolution of this symptom complex usually is subacute over days. Focal findings of hemiparesis or other cerebellar neurological signs have been estimated to occur in 42% (13). The absence of focal findings, however, does not exclude the possibility of *Nocardia* brain abscess.

Nocardia typically is an opportunistic infection disseminated to the nervous system from a pulmonary source. Clinically evident and obvious pulmonary infection has been suggested to be present in 66% to 88% of patients (13,14). Associated cutaneous infection with nodules has been found in approximately 20%. Pulmonary or cutaneous site therefore may serve as a useful adjunct for microbiological testing outside of the CNS.

Because this bacterium is hematogenously disseminated to the CNS, the location of the abscess frequency is 10 times more likely to be supratentorial as infratentorial. This is proportional to cerebral blood flow. The typical location in the cerebral hemispheres to be involved is the gray/white matter junction. Imaging with CT scanning or MRI scanning will often show multiple or multiloculated brain abscess with ring enhancement after contrast is given. It has been estimated that abscesses are multiple in 38% of cases (13). The appearance of *Nocardia* brain abscess is otherwise nonspecific when compared with other forms of infectious brain abscess. As in other circumstances, MRI scan of the head is much more sensitive than CT scan in detecting multiple abscesses.

In general, CSF examination is not helpful in the diagnosis of cerebral abscess from *Nocardia*. The main indication for CSF is to exclude other forms of infection. Again, caution needs to be exercised before examining spinal fluid in suspected brain abscess. In *Nocardia* brain abscess, where spinal fluid has been obtained, it is often normal. In a minority of cases, there is a mild elevation of protein and cell count with a predominance of lymphocytes.

The diagnosis of *Nocardia* brain abscess is difficult without direct culture from brain. A high index of suspicion is indicated when pulmonary infection with *Nocardia* is known. Skin nodule culture may provide further systemic dissemination evidence and by inference imply that brain abscess found on neuroimaging may have a similar microbiology. CT scan or MRI scan–directed stereotactic biopsy is probably the technique of choice for establishing CNS abscess infection. The most common species found in the nervous system is *Nocardia asteroides*. Rarely, *Nocardia brasiliensis* can be isolated (14).

Neuropathology of brain abscess is dictated by the temporal evolution of the abscess. In more acute or subacute cases, there is a predominance of necrosis and polymorphonuclear reaction. However, if the course has been subacute to chronic, then a more granulomatous histologic reaction can be found. Though the organism is weakly acid fast and Gram positive, the stains on histologic tissue are difficult to interpret. The best stain to identify organisms present in the tissue is methenamine silver preparation. The presence of silver staining branching filamentous bacteria in the area of histologic brain abscess is diagnostic of *Nocardia*. This finding should be distinguished from *Actinomycosis*, another branched bacterial form. That organism forms sulfur granules in tissue. Similar granules are not formed by *Nocardia*.

Fungal Infections

Aspergillus fumigatus

Aspergillosis of the nervous system is a common transplant infection. In the transplant population, it is the most common neurological infection responsible for mortality.

The most common clinical presentation for CNS aspergillosis is fever associated with change in level of consciousness. Unfortunately, this complex of symptoms is nonspecific. Virtually all the patients who have CNS aspergillosis eventually develop change in level of consciousness. The interpretation of fever and reduction in level of consciousness is complex because other associated toxic or metabolic phenomena commonly coexist with underlying infections. These include hepatic encephalopathy, uremic encephalopathy, gastrointestinal bleeding, sepsis, or coincidental multiple infections systemically. However, CNS aspergillosis must be considered in the differential diagnosis of any transplant patient with an acute or subacute decline in level of consciousness, particularly if it occurs coincidentally with fever.

Another common feature of presentation is seizures. The seizures may be focal or generalized from onset. In several series the incidence of seizures at presentation ranges from 15% to 40% (15–18). Because the pathology of the infection most commonly affects the subcortical gray/white matter junction, it is easy to induce cortical irritability and associated seizures coincident with the onset of infection.

Headache is sometimes a difficult symptom to elicit in patients who are otherwise often systemically very ill. However, it is recorded as a symptom in at least 10% of patients with CNS aspergillosis. A rare cause for explosive onset headache associated with CNS aspergillosis is subarachnoid hemorrhage from ruptured mycotic aneurysm secondary to aspergillosis infection of cerebral blood vessels. Manifestations of this syndrome are abrupt loss of consciousness often associated with frank meningismus and bloody spinal fluid.

CNS aspergillosis can occur after transplantation of liver, kidney, lung, heart, or bone marrow. Although *Aspergillus* can complicate any form of solid organ transplantation, experience suggests that the association with liver transplantation is overrepresented (15,18). Other complications of organ transplantations with solid organ failure, sepsis, or CNS toxicity from systemically administered drugs may be coincidental and complicate the interpretation of clinical data regarding these patients.

The timing of the dissemination of aspergillosis to the nervous system after transplantation may be early or late (Table 1). Infection usually does not occur within the first week after transplantation because the patient does not yet develop dissemination of *Aspergillus* from invasive disease involving the primary site of infection, either the lung or the cranial sinus. The infection may occur within the first month after transplantation and often in the context of complicated pulmonary illness, particularly with respiratory distress or respiratory-associated infection. However, CNS aspergillosis can also occur as a late consequence of transplantation, typically in association with other systemic disease. Respiratory distress is by far the most common associated systemic symptom associated with invasive lung disease, which is often present at the time of CNS dissemination.

Fever is common and occurs in most patients but is not inevitably present. In addition, fever is sometimes ascribed to coincident other infections of bacterial sepsis or viral infections complicating the transplantation systemically. Overall and by far the most common neurological sign is a decreased level of consciousness. The reduction in level of consciousness may be entirely nonfocal, without associated focal neurological findings to clue the examiner into an expanding mass, or multifocal injury to the brain. Declining level of consciousness occurs acutely or subacutely. The evolution of the abrupt change in consciousness is the most common reason for neurological consultation.

Focal neurological signs may not be present on physical exam to clue the examiner that a focal *Aspergillus* brain abscess is responsible for the reduced level of consciousness. Focal findings on physical examination of hyperreflexia, hemiparesis, unilateral Babinski sign, cerebellar dysfunction, brain stem dysfunction, or cranial nerve abnormalities are present in approximately one-half of patients at physical examination (15–17). Meningeal irritation signs with nuchal rigidity, Kernig's or Brudzinski's signs are only present in 10% to 15% of patients. Again, subarachnoid hemorrhage from mycotic aneurysm rupture, though rare, is typically associated with meningeal irritation signs.

Rare spinal cord involvement, particularly with meningeal aspergillosis, has been reported. It may occur in 10% to 20% pathologically at autopsy. However, clinically, spinal cord involvement is difficult to diagnose in a patient with a depressed level of consciousness from associated cerebral involvement. Spinal cord invasion in isolation is rare.

Patients with CNS aspergillosis have a remote site of infection with secondary dissemination to the nervous system. This is most often pulmonary. Pulmonary parenchymal disease is often diagnosed before CNS dissemination occurs. Pulmonary parenchymal diseases include nodular densities on the chest x-ray, bilateral pulmonary infiltrates, cavitary lesions, or pulmonary effusions. If there is a sudden change in level of consciousness, it is important to examine for evidence of pulmonary infection and to suspect CNS aspergillosis.

Cranial sinus disease can also serve as a primary nidus for aspergillosis infection. Dissemination may occur in this circumstance either through hematogenous route, as with pulmonary disease, or via direct invasion of the brain through communicating venous channels.

Because CNS disease occurs often as a part of systemic dissemination, other evidence of multiple organ dissemination may also be present. The most visible and easily diagnosable sign is dissemination to the skin. Biopsy of skin lesions showing aspergillosis is highly suggestive that there is also coincident CNS dissemination of aspergillosis when the clinical picture of encephalopathy and fever is present.

Imaging changes of CNS aspergillosis reflect the multifocal nature and hematogenous dissemination of the organism. The lesions in the brain are most commonly in the cerebral hemispheres and are commonly multiple. They can also occur in the cerebellum or in the brain stem. CT scanning of the head is less sensitive than MRI scan in detecting multiple lesions. The lesions appear on both the CT scan or MRI as focal or multifocal lesions with a predilection for the gray/white matter junction. They can often be interpreted as infarcts. They are frequently associated with edema and mass effect, though this may be mild. MRI scan is more sensitive than CT scan in distinguishing stroke from the cerebritis associated with aspergillosis. The edema associated with cerebritis or early abscess formation will obey the gray/white matter junction boundary. Gadolinium or CT contrast ring enhancement is often present because of breakdown in the blood/brain barrier that occurs with early cerebritis or abscess formation.

CT scan is particularly sensitive to hemorrhage in the brain, and because of the vascular invasive nature of aspergillosis, there can be a hemorrhagic component frequently present on CT scan. The presence of a hemorrhagic lesion or multiple lesions associated with reduction in level of consciousness and fever is highly suggestive of CNS aspergillosis. Because MRI is less sensitive than CT scanning to hemorrhage, CT head scan may be preferable as an initial screening assessment in suspected cases.

CSF sampling may be dangerous because of mass effect and risk of herniation in transplant patients. Often patients may have mass effect from hemorrhage or abscess formation without focal signs putting the patient at risk for herniation if spinal fluid examination is attempted. The reason to obtain spinal fluid in this circumstance is to exclude the possibility of other types of infection, especially meningitis of other causes. Imaging should always be obtained first if possible with CT or MRI head scan.

CSF parameters may be normal in CNS aspergillosis. However, in approximately half of the patients, the spinal fluid protein is elevated. Likewise, spinal fluid cell count may be elevated in one-fourth to one-half of patients. It is typically mononuclear, though polymorphonuclear cells, or red blood cells can also be found in the CSF.

Microbiology of spinal fluid is not helpful because aspergillosis cannot be grown from spinal fluid in most cases of CNS aspergillosis. Presumably, this represents the fastidious nature of the organism and lack of spread through spinal fluid pathways. Again, microbiology for other organisms is the main reason to obtain spinal fluid. Brain biopsy is the only direct way to prove the diagnosis. However, preliminary or tentative diagnosis can be made, based on culture or stain of aspergillosis from a site such as lung parenchyma, pleural fluid, or skin biopsy. Because these sites are either primary or part of dissemination, a presumptive diagnosis with a correct clinical circumstance can be made without invasive CNS biopsy.

Hemorrhagic cerebritis is the most common associated pathological change at biopsy or autopsy (Fig. 1). The cerebritis is necrotizing and the organism shows a vascular invasive character. The lesions are often angiocentric or show evidence of frank vasculitis associated with fungal invasion of blood vessel walls (Fig. 2). Commonly, leptomeningeal blood vessels will also be affected in areas near the involvement of the cortex and gray/white matter junction. Again, frank vasculitis with mycotic aneurysm formation can rarely be observed. The cerebritis by the time of autopsy is typically multifocal even if clinical or imaging studies were unifocal. Solitary lesions are only present in 10% to 20% of cases at autopsy. Spinal cord involvement can also be found incidentally at autopsy and is associated particularly with leptomeningitis at the level of the cord involved.

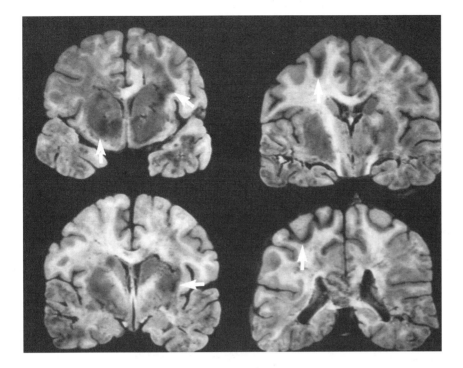

Figure 1. Gross coronal section of brain from a liver transplant patient with cerebral aspergillosis. The coronal sections show multiple necrotizing abscesses concentrated in the basal ganglia, white matter, and some near the gray/white junction of the cerebral hemispheres (white arrows). There is slight hemorrhagic discoloration.

Cryptococcus neoformans

Cryptococcal infection in transplantation is a common reason for CNS infection. Cryptococcal meningitis is the most common presentation. Cryptococcus has a strong predilection for dissemination to the nervous system with nervous system infection, particularly the meningeal surfaces. Polysaccharide capsules surrounding the organism produce unique pathological and radiographic changes in the brain of infected patients.

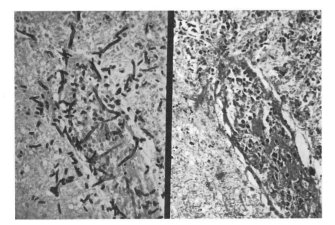

Figure 2. Photomicrograph of aspergillosis cerebritis. The right half of the picture showed a hematoxylin and eosin photomicrograph of a necrotizing cerebritis caused by aspergillosis. The brain parenchyma as well as the blood vessel wall are affected. The left panel is a silver stain for fungus demonstrating hyphae invading the blood vessel wall as well as the brain parenchyma. *Aspergillus* has a strong vascular invasive tendency, as shown (original magnification 100×).

The presenting symptoms of cryptococcal meningitis are usually a subacute or chronic meningitis. The variability in the clinical symptoms is influenced by the severity of immune suppression. The most common symptoms are fever and headache. However, those symptoms may be absent in flagrant cryptococcal meningitis, particularly when there is little spinal fluid inflammatory response. Subacute cognitive decline without headache or fever can occur. Therefore a high index of suspension for cryptococcal meningitis is warranted in transplant patients.

The incidence of cryptococcal meningitis in solid organ transplantation has been estimated to be 1% or less (1,19,20). However, cryptococcal meningitis is the second most common CNS infection in transplantation. Cryptococcal meningitis requires immunosuppression and therefore occurs more than 1 month after transplantation and usually more than 6 months after transplantation (21). The mean latency of occurrence after liver transplant ranges from 60 days to 3.5 months (20,22).

The neurological examination is typically nonfocal, with confusion and declining mental status usually being the first signs of neurological consequence. Stiff neck is variably present and is only found in one-third (22). Other parts of the neurological examination are usually not helpful. Though the imaging of the brain may show focal abnormalities with local brain invasion by the organism, focal deficits on clinical examination are difficult to find.

Cryptococcus enters the immunosuppressed patient through a pulmonary route. Therefore primary pulmonary symptoms may be prominent in association with CNS dissemination. However, because of immunosuppressed state, dissemination to extrapulmonary sites may occur with relatively few symptoms. Other sites of involvement include skin and occasionally articular surfaces, causing a septic arthritis (19). Dissemination to extrapulmonary sites attests to the invasiveness of disease and should raise the index of suspicion for CNS dissemination.

The most sensitive imaging technique for evaluating cryptococcal meningitis is MRI scan of the head. It is most useful in excluding focal mass abnormalities. Most commonly, MRI scan of the head is entirely normal with cryptococcal meningitis. However, if the meningeal inflammation is significant or the cryptococcal infection has been present for a longer period of time, diffuse or even focal meningeal enhancement may be seen with gadolinium administration on MRI scan of the head. The most common imaging abnormality when one is seen associated with cryptococcal meningitis is nonenhancing microabscesses, particularly in the area of the basal ganglia, or less commonly in the cerebellum. Cryptococcal organisms can cause direct infection of the brain by dissection along the penetrating blood vessels, particularly at the base of the brain, and leads to the nonenhancing abscesses. Nonenhancement on MRI scan is thought to be secondary to the lack of inflammatory response to the *Cryptococcus* capsule.

The most common abnormality associated with cryptococcal meningitis is increased intracranial pressure. Therefore measuring opening pressure should not be ignored at the time of lumbar puncture. Pleocytosis with predominance of lymphocytes in the range of 10–200 cells/mm^2 are the most common. Low CSF glucose is seen in approximately 40% of patients. Occasionally, particularly if meningitis has been more acute and the patient

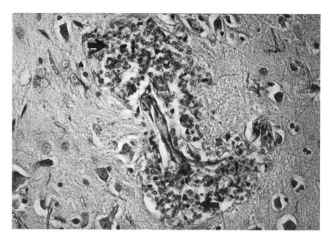

Figure 4. Higher magnification of an example of cryptococcal meningitis involving the perivascular spaces of the gray matter. Yeast cryptococcal organisms are clustered around the surface of the blood vessels leading to widening of the perivascular spaces (original magnification 400×, LFB-PAS stain).

has relative immunopreservation, polys can predominate the spinal fluid cellular reaction. Spinal fluid findings can sometimes be entirely normal. This includes a normal protein level. Patients who are severely immunosuppressed with cryptococcal meningitis can occasionally have more cryptococcal organisms identified per microliter of spinal fluid than white blood cells.

Cryptococcus can be cultured from the spinal fluid, but direct culture is less sensitive than examination for cryptococcal antigen. The polysaccharide capsule of cryptococcus serves as a useful means for identification of the organism in clinically significant cryptococcal meningitis. The cryptococcal antigen is present by routine antigen assay in 95% to 99% of patients with cryptococcal meningitis.

The neuropathology of cryptococcal meningitis is relatively unique. The subarachnoid space is often filled with the organism. However, cryptococcus also has a predilection for dissecting along the perivascular spaces, particularly at the base of the brain. The invasion of the Virchow-Robin spaces by the organism is associated with formation of microabscesses and is often only appreciated at autopsy (Fig. 3). These gelatinous-appearing microabscesses are filled with cryptococcal organisms and their capsules, and may be multiple (Fig. 4).

Candida

Brain infection with *Candida* can occur as an opportunistic infection associated with transplantation. *Candida* can present as either meningitis, brain abscess (which can be multiple), or rarely, mycotic aneurysm with presentation of subarachnoid hemorrhage. *Candida* infection of

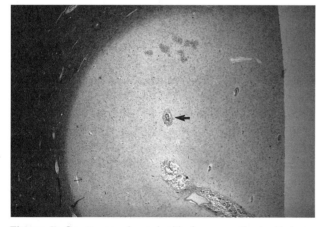

Figure 3. Cryptococcal meningitis from a patient with bone marrow transplant. There is dissection of cryptococcal organisms down the Virchow-Robin space evident on this low-magnification histologic section from the brain. The gray matter is to the right, and the white matter is more darkly stained to the left with luxol fast blue. Along the blood vessels in the gray matter, there is apparently increased cellularity. These represent cryptococcal organisms dissecting down the Virchow-Robin spaces (original magnification 25×, LFB-PAS stain).

the CNS usually occurs in the circumstance of systemic candidiasis and invasive disease in other organs.

Candidiasis presenting with meningitis typically involves fever, headache, and nausea and vomiting. Clinical presentation is similar to other forms of meningitis and must be distinguished from bacterial meningitis. Its fulminant onset often mimics bacterial meningitis, though underlying immunosuppression can make the degree of fever and headache significantly less than in nonimmunosuppressed patients.

Patients with *Candida* brain abscess typically present with a diffuse encephalopathy. This is because the abscesses are typically multiple and often small. The clue that the patient has brain abscess from *Candida* is the presence of superimposed focal neurological deficits associated with the encephalopathy.

Rarely, *Candida* can present as a subarachnoid hemorrhage secondary to rupture of a mycotic aneurysm. In that circumstance, the presenting symptoms are sudden explosive onset of headache and loss of consciousness (23,24).

Candida is probably the most common fungal infection to occur in the first 60 days after transplantation. One study estimated that 0.3% to 1% of patients will develop a brain abscess in the post-transplant period (25). *Candida* was the second most common cause for brain abscess. Bone marrow transplantation is the most common transplant associated with candidiasis (26). It is estimated that 12.5% of bone marrow transplant patients will have systemic candidal infection (27). However, candidal infection of the nervous system can also occur after renal transplantation (23), liver transplantation (20), or heart transplantation (25).

For meningitis the most common presenting sign is meningismus and reduction in level of consciousness. Fever is also present in more than 50%. Brain abscess, whether it be single or more commonly multiple, is often associated with some focal neurological deficit on physical examination. However, the most common clinical signs are those of reduced level of consciousness, which makes precise determination about focal neurological deficit difficult. Therefore an index of suspicion of candidal abscess should be high with any depression and level of consciousness associated with the post-transplant period. This is especially important if there is systemic evidence of candidal infection.

Candidal infection of the nervous system is typically associated with *Candida* fungal dissemination through the bloodstream. Fungemia by blood cultures is present in 70% of patients with neurological infection. Systemic invasive disease of solid organs also raises the likelihood that neurological symptoms are secondary to nervous system invasion as well. Other factors that have been associated with candidal infection, including that of the nervous system, are the use of triple antibiotics, the use of corticosteroids, IV indwelling catheters, and hyperglycemia associated with diabetes.

As with other brain abscesses, *Candida* brain abscess typically appears as a ring-enhancing lesion. It is usually smaller than other causes for brain abscess, and therefore multiple small lesions should raise the index of suspicion for the possibility of candidiasis. Meningitis associated with candidal infection may not produce any abnormality on the CT or MRI scan.

MRI scan imaging of the head is superior to CT scan imaging in demonstrating small abscesses. MRI also helps to establish the multiplicity of infection. Because of the hematogenous dissemination of the fungus to the brain, the typical location for the ring-enhancing lesions will be at the gray/white matter junction. However, *Candida* can be found in gray matter as well as deeper white matter structures.

CSF sampling is dangerous in patients who have mass effect. Depressed level of consciousness may suppress the ability to detect focal neurological signs before a spinal fluid examination. Therefore imaging is required before doing spinal tap in suspected cases of *Candida* meningitis or brain abscess.

If brain abscess mass effect is excluded, and spinal fluid examination is carried out, candidal meningitis is typically associated with a marked pleocytosis. The CSF will average as many as 600 white blood cells per microliter (28). CSF glucose is typically depressed also if there is a significant pleocytosis.

In the rare circumstance where *Candida* causes a mycotic aneurysm and presents with subarachnoid hemorrhage, the spinal fluid is bloody, as in other cases of subarachnoid hemorrhage (23,24).

Fungal stains on the CSF for yeast forms of *Candida* have approximately a 17% yield (29). CSF culture is required for diagnosis of *Candida* meningitis. However, it is incompletely sensitive and may be positive in only 50% to 60% of meningitis infections (28,29). Although still in developmental stages, the polymerase chain reaction (PCR) on CSF may prove beneficial for diagnosis in the future.

Candida meningitis is associated with a marked pleocytosis in the subarachnoid space at pathology. A combination of lymphocytes and polymorphonuclear leukocytes is present in the subarachnoid space. The degree of polymorphonuclear leukocyte reaction usually depends on the acuteness of the infection.

More typically, multiple brain abscesses are found at pathology. These usually have the appearance of multiple microabscesses in a perivascular distribution and occur most commonly at the gray/white matter junction, but any site is possible (23).

The combination of yeast and hyphae destroying brain tissue and associated with brain inflammation is strongly suggestive of candidal infection. *Candida* yeast and hyphoforms can be seen on silver stains of brain parenchyma, and sometimes with periodic acid Schiff stain.

Other Fungi

Rhizopus or *Mucor* can cause a rhinocerebral meningoencephalitis in immunosuppressed patients. Though these classically occur in patients with diabetes, they have also been reported in transplant patients. All forms of transplantation have been associated with these opportunistic infections, including bone marrow transplantation (30), cardiac transplantation (31), and renal transplantation patients (32). Like *Rhizopus* or *Mucor* in diabetes, infection usually begins as a mucous membrane, nasal, oral, or sinus infection that progresses to involve the orbit and base of the brain through the skull, invading through the sinuses. Surgical debridement of the necrotizing tissue is usually diagnostic, demonstrating nonseptate branched hyphae on pathology. Culture will demonstrate sporangiphore-bearing organisms (32). These cases are usually fatal.

Brain abscesses have also been reported with assorted invasive fungal infections. Treatment of *Dactylaria gallopava* (33) brain abscess has been reported to be successful in a liver transplant recipient. Necrotizing cerebritis has been described from a dematiacious fungus, *Cladophialophora bantiana* (34).

Viral Infections

Progressive Multifocal Leukoencephalopathy

Progressive multifocal leukoencephalopathy (PML) is an opportunistic viral infection of the myelin-forming cells of the CNS (35). The virus that causes PML, JC virus, selectively infects and destroys oligodendrocytes in patients who are immunosuppressed with a T-cell defect. Progressive lysis of oligodendrocytes leads to multifocal demyelination in the brain and associated progressive neurological deficits.

PML typically presents as a unifocal neurological syndrome with the clinical manifestations reflecting the focal involvement of either the cerebral cortex, brain stem, or cerebellum. The cerebral cortex is approximately 10 times more commonly affected than the brain stem or cerebellum. Interestingly, optic nerves or the spinal cord are clinically never affected by this demyelinating virus.

The most common presentations of PML are as visual deficits, hemiparesis, or frontal lobe dementia. Clinically, focal cortical syndromes associated with PML evolve subacutely, usually over days to weeks. These include hemiparesis with unilateral weakness, visual disturbance from hemianopsia, hemisensory deficit with unilateral numbness, aphasia associated with involvement of the subcortical white matter of the speech areas, or less commonly, focal pain syndrome unilaterally affecting limbs unilaterally. Because of PML's discrete nature, an upper or lower limb can be affected in isolation. A second cerebral presentation of PML is that of frontal lobe dementia with behavioral changes without focal neurological find-

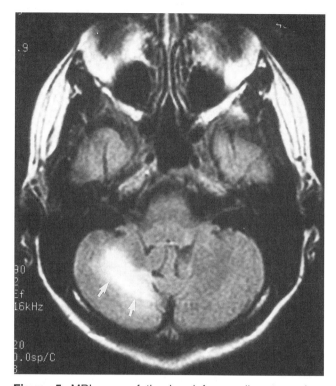

Figure 5. MRI scan of the head from a liver transplant patient with progressive multifocal leukoencephalopathy. Patient had PML involving the right cerebellar hemisphere and had right cerebellar signs. The MRI scan shows increased T2 signal in the right cerebellar hemisphere white matter. There is no mass effect, and no enhancement was present on other images after gadolinium injection. There is no involvement of the gray matter (FLAIR sequence).

ings. This may be manifest as abulia or as inappropriate disinhibited behavior only.

Finally, if the brain stem or cerebellum is affected, cerebellar syndromes are produced that are often unilateral or midline. If unilateral, they tend to cause clumsiness or incoordination of limbs on one side of the body (Fig. 5). Falls, imbalance, dysequilibrium, and gait disturbance are more common with midline lesions. Nystagmus associated with cerebellar injury can cause blurred vision, and dysarthria can be present because of incoordination of speech. When the brain stem is involved, contralateral hemiparesis or hemisensory deficit associated with unilateral cranial nerve deficit occurs.

Uncommonly, PML, which pathologically causes lesions at the gray/white matter junction of the cerebral hemisphere, can be associated with seizures. It has been estimated that approximately 5% of patients with progressive multifocal leukoencephalopathy will have seizures as a presenting or early clinical manifestation of their disease.

The type of transplant the patient has undergone does not predict the likelihood of PML as a complication. In the Mayo Clinic experience, we have cared for patients with PML who have had renal, liver, or heart transplant

(36). Of significance, however, the timing of the onset of the neurological syndrome is usually late after transplant. It typically occurs more than 6 months after transplant and often can occur several years later. The sustained immunosuppressed state best predicts the possibility of PML. Thus if bone marrow transplant is successful, this form of transplantation may prevent the prolonged T-cell defect necessary for clinical PML. The delay in the onset of PML after other organ transplantation is multifactorial. The virus is typically a reactivation infection, though there is controversy about whether that reactivation occurs systemically and is associated with dissemination to the CNS at the time of immunosuppression or whether there is latency in the brain and reactivation at the time of the immunosuppression. JC virus, the etiologic agent, is a weak opportunistic pathogen and a true slow virus. However, once infection begins, the progression is subacute. Typically, the neurological syndrome will evolve over days to a few weeks. Occasionally, the presentation can be rather abrupt and strokelike, but in that circumstance, there will be continued worsening of the neurological syndrome with serial examination.

It is not recognized that the type of immunosuppressant associated with transplantation is important in the pathogenesis of the disease. The T-cell defect of transplant immunosuppression is shared among not only transplant patients but patients who have PML associated with other causes such as AIDS, leukemia or lymphoma, or collagen vascular disease with associated exogenous immunosuppression.

PML is a noninflammatory CNS infection. Therefore the disease is not associated with fever or meningeal signs of nuchal rigidity. Consciousness is usually preserved, particularly at the onset of the illness. However, focal neurological signs emerge associated with the focal symptoms outlined earlier. Hemiparesis, when it occurs, is often associated with prominent spasticity, hyperreflexia, and extensor toe signs, as in other white matter disease of the brain. Visual symptoms associated with occipital lobe lesions produce a hemianopsia typically. Other cortical visual syndromes can occur such as alexia without agraphia or visual agnosias. When the parietal lobes are affected, cortical sensory loss occurs. Joint position sense, graphesthesia, two-point discrimination, and stereognosis are prominently affected out of proportion to pin, touch, and temperature. Nondominant parietal lobes can also be affected and produce cortical neglect syndromes with visual spatial disorientation, constructional apraxia, dressing apraxia, or agnosia. Language deficits, either expressive or receptive aphasia, can be produced when the dominant cerebral hemisphere is affected. Despite the name multifocal, the lesions usually initially evolve as unifocal disturbances so change in level of consciousness is uncommon at presentation.

When the frontal lobes are affected, behavior manifestations may be the only clinical abnormality. Typically, this affects motivational aspects of behavior rather than memory. The symptom complex is typically subcortical, affecting motivational aspects of behavior with apathy, change in social interaction, change in social interest, slowing of mentation, lack of initiative, and less spontaneity. Patients often appear depressed. The telling symptom complex, however, is that this is an inexorably progressive syndrome.

Transplantation patients develop progressive multifocal leukoencephalopathy (PML) after chronic immunosuppressive therapy. Therapy is usually successful in controlling rejection at the time of developing PML. There is no clinical evidence of a systemic viral syndrome when PML affects the brain. Sensitive techniques such as PCR can detect the shedding of JC virus in urine of patients with progressive multifocal leukoencephalopathy (37). However, there is a high incidence of shedding JC virus in transplant patients without PML, and therefore the finding is nonspecific. Also, patients can have PCR-based positive assays of blood for JC virus without clinical PML.

CT scanning of the head can be helpful in this disease but is relatively insensitive to demyelinating disorders. MRI imaging of the head is very helpful in that it is a sensitive and relatively specific means for demonstrating lesions of progressive multifocal leukoencephalopathy. Because PML is a myelin-destructive process, an associated visualizable lesion is seen on MRI scan when there is clinical deficit. Though MRI scan may show nonspecific abnormalities that may mimic PML, normal findings on head MRI scan essentially exclude the diagnosis of PML.

The characteristic MRI finding in PML lesions is increased T2 signal in focal areas affecting the gray/white matter junction (see Fig. 5). The gray matter is spared, and the T2 signal follows the cortical gyral pattern, contrasting the abnormally bright affected white matter against normal cortical gray matter. Typically, little or no mass effect is associated with this focal abnormality. Gadolinium contrast produces little or no enhancement. There may be a small peripheral rim of indiscreet enhancement with these lesions. Only very rarely is marked enhancement associated with this syndrome. Therefore MRI is a very sensitive diagnostic test for PML. Specificity is relatively high in the correct circumstance, but focal infiltrative gliomas and lymphoma can rarely produce a similar appearance on MRI scan.

CSF parameters in progressive multifocal leukoencephalopathy are typically noninflammatory (38). That is, cell count, protein, and glucose are usually normal. Typically, patients are immunosuppressed who have this infection and are unable to mount a significant cellular reaction in the spinal fluid. However, the more immunopreserved the patient, the greater the likelihood of pleocytosis. An elevated CSF cell count can be found in approximately 20% of patients. Usually, the cell count is <20 cells/µl in the spinal fluid. If there are more than 20 cells/µl in the spinal fluid, this would call into question the diagnosis of progressive multifocal leukoencephalopathy or suggest a coincident second infection. CSF protein is typically normal. Minimal elevations of CSF protein to <70 mg% are acceptable and entirely compatible with the diagnosis of PML. CSF glucose is typically normal.

JC virus, the etiologic agent of PML, is not culturable from spinal fluid. Therefore viral cultures are no additional help except to exclude the possibility of other infections.

JC virus infection causing PML is a reactivation infection. Therefore serology is not helpful. Seventy percent of the normal adult population carry antibodies in the serum without PML. Asymptomatic urinary shedding of JC virus occurs particularly after immunosuppression has begun without PML. This is often associated with a coincident elevation of serum antibody levels.

PCR performed on the spinal fluid for JC virus is the most helpful test available for noninvasively confirming the diagnosis of PML (38). Seventy to ninety percent of patients who have progressive multifocal leukoencephalopathy will have a positive CSF result by PCR when looking for JC virus (JCV). This presence of viral DNA in the spinal fluid is specific. The biggest problem with PCR amplification as a diagnostic technique is the incomplete sensitivity. Therefore PCR amplification that is negative for JCV does not exclude the diagnosis of PML. The other problem with regard to PCR analysis is that PCR amplification is vulnerable to contamination. Therefore laboratories that perform PCR must be scrupulous in dealing with the issues of contamination, and routinely run both positive and negative controls to ensure that a positive result is not spurious.

CSF serology for JCV antibodies is not helpful. Again, passive diffusion from blood makes the presence of antibody nonspecific. In questionable cases of PML, brain biopsy is a very helpful adjunct in confirming the diagnosis. The lesions are easily localizable by MRI scan of the head. The biopsy should be performed at the advancing edge of the abnormal white matter lesion, as virus may be absent from the center of the abnormal lesion seen on imaging.

Characteristically, the pathological study shows enlarged inclusion bearing oligodendrocytes, which are diagnostic of the disease (39,40). Another diagnostic histologic finding is the formation of bizarre astrocytes.

Because brain biopsy is sometimes performed with only very small fragments of brain available for analysis, characteristic pathological features might not be seen. Electron microscopy is of additional help but suffers from sampling error. When electron microscopy is positive, 40-nm-diameter virons of JC virus fill the oligodendrocyte nuclei of infected brain.

The most useful test performed on brain biopsy for confirmation of diagnosis is *in situ* hybridization for JC virus (39,40). This technique allows a wide sampling of multiple cells in the brain biopsy specimen. It is also highly reliable and sensitive. It may demonstrate viral DNA in cells that do not have the typical pathological change, which might be missed by routine pathology. *In situ* hybridization can be done by nonradioactive means. Positive results are diagnostic with 100% specificity. Sensitivity is still affected by sampling, but this technique is less prone to sampling error than electron microscopy.

Herpes Simplex Virus

Herpes simplex virus infection is common in the circumstance of immunologic suppression associated with transplantation. Despite the fact that herpes simplex stomatitis and pharyngitis or esophagitis occur in 11% in transplant recipients (41), dissemination to the nervous system is infrequent. There is still some controversy as to whether the focal expression of herpes simplex encephalitis seen in the normal population with predilection for the mesial, temporal, and inferior frontal lobes of the brain occurs in immunosuppressed individuals and particularly in the transplant population. It is unknown if herpes encephalitis occurs more frequently in transplant patients than in the population at large. The systemic manifestations of herpes simplex dissemination in transplant patients can sometimes overshadow neurological manifestations when they occur. Neurological infection with encephalitis in adults is usually due to herpes simplex virus type 1 (HSV-1).

Herpes simplex encephalitis or meningoencephalitis usually presents with headache, fever, seizures, or a declining level of consciousness. The degree of fever and stiff neck is dependent on a degree of immunosuppression. In the bone marrow transplant population, the most common transplantation group affected by this infection, the degree of immunosuppression present may preclude mounting a substantial systemic febrile response.

Herpes simplex infection involving the nervous system most commonly occurs in bone marrow transplantation. It is infrequent in solid organ transplantation, though reported. In this circumstance, herpes simplex represents a reactivation infection. However, whether the brain infection arises from reactivation from the trigeminal ganglion or the brain itself is still controversial (42).

The most common presenting manifestation of herpes simplex encephalitis or meningoencephalitis is seizures. Second is declining level of consciousness. Focal signs of hemiparesis are rare presenting signs but may be found after evaluation of a patient having seizures or who is obtundent from encephalitis. Fever is variable. The presence of stiff neck depends on degree of immunosuppression.

Herpes simplex virus type 2, when it disseminates to the nervous system, typically produces a meningitis without focal signs or imaging. Genital or perirectal cutaneous coincident eruption may be the clue to this viral infection.

Herpes labialis and pharyngitis secondary to HSV-1 are common with other coincident CNS pathogens. Therefore the presence of these systemic manifestations does not necessarily suggest the encephalitic process in the transplant patient is due to herpes. Therefore a clinician needs to be vigilant in looking for other pathogens in the nervous system with these nonspecific systemic manifestations of herpes simplex.

Herpes simplex can also be associated with systemic viremia and a generalized viral rash during dissemination to the nervous system. Herpes simplex pneumonitis or hepatitis are rare systemic accompaniments.

MRI scan of the head is very sensitive to this focal parenchymal abnormality and is a useful adjunct in diagnosis. However, the destruction that sometimes occurs with herpes simplex encephalitis in the mesial temporal structures can sometimes be confused with early bacterial cerebritis, bacterial abscess, or even cerebral infarct.

The CSF is usually abnormal with herpes simplex encephalitis. The laboratory analysis usually shows an elevation of CSF protein and an elevated number of CSF cells. The cellular reaction is usually lymphocytic, but its severity again will vary, depending on the degree of immunosuppression of the individual patient. The CSF glucose is usually normal.

Herpes simplex virus is rarely culturable from the spinal fluid. The most sensitive and specific means for detection of herpes simplex in the CSF is by PCR methods that detect small amounts of virus in the CSF (43,44). This is a highly sensitive technique with more than 90% positive results in reliable laboratories. PCR always has the risk of false-positive results from a contamination occurring in handling the specimen or in the laboratory where the assay is performed. Therefore clinical correlation of PCR results is very important.

There are relatively few pathological studies on diffuse herpes simplex virus infection of the brain in immunosuppressed patients (45). When they have been done, the findings have been largely nonspecific and have shown neuronal loss, hemorrhagic necrosis, and less parenchymal inflammation with lymphocytic perivascular infiltrates than in nonimmunosuppressed patients. A prominent microglial reaction in the parenchyma is common. Because of the immunosuppression, the usual hemorrhagic, necrotic, pathological change that occurs with immunologically preserved herpes simplex encephalitis is often absent. However, some patients with herpes simplex encephalitis with mesial, temporal, and inferior frontal involvement may have disease indistinguishable from that which occurs in immunologically preserved individuals. Immunohistochemistry for herpes simplex virus is very useful in this circumstance to identify parenchymal involvement. Viral antigens are commonly detected in neurons and their processes. Oligodendrocytes and astrocytes can also be infected. Other techniques, including *in situ* hybridization and electron microscopy, may be useful adjunctive pathological techniques for identifying herpes simplex virus and for infected parenchymal tissue.

Varicella-zoster Virus

Varicella-zoster virus is a common complication of transplantation, particularly in bone marrow transplantation. However, the neurological complications of zoster are less well described and documented, particularly in transplant patients. Because this viral infection is often treated and may be self-limited, the neurological consequences of infection are underappreciated.

Typical herpes zoster presenting with dermatomal distribution pain and rash is very common in transplant recipients. Relatively few statistics exist about to describe how many actually disseminate, but one series (46) suggested that one-third of patients with zoster will have dissemination to either a visceral organ or the CNS. If meningoencephalitis is the main manifestation of disease, headache, fever, and obtundation are the main manifestations. Similarly, seizures are common.

Most transplant-related zoster infections occur in bone marrow transplant patients. Up to one-third of children (47) and 20% of adults (46) will have zoster following bone marrow transplantation. Most will occur in the first 18 months following transplantation. The mean latency of time between bone marrow transplantation and zoster is 96 days (47).

When herpes zoster is disseminated to the CNS and causes a meningoencephalitis, obtundation, fever, and stiff neck are the most common manifestations (48). The degree of immunosuppression, however, may modify the degree of stiff neck.

A number of other neurological complications have been reported associated with herpes zoster infection, though not necessarily in association with transplantation. However, because of the immune compromise state of transplant recipients, it is likely that these complications may also occur in transplant recipients. These include direct zoster involvement of the spinal cord with myelopathy (49), segmental zoster weakness with focal motor findings on physical examination (50), and stroke secondary to granulomatis vasculitis following zoster ophthalmicus (51).

Cutaneous dissemination of zoster raises the suspicion for the possibility of dissemination to the CNS by zoster virus. Again, dissemination to lung or liver provides evidence of more widespread disease.

Little is reported about the imaging association with meningoencephalitis and varicella-zoster virus. With the post zoster ophthalmicus stroke syndrome, ipsilateral stroke to the side of the zoster ophthalmicus has been reported. A rarer complication that has been reported pathologically primarily is the leukoencephalitis with multifocal involvement of the white matter (52).

With CNS dissemination and meningoencephalitis, varicella-zoster virus can elicit a pleocytosis and a modest elevation of CSF protein. The CSF reaction is typically lymphocytic. CSF glucose is typically normal.

Varicella-zoster virus is notoriously difficult to culture, and this is especially true in attempting to culture virus from CSF. However, varicella-zoster virus has been detected in the CSF in association with varicella-zoster meningoencephalitis and myelitis when detected by PCR technique. Sensitivity for this technique in varicella-zoster-associated neurological complications is uncertain, but future studies may prove this to be the diagnostic method of choice.

Cytomegalovirus

Though cytomegalovirus (CMV) is a serious and frequent pathogenic infection in transplant recipients, dissemination to the nervous system is rarely documented (53). The severe CMV ventriculoencephalitis and ascending polyradiculopathy documented in AIDS patients have not been recognized in the transplant recipient population (54).

Ventriculoencephalitis as described in AIDS (54) is an encephalopathic illness associated with change in sensorium, poor attention, frank delirium, and, eventually, declining level of consciousness. Headache, cranial nerve palsy, and stiff neck are common accompaniments. However, the clinical signs and symptoms corresponding to what has been described as microglial encephalitis due to CMV are poorly defined (54).

Bone marrow transplantation is the most common type of transplant associated with CMV infection disseminating to the brain (53,54). However, CMV infection in the nervous system has been noted in kidney, liver, and heart transplant recipients (55).

The systemic manifestations of widespread CMV infection are much more severe than those that infect the brain. Pneumonitis, hepatitis, renal infection, infection of the gastrointestinal tract, and CMV retinitis are all well documented among transplant recipients.

The ventriculoencephalitis associated with AIDS has been described to have a characteristic MRI appearance with periventricular subependymal gadolinium enhancement because of the subependymal infection that occurs. However, the microglial nodule encephalitis associated with CMV infection in the brain has not been associated with a specific radiographic change on the MRI scan in transplant patients.

Because the clinical circumstances of CMV infection in the brain are somewhat incompletely described, the spinal fluid abnormalities and the range of qualitative changes are unclear. In AIDS-related ventriculoencephalitis, there is a striking pleocytosis of the spinal fluid, commonly with a polymorphonuclear reaction and low CSF glucose. Similar kinds of changes have not been clearly documented in the transplant recipient population with CMV infection.

PCR detection of CMV DNA from spinal fluid in patients with CMV infections has been described as positive (54,56). CMV culture is usually negative. Therefore PCR should be regarded as the standard for detection of CMV in the spinal fluid. However, its precise sensitivity and specificity in the circumstance of transplant recipient infection have not been fully evaluated.

The pathological changes associated with CMV infection in the brain in transplant recipients have been subtle multifocal microglial nodule encephalitis (53,54). One report also suggested that a leptomeningitis may also be associated with CMV infection in the brain (55).

Human Herpesvirus 6

Human herpesvirus 6 (HHV-6), first described in association with AIDS patients, has been increasingly recognized as a CNS pathogen in patients with organ transplantation. Sensitive techniques using PCR as well as immunohistochemical staining have shown this virus to be present in the brain in normal controls as well as patients with multiple sclerosis (57). Therefore the potential mechanism for CNS infection in the circumstance of immunosuppression is reactivation from a latent brain infection.

Fever, headache, and focal neurological symptoms have all been reported as manifestations of HHV-6. Typically, headache, fever, and obtundation are the most common neurological symptoms associated with HHV-6 systemic viremia. Whether this represents primary infection in the nervous system or is simply a neurological symptom that stems from systemic factors remains to be established (58). An interesting accompaniment of HHV-6 infection is its propensity for developing very high fever despite immunosuppression.

HHV-6 has been described as an infection after bone marrow, liver, and kidney transplantation (58–60). The incidence of systemic infection has been estimated at 30% to 50% (59). It is unknown what the spectrum of systemic infection produces and how often nervous system invasion occurs after organ transplantation.

Seizures or focal neurological signs may be present in HHV-6 encephalitis (60,61). There has been a lack of clear clinical/pathological studies correlating focal involvement of brain and neurological signs. Focal seizures, however, have been described, and focal pathological cerebral involvement has been seen on imaging and at pathology.

Results of imaging of CNS in HHV-6 infection, particularly with MRI studies, have been inconsistent. Some patients with HHV-6 infection have been reported to have focal white matter abnormality (62). The lesions have been similar to those described with demyelinating multiple sclerosis except that they tend to extend into gray matter structures. Whether similar imaging characteristics will be delineated in patients with transplantation infection remains to be described.

The CSF associated with HHV-6 infection has been mildly abnormal with elevations of protein and mild elevation of cell count, with predominance of lymphocytes (60,61,63).

CSF culture has been of limited value in isolating HHV-6 in suspected cases of HHV-6. PCR techniques amplifying virus-specific sequences from the spinal fluid have been the predominant method used to associate virus with infections in the nervous system (59,61). Because the HHV-6 is a reactivation of latent infection, positive serum serology may not predict any association with nervous system invasion.

A subacute leukoencephalitis with plaquelike demyelination has been associated with HHV-6 in nonimmunosuppressed patients (62,63). Detailed pathological analysis of transplant neurological infection is lacking. Whether HHV-6 is a prominent pathogen in human transplantation awaits detailed and more extensive reporting with pathological confirmation.

Parasitic Infections

Toxoplasmosis

Toxoplasma gondii was known as a rare infection of transplant recipients in the pre-AIDS era (64). Toxoplasmosis has become a much more easily recognized cause for brain abscess because of its high frequency in the AIDS population. It is the most common CNS opportunistic infection in AIDS. However, in the transplantation population, it remains an infrequent but important cause for a brain abscess. This organism's strong predilection for the CNS is poorly understood.

Headache, obtundation, focal neurological symptoms, fever, and seizures are the most common manifestations of toxoplasmosis. Headache is nonspecific and often nonfocal. Obtundation occurs often because of multiplicity of abscess formation. Focal neurological symptoms evolve subacutely, usually over days. Fever is present in more than 50% of patients. Seizures tend to occur as focal onset motor seizures, but any form of seizures, including generalized seizures from onset, may theoretically be produced. Rarely, toxoplasmosis can selectively affect the spinal cord. The symptoms of toxoplasmosis in the spinal cord are usually masked by coincident symptoms involving the brain (65).

CNS toxoplasmosis occurs most often in bone marrow transplantation (66,67). The incidence in one study has been estimated at 0.3% of all bone marrow transplant patients (67). However, other solid organ transplant patients are vulnerable to toxoplasmosis, including kidney (68), heart (31), and liver (65) recipients.

Typically, the neurological syndrome evolves more than 1 month after the transplantation. This is because toxoplasmosis typically causes CNS invasion and infection from a latent state. Occasionally, it can occur as a primary infection even coming from the transplanted organ (65). Also, toxoplasmosis requires significant immunosuppression. It typically occurs in the first 6 months after transplantation but can occur more than 12 months after transplantation.

As with other causes for brain abscess, declining level of consciousness is the most common sign. The change in level of consciousness is frequently accompanied by a focal neurological deficit on physical examination. Increased intracranial pressure can occur because of multiplicity of abscess formation in the same patient. Also, toxoplasmosis has a predilection for the periventricular location, where it can cause obstructive hydrocephalus by occluding spinal fluid pathways.

Toxoplasma gondii has a strong predilection for the brain. However, other organs can be involved and can include the chorioretinal membranes of the eye, myocardium, and the lung. Also, the liver can contain organisms. Association with the clinical syndrome of brain abscess or neuroimaging evidence of brain abscess is strongly suggestive of cerebral toxoplasmosis.

Toxoplasmosis causes multiple brain abscesses. These tend to be grouped on imaging in a periventricular location involving deep white matter and gray matter structures more commonly than superficial cortex or more superficial white matter of the cerebral hemispheres. Though brain stem and cerebellum can be affected, cerebral hemispheres are more commonly involved. The appearance of multiple abscesses simultaneously is suggestive of toxoplasmosis but is not specific. The lesions of toxoplasmosis abscesses are typically associated with ring enhancement on both CT scanning and MRI scanning of the brain. Disappearance of brain abscesses occurring after empiric therapy for toxoplasmosis is strongly suggestive of toxoplasma abscess formation. Response to empiric therapy should appear radiographically by 10 days on CT scan or MRI scan of the brain.

CSF acquisition may be hazardous in association with *Toxoplasma* brain abscesses because of the risk of obstructive hydrocephalus. Therefore imaging should always be performed before testing spinal fluid. Seropositivity in the spinal fluid is helpful for confirmation of diagnosis if CSF can be obtained safely. However, negative CSF serology for toxoplasmosis does not exclude the possibility of *Toxoplasma* as being responsible for the brain abscesses.

Toxoplasma gondii is an obligate intracellular parasite. It usually is ubiquitous in the environment and is acquired relatively early in life by most of the population; therefore positive serology does not prove the diagnosis of cerebral toxoplasmosis in the clinical circumstance of multiple brain abscesses. However, pretransplant negative serology for toxoplasmosis is a strong argument against

Toxoplasma infection. Conversion from pretransplant seronegative status to seropositive status in the posttransplant period is associated with clinically significant disease. Pretransplant seropositive bone marrow transplant patients will often become seronegative during the first months following transplant.

The best means for establishing microbiology in indeterminate brain abscesses is stereotactic brain biopsy. Pathological evaluation is enhanced with immunohistochemical staining for toxoplasma antigens in pathological material. PCR techniques are under investigation, but sensitivity and specificity are not yet established.

The pathology of *Toxoplasma* brain abscesses are nonspecific. The inflammatory infiltrates associated with abscess formation are typically perivascular in location. They tend to have a predominance of lymphocytes, but significant necrosis occurs particularly in a perivascular distribution. On routine staining, tachyzoites, which are the free organisms in the tissue, or bradyzoites, which are encysted collections of organisms, can sometimes be seen. These findings are diagnostic when present, but routine pathological evaluation will often miss the presence of organisms, mostly because there is little contrast between background tissue staining and organisms present in the tissue. Immunostaining against *Toxoplasma* antigens is very helpful in enhancing sensitivity, particularly when dealing with small stereotactic biopsies of brain.

REFERENCES

1. Estol CJ, Lopez O, Brenner RP, Martinez AJ. Seizures after liver transplantation: a clinicopathological study. *Neurology* 1989;39:1297–1301.
2. Martinez AJ, Estol CJ, Faris AA. Neurologic complications of liver transplantation. *Neurol Clin* 1988;6:327–348.
3. Conti DJ, Rubin RH. Infections of the central nervous system in organ transplant recipients. *Neurol Clin* 1988;6:241–278.
4. Davis DG, Patchell RA. Neurologic complications of bone marrow transplantation. *Neurol Clin* 1988;6:377–387.
5. Chang J, Powles R, Mehta J, Paton N, Treleaven J, Jamison B. Listeriosis in bone marrow transplant recipients: incidence, clinical features, and treatment. *Clin Infect Dis* 1995;21:1289–1290.
6. Long SG, Legland MJ, Milligan DW. *Listeria* meningitis after bone marrow transplantation. *Bone Marrow Transplant* 1983;12:537–539.
7. Peeters A, Waer M, Michielsen P, Verbist L, Carton H. Listeria monocytogenes meningitis. *Clin Neurol Neurosurg* 1989;91:29–36.
8. Southwick FS, Purich DL. Intracellular pathogenesis of listeriosis. *N Engl J Med* 1996;334:770–776.
9. Brown RH, Sobel R. *Listeria monocytogenes* rhombencephalitis; case record 37–1989. *N Engl J Med* 1989;321:734–750.
10. Kennard C, Howard AJ, Scholtz C, Swash C. Infection of the brain stem by *Listeria monocytogenes. J Neurol Neurosurg Psychiatry* 1979;42:931–933.
11. Larner DJ, Conway MA, Mitchell RG, Forfar JC. Recurrent *Listeria monocytogenes* meningitis in a heart transplant recipient. *J Infect* 1989;19:263–266.
12. Davies RS, Burgin M. MRI appearances of *Listeria* rhombencephalitis. *Australas Radiol* 1996;40:354–356.
13. Mamelak AN, Obana WG, Flaherty JF, Rosenblum ML. Nocardial brain abscess: treatment strategies and factors influencing outcome. *Neurosurgery* 1994;35:622–631.
14. Ardnino RC, Johnson PC, Miranda AG. Nocardiosis in renal transplant recipients undergoing immunosuppression with cyclosporine. *Clin Infect Dis* 1993;16:505–512.
15. Boes B, Bashir R, Boes C, Hohn F, McConnell JR, McComb R. Central nervous system aspergillosis. *J Neuroimaging* 1994;4:123–129.
16. Beal MF, O Carroll CP, Kleinman GM, Grossman RI. Aspergillosis of the nervous system. *Neurology* 1982;32:473–479.
17. Walsh TJ, Hier DB, Caplan LR. Aspergillosis of the central nervous system: clinicopathological analysis of 17 patients. *Ann Neurol* 1985;18:574–582.
18. Torre-Cisneros J, Lopez OL, Kusne S, et al. CNS aspergillosis in organ transplantation: a clinicopathologic study. *J Neurol Neurosurg Psychiatry* 1993;56:188–193.
19. Singh N, Gayowski T, Wagener MM, Marino IR. Clinical spectrum of invasive cryptococcosis in liver transplant recipients receiving tacrolimus. *Clin Transplant* 1997;11:66–70.
20. Patel R, Portela D, Badley AD, et al. Risk factors of invasive *Candida* and non-*Candida* fungal infections after liver transplantation. *Transplantation* 1996;62:926–934.
21. Schröter GPJ, Temple DR, Husberg BJ, Weil R. Stanzl TE. Cryptococcosis after renal transplantation: report of ten cases. *Surgery* 1976;79:268–277.
22. Tabborn N, Rayes J, Kusne S, Martin M, Fung J. Cryptococcal meningitis after liver transplantation. *Transplantation* 1996;61:146–149.
23. Lipton SA, Hickey WF, Morris JH, Loscalzo J. Candidal infection in the central nervous system. *Am J Med* 1984;76:101–108.
24. Wijdicks EF, deGroen PC, Wiesner RH, Krom RA. Intracerebral hemorrhage in liver transplant recipients. *Mayo Clin Proc* 1995;70:443–446.
25. Selby R, Ramisey CB, Single R, et al. Brain abscess in solid organ transplant recipients receiving cyclosporine based immunosuppression. *Arch Surg* 1997;132:304–310.
26. Costagnola E, Bucci B, Montinero E, Viscoli C. Fungal injections in patients undergoing bone marrow transplantation: an approach to a rational management protocol. *Bone Marrow Transplant* 1996;18[Suppl 2]:97–106.
27. Verfaille C, Weisdorf D, Haake R, Hostetter M, Ramsay NK, McGlave P. *Candida* infection in bone marrow transplant recipients. *Bone Marrow Transplant* 1991;8:177–184.
28. Bayer AS, Edwards JE, Seidel JS, Guze LB. *Candida* meningitis. Report of seven cases and reviews of the English literature. *Medicine* 1976;55:477–486.
29. Voice RA, Bradley SF, Sangeorzan JA, Kaufman CA. Chronic *Candida* meningitis: an uncommon manifestation of candidiasis. *Clin Infect Dis* 1994;19:60–66.
30. Hyatt DS, Young YM, Haynes KA, Taylor JM, McCarthy DM, Rogers TR. Rhinocerebral mucormycosis following bone marrow transplantation. *J Infect* 1992;24:67–71.
31. Britt RH, Enzmann DR, Remington JS. Intracranial infection in cardiac transplant recipients. *Ann Neurol* 1983;9:107–119.
32. Hammer GS, Bottone EJ, Hirschman SZ. Mucormycosis in a transplant recipient. *Am J Clin Pathol* 1975;64:389–398.
33. Vukmir RB, Kusne S, Linden P, et al. Successful therapy for cerebral phaeohyphomycosis due to *Dactylaria gallopava* in a live transplant recipient. *Clin Infect Dis* 1994;19:714–719.
34. Emmens RK, Richardson D, Thomas W, et al. Necrotizing cerebritis in an allogenic bone marrow transplant recipient due to *Cladophialophora bantiana. J Clin Microbiol* 1996;34:1330–1332.
35. Aksamit AJ. Progressive multifocal leukoencephalopathy, a review of the pathology and pathogenesis. *Microsc Res Tech* 1995;32:302–311.
36. Aksamit AJ, Okazaki H, Proper J, deGroen PC. Cyclosporine-related leukoencephalopathy and progressive multifocal leukoencephalopathy in a liver transplant recipient. *Transplantation* 1995;60:874–876.
37. Marshall WF, Telenti A, Proper J, Aksamit AJ, Smith TF. Survey of urine from transplant recipients for polyoma virus JC and BK using the polymerase chain reaction. *Mol Cell Probes* 1991;5:125–128.
38. Aksamit AJ. Cerebrospinal fluid in the diagnosis of central nervous system infections. In: Roos K, ed. *Central nervous system infectious diseases and therapy.* New York: Marcel Decker; 1997:731–745.
39. Aksamit AJ, Sever JL, Major ED. Progressive multifocal leukoencephalopathy: JC virus detection by *in situ* hybridization compared with immunohistochemistry. *Neurology* 1986;36:499–504.
40. Aksamit AJ. Nonradioactive *in situ* hybridization in progressive multifocal leukoencephalopathy. *Mayo Clin Proc* 1993;68:899–910.
41. Paya CV, Hermans PE, Washington JA, et al. Incidence, distribution and outcome of episodes of infections in 100 orthotopic liver transplantations. *Mayo Clin Proc* 1989;64:555–564.
42. Baringer JR, Pisani P. Herpes simplex virus genomes in human nervous system tissue analyzed by polymerase chain reaction. *Ann Neurol* 1994;36:823–829.

43. Aurelius E, Johansson B, Sköldenberg B, Staland A, Forsgren M. Rapid diagnosis of herpes simplex encephalitis by nested polymerase chain reaction assay of cerebrospinal fluid. *Lancet* 1991;337: 189–192.

44. Rowley AH, Whitley RJ, Lakeman FD, Wolinsky SM. Rapid detection of herpes simplex virus DNA in cerebrospinal fluid of patients with herpes simplex encephalitis. *Lancet* 1990;335:440–441.

45. Price R, Chernik NL, Horta-Barbosa L, Posner JB. Herpes simplex encephalitis in an anergic patient. *Am J Med* 1973;54:222–228.

46. Han CS, Miller W, Haake R, Weisdorf D. Varicella zoster infection after bone marrow transplantation: incidence, risk factors and complications. *Bone Marrow Transplant* 1994;13:277–283.

47. Kawasaki H, Takayama J, Ohira M. Herpes zoster infection after bone marrow transplantation in children. *J Pediatr* 1996;128:353–356.

48. Thomas JE, Howard FM. Segmental zoster paresis—a disease profile. *Neurology* 1972;22:459–466.

49. Gilden DH, Beinlich BR, Rubenstein EM, et al. Varicella-zoster virus myelitis. *Neurology* 1994;44:1818–1823.

50. Hughes BA, Kimmel DW, Aksamit AJ. Herpes zoster-associated meningoencephalitis in patients with systemic cancer. *Mayo Clin Proc* 1993;68:652–655.

51. MacKenzie RA, Forbes GS, Karnes WE. Angiographic findings in herpes zoster arteritis. *Ann Neurol* 1981;10:458–464.

52. Horten B, Price RW, Jimenez D. Multifocal varicella-zoster virus leukoencephalitis temporally remote from herpes zoster. *Ann Neurol* 1981;9:251–266.

53. Graus F, Saiz A, Sierra J, Arbaiza D, Rovira M, Carreras E, Tolosa E, Rozman C. Neurologic complications of autologous and allogenic bone marrow transplantation in patients with leukemia: a comparative study. *Neurology* 1996;46:1004–1009.

54. Arribas JR, Storch GA, Clifford DB, Tselis AC. Cytomegalovirus encephalitis. *Ann Intern Med* 1996;125:577–587.

55. Montero CG, Martinez AJ. Neuropathology of heart transplantation: 23 cases. *Neurology* 1986;36:1149–1154.

56. Levy R, Najioullah F, Thouvenst D, Bosshard S, Aymard M, Lina B. Evaluation and comparison of PCR and hybridization methods for rapid detection of cytomegalovirus in clinical samples. *J Virol Methods* 1996;62:103–111.

57. Challoner PB, Smith KT, Parker JD, et al. Plaque-associated expression of human herpesvirus 6 in multiple sclerosis. *Proc Natl Acad Sci* 1995;92:7440–7444.

58. Singh N, Carrigan DR, Gayowski T, Singh J, Marino IR. Variant B human herpesvirus-6 associated febrile dermatosis with thrombocytopenia and encephalopathy in a liver transplant recipient. *Transplantation* 1995;60:1355–1357.

59. Singh N, Carrigan DR. Human herpesvirus 6 in transplantation: an emerging pathogen. *Ann Intern Med* 1996;124:1065–1071.

60. Drobyski WR, Knox KK, Majewski D, Carrigan DR. Fatal encephalitis due to variant B human herpesvirus 6 infection in a bone marrow transplantation recipient. *N Engl J Med* 1994;330:1356–1360.

61. McCullers JA, Lakeman FD, Whitley RJ. Human herpesvirus 6 is associated with focal encephalitis. *Clin Infect Dis* 1995;21:571–576.

62. Carrigan DR, Harrington D, Knox KK. Subactue leukoencephalitis caused by CNS infection with human herpesvirus 6 manifesting as acute multiple sclerosis. *Neurology* 1996;46:145–148.

63. Novoa LJ, Nagra RM, Nakawatase T, Edwards-Lee T, Tourtellotte WW, Cornford ME. Fulminant demyelinating encephalomyelitis associated with productive HHV-6 infection in an immunocompetent adult. *J Med Virol* 1997;52:301–308.

64. Ruskin J, Remington JS. Toxoplasmosis in the compromised host. *Ann Intern Med* 1976;84:193–199.

65. Mayes JT, O Connor BJ, Avery R, Costillami R, Carey W. Transmission of *Toxoplasma gondii* infection by liver transplantation. *Clin Infect Dis* 1995;21:511–515.

66. Chandrasekar PH, Momin F. Disseminated toxoplasmosis in marrow recipients: a report of three cases and a review of the literature. *Bone Marrow Transplant* 1997;19:685–689.

67. Slavin MA, Meyers JD, Remington JS, Hackman RC. *Toxoplasma gondii* infection in marrow transplant recipients: a 20-year experience. *Bone Marrow Transplant* 1994;13:549–557.

68. Renault E, Georges E, Biara MF, et al. Toxoplasmosis in kidney transplant recipients: report of six cases and review. *Clin Infect Dis* 1997;24:625–634.

Transplant Infections edited by
Raleigh A. Bowden, Per Ljungman, and Carlos V. Paya.
Lippincott–Raven Publishers, Philadelphia © 1998

CHAPTER 11

Management of the Febrile Patient in Hematopoietic Stem Cells and Solid Organ Transplant Recipients

Ben E. De Pauw, Raleigh A. Bowden, and Carlos V. Paya

The occurrence of fever following both hematopoietic stem cell transplantation (HCT) and solid organ transplantation (SOT) is important and is a common complicating event that requires prompt evaluation and management. Although fever during neutropenia is an event most commonly complicating the HCT setting, fever in the absence of neutropenia occurs frequently in both settings. The urgency of evaluation and prompt institution of therapy depends in large part on when the fever occurs relative to the transplant procedure.

Not all fever occurring in either transplant setting is due to infection. A careful history, physical exam, and thorough knowledge of the organisms that are likely to occur during each time period following transplant will not only assist in selecting the appropriate diagnostic approaches but increase the likelihood of identifying the cause of the fever and allowing for initiation of appropriate, often life-saving therapy.

Evaluation of the febrile patient in both the HCT and SOT setting involves similar overall approaches. A detailed discussion of the diagnosis of specific types of infection can be found elsewhere in this book. It is imperative to have a standardized approach to the microbiological evaluation of the transplant patient with fever or a suspected infection. Surveillance cultures are theoretically attractive for the early identification of resistant bacterial or fungal organisms that may require specific antimicrobial therapy, but in general their cost-effectiveness is questioned (1).

Particularly in the first 3 months after transplant, every febrile patient should be evaluated with blood cultures, a chest radiograph, and in some cases an examination of the urine for bacteria, fungi, and viral infections. Bacterial/fungal blood cultures should be repeated daily in the persistently febrile patient until a cause has been identified and eliminated from the blood with appropriate therapy. The use of preferably two 10-ml samples of blood—one from the central intravenous catheter, if one is in place, and one from a separate vein, if possible—with an interval of at least 30 minutes will reliably detect most episodes of bacteremia. Either lysis centrifugation or an automated blood culture system will optimize the recovery of yeasts from blood (see Chapter 7). For patients with suspected wound or soft-tissue infections, it is always preferable to obtain tissue samples. Swab samples of nonsterile aspirates are less helpful but may be collected when more invasive culturing is impossible. Immediate transportation to the laboratory is critical in optimizing results. Tissue specimens are to be processed for histologic examination, Gram stain, and routine aerobic and anaerobic culture. Technical personnel should be aware not to discard sputum samples on the basis of low numbers of leukocytes. Bronchoalveolar lavage (BAL) constitutes an accurate alternative to lung biopsy as a means of diagnosing many infections in a patient with pulmonary infiltrates. Smears, cultures, and special stains of BAL material for the possible presence of bacteria, viruses, and fungi should always be performed, and may need to include evaluation for *Pneumocystis carinii*, *Legionella* spp., tuberculosis, and *Nocardia* spp.

Serodiagnosis for most infections in the transplant setting is of limited use in the acutely ill transplant patient and is limited by the lag time between the infection and

BEDP: From University Hospital, St. Radboud, Nijmegen, The Netherlands. RAB: From Fred Hutchinson Cancer Research Center, University of Washington, Seattle, WA. CVP: From The Mayo Clinic, Rochester, MN 55905.

the immunologic response and by the immunosuppressive state that might prohibit proliferation of the antibody. Special diagnostic approaches specific to each transplant type and time period following transplant will be discussed later.

This chapter will discuss the differential diagnosis of fever in the HCT setting and after SOT. Many of the risk factors for fever and infection in the HCT are similar for SOT and change with each sequential time period following the specific transplant type.

MANAGEMENT OF FEVER FOLLOWING HCT: GENERAL PRINCIPLES

HCT, approximately 35 years ago considered an experimental preterminal procedure for treatment refractory patients, has now been accepted as a life-saving option for a wide array of diseases, particularly severe aplastic anemia, many hematologic malignancies, and immune deficiencies. However, modern conditioning regimens will destroy virtually every component of the host defense mechanisms and, despite all preventive measures and prophylactically administered antibiotics, fever has remained a common occurrence in patients who undergo HCT. Thus, particularly because HCT has become an elective intervention in the majority of cases, knowledge about the possible complications and an adequate antiinfective strategy are mandatory for HCT centers that offer these patients care. This ideally implies a close cooperation among everyone involved, including nurses, hematologists, microbiologists, radiologists, pulmonologists, and pathologists.

The types and severity of infections after HCT differ according to a variety of factors: type of transplant, degree of donor/recipient match, manipulation of donor T-lymphocytes in the marrow graft, type of graft-versushost disease (GVHD) prophylaxis, and medical history of the patient. Immunodeficiency is less profound in syngeneic and autologous HCT, although marrow-purging regimens, if applied, generally delay recovery of the immune function in the latter. Autologous HCT is accompanied by less peritransplant mortality, which in general occurs with one-third the frequency of that observed during an allogeneic transplantation procedure, mainly due to fewer fatal infections. When peripheral stem cells, either allogeneic or autologous, are used, the risk for infection may be lower than when marrow is used as the stem cell source because this technique has the major advantage of a considerably shorter duration of the ensuing neutropenia (2).

An infectious cause of a fever can only be confirmed microbiologically or clinically in between 30% and 50% of cases. As a result of the extensive tissue damage by the conditioning regimen, the use of potentially pyrogenic drugs, the frequent administration of blood products, and

the occurrence of GVHD, the source of fever remains undetermined in a many cases. Even the presence of chills or rigors does not appear to correlate with an eventual diagnosis of bacteremia. Such noninfectious fevers may lead to the overuse of antibiotics, and noninfectious causes of fever should be in the differential diagnosis.

Defense Mechanisms and Infection After HCT

Infection results from a negative balance between the host defense system and the virulence of invading micro-organisms. In normal individuals, physical barriers consisting of skin and mucous membranes, granulocytes, and other components of the cellular and humoral immune system provide an adequate protection against pathogenic micro-organisms. Any qualitative or quantitative defect that results from conditioning regimens predisposes to infection. In principle, a specific deficiency increases the patient's susceptibility to those pathogens whose eradication depends on that particular host defense mechanism. Nevertheless, the pattern of infectious complications during a given episode after the transplant procedure is quite unpredictable because simultaneous impairment of different defense systems is a rule rather than an exception. Furthermore, impairments change constantly over time, and various defects prevail at different times, influenced by course of the transplant and therapeutic interventions (Table 1). Bacteremia accounts for the vast majority of culture-documented bacterial infections, but viruses, particularly CMV and respiratory viruses, as well as fungi are important causes of fever. Worldwide there is presently no single predominant pathogen; the variations between centers are considerable and depend on differences in conditioning regimens, prophylactic antibacterial and antifungal agents, management of central venous catheters, hospital environment, climate, and so on.

Granulocytes

Granulocytopenia is probably the most important primary risk factor for bacterial and fungal infection, there being an inverse correlation between the number of circulating granulocytes and the frequency of infection. Virtually all patients with a granulocyte count of less than $100/mm^3$ for more than 3 weeks will develop fever. Even when the neutrophils increase in number, they are initially less efficient. They exhibit reduced mobility and are rather indifferent to chemotactic stimuli in conjunction with a lower ability for phagocytosis and killing. Moreover, as a result of fewer numbers or qualitatively defective granulocytes, the inflammatory response is muted with absence of characteristic signs and symptoms of infection that hampers early clinical recognition (3).

TABLE 1. *Sequence of infective events in relation to the phases of allogeneic HCT*

	Early phase	Mid-recovery phase	Late phase
Host defense mechanisms without GVHD			
Integument			
Skin	Damaged	Damaged	Intact
Mucous membranes	Severely damaged	Damaged	Intact
Phagocytes	Absent	Deficient	Normal
Humoral immunity	Normal	Decreased	Severely decreased
Cellular immunity	Slightly decreased	Decreased	Decreased
Host defense mechanisms with GVHD			
Integument			
Skin	Damaged	Damaged	Damaged
Mucous membranes	Damaged	Severely damaged	Damaged
Phagocytes	Absent	Deficient	Normal
Humoral immunity	Normal	Decreased	Severely decreased
Cellular immunity	Slightly decreased	Severely decreased	Severely decreased
Prevalent infections			
Mucositis	Herpes/streptococci	Herpes/yeast	Herpes/yeast
Lung	Gram-negative rods	Cytomegalovirus	Pneumococci
	Aspergillus	*Aspergillus*	Viruses/*Pneumocystis*
Blood	Streptococci/staphylococci	Staphylococci	Pneumococci
	Gram-negative rods/yeast	Yeast	Meningococci

Integument

The protective effect of the skin is commonly compromised by the inevitable use of high doses of chemotherapy, irradiation, herpesvirus infection, intravenous catheters, and at later stages, GVHD in allogeneic HCT recipients. Needles and intravascular catheters provide a nidus for local infection and a portal of entry into the bloodstream. Many of the bacteremias that occur during a HCT procedure are related to these indwelling venous catheters. Colonization of indwelling catheters with staphylococci is virtually universal (4). This represents a diagnostic dilemma, particularly in the context of a persistently febrile neutropenic patient, because bacteremia might only reflect colonization rather than systemic infection. When an intravenous catheter is present and bacteremia has been documented, the significance of such a culture remains controversial as to whether this represents true bloodstream infection or a contamination from the catheter. We currently have no way to reliably distinguish a contaminant from a true positive blood culture, and in general, all such positive blood cultures should be treated. Some advocate drawing simultaneous blood cultures from the catheter and a peripheral site, but many centers do not perform peripheral blood cultures in patients with central catheters in place. Coexistent hemorrhagic diathesis enhances the risks of catheter-related and other skin infections.

Although coagulase-negative staphylococci are currently the predominant Gram-positive bacterial isolates, some centers have reported the increasing importance of other Gram-positive organisms. In a review of 832 bone marrow transplant patients the incidence of viridans streptococci bacteremia was 15% (5). With increasingly intensive conditioning regimens and associated mucositis and the direct correlation between the rate of positive blood cultures and the severity of damage to the mucosal surface, it is questionable whether viridans streptococci are true pathogens in all cases or whether they simply represent an epiphenomenon (6). Interestingly, infections by viridans streptococci are principally seen in patients who receive prophylactically oral quinolones, which induce preferential presence of these organisms on the damaged mucous membranes (7,8). Considering this mucosal damage, it is not surprising that *Clostridium perfringens* and *Clostridium septicum* septicemia, classically with massive hemolysis and diffuse intravascular coagulation, have also been reported (9,10). Serious infections caused by *Stomatococcus mucilaginosus*, a Gram-positive coccus that belongs to the normal flora of the human oral cavity and that is similar in many respects to *Staphylococcus* spp., have been described (11).

Colonization Resistance

The protective effect of the indigenous microbial flora, or so-called colonization resistance, is more or less controversial. Epidemiologic studies have demonstrated that colonization with *Klebsiella*, *Proteus*, and *Pseudomonas* spp. is more likely to result in infection than is that with *Escherichia coli* (12). There is some evidence to suggest that normal flora, presumably anaerobes, impede colonization by more virulent exogenous aerobic Gram-negative bacilli and yeasts (13). Colonization of the gut is influenced by treatment with antibiotics and a variety of other environmental factors, including food, water, air, and contacts with visitors or medical personnel. In addition, treatment-induced mucositis, in combination with other disturbances of local host defenses, such as diminished quality and quantity of the saliva, and presumably altered epithelial binding sites for micro-organisms, contributes to the microbial shift (14). Drugs that are H$_2$-receptor antagonists and, similarly, antacids should not be prescribed unless absolutely necessary, because they will induce achlorhydria, which facilitates colonization of the gut by Gram-negative bacilli and organisms like *Listeria monocytogenes*. Other well-known examples of infectious complications associated with disturbance of the normal microbial equilibrium are the appearance of oropharyngeal yeast infections and pseudomembranous colitis due to *Clostridium difficile* after treatment with broad-spectrum antibacterials.

Other Factors

Severe impairment of the cellular and humoral immunity is an inherent consequence of the aggressive conditioning regimens. It is obviously more profound following HCT where T-cell depletion has been used. Additional serious defects in the cellular and humoral immunity are caused by the use of corticosteroids, antithymocyte globulin, cyclosporine, and methotrexate to protect against GVHD and/or rejection of the graft. On the other hand, patients with poorly controlled acute and chronic GVHD have even more extended periods of immunodeficiency and a corresponding increased risk of infection. Viral infections, particularly caused by the herpesviruses, play a more prominent role after HCT than with other organ allograft recipients, presumably because of the reduction of virus-specific immunity by HCT conditioning. It appears that GVHD increases both the incidence and severity of virus infections. Long-lasting depletion of IgA, IgG (important for the humoral reaction to bacterial polysaccharide antigens), and IgM results in an attenuated response to antigenic stimuli (15,16).

EVALUATION PRIOR TO HCT

Some patients may be actively infected when they are referred for HCT, and this may have direct consequences because the immunosuppression associated with HCT will impair the patient's ability to contain specific infections. Tuberculosis, toxoplasmosis, CMV, and other herpesviruses have a strong tendency for reactivation under these circumstances. Therefore the history of the patients with regard to previous infections should be obtained, as it might reveal important information for the risk of infectious complications during the aplastic phase after the transplantation. For bacterial infection, this information has no apparent predictive value. An infected transplant candidate should be excluded from transplantation unless

the infection can be controlled adequately by appropriate antimicrobial therapy and adjunctive measures prior to the onset of conditioning. Serological screening for a variety of infectious processes is therefore an important part of the pretransplant evaluation (Table 2).

Because the types of infection early in the granulocytopenic period differ from the late infectious complications, it has become common practice to divide the typical course of febrile episodes in the HCT recipient into different time periods. The sequence of risk factors determines to a large extent the sequence of infectious events (17,18). The spectrum of pathogens, their frequency, and the severity of infection during the preengraftment period are comparable in the various transplant types that share profound neutropenia and severe mucosal damage, whereas the infectious complications in the mid-recovery periods are less frequent after an autologous or syngeneic transplant as a direct consequence of the absence of GVHD.

Early Phase From Conditioning Until Engraftment

Regardless of the conditioning regimen, a period of profound granulocytopenia and mucosal damage invariably develops within a few days. Initially, the situation in HCT recipients is strikingly similar to that of patients undergoing remission-induction or consolidation treatment for acute leukemia. The most significant causes of infection-related fever during this period are bacterial and, to a lesser extent, fungal. A significant portion of bacteremia, including Gram-negative bacilli, and candidemia occurs during the first weeks after transplantation. Thereafter the number of positive blood cultures gradually decreases and stays relatively constant after the fourth week. The central intravenous catheter should always be considered a potential risk for bacterial infection as long as the catheter remains in place. Without prophylactic acyclovir, herpes simplex virus (HSV) is the prevalent infection within 30 days after HCT but is rarely itself a cause of significant fever. HSV excretion is seen in 80% of all transplant recipients (19). It is frequently difficult to distinguish this viral infection clinically from oral mucositis caused by radiation and chemotherapy without the help of the diagnostic laboratory. Noninfectious causes of fever

TABLE 2. *Microbiological screening of the patients before transplantation*

- History of infections during previous life and possible previous neutropenic episodes
- Surveillance cultures of feces, throat, nose, axilla, and groin
- Serological testing for cytomegalovirus; herpes simplex; Epstein-Barr virus; Varicella-zoster virus; hepatitis A, B, and C virus; human immunodeficiency virus; *Toxoplasma gondii;* lues
- *Strongyloides stercoralis* (in endemic areas)

have been difficult to quantitate but include fever associated with tissue damage (e.g., caused by conditioning therapy, drug fever, pulmonary atelectasis, etc.).

The spectrum of organisms responsible for bacterial infections during the early post-HCT period does, in fact, not differ significantly from the spectrum encountered during remission induction and consolidation treatment of acute leukemia. Therefore in view of their pathogenicity with a possibly rapidly fatal course of infection, enteric pathogens—including *Escherichia coli*, *Klebsiella*, and in some centers *Pseudomonas* spp.—remain among the primary pathogens to be covered by an empirical antimicrobial regimen. Numerous antibiotics, given alone or in combination, have been tested for this purpose, but no superior regimen has been established. Aminoglycoside-related nephrotoxicity poses a problem in patients who receive cyclosporine concomitantly. Although this nephrotoxicity is usually mild and reversible, it regularly necessitates dose reductions of cyclosporine that in turn could compromise control of GVHD. Double β-lactam combinations have rather high sodium contents and may delay marrow recovery (20). Studies comprising a sufficient number of serious infections in high-risk patients, such as those treated for hematologic malignancies or undergoing HCT, have shown equivalent efficacy of monotherapy in comparison with more traditional aminoglycoside-containing combinations (21–24). Single-agent empiric therapy is easier to administer, is associated with fewer adverse events, is more cost-effective, and can be safely co-administered with cyclosporine (25,26). Carbapenems provide a reasonable alternative to the ceftazidime and cefepime, but concomitant treatment with drugs such as ganciclovir and cyclosporine may predispose to development of seizures in imipenem-cilastatin recipients. Meropenem has no distinctive propensity for inducing seizures and appears to be an attractive candidate for empiric treatment of febrile bone marrow transplant patients (23,27). The risk of emergence of resistant strains with monotherapy is limited if appropriate doses are given, especially when a quinolone is used for prophylactic purposes. Based on these facts, empirical treatment with a single broad-spectrum β-lactam with a spectrum that includes *Pseudomonas aeruginosa* should be considered an attractive alternative option, especially in centers where *Pseudomonas* has not been a problem. Because there is an obvious variation in the prevalent pathogens from hospital to hospital, the choice of a basic empiric regimen should be guided by hospital sensitivity patterns.

Different types of infection are associated with distinct causative pathogens and different prognosis (28,29). Hence, despite the common lack of physical signs and symptoms, it is important to conduct a careful physical examination with special attention to oropharynx, lungs, venous access devices, and perianal areas, and to use the available modern imaging techniques at regular intervals. In certain patients, it is probably prudent to consider supplementing empirical schemes with a more specific antibiotic to accomplish an optimal antibiotic cover.

A change from Gram-negative to Gram-positive bacteria as the predominant causative organisms has occurred over the past two decades. This phenomenon is related to increased mucosal damage and liberal use of central venous catheters in conjunction with the employment of prophylactic antibacterial agents as a key factor (7). In fact, none of the common empirical regimens are yet the optimal choice for treating infection with Gram-positive cocci, including coagulase-negative staphylococci. Incorporation of antibiotics with better Gram-positive coverage into the initial regimen remains controversial but is generally not recommended (30). Adaptation of the empirical regimen with antimicrobials such as penicillin to treat mucositis where the risk of viridans streptococci is high may be appropriate in some centers, although the addition of clindamycin to ceftazidime failed to influence the clinical course of fever even though all the streptococci were rapidly eradicated from the blood (31). Similarly, patients with a catheter-associated infection or other infections of the skin and soft tissues might benefit from early addition of a glycopeptide. However, empiric use of a glycopeptide is controversial because early mortality due to infections with these organisms is very low. Indeed, from the results of several prospective studies, there appears to be no need for a glycopeptide as part of the front-line therapeutic regimen unless there is reason to suspect the presence of a methicillin-resistant *Staphylococcus aureus* on the basis of local patterns of resistance (32–34). Because glycopeptides otherwise do not contribute to the ultimate chances of survival, these drugs can be added later when Gram-positive bacteria have been isolated or in the case of clinical deterioration (35). Besides, a variety of other Gram-positive bacteria such as *Corynebacterium jeikeium* and *Stomatococcus mucilaginosus*, and Gram-negative bacilli (e.g., *Enterobacter cloacae*, *Acinetobacter* spp. and *Stenotrophomonas maltophilia*) are capable of initiating tissue infection around the exit site and tunnel of a central intravenous catheter. Catheter removal should be considered for any persistent blood culture after 48 hours of appropriate therapy and/or the failure of the patient to have an adequate clinical response (i.e., defervescence of fever, resolution of other associated symptoms).

Modification of the Empirical Regimen During Neutropenia

When a clinician feels compelled to change an antibiotic regimen in a persistently febrile patient, it is important to realize that the median duration of fever in serious, established infections is 4 or 5 days, even with adequate antibiotic therapy (21,24,32). Persistent or relapsing fever is not a trivial item because the response rate to the empirically administered antibiotics is usually lower after HCT than in leukemia patients who undergo remission induction or consolidation chemotherapy courses. Moreover, the profound immunosuppression renders the HCT patient susceptible to many different infectious agents, both concomitantly and consecutively. This lower response rate to empirical treatment of neutropenia-associated fever is due to a higher incidence of nonbacterial infections and noninfectious causes or possibly the greater proportion of Gram-positive isolates that are relatively more resistant to the standard regimens. However, in many cases, premature modifications are made without any evidence of clinical deterioration, persistence of a pathogen, or development of a new site of infection (Table 3). The temptation to escalate therapy by adding more drugs becomes almost irresistible when cultures fail to yield a pathogen and fever persists. However, an intentional approach involving modification of the antimicrobial regimen every 2 or 3 days according to a predetermined schedule until the patient becomes afebrile is not advised because it ignores the individual differences between various febrile neutropenic patients. It can also instill a false sense of security precisely because the regimens chosen offer an increasing spectrum of activity, encouraging the false confidence that further attempts at diagnosis can be abandoned. Rather than improving the outcome, liberal use of antibiotics actually increases the risk of organ toxicity, the development of resistance, and excessive costs (36).

Decisions on antimicrobial therapy after the neutropenic period have to be tailored to meet the need of an individual patient and should be based, as much as possible, on the results of diagnostic procedures. For instance, treatment failures are commonly encountered in infections related to right atrial tunneled central catheter. Glycopeptides such as vancomycin and teicoplanin are, indeed, a reasonable choice for this purpose, whereas prescribing glycopeptides for persisting fever alone is disappointing in more than 80% of patients (36). Vancomycin usage has decreased dramatically in many centers as the concern regarding vancomycin-resistant enterococci increases.

Candida and *Aspergillus* spp. may also be responsible for fevers and documented superinfections in granulocytopenic HCT recipients receiving broad-spectrum antimicrobial agents. The propensity of yeasts to adhere to mucosal surfaces or intravascular catheters is an important etiologic factor for development of invasive fungal infections. *Candida albicans* is still the predominant pathogen in disseminated candidal infections, but *Candida tropicalis*, *C. glabrata*, *C. krusei*, and *C. parapsilosis* (the latter often in association with central venous lines) are increasingly encountered. All species have to be considered as potential pathogens in these patients and treated accordingly with parenteral antifungal agents.

Pulmonary infiltrates may be of either infectious or noninfectious etiology during this period (37). Noninfectious causes include infiltrates caused by the adverse effects of cytotoxic therapy or irradiation, pulmonary edema, or pulmonary hemorrhage. Establishment of a definitive diagnosis is very difficult because of the challenges of performing a successful diagnostic procedure in an often critically ill patient population. In about 10% of cases of viridans streptococcal septicemia, an adult respiratory distress syndrome may evolve with a mortality of around 60% despite aggressive supportive therapy. The pathophysiology of this serious complication is not clear

TABLE 3. *Algorithm for antibiotic treatment before granulocyte recovery*

Empiric therapy at onset of fever:
  Cephalosporin or carbapenem with anti-*Pseudomonas* activity
Evaluate after 3 days:
  Improvement:
    Continue regimen until the patient has recovered neutrophil count or has remained afebrile and symptom-free for 7 days
  No improvement:
    Positive culture

Gram-negative:	Add aminoglycoside and change beta-lactam if isolate is not susceptible
Gram-positive:	Add teicoplanin or vancomycin
	Consider amoxicillin and/or corticosteroids in case of viridans streptococci
Fungus:	Add amphotericin B
	Consider hematopoietic growth factor in case of molds

    Focus of infection without positive culture—further diagnostic procedures needed

Skin, soft tissue:	Add teicoplanin or vancomycin
Lung:	Add amphotericin B
Abdomen:	Reconsider anaerobic cover if evidence of bowel obstruction/perforation

  No positive culture and

no focus of infection:	Emphasis on daily physical exams, cultures, and diagnostic procedures
	Consider noninfectious cause of fever
	Add teicoplanin or vancomycin if there is strong suspicion of infection
	Consider amphotericin B

(5). It likely involves several factors, including both the effects of the streptococcal infection and preexisting tissue damage. Therefore corticosteroids rather than supplementary antibiotics should be considered to manage patients affected by this complication (38). When a new infiltrate appears and progresses in patients who remain granulocytopenic or on broad-spectrum antibiotics, particularly in conjunction with chest pain, a fungal pneumonia by *Aspergillus fumigatus* is the leading diagnostic consideration (39,40). The finding of *Aspergillus* spp. in a BAL specimen or even in sputum in these patients is closely correlated with *Aspergillus* pneumonia (41). Conversely, a negative finding cannot be regarded as sufficient evidence against a possible fungal pneumonia because as many as 50% of BAL in HCT patients who are subsequently proven to have aspergillosis are negative.

Dysphagia or odynophagia may be due to chemotherapy or gastric reflux, but esophagitis is of infectious origin in many cases, *Candida* spp. being the most likely causative organisms (42). Fungal sinusitis may begin as a small, necrotic, crusted lesion but can progress rapidly to involve the paranasal sinuses. *Aspergillus* spp. lead the list of etiologic agents of the rhinocerebral syndrome, with *Phycomycetes* being less common pathogens.

Other fungi, such as *Phycomycetes*, *Mucor*, *Fusarium* spp., *Pseudallescheria boydii*, and *Malassezia furfur*, are occasionally encountered. The very high mortality associated with fungal infections after HCT is, at least in part, related to the lack of adequate diagnostic techniques. Although the exact incidence is unknown, it has been shown that more than 30% of patients who received allogeneic transplants have invasive fungal infection at the time of autopsy (43). Treatment is usually not initiated until the later stages of infection, and the currently available antifungal agents are not very effective in this setting. By consequence, if a patient is persistently febrile for more than 5 days and is doing poorly on broad-spectrum antibacterial therapy, and if no causative micro-organism can be found, it has become standard practice to add empiric intravenous amphotericin B to the patient's empirical regimen (44,45). Such an approach has been shown to reduce fungal infections but is less than an ideal solution, because it leads to overuse of amphotericin B, which is nephrotoxic. Such nephrotoxicity may lead to compromising the dose of cyclosporine that can be used to prevent GVHD. On the other hand, it must be emphasized that patients who are at high risk of an invasive fungal infection might profit from a very early institution of systemic antifungals in a preemptive fashion. This pertains to essentially the same category of patients who are the principal candidates for antifungal prophylaxis. Although the detection of circulating fungal antigens may correlate with invasive disease, the value of such a test is still considered experimental (46). In the near future, the rapidly evolving and promising techniques in molecular biology, such as the polymerase chain reaction, may enhance the possibilities of establishing a definitive diagnosis in an earlier stage of the infection (47). Imaging techniques such as the use of computed tomography are important for the diagnosis of aspergillosis (48).

Amphotericin B deoxycholate, at a starting dose of 0.5–1.0 mg/kg/day for suspected candidal infection and 1.0–1.5 mg/kg/day for suspected mold infection, remains the first choice for treatment of invasive fungal infections. Therapy is generally continued until the neutrophil count returns to greater than 500/mm^3; discontinuation of antifungal therapy after 7 days of responding to therapy and remaining afebrile before the recovery of counts has been proposed by some (30). In patients with an impaired kidney function and in those who receive concomitantly other possibly nephrotoxic drugs, 0.7 mg/kg/day is recommended. If the serum creatinine exceeds two times the baseline level, treatment should be interrupted for 1 or 2 days to allow for recovery of the kidney function. Thereafter amphotericin B has to be reinstituted at a dose of 0.5 mg/kg/day with doses increasing daily to the maximally tolerated level under monitoring of the serum creatinine level. Because amphotericin B is frequently poorly tolerated by recipients of allogeneic HCT, lipid preparations of amphotericin B are more and more valued as safer, though expensive, alternatives (49–51). They are undoubtedly better tolerated than conventional amphotericin B and allow for prescription of higher daily doses. However, it is questionable whether a higher dose will produce superior results. A recent trial by the European Organization for Research and Treatment of Cancer (EORTC)'s Invasive Fungal Infection Group learned that a dose of 1 mg/kg/day of liposomal amphotericin B was as effective as 4 mg/kg/day in treating invasive aspergillosis (52). Fluconazole in high doses offers a reasonable alternative for invasive candidal infections (53,54). The opportunity to manage chronic disseminated candidiasis with fluconazole in an outpatient setting is both convenient and cost-effective (54–56).

Middle Phase: From Engraftment Until Day 100 After HCT

Infectious complications in HCT recipients are determined by the pace of gradual reconstitution of the immune system. During the mid-recovery phase, covering the interval between successful engraftment and 3 months after transplantation, fever may still be common. The major immunocompromising factors after the initial phase of an allogeneic HCT is GVHD, a prominent cause of fever itself, and its treatment. The occurrence of GVHD results in increased incidence of fever in the allogeneic compared with the syngeneic or autologous transplant settings during the period after engraftment. Acute GVHD may also result in ulceration of the gastrointestinal tract, which allows pathogens to enter the bloodstream from the intestine, compounded by effect on granulocyte function (57). Among the serious infections that cause fever during this time are those caused by viruses, particularly CMV and respiratory viruses. Persistent bacteria as well as non-bacterial pathogens, principally fungi, continue to be major causes of fever in those patients with severe GVHD or in those who remain granulocytopenic. In addition, when the neutrophil count recovers, occult infections, such as hepatosplenic candidiasis, may become manifest.

Viral Infections

The most prominent and ominous febrile syndrome after engraftment is that which occurs with interstitial pneumonia. Interstitial pneumonia occurs in approximately 40% of all allogeneic HCT recipients and in 15% of syngeneic recipients prior to prophylaxis with ganciclovir (37). The reported mortality ranges from 50% to 80%. The initial clinical presentation of interstitial pneumonia manifestation consists of fever, nonproductive cough, dyspnea, and either diffuse bilateral interstitial infiltrates or bibasilar infiltrates that subsequently progress to diffuse infiltrates.

Various viruses are known to cause severe lung injury in HCT patients. These include adenovirus (58), influenza virus, parainfluenza virus, respiratory syncytial virus (59), and, in particular, CMV prior to the use of ganciclovir prophylaxis. Historically, CMV has been associated with 50% to 70% of interstitial pneumonias, with an overall incidence of approximately 40% in patients developing GVHD after an allogeneic bone marrow transplant (60). Analysis of BAL fluid with centrifugation cultures for diagnostic purposes in case of a pneumonitis yields sensitivity and specificity of >95% and therefore provides an accurate alternative to a more dangerous open lung biopsy. CMV pneumonitis after autologous or syngeneic HCT is much less common, showing rates of only 1% to 2%, but when it occurs, it is as severe as after allogeneic HCT and carries a similarly high mortality (61). Preemptive administration of ganciclovir to patients who have high or increasing CMV titers in BAL or in blood specimens prior to the development of any clinical symptom of CMV disease has been shown to reduce the probability of subsequent pneumonitis significantly and has become a widely accepted approach (62,63).

Adenovirus, rotavirus, and coxsackievirus may cause infectious gastroenteritis during this phase of allogeneic HCT. Symptoms such as nasal discharge and otitis media, distinctly unusual in CMV infection, are the usual presenting symptoms of respiratory syncytial virus and other community-acquired respiratory viruses. The apparent increase in viral pathogens during the last decade may represent, at least in part, the availability of better isolation and diagnostic techniques.

Other Infections

An organism deserving special attention is *Listeria monocytogenes*, which can cause central nervous system infection and bacteremia after HCT (64). *Legionella*

pneumophila infections depend on the presence of the organism in the nosocomial environment, and if no quinolone prophylaxis is being used, they may occur throughout the entire transplant period, often presenting with atypical symptoms or duration of infection due to coexisting neutropenia. Management of these bacterial infections is based on isolation of the specific organism.

Given the severity of immunosuppression after HCT one might expect to see infections caused by *Mycobacterium tuberculosis*, *Cryptococcus neoformans*, *Toxoplasma gondii*, *Mycoplasma pneumonia*, and *Nocardia* spp. *Pneumocystis carinii* rarely occurs if adequate prophylaxis is given, but when an infection does occur, it requires high doses of intravenous trimethoprim-sulfamethoxazole and is characterized by a considerable relapse rate. Parasites like *Strongyloides stercoralis*, *Leishmania* spp., and *Trypanosoma cruzi* are found in many parts of the world and may be encountered in HCT recipients in endemic areas. Fever accompanied by atypical rashes or mucocutaneous lesions, lymphadenopathy, and hepatosplenomegaly, respectively, demand specific microbiological investigations to exclude the possibility that one of these micro-organisms is responsible for the actual signs and symptoms of infection (65).

Late Phase: Infections Following Day 100 After HCT

Approximately 3 months after allogeneic HCT, a recovery of orderly immune function has taken place in most patients, particularly those without GVHD. Following day 100 after HCT, the incidence and severity of infections are linked to the presence or absence of chronic GVHD. Chronic GVHD is a multisystem disease that may involve skin, mucosa, gastrointestinal tract, liver, skeletal muscle, and serosal surfaces, and resembles connective tissue disorders such as scleroderma. Fever in patients with chronic GVHD is common. Chronic GVHD is associated with long-lasting deficiency of humoral and cellular immunity. Common infectious complications include sinopulmonary infections related to IgA deficiency and sicca syndrome. Furthermore, antigen-specific responses, such as T-cell responses to various viral antigens, or antibody production to bacterial antigens, such as pneumococcal polysaccharide, usually take longer to recover in patients with chronic GVHD.

Varicella-zoster virus (VZV) infection develops in about 30% of all patients, including autologous HCT recipients (66), and in 45% of patients with chronic GVHD (67) who survive for at least 6 months. Median time of onset is 4–5 months after transplant with a disseminated infection at the outset in approximately a quarter of cases. Disseminated infection is more likely to be associated with fever than localized VZV. Before antiviral chemotherapy was available, up to 10% of HCT recipients with VZV infection died as a result of visceral dissemination. Fortunately, acyclovir proved to be superior treatment, although even the use of high-dose oral acy-clovir should be discouraged for treatment of established infections because peak concentrations achieved are often lower than the concentration required to inhibit many VZV. This is related to the poor absorption of only 15% of oral acyclovir, as well as to the lower susceptibility of VZV in comparison to herpes zoster. Hence acyclovir should be given intravenously in high doses in allogeneic HCT patients. With the arrival of the newer acyclovir derivatives, such as valaciclovir, that attain higher plasma concentrations than acyclovir, oral treatment may become available in the near future, but presently the efficacy of such an approach has been insufficiently documented in HCT patients.

Long-term survivors may develop abnormalities of hepatic enzymes associated with fever, occasionally accompanied by symptomatic jaundice. Hepatitis C virus (HCV) is likely responsible for most of these cases with a clinical picture that resembles non-A, non-B hepatitis. The long-term prospects of HCV infection remain to be defined and are discussed more fully in Chapter 22. In a nontransplant population, half of patients with HCV develop chronic infection, about 10% develop chronic active hepatitis, and about 5% get cirrhosis. Because all blood products are now routinely screened to eliminate those that may harbor the HCV, it is hoped that the morbidity from HCV will be reduced.

Late CMV may be encountered in 15% of patients with chronic GVHD (68). Adenovirus is recovered from approximately 5% of patients and is a rare cause of interstitial pneumonitis, diarrhea, or even disseminated infection (58). Infections by a variety of other viruses—including human herpesvirus 6 (HHV6), rotaviruses, influenza, parainfluenza, and coxsackievirus—can also arise, partly depending on seasonal variations and communicable events in the community at large. Among allogeneic HCT recipients, human herpesvirus 6 has been linked to interstitial pneumonitis, rash, encephalitis, and bone marrow suppression (69–72). Excretion of the Epstein-Barr virus (EBV) in saliva has been noted in approximately 60% of allogeneic HCT patients, but clinical manifestations are usually not apparent in HCT recipients. Conversely, it must be stressed that *Pneumocystis carinii* infections may emerge in patients with chronic GVHD after cessation of prophylaxis with trimethoprim-sulfamethoxazole.

Months, if not years, after successful engraftment, encapsulated organisms like meningococci, *Haemophilus influenzae* type B, *Staphylococcus aureus*, and the notorious *Streptococcus pneumoniae* have been shown to be responsible for rapidly fatal bacteremias and life-threatening respiratory infections. The well-known high incidence of pneumococcal infections can be attributed to the inability to make opsonizing antibody in functionally asplenic subjects even after antigenic reexposure (73) and affects patients without any sign of GVHD. Remarkably, the capsular types of *S. pneumoniae* involved appear to be those that are poorly immunogenic even in the normal host. Some of the immune responses have been shown to require antigenic reexposure in the form of active infection, although even recurrent pneumococcal infection may not be sufficient to elicit specific antibody production in some patients. This is confirmed by the fact that patients with GVHD have subnormal antibody responses to pneumococcal vaccination. Pneumococcal infections have a high mortality because the onset is insidious and infection may be well beyond cure by the time the patient consults the general practitioner or the hospital. Although not substantiated by randomized studies, it seems prudent to protect patients with chronic GVHD with prophylactic oral penicillin or trimethoprim-sulfamethoxazole, especially after a previous pneumococcal infection. However, vigilance remains warranted because breakthrough pneumococcal infections as well as resistant pneumococci have occurred. Alternatively, patients may benefit from education regarding this risk and should be advised to begin antibiotics immediately at the first sign of fever or other suspicious complaints, in addition to consulting their general practitioner or specialist as soon as possible.

MANAGEMENT OF FEVER IN SOLID ORGAN TRANSPLANT RECIPIENTS: GENERAL PRINCIPLES

Fever following SOT is a common and potentially life-threatening occurrence. The immunosuppression state that is present during the initial months following SOT is extremely effective in suppressing the soluble mediators that lead to fever, and thus a febrile episode during this period most likely reflects a significant underlying cause. The etiology of fever following SOT can be arbitrarily subdivided into infectious and noninfectious. Although the infectious etiologies that develop following SOT are common to those in other immunocompromised individuals, noninfectious etiologies of febrile syndromes may be unique to certain types of SOT. For an orderly discussion of the evaluation and management of febrile episodes in SOT, the post-transplant period is divided into time periods that include the following: pretransplantation, immediate post-transplantation (first 10 days), and early post-transplantation (10 days to 3 months) (74,75).

Pretransplantation Evaluation Prior to SOT

It is well established that any febrile episode that develops in a potential organ recipient may represent an underlying infectious process that may ultimately become a contraindication for proceeding with transplantation, especially when some of these patients are already immunosuppressed secondary to their organ failure (e.g., liver or renal transplant candidates).

Common infectious etiologies that may develop prior to transplantation are due, in decreasing order of frequency, to bacterial, fungal, and viral micro-organisms. Among the bacterial infections that need to be considered, these are usually specific to the type of organ failure for which the patient requires transplantation. Pretransplant liver recipients commonly develop recurrent colangitis, whose sole clinical manifestation may be intermittent febrile episodes in the absence of documented bacteremias, especially for patients with end-stage liver disease secondary to biliary defects such as primary sclerosing colangitis or primary biliary cirrhosis. The clinical response of the febrile episode to the empirical use of broad-spectrum antibacterial agents in these patients supports the presumed diagnosis. The high frequency of recurrent febrile episodes has led to the common practice of placing these patients in suppressive bacterial antibiotic regimens, such as rotating cycles of sulfamethoxazole/trimethoprim, quinolones, or ampicillin/sulbactam (76). Unfortunately, the continuous use of broad-spectrum antibiotics will predispose these patients to fungal infections such as those caused by *Candida* spp., leading to antibiotic resistance. Because of the diffuse and microscopic structures of the biliary tree in these pretransplant patients, there is no indication for percutaneous biliary drainage.

Febrile syndromes can be observed in patients awaiting lung transplantation, especially those with cystic fibrosis and chronic diffuse bronchiectasis. The natural history of these underlying lung diseases is that of chronic and recurrent respiratory tract infections (pneumonia or bronchitis). Thus, as is the case for preliver transplant recipients, potential lung recipients are usually placed on chronic suppressive antibacterial therapy in an attempt to eliminate colonization infection with, for example, Gram-negative bacteria such as with *Pseudomonas* spp. As discussed, for preliver transplant recipients, a judicious use of antibiotics is warranted because overuse will predispose patients to later antibiotic resistance, drug allergies, and more important, supercolonization with fungal agents such as *Candida* spp.

A third group of patients that commonly develop febrile episodes while awaiting SOT are those with underlying severe diabetes, as is usually the case in prepancreas or kidney/pancreas transplantation. Intermittent fever due to urinary tract infections is not infrequent, and thus specific identification of the micro-organism(s) present in the urine, rather than empirical use of antibiotics, is necessary to provide a focused and narrow choice of antibacterial therapy. Moreover, these patients are usually colonized with candidal organisms, and a short course of antifungal therapy with, for example, fluconazole (in the case of *Candida albicans*) is recommended even though patients may be asymptomatic. Antifungal therapy helps sterilize the urine at the time of pancreas transplantation and reduces complications associated with anastomosing the pancreatic duct into the bladder.

Although rare, noninfectious etiologies can be a cause of intermittent febrile episodes pre-SOT. For example, in patients with cardiac or hepatic amyloidosis who are awaiting heart and/or liver transplantation, noninfectious fever is not uncommon. Usually, these patients undergo a routine infectious disease evaluation of such febrile episodes that usually yields negative results. Nevertheless, the transplantation of the diseased organ is sufficient to eliminate this chronic and intermittent type of unexplained fever. Lastly, patients with chronic active hepatitis awaiting liver transplantation may have low-grade intermittent fevers that also resolve following liver transplantation.

Recommendations for routine infectious disease evaluation prior to SOT have been summarized (74).

Immediate Early Post-transplantation Period (First 10 Days)

Infectious complications leading to fever during the first ten days following SOT are usually not related to immunosuppression, but rather to bacterial infections that arise during the intensive hospitalization period. As such, nosocomial or aspiration pneumonias, catheter-related sepsis, or surgical wound infections are the most frequent infectious etiologies toward which evaluation should be directed (74). However, due to the increased chance of noninfectious etiologies leading to febrile episodes, it is mandatory that empirical antibiotics are not immediately started unless either a clear documentation of microbial infection is established or the patient is hemodynamically unstable.

Among the noninfectious etiologies that can lead to febrile episodes during the first 10 days post-SOT are those related to surgical complications such as intra-abdominal hematomas secondary to bleeding of the vascular or nonvascular graft anastomosis, most commonly seen in liver transplant recipients (74). Drug fever secondary to the antibiotic prophylactic regimen administered perioperatively may be also responsible for a febrile episode during the first 1 or 2 days following transplantation. A third cause of noninfectious febrile episode is related to the use of antilymphocyte immunoglobulins. Some solid organ transplant centers administer anti-T-cell antibodies such as OKT3 as the immunosuppressive induction regimen. A main side effect of this antibody is the release of pyrogenic cytokines such as IL1 or TNF, and thus in some patients significant febrile episodes can develop following the first or second dose of OKT3 (77). Although premedication may decrease this incidence, in some patients it is necessary to avoid the use of OKT3 and provide other immunosuppressive medications. It is also during this time period that a number of antimicrobial agents are first introduced as part of the long-term antimicrobial prophylaxis program, some of which may lead to drug fever. Trimethaprim-sulfamethoxazole, which is frequently utilized in the prevention of bacterial and *Pneumocystis carinii* infection, needs to be frequently considered in this situation.

Early Post-transplantation Period (10 Days–3 Months)

During the second to the fourth week following SOT, both allograft rejection and infectious complications secondary to T-cell immunodeficiency frequently develop, therefore resulting in a significant number of febrile episodes. Among the most common infectious complications that need to be considered are those related to bacterial infection and, to a lesser degree, those caused by *Candida* spp. In liver transplant recipients, biliary anastomosis leaks result in peritonitis (sterile peritonitis if the bile fluid is noncontaminated, or bacterial, if this was colonized). Perihepatic abscesses and/or bacterial/fungal peritonitis without a biliary leak also need to be considered (78). In the case of pancreas kidney transplants, a similar situation is present with regard to perigraft infections (79); for heart/lung or lung transplant recipients, complications arising from the tracheo-bronchial anastomosis or mediastinal wound infection may develop (80). The diagnostic work-up and specific management of these etiologies are discussed in Chapter 4 of this book. To stress the potential danger of starting empirical antibiotics in these patients, it is important to realize that establishment of the microbial diagnosis needs to be made to provide a narrow, focused, and limited antibacterial regimen.

A significant number of individuals will develop febrile episodes that are not related directly to infections. The incidence of acute allograft rejection (which is different from the hyperacute allograft rejection that develops within the first few hours following renal and other types of SOT) peaks during the second and third weeks following transplantation. It is during this time that the high degree of immunosuppression is slowly being tapered and in which an immune response may have developed against the allograft. An aggressive diagnostic work-up to exclude or document allograft rejection by means of tissue biopsy should be pursued. Unless the patient is hemodynamically unstable, it is preferable to await the results from these biopsies to formally exclude rejection before assuming the fever is due to infection. If rejection is excluded with a high degree of certainty, then it is up to the individual physician to decide whether broad-spectrum antibiotics are needed or to wait for defined microbiological etiology. Treatment of allograft rejection with, for example, OKT3 may also lead to febrile episodes (77).

Infectious febrile syndromes are common during the early part of the second month after SOT, especially those caused by fungal and viral infections. Herpesviruses such as CMV, EBV, and to a lesser extent HHV-6 are common causes of fever. A more effective utilization of anti-CMV prophylactic regimens has decreased its incidence and changed its natural history,

and hence, timing of appearance post-SOT (81). The diagnostic work-up and management of CMV are discussed in Chapter 5. A high index of suspicion of EBV infection needs to be maintained in patients who are EBV-seronegative and have received an EBV-seropositive organ (82,83). Syndromes resembling atypical infectious mononucleosis (prolonged febrile episodes with arthralgias and malaise without lymphadenopathy or atypical lymphocytosis in peripheral smear) are common manifestations of EBV infection. More important, EBV-induced lymphoma may occur as early as 6–8 weeks following SOT, especially in EBV-seronegative patients. An aggressive diagnostic work-up to exclude EBV-induced lymphoma is of importance, for if immunosuppresion is not reduced, these patients may quickly progress into monoclonal and monomorphic types of lymphoma (see discussion in Chapter 18).

Candidal infections and those caused by *Aspergillus* spp. are common between the fourth and tenth week after SOT. It is therefore important that individual patients presenting with a febrile episode and in whom rejection has been excluded be evaluated for deep fungal infections. Multiple studies have addressed specific risk factors that predispose SOT recipients to fungal infections (84). This is extremely important because of the relative lack of sensitivity of current diagnostic techniques for the early diagnosis of these infections.

Another infectious cause of low-grade fever that develops during the first 2–3 months after SOT is that of hepatitis secondary to hepatitis C virus (HCV). Such complication is normally seen in liver transplant recipients who were transplanted for HCV-induced cirrhosis, and occasionally in renal transplant recipients who were HCV-infected pretransplantation (85). Chronic bacterial infections such as those caused by atypical microbacteria, or infections with dimorphic fungi such as *Histoplasma* or *Blastomyces*, can present with low-grade febrile episodes. Lastly, and as for any other type of immunocompromised patient, infection with common respiratory viruses, streptococcal pharyngitis, and so on, may have a more severe clinical manifestations in SOT recipients, and fever may be the first and most significant symptom.

Noninfectious etiologies presenting as febrile symptoms that can develop during the second to third month after SOT are less common than infectious ones. As mentioned before for the early post-transplant period, allograft rejection and drug reactions need to be considered as the main etiologies to exclude during a febrile episode. Chronic, rather than acute, allograft rejection is usually manifested by abnormalities of the transplanted graft function rather than by fever. However, it is possible to observe chronic liver rejection such as the vanishing bile duct syndrome develop in conjunction with low-grade fever caused by obstructing colangitis. Similarly, lung graft failure can begin with recurrent bouts of pneumonitis and/or bronchitis.

Beyond the 6 months of a successful SOT recipient, it is unusual to observe many febrile episodes. If they were to develop, the same differential diagnosis pertaining to opportunistic or severe community acquired infections and to late allograft rejection need to be considered, and the appropriate diagnostic and management work-up must be done.

REFERENCES

1. Donnelly JP. Bacterial complications of transplantation: diagnosis and treatment. *J Antimicrob Chemother* 1995;36[Suppl. B]:59–72.
2. Hartmann O, Le Corroller AG, Blaise D, et al. Peripheral blood stem cell and bone marrow transplantation for solid tumors and lymphomas: hematologic recovery and costs. A randomized, controlled trial. *Ann Intern Med* 1997;126:600–607.
3. Sickles EA, Greene WH, Wiernik PH. Clinical presentation of infection in granulocytopenic patients. *Arch Intern Med* 1975;135:715–719.
4. Raad II, Bodey GP. Infectious complications of indwelling vascular catheters. *Clin Infect Dis* 1992;15:197–210.
5. Villablanca JG, Steiner M, Kersey J, et al. The clinical spectrum of infections with viridans streptococci in bone marrow transplant recipients. *Bone Marrow Transplant* 1990;6:387–393.
6. Classen DC, Burke JP, Ford CD, et al. *Streptococcus mitis* sepsis in bone marrow transplant patients receiving oral antimicrobial prophylaxis. *Am J Med* 1990;89:441–446.
7. De Pauw BE, Donnelly JP, De Witte T, Novakova IRO, Schattenberg A. Options and limitations of long-term oral ciprofloxacin as antibacterial prophylaxis in allogeneic bone marrow transplant recipients. *Bone Marrow Transplant* 1990;5:179–182.
8. Elting LS, Bodey GP, Keefe BH. Septicemia and shock syndrome due to viridans streptococci: a case control study of predisposing factors. *Clin Infect Dis* 1992;14:1201–1207.
9. Stamm WE, Tompkins LS, Wagner KF, et al. Infection due to *Corynebacterium* species in marrow transplant recipients. *Ann Intern Med* 1979;91:167–173.
10. Pouwels MJM, Donnelly JP, Raemaekers JMM, Verweij PE, De Pauw BE. *Clostridium septicum* sepsis and neutropenic enterocolitis in a patient treated with intensive chemotherapy for acute myeloid leukemia. *Ann Hematol* 1997;74:153–157.
11. Weers-Pothof G, Novakova IRO, Donnelly JP, Muytjens HL. Bacteraemia caused by *Stomatococcus mucilaginosus* in a granulocytopenic patient with acute lymphocytic leukaemia. *Neth J Med* 1989;35:143–146.
12. Fainstein V, Rodriguez V, Turck M, et al. Patterns of oropharyngeal and fecal flora in patients with acute leukemia. *J Infect Dis* 1981;144:82–86.
13. Van der Waaij D, Berghuis-De Vries JM, Lekkerker-Van der Wees JEC, et al. Colonization resistance of the digestive tract in conventional and antibiotic-treated mice. *J Hygiene* 1971;69:405–411.
14. Sotiropoulos SV, Jackson MA, Woods GM, et al. Alpha-streptococcal septicemia in leukemic children treated with continuous or large dosage intermittent cytosine arabinoside. *Ped Infect Dis J* 1989;8:755–758.
15. Aucouturier P, Barra A, Intrator L. Long-lasting IgG subclass and antibacterial polysaccharide antibody deficiency after allogeneic bone marrow transplantation. *Blood* 1987;70:779–785.
16. Al-Eid MA, Tutschka PJ, Wagner HN Jr. Functional apslenia in patients with chronic graft-versus-host disease: concise communication. *J Nucl Med* 1983;24:1123–1126.
17. Van der Meer JWM, Guiot HFL, Van den Broek PJ, Van Furth R. Infections in bone marrow transplant recipients. *Semin Hematol* 1984;21:123–140.
18. Wingard JR. Advances in the management of infectious complications after bone marrow transplantation. *Bone Marrow Transplant* 1990;6:371–386.
19. Meyers JD, Flournoy N, Thomas ED. Infection with herpes simplex virus and cell-mediated immunity after marrow transplant. *J Infect Dis* 1980;142:338–346.
20. Kibbler CC, Prentice HG, Sage RJ, Hoffbrand AV, Brenner MK, Noone P. Do double β-lactam combinations prolong neutropenia in patients undergoing chemotherapy or bone marrow transplantation for hematological disease? *Antimicrob Agents Chemother* 1989;33:503–507.
21. De Pauw BE, Deresinski SC, Feld R, Lane-Allman EF, Donnelly JP. Ceftazidime compared with piperacillin and tobramycin for the empiric treatment of fever in neutropenic patients with cancer—a multicenter randomized trial. *Ann Intern Med* 1994;120:834–844.
22. Freifeld AG, Walsh T, Marshall D, et al. Monotherapy for fever and neutropenia in cancer patients: a randomized comparison of ceftazidime versus imipenem. *J Clin Oncol* 1995;13:165–176.
23. De Pauw BE, for the Meropenem Study Group of Leuven-London-Nijmegen. Meropenem and ceftazidime are equally effective as single agents for empirical therapy of the febrile neutropenic patient. *J Antimicrob Chemother* 1995;36:185–200.
24. Cometta A, Calandra T, Gaya H, et al. Monotherapy with meropenem versus combination therapy with ceftazidime plus amikacin as empiric therapy for fever in granulocytopenic patients with cancer. *Antimicrob Agents Chemother* 1996;40:1108–1115.
25. Verhagen C, De Pauw BE, De Witte T, Holdrinet RSG, Janssen JTP, Williams KJ. Ceftazidime does not enhance cyclosporine A nephrotoxicity in febrile bone marrow transplant patients. *Blut* 1986;53:333–339.
26. Eggiman P, Glauser MP, Aoun M, Meunier F, Calandra T. Cefepime monotherapy for empirical treatment of fever in granulocytopenic patients. *J Antimicrob Chemother* 1993;32:151–163.
27. Del Favero A. Clinically important aspects of carbapenem safety. *Curr Opin Infect Dis* 1994;7[Suppl. 1]:S38–42.
28. Novakova IRO, Donnelly JP, De Pauw B. Potential sites of infection that develop in febrile neutropenic patients. *Leuk Lymph* 1993;10:461–467.
29. Donnelly JP, Novakova IRO, Raemaekers JMM, De Pauw BE. Empiric treatment of localized infections in the febrile neutropenic patients with monotherapy. *Leuk Lymph* 1993;9:193–203.
30. Hughes WT, Armstrong D, Bodey GP, et al. 1997 guidelines for the use of antimicrobial agents in neutropenic patients with unexplained fever. *Clin Infect Dis* 1997;25:551–573.
31. Donnelly JP, Muus P, Horrevorts AM, Sauerwein RW, De Pauw BE. Failure of clindamycin to influence the course of severe oromucositis associated with streptococcal bacteraemia in allogeneic bone marrow transplant recipients. *Scand J Infect Dis* 1993;25:43–50.
32. Ramphal R, Bolger M, Oblon DJ, et al. Vancomycin is not an essential component of the initial empiric treatment regimen for febrile neutropenic patients receiving ceftazidime—a randomized prospective study. *Antimicrob Agents Chemother* 1992;36:1062–1067.
33. Novakova IRO, Donnelly JP, De Pauw BE. Ceftazidime as monotherapy or combined with teicoplanin for initial empiric treatment of presumed bacteremia in febrile granulocytopenic patients. *Antimicrob Agents Chemother* 1991;35:672–678.
34. The EORTC International Antimicrobial Therapy Cooperative Group and National Cancer Institute of Canada. Vancomycin added to empirical combination antibiotic therapy for fever in granulocytopenic cancer patients. *J Infect Dis* 1991;163:951–958.
35. Novakova IRO, Donnelly JP, Verhagen CS, et al. Teicoplanin as modification of initial empirical therapy in febrile granulocytopenic patients. *J Antimicrob Chemother* 1990;25:985–993.
36. De Pauw BE, Dompeling EC. Antibiotic strategy after the empiric phase in patients treated for a hematological malignancy. *Ann Hematol* 1996;72:273–279.
37. Meyers JD, Flournoy N, Thomas ED. Nonbacterial pneumonia after allogeneic marrow transplantation. *Rev Infect Dis* 1982;4:1119–1132.
38. Dompeling EC, Donnelly JP, Raemaekers JMM, De Pauw BE. Preemptive administration of corticosteroids prevents the development of ARDS associated with *Streptococcus mitis* bacteremia following chemotherapy with high-dose cytarabine. *Ann Hematol* 1994;69:69–72.
39. Gerson GL, Talbot GH, Hurwitz S, et al. Prolonged granulocytopenia: the major risk factor for invasive pulmonary aspergillosis in patients with acute leukemia. *Ann Intern Med* 1984;100:345–351.
40. Wingard JR, Beals SU, Santos GW, Merz WG, Saral R. *Aspergillus* infections in bone marrow transplant recipients. *Bone Marrow Transplant* 1987;2:175–181.
41. Yu VL, Muder RR, Poorsattar A. Significance of isolation of *Aspergillus* from the respiratory tract in diagnosis of invasive pulmonary aspergillosis: results from a three-year prospective study. *Am J Med* 1986;81:249–254.
42. McDonald GB, Sharma P, Hackman RC, Meyers JD, Thomas ED. Esophageal infections in immunosuppressed patients after marrow transplantation. *Gastroenterology* 1985;88:1111–1117.
43. Bodey GP, Bueltman B, Duguid W, et al. Fungal infections in cancer

patients: an international autopsy survey. *Eur J Clin Microbiol Infect Dis* 1992;11:99–109.

44. Pizzo PA, Robichaud KJ, Gill FA, Witebsky FG. Empiric antibiotic and antifungal therapy for cancer patients with prolonged fever and granulocytopenia. *Am J Med* 1982;2:101–110.

45. EORTC International Antimicrobial Therapy Cooperative Group. Empiric antifungal therapy in febrile neutropenic patients. *Am J Med* 1989;86:668–672.

46. Rodgers TR, Haynes KA, Barnes RA. Value of antigen detection in predicting invasive pulmonary aspergillosis. *Lancet* 1990;330:1210–1213.

47. Verweij PE, Latge JP, Rijs AJMM, et al. Comparison of antigen detection and PCR assay with bronchoalveolar lavage fluid for diagnosing invasive aspergillosis in patients receiving treatment for hematological malignancies. *J Clin Microbiol* 1995;33:3150–3153.

48. Caillot D, Casanovas O, Bernard A, et al. Improved management of invasive pulmonary aspergillosis in neutropenic patients using early thoracic computed tomographic scan and surgery. *J Clin Oncol* 1997; 15:139–147.

49. Ringden O, Andstrom E, Remberger M, Svahn BM, Tollemar J. Safety of liposomal amphotericin B (Ambisome) in 187 transplant recipients treated with cyclosporin. *Bone Marrow Transplant* 1994;14[Suppl. 5]: S10–14.

50. Oppenheim BA, Herbrecht R, Kusne S. The safety and efficacy of amphotericin B colloidal dispersion in the treatment of invasive mycoses. *Clin Infect Dis* 1995;21:1145–1153.

51. Lister J. Amphotericin B lipid complex (Abelcet) in the treatment of invasive mycoses: the North American experience. *Eur J Haematol* 1996;56[Suppl. 57]:18–23.

52. Ellis M, Spence D, Meunier F, et al. Randomised multicentre trial of 1 mg/kg (LD) versus 4 mg/kg (HD) liposomal amphotericin B (Ambisome) (LAB) in the treatment of invasive aspergillosis (IA). 36th Interscience Conference on Antimicrobial Agents and Chemotherapy. New Orleans, 1996.

53. Anaissie EJ, Darouiche RO, Abi-Said D, et al. Management of invasive candidal infections: results of a prospective, randomized, multicenter study of fluconazole versus amphotericin B and a review of the literature. *Clin Infect Dis* 1996;23:964–972.

54. De Pauw BE, Raemaekers JMM, Donnelly JP, et al. An open study on the safety and efficacy of fluconazole in the treatment of disseminated *Candida* infections in patients treated for a hematological malignancy. *Ann Hematol* 1995;70:83–87.

55. Anaissie E, Bodey GP, Kantarjian H, et al. Fluconazole therapy for disseminated candidiasis in patients with leukemia and prior amphotericin B therapy. *Am J Med* 1991;91:143–150.

56. Kaufman CA, Bradley SF, Ross SC, Weber DR. Hepatosplenic candidiasis: successful treatment with fluconazole. *Am J Med* 1991;91: 137–141.

57. Meyers JD. Infection in bone marrow transplant recipients. *Am J Med* 1986;81[Suppl. 1A]:27–38.

58. Shields AF, Hackman RC, Fife KH, Corey L, Meyers JD. Adenovirus infections in patients undergoing bone marrow transplantation. *N Engl J Med* 1985;312:529–533.

59. Hertz MI, Englund JA, Snover D, Bitterman PB, McGlave PB. Respiratory syncytial virus-induced acute lung injury in adult patients with bone marrow transplants: a clinical approach and review of the literature. *Medicine* 1990;68:269–281.

60. Meyers JD, Flournoy N, Thomas ED. Risk factors for cytomegalovirus infection after human marrow transplant. *J Infect Dis* 1986;153: 478–488.

61. Wingard JR, Chen DY-H, Burns WH, et al. Cytomegalovirus infection after autologous bone marrow transplantation: comparison to infection after allogeneic bone marrow transplantation. *Blood* 1988;71:143–147.

62. Goodrich JM, Mori M, Gleaves CA, et al. Early treatment with ganciclovir to prevent cytomegalovirus disease after allogeneic bone marrow transplantation. *N Engl J Med* 1991;325:1601–1607.

63. Schmidt GM, Horak DA, Niland JC, et al. A randomised, controlled trial of prophylactic ganciclovir for cytomegalovirus pulmonary infection for recipients of allogeneic bone marrow transplant. *N Engl J Med* 1991;324:1005–1011.

64. Chang J, Powles R, Mehta J, Paton S, Treleaven J, Jameson B. Listeriosis in the bone marrow transplant recipient. *Clin Infect Dis* 1995: 1289–1290.

65. Fishman JA. Pneumocystis carinii and parasitic infections in transplantation. *Infect Dis Clin* 1995;85:95–97.

66. Schuchter LM, Wingard JR, Piantadosi S, et al. Herpes zoster infection after autologous bone marrow transplantation. *Blood* 1989;74:1424–1427.

67. Locksley RM, Flournoy N, Sullivan K, et al. Infection with varicella-zoster virus in immunocompromised patients. *J Infect Dis* 1986; 153:840–847.

68. Boeckh M, Riddell SR, Cunningham T, et al. Increased incidence of late CMV disease in allogeneic marrow transplant recipients after ganciclovir prophylaxis is due to a lack of CMV-specific T cell responses. 38th Annual Meeting of the American Society of Hematology. Orlando, 1996:302a.

69. Carrigan DR, Drobyski WR, Russler SK, Tapper MA, Knox KK, Ash RC. Interstitial pneumonitis associated with human herpesvirus 6 after marrow transplantation. *Lancet* 1991;338:147–149.

70. Yoshikawa T, Suga S, Asano Y, et al. Human herpesvirus 6 in bone marrow transplantation. *Blood* 1991;78:1381–1384.

71. Drobyski WR, Knox KK, Majewski BS, Carrigan DR. Brief report: fatal encephalitis due to variant B human herpesvirus 6 in a bone marrow transplant recipient. *N Engl J Med* 1994;330:1356–1360.

72. Drobyski WR, Dunne WM, Burd EM, et al. Human herpesvirus 6 (HHV-6) infection in allogeneic bone marrow transplant recipients: evidence of a marrow suppressive role for HHV-6 *in vivo*. *J Infect Dis* 1993;167:735–739.

73. Winston DJ, Schiffman G, Wang DC, et al. Pneumococcal infections after human bone marrow transplantation. *Ann Intern Med* 1979,91: 835–841.

74. Patel R, Paya CV. Infections in solid-organ transplant recipients. *Clin Microbiol Rev* 1997;10(1):86–124.

75. Rubin RH. Infection in the organ transplant recipient. In: Rubin RH, Young LS, eds. *Clinical approach to infection in the compromised host*, 3rd ed. New York: Plenum; 1994:629–705.

76. Van den Hazel SJ, Speelman P, Tytgat GN, van Leuwen DJ. Successful treatment of recurrent cholangitis with antibiotic maintenance therapy. *Eur J Clin Microbiol Infect Dis* 1994;13(8):662–665.

77. Cosimi AB, Colvin RB, Burton RC. Use of monoclonal antibodies to T-cell subsets for immunologic monitoring and treatment in recipients of renal allografts. *N Engl J Med* 1981;305:308–314.

78. Kusne S, Dummer JS, Singh N, et al. Infections after liver transplantation: an analysis of 101 consecutive cases. *Medicine* 1988;67(2): 132–143.

79. Lumbreras C, Fernandez I, Velosa J, Munn S, Sterioff S, Paya CV. Infectious complications following pancreas transplantation: incidence, microbiological and clinical characteristics, and outcome. *Clin Infect Dis* 1995;20:514–520.

80. Dummer JS, Montero CG, Griffith BP, Hardesty RL, Paradis IL, Ho M. Infections in heart-lung transplant recipients. *Transplantation* 1986;41(6):725–729.

81. Patel R, Snydman DR, Rubin RH, et al. Cytomegalovirus prophylaxis in solid organ transplantation. *Transplantation* 1996;61:1279–1289.

82. Walker RC, Marshall WF, Strickler JG, et al. Pretransplantation assessment of the risk for lymphoproliferative disorder. *Clin Infect Dis* 1995;20:1346–1355.

83. Patel R, Portela DF, Bradley AD, et al. Risk factors of invasive *Candida* and non-*Candida* fungal infections following liver transplantation. *Transplantation* 1996;62:926–934.

84. Katkov WN, Rubin RH. Liver disease in the organ transplant recipient: etiology, clinical impact, and clinical management. *Transplant Rev* 1991;5:200–208.

85. Randhawa PS, Martin RS, Starzl TE, Demetris AJ. Epstein-Barr virus associated syndromes in immunosuppressed liver transplant recipients. *Am J Surg Pathol* 1990;14:538–547.

Transplant Infections edited by
Raleigh A. Bowden, Per Ljungman, and Carlos V. Paya.
Lippincott–Raven Publishers, Philadelphia © 1998

CHAPTER 12

Gram-Positive Bacterial Infections

Dan Engelhard and Nina Geller

Gram-positive bacteria cause significant morbidity and mortality in bone marrow and solid organ transplant (SOT) recipients (1–7). The proliferation of Gram-positive pathogens can be attributed in part to the extensive use of central venous catheters (CVCs) and to strategies such as prophylaxis and selective gut decontamination, which are directed primarily toward preventing Gram-negative bacterial infections.

Gram-positive pathogens are implicated in post-transplantation infections, both in the short and long term. They are isolated in postoperative focal infections in solid organ recipients, mainly liver transplant recipients (5), and in bacteremia in solid organ and bone marrow recipients (5,8). In the long term, they constitute a threat in the solid organ recipient because of ongoing immunosuppressive therapy, and in the bone marrow transplant (BMT) recipient, especially in those with graft-versus-host disease (GVHD), because of the slow recovery of the recipient's immune system (1).

A principal source of Gram-positive pathogens is the patient's own flora, with the site varying by pathogen: skin for coagulase-negative staphylococcus (CNS) and *Staphylococcus aureus*; the oral cavity for *Streptococcus viridans*; the gastrointestinal tract for enterococci; and the upper respiratory tract for *Streptococcus pneumoniae*. Pathogens can also be transmitted via an infected donor organ (9), and, rarely, during BMT transplantation, by contaminated marrow that has been manipulated *in vitro* (10).

This chapter will focus on the role of these bacteria in transplant infections and the increasing emergence of multiply resistant strains among Gram-positive pathogens.

ENTEROCOCCI

Introduction

Enterococci are Gram-positive facultative anaerobes which are seen microscopically as singles, pairs, and short chains and are part of the normal flora (commensals) of the GI tract. They are the second most common cause of all nosocomial infections in the United States (11,12). *Enterococcus faecalis* constitutes 80% to 90% and *E. faecium*, 5% to 10% of organisms isolated in clinical microbiological laboratories, with the frequency of *E. faecium*, particularly multiply resistant strains, increasing, especially in the transplant population (5,13). In addition, at least 10 other species have been isolated from colonized stool in man and from patients with enterococcal infections.

In transplant recipients, enterococcal infections are usually nosocomial and generally occur as invasive infections in the immediate post-transplant period. However, they are also a source of later infections, especially in liver transplant recipients (5,14).

The most important issue over the last decade regarding enterococci has been the emergence of glycopeptide resistance. Resistant enterococci are becoming a common intestinal colonizer among transplant recipients (12) and sometimes cause invasive infection, either as a single pathogen or as part of a polymicrobial infection.

Epidemiology

Enterococci are found in diverse environments as they flourish under harsh conditions in soil, food, water, and a wide variety of animals. Infection in transplant recipients may be acquired endogenously via their own flora or exogenously from environmental sources. The gastrointestinal tract is the major habitat of enterococci, and they are commonly found at intra-abdominal wounds as part of polymicrobial flora. Enterococci are a frequent cause of bacteremia subsequent to urinary tract infection (UTI),

From the Department of Pediatrics, Hadassah University Hospital, Jerusalem 91120, Israel.

intra-abdominal infection, cholangitis, and infection of intravenous or intra-arterial lines.

The emergence of resistant strains of enterococci has led to the investigation of the means and patterns of their transmission. Transmission is both between patients and via the hands of medical staff who frequently harbor resistant enterococci in their gastrointestinal tract that may be responsible for colonization in their patients (13).

The ability of E. faecium to resist desiccation was demonstrated in a liver transplant unit by the isolation of resistant E. faecium on equipment in storage, especially on hemodynamic monitoring devices and pumps. This finding is consistent with the supposition that they were indeed the means of transmission despite the absence of vancomycin-resistant E. faecium isolates from the hands of the staff (15). Outbreaks of nosocomially transmitted vancomycin-resistant E. faecium have been reported in both liver transplant recipients (16) and BMT recipients (17).

Although stool colonization with high numbers of vancomycin-resistant enterococci strains can be found, there are few descriptions of disease caused by these strains (18). It has been suggested that antibiotic selective pressure may contribute to colonization (19), a contention that is supported by the observation that neutropenic BMT recipients who receive long-term therapy with cephalosporins and aminoglycosides, which do not exert an antienterococci effect, are at increased risk for E. faecalis septicemia (8).

Incidence

Enterococcal infections are more common in liver transplant recipients than in other solid organ or BMT recipients. In a study of 284 adult liver transplant recipients, 159 (56%) experienced bacterial infections, of which 28% were caused by either E. faecium or E. faecalis (5); in another study, of 405 liver transplant recipients, 13% had enterococcal bacteremia (20); and in pediatric liver transplant recipients with infections, 19% of all isolates were enterococci (21). In a study of vancomycin-resistant enterococci, six different enterococcal species were isolated from the stool of 63% of 49 pediatric liver transplant recipients; however, only three patients developed infections (two urinary tract and one peritonitis) all of which were due to vancomycin-resistant (MIC 7-8) E. faecium (22). In two groups of cardiac transplant recipients, each having received a different immunosuppresive therapy regimen, enterococci were isolated from various sites of infection in 16% and 11% of the 38 and 72 patients, respectively (6). In renal transplant recipients, E. faecalis is the major pathogen, causing 21% of UTIs (23). And, in our BMT unit, 7% (16/242) of the patients experienced nosocomial E. faecalis infections (a third of them polymicrobial) during the post-BMT hospitalization period (8).

Contrary to the predominance by E. faecalis over E. faecium in the general population, the frequency of E. faecium may exceed that of E. faecalis in transplant recipient infections, especially in liver transplant recipients. In one liver transplantation center, bacteremia with E. faecium was 2.5 times more frequent than E. faecalis (5), but in another, there were approximately 3 times more E. faecalis isolates than E. faecium (20). In patients with hematologic malignancies, two-thirds of whom had undergone BMT or peripheral-blood stem cell transplants, bacteremia due to E. faecium predominated over that due to E. faecalis (24). In our BMT recipients, E. faecalis was the sole enterococcal pathogen causing invasive infection (8).

Onset of Infection

In liver transplant recipients, bacteremia episodes due to E. faecalis generally occur within the first 4 weeks following transplantation, while one-half of those due to E. faecium occur within the first 4 weeks, and the other half occur later (5). Enterococcal bacteremia in cardiac transplant recipients and intra-abdominal infections in liver transplant recipients usually occur within the first few weeks following transplantation (21,25). In renal transplant recipients, bacterial infections, including those caused by enterococci, the most common Gram-positive bacterial pathogens, occur most frequently during hospitalization for transplantation (26). In addition, in the months following renal transplantation, enterococci are the major pathogens causing UTI (23).

In our center, nosocomial E. faecalis bacteremia occurred on days $^-3$ to $^+51$ post-BMT (median, $^+21$ days). The onset of polymicrobial perianal infection including Enterococcus, an infrequent post-BMT complication, ranges from 2 to 375 (mean 86) days post-BMT, with those episodes involving abscesses tending to occur later (27).

Vancomycin-resistant E. faecium bacteremia in liver transplant recipients occurs significantly later during hospitalization (median 43 days) than that with vancomycin-susceptible (median 24 days) (16). It is possible that the later onset of infection with vancomycin-resistant strains may be attributable to acquisition of resistance by the enterococci during the hospitalization period. Stool colonization with vancomycin-resistant enterococci in liver transplant recipients shows a steady increase during the first month following liver transplantation (22), and, in 75% of organ transplant recipients (kidney, liver, heart, lung, and kidney plus pancreas), vancomycin-resistant enterococci were isolated within 6 months (mean 30 days) following transplantation (18).

Clinical Manifestations

Enterococci cause bacteremia, including that associated with the use of intravascular devices, and a variety of focal infections, some of which are typical of particular types of transplantation. In liver transplant recipients, enterococcal infection occurs at a wide variety of sites: the urinary tract (most common), intra-abdomen (frequently multibacterial), bloodstream (as bacteremia), surgical wound, bile duct (cholangitis), the chest, and liver (abscess) (5,21). Enterococcal endocarditis may be sequential to intra-abdominal infection (16). Enterococcal bacteremias are frequently polymicrobial, one series reporting 49% as polymicrobial (20). In liver transplant recipients, bacteremia due to vancomycin-resistant *E. faecium* differs significantly from that due to vancomycin-susceptible *E. faecium*. Vancomycin-resistant *E. faecium* has been isolated far more frequently as a sole blood pathogen than vancomycin-susceptible *E. faecium*. Vancomycin-resistant *E. faecium* has required more frequent invasive interventions for intra-abdominal and intrathoracic infection, has been a more frequent cause of recurrent bacteremia and recurrent infection at the primary site, has been found in a higher percentage of patients with enterococcal infection at autopsy, and has been more frequently implicated in *Enterococcus*-associated mortality (16).

In heart transplant recipients, nosocomial enterococci infections include pneumonia, urinary tract and wound infections, bacteremia associated with the use of intravascular devices (6,25), and mediastinitis (28). Glycopeptide-resistant *E. faecalis* catheter-related endocarditis has also been reported in a transplanted heart (29). *E. faecalis* has been found as the major pathogen causing UTI during the first 6 months following renal transplantation (23). Enterococci show a propensity to adhere to renal epithelial cells and heart valves, contributing to their causal role in UTIs and endocarditis (13). In addition, *Enterococcus* has been identified as the cause of infection around joint replacements in a renal transplant recipient (30).

In BMT recipients, *E. faecalis* was found to be a significant pathogen in exit site infection, colonization, catheter-related septicemia, and septicemia of unknown origin (8). It can also cause catheter-related right-sided endocarditis (31). An infrequent complication in BMT recipients is polymicrobial perianal infection including *Enterococcus* (27).

Outcome

Enterococci synergize with other bacteria, leading to increased morbidity and mortality. However, because they are frequently involved in polymicrobial bacteremia, it is difficult to determine their independent contribution. Furthermore, they may be an indicator of severe underlying disease rather than the immediate cause of death (13).

In our BMT recipients, the outcome of vancomycin-sensitive *E. faecalis* bacteremia was favorable. The sole patient with *E. faecalis* who died had polymicrobial bacteremia with an additional three Gram-negative Enterobacteriaceae (8).

High rates of refractory infection, serious morbidity, and attributable death, which are exacerbated by the lack of effective antimicrobial therapy, occur with infections due to vancomycin-resistant *E. faecium* (VREF) in transplant recipients as in the nontransplant population (16,32,33). In recipients of liver transplantation with VREF, *E. faecium*-associated death was reported as 46% (26/54), versus 25% (12/48) in those with vancomycin-susceptible *E. faecium* (16). Another study reported 75% mortality in liver transplant recipients: all nine patients with polymicrobial bacteremia, including both VREF and Gram-negative bacteria, died; but all three patients with bacteremia with VREF alone survived (19). In a renal transplantation center, *Enterococcus* has been found to be the most common Gram-positive pathogen associated with death (34). In a mixed population of organ transplant recipients (kidney, liver, heart, lung, and kidney plus pancreas), a 25% mortality, half of which was directly attributable to vancomycin-resistant enterococcal infection, was reported (18).

Factors Associated with Enterococcal Infection and Its Outcome

A number of factors have been found to be associated with enterococcal infections in transplant recipients. In liver transplant recipients, administration of prophylactic antilymphocyte antibodies (21) and acute rejection have been associated with enterococcal infection (5); Roux-en-Y choledochojejunostomy, a cytomegalovirus-seropositive donor, biliary stricturing, primary sclerosing cholangitis, symptomatic cytomegalovirus infection, and prolonged transplantation time with enterococcal bacteremia (20). Vancomycin resistance, shock, and liver failure have been identified as independent risk factors for *Enterococcus*-associated mortality in liver transplant recipients (16) and associated with increased mortality due to VREF in patients undergoing hemodialysis or being admitted to the ICU preoperatively (19). In heart transplant recipients, a somewhat greater frequency of enterococcal infection has been seen in those who had been treated with the immunosuppressive therapy of a combination of azathioprine, rabbit antithymocyte globulin, and corticosteroids (16%) than with cyclosporine plus corticosteroids (11%); the respective rates with lung infection were 8% and 1% (6). In our center, post-BMT *E. faecalis* bacteremia has been associated with prolonged neutropenia and acute GVHD (8).

Antimicrobial Resistance

Enterococci have intrinsic or acquired resistance to aminoglycosides, β-lactams, lincosamides and trimethoprim-sulfamethoxazole (TMP-SMZ), fluoroquinolones, macrolides, rifampin, tetracyclines, and more recently, also to glycopeptides. Glycopeptide resistance is ubiquitous in enterococci which are frequently involved in multiply resistant polymicrobial bacteremia in transplant recipients, principally liver transplant recipients (13).

In contrast to findings in Europe, a study in the United States failed to find evidence of VanA- or VanB-type vancomycin-resistant *Enterococcus* in the community or among environmental sources, and suggested that chickens who ingested glycopeptides were not a likely source of vancomycin-resistant *Enterococcus* in patients (35). A possible association, a genetic linkage, between vancomycin- and gentamicin-resistant genes has been suggested by their presence in the same plasmid of an *E. durans* isolate. Although *E. durans* isolates are an infrequent cause of infection in humans, they could play an important role in the dissemination of resistant genes (36). In an adult liver transplantation unit, vancomycin-resistant *E. faecium* isolates were detected only subsequent to the prior presence of gentamicin-resistant *E. faecium*; they increased from 19% to 83% over a one-year period (15).

Factors Associated with Glycopeptide Resistance

Factors found common to SOT recipients in whom vancomycin-resistant enterococci were cultured were prolonged hospitalization, the presence of invasive devices (such as foley catheters and central lines) or invasive procedures, increased immunosuppression for rejection, and prior administration of antibiotics, especially vancomycin (18).

A number of risk factors for acquisition of nosocomial vancomycin-resistant *E. faecium* infections in orthotopic liver transplant recipients have been identified: many more antibiotics having been administered preoperatively, greater likelihood of having received vancomycin therapy preoperatively, having been hospitalized in the intensive care unit (ICU) preoperatively, prolonged stay in the surgical ICU postoperatively, and surgical reexploration (19).

Vancomycin-dependent Enterococci

Another problem with enterococci, though rare, is the development of vancomycin-dependent strains, that is, particular enterococcal strains that do not grow in the absence of vancomycin. It is hypothesized that the normal D-ala ligase is not expressed in the vancomycin-dependent strain so survival of the strain is dependent on expression of the VanB ligase, which produces a depsipeptide precursor that is resistant to vancomycin binding. The presence of a vancomycin-dependent *E. faecium* strain in a small-bowel plus liver transplant recipient with polymicrobial bacteremia while the patient was receiving amikacin, imipenem, and vancomycin has been reported. Awareness of the existence of these strains is important, especially when clinical and microbiological data are consistent with infection due to a fastidious or nutritionally deficient organism (37).

Management

Treatment of enterococcal infections is complicated by the unusual patterns of susceptibility and resistance frequently exhibited by enterococci and by the necessity for specialized techniques required for demonstrating true susceptibility in the clinical microbiology laboratory. In addition, reports on the isolate's susceptibility to specific drugs may be misleading because the standard acceptable level of susceptibility appropriate for use of the specific drug is not indicated (13).

In general, a penicillin is the antibiotic of choice for susceptible strains of enterococci. Vancomycin or teicoplanin are the alternatives for patients allergic to penicillin or organisms with high levels of penicillin resistance (13,38). For *E. faecalis* endocarditis, treatment with the following synergistic antibiotics has been suggested: penicillin and streptomycin, penicillin and gentamicin, or vancomycin and streptomycin. These combinations are used because the penicillins, the cephalosporins, vancomycin, and the aminoglycosides are usually only bacteriostatic against enterococci, and relapse is common in patients with enterococcal endocarditis when a single drug is used (39).

The treatment for infections with vancomycin-resistant enterococci poses a very difficult problem. Despite the usual inclusion of chloramphenicol or doxycycline in the treatment of vancomycin-resistant enterococcal infection (40,41), they may not be beneficial. For example, in a cohort of liver transplant recipients, in whom 93% of vancomycin-resistant *E. faecium* isolates were susceptible to chloramphenicol, mortality was not reduced when it was used as monotherapy for severely ill patients, including those with bacteremia (19). Very-high-dose continuous infusion of ampicillin/sulbactam plus gentamicin was found successful in one study of liver transplant recipients. Although none of the strains produced β-lactamase, it was suggested that sulbactam may have had an unexplained beneficial effect against some enterococci (42). Highly vancomycin-resistant *E. faecium* strains have been found sensitive to pristinamycin. However, administered orally, it has been shown ineffective in liver transplant recipients with serious intra-abdominal infections or recurrent bacteremias (43).

Two new oxazolidinone antimicrobial agents have been found successful, *in vitro*, in inhibiting all isolates of enterococci, including strains resistant to vancomycin, ampicillin, and minocycline despite their activity being primarily bacteriostatic (44). If pharmacokinetic characteristics and safety are demonstrated, they could become useful in the arsenal of multiresistant enterococcal infection treatment.

Prevention

Control measures—education of physicians, nursing and environmental services personnel, strict adherence to handwashing procedures, compliance with gloves and gown barrier precautions, environmental surface cleaning, and placement of large isolation precaution signs on the door to each patient's room—can be expected to reduce the incidence of glycopeptide-resistant enterococcal infections (17,45).

Prophylactic antibiotics are used at different times with regard to the transplantation—pretransplantation, peritransplantation, and/or post-transplantation—and as preemptive therapy to prevent infections, including those caused by enterococci. Selective bowel decontamination with a variety of nonabsorbable antibacterial agents (e.g., gentamicin and polymyxin B combined with nystatin or amphotericin B) is used in liver transplantation and in some BMT centers. Some BMT centers use prophylactic quinolones with or without penicillin. Perioperative antibacterial prophylaxis (e.g., with cefazolin or ampicillin-sulbactam) has become standard practice in organ transplantation (3). Post-transplantation prophylactic TMP-SMZ has been shown effective in reducing the incidence of enterococcal infection in renal transplant recipients (26) and is also used with other transplantations (3). Preemptive therapy with the addition of drugs such as vancomycin plus aztreonam or ampicillin-sullbactam is administered whenever liver biopsy is performed or biliary tract manipulation is undertaken (3).

Currently, however, the emergence of antimicrobial-resistant pathogens, especially multiply resistant strains, raises questions regarding the use of prophylaxis and complicates the determination of empiric regimens for nosocomial infections. Efforts should be directed toward preventing the emergence of resistant strains and eliminating unnecessary administration of prophylactic and therapeutic antibiotics, including glycopeptides.

COAGULASE-NEGATIVE STAPHYLOCOCCI

Introduction

All staphylococci are members of the Micrococcacae family, produce catalase, and divide in irregular clusters to produce packets of cells. Of the 32 species of human coagulase-negative staphylococci (CNS), 15 are indigenous to humans. Once considered harmless commensals, nonpathogenic bacteria living on the skin and mucous membranes, they have become increasingly significant clinically, causing substantial morbidity and, at times, contributing to mortality.

Transplant recipients with a CVC are especially vulnerable to coagulase-negative staphylococcal infections. Indeed, CNS have become the most common cause of nosocomial bacteremia in BMT recipients, both during and following the neutropenic period (2,46,47). They are also common pathogens in SOT recipients, especially early post-transplantation, when patients are hospitalized in intensive care units (3,5–8).

Epidemiology

Staphylococcus epidermidis, comprising 65% to 90% of all CNS isolated, is the most prevalent and persistent species on human glabrous skin and mucous membranes, with *S. hominis* the next most common. Virtually all *S. epidermidis* infections are hospital-acquired while all *S. saprophyticus* infections, primarily UTIs, are community acquired (48). Colonization in patients and hospital staff precedes infection with antibiotic-resistant *S. epidermidis,* which probably gains access to indwelling foreign bodies by direct inoculation during insertion of the device or later, via the CVC exit site.

Incidence

In our study of 242 BMT recipients, 15% experienced CNS infections, half of which were bacteremia (46). Another study reported that 12% of BMT recipients had CNS bacteremia (49). Three percent of our patients had an exit site infection with CNS (46), which constituted 29% of all pathogens causing exit site infection, compared with the 42% of exit site isolates in the other study (49). In liver transplant recipients, CNS have caused 12% of bacterial infectious episodes, mainly as bacteremia or wound infections, most occurring early post-transplantation (5). *S. epidermidis* was found responsible for 21% (10/47) of septicemia episodes following heart transplantation (7).

Clinical Manifestations

CNS cause surgical wound infections and infections associated with lines, including CVC bacteremia, CVC local infections, and drains-associated peritonitis. CNS bacteremia usually runs a relatively benign clinical course, without metastatic blood spreading infections, and mortality is rare (5,46). In heart transplant recipients, there have been reports of CNS endocarditis with a favorable outcome (50) and of a CNS surgical wound infection months post-transplantation (51). Following liver transplantation, CNS colonization of the biliary tree can occur, and may cause infection when a biopsy or biliary tract manipulation is performed (3).

CVC Factors Associated with CNS Infections

Biomaterial implants are markedly susceptible to staphylococcal infections (52). Adherence of the bacteria to the catheter surface depends on the host, the microbial factors, and the catheter material (53). *In vitro* colonization has been found to occur within 6 hours of a catheter's being suspended in a buffer containing CNS (54). Most CNS infecting intravascular lines produce an extracellular fibrous matrix, slime, which may exacerbate colonization. It has been suggested that fibronectin, fibrinogen, or fibrin as well as other host proteins coating the catheter surfaces may also play a role (52).

Antimicrobial Resistance and Factors Associated with Its Development

CNS in nosocomial infections are usually multiply antibiotic resistant, with up to more than 80% resistant to methicillin and all β-lactam antibiotics and more than 50% resistant to erythromycin, clindamycin, trimethoprim, gentamicin, chloramphenicol, and tetracycline (48). As expected, infections with methicillin-resistant CNS tend to occur later in the hospitalization period than those with methicillin-sensitive bacteria (46). Resistance to antibiotics such as penicillin, macrolides, lincosamides, tetracyclines, chloramphenicol, trimethoprim, and aminoglycosides has been associated with specific plasmids. Certain aminoglycoside-resistant plasmids found in *S. epidermidis* can be transferred to other *S. epidermidis* by conjugation. These conjugative plasmids can also encode resistance to penicillin, trimethoprim, and disinfectants, and can mobilize the transfer of plasmids encoding resistance to macrolides, lincosamides, and chloramphenicol. Conjugative resistance transfer may help explain the rapid increase in resistance seen among hospital-associated *S. epidermidis* isolates and probably is also a reflection of the selection pressure of widespread antibiotic use in the hospital (48).

Management

The recommended treatment for methicillin-sensitive CNS is cloxacillin or first-generation cephalosporins, and for methicillin-resistant CNS, glycopeptides. The worldwide emergence of methicillin-resistant CNS has led many centers to include a glycopeptide—vancomycin or teicoplanin—in the initial empiric antimicrobial therapy regimen administered to BMT recipients, especially during the periods of febrile neutropenia. We, as some others, are reluctant to use glycopeptide empirically because of the risk of development of glycopeptide-resistant enterococci, its potential toxicity, and because coagulase-negative staphylococcal bacteremia usually runs a relatively benign clinical course (46). However, when there is clinical deterioration during the neutropenic period while the patient is receiving broad-spectrum antibiotics, addition of vancomycin should be considered. Empiric therapy for nosocomial tunnel infection or CVC-associated thrombophlebitis should include a glycopeptide in addition to removal of the CVC. Patients with catheter-related CNS bacteremia can be treated successfully without catheter removal (46,53).

The high frequency (>80%) of CNS as contaminants in blood cultures continues to pose a problem (46). True CNS bacteremia is defined as two consecutive positive blood cultures (one or two bottles) with CNS exhibiting the same sensitivity pattern (46). Ultimately, the decision whether to treat the patient with antibiotics until there is a second positive culture is based on clinical assessment, including presence of fever or local signs of infection.

Prevention

Careful attention to sterile technique in the management of CVC and other lines is mandatory for eliminating infection with CNS. Antibodies against the polysaccharide surface antigen, which are on almost all *S. epidermidis* clinical specimen isolates, have been found to prevent *S. epidermidis* infections on foreign bodies and endocarditis in an animal model, but they are not yet used clinically (48).

Although there are data suggesting that daily prophylactic IV teicoplanin or vancomycin, initiated at central line insertion, reduces the incidence of CNS infection in patients receiving intense chemotherapy for hematologic malignancies (55), use of these drugs is not recommended. Nevertheless, administration of antistaphylococcal drugs for 24 hours periprocedure for CVC insertion is recommended.

In liver transplant centers, drugs such as vancomycin plus aztreonam or ampicillin-sulbactam are used periprocedure for liver biopsy or biliary tract manipulation, as there may be CNS and/or other Gram-negative bacteria colonization of the biliary tree following transplantation (3).

STAPHYLOCOCCUS AUREUS

Introduction

Staphylococcus aureus occurs microscopically as single, pairs, and short chains and has a strong tendency to form clusters. Man is colonized by *S. aureus*, mainly in the nasopharynx and on the skin. *S. aureus* infections occur in transplant recipients, primarily as wound infections and bacteremia, with or without bloodstream metastatic infections, which include arthritis, osteomyelitis, meningitis, endocarditis, pericarditis, lung abscess, and pyomyositis (25,48,56). *S. aureus* CVC-related focal infections include exit site and tunnel infections and thrombophlebitis (8).

Incidence

The incidence of *S. aureus* infections in liver transplant recipients ranges from 8% to 23%, with wound infections predominating, followed, in frequency, by bacteremia and chest infections (4,5,21,57–59). In one large series of 284 liver transplant recipients, there were 59 *S. aureus* episodes, 83% occurring early (during the first 4 weeks post-transplantation) and the remainder occurring later

(5). *S. aureus* early infections, within the first month following heart transplantation, are common, and include pneumonia, UTI, wound infections, and bacteremia (25). *S. aureus* is the most common Gram-positive bacterial pathogen causing infections during the first 2 weeks post-lung transplantation (60). It caused bacteremia in 2% of 651 heart transplant recipients—11 of 47 (23%) of all episodes of bacteremia (7). In our BMT center, *S. aureus* caused nosocomial bacteremia episodes in 4% (9/242) of transplant recipients (8), similar to the 3% to 5% reported by other centers (49,61). Exit site infection occurred in 5% of our BMT recipients, constituting 13% of all CVC exit site infectious episodes (8).

Transmission

Methicillin-resistant *S. aureus* (MRSA) nosocomial pathogens are transmitted via an infected or colonized patient or by a colonized health care worker. The infected organ donor can also be a source of infections. In one series of lung transplantations, in which *S. aureus* was found in 41% of donor bronchial cultures, half of the recipients developed *S. aureus* infections, and all recovered (60).

Clinical Manifestations

The most common manifestations of *S. aureus* infection in SOT recipients are pneumonia, wound infections, and bacteremia. *S. aureus* is the most common Gram-positive pathogen causing bacterial pneumonia in the first 3 months following SOT (5,62). In many cases, *S. aureus* bacteremia is consequential to a local infection, such as wound infection or pneumonia.

In liver transplant recipients, postoperative wound infection was by far the most common type of *S. aureus* infection, followed by bacteremia and chest infection (5). Other manifestations of *S. aureus* infections in liver transplant recipients have occasionally been seen: an infected hematoma in a patient with choledochojejunostomy within 1 week following a liver biopsy (63) and an infected false hepatic artery aneurysm post-transplantation (64). In a study of 361 heart transplant recipients, *S. aureus* was the most frequent cause (in five of nine patients) of bacterial mediastinal abscess or mediastinitis (65), and there are reports of post–heart transplantation *S. aureus* endocarditis and pericarditis (66). *S. aureus* endocarditis has also been reported in a heart-lung transplant recipient (67), and mediastinitis in a lung transplant recipient (68). In renal transplant recipients, *S. aureus* has been known to cause UTI months following transplantation (69).

In our BMT recipients, *S. aureus* was a significant pathogen in CVC exit site and tunnel infections. However, a relatively low incidence of *S. aureus* CVC-related bacteremia (two episodes in 242 patients) suggests that *S. aureus* may adhere to the catheter much less readily than CNS or even *E. faecalis* (8).

Staphylococcal scalded skin syndrome may mimic acute GVHD in BMT recipients (70).

Outcome

S. aureus pneumonia and bacteremia can be fatal in SOT (62) and BMT recipients (61). All nine of our BMT recipients with *S. aureus* bacteremia survived (8), unlike in another center, where all three of the BMT recipients with *S. aureus* bacteremia died (61). In renal transplant recipients, *S. aureus* has been found to be the most common Gram-positive bacteria, constituting 10% of all organisms detected at or near the time of death (34).

Drug Resistance

In the community, *S. aureus* is methicillin-sensitive, but MRSA is common in hospitals, leading to MRSA nosocomial infections. *S. aureus* strains resistant to ciprofloxacin and other quinolones are found in lung transplant recipients with cystic fibrosis because of their routine use (71).

Treatment

The recommended antimicrobial therapy for infections with methicillin-sensitive strains of *S. aureus* is a semisynthetic penicillin, such as oxacillin, methicillin, or nafcillin, and for MRSA, a glycopeptide (vancomycin or teicoplanin). In cases of benign penicillin allergy, first- or second-generation cephalosporins are administered. Ciprofloxacin has been described as an effective therapy in renal transplant patients with UTI, including *S. aureus* UTI (69). Rifampin or gentamicin are usually added in severe *S. aureus* infections, especially endocarditis.

Prevention

In BMT recipients, antistaphylococcal drugs such as cefazolin are administered 24 hours periprocedure when a CVC is inserted. Perioperative prophylaxis with regimens, such as cefazolin (for up to 3 days post-transplantation), directed mainly against Gram-positive pathogens, has been shown effective in preventing wound infections in renal transplant recipients and become standard practice in all types of SOTs (3). Prophylaxis with TMP-SMZ, which is well tolerated, significantly reduces the post–renal transplantation incidence of UTI and bloodstream infections with *S. aureus* and other pathogens (26).

Efforts should be made to identify the pathogens carried by potential transplantation donors and recipients and, if possible, active infections should be eradicated prior to transplantation.

STREPTOCOCCUS VIRIDANS

Introduction

Streptococcus viridans are facultatively anaerobic, Gram-positive cocci. There are many clinically significant species that are part of the normal microflora, found mainly in the oral cavity, but also in the upper respiratory tract, gastrointestinal tract, and female genital tract. Their ability to adhere to and propagate on cardiac valves may lead to endocarditis. In the immunocompromised host, *S. viridans* bacteremia occurs mainly during neutropenia, and therefore, BMT recipients, but not SOT recipients, are at special risk. *S. viridans*, mainly *S. mitis* and *S. sanguis*, have become among the most common pathogens found following BMT (10,72–75).

Incidence

S. viridans is isolated from blood and/or CSF in 11% to 15% of patients undergoing BMT, mainly during the neutropenic period (74,75). In our center, *S. viridans* septicemia occurred in 23 of the 209 subjects (11%) with underlying malignant disease, all during the first 2 weeks post-BMT, at the time of profound neutropenia with concomitant mucositis. In 20 of these 23 patients, *S. viridans* septicemia occurred at onset of febrile neutropenia, within 5 days post-BMT, whereas in three, onset occurred on day 11 post-BMT (75). In another study, 78% of the invasive infections occurred within 15 days of the transplantation, usually during profound neutropenia (74). *S. viridans* is an infrequent cause of bacteremia in SOT recipients. For example, in one study, only one of 53 liver transplant recipients experienced *S. viridans* bacteremia (4), and in another, only one of 284 liver transplant recipients had "*Streptococcus spp.*" bacteremia (5).

Clinical Manifestations and Outcome

Septicemia is the most common manifestation of *S. viridans* infection in BMT recipients. The majority of *S. viridans* septicemic patients have fever alone, without other clinical manifestations. *S. viridans* can, however, cause septic shock, neurological manifestations, pneumonia and adult-type respiratory distress syndrome (ARDS) with occasional fatalities (74,76). In one BMT study, mortality with *S. viridans* septicemia was 6% (7/123) (74), and in our BMT center, 9% (2/23) (75).

S. viridans peritonitis has been reported following liver transplantation (4). In SOT recipients, *S. viridans* infection has contributed to a fatal outcome. For example, a case of *S. viridans* pneumonia with ARDS in a liver transplant recipient (57) and one with *S. viridans* septicemia with *Pneumocystis carinii* pneumonia in a renal transplant recipient were fatal (77).

Risk Factors

It has been suggested that several highly interrelated risk factors—neutropenia, oral mucositis, Herpes simplex virus (HSV) infection, antibiotic prophylaxis, use of antacids or histamine type 2 (H_2) receptor antagonists (e.g., cimetidine)—coexist in the infected patient, can affect each other, and increase the risk for *S. viridans* septicemia in BMT recipients and other patients with cancer (74,75,78–82).

S. viridans normally constitutes most of the oral bacterial flora. Mucositis, an inevitable side effect of the conditioning regimen, probably facilitates entry of *S. viridans* into the bloodstream (78). With the absence of neutrophils, the major defense mechanism for protection against bacteria that have entered the blood system is lacking, and septicemia develops.

In our BMT center, only patients transplanted for malignant disease developed *S. viridans* septicemia (75). In another center, where *S. viridans* was also found in patients with nonmalignant diseases, acute lymphocytic leukemia was found to be a significant risk factor (74). Inclusion of cytosine arabinoside in the conditioning regimen was identified as a significant risk factor for *S. viridans* infection in BMT recipients in our center (75). The effect of age (adults versus children) as a risk factor for *S. viridans* septicemia is controversial (73–75).

Contamination with *S. viridans* during BMT can result as a consequence of *in vitro* manipulation of marrow (10).

Antibiotic Resistance

Most *S. viridans* isolates are susceptible to a very low concentration of penicillin G (MIC of 0.1 µg/ml or less). Ten to twenty percent of the strains are relatively resistant to penicillin (MIC >0.1 to <4.0 µg/ml). Emergence of strains of *S. viridans* that are highly resistant to penicillin (MIC ≥ 4.0 µg/ml) is of concern, particularly in some geographic areas, such as South Africa, where they are prevalent (83). Resistance is mediated by alterations in the penicillin binding proteins, similar to the mechanism of resistance in *S. pneumoniae*. Most *S. viridans* strains are resistant to TMP-SMZ (75,80). Ceftriaxone, the carbapenems (imipenem and meropenem), and the glycopeptides (vancomycin and teicoplanin) have demonstrated effective *in vitro* activity against *S. viridans* (83).

Treatment

For penicillin-sensitive strains, a penicillin is the drug of choice. For serious infections, such as endocarditis, combination therapy of a penicillin plus an aminoglycoside is recommended, especially for relatively resistant strains. For highly penicillin-resistant strains, therapy with a glycopeptide is administered.

There is controversy as to whether either vancomycin or teicoplanin should be included in the initial empiric antimicrobial therapy in febrile neutropenia in BMT recipients and other patients with malignant diseases (74,75,81,84,85). There have been fatalities with *S. viridans* despite administration of vancomycin (74). In our center, glycopeptides are not included in the initial empiric antimicrobial therapy during febrile neutropenia, an approach which would seem justified by the relatively benign course of *S. viridans* septicemia at the onset of febrile neutropenia. The risk of developing glycopeptide-resistant bacteria may be too high to warrant its routine use in all patients with febrile neutropenia. In addition, the possible toxicity of glycopeptides should be taken into account, especially when other nephrotoxic drugs, such as cyclosporine A, aminoglycosides, or amphotericin B, are administered concurrently. However, administration of empiric glycopeptide should be considered if the patient deteriorates during the second week of the profound neutropenia; as in breakthrough *S. viridans* bacteremia, penicillin-resistant strains should be expected.

Prophylaxis

To diminish the risk of oral sources of infection following the BMT, especially during the neutropenic period, required dental treatment should be performed and oral hygiene instructions given 3–4 weeks before the BMT. There should be daily oral rinse with antiseptic solution throughout the neutropenic period.

The addition of penicillin V to fluoroquinolone prophylaxis in granulocytopenic patients, including BMT recipients, has been shown to effectively reduce the incidence of febrile episodes and bacteremia, especially that due to streptococci (86). However, no significant differences in mortality due to infections were found with its administration. Its use remains controversial because of the concern raised by the risk of emerging resistance.

STREPTOCOCCUS PNEUMONIAE

Introduction

Streptococcus pneumoniae, a Gram-positive diplococcus, causes significant morbidity and mortality in all age groups, with children, the elderly, and immunocompromised patients being especially vulnerable. Transplant recipients are at a high risk for pneumococcal invasive infections (bacteremia and meningitis) and pneumococcal respiratory infections (87–90). In addition, heart transplant recipients are especially vulnerable to pneumococcal endocarditis (90), liver transplant recipients, to pneumococcal peritonitis (88), and renal transplant recipients to pneumococcal UTI (91). Although pneumococcal infection may occur during hospitalization for the transplantation procedure, it typically, and more commonly,

occurs as a community-acquired infection, months or years following the transplantation.

Incidence

The incidence of *S. pneumoniae* infections varies by type of transplant, with BMT recipients experiencing considerably higher rates of infection than SOT recipients. Although, in an immunocompetent host, *S. pneumoniae* causes primary bacteremia more frequently in infants and the elderly, all age groups of transplant recipients are vulnerable.

In the 1970s, prior to the era of long-term administration of prophylactic antibiotics, pneumococcal infection occurred in as many as 27% of long-term BMT survivors, especially in patients with chronic GVHD (87). Currently, even with the use of prophylactic TMP-SMZ and oral penicillin in high-risk patients, *S. pneumoniae* continues to be the most common pathogen in the long-term post-BMT period and a significant threat causing invasive, sometimes fatal, infections. It has been suggested that the susceptibility of BMT recipients to pneumococcal disease may be related to lowered concentrations of specific antibodies post-BMT and to decreased ability to produce specific antibodies in response to the pneumococcal antigen (92). In addition, median titers of specific IgG, IgG_1, and IgG_2 pneumococcal antibodies post-BMT fall significantly from pretransplantation levels (93).

Four percent of heart transplant recipients have been found to experience pneumococcal infection, principally pneumonia and bacteremia, over an almost 3-year period (90). Similarly, 4% of liver transplant recipients experienced pneumonia and bacteremia (4).

Seven percent of renal transplantation recipients with functioning allografts have been found to have experienced post-transplantation pneumococcal infections, including pneumonia, bacteremia, and meningitis (89). Renal transplant recipients undergoing splenectomy prior to, or concomitant with, transplantation are at even greater risk for *S. pneumoniae* infection (94). Renal transplant recipients have a tendency to develop pneumococcal UTI. *S. pneumoniae* grew in 5% of renal transplant recipients' urine samples compared with less than 1% of urine samples of a nontransplanted group (91).

Clinical Manifestations

Although bacteremia and meningitis are of special concern in transplant recipients, *S. pneumoniae* also causes infections of the middle ear, sinuses, trachea, bronchi, and lungs by direct spread from the nasopharyngeal site of colonization, and in the bones, joints, and peritoneal cavity by hematogenous spread.

In BMT recipients, pneumococcal infection is manifested as meningitis and fulminant, often fatal, sepsis, months or years following transplantation (87). In addition, *S. pneumoniae* is the most common pathogen causing late post-BMT bacterial pneumonia (76).

S. pneumoniae is the most common Gram-positive pathogen causing bacterial pneumonia more than 3 months following SOT (62). Liver transplant recipients experience *S. pneumoniae* infections as peritonitis, pneumonia, and bacteremia (88). Although less frequent than *S. pneumoniae* pneumonia or bacteremia, endocarditis is a typical clinical manifestation of pneumococcal infection in heart transplant recipients (90). In renal transplant recipients, pneumonia is the most common manifestation of *S. pneumoniae*, which also causes bacteremia and UTI.

Outcome

Respiratory infections with *S. pneumoniae* usually have a favorable outcome, but invasive disease is frequently fatal. In a current ongoing, not yet completed study by the Infectious Disease Working Party of the European BMT, nine of 40 (22.5%) BMT recipients with invasive pneumococcal infections (bacteremia and/or meningitis) died (Engelhard, unpublished data). Mortality from pneumococcal pneumonia following organ transplantation is relatively low (62), even following lung transplantation (95).

Drug Resistance

Many strains of *S. pneumoniae* have gradually become increasingly resistant to penicillin, the standard drug for treating pneumococcal infection for almost 50 years (96). Penicillin-resistant strains, to a much greater extent than penicillin-susceptible strains, develop multiple resistance to other antimicrobials such as β-lactams, tetracycline, chloramphenicol, erythromycin, and TMP-SMZ (97). In the mid-1990s, clinical isolates resistant to third-generation cephalosporins were identified, but their proliferation among transplant recipients has not yet been determined. Thus, specimens for culture should be obtained promptly and antibiotic susceptibility of pneumococcal isolates tested routinely.

Management

As antibiotic resistance varies considerably geographically, appropriate treatment should be determined locally. Penicillin is the drug of choice for susceptible strains of *S. pneumoniae*. Intravenous cephalosporin is recommended as the initial empiric antibiotic for management of outpatients suspected of pneumococcal sepsis, as well as for those with segmental or lobar pneumonia. For suspected pneumococcal meningitis, a third-generation cephalosporin should be used, and in centers where third-generation cephalosporin-resistant *S. pneumoniae* has developed, vancomycin should be added (96).

Prevention

There are two approaches to prevention of pneumococcal infection: (a) administration of prophylactic antibiotics and (b) enhancement of the host-specific immune response by passive or active immunization.

Antibiotic Prophylaxis

Prophylactic administration of TMP-SMZ against *Pneumocystis carinii,* used in transplant recipients, is also active against some strains *S. pneumoniae*. Long-term penicillin prophylaxis against pneumococcal infections has been practiced in a number of BMT centers, especially for patients with chronic GVHD. However, this regimen has not been shown to ensure protection against *S. pneumoniae* (98). In addition, the effect of long-term penicillin prophylaxis on the development of drug resistance in transplant recipients has not been determined; in children with sickle cell disease, resistance was shown to have developed during prolonged use of prophylactic penicillin (99).

Passive Immunization

Infusion of normal human globulin has been found to protect against pneumococcal infection in children with HIV infection and in adults with lymphoma (96). Its applicability to transplant recipients remains unknown and, as pneumococcal infections may occur many years subsequent to the transplantation, the cost-effectiveness of this approach needs to be considered.

Active Immunization

Pneumococcal vaccination with 14-valent pneumococcal vaccine has shown limited antibody response in BMT recipients receiving corticosteroids and having been vaccinated less than 7 months post-transplantation. However, in patients not receiving corticosteroids and being vaccinated more than 7 months post-transplantation, antibody responses improve with time post-transplantation (100). The immune response of pediatric BMT recipients administered the 23-polyvalent pneumococcal capsular polysaccharide vaccine 1 or more years or more following BMT has not been significantly different from that of controls, except for IgG_2 receptor antibodies. However, because of the lower preimmunization levels, transplant recipients have not achieved as high postimmunization specific antibody titers as normal children's in any immunoglobulin class or subclass. Splenectomy or the presence of chronic GVHD has not been found to have affected either the preimmunization specific antibody levels or the response to immunization. Immunization of the donor before bone marrow harvest has not influenced the specific antibody level 1 or more years post-transplantation. It has been assumed that the lack of specific antibodies and the poor IgG$_2$ response to pneumococcal antigens may have contributed to infections occurring during the late post-transplantation period (93).

The interval post-transplant has been shown to be the major factor influencing the recovery of immune reactivity to polysaccharide antigens. In a recent study, all children vaccinated more than 2 years post-BMT responded to pneumococcal polysaccharides, 50% of those vaccinated 1–2 years post-BMT and 20% to 30% of those vaccinated 6 months to 1 year post-BMT. As in the previous study, GVHD was not strongly associated with antibody response (101).

The immune response achieved by heart and liver transplant recipients administered 23-valent vaccine of capsular polysaccharides during therapeutic immunosuppression post-transplantation was found comparable to that in healthy subjects (102). In renal transplant recipients, 14-valent pneumococcal vaccine has been shown to generate functional antibody response and found safe (103).

The 23-valent pneumococcal polysaccharide vaccine is recommended for BMT and organ transplant recipients (104). As the vaccine is more effective when administered prior to initiation of immunosuppressive therapy, it is recommended that potential SOT recipients be vaccinated at least 2 weeks prior to the transplantation (105,106). For BMT recipients, the 23-valent vaccine is recommended at 1 year post-transplantation (107). It is further recommended that transplant recipients be revaccinated: children ten years old or younger, three years subsequent to previous vaccination; children over ten years and adults, six or more years after the first dose (105,106).

Effective conjugated pneumococcal vaccines for transplant recipients are being developed. Greatly improved specific immune response is anticipated, with significant reduction in morbidity and mortality resulting from *S. pneumoniae* infection.

REFERENCES

1. Engelhard D, Marks MI, Good RAE. Infections in bone marrow transplant recipients. *J Pediatr* 1986;108:335–346.
2. Walter EA, Bowden RA. Infection in the bone marrow transplant recipient. *Infect Dis Clin North Am* 1995;4:823–847.
3. Rubin HR, Tolkoff-Rubin, NE. Antimicrobial strategies in the care of organ transplant recipients. *Antimicrob Agents Chemother* 1993;374:619–624.
4. Paya CV, Hermans PE, Washington II J, et al. Incidence, distribution, and outcome of episodes of infection in 100 orthotopic liver transplantations. *Mayo Clin Proc* 1989;64:555–564.
5. Wade JJ, Rolando N, Hayllar K, Philpott-Howard J, Casewell MW, Williams R. Bacterial and fungal infections after liver transplantation: an analysis of 284 patients. *Hepatology* 1995;21(5):1328–1336.
6. Hofflin JM, Potasman I, Baldwin JC, Oyer PE, Stinson EB, Remington JS. Infectious complications in heart transplant recipients receiving cyclosporine and corticosteroids. *Ann Intern Med* 1987;106:209–216.
7. Grossi P, DeMaria R, Caroli A, Zaina MS, Minoli L, on behalf of the Italian Study Group on Infections in Heart Transplantation. Infections

in heart transplant recipients: the experience of the Italian heart transplantation program. *J Heart Lung Transplant* 1992;11:847–866.
8. Elishoov H, Or R, Strauss N, Engelhard D. Nosocomial colonization, septicemia, and Hickman/Broviac catheter-related infections in bone marrow transplantation recipients—a 5-year prospective study. *Medicine* 1998;77 (2):83–101.
9. Lammermeier DE, Sweeney MS, Haupt HE, Radovancevic B, Duncan JM, Frazier OH. Use of potentially infected donor hearts for cardiac transplantation. *Ann Thorac Surg* 1990;50(2):222–225.
10. Henslee J, Bostrom B, Weisdorf D, Ramsay N, McGlove P, Kersey J. Streptococcal sepsis in bone marrow transplantation. *Lancet* 1984;1:393 (Letter).
11. Jett BD, Huycke MM, Gilmore MS. Virulence of enterococci. *Clin Microbiol Rev* 1994;7:462–478.
12. Morris JG Jr, Shay DK, Hebden JN, et al. Enterococci resistant to multiple antimicrobial agents, including vancomycin. Establishment of endemicity in a university medical center. *Ann Intern Med* 1995;123(4):250–259.
13. Moellering RC. *Enterococcus* species, *Streptococcus bovis*, and *Leuconostoc* species. In: Mandell GL, Douglas JE, Dolin R, eds. *Principles and practice of infectious diseases*, 4th ed. New York: Churchill Livingstone; 1995:1826–1835.
14. Raakow R, Bechstein WO, Kling N, et al. The importance of late infections for the long-term outcome after liver transplantation. *Transpl Int* 1996;9[Suppl 1]:S155–S156.
15. Wade JJ. The emergence of *Enterococcus faecium* resistant to glycopeptides and other standard agents—a preliminary report. *J Hosp Infect* 1995;30[Suppl]:483–493.
16. Linden PK, Pasculle AW, Manez R, et al. Differences in outcomes for patients with bacteremia due to vancomycin-resistant *Enterococcus faecium* or vancomycin-susceptible *E. faecium*. *Clin Infect Dis* 1996;22(4):663–670.
17. Chadwick PR, Oppenheim BA, Fox A, Woodford N, Morgenstern GR, Scarffe JH. Epidemiology of an outbreak due to glycopeptide-resistant *Enterococcus faecium* on a leukaemia unit. *J Hosp Infect* 1996;34(3):171–182.
18. Sastry V, Brennan PJ, Levy MM, et al. Vancomycin-resistant enterococci: an emerging pathogen in immunosuppressed transplant recipients. *Transplant Proc* 1995;27(1):954–955.
19. Papanicolaou GA, Meyers BR, Meyers J, et al. Nosocomial infections with vancomycin-resistant *Enterococcus faecium* in liver transplant recipients: risk factors for acquisition and mortality. *Clin Infect Dis* 1996;23(4):760–766.
20. Patel R, Badley AD, Larson-Keller J, et al. Relevance and risk factors of enterococcal bacteremia following liver transplantation. *Transplantation* 1996;61(8):1192–1197.
21. George DL, Arnow PM, Fox A, et al. Patterns of infection after pediatric liver transplantation. *Am J Dis Child* 1992;146(8):924–929.
22. Green M, Barbadora K, Michaels M. Recovery of vancomycin-resistant gram-positive cocci from pediatric liver transplant recipients. *J Clin Microbiol* 1991;29(11):2503–2506.
23. Bantar C, Fernandez-Canigia L, Diaz C, et al. Clinical, epidemiologic, and microbiologic study of urinary infection in patients with renal transplant at a specialized center in Argentina. *Arch Esp Urol* 1993;46(6):473–477.
24. Suppola JP, Volin L, Valtonen VV, Vaara M. Overgrowth of *E. faecium* in the feces of patients with hematologic malignancies. *Clin Infect Dis* 1996;23:694–697.
25. Gentry LO. Cardiac transplantation and related infections. *Semin Respir Infect* 1993;8(3):199–206.
26. Fox BC, Sollinger HW, Belzer FO, Maki DG. A prospective, randomized, double-blind study of trimethoprim-sulfamethoxazole for prophylaxis of infection in renal transplantation: clinical efficacy, absorption of trimethoprim-sulfamethoxazole, effects on the microflora, and the cost-benefit of prophylaxis. *Am J Med* 1990;89(3):255–274.
27. Cohen JS, Paz IB, O'Donnell MR, Ellenhorn JD. Treatment of perianal infection following bone marrow transplantation. *Dis Colon Rectum* 1996;39(9):981–985.
28. Albat B, Trinh-Duc P, Boulfroy D, Picard E, Wintrebert P, Thevenet A. Mediastinitis in heart transplant recipients: successful treatment by closed local irrigation. *Cardiovasc Surg* 1993;1(6):657–659.
29. Venditti M, Biavasco F, Varaldo PE, et al. Catheter-related endocarditis due to glycopeptide-resistant *Enterococcus faecalis* in a transplanted heart. *Clin Infect Dis* 1993;17(3):524–525 (Letter).

30. Tannenbaum DA, Matthews LS, Grady-Benson JC. Infection around joint replacements in patients who have a renal or liver transplantation. *J Bone Joint Surg Am* 1997;79(1):36–43.

31. Martino P, Micozzi A, Venditti M, et al. Catheter-related right-sided endocarditis in bone marrow transplant recipients. *Rev Infect Dis* 1990;12(2):250–257.

32. Edmond MB, Ober JF, Weinbaum DL, et al. Vancomycin-resistant *Enterococcus faecium* bacteremia: risk factors for infection. *Clin Infect Dis* 1994;20:1126–1133.

33. Patterson JE, Sweeney AH, Simms M, et al. An analysis of 110 serious enterococcal infections. Epidemiology, antibiotic susceptibility and outcome. *Medicine (Baltimore)* 1995;74:191–200.

34. Scroggs MW, Wolfe JA, Bollinger RR, Sanfilippo F. Causes of death in renal transplant recipients. A review of autopsy findings from 1966 through 1985. *Arch Pathol Lab Med* 1987;111(10):983–987.

35. Coque TM, Tomayko JF, Ricke SC, Okhyusen PC, Murray BE. Vancomycin-resistant enterococci from nosocomial, community, and animal sources in the United States. *Antimicrob Agents Chemother* 1996;40(11):2605–2609.

36. Cercenado E, Unal S, Eliopoulos CT. Characterization of vancomycin resistance in *Enterococcus durans*. *J Antimicrob Chemother* 1995;36: 821–825.

37. Green M, Shlaes JH, Barbadora K, Shlaes DM. Bacteremia due to vancomycin-dependent *Enterococcus faecium*. *Clin Infect Dis* 1995; 20(3):712–714.

38. Donnelly JP. Bacterial complications of transplantation: diagnosis and treatment. *J Antimicrob Chemother* 1995;36 Suppl B:59–72.

39. Sande MA, Scheld WM. Combination antibiotic therapy of bacterial endocarditis. *Ann Intern Med* 1980;92:390–395.

40. Norris AH, Reilly JP, Edelstein PH, Brennan PJ, Schusterr MG. Chloramphenicol for the treatment of vancomycin-resistant enterococcal infections. *Clin Infect Dis* 1995;20:1137–1144.

41. Moreno F, Jorgensen JH, Weiner MH. An old antibiotic for new multiple-resistant *Enterococcus faecium*? *Diagn Microbiol Infect Dis* 1994;20:41–43.

42. Mekonen ET, Noskin GA, Hacek DM, Peterson LR. Successful treatment of persistent bacteremia due to vancomycin-resistant, ampicillin-resistant *Enterococcus faecium*. *Microb Drug Resist* 1995;1(3): 249–253.

43. Wade JJ, Rolando N, Williams R, Caswell MW. Serious infections caused by multiply-resistant *Enterococcus faecium*. *Microb Drug Resist* 1995;1(3):241–243.

44. Eliopoulos GM, Wennersten CB, Gold HS, Moellering RC, Jr. In vitro activities of new oxazolidinone antimicrobial agents against enterococci. *Antimicrob Agents Chemother* 1996;40(7):1745–1747.

45. Bodnar UR, Noskin GA, Suriano T, Cooper I, Reisberg B, Peterson L. Use of In-house studies of molecular epidemiology and full species identification for controlling spread of vancomycin-resistant E. faecalis isolates. *J Clin Microbiol* 1996;34(9):2129–2132.

46. Engelhard D, Elishoov H, et al. Nosocomial coagulase-negative staphylococcal infections in bone marrow transplantation recipients with central vein catheter—a 5-year prospective study. *Transplantation* 1996;61(3):430–434.

47. Meyers JD. Infection in bone marrow transplant recipients. *Am J Med* 1986;81[Suppl 1A]:27–38.

48. Wadvogel FA. Staphylococcal aureus (including toxic shock syndrome). In: Mandell GL, Douglas JE, Dolin R, eds. *Principles and practice of infectious diseases*, 4th ed. New York: Churchill Livingstone; 1995:1754–1777.

49. Petersen FB, Clift RA, Hickman RO, et al. Hickman catheter complications in marrow transplant recipients. *J Parenter Enteral Nutr* 1986;10(1):58–62.

50. Stewart MJ, Huwez F, Richens D, Naik S, Wheatley DJ. Infective endocarditis of the tricuspid valve in an orthotopic heart transplant recipient. *J Heart Lung Transplant* 1996;15(6):646–649.

51. Hosenpud JD, Hershberger RE, Pantely GA, et al. Late infection in cardiac allograft recipients: profiles, incidence, and outcome. *J Heart Lung Transplant* 1991;10(3):380–38.

52. Vaudaux P, Pittet D, Haeberli A, et al. Host factors selectively increase staphylococcal adherence on inserted catheters: a role for fibronectin and fibrinogen or fibrin. *J Infect Dis* 1989:160(5):865–875.

53. Raad II, Bodey GP. Infectious complications of indwelling vascular catheters. *Clin Infect Dis* 1992;15:197–210.

54. Peters G, Locci PG, Pulvere G. Adherence and growth of coagulase-negative staphylococci on surfaces of intravenous catheters. *J Infect Dis* 1982;146:479–486.

55. Lim SH, Smith MP, Machin SJ, Goldstone AH. A prospective randomized study of prophylactic teicoplanin to prevent early Hickman catheter–related sepsis in patients receiving intensive chemotherapy for haematological malignancies. *Eur J Haematol* 1993;51[Suppl.54]: 10–13.

56. Holzel H, de Saxe M. Septicaemia in paediatric intensive-care patients at the Hospital for Sick Children, Great Ormond Street. *J Hosp Infect* 1992;22(3):185–195.

57. Saint-Vil D, Luks FI, Lebel P, et al. Infectious complications of pediatric liver transplantation. *J Pediatr Surg* 1991;26(8):908–909.

58. Lumbreras C, Lizasoain M, Moreno E, et al. Major bacterial infections following liver transplantation: a prospective study. *Hepatogastroenterology* 1992;39(4):362–365.

59. Falagas ME, Snydaman DR, Griffith J, Werner BG. Exposure to cytomegalovirus from the donated organ is a risk factor for bacteremia in orthotopic liver transplant recipients. Boston Center for Liver Transplantation CMVIG Study Group. *Clin Infect Dis* 1996;23: 468–474.

60. Deusch ED, End A, Grimm M, Graninger W, Klepetko W, Wolner E. Early bacterial infections in lung transplant recipients. *Chest* 1993; 104(5):1412–1416.

61. Heimdahl A, Mattson T, Dahllöf G, Lönnquist B, Ringden O. The oral cavity as a port of entry for early infections in patients treated with bone marrow transplantation. *Oral Surg Oral Med Oral Pathol* 1989; 68:711–716.

62. Mermel LA, Maki DG. Bacterial pneumonia in solid organ transplantation. *Semin Respir Infect* 1990;5(1):10–29.

63. Bubak ME, Porayko MK, Krom RAF, Wiesner RH. Complications of liver biopsy in liver transplant patients: increased sepsis associated with choledochojejunostomy. *Hepatology* 1991;14(6):1063–1065.

64. Fichelle JM, Colacchio G, Castaing D, Bismuth H. Infected false hepatic artery aneurysm after orthotopic liver transplantation treated by resection and reno-hepatic vein graft. *Ann Vasc Surg* 1997;11(3): 300–303.

65. Baldwin RT, Radovancevic B, Sweeney MS, Duncan JM, Frazier OH. Bacterial mediastinitis after heart transplantation. *J Heart Lung Transplant* 1992;11:545–549.

66. Davies RA, Newton G, Masters RG, Saginur R, Struthers C, Walley VM. Bacterial pericarditis after heart transplantation: successful management of two cases with catheter drainage and antibiotics. *Can J Cardiol* 1996;12(7):641–644.

67. Hasan A, Hamilton JR, Au J, et al. Surgical management of infective endocarditis after heart-lung transplantation. *J Heart Lung Transplant* 1993;12(2):330–332.

68. Dauber JH, Paradis IL, Dummer JS. Infectious complications in pulmonary allograft recipients. *Clin Chest Med* 1990;2(11):291–308.

69. Grekas D, Thanos V, Dioudis C, Alivanis P, Tourkantonis A. Treatment of urinary tract infections with ciprofloxacin after renal transplantation. *Int J Clin Pharmacol Ther Toxicol* 1993;31(6):309–311.

70. Goldberg NS, Ahmed T, Robinson-B, Ascensao J, Horowitz H. Staphylococcal scalded skin syndrome mimicking acute graft-vs-host disease in a bone marrow transplant recipient. *Arch Dermatol* 1989; 125(1):85–87.

71. Hoiby-N. Cystic fibrosis and endobronchial pseudomonas infection. *Curr Opin Pediatr* 1993;5(3):247–254.

72. Ringden O, Heimdahl A, Lonnqvist B, Malmborg A, Wilczek H. Decreased incidence of viridans streptococcal septicemia in allogeneic bone marrow transplant recipients after the introduction of acyclovir. *Lancet* 1984;1:744 (Letter).

73. Mascret B, Maraninchi D, Gastaut JA et al. Risk factors for streptococcal septicemia after marrow transplantation. *Lancet* 1984;1: 1185–1186 (Letter).

74. Villablanca JG, Steiner M, Kersey J, et al. The clinical spectrum of infections with viridans streptococci in bone marrow transplant patients. *Bone Marrow Transplant* 1990;6:387–393.

75. Engelhard D, Elishoov H, Or R, et al. Cytosine arabinoside as a major risk factor for *Streptococcus viridans* septicemia following bone marrow transplantation: a 5-year prospective study. *Bone Marrow Transplant* 1995;16(4):565–570.

76. Lossos IS, Breuer R, Or R, et al. Bacterial pneumonia in recipients of bone marrow transplantation—a five-year prospective study. *Transplantation* 1995;60;672–678.

77. Ludwin D, Quinonez G, Chernesky MA, et al. Polyclonal B cell hyperplasia associated with Epstein-Barr virus causing acute renal allograft failure. *Clin Nephrol* 1985;24(3):151–154.

78. Weisman SJ, Scoopo FJ, Johnson GM, Altman AJ, Quinn JJ. Septicemia in pediatric oncology patients: the significance of viridans streptococcal infections. *J Clin Oncol* 1990;8:(3):453–459.

79. Elting LS, Bodey GP, Keefe BH. Septicemia and shock syndrome due to viridans streptococci: a case-control study of predisposing factors. *Clin Infect Dis* 1992;14:1201–1207.

80. Cohen J, Donnelly JP, Worsley AM, Catovsky D, Goldman JM, Galton DA. Septicaemia caused by viridans streptococci in neutropenic patients with leukemia. *Lancet* 1983;2:1452–1454.

81. Guiot HFL, van der Meer JWM, van den Broek PJ, Willemze R, van Furth R. Prevention of viridans-group streptococcal septicemia in oncohematologic patients: a controlled comparative study on the effect of penicillin G and cotrimoxazole. *Ann Hematol* 1992;64: 260–265.

82. Classen DC, Burke JP, Ford CD et al. *Streptococcus mitis* sepsis in bone marrow transplant patients receiving oral antimicrobial prophylaxis. *Am J Med* 1990;89:441–446.

83. Johnson CC, Tunkel AR. Viridans streptococci and group C and G streptococci. In: Mandell GL, Douglas JE, Dolin R, eds. *Principles and practice of infectious diseases*, 4th ed. New York: Churchill Livingstone; 1995:1845–1861.

84. Valteau D, Hartmann O, Brugieres L, et al. Streptococcal septicaemia following autologous bone marrow transplantation in children with high-dose chemotherapy. *Bone Marrow Transplant* 1991;7:415–419.

85. Pizzo PA. Management of fever in patients with cancer and treatment-induced neutropenia. *N Engl J Med* 1993;328:1323–1332.

86. Anonymous. Reduction of fever and streptococcal bacteremia in granulocytopenic patients with cancer. A trial of oral penicillin V or placebo combined with pefloxacin. International Antimicrobial Therapy Cooperative Group of the European Organization for Research and Treatment of Cancer. *JAMA* 1994;272(15):1183–1189.

87. Winston DJ, Schiffman G, Wang DC, et al. Pneumococcal infections after human bone-marrow transplantation. *Ann Intern Med* 1979; 91(6):835–841.

88. Winston DJ, Emmanouillides C, Busuttil RW. Infections in liver transplant recipients. *Clin Infect Dis* 1995;21:1007–1089.

89. Linnemann CC Jr, First MR. Risk of pneumococcal infections in renal transplant patients. *JAMA* 1979;241(24):2619–2621.

90. Amber IJ, Gilbert EM, Schiffman G, Jacobson JA. Increased risk of pneumococcal infections in cardiac transplant recipients. *Transplantation* 1990;49(1):122–125.

91. Garcia Curiel A. Bacteriuria caused by *Streptococcus pneumoniae*. *Enferm Infecc Microbiol Clin* 1989;(7):377–379.

92. Giebink GS, Warkentin PI, Ramsay NK, Kersey JH. Titers of antibody to pneumococci in allogeneic bone marrow transplant recipients before and after vaccination with pneumococcal vaccine. *J Infect Dis* 1986;154(4):590–596.

93. Lortan JE, Vellodi A, Jurges ES, Hugh-Jones K. Class- and subclass-specific pneumococcal antibody levels and response to immunization after bone marrow transplantation. *Clin Exp Immunol* 1992;88(3): 512–519.

94. Bourgault AM, Van Scoy RE, Wilkowski CJ, Sterioff S. Severe infection due to *Streptococcus pneumoniae* in asplenic renal transplant patients. *Mayo Clin Proc* 1979;54(2):123–126.

95. Chaparro C, Maurer JR, Chamberlain D, et al. Causes of death in lung transplant recipients. *J Heart Lung Transplant* 1994;13(5): 758–766.

96. Musher DM. Streptococcus pneumoniae. In: Mandell GL, Douglas JE, Dolin R, eds. *Principles and practice of infectious diseases,* 4th ed. New York: Churchill Livingstone; 1995:1811–1826.

97. Centers for Disease Control. Isolation of multiply antibiotic-resistant pneumococci. *Morb Mortal Wkly Rep* 1985;34:545.

98. D'Antonio D, Di Bartolomeo P, Iacone A, et al. Meningitis due to penicillin-resistant *Streptococcus pneumoniae* in patients with chronic graft-versus-host disease. *Bone Marrow Transplant* 1992;9(4): 299–300.

99. Woods GM, Jorgensen JH, Waclawiw-MA, et al. Influence of penicillin prophylaxis on antimicrobial resistance in nasopharyngeal *S. pneumoniae* among children with sickle cell anemia. The ancillary nasopharyngeal culture study of prophylactic penicillin study II. *J Pediatr Hematol Oncol* 1997;19(4):327–33.

100. Winston DJ, Ho WG, Schiffman G, Champlin RE, Feig SA, Gale RP. Pneumococcal vaccination of recipients of bone marrow transplants. *Arch Intern Med* 1983;143(9):1735–1737.

101. Avanzini MA, Carra AM, Maccario R, et al. Antibody response to pneumococcal vaccine in children receiving bone marrow transplantation. *J Clin Immunol* 1995;15(3):137–144.

102. Dengler TJ, Strnad N, Zimmermann R, et al. Pneumococcal vaccination after heart and liver transplantation. Immune responses in immunosuppressed patients and in healthy controls. *Dtsch Med Wochenschr* 1996;121(49):1519–1525.

103. Arnold WC, Steele RW, Rastogi SP, Flanigan WJ. Response to pneumococcal vaccine in renal allograft recipients. *Am J Nephrol* 1985;5(1):30–34.

104. Morbidity and mortality weekly report. Prevention of pneumococcal disease: recommendations of the Advisory Committee on Immunization Practices (ACIP). *MMWR* 1997;46(RR-8):1–24.

105. American College of Physicians Task Force of Adult Immunization and the Infectious Diseases Society of America. *Guide for adult immunization*, 3rd ed. Philadelphia: American College of Physicians; 1991.

106. American Academy of Pediatrics. Pneumococcal infections. In: Peter G, ed. *1997 red book: report of the Committee on Infectious Diseases*, 24th ed. Elk Grove Village, IL: American Academy of Pediatrics; 1997:417–418.

107. Ljungman P, Cordonnier C, de Bock R, et al, for the Infectious Diseases Working Party of the EBMT. Immunizations after bone marrow transplantation; results of a European survey and recommendations from the Infectious Diseases Working Party of the European Group for Bone Marrow Transplantation. *Bone Marrow Transplant* 1995; 15(3):455–460.

Transplant Infections edited by
Raleigh A. Bowden, Per Ljungman, and Carlos V. Paya.
Lippincott–Raven Publishers, Philadelphia © 1998

CHAPTER 13

Gram-Negative Infections

Randall C. Walker

Early in the history of transplantation, infections from Gram-negative bacteria were an important cause of early mortality both in bone marrow transplant (BMT) and in solid organ transplant (SOT) recipients (1–4). This obvious hazard is the basis for various strategies involving antibiotic prophylaxis, selective decontamination, and empirical and preemptive therapy, which will be discussed in this chapter. However, the reduction of the frequency and severity of Gram-negative infections in the transplant recipient should not be characterized as the result of antibiotic practices alone (2,5). Moreover, the problem of Gram-negative infections remains significant and may be evolving to a qualitatively different problem involving fewer normal flora and increasingly involving nosocomial and opportunistic Gram-negative pathogens (6,7). In addition, as long-term survival in the transplant recipient increases, the possibility of unusual opportunistic Gram-negative infections and of unusual presentations of more common Gram-negative pathogens will likely increase (8).

EARLY EXPERIENCE

Before current practice methods, including prophylaxis and selective decontamination, the risk of Gram-negative infection in transplant recipients was very high. In kidney transplant patients in the 20 years before 1986, infections caused 93 of 116 autopsy-reviewed deaths, and 72 of these involved Gram-negative bacteria (1). In early liver transplant series, the frequency of Gram-negative bacterial infection was as high as 66% among all liver recipients and was the main cause of early mortality (e.g., 11 of 17 who died in the first month) (9,10).

Early prophylaxis strategies in BMT were adopted from those used for the neutropenia of leukemia treatment. In this population, 13 of 33 neutropenic patients

given placebo for prophylaxis had Gram-negative infection (12 of these 13 had bacteremia and all but two involved enteric Gram-negative bacteria). This compared with only four of 35 of those receiving norfloxacin as prophylaxis (three of these had *Pseudomonas bacteremia*) (11).

Gram-negative bacteremia in placebo-controlled studies of BMT patients has been found to be at least as frequent (five of 11, or 45%) as in the neutropenia of acute leukemia treatment (12), with most prophylaxis studies in BMT patients no longer containing a placebo-controlled arm (13).

Practices have evolved in many ways since then. But these high historical rates of serious Gram-negative infection should not be forgotten, when current experience demonstrates rates of Gram-negative bacteremia of (a) 1.5% (seven of 536) among neutropenic patients receiving a quinolone (14); (b) less than 2% (two of 145) liver transplant patients receiving selective bowel decontamination (15); and (c) one of 60 kidney transplant patients receiving trimethoprim sulfamethoxazole prophylaxis (16). These practices have therefore been exported to other transplantation procedures, including (a) autologous BMT (17); (b) lung transplantation (18); and (c) small intestine transplantation (19).

Although studies of Gram-negative prophylaxis and/or decontamination are no longer placebo-controlled but involve comparisons of alternative active regimens, it is important to consider the evidence for other contributions to the lower frequency of Gram-negative infection in these patients.

Improvements in the precision and effectiveness of immunosuppression appear to have affected Gram-negative infection rates. For example, the introduction of cyclosporine A in kidney transplantation was associated with a decreased risk of predominantly Gram-negative bacterial infection from 52% to 34% (20). However, the introduction of FK506 may be associated with an increased risk for intracellular Gram-negative bacilli such

From the Division of Infectious Diseases, Mayo Clinic, Rochester, MN 55905.

as *Legionella* (6). Similarly, splenectomy, a procedure performed to modify the immune response but no longer performed in patients undergoing kidney transplantation, was associated with a higher risk for sepsis, including probable *Haemophilus influenzae* infection (21) but possibly also enteric bacteria (22).

Improvements in microbiological surveillance methods of transplant patients (23–26) and in hospital infection control (27) can detect potentially resistant Gram-negative organisms before they cause disease and can limit the spread of these organisms in transplant units.

Microbiological surveillance can, in addition, make the choice of empirical or preemptive antibiotic therapy of the transplant patient more appropriate (28). The judicious use of antimicrobials with unique activity against highly resistant Gram-negative organisms can help ensure that these agents will remain useful for the transplant population (29).

Advances in the procedures used to harvest and preserve and/or process transplant tissue can also reduce the risk of contamination of the graft, which can lead to Gram-negative infection in recipients of allogeneic and autologous bone marrow and solid organs (30–39).

Cytomegalovirus is a problem of varying degrees and severity among bone marrow and SOT patients. Cytomegalovirus infection, especially primary infection, is associated with higher rates of colonization and infection with Gram-negative bacteria in transplant patients (40–43). Progress in the prevention and treatment of cytomegalovirus could therefore also affect the rate of Gram-negative infection.

Together, all these nonprophylaxis dimensions of transplantation contribute to the moving target of Gram-negative infection risk in the transplant recipient. Obviously, other advances in the prevention, diagnosis, and treatment of Gram-negative infection in hospitalized patients in general will also benefit the transplant recipient.

PROCEDURE-SPECIFIC CONSIDERATIONS

To differentiate transplant procedures according to considerations for Gram-negative infection, three basic questions can be asked: (a) What are the Gram-negative pathogens and where do they come from? (b) What host defense mechanisms that would ordinarily prevent Gram-negative infection are impaired in the particular transplant recipient? (c) Based on the answers to the first two questions, when will the patient be at greatest risk for a particular pathogen?

The Pathogens

The Gram-negative bacteria that cause disease in transplant patients have three main sources: (a) endogenous flora; (b) exogenous bacteria that colonize anatomically compromised structures; (c) exogenous pathogens that gain access to the host by crossing normal or impaired barriers (Table 1).

The endogenous Gram-negative flora vary by anatomic location. In the upper respiratory tract, *Haemophilus influenzae* or *Moraxella catarrhalis* may, in small quantities, be among the usual flora. In the mouth, oral anaerobic Gram-negative bacilli such as capnocytophagis may be among the usual flora. In the lower intestinal tract, some "usual" flora among the Enterobacteriaceae may nonetheless harbor rather extraordinary antimicrobial resistance profiles such as hyper-β-lactamase-producing *Klebsiella* or chromosomal-inducible β-lactamase-producing *Enterobacter* species. Even *E. coli* can be resistant to antimicrobials that were considered adequate empirical coverage just a few years ago (44). This obviously raises concern about the long-term utility of current prophylaxis strategies.

When an organ is compromised, usual flora from another anatomic location and completely exogenous organisms may colonize the compromised structure. Examples of this include colonization of the sinuses and lower airways of patients with cystic fibrosis by *Pseudomonas aeruginosa* and *Pseudomonas cepacia* (45–48); airway colonization of tracheal secretions in a patient requiring long-term mechanical ventilation (49); colonization of the throat and mouth when patients are debilitated and bedridden; urinary tract colonization associated with indwelling catheters; and nonhealing wounds or ulcers that can become colonized with exogenous Gram-negative bacteria such as *Xanthomonas maltophilia*.

Exogenous pathogens can cause disease in normal hosts even if the portal-of-entry organ is not compro-

TABLE 1. *Important Gram-negative pathogens in transplant recipients*

Source/route	Organism
Usual flora	
Upper respiratory tract	*H. influenzae*
Mouth	Capnocytophaga
Gut	Enterobacteriacae
Exogenous colonizers of compromised anatomic structures	
	Pseudomonas aeruginosa
	Pseudomonas cepacia
	Stenotrophomonas (Xanthomonas) maltophilia
	Acinetobacter spp.
Exogenous pathogens	
Respiratory portal	*Legionella* spp.
Enteric portal	*Salmonella* spp.
	Vibrio
	Shigella
	Brucellosis
Cutaneous portal	*Vibrio vulnificus*
	Bartonella
	Aeromonas

mised, but the transplant recipient is even more susceptible to these infections and will have more severe forms. Examples of these exogenous infections include *Legionella* infection; *Salmonella* infection, including *Salmonella typhi* and non-*typhi* species; *Vibrios* infection; brucellosis; and *Bartonella* infections.

Host Defenses Against Gram-Negative Infection

There are several different types of normal host defenses against Gram-negative infection whose absence becomes evident in specific transplantation groups.

Humoral immunity is an important defense against encapsulated respiratory Gram-negative pathogens such as *Haemophilus influenzae* (50). Humoral immunity but may also play a role—combined with normal splenic function—against enteric bacteria such as *E. coli* and *Klebsiella* (22,51) as well as against *Pseudomonas aeruginosa* (51,52).

Both the autologous and the allogeneic BMT recipient will have impaired humoral immunity for 6 and 12 or more months, respectively. Chronic graft-versus-host disease (GVHD) and its treatment will also delay the return of humoral immunity; these may include IgG subclass deficiencies (53–55). Even when immune globulins are measured and in normal quantitative ranges, immune globulin regulation and function remain impaired (56).

Cellular immunity against Gram-negative bacteria is predominantly based on neutrophil number and function, particularly as a defense against enteric Gram-negative bacilli and *Pseudomonas aeruginosa* (57). However, macrophage/monocyte-dependent immunity appears, as evidenced by patients who lack it (including SOT patients and allogeneic BMT patients on therapy for GVHD), to confer protection against intracellular Gram-negative infection such as *Legionella* and *Salmonella* (58,59).

Not all cellular-based immunity circulates. Tissue-based cellular immunity in the lung, liver, and intestine is

TABLE 2. *Time-dependent impairment of host defenses against Gram-negative infection associated with various transplantation procedures*

		Immune system			Anatomic barrier	
		Cellular				
		Circulating				
Host defense impairment	Humoral	Neutrophil	Macrophage/ monocyte	Tissue-based cellular-immunity	Temporary disruption	Permanent alteration
Typical pathogen	*H. influenzae*	Entero-bacteriaceae *Pseudo-monas*	*Legionella* *Salmonella*	Usual flora and colonizing Gram-negative bacteria	Usual flora and colonizing Gram-negative bacteria	Colonizing Gram-negative bacteria
Procedure Autologous BMT	6+ months	2–4 weeks	6 months		Oral and GI mucositis– 4 weeks	
Allogeneic BMT	12+ months	3–4 weeks	Lifelong Rx for (GVH)	GVH—bowel, sinus, lung	Oral and GI mucositis— 4–6 weeks	CGVH—bowel, sinus, lung
Kidney and kidney/ pancreas	Minor (including preexisting uremia)	0	Lifelong (chronic immuno-suppression)	0	Surgical wound, urinary catheter, endotracheal intubation	Heterotopic Tx
Liver	Minor (including preexisting liver failure)	0	Lifelong chronic suppression	Decreased hepatic clearance of mesenteric bacteremia (3 weeks)	Surgical wound, urinary catheter, endotracheal intubation	Biliary strictures; choledocho-jejunostomy
Small intestine	Minor (preexisting protein loss)	0	Lifelong chronic suppression	Chronic reduction of intestinal lymphoid and macrophage function	Surgical wound, urinary catheter, endotracheal intubation	0
Heart	Minor (benefit from preTX Hib vaccines)	0	Lifelong chronic suppression	0	Surgical wound, urinary catheter, endotracheal intubation	0
Lung	Minor	0	Lifelong chronic suppression	Pulmonary alveolar macrophage	Surgical wound, urinary catheter, endotracheal intubation	Airway stenosis (anastomosis), loss of lymphatic airway, scarring from ch. rejection

an important safeguard against Gram-negative infection (18,60,61). Similarly, local mucosal humoral immunity conferred by secretory IgA also appears to contribute to normal defenses against Enterobacteriaceae (62).

Intact cutaneous and mucosal boundaries prevent Gram-negative infection in the normal host, and these boundaries are necessarily compromised by the surgical procedure of the organ transplant itself, by the tumor-ablative chemoradiotherapy given prior to a marrow transplant or stem cell rescue, and by the CGVHD that affects the bowel, lung, and skin in the allogeneic BMT patient (63–67).

Finally, the transplant procedure otherwise may permanently alter certain anatomic structures and functions that can predispose it to colonization by endogenous and exogenous flora. This includes the heterotopic placement of kidney and kidney/pancreas transplants and the risk for urinary tract infection (68–71); the choledochojejunostomy required in some liver transplant patients (72,73); the problem of biliary strictures that any liver transplantation patient is at risk for (74); and, in the lung transplant recipient, the loss of lymphatic drainage and the development of airway stenoses at the anastomosis site (18,75).

Procedure- and Time-Dependent Risks

The variables discussed in the preceding two sections change over time (Table 2). In general, enteric and nosocomial Gram-negative infections pose their greatest risk in the first month following transplantation, when neutrophil function and/or anatomic barriers are most impaired in both the BMT and SOT patient. This would include pneumonia, sepsis, urinary tract infection, wound infection, and deep surgical site infection.

The increased risk for intracellular Gram-negative infection persists for the life of SOT and allogeneic BMT patients (8,43,76–81).

TRANSPLANT-PROCEDURE-SPECIFIC ISSUES IN PATIENT MANAGEMENT FOR GRAM-NEGATIVE INFECTION

Bone Marrow Transplantation

Both the allogeneic BMT patient and the autologous BMT/stem cell rescue patient have, as their principal risk for Gram-negative infection early following transplantation, neutropenia- and chemoradiation-induced mucositis involving the gastrointestinal tract (4,63,82). This risk has been addressed in several ways: protective isolation, selective decontamination, prophylactic antibiotics, empirical treatment of neutropenic fever, granulocyte stimulation, and therapeutic use of granulocyte transfusions.

Individuals who come into contact with neutropenic patients should obviously wash their hands meticulously (4). These patients may further benefit from restricted diets for neutropenic patients (e.g., omitting uncooked vegetables). There is evidence that total bowel decontamination combined with strict protective isolation that includes HEPA-filtration or laminar-airflow rooms can decrease the risk of bacterial infection in neutropenic BMT patients (4,83–86). However, this practice is difficult to execute in many centers (4) and has not always been found to be superior to transplantation without protective isolation (17,87).

In the neutropenic BMT patient, selective bowel decontamination with nonabsorbable antibiotics may be better than placebo but is not as effective in preventing Gram-negative bacterial infection as absorbable antibiotics (88).

It has been more difficult to determine differences between various types of absorbable antibiotics. However, fluoroquinolones appear superior to trimethoprim sulfamethoxazole in preventing Gram-negative infection and febrile episodes (13). Ciprofloxacin prophylaxis also appears to be associated with a faster neutrophil recovery than trimethoprim sulfamethoxazole (13,89). Ciprofloxacin, which achieves higher blood levels, also appears to me more effective than norfloxacin and is concentrated predominantly in the gastrointestinal tract and urinary system (90).

Because of the risk of Gram-positive sepsis in neutropenic BMT patients, specific Gram-positive prophylaxis is now added to fluoroquinolone regimens (14,91–94). These prophylactic strategies, of course, do not prevent all episodes of febrile neutropenia, nor do they obviate the need to institute empirical intravenous antibiotic therapy for Gram-negative infection if fever emerges while on the prophylactic regimen. However, modifications in the conventional empirical intravenous antibiotic regimen for neutropenic fever in BMT, in combination with oral quinolone prophylaxis, have been evaluated (57,95,96).

In one study, a short course of intravenous antibiotics for 72 hours comprising an aminoglycoside, an antipseudomonal β-lactam agent and vancomycin were used for the empirical treatment of a neutropenic patient with fever and was given concurrently with the prophylactic ciprofloxacin that the patient had already been receiving. Two-thirds of such BMT patients with neutropenic fever responded to this addition of empirical intravenous antibiotics; and three-fourths of these responders, in turn, had no recurrence of the fever after the 72-hour empirical intravenous antibiotic course was stopped. The one-third of patients who did not respond to these intravenous empirical antibiotics then had the intravenous antibiotics discontinued (but did continue on ciprofloxacin) and were treated empirically with amphotericin B. Three-fourths of this group responded to the amphotericin B (96). The continuous use of quinolone prophylaxis in this way may permit the strategic use of sequential antibacterial, then antifungal empirical therapy to determine a probable cause of neutropenic fever without increasing the risk of mortality from Gram-negative infection.

However, as an alternative to oral quinolone prophylaxis, a more aggressive prophylactic antibiotic strategy involving intravenous antibiotics (e.g., ceftazidime plus teicoplanin, for Gram-negative and Gram-positive prophylaxis, respectively) has been adopted in some centers (97). Empirical treatment of febrile neutropenic episodes in BMT patients has also been modified to facilitate outpatient therapy, using once daily aminoglycoside and glycopeptide intravenous antibiotics (98,99).

The duration of antibacterial therapy in a neutropenic BMT patient depends on many factors: whether a pathogen is found; the underlying disease of the patient; and the time at which the neutrophil returns to greater than 500/mm^3 (100).

Numerous studies have shown that colony stimulating factor can shorten the duration of neutropenia by about 7 days in BMT patients (4,101–103). Not every BMT patient is a candidate for this type of therapy (e.g., those patients whose primary disease, such as acute myelogenous leukemia, might be stimulated by the growth factor). Although no survival benefit has yet been found with the use of these factors, the frequency of febrile neutropenia and documented Gram-negative infection has been decreased. The optimal timing of administration has not been determined, and these agents may prove to be optimally used in febrile neutropenic patients (104,105).

For patients with neutropenic fever, granulocyte transfusions have been reconsidered as a therapeutic possibility, with the use of granulocyte colony stimulating factor in the normal donors of the white blood cells as a means to increase the number of white blood cells in the transfusion product. Preliminary experience has suggested a benefit may be possible if these granulocyte transfusions are used before sepsis evolves to multiorgan failure (106).

SOLID ORGAN TRANSPLANTATION

Beyond the general risks of prolonged hospitalization, intubation, surgical wound, and indwelling catheters—which are shared by all SOT patients—each type of SOT procedure carries different degrees and types of risk for Gram-negative bacterial infection.

Kidney Transplantation

Early kidney transplantation experience was often complicated by Gram-negative infection. Between 1966 and 1985, 72 of 116 autopsy-available deaths in one center were from Gram-negative infection, primarily pneumonia (43 patients), but also sepsis (32 patients) and peritonitis (11 patients) (1).

Long-term prophylaxis after kidney transplantation with trimethoprim sulfamethoxazole has greatly reduced this risk, with the rate of Gram-negative infection dropping from 46/132 in a placebo-controlled group to 4/132 in a treatment group receiving trimethoprim sulfamethoxazole at a dose of 320/1,600 mg daily (16). This also prevents *Pneumocystis carinii* and *Listeria* infection. The efficacy of trimethoprim sulfamethoxazole in this population appears to make unnecessary other specific topical antimicrobial prophylaxis measures (e.g., intravesical antibiotic solution) (107).

The use of trimethoprim sulfamethoxazole does not appear to eliminate from the enteric tract the usual species of Enterobacteriaceae that constitute its normal flora; however, this prophylaxis may be associated with development of antimicrobial resistance by these normal flora organisms (108). Patients who develop signs of possible enteric Gram-negative infection (e.g., urinary tract infection) while receiving trimethoprim sulfamethoxazole prophylaxis should therefore receive another agent for empirical therapy pending identification and susceptibility testing of the pathogen.

Other Gram-negative infections that occur specifically in a kidney transplant recipient include infected lymphoceles (109,110), wound infections, and infected peritransplant fluid collections (often nosocomial Gram-negative bacteria that are resistant to perioperative antibiotic prophylaxis) (111,112). Rarely, acute focal bacterial nephritis mimicking rejection can occur (68,113). Urease-splitting *Proteus mirabilis* urinary tract infection can induce struvite stone infection in the renal allograft (114).

Pancreas Transplantation

The anatomic changes from pancreas transplantation with or without a concurrent kidney transplant are greater than from kidney transplantation alone. The pancreas is usually placed in the iliac fossa with the iliac artery and vein as vasculature anastomoses. The pancreatic ductal system is drained by way of an anastomosis using a patch or segment of the duodenum around the ampulla of water into the bladder (115). This altered anatomy and the diabetes of the recipient predispose the kidney/pancreas transplant patient to a higher rate of surgical site infection compared with kidney transplantation alone (up to 30%, half of these from Gram-negative bacterial infection, in pancreas recipients compared with only 4% to 10% in kidney-alone transplant recipients) (69). Urinary tract infections are at least two times more common in pancreas transplantation than in kidney transplantation (16,69), although early removal of indwelling catheters is associated with a reduced risk of urinary tract infection in both procedures.

A unique Gram-negative bacterial infection that complicates pancreas transplantation is infection in the pancreatic duct itself. Gram-negative bacteria appear to grow more easily in pancreatic juice than Gram-positive organisms. Some antibacterial agents achieve better concentration in pancreatic juice than others (e.g., ampicillin sulbactam may be superior than cephalosporins, imipenem, and aminoglycosides). Prolonged treatment for 5 or more weeks may be needed when infection of the pancreatic duct occurs (70).

In a kidney/pancreas or a pancreas-alone transplant procedure, programs using selective bowel decontamination around the time of transplantation, in addition to trimethoprim sulfamethoxazole prophylaxis, Gram-negative organisms have been reported to account for a small minority of bacterial infection (71).

Liver Transplantation

Among SOT patients, liver transplant patients have the greatest risk for Gram-negative bacteria infection. The obvious risks for this include the transient loss of hepatic macrophage function that normally serves as a filter of Gram-negative bacteria in the mesenteric circulation; biliary anastomoses, leaks, and strictures; manipulation of the intestines with the procedure that may increase translocation of bacteria across the intestine; preexisting ascites; and portal hypertension before transplantation (81,116–118).

In the first 2 months after liver transplantation, Gram-negative bacteria are frequent causes of intra-abdominal infection and bacteremia. Early reports in programs not using selective bowel decontamination identify Gram-negative sepsis as the main cause of early mortality (i.e., the first 60 days following transplant) (119). However, the contribution of Gram-negative infection to this early infection rate appears to drop from as high as 66% (9) to as low as 5% when selective bowel decontamination is used (15,120–123). A randomized, prospective study demonstrated that, among patients who had taken selective bowel decontamination treatment for at least 3 days before transplantation, there were fewer Gram-negative infections in "key sites" (primary bloodstream, abdomen, wound, and lungs), dropping from 36% (12 of 33) in the placebo group to 23% (6 of 26) in a treatment group (124).

No prospective, randomized, controlled study has confirmed a decrease in mortality from infection that can be attributed to the use of selective bowel decontamination. The success of the regimen may depend on the compliance of patients who need to take the treatment at least 3 days before aerobic Gram-negative bacteria are eliminated from the alimentary canal (125).

The use of historical controls may overestimate the benefit of selective bowel decontamination seen in non-controlled studies. For example, prolonged duration of surgery and the number of cellular blood products used during surgery may be independent risk factors for early bacterial infection (9,81,126). As experience in transplantation in a center improves, these variables will differ in historical controls.

Moreover, selective bowel decontamination does not prevent infection by Gram-positive organisms. The frequency of infection by Gram-positive organisms appears to be greater in programs using selective bowel decontamination than in those not using selective bowel decontamination (127). These include potentially virulent pathogens such as *Staphylococcus aureus* and *Enterococcus faecium*.

Early post-transplantation pneumonia from Gram-negative bacteria can occur in 10% to 15% of liver transplant patients (6,128). Selective bowel decontamination appears to reduce the colonization of airways by aerobic Gram-negative bacteria. However, the rate of systemic endotoxemia among intubated patients in an intensive care unit was not found to be affected by selective bowel decontamination in one controlled study (129).

Moreover, selective bowel decontamination regimens will not prevent *Legionella* infection (discussed later), which, with *Pseudomonas* infection, may be increasing in frequency among liver transplant patients despite the use of selective bowel decontamination (6,7).

Late biliary complications (strictures and leaks) are common (approximately 15%) after liver transplantation. Except for those associated with hepatic artery thrombosis, these complications do not cause excess mortality (74). They often require further manipulation of the biliary system with stents and drains. If the biliary system is colonized with Gram-negative bacteria (as might be expected in the late post-transplantation period, when selective bowel decontamination is no longer used), prophylactic Gram-negative bacterial antibiotic coverage may be needed for these procedures.

The liver transplant patients who require choledochojejunostomy (e.g., those with primary sclerosing cholangitis) have been studied to see if there has been an increased risk for sepsis after liver biopsy. The presence of occult biliary obstruction (evident on ERCP but not on ultrasound) can predispose these patients to Gram-negative bacteremia after liver biopsy. The "occult" nature of this type of obstruction may account for the variations in reported risks for these procedures in these patients (72,73).

Heart Transplantation

Heart transplant patients are at less risk for Gram-negative bacteria infection than liver transplant patients (130). However, Gram-negative pneumonia early following cardiac transplantation is still a significant hazard, occurring in 5% to 10% of patients, and can be fatal in as many as 20% of these patients who do develop Gram-negative pneumonia (131,132). Prolonged mechanical ventilation, the age of the recipient, and donor ischemia time all appear to contribute to this risk (78,133–135).

Uncommon infections that are more specific to heart transplant patients include infected aortic arch, pseudoaneurysm, endocarditis, mediastinitis, pericarditis, and infection in the mechanical ventricular assist devices that are used pretransplantation. The pathogens in these infections tend to be Gram-positive (especially *Staphylococcus aureus*) organisms, although *Hemophilus* or nosocomial Gram-negative pathogens (e.g., *Pseudomonas aeruginosa, Serratia, Enterobacter* spp.) can occur (136–145).

The heart transplant patient will receive trimethoprim sulfamethoxazole for *Pneumocystis carinii* prophylaxis; otherwise, no specific measures to prevent Gram-negative bacteria infections in these patients have been recommended.

The heart transplant recipient may be at particular risk for bacteremia, sepsis, and/or mediastinitis following transplantation as a result of direct transmission of pathogens with the graft from a donor with positive blood cultures at the time of transplantation (146). These complications appear to occur more frequently if the donor has positive blood cultures for Gram-negative bacteria compared with Gram-positive bacteria and can be fatal. Despite this risk of known Gram-negative infection in the donor, critically ill patients have been the recipients of such organs because of the overall shortage of donors. With appropriate perioperative antibiotic therapy, this practice may be safe when heart transplant candidates have an immediate need for transplantation (147). Similarly, heart transplant candidates may themselves develop serious bacterial infection while awaiting transplantation. These patients have often spent weeks in the hospital environment and may not survive an extended wait for a suitable donor. Despite the unstable condition of these potential recipients, transplantation has been completed successfully without an obvious risk for increased mortality (compared with potential recipients without a serious infection in the week preceding transplantation) (148).

The level of immunosuppression heart transplant recipients require to avoid and treat rejection is greater than that with kidney and liver transplantation. Nevertheless, the possibility of optimizing the level of immunosuppression that a specific heart transplant patient requires has been addressed as a way of reducing risk for infection, including Gram-negative infection (149,150). Reduction in the use of steroids and azathioprine has been the principal measure to accomplish this. Prospective studies are needed to confirm this impression, as the reported 2-year actuarial infection-free survival (13% to 25%) has not differed significantly between programs that did or did not attempt such approaches of reduced immunosuppression (80,151).

Lung Transplantation

Among SOT recipients, the lung transplant recipient has the greatest risk for Gram-negative bacterial pneumonia early following transplantation. Pneumonia from Gram-negative bacteria is also the most common cause of mortality in the first month after transplantation (18,130,152,153). As many as 20% to 25% of lung transplant patients will develop bacterial pneumonia, most of these from Gram-negative bacilli in the first 3 months after transplantation.

Depending on the indication for lung transplantation, single-lung, heart/double-lung, double-lung, or bilateral sequential single-lung transplantation may be performed (154–159). It is difficult to make direct comparisons among these procedures, but there is a concern that cystic fibrosis patients carry a greater risk for Gram-negative pneumonia compared with patients with other types of lung disease. Regardless of the preexisting disease, aggressive optimization of antibiotic therapy based on susceptibility testing of respiratory isolates from the recipient and donor respiratory tracts is necessary in the treatment of early pneumonia after lung transplantation (152,160–162).

The patient with cystic fibrosis is a particular challenge. Although the chronically infected lungs are removed, the paranasal sinuses remain colonized with resistant strains of *Pseudomonas aeruginosa* and *Pseudomonas cepacia* (48). The same strains of these organisms in a patient's airways before transplant can be found in the airways of the patient following transplant (45,47,163). The sinuses therefore likely represent a reservoir of antibiotic-resistant bacteria that can recolonize the transplanted lungs. Pretransplant sinus surgery as a measure to reduce the risk of pneumonia after transplantation has been advocated (48). However, the recipient trachea, in addition to the sinuses, may be a reservoir for resistant bacteria in the cystic fibrosis lung transplant recipients. Therefore sinus surgery alone will not eliminate this risk for recolonization with resistant bacteria (45,160).

Pseudomonas cepacia is less common than *P. aeruginosa* in colonizing the cystic fibrosis patient before transplant (19% versus 89%), but because it is more resistant to antibiotics it is more likely to be the cause of early death among patients who have it (approximately 20% to 30% versus less than 10%) (154,160). If lung function is satisfactory, even these resistant organisms are amenable to combination antibiotic therapy that may include aerosolized aminoglycoside administration. *Pseudomonas cepacia* can also complicate lung transplantation with empyema (164,165).

The development of airways stenosis after lung transplantation is an infrequent (<10%) complication, but when it occurs it is often associated with bacterial pneumonia, usually *Pseudomonas aeruginosa* (75). This complication is amenable to stent placement and antibiotic therapy but may be fatal despite these measures (75,166).

A potential lung transplant candidate may be dependent on mechanical ventilator support prior to transplantation. The contribution of this risk to the outcome of transplantation is multifactorial; however, the possibility of colonization of the potential recipient's airways with nosocomial bacteria does not appear to be a major hazard and by itself would not be a contraindication to transplantation (46,49).

Most lung donors will not have been on ventilator support long enough to become colonized with nosocomial

Gram-negative bacteria prior to transplantation. Usual oral flora, including *Streptococcus viridans* and *Candida,* may—if found in the donor trachea with cultures taken at transplantation—be a risk for early pneumonia following transplantation, although the pneumonia isolates will not be the same (162).

The long-term management of lung transplant recipients includes the use of trimethoprim sulfamethoxazole for *Pneumocystis carinii* prophylaxis (18). This may also help prevent infection from susceptible Gram-negative bacteria- including *Hemophilus influenzae, Moraxella catarrhalis,* and some enteric aerobic Gram-negative bacteria such as *E. coli* and *Klebsiella.* However, when an acute infection develops in a lung transplant patient who is taking trimethoprim sulfamethoxazole at the lower *Pneumocystis carinii* pneumonia prophylaxis doses, it should be assumed that any Gram-negative pathogen will be *resistant* to trimethoprim sulfamethoxazole until susceptibility testing proves otherwise. Empirical therapy should therefore include coverage for possible antibiotic-resistant Gram-negative bacteria. In patients with airway stenosis associated with *Pseudomonas aeruginosa* colonization or in patients with a single native lung that has obstructive airway disease and that is colonized, this empirical therapy can be based on the results of surveillance sputum or throat cultures (75,155).

Early poorly controlled severe rejection will likely result in obliterate bronchiolitis and fibrosis (167,168). Therefore it is difficult to attempt reduced immunosuppression in the lung transplant patient as a measure to reduce the risk of infection. The use of tacrolimus (FK506) instead of cyclosporine may be associated with a lower rate of bacterial infection but a higher rate of fungal infection in lung transplantation (169). There is not yet enough experience in lung transplantation, but in liver transplant patients on tacrolimus, an increased rate of *Legionella* infection has been observed (6).

PROBLEMATIC PATHOGENS

Salmonellosis

Salmonella organisms are, like *Legionella,* also intracellular, and their immunologic control requires monocyte and macrophage function, both of which are impaired in transplant recipients (59,170–173).

The SOT recipient is perhaps at a 20 times greater risk for developing *Salmonella* infection than the general population. The actual rate in the general population will be greater in tropical regions (25). Both *Salmonella typhi* and nontyphoidal *Salmonella* infections occur at an increased rate with more complications in SOT patients compared with the general population. Complicated *Salmonella* infections in BMT recipients have also been reported (59,172,174).

Contrary to normal hosts, who usually only develop intestinal disease, the most common presentation of *Salmonella* in transplant recipients is bacteremia (approximately 60%) (59). This may occasionally represent an intravascular focus of infection such as a mycotic aneurysm or an infected prosthetic vascular graft used for dialysis, either of which should be suspected if bacteremia persists despite antimicrobial therapy (175,176). Extraintestinal complications of salmonellosis are also more common (approximately 35%) in transplant recipients compared with normal hosts and have included pneumonia, pleural effusion, septic thrombophlebitis, orchitis, sinusitis, pyelonephritis, arthritis, osteomyelitis, and prosthetic vascular graft infection. Persistent or relapsing bacteriuria in a renal transplant recipient may be caused by infection in the native kidneys, requiring nephrectomy for cure (172). Persistent or relapsing *Salmonella* bacteremia warrants further clinical evaluation for an occult focus of infection that might require surgery or drainage (25).

Surveillance stool cultures and urine cultures before transplantation are useful in identifying patients who are asymptomatic before transplantation and who therefore need eradication of a possible focus of *Salmonella* before transplantation (172).

Trimethoprim sulfamethoxazole prophylaxis, which is used for *Pneumocystis carinii* pneumonia, may prevent *Salmonella* infection in transplant recipients. However, just as important as prophylaxis is the education of the transplant patient to prevent exposure to *Salmonella* as well as exposure to other enteric pathogens. The same instructions given to patients infected with human immunodeficiency virus to prevent exposure to enteric pathogens can also be given to transplant recipients (177).

These recommendations include the following:

1. Food
   a. Avoid raw or undercooked eggs and egg products, poultry, meat, or seafood; avoid unpasteurized dairy products and soft cheeses.
   b. Poultry and meat should be well cooked and not pink in the middle.
   c. Produce should be washed thoroughly before being eaten.
   d. Avoid cross-contamination of foods via hand and utensils during food preparation.
   e. Reheat "ready-to-eat" foods such as cold cuts until they are steaming hot before eating.
2. Pets
   a. Avoid contact with pets with diarrhea and have the animal examined by a veterinarian.
   b. Avoid pets <6 months of age, especially if they have diarrhea.
   c. Wash hands after handling pets.
   d. Avoid contact with reptiles (e.g., snakes, lizards, iguanas, and turtles) because of the risk of salmonellosis.

3. Travel

During travel to developing countries, avoid food and beverages that may be contaminated, especially raw fruits and vegetables, raw or undercooked seafood or meat, tapwater or ice made with tapwater, unpasteurized mild or dairy products, and items sold by street vendors (178).

Other Enteric Pathogens

SOT recipients are at increased risk for serious *Vibrio vulnificus* infection, which can cause sepsis as well as fulminant soft-tissue infection after ingestion of contaminated raw oysters and shellfish or after exposure of open wounds to saltwater environments (179). These hazards are also important to emphasize to the transplant recipient. Similarly, the transplant recipient will be at increased risk of soft-tissue infection (myonecrosis) and sepsis from contact with fresh water that is contaminated with *Aeromonas hydrophila* (180).

Other enteric pathogens such as *Plesiomonas shigelloides* (181). and *Campylobacter* (178) can also cause sepsis and extraintestinal disease in transplant recipients.

Transplant recipients should be advised to seriously consider the potential risks of cat ownership. Those who elect to acquire a cat should adopt or purchase a healthy and older (>1 year) animal. Rough play with a cat should be avoided; cat-associated wounds should be washed promptly; and cats should not be allowed to lick open cuts or wounds of the transplant recipient (177).

Capnocytophaga

Capnocytophaga is a Gram-negative, facultatively anaerobic bacteria that is part of the normal flora of the oral cavity. Prolonged neutropenia and the mucositis of chemoradiation therapy are the principal risk factors for bacteremia with *Capnocytophaga*. This possibility should be considered in BMT patients with these risk factors and fever. Suppurative metastatic infection to organs and tissues can occur. Occasionally, these organisms are resistant to β-lactam agents, with clindamycin appearing to be the most effective antibiotic against *Capnocytophaga* (182).

Stenotrophomonas (Xanthomonas) maltophilia

Stenotrophomonas (Xanthomonas) maltophilia is occasionally identified as a colonizer of surgical wounds and as a colonizer of endotracheal tubes and airways of intubated patients. However, it can cause bacteremia and septic complications in compromised hosts, including transplant recipients. The mortality from *S. maltophilia* bacteremia is significant (approximately 20%), which can occur despite therapy with an effective antimicrobial agent. This organism is typically resistant to β-lactam agents and aminoglycosides but usually susceptible to trimethoprim sulfamethoxazole. Combination therapy with at least one other active agent (e.g., minacycline or ticarcillin clavulanic acid) should be considered in the transplant patient with *S. maltophilia* bacteremia (183,184).

Other Unusual Pathogens and Syndromes

Besides *S. maltophilia*, other glucose nonfermenting Gram-negative bacilli can cause serious disease in BMT and SOT recipients. These organismis include *Pseudomonas putida, Sphingomonas paucimobilis,* and *Alcaligenes xylosoxidans*. Many of these cases are catheter-associated bacteremia that require catheter removal in addition to antibiotic therapy for cure (184,185).

Necrotizing Soft-Tissue Infections

In addition to the "typical" soft-tissue infections caused by *Vibrios vulnificus* and *Aeromonas hydrophila*, discussed previously, atypical soft-tissue infections involving Gram-negative bacteria can occur in transplant patients. *Ecthyma gangrenosum*, due to bacteremia with *Pseudomonas aeruginosa*, can occur in SOT recipients even in the absence of neutropenia (186). Also somewhat atypically, enteric Gram-negative bacteria—such as *E. coli*—can cause necrotizing fasciitis in neutropenic transplant recipients (187).

ANTIMICROBIAL RESISTANCE OF GRAM-NEGATIVE BACTERIA IN TRANSPLANT PATIENTS

Transplant patients have several risk factors for infection caused by antimicrobial resistant Gram-negative bacteria.

First, anatomic abnormalities of organs and tissues before transplant will result in the eventual colonization of these structures by resistant bacteria. The clearest example of this is provided by the lung transplant candidate with bronchiectasis. If the patient has cystic fibrosis, then the lungs and upper respiratory tract will also be colonized with *Pseudomonas aeruginosa* and possibly *P. cepacia*. However, in a recent retrospective review at a single center, the organisms present in the lung transplant candidate prior to transplantation were not the primary cause of mortality after transplantation (188). As previously stated, careful evaluation, including microbiological cultures and susceptibility testing of colonizing isolates before transplantation, can provide information that will optimize antibiotic management in the immediate post-transplant period.

Second, long-term antibiotic prophylaxis has been associated with infection by resistant Gram-negative bacteria that were resistant to the prophylactic agent (108).

This would be more likely to occur if the patient continues to have, or develops, post-transplantation abnormal anatomic structures such as biliary strictures, tracheal or bronchus anastomotic strictures, or ureteral strictures after liver, lung, or kidney transplantation, respectively. There is therefore limited long-term success with the use of prophylaxis to prevent stricture-associated infection in the absence of treatment for the stricture problem itself.

The risk of prophylactic antibiotic resistance emerging in BMT recipients is lower than in organ transplant recipients because of the lack of anatomic abnormalities. However, even in BMT patients receiving fluoroquinolone prophylaxis, resistance to the quinolones is now being reported (44). The historical period of a reduced frequency of Gram-negative infection in BMT patients that was made possible by quinolone prophylaxis may be over soon.

Third, antibiotic resistance in Gram-negative bacterial infections in transplant patients results from the high inoculum of organisms that develop and persist when infections cannot be adequately drained or debrided. Again, large intra-abdominal fluid collections and biliary strictures in liver transplant recipients are the clearest example of this. One of the first case reports of *Enterobacter* resistance to cefepime, a fourth-generation cephalosporin that was expected to retain high activity against this organism, developed in a liver transplant patient with liver abscesses and biliary strictures (189,190).

Finally, transplant patients are at risk for nosocomial Gram-negative bacterial infections. The antimicrobial resistance of nosocomial Gram-negative bacteria varies between institutions and is a function of antimicrobial usage patterns in each hospital. Such variability may also depend on the type of care unit the transplant patient is in. It is therefore important that clinicians know the resistance patterns in their own hospital, especially when selecting empirical therapy of a critically ill transplant patient. Appropriate management of transplant recipients includes reducing unnecessarily broad antibiotic use, as directed by the results of cultures, to reduce the selective pressure for antibiotic resistance in the hospital setting.

REFERENCES

1. Scroggs MW, Wolfe JA, Bollinger RR, et al. Causes of death in renal transplant recipients. A review of autopsy findings from 1966 through 1985. *Arch Pathol Lab Med* 1987;111(10):983–987.
2. Garibaldi RA. Infections in organ transplant recipients. *Infect Control* 1983;4(6):460–464.
3. Copeland JG, Mammana RB, Fuller JK, et al. Heart transplantation. Four years' experience with conventional immunosuppression. *JAMA* 1984;251(12):1563–1566.
4. Serody JS, Shea TC. Prevention of infections in bone marrow transplant recipients. *Infect Dis Clin North Am* 1997;11(2):459–477.
5. Wingard JR. Advances in the management of infectious complications after bone marrow transplantation. *Bone Marrow Transplant* 1990; 6(6):371–383.
6. Singh N, Gayowski T, Wagener M, et al. Pulmonary infections in liver transplant recipients receiving tacrolimus. Changing pattern of microbial etiologies. *Transplantation* 1996;61(3):396–401.
7. Korvick JA, Marsh JW, Starzl TE, et al. *Pseudomonas aeruginosa* bacteremia in patients undergoing liver transplantation: an emerging problem. *Surgery* 1991;109(1):62–68.
8. Donnelly JP. Bacterial complications of transplantation: diagnosis and treatment. *J Antimicrob Chemother* 1995;36[Suppl B}:59–72.
9. Paya CV, Hermans PE. Bacterial infections after liver transplantation. [Review] *Eur J Clin Microbiol Infect Dis* 1989;8(6):499–504.
10. Cuervas-Mons V, Millan I, Gavaler JS, et al. Prognostic value of preoperatively obtained clinical and laboratory data in predicting survival following orthotopic liver transplantation. *Hepatology* 1986;6(5): 922–927.
11. Karp JE, Merz WG, Hendrickson C, et al. Oral norfloxacin for prevention of gram-negative bacterial infection in patients with acute leukemia and granulocytopenia. *Ann Intern Med* 1987;106:1–7.
12. Lew MA, Kehoe K, Ritz J, et al. Prophylaxis of bacterial infections with ciprofloxacin in patients undergoing bone marrow transplantation. *Transplantation* 1991;51(3):630–636.
13. Lew MA, Kehoe K, Ritz J, et al. Ciprofloxacin versus trimethoprim sulfamethoxazole for prophylaxis of bacterial infections in bone marrow transplant recipients: a randomized, controlled trial. *J Clin Oncol* 1995;13(1):239–250.
14. Anonymous. Reduction of fever and streptococcal bacteremia in granulocytopenic patients with cancer. A trial of oral penicillin V or placebo combined with pefloxacin. International Antimicrobial Therapy Cooperative Group of the European Organization for Research and Treatment of Cancer. *JAMA* 1994;272(15):1183–1189.
15. Wiesner RH. The incidence of gram-negative bacterial and fungal infections in liver transplant patients treated with selective decontamination. *Infection* 1990;18[Suppl 1]:S19–S21.
16. Fox BC, Sollinger HW, Belzer FO, et al. A prospective, randomized, double-blind study of trimethoprim-sulfamethoxazole for prophylaxis of infection in renal transplantation: clinical efficacy, absorption of trimethoprim-sulfamethoxazole, effects on the microflora, and the cost-benefit of prophylaxis. *Am J Med* 1990;89(3):255–274.
17. Dekker AW, Verdonck LF, Rozenberg-Arska M. Infection prevention in autologous bone marrow transplantation and the role of protective isolation. *Bone Marrow Transplant* 1994;14(1):89–93.
18. Dauber JH, Paradis IL, Dummer JS. Infectious complications in pulmonary allograft recipients. [Review] *Clin Chest Med* 1990;11(2): 291–308.
19. Todo S, Tzakis A, Reyes J, et al. Small intestinal transplantation in humans with or without the colon. *Transplantation* 1994;57(6): 840–848.
20. D'Ivernois C, Dupon M, Dartigues JF, et al. Decreased incidence of infection after renal transplantation with the use of cyclosporine. European *J Clin Microbiol Infect Dis* 1991;19(11):911–916.
21. Alexander JW, First MR, Majeski JA, et al. The late adverse effect of splenectomy on patient survival following cadaveric renal transplantation. *Transplantation* 1984;37(5):467–470.
22. Thalhamer J, Pimpl W, Pattermann M. The role of the spleen and splenic autotransplants in clearing experimental bacteremia caused by the gram-negative bacterium *Escherichia coli. Res Exp Med* 1986; 186(3):229–238.
23. Galili D, Tagger N, Sela MN, et al. Surveillance of oral cultures for Enterobacteriaceae during bone marrow transplantation. *Eur J Cancer* 1995;31B(1):58–62.
24. Paya CV, Hermans PE, Washington JA. Incidence, distribution, and outcome of episodes of infection in 100 orthotopic liver transplantations. *Mayo Clin Proc* 1989;64(5):555–564.
25. Patel R, Paya CV. Infections in solid organ transplant recipients. *Clin Microbiol Rev* 1997;10(1):86–124.
26. LaRocco MT, Burgert SJ. Infection in the bone marrow transplant recipient and role of the microbiology laboratory in clinical transplantation. *Clin Microbiol Rev* 1997;10(2):277–297.
27. Kibbler CC. Infections in liver transplantation: risk factors and strategies for prevention. *J Hosp Infect* 1995;30[Suppl]:209–217.
28. Rubin RH, Tolkoff-Rubin NE. Antimicrobial strategies in the care of organ transplant recipients. *Antimicrob Agents Chemother* 1993; 37(4):619–624.
29. Giamarellou H, Antoniadou A. The effect of monitoring of antibiotic use on decreasing antibiotic resistance in the hospital. Ciba Foundation Symposium 207:76–86, discussion 86–92, 1997.
30. Taylor GD, Kirkland T, Lakey J, et al. Bacteremia due to transplanta-

tion of contaminated cryopreserved pancreatic islets. *Cell Transplant* 1994;3(1):103–106.

31. D'Antonio D, Iacone A, Fioritoni G, et al. Detection of bacterial contamination in bone marrow graft. *Haematologica* 1991;76[Suppl 1]:44–45.

32. Buchholz B, Zastrow F, Valenzuela A, et al. How to detect bacterial contamination prior to transplantation. *Scand J Urol Nephrol* 1985;92:45–47.

33. Schwella N, Zimmerman R, Heuft HG. Microbiologic contamination of peripheral blood stem autografts. *Vox Sanguinis* 1994;67(1):32–35.

34. Espinosa MT, Fox R, Creger RJ. Microbiologic contamination of peripheral blood progenitor cells collected for hematopoietic cell transplantation. *Transfusion* 1996;36(9):789–793.

35. Rowley SD, Davis J, Dick J. Bacterial contamination of bone marrow grafts intended for autologous and allogeneic bone marrow transplantation: incidence and clinical significance. *Transfusion* 1988;28(2):109–112.

36. Spees EK, Light JA, Oakes DD, et al. Experiences with cadaver renal allograft contamination before transplantation. *Br J Surg* 1982;69(8):482–485.

37. Gottesdiener KM. Transplanted infections: donor-to-host transmission with the allograft. *Ann Intern Med* 1989;110(12):1001–1016.

38. Bijnen AB, Weimar W, Bijlstra AM, Jeekel J. Infections after transplantation of a contaminated kidney. *Scand J Urol Nephrol* 1985;92:49–51.

39. Lazarus HM, Magalhaes-Silverman M, Fox RM, et al. Contamination during in vitro processing of bone marrow for transplantation: clinical significance. *Bone Marrow Transplant* 1991;7(3):241–246.

40. Mackowiak PA, Goggans M, Torres W, et al. Relationship between cytomegalovirus and colonization of the oropharynx by gram-negative bacilli following renal transplantation. *Epidemiol Infect* 1991;107(2):411–420.

41. Smyth RL, Scott JP, Borysiewicz LK, et al. Cytomegalovirus infection in heart-lung transplant recipients: risk factors, clinical associations, and response to treatment. *J Infect Dis* 1991;164(6):1045–1050.

42. Falagas ME, Snydman DR, Griffith J, et al. Exposure to cytomegalovirus from the donated organ is a risk factor for bacteremia in orthotopic liver transplant recipients. Boston Center for Liver Transplantation CMVIG Study Group. *Clin Infect Dis* 1996;23(3):468–474.

43. Paya CV, Wiesner RH, Hermans PE, et al. Risk factors for cytomegalovirus and severe bacterial infections following liver transplantation: a prospective multivariate time-dependent analysis. *J Hepatol* 1993;18(2):185–195.

44. Palau J, Lopez-Aldeguer J, Garcia-Boyer R, et al. Role of ciprofloxacin prophylaxis in the re-emergence of *E. coli* as a significant pathogen causing bacteremia in neutropenic patients with hematologic malignancies. Abstract C-16 37th ICAAC, Toronto 1997.

45. Walter S, Gudowius P, Bosshammer J, et al. Epidemiology of chronic *Pseudomonas aeruginosa* infections in the airways of lung transplant recipients with cystic fibrosis. *Thorax* 1997;52(4):318–321.

46. Kurland G. Pediatric lung transplantation: indications and contraindications. [Review] *Semin Thorac Cardiovasc Surg* 1996;8(3):277–285.

47. Steinbach S, Sun L, Jiang RZ, et al. Transmissibility of Pseudomonas cepacia infection in clinic patients and lung-transplant recipients with cystic fibrosis. *N Engl J Med* 1994;331(15):981–987.

48. Davidson TM, Murphy C, Mitchell M, et al. Management of chronic sinusitis in cystic fibrosis. *Laryngoscope* 1995;105(4 pt 1):354–358.

49. Flume PA, Egan TM, Westerman JH, et al. Lung transplantation for mechanically ventilated patients. *J Heart Lung Transplant* 1994;13(1 pt 1):15–21.

50. Parkkali T, Ruutu T, Stenvik M, et al. Loss of protective immunity to polio, diphtheria, and Haemophilus influenzae type b after allogeneic bone marrow transplantation. *APMIS* 1996;104(5):383–388.

51. Kalhs P, Panzer S, Kletter K, et al. Functional asplenia after bone marrow transplantation. A late complication related to extensive chronic graft-versus-host disease. *Ann Intern Med* 1988;109(6):461–464.

52. Gottlieb DJ, Cryz SJ, Furer E, et al. Immunity against *Pseudomonas aeruginosa* adoptively transferred to bone marrow transplant recipients. *Blood* 1990;76(12):2470–2475.

53. Aucouturier P, Barra A, Intrator L, et al. Long lasting IgG subclass and antibacterial polysaccharide antibody deficiency after allogeneic bone marrow transplantation. *Blood* 1987;70(3):779–785.

54. Sheridan JF, Tutschka PJ, Sedmak DD, et al. Immunoglobulin G subclass deficiency and pneumococcal infection after allogeneic bone marrow transplantation. *Blood* 1990;75(7):1583–1586.

55. Tutschka PJ. Infections and immunodeficiency in bone marrow transplantation. *Pediatr Infect Dis J* 1988;7[Suppl 5]:S22–S29.

56. Sullivan KM. Immunoglobulin therapy in bone marrow transplantation. *Am J Med* 1987;83(4A):34–45.

57. Klastersky J. Febrile neutropenia. *Curr Opin Oncol* 1993;5(4):625–632.

58. Stout JE, Yu VL. Legionellosis *N Engl J Med* 1997;377:682–687.

59. Samra Y, Shaked Y, Maier MR. Nontyphoidal salmonellosis in renal transplant recipients: report of five cases and review of the literature. [Review] *Rev Infect Dis* 1986;8(3):431–440.

60. Shaked A, McDiarmid SV, Harrison RE, et al. Hepatic artery thrombosis resulting in gas gangrene of the transplanted liver. *Surgery* 1992;111(4):462–465.

61. Magnan A, Mege JL, Reynaud M, et al. Monitoring of alveolar macrophage production of tumor necrosis factor-alpha and interleukin-6 in lung transplant recipients. Marseille and Montreal Lung Transplantation Group. *Am J Respir Crit Care Med* 1994;150(3):684–689.

62. Garfunkel AA, Tager N, Chausu S, et al. Oral complications in bone marrow transplantation patients: recent advances. *Israel J Med Sci* 1994;30(1):120–124.

63. Walter EA, Bowden RA. Infection in the bone marrow transplant recipient. *Infect Dis Clin North Am* 1995;9(4):823–847.

64. Ferretti GA, Ash RC, Brown AT, et al. Control of oral mucositis and candidiasis in marrow transplantation: a prospective, double-blind trial of chlorhexidine digluconate oral rinse. *Bone Marrow Transplant* 1988;3(5):483–493.

65. Bianco JA, Pepe MS, Higano C, et al. Prevalence of clinically relevant bacteremia after upper gastrointestinal endoscopy in bone marrow transplant recipients. *Am J Med* 1990;89(2):134–136.

66. Callum JL, Brandwein JM, Sutcliffe SB, et al. Influence of total body irradiation on infections after autologous bone marrow transplantation. *Bone Marrow Transplant* 1991;8(4):245–251.

67. Heimdahl A, Mattsson T, Dahllof G, et al. The oral cavity as a port of entry for early infections in patients treated with bone marrow transplantation. *Oral Surg Oral Med Oral Pathol* 1989;68(6):711–716.

68. Goya N, Tanabe K, Iguchi Y, et al. Prevalence of urinary tract infection during outpatient follow-up after renal transplantation. *Infection* 1997;25(2):101–105.

69. Smets YF, van der Pijl JW, van Dissel JT, et al. Infectious disease complications of simultaneous pancreas kidney transplantation. *Nephrol Dial Transplant* 1997;12(4):764–771.

70. Bonatti H, Steurer W, Konigsrainer A, et al. Infection of the pancreatic duct following pancreas transplantation with bladder drainage. *J Chemother* 1995;7(5):442–445.

71. Lumbreras C, Fernandez I, Velosa J, et al. Infectious complications following pancreatic transplantation: incidence, microbiological and clinical characteristics, and outcome. *Clin Infect Dis* 1995;20(3):514–520.

72. Bubak ME, Porayko MK, Krom RA, et al. Complications of liver biopsy in liver transplant patients: increased sepsis associated with choledochojejunostomy. *Hepatology* 1991;14(6):1063–1065.

73. Ben-Ari Z, Neville L, Rolles K, et al. Liver biopsy in liver transplantation: no additional risk of infections in patients with choledochojejunostomy. *J Hepatol* 1996;24(3):324–327.

74. Koivusalo A, Isoniemi H, Salmela K, et al. Biliary complications in one hundred adult liver transplantations. *Scand J Gastroenterol* 1996;31(5):506–511.

75. Higgins R, McNeil K, Dennis C, et al. Airway stenoses after lung transplantation: management with expanding metal stents. *J Heart Lung Transplant* 1994;13(5):774–778.

76. Lossos IS, Breuer R, Or R, et al. Bacterial pneumonia in recipients of bone marrow transplantation. A five-year prospective study. *Transplantation* 1995;60(7):672–678.

77. Arnow PM. Infections following orthotopic liver transplantation. [Review] *HPB Surg* 1991;3(4):221–232.

78. Miller JW, Naftel DC, Bourge RC, et al. Infection after heart transplantation: a multi-institutional study. Cardiac Transplant Research Database Group. *J Heart Lung Transplant* 1994;13(3):381–392.

79. Barkholt L, Ericzon BG, Tollemar J, et al. Infections in human liver recipients: different patterns early and late after transplantation. *Transplant Int* 1993;6(2):77–84.

80. Hosenpud JD, Hershberger RE, Pantely GA, et al. Late infection in

cardiac allograft recipients: profiles, incidence, and outcome. *J Heart Lung Transplant* 1991;10(3):380–386.

81. George DL, Arnow PM, Fox AS, et al. Bacterial infection as a complication of liver transplantation: epidemiology and risk factors. *Rev Infect Dis* 1991;13(3):387–396.

82. Kirk JL, Greenfield RA, Slease RB, et al. Analysis of early infectious complications after autologous bone marrow transplantation. *Cancer* 1988;62(11):2445–2450.

83. Moller J, Skinhoj P, Hoiby N. Microbial colonization and infectious complications in bone marrow transplant recipients treated in strict protective isolation. *Scand J Infect Dis* 1984;16(1):43–50.

84. Heidt PJ. Management of bacterial and fungal infections in bone marrow transplant recipients and other granulocytopenic patients. *Cancer Detect Preven* 1988;12(1-6):609–619.

85. Petersen FB, Buckner CD, Clift RA, et al. Infectious complications in patients undergoing marrow transplantation: a prospective randomized study of the additional effect of decontamination and laminar air flow isolation among patients receiving prophylactic systemic antibiotics. *Scand J Infect Dis* 1987;19(5):559–567.

86. Schmeiser T, Kurrle E, Arnold R, et al. Antimicrobial prophylaxis in neutropenic patients after bone marrow transplantation. *Infection* 1988;16(1):19–24.

87. Russell JA, Poon MC, Jones AR, et al. Allogeneic bone-marrow transplantation without protective isolation in adults with malignant disease. *Lancet* 1992;339(8784):38–40.

88. Gluckman, E, Roudet C, Hirsch I, et al. Prophylaxis of bacterial infections after bone marrow transplantation. A randomized prospective study comparing oral broad-spectrum nonabsorbable antibiotics (vancomycin-tobramycin-colistin) to absorbable antibiotics (floxacin-amoxicillin). *Chemotherapy* 1991;37[Suppl 1]:33–38.

89. Imrie KR, Prince HM, Couture F, et al. Effect of antimicrobial prophylaxis on hematopoietic recovery following autologous bone marrow transplantation: ciprofloxacin versus co-trimoxazole. *Bone Marrow Transplant* 1995;15(2):267–270.

90. Anonymous. Prevention of bacterial infection in neutropenic patients with hematologic malignancies: A randomized, multicenter trial comparing norfloxacin with ciprofloxacin. The GIMEMA Infection Program. Gruppo Italiano Malattie Ematologiche Maligne dell'Adulto. *Ann Intern Med* 1991;115(1):7–12.

91. Broun ER, Wheat JL, Kneebone PH, et al. Randomized trial of the addition of gram-positive prophylaxis to standard antimicrobial prophylaxis for patients undergoing autologous bone marrow transplantation. *Antimicrob Agents Chemother* 1994;38(3):576–579.

92. Engelhard D, Elishoov H, Or R, et al. Cytosine arabinoside as a major risk factor for Streptococcus viridans septicemia following bone marrow transplantation: a 5-year prospective study. *Bone Marrow Transplant* 1995;16(4):565–570.

93. Martino R, Manteiga R, Sanchez I, et al. Viridans streptococcal shock syndrome during bone marrow transplantation. *Acta Haematologica* 1995;94(2):69–73.

94. DePauw BE, Donnelly JP, DeWitte T, et al. Options and limitations of long-term oral ciprofloxacin as antibacterial prophylaxis in allogeneic bone marrow transplant recipients. *Bone Marrow Transplant* 1990;5(3):179–182.

95. DePauw BE, Deresinsk SC, Feld R, et al. Ceftazidime compared with piperacillin and tobramycin for the empiric treatment of fever in neutropenic patients with cancer. A multicenter randomized trial. The Intercontinental Antimicrobial Study Group. *Ann Intern Med* 1994; 120(10):834–844.

96. Mahendra P, Jacobson SK, Ager S, et al. Short-course intravenous antibiotics with oral quinolone prophylaxis in the treatment of neutropenic fever in autologous bone marrow or peripheral blood progenitor cell transplant recipients. *Acta Haematologica* 1996;96(2):64–67.

97. Avril M, Hartmann O, Valteau-Couanet D, et al. Anti-infective prophylaxis with ceftazidime and teicoplanin in children undergoing high-dose chemotherapy and bone marrow transplantation. *Pediatr Hematol Oncol* 1994;11(1):63–73.

98. Gilbert C, Meisenberg B, Vredenburgh J, et al. Sequential prophylactic oral and empiric once-daily parenteral antibiotics for neutropenia and fever after high-dose chemotherapy and autologous bone marrow support. *J Clin Oncol* 1994;12(5):1005–1011.

99. Viscoli C, Dudley M, Ferrea G, et al. Serum concentrations and safety of single daily dosing of amikacin in children undergoing bone marrow transplantation. *J Antimicrob Chemother* 1991;27[Suppl C]: 113–120.

100. Hughes WT, Armstrong D, Bodey GP, et al. Guidelines for the use of antimicrobial agents in neutropenic patients with unexplained fever. *Clin Infect Dis* 1997;25:551–573.

101. Saarinen UM, Hovi L, Juvonen E, et al. Granulocyte colony-stimulating factor after allogeneic and autologous bone marrow transplantation in children. *Med Pediatr Oncol* 1996;26(6):380–386.

102. Vose JM, Bierman PJ, Kessinger A, et al. The use of recombinant human granulocyte-macrophage colony stimulating factor for the treatment of delayed engraftment following high dose therapy and autologous hematopoietic stem cell transplantation for lymphoid malignancies. *Bone Marrow Transplant* 1991;7(2):139–143.

103. Link H, Boogaerts MA, Carella AM, et al. A controlled trial of recombinant human granulocyte-macrophage colony-stimulating factor after total body irradiation, high-dose chemotherapy, and autologous bone marrow transplantation for acute lymphoblastic leukemia or malignant lymphoma. *Blood* 1992;80(9):2188–2195.

104. Torres Gomez A, Jimenez MA, Alvarez MA, et al. Optimal timing of granulocyte colony-stimulating factor (G-CSF) administration after bone marrow transplantation. A prospective randomized study. *Ann Hematol* 1995;71(2):65–70.

105. Vey N, Molnar S, Faucher C, et al. Delayed administration of granulocyte colony-stimulating factor after autologous bone marrow transplantation: effect on granulocyte recovery. *Bone Marrow Transplant* 1994;14(5):779–782.

106. Grigg A, Vecchi L, Bardy P, et al. G-CSF stimulated donor granulocyte collections for prophylaxis and therapy of neutropenic sepsis. *Austral NZ J Med* 1996;26(6):813–818.

107. Salmela K, Eklund B, Kyllonen L, et al. The effect of intravesically applied antibiotic solution in the prophylaxis of infectious complications of renal transplantation. *Transplant Int* 1990;3(1):12–14.

108. Wells CL, Podzorski RP, Peterson PK, et al. Incidence of trimethoprim sulfamethoxazole resistant Enterobacteriaceae among transplant recipients. *J Infect Dis* 1984;150(5):699–706.

109. Ridge JA, Manco-Johnson ML, Weil R 3d: Ultrasonographic diagnosis of infected lymphocele after kidney transplantation. *Eur Urol* 1987;13(1-2):31–34.

110. Indudhara R, Menon M, Khauli RB. Post-transplant lymphocele presenting as "acute abdomen." *Am J Nephrology* 1994;14(2):154–156.

111. Judson RT. Wound infection following renal transplantation. *Austral NZ J Surg* 1984;54(3):223–224.

112. Lorber MI, Campbell DA Jr, Konnak JW, et al. Etiology and management of early and late peritransplant infections. *J Urol* 1982;127(5): 870–872.

113. Yang CW, Kim YS, Yang KH, et al. Acute focal bacterial nephritis presented as acute renal failure and hepatitic dysfunction in a renal transplant recipient. *Am J Nephrol* 1994;14(1):72–75.

114. Hess B, Metzger RM, Ackermann D, et al. Infection-induced stone formation in a renal allograft. *Am J Kidney Dis* 1994;24(5):868–872.

115. Bentley FR, Garrison RN. Superior results with combined kidney-pancreas transplants. *Am Surgeon* 1992;58(2):136–140.

116. Bac DJ. Spontaneous bacterial peritonitis: an indication for liver transplantation? [Review] *Scand J Gastroenterol* 1996;218[Suppl]: 38–42.

117. Altman C, Grange JD, Amiot X, et al. Survival after a first episode of spontaneous bacterial peritonitis. Prognosis of potential candidates for orthotopic liver transplantation. *J Gastroenterol Hepatol* 1995;10(1): 47–50.

118. Rolando N, Philpott-Howard J, Williams R, et al. Bacterial and fungal infection in acute liver failure. [Review] *Semin Liver Dis* 1996;16(4): 389–402.

119. Cuervas-Mons V, Julio Martinez A, Dekker A, et al. Adult liver transplantation: an analysis of the early causes of death in 40 consecutive cases. *Hepatology* 1986;6(3):495–501.

120. Gorensek MJ, Carey WD, Washington JA 2d. Selective bowel decontamination with quinolones and nystatin reduces gram-negative and fungal infections in orthotopic liver transplant recipients. *Cleveland Clin J Med* 1993;60(2):139–144.

121. Wiesner RH, Hermans PE, Rakela J, et al. Selective bowel decontamination to decrease gram-negative aerobic bacterial and *Candida* colonization and prevent infection after orthotopic liver transplantation. *Transplantation* 1988;45(3):570–574.

122. Lumbreras C, Lizasoain M, Moreno E, et al. Major bacterial infections following liver transplantation: a prospective study. *Hepato-Gastroenterol* 1992;39(4):362–365.

123. Steffen R, Reinhartz O, Blumhardt G, et al. Bacterial and fungal col-

onization and infections using oral selective bowel decontamination in orthotopic liver transplantations. *Transplant Int* 1994;7(2): 101–108.

124. Arnow PM, Carandang GC, Zabner R, et al. Randomized controlled trial of selective bowel decontamination for prevention of infections following liver transplantation. *Clin Infect Dis* 1996;22(6):997–1003.

125. Arnow PM. Prevention of bacterial infection in the transplant recipient. The role of selective bowel decontamination. [Review] *Infect Dis Clin North Am* 1995;9(4):849–862.

126. Hadley S, Samore MH, Lewis WD, et al. Major infectious complications after orthotopic liver transplantation and comparison of outcomes in patients receiving cyclosporine or FK506 as primary immunosuppression. *Transplantation* 1995;59(6):851–859.

127. Wade JJ, Rolando N, Hayllar K, et al. Bacterial and fungal infections after liver transplantation: an analysis of 284 patients *Hepatology* 1995;21(5):1328–1336.

128. Afesssa B, Gay PC, Plevak DJ, et al. Pulmonary complications of orthotopic liver transplantation. *Mayo Clin Proc* 1993;68(5):427–434.

129. Bion JF, Badger I, Crosby HA, et al. Selective decontamination of the digestive tract reduces gram-negative pulmonary colonization but not systemic endotoxemia in patients undergoing elective liver transplantation. *Crit Care Med* 1994;22(1):40–49.

130. Mermel LA, Maki DG. Bacterial pneumonia in solid organ transplantation. *Semin Respir Infect* 1990;5(1):10–29.

131. Cooper DK, Lanza RP, Oliver S, et al. Infectious complications after heart transplantation. *Thorax* 1983;38(11):822–828.

132. Green M, Wald ER, Fricker FJ, et al. Infections in pediatric orthotopic heart transplant recipients. *Pediatr Infect Dis J* 1989;8(2):87–93.

133. Prieto M, Lake KD, Pritzker MR, et al. OKT3 induction and steroid-free maintenance immunosuppression for treatment of high-risk heart transplant recipients. *J Heart Lung Transplant* 1991;10(6):901–911.

134. Smart FW, Naftel DC, Costanzo MR, et al. Risk factors for early, cumulative, and fatal infections after heart transplantation: a multi-institutional study. *J Heart Lung Transplant* 1996;15(4):329–341.

135. Foerster A, Abdelnoor M, Geiran O, et al. Morbidity risk factors in human cardiac transplantation. Histoincompatibility and protracted graft ischemia entail high risk of rejection and infection. *Scand J Thorac Cardiovasc Surg* 1992;26(3):169–176.

136. Fischer SA, Trenholme GM, Costanzo MR, et al. Infectious complications in left ventricular assist device recipients. *Clin Infect Dis* 1997;24(1):18–23.

137. Baldwin RT, Radovancevic B, Sweeney MS, et al. Bacterial mediastinitis after heart transplantation. *J Heart Lung Transplant* 1992;11(3 pt 1):545–549.

138. Slater D, Ganzel BL, Keller M, et al. Repair of infected pseudoaneurysm with aortic arch replacement after orthotopic heart transplantation. *J Heart Transplant* 1990;9(3 pt 1):230–235.

139. Quirce R, Serano J, Arnal C, et al. Detection of mediastinitis after heart transplantation by gallium-67 scintigraphy. *J Nuclear Med* 1991;32(5):860–861.

140. Holman WL, Murrah CP, Ferguson ER, et al. Infections during extended circulatory support: University of Alabama at Birmingham experience 1989 to 1994; *Ann Thorac Surg* 1996;61(1):366–371.

141. McCarthy PM, Schmitt SK, Vargo RL, et al. Implantable LVAD infections: implications for permanent use of the device. *Ann Thorac Surg* 1996;61(1):359–365.

142. Davies RA, Newton G, Masters RG, et al. Bacterial pericarditis after heart transplantation: successful management of two cases with catheter drainage and antibiotics. *Can J Cardiol* 1996;12(7):641–644.

143. Herrmann M, Weyand M, Greshake B, et al. Left ventricular assist device infection is associated with increased mortality but is not a contraindication to transplantation. *Circulation* 1997;95(4): 814–817.

144. McGiffin DC, Galbraith AJ, McCarthy JB, et al. Mycotic false aneurysm of the aortic suture line after heart transplantation. *J Heart Lung Transplant* 1994;13(5):926–928.

145. Copeland JG, Riley JE, Fuller J. Pericardiectomy for effusive constrictive pericarditis after heart transplantation. *J Heart Transplant* 1986;5(2):171–172.

146. Bull DA, Stahl RD, McMahan DL, et al. The high risk heart donor: potential pitfalls. *J Heart Lung Transplant* 1995;14(3):424–428.

147. Lammermeier DE, Sweeney MS, Haupt HE, et al. Use of potentially infected donor hearts for cardiac transplantation. *Ann Thorac Surg* 1990;50(2):222–225.

148. Anguita M, Arizon JM, Valles F, et al. Results of heart transplantation

in recipients with active infection. *J Heart Lung Transplant* 1993; 12(5):808–809.

149. Reid KR, Menkis AH, Novick RJ, et al. Reduced incidence of severe infection after heart transplantation with low-intensity immunosuppression. *J Heart Lung Transplant* 1991;10(6):894–900.

150. Livi U, Luciani GB, Boffa GM, et al. Clinical results of steroid-free induction immunosuppression after heart transplantation. *Ann Thorac Surg* 1993;55(5):1160–1165.

151. Grattan MT, Moreno-Cabral CE, Starnes VA, et al. Eight-year results of cyclosporine-treated patients with cardiac transplants. *J Thorac Cardiovasc Surg* 1990;99(3):500–509.

152. Deusch E, End A, Grimm M, et al. Early bacterial infections in lung transplant recipients. *Chest* 1993;104(5):1412–1416.

153. Chaparro C, Maurer JR, Chamberlain D, et al. Causes of death in lung transplant recipients. *J Heart Lung Transplant* 1994;13(5):758–766.

154. Egan TM, Detterbeck FC, Mill MR, et al. Improved results of lung transplantation for patients with cystic fibrosis. *J Thorac Cardiovasc Surg* 1995;109(2):224–234.

155. Speziali G, McDougall JC, Midthun DE, et al. Native lung complications after single lung transplantation for emphysema. *Transplant Int* 1997;10(2):113–115.

156. Hasan A, Corris PA, Healy M, et al. Bilateral sequential lung transplantation for end stage septic lung disease. *Thorax* 1995;50(5): 565–566.

157. Egan TM, Westerman JH, Lambert CJ Jr, et al. Isolated lung transplantation for end-stage lung disease: a viable therapy. *Ann Thorac Surg* 1992;53(4):590–595.

158. Ramirez JC, Patterson GA, Winton TL, et al. Bilateral lung transplantation for cystic fibrosis. The Toronto Lung Transplant Group. *J Thorac Cardiovasc Surg* 1992;103(2):287–293.

159. Dennis CM, McNeil KD, Dunning J, et al. Heart-lung-liver transplantation. *J Heart Lung Transplant* 1996;15(5):536–538.

160. Flume PA, Egan TM, Paradowski LJ, et al. Infectious complications of lung transplantation. Impact of cystic fibrosis. *Am J Respir Crit Care Med* 1994;149(6):1601–1607.

161. Dummer JS, Montero CG, Griffith BP, et al. Infections in heart-lung transplant recipients. *Transplantation* 1986;41(6):725–729.

162. Zenati M, Dowling RD, Dummer JS, et al. Influence of the donor lung on development of early infections in lung transplant recipients. *J Heart Transplant* 1990;9(5):502–508.

163. Saiman L, Mehar F, Niu WW, et al. Antibiotic susceptibility of multiply resistant Pseudomonas aeruginosa isolated from patients with cystic fibrosis, including candidates for transplantation. *Clin Infect Dis* 1996;23(3):532–537.

164. Noyes BE, Michaels MG, Kurland G, et al. *Pseudomonas cepacia* empyema necessitatis after lung transplantation in two patients with cystic fibrosis. *Chest* 1994;105(6):1888–1891.

165. Herridge MS, de Hoyos AL, Chaparro C, et al. Pleural complications in lung transplant recipients. *J Thorac Cardiovasc Surg* 1995;110(1): 22–26.

166. Shennib H, Noirclerc M, Ernst P, et al. Double-lung transplantation for cystic fibrosis. The Cystic Fibrosis Transplant Study Group. *Ann Thorac Surg* 1992;54(1):27–31.

167. Scott JP, Higenbottam TW, Sharples L, et al. Risk factors for obliterative bronchiolitis in heart-lung transplant recipients. *Transplantation* 1991;51(4):813–817.

168. Mallory, GB Jr. Major medical complications of lung transplantation: a pediatric perspective. [Review] *Semin Thorac Cardiovasc Surg* 1996;8(3):305–312.

169. Keenan RJ, Konishi H, Kawai A, et al. Clinical trial of tacrolimus versus cyclosporine in lung transplantation. *Ann Thorac Surg* 1995; 60(3):580–584.

170. Dhar JM, Al-Khadel AA, Al-Sulaiman M, et al. Non-typhoid *Salmonella* in renal transplant recipients: a report of twenty cases and a review of the literature. *Q J Med* 1991;78:235–250.

171. Wheat LJ, Rubin RH, Harris NL, et al. Systemic salmonellosis in patients with disseminated histoplasmosis. Case for "macrophage blockage" caused by *Histoplasma capsulatum*. *Arch Intern Med* 1987;147(3):561–564.

172. Berk MR, Meyers AM, Cassal W, et al. Non-typhoidal salmonella infections after renal transplantation. A serious clinical problem. *Nephron* 1984;37(3):186–189.

173. Huang JY, Huang CC, Lai MK, et al. *Salmonella* infection in renal transplant recipients. *Transplant Proc* 1994;26:2147.

174. Hashino S, Imamura M, Tanaka J, et al. Renal *Salmonella enteritidis*

abscess in a patient with severe aplastic anemia after allogeneic stem cell transplantation. *Bone Marrow Transplant* 1996;18(4):807–808.

175. Smith EJ, Milligan SL, Filo RS. Salmonella mycotic aneurysm after renal transplantation. *Southern Med J* 1981;74(11):1399–1401.

176. Bogers AJ, van't Wout JW, Cats VM, et al. Mediastinal rupture of a thoracoabdominal mycotic aneurysm caused by *Salmonella typhimurium* in an immunocompromised patient. *Eur J Cardio-Thorac Surg* 1987;1(2):116–118.

177. US Public Health Service/Infectious Diseases Society of America Guidelines for the Prevention of Opportunistic Infections in Persons Infected with HIV. *MMWR* 1997;46(RR-12):1–31.

178. Rao KV, Ralston RA. Meningitis due to *Campylobacter fetus intestinalis* in a kidney transplant recipient. A case report. *Am J Nephrology* 1987;7(5):402–403.

179. Ali A, Mehra MR, Stapleton DD, et al. *Vibrio vulnificus* sepsis in solid organ transplantation: a medical nemesis. *J Heart Lung Transplant* 1995;14(3):598–600.

180. Moses AE, Leibergal M, Rahav G, et al. *Aeromonas hydrophila* myonecrosis accompanying mucormycosis five years after bone marrow transplantation. [Review] *Eur J Clin Microbiol Infect Dis* 1995; 14(3):237–240.

181. Lee AC, Yuen KY, Ha SY, et al. *Plesiomonas shigelloides* septicemia; case report and literature review. [Review] *Pediatr Hematol Oncol* 1996;13(3):265–269.

182. Bilgrami, S, Bergstrom SK, Peterson DE, et al. Capnocytophagia

bacteremia in a patient with Hodgkin's disease following bone marrow transplantation: case report and review. [Review] *Clin Infect Dis* 1992;14(5):1045–1049.

183. Muder RR, Harris AP, Muller S, et al. Bacteremia due to *Stenotrophomonas* (*Xanthomonas*) *maltophilia*: a prospective, multicenter study of 91 episodes. *Clin Infect Dis* 1996;22(3):508–512.

184. Martino R, Martinez C, Pericas R, et al. Bacteremia due to glucose non-fermenting gram-negative bacilli in patients with hematological neoplasias and solid tumors. *Eur J Clin Microbiol Infect Dis* 1996; 15(7):610–615.

185. Cover TL, Appelbaum PC, Aber RC. *Pseudomonas paucimobilis* empyema after cardiac transplantation. *South Med J* 1988;81(6): 796–798.

186. Collini FJ, Spees EK, Munster A, et al. *Ecthyma gangrenosum* in a kidney transplant recipient with *Pseudomonas* septicemia. *Am J Med* 1986;80(4):729–734.

187. Murphy JJ, Granger R, Blair GK, et al. Necrotizing fasciitis in childhood. *J Pediatr Surg* 1995;30(8):1131–1134.

188. Kanj SS, Tapson V, David RD, et al. Infections in patients with cystic fibrosis following lung transplantation. *Chest* 1997;112(4):924–930.

189. Sanders C. Cefepime: the next generation? *Clin Infect Dis* 1993;17: 369–379.

190. Limaze A, Gautom RK, Black D, Fritsche TR. Rapid emergence of resistance to cefepime during treatment. *Clin Infect Dis* 1997;25: 339–340.

Transplant Infections edited by
Raleigh A. Bowden, Per Ljungman, and Carlos V. Paya.
Lippincott–Raven Publishers, Philadelphia © 1998

CHAPTER 14

Typical and Atypical Mycobacterium

Vivek Roy and Daniel Weisdorf

INTRODUCTION

Bacteriology

Mycobacteria are a group of organisms that share the staining characteristic referred to as *acid fastness*. These include the organisms causing tuberculosis (*Mycobacterium tuberculosis* and *M. bovis*) and a variety of other mycobacterial species of varying pathogenicity and clinical importance. The term *acid-fast bacilli* (AFB) is, practically speaking, the identifying feature of mycobacteria, although some other microbial agents, notably nocardia, are variably acid-fast.

From a clinical standpoint, mycobacteria can be divided into two broad classes: those causing tuberculosis (*M. tuberculosis* and *M. bovis*) and the rest. These organisms are also referred to as typical and atypical mycobacteria, respectively. The atypical mycobacteria have also been called anonymous mycobacteria, or Mycobacteria Other Than Tuberculosis (MOTT). *M. tuberculosis* can be differentiated from other mycobacteria by their *in vitro* culture characteristics as they grow slowly, lack pigment, produce niacin, and are usually sensitive to isoniazid (INH). The atypical mycobacteria are usually niacin negative, produce heat-resistant catalase in large amounts, and are highly resistant to INH. In stained preparation, *M. tuberculosis* demonstrates serpentine cord formation, whereas nontuberculous atypical mycobacteria orient randomly. Using culture characteristics of mycobacteria, Timpe and Runyon proposed a useful method of classification based on colony characteristics, rate of growth in culture, and pigment production (1,2). The four major groups are referred to as photochromogens, scotochro-

mogens, nonchromogens, and rapidly growing mycobacteria. Recently, more sophisticated methods have been used to speciate mycobacteria in culture. These include DNA hybridization methods using highly specific DNA probes, or computer-assisted gas liquid chromatography (3,4). These techniques can readily speciate mycobacteria but are time and labor intensive, require pure cultures, and are available only in specialized laboratories.

Epidemiology and Pathogenesis

Mycobacterium tuberculosis is an aerobic, non-spore-forming, nonmotile, slow-growing bacillus with a lipid-rich cell wall. Humans are the only known reservoir of this organism. Almost all infections are due to inhalation of infectious particles aerosolized by coughing, sneezing, or talking. *M. tuberculosis* can survive only for very short periods outside the human body. Fomites, therefore, are rarely responsible for transmitting infection. *M. tuberculosis* is rarely, if ever, a commensal. Isolation of *M. tuberculosis* from pathological specimens should therefore always be considered evidence of infection.

Atypical mycobacteria are free-living organisms that are ubiquitous in nature. They have been found in soil, water, domestic and wild animals, milk, and fruit products. They have been known to colonize body surfaces and secretions, and frequently can contaminate clinical specimens from the environment (5–8). Therefore, unlike *M. tuberculosis* in which isolation of even a single colony is considered evidence of infection and always clinically significant, atypical mycobacterial species may colonize body surfaces and secretions for prolonged periods without causing disease. The differentiation between contamination, colonization, and disease can often be difficult. Guidelines have been proposed to facilitate such decision making (9,10). A clinical syndrome consistent with atypical mycobacterial infection, isolation of a species known to cause human disease, culture of the pathogen from a normally sterile site such as cerebrospinal fluid or liver

V R: From the Division of Hematology-Oncology, Bone Marrow Transplantation Program, Department of Medicine, University of Oklahoma Health Sciences Center, Oklahoma City, OK 73104. DW: From the Division of Hematology, Oncology and Transplantation, Department of Medicine, University of Minnesota Medical School, Minneapolis, MN 55455.

biopsy and/or repeated isolation of potential pathogens are strong arguments in favor of their clinical significance.

Host immunity plays an important role in the pathogenesis of tuberculosis infections. In the presence of normal host immune function, organization of lymphocytes, macrophages, and Langerhans' giant cells results in granuloma formation and containment of infection. When the host immunity is compromised, tissue reaction can be minimal or nonexistent and uncontrolled proliferation of mycobacteria can continue without granuloma formation. Patients undergoing bone marrow or solid organ transplantation require potent and often prolonged immunosuppressive therapy. These patients are therefore at increased risk of a variety of infections, including mycobacterial infections. Furthermore, because the host response to these infections is modified, these patients may often present with atypical features, making diagnosis difficult.

BONE MARROW TRANSPLANTS

Epidemiology of Mycobacterial Infections in BMT Recipients

Patients receiving allogeneic or autologous transplant are severely immunocompromised as a result of their underlying condition, pretransplant chemotherapy and radiation therapy, and graft-versus-host disease (GVHD). A high incidence of a variety of infections has been described in these patients. However, the literature describing mycobacterial infections in bone marrow transplant (BMT) recipients is relatively sparse, and studies have not consistently shown a high incidence of mycobacterial infections. The literature regarding the epidemiology of mycobacterial infections in BMT recipients is summarized in Table 1.

Navari and colleagues (11) reported seven mycobacterial infections in their series of 682 patients (about 1%) with acute leukemia who received allogeneic marrow grafts. There were four pulmonary and three extra-pulmonary infections with *M. tuberculosis* or atypical mycobacteria. In a report from M.D. Anderson Hospital published in 1984, Kurzrock and colleagues (12) reported three patients with mycobacterial infections in a series of 90 (3.3%) allogeneic marrow transplants for hematologic malignancies or aplastic anemia. There were two infections with *M. tuberculosis* and one with *M. avium-intracellulare* (MAI). The two patients with *M. tuberculosis* infections were from Latin America, a high-prevalence area for tuberculosis. The authors emphasized difficulties in making a specific diagnosis due to unusual presentations, often involving more than one pathogen.

In a recent study from the University of Minnesota (13), we reviewed our experience with mycobacterial infections following BMT over a 20-year period. Eleven mycobacterial infections were diagnosed out of 2,241 (0.49%) recipients of allogeneic (nine of 1,486) or autologous (two of 755) marrow transplants. There were two patients with *M. tuberculosis*, two with MAI, and seven with infections due to rapid-growing atypical mycobacteria (*M. fortuitum* or *M. chelonae*). There have been several additional case reports of both typical and atypical mycobacterial infections in BMT recipients (14–16). These reports emphasize the variety of unusual presentations of mycobacterial infection in BMT patients and the generally successful treatment outcome with appropriate therapy.

The incidence of mycobacterial infections in BMT patients, although higher than that in the general popula-

TABLE 1. *Clinical reports of mycobacterial infections after bone marrow transplantation*

	Reference		
	Navari et al. (11)	Kurzrock et al. (12)	Roy et al. (13)
Patients, N =	682	90	2241
Mycobacterial infections (%)	7 (1%)	3 (3.3%)	11 (0.49%) 9 of 11 Allo. recipients
Sex (M/F)	5/2	3/0	6/5
Transplant type	Allo. BMT	Allo. BMT	Allo. BMT (1486)
			Auto. BMT (755)
Organism:			
M. tuberculosis	2	2	2 (both Allo.)
Atypical Mycobacteria	5	1	9 (7 Allo., 2-Auto.)
Site of infection:			
Pulmonary only	4	3	2
Nonpulmonary or disseminated	3	—	9
Interval from transplant	2–3 m	2–11 m	All <100 days
Co-morbidity at time of Mycobacterial infection	NR	All had acute or chronic GVHD	5 (GVHD, prolonged neutropenia ± bacterial infection
Infection outcome	6/6 treated resolved	NR	9/9 treated resolved

Allo, allogeneic; Auto, autologous; BMT, bone marrow transplant; GVHD, graft-versus-host disease; Myc, mycobacteria; NR, not reported.

tion, is not as high as that seen in organ transplant recipients or in patients with AIDS. This may be due, at least in part, to prolonged duration of immunosuppression in the latter groups of patients compared with the usual BMT patient. Marrow allograft recipients typically recover adequate immune function in 9–12 months, unlike organ transplant recipients or AIDS patients, who experience immune suppression for several years or throughout their lives. Therefore the transient immune compromise in BMT patients may induce only a limited risk of infection compared with organ allografts or AIDS patients.

Clinical Manifestations and Diagnosis of Mycobacterial Infections in BMT Recipients

Atypical presentations make recognition of mycobacterial infections in BMT recipients difficult. These patients are severely immunocompromised and often neutropenic, which can mask febrile response and obscure a granulomatous reaction. Presenting features are nonspecific and related to the site of infection. In our review of mycobacterial infections in 2,241 transplant recipients over a 20-year period at the University of Minnesota (13), the clinical manifestations of mycobacterial infection included unexplained fever, pulmonary infiltrates, osteomyelitis, or central venous catheter tunnel inflammation. The most common manifestation of mycobacterial infection in our patients was central venous catheter-related infection, which occurred in 6 of 11 patients. All central venous catheter-related infections were due to atypical, rapid-growing mycobacteria.

Invasive procedures may be required to obtain diagnostic material for culture or histopathology. Because laboratory diagnosis of mycobacterial infection requires specific cultures, often held for prolonged periods (3,4), a high index of suspicion is required to specifically request appropriate diagnostic studies to identify these infections. BMT recipients often have coexisting multiple infectious pathogens, which can mask the existence or the significance of mycobacterial isolates. Although mycobacterial infections are uncommon in BMT patients, they should be considered in all apparently affected BMT recipients, particularly those at high risk because of previous tuberculosis exposure, positive purified protein derivative (PPD) skin test, residence in endemic area, or ethnic background.

Treatment of Mycobacterial Infections in BMT Recipients

As in non-BMT patients, the treatment of tuberculosis in BMT recipients is with a combination of antimycobacterial agents. Isoniazid (INH) and rifampin are almost always used for 12–18 months, with additional one or two drugs for the initial 2–4 months. We and others have reported that despite continuing immunosuppression, BMT recipients with tuberculosis respond to standard antimycobacterial therapy (11–13,15), but extensive data on clinical and bacteriological responses are not available. It is important to remember that atypical mycobacteria are often not susceptible to the agents typically used to treat tuberculosis. Furthermore, drug susceptibilities of atypical mycobacteria are often unpredictable. Therefore *in vitro* drug sensitivity assays should always be performed and treatment revised if resistance to any of the drugs being used is demonstrated.

Drug-resistant tuberculosis has been reported in many endemic areas and in patients with AIDS. As yet there have been no reports of drug-resistant tuberculosis in BMT recipients, but that possibility should be kept in mind when the patient comes from an endemic area with a high incidence of drug-resistant tuberculosis. Certain drugs used to treat tuberculosis can have important side effects and drug interactions in BMT patients. INH may cause transplant-related liver toxicity and often needs to be discontinued in the immediate post-transplant period. Rifampin, a hepatic P-450 enzyme inducer, can accelerate cyclosporine metabolism, resulting in subtherapeutic levels and increasing the risk of GVHD or graft rejection.

Prophylaxis of Mycobacterial Infections in BMT Recipients

High-risk patients can be readily identified during pretransplant evaluation based on history of previous exposure to tuberculosis, PPD skin reactivity, or residence in endemic areas. Previous Bacille Calmette Guerin (BCG) immunotherapy has been reported to result in reactivation following transplant (11). INH chemoprophylaxis has been suggested for patients with previous BCG vaccination (11), but there is scant definitive data to quantify the risk posed by previous BCG vaccination, or the benefit of INH chemoprophylaxis. Optimal prophylaxis for high-risk patients remains unclear. Patients identified to be PPD reactive during pretransplant evaluation are often placed on INH chemoprophylaxis, starting before transplant and continuing during the transplant period. However, the efficacy of this approach has not been critically evaluated in the BMT setting, and the duration of needed therapy is unknown. Potential problems with INH therapy include liver toxicity, neuropathy, and drug interaction with cyclosporine. INH therapy often needs to be interrupted in BMT patients who develop liver function abnormalities, a particularly common problem in the transplant setting. A clinical strategy of aggressive surveillance in high-risk patients, maintenance of high index of suspicion, early diagnosis, and prompt treatment is most likely to be effective in limiting morbidity and mortality from mycobacterial infections in BMT recipients.

SOLID ORGAN TRANSPLANTS

Immune Defects in Solid Organ Transplant Recipients

Several factors contribute to the high incidence of infection in solid organ transplant recipients. These patients are often immunosuppressed because of their underlying condition (e.g., uremia, liver failure, and/or malnutrition). In addition, therapeutic immunosuppression to prevent graft rejection is probably the most important factor contributing to infection in transplant recipients (17). Although agents differ in their mechanism of action and the aspects of immune function primarily affected by them, all agents have increased infection risk as one of their major side effects. The ideal immunosuppressive agent, which would prevent graft rejection while preserving antimicrobial immunity, is unavailable.

Corticosteroids are commonly included in most immunosuppressive regimens to prevent graft rejections. The spectrum of host defense defects induced by corticosteroids includes suppression of macrophage function, blunting of acute inflammation, inhibition of T-cell activation cascade leading to impaired cellular immunity, and impaired antibody production (18–20). Corticosteroid effects appear to be dose dependent, although a threshold dose below which immune function is not affected is not apparent (21,22). Azathioprine, a purine analog, is commonly part of immunosuppressive regimens to prevent organ allograft rejection. After *in vivo* conversion to 6- mercaptopurine, it inhibits purine nucleotide synthesis, thereby preventing antigen-induced lymphocyte proliferation and leading to impaired NK cell activity, generation of cytotoxic T cells, and antibody production by B cells (23). In addition, azathioprine is myelosuppressive and the resulting leukopenia further adds to the infection risk.

Cyclosporine A, introduced in the early 1980s, has had a major impact on the prevention of graft rejection and improvement in graft survival rates. Unlike corticosteroids and cytotoxic agents, cyclosporine has a narrowly focused effect on T-helper cells and spares cytotoxic T-cell function (24). Its major action is to block the antigen-induced T-cell expression of lymphokines, including IL-2, IL-3, IL-4, Interferon-γ, and TNF-α (25,26). NK cells and macrophages are unaffected by cyclosporine. Unlike azathioprine and other cytotoxic agents, cyclosporine does not result in bone marrow suppression.

Patients receiving cyclosporine-containing immunosuppressive regimens are at a lower infection risk than those receiving noncyclosporine immunosuppressive regimens (27,28). The risk of mycobacterial infections in cyclosporine-treated patients also appears to be less than that in noncyclosporine-treated patients (29),

although randomized comparative studies reporting risks of mycobacterial infections are not available. FK506 (tacrolimus) is nearly 10 times more potent than cyclosporine and has a similar mechanism of action. The risk of infection in FK506-treated patients is expected to be similar to that in cyclosporine-treated patients.

Antilymphocyte globulin (ALG), antithymocyte globulin (ATG), and more recently monoclonal anti-T-cell antibodies (OKT3) have been used for treatment of graft rejection. A significant increase in the incidence of bacterial and viral infections has been reported with the use of these agents. However, specific data about the effect of these agents on mycobacterial infections are not available (30,32).

Epidemiology of Mycobacterial Infections in Organ Transplant Recipients

The literature regarding epidemiology of mycobacterial infections in organ transplant recipients is summarized in Table 2.

In contrast to BMT patients, solid organ transplant recipients typically remain immunosuppressed for long periods of time or for life. Consistent with this is the observation that mycobacterial infections generally occur later in organ transplant patients compared with patients who receive BMT. Infections were diagnosed a mean of 48 months after transplant, with rare infections reported as late as 269 months following transplant (33,34). This contrasts with the experience in BMT patients, where almost all infections occur early in the course of the transplant (13). A higher incidence of *M. tuberculosis* and nontubercular mycobacterial infections has been reported in renal transplant recipients than in the general population. A 0.5% to 0.7% incidence of tuberculosis was reported from three U.S. renal transplant centers (35–37) in comparison to the incidence in the general population of 0.01% (38). In contrast, much higher incidences, between 3.5% and 11.8%, have been reported from centers in areas endemic for tuberculosis (39–41). Patients undergoing liver or heart transplantation also have higher rates of mycobacterial infections than the general population; the reported incidences varied between 0.95% and 2.7% (29,33,34). Nontuberculous mycobacterial infections after solid organ transplants have been reported mainly as case reports, which prevents a reliable estimation of the incidence of such infections in these patients. These are usually caused by *M. avium-intracellulare* (MAI), *M. kansasi*, *M. chelonae*, *M. fortuitum*, and rarely other species (29,33). Diagnosis is most frequent within the first year following transplant but can be as late as 11 years following transplant (mean 3.5 years) (29). Patients present with isolated pulmonary infections, cutaneous lesions, tenosynovitis, joint infections, or infection of surgical wounds (29,33).

TABLE 2. *Summary of reports of mycobacterial infections after solid organ transplantation*

Reference	Delaney (37)	Qunibi* (40)	Hall* (43)	Malhotra* (39)	Sakhuja* (41)	Munoz (34)	Novick (29)	Meyers (42)
Patients N =	1097	403	487	95	305	144	502	550
Mycobacterial infections N (%)	10(0.9%)	14(3.5%)	22(4.5%)	9(9.5%)	36(11.8%)	3(2%)	14(2.8%)	5(0.9%)
Sex (M/F)	NR	11/3	14/7 (M. Tb only reported)	9/0	31/5	2/1	13/1	3/2
Transplant	Renal	Renal	Renal	Renal	Renal	Heart	Heart	Liver
Organism:								
M. tuberculosis	6	14	21	9	36	3	0	5
Atypical mycobacteria	4	—	1	—	—	0	14	0
Site of infection:								
Pulmonary only	4	4	16	5	15	2	4	1
Nonpulmonary or disseminated	6	10	5	4	14 (+7 FUO)	1	10	4
Interval from transplant	NR	1–84 m	2–74 m (median 14 m)	2–32 m	median 1 yr.	50–102 d	86 d– 11.5 year.	2–57 m
Co-morbidity at time of mycobacterial infection	1 HIV+, 4 (acute rejection)	NR	9 (recent increase in immune suppression)	NR	NR	2 (acute) rejection	↑incidence of rejection episodes	4 (rejection)
Infection outcome	7 R, 3 URD	12 R, 1D, 1URD,	1 NT, 1 D, 3 URD, 12 R, 5 NR	2 PMDx, 2 URD, 5 R	2 D, 5 URD, 18 R, 11 LTF	3 R	1D, 12/12 treated R, 1 NT	2 D, 3R

D, death related to mycobacterial infection; FUO, fever of unknown origin; LTF, lost to follow up; Myc, mycobacteria; NR, not reported; NT, not treated; PMDx, postmortem diagnosis; R, resolved; URD, death unrelated to mycobacterial infection.

*Indicates report from an area of high prevalence rate of tuberculosis.

Clinical Manifestations and Diagnosis of Mycobacterial Infections in Organ Transplant Recipients

Tuberculosis and atypical mycobacterial infections often present with unusual features in immunocompromised patients. Patients often present with nonlocalized, systemic symptoms. Studies of tuberculosis in organ transplant recipients consistently show a high proportion of patients, up to 63%, with nonpulmonary or disseminated tuberculosis (39–42). Extra-pulmonary presentations include meningitis, peritonitis, lymphadenopathy, liver abscess, DIC, pericarditis, and renal tuberculosis (40,41,43,44). In one study 20% of renal transplant patients had a fever of unknown origin (41). Some patients may be asymptomatic and infection may be diagnosed incidentally, or rarely, at post-mortem examination (39).

Because of nonspecific clinical manifestations, the diagnosis of mycobacterial infections in organ transplant recipients can be difficult. Patients receiving immunosuppressive therapy have a blunted inflammatory response, so that characteristic granulomatous reaction to mycobacteria may not be seen. Patients may often have coexistent infectious and noninfectious complications that can add to the difficulty in diagnosis (34,40). A high index of suspicion is therefore crucial for appropriate

diagnostic work-up to be performed. Invasive procedures often may be necessary to obtain diagnostic material (33,43,45).

Treatment of Mycobacterial Infections in Organ Transplant Recipients

As in the general population, treatment of tuberculosis in organ transplant recipients involves therapy with combination antituberculous agents. Most centers use a combination of isoniazid and rifampin for at least 12 months. One or two additional drugs, such as ethambutol or pyrazinamide, are often included in the treatment program for the first 2–3 months (35,39,40). Optimal duration of antituberculous therapy in these patients is controversial. Therapy is usually given for 12–18 months. Limited experience suggests that, similar to therapy in immunocompetent hosts, shorter treatment duration may be adequate. Successful outcomes with a 9-month regimen have been reported in renal transplant patients with localized pulmonary tuberculosis (41,46).

Multidrug-resistant tuberculosis has been reported in several endemic areas and in HIV-infected patient populations around the world, including the United States. Although drug-resistant tuberculosis has not been reported in transplant recipients in the United States, drug-resistant tuberculosis in transplant recipients has been described. A renal transplant center in India reported a high incidence of primary drug-resistant tuberculosis. INH resistance was seen in seven of 23, and rifampin resistance in five of 23 *M. tuberculosis* isolates from 727 renal allograft recipients (47). This suggests that multidrug-resistant infections are likely in patients who come from communities harboring a large reservoir of drug-resistant *M. tuberculosis*. Patients residing in areas where drug-resistant tuberculosis rates are high should commence treatment with four antituberculous drugs such as INH, rifampin, ethambutol, and pyrazinamide until antimicrobial susceptibility results are available. The duration of therapy should be prolonged up to 18–24 months in patients with drug-resistant tuberculosis (48,49).

INH can cause significant hepatotoxicity in transplant patients, necessitating its discontinuation (39,41). Hepatotoxicity may be a particular problem in liver transplant recipients (50). Rifampin, a hepatic P-450 microsomal enzymes inducer, increases the clearance of prednisone and cyclosporine, lowering their effective blood levels and thereby increasing risk of rejection. Maintenance of therapeutic cyclosporine levels requires increasing cyclosporine dose by a factor of 3–5, a costly approach. An alternative strategy is to use nonrifampin-containing regimens that generally need to be administered for longer periods of time. Comparative efficacy data on which to base recommendations regarding choice of therapy of tuberculosis in organ graft recipients are unavailable. The clinical setting, frequency of drug resistance in the community, and *in vitro* sensitivities should guide therapy.

In general, antituberculous therapy in transplant patients is effective despite continuing immunosuppression (13,34,39). However, mortality from tuberculous infections in transplant patients has been reported (40–42). The role of temporarily reducing immunosuppression to facilitate antituberculous response has been discussed in the literature without consensus. Some authors recommend routinely decreasing immunosuppression until patients' febrile illness resolves (50). Several investigators, however, report successful treatment of tuberculosis despite continuing immunosuppression (34,39,41).

Prophylaxis of Mycobacterial Infections in Organ Transplant Recipients

PPD skin test positivity and residence in an area endemic for tuberculosis identify a group of patients at high risk for developing tuberculosis. However, because only a minority of patients, even from areas of high endemicity, develop clinical infection, chemoprophylaxis of the whole population will involve unnecessary treatment for the vast majority of such patients and cannot be recommended. Many authors recommend chemoprophy-

laxis with INH for all PPD-positive patients (35,40,42). INH prophylaxis has been shown to prevent tuberculosis in a recent double-blind randomized trial in transplant recipients (51). However, because up to 80% of transplant candidates may be anergic (40,42), PPD testing is an imperfect identifier of high-risk patients. Transmission of tuberculosis by the transplanted organ has also been documented (53,54). Quinibi and colleagues suggest INH prophylaxis for PPD-negative recipients of organs from PPD-positive donors (40). Potential problems with INH prophylaxis include risk of drug-induced hepatitis (especially in older individuals), drug interaction with cyclosporine, and possibility of selecting out INH-resistant organisms.

Because of the lifelong immunosuppression in solid organ transplant recipients, post-treatment prophylaxis with INH has been proposed by some investigators (43). However, reports of successful treatment in most patients, without a significant incidence of late recurrences, argues against the need for post-treatment prophylaxis (34, 39,41).

REFERENCES

1. Timpe A, Runyon EH. Relationship of atypical acid fast bacilli to human disease. *J Lab Clin Med* 1954;44:202–209.
2. Runyon EH. Anonymous mycobacteria in pulmonary disease. *Med Clin North Am* 1959;43:273–290.
3. Johnston RF, Wildrick KH. The impact of chemotherapy on the care of patients with tuberculosis. *Am Rev Respir Dis* 1974;109:636–664.
4. Peterson EM, Lu R, Floyd C, Nakasone A, Friedly G, de la Maza LM. Direct identification of *Mycobacterium tuberculosis*, *Mycobacterium avium* and *Mycobacterium intracellulare* from amplified primary cultures in BACTEC media using DNA probes. *J Clin Microbiol* 1989;27(7):1542–1547.
5. Good RC, Snider DEJ. Isolation of nontuberculous mycobacteria in the united states, 1980. *J Infect Dis* 1982;146:829–833.
6. Gruft H, Falkinham JO, Parker BC. Recent experience in epidemiology of disease caused by atypical mycobacteria. *Rev Infect Dis* 1981; 3:990–996.
7. Woods GL, Washington JA. Mycobacteria other than *Mycobacterium tuberculosis*: review of microbiologic and clinical aspects. *Rev Infect Dis* 1987;9:275–294.
8. Wolinsky E. Nontuberculous mycobacteria and associated diseases. *Am Rev Respir Dis* 1979;119:107–159.
9. Ahn CH, McLarty JW, Ahn SS, Ahn SI, Hurst GA. Diagnostic criteria for pulmonary disease caused by *Mycobacterium kansasi* and *Mycobacterium intracellulare*. *Am Rev Respir Dis* 1982;125(4): 388–391.
10. Wallace RJ Jr, O Brien R, Glassroth J, Raleigh J, Dutt A. Diagnosis and treatment of disease caused by nontuberculous mycobacteria. *Am Rev Respir Dis* 1990;142(4):940–953.
11. Navari RM, Sullivan KM, Springmeyer SC, et al. Mycobacterial infections in marrow transplant patients. *Transplantation* 1983;36(5): 509–513.
12. Kurzrock R, Zander A, Vellekoop L, Kanojia M, Luna M, Dicke K. Mycobacterial pulmonary infections after allogeneic bone marrow transplantation. *Am J Med* 1984;77:35–40.
13. Roy V, Weisdorf D. Mycobacterial infections following bone marrow transplantation. A 20 year retrospective review. *Bone Marrow Transplant* 1997;19:467–470.
14. Beckassy AN, Miorner H, hagerstrand I, Anders F. Graft failure disclosing disseminated *Mycobacterium avium-intracellulare* infection. *Bone Marrow Transplant* 1992;10:476–476.
15. Martino R, Martinez C, Brunet S, Sureda A, Lopez R, Domingo-Albos A. Tuberculosis in bone marrow transplant recipients: report of two

cases and review of literature. *Bone Marrow Transplant* 1996;18:809–812.

16. Toren A, Ackerstein A, Gazit D, et al. Oral tuberculosis following autologous bone marrow transplantation for Hodgkin's disease with interleukin-2 and α-interferon. *Bone Marrow Transplant* 1996;18:209–210.

17. Ho M. Infection and organ transplantation. In: Gelman S, ed., *Anesthesia and organ transplantation.* Philadelphia: WB Saunders; 1987:49–60.

18. Hayes BF, Fauci AS. The differential effect of *in vivo* hydrocortisone on the kinetics of subpopulations of human peripheral blood-derived lymphocytes. *Blood* 1975;46:235–243.

19. Vernon-Roberts B. The effect of steroid hormones on macrophage activity. [Review] *Int Rev Cytol* 1969;25:131–159.

20. Saxon A, Stevens RH, Ramer SJ, Clements AJ, Yu DT. Glucocorticoids administered *in vivo* inhibit human suppressor T-lymphocyte function anddiminish B lymphocyte responsiveness in *in vitro* immunoglobulin synthesis. *J Clin Invest* 1978;61(4):922–930.

21. Anderson RJ, Schaffer LA, Olin DB, Eickhoff TC. Infectious risk factors in the immunosuppressed host. *Am J Med* 1973;54(4):453–460.

22. Gustafson TL, Schaffner W, Lavely GB, Stratton CW, Johnson HK, Hutcheson RHJ. Invasive aspergillosis in renal transplant recipients: correlation with corticosteroid therapy. *J Infect Dis* 1983;148(2):230–238.

23. Winkelstein A. The effects of Azathioprine and 6 MP on immunity. [Review] *J Immunol* 1979;1(4):429–454.

24. Kahan BD, Van Buren CT, Flechner SM, et al. Clinical and experimental studies with cyclosporin in renal transplantation. *Surgery* 1985;97(2):125–140.

25. Kronke M, Leonard WJ, Depper JM, et al. Cyclosporin A inhibits T-cell growth factor gene expression at the level of mRNA transcription. *Proc Natl Acad Sci USA* 1984;81(16):5214–5218.

26. Emmel EA, Verweij CL, Durand DB, Higgins KM, Lacy E, Crabtree GR. Cyclosporin specifically inhibits the function of nuclear proteins involved in T-cell activation. *Science* 1989;246(4937):1117–1120.

27. Najarian JS, Fryd DS, Strand M, et al. A single institution, randomized, prospective trial of cyclosporin versus azathioprine- antilymphocyte globulin for immunosuppression in renal allograft recipients. *Ann Surg* 1985;201(2):142–157.

28. Canadian Multicenter Transplant Study Group. A randomized clinical trial of cyclosporin in cadaveric renal transplantation. *N Engl J Med* 1983;309:809–815.

29. Novick RJ, Moreno-Cabral CE, Stinson EB, et al. Nontuberculous mycobacterial infections in heart transplant recipients: a seventeen-year experience. *J Heart Transplant* 1990;9:357–363.

30. Mason JW, Stinson EB, Hunt SA, Schroder JS, Rider AK. Infections after cardiac transplantation: relation to rejection therapy. *Ann Intern Med* 1976;85(1):69–72.

31. Peterson PK, Balfour HH Jr, Fryd DS, Furguson R, Kronenberg R, Simmons RL. Risk factors in the development of cytomegalovirus-related pneumonia in renal transplant recipients. *J Infect Dis* 1983;148(6):1121.

32. Singh N, Dummer JS, Kusne S, et al. Infections with cytomegalovirus and other herpesviruses in 121 liver transplant recipients: transmission by donated organ and the effect of OKT3 antibodies. *J Infect Dis* 1988;158:124–131.

33. Patel R, Roberts GD, Keating MR, Paya CV. Infections due to nontuberculous mycobacteria in kidney, heart, and liver transplant recipients. *Clin Infect Dis* 1994;19:263–273.

34. Munoz P, Palomo J, Munoz R, Rodriguez-Creixems M. Tuberculosis in heart transplant recipients. *Clin Infect Dis* 1995;21:398–402.

35. Lloveras J, Peterson PK, Simmons RL, Najarian JS. Mycobacterial infections in renal transplant recipients. Seven cases and a review of literature. *Arch Intern Med* 1982;142:888–892.

36. Lichtenstein IH, MacGregor RR. Mycobacterial infections in renal transplant recipients: report of five cases and review of literature. *Rev Infect Dis* 1983;5(2):216–226.

37. Delaney V, Sumrani N, Hong JH, Sommer B. Mycobacterial infections in renal allograft recipients. *Transplant Proc* 1993;25(3):2288–2289.

38. Jereb JA, Kelly GD, Dooley SWJ, Cauthen GM, Snider DEJ. Tuberculosis morbidity in the united states: final data, 1990. *MMWR CDC Surveillance Summaries* 1991;40(3):23–26.

39. Malhotra KK, Dash SC, Dhawan IK, Bhuyan UN, Gupta A. Tuberculosis and renal transplantation—observations from an endemic area of tuberculosis. *Postgrad Med J* 1986;62:359–362.

40. Qunibi WY, Al-Sibai MB, Taher S, et al. Mycobacterial infections after renal transplantation—report of seven cases and review of the literature. *Q J Med* 1990;77(14):1039–1060.

41. Sakhuja V, Jha V, Verma PP, Joshi K, Chugh KS. The high incidence of tuberculosis among renal transplant recipients in India. *Transplantation* 1996;61(2):211–215.

42. Meyers BR, Halpren M, Sceiner P, Mendelson MH, Neibart E, Miller C. Tuberculosis in liver transplant patients. *Transplantation* 1994;58(3):301–306.

43. Hall CM, Willcox PA, Swanepoel CR, Kahn D, van Zyl Smit R. Mycobacterial infection in renal transplant recipients. *Chest* 1994;106(2):435–439.

44. Wong LL, Levin BS, Collins GM, Bry WI. Unusual manifestations of tuberculosis in cyclosporin-treated renal transplant recipients. *Clin Transplant* 1993;7:18–24.

45. John GT, Juneja R, Mukundan U, et al. Gastric aspiration for diagnosis of pulmonary tuberculosis in adult renal allograft recipients. *Transplantation* 1996;61(6):972–973.

46. Riska H, Gronhagen-Riska C, Ahonen J. Tuberculosis in renal allograft transplantation. *Transplant Proc* 1987;19:4096–4097.

47. John GT, Mukundan U, Vincent L, Jacob CK, Shastry JC. Primary drug resistance to mycobacterium tuberculosis in renal transplant recipients. *Natn Med J India* 1995;8(5):211–212.

48. Advisory Council for the Elimination of Tuberculosis. Initial therapy for tuberculosis in the era of multidrug resistance. Recommendations. *MMWR* 1993;42:1.

49. Iseman MD. Treatment of multidrug resistant tuberculosis. *N Engl J Med* 1993;329(11):784–91.

50. Higgins RSD, Kusne S, Reyes J, et al. *Mycobacterium tuberculosis* after liver transplantation: management and guidelines for prevention. *Clin Transpl* 1992;6:81–90.

51. John GT, Thomas PP, Jeyaseelan L, Jacob CK, Shastry JC. A double-blind randomized controlled trial of primary isoniazid prophylaxis in dialysis and transplant patients. *Transplantation* 1994;57(11):1683–1684.

52. Mcwhinney N, Khan O, Williams G. Tuberculosis in patients undergoing maintenance hemodialysis and renal transplantation. *Br J Surg* 1981;68:408–411.

53. Gottesdiener KM. Transplanted infections: donor to host transmission with the allograft. [Review] *Ann Intern Med* 1989;110:1001–1016.

54. Peters TG, Reiter CG, Boswell R. Transmission of tuberculosis by kidney transplantation. *Transplantation* 1984;38(6):514–516.

Transplant Infections edited by
Raleigh A. Bowden, Per Ljungman, and Carlos V. Paya.
Lippincott–Raven Publishers, Philadelphia © 1998

CHAPTER 15

Other Bacterial Infections

Steven M. Standaert and J. Stephen Dummer

The purpose of this chapter is to discuss important but less frequent bacterial infections that occur after transplantation. Some of these infections are caused by pathogens such as *Listeria monocytogenes* or *Norcadia* species that have long been recognized as important agents causing disease in transplant patients and other compromised hosts. Others are pathogens such as *Mycoplasma hominis* or *Rhodococcus* species that are rarely encountered but appear to have a predilection for patients with impaired immunity and to present interesting challenges in diagnosis or management. Finally, the chapter will discuss some emerging pathogens, such as *Helicobacter pylori* or *Bartonella* species, for which there is a small but evolving literature regarding their role in transplantation. For most of the pathogens described here, infection after solid organ transplantation is more widely reported than infection after bone marrow transplantation.

GRAM-POSITIVE ORGANISMS

Listeria monocytogenes

Listeria monocyotgenes is a motile, Gram-positive bacillus that is widespread throughout nature and has been isolated from tapwater, sewage, and several mammals and birds. The organism can be found in many different foods, including fresh vegetables, fish, poultry, meats, and all dairy products, especially raw milk and cheeses (1). An unusual property of the organism is its ability to grow at refrigerator temperature, which adds to the difficulty of controlling transmission from food. A laboratory process called cold enrichment takes advantage of this characteristic and can be successful in recovering the organism from samples where it is present only in small quantities.

Many individuals have asymptomatic carriage of *L. monocyotgenes* in the gastrointestinal tract; the bacteria has been cultured from the feces of 5% to 20% of healthy renal transplant recipients (1–3). Clinical infection is thought to arise from ingestion of contaminated food, but in most cases no definitive food source is identified. Endogenous infection from the gut of asymptomatic carriers is also considered likely, especially in immunocompromised hosts. Direct person-to-person transmission may be an occasional mode of transmission (4,5). Clinical infections occur during all seasons, with a preponderance of cases between July and October (3).

Several food-borne outbreaks of listeriosis have been reported (3,6,7), and it is felt that many cases that appear to be sporadic may in fact be linked to larger, undetected common-source outbreaks. Rates of infection are highest among newborn infants, pregnant women, and adults more than 60 years of age. Among nonperinatal infections, 70% occur in patients with hematologic malignancies, in patients with acquired immunodeficiency syndrome (AIDS), in organ transplant recipients, or in other patients taking immunosuppresive medications (8).

L. monocyotgenes is the leading cause of acute meningitis following renal transplantation (3,9). Listeriosis has also been reported following heart (10–14) and liver (15,16) transplantation. In the solid organ transplant setting most infections occur within 2–3 months after transplantation or shortly after treatment for organ rejection. Several cases, however, have been reported many years after solid organ transplantation, when doses of immunosuppresive medications are at their lowest (3,17). In contrast to solid organ transplant recipients, listeriosis appears to be a relatively rare infectious complication in bone marrow transplant recipients (18–21).

The initial manifestations of *Listeria* infection in transplant patients include fever with diarrhea, abdominal cramps, nausea, and vomiting. The presentation may be very acute or include a prodrome of milder symptoms lasting 2–7 days. Almost all transplant patients with

From the Division of Infectious Diseases, Department of Medicine, the Department of Surgery and the Transplant Center, Vanderbilt University School of Medicine, Nashville, TN 37232.

proven infection have bacteremia, and two-thirds have meningitis (22). Meningeal symptoms and other signs of central nervous system (CNS) involvement may be subtle, despite laboratory evidence of meningitis. Focal neurological signs are less common than diffuse signs, such as personality changes or forgetfulness. For this reason lumbar puncture should be performed in solid organ recipients with any hint of CNS involvement. Because of severe thrombocytopenia and the relative rarity of this infection in bone marrow transplant recipients, the decision to perform a lumbar puncture in these patients should be made on a more individual basis.

Examination of the cerebrospinal fluid (CSF) usually reveals a pleocytosis with less than 1,000 white cells, and a mixture of neutrophils and lymphocytes. It is common to find an elevated CSF protein and decreased CSF glucose, although these parameters may also be normal, particularly early in the illness. *L. monocytogenes* has been cultured from completely normal CSF. The organism is only occasionally visualized on Gram's stain of CSF, but centrifugation of the sample may increase the yield. Clinical isolates of *L. monocytogenes* are frequently misidentified as either diphtheroids or streptococcal species. In a compatible clinical situation, such reports should heighten the suspicion of listerial infection and prompt empiric therapy while awaiting definitive identification.

L. monocytogenes has a tropism for brain tissue and can cause several forms of CNS infection in addition to meningitis, including cerebritis, encephalitis, and brain abscess. An unusual form of listerial encephalitis involves the brainstem (rhomboencephalitis) and produces movement disorders, facial nerve palsies, and hemiparesis. Direct parenchymal invasion in the form of cerebritis or brain abscess is more common among transplant recipients than normal hosts (3). Listerial brain abscesses differ from other bacterial brain abscesses by a tendency to involve the brain stem, the presence of meningitis in 25% of patients, and the almost universal presence of bacteremia. The mortality rate for listeriosis in patients with CNS involvement is approximately 30%, but only 3% when bacteremia alone is present (3,22). Several forms of localized listerial infection have also been reported in transplant patients, including peritonitis (17), arthritis (23), and endophthalmitis (24). In contrast to normal hosts, however, listerial endocarditis is distinctly unusual in transplant patients (3).

There have been no controlled studies evaluating the treatment for listeriosis in any patient population. Recommendations are based upon the *in vitro* activity of antibiotics, animal studies, and clinical observation. The therapy of choice is high-dose penicillin or ampicillin with or without an aminoglycoside (8,25). Ampicillin is probably the preferable agent in transplant patients with reduced renal function, because of its excretion via the hepatobiliary route. *In vitro* and animal data support synergistic activity of ampicillin and aminoglycosides

against *L. monocytogenes*; for this reason the combination is often recommended in severe infection and in compromised hosts (26). The use of intrathecal gentamicin was more common in the past. However, because CNS listerial infection commonly involves the ventricles and the brain parenchyma, this form of therapy, other than by direct intraventricular instillation, would not be expected to be effective and cannot be recommended. Trimethoprim-sulfamethoxazole (TMP-SMX) has excellent activity and is a reasonable alternative (25). Infection may be effectively prevented by TMP-SMX prophylaxis (27). There are limited data on the use of the macrolides, tetracyclines, and vancomycin, and these agents cannot be recommended for routine use (8). Cephalosporins and fluoroquinolones should be avoided, as they have little to no activity against *Listeria*. Therapy with chloramphenicol, despite its good *in vitro* activity, has been associated with an unacceptable rate of failure or relapse, and the possible side effects of aplastic anemia exclude this agent as an appropriate therapy. Transplant recipients are at higher risk for recurrence or reinfection (13,16,28) than other patients and should receive a minimum of 3 weeks of therapy for bacteremia or meningitis and longer courses in the case of brain abscess.

Nocardia

Nocardia organisms are aerobic Gram-positive rods, which have a typical appearance of filamentous, branching chains on clinical microscopy of specimens. The organism has been isolated from soil and decaying organic material throughout the world, and human infection usually results from the inhalation of airborne bacilli or the traumatic inoculation of organisms into the skin.

Infection due to *Nocardia* species was first described in transplant recipients in the 1960s (29). By 1976, Beaman and co-workers estimated that transplant recipients accounted for 13% of the cases of nocardiosis occurring in the United States (30). Two decades later, Beaman estimated that the proportion of cases accounted for by transplant recipients had increased to 22% (31). Much of this increase was accounted for by the rapid expansion of heart and liver transplantation after 1980. Recently, Wilson and her co-workers summarized previous reports of nocardial infection in solid organ recipients. The reported frequency of nocardiosis in renal transplant recipients varied from none to 20%, with a mean of 2.8%. Most large series had an incidence between 1% and 4% (29). There are relatively few descriptions of *Nocardia* infection after liver transplantation, and rates of infection have varied from none to 3.7% (32,33). *Nocardia* infection may be more common in heart transplant recipients, at least based on high rates reported before the introduction of cyclosporine from cardiac transplant units at Stanford (13%) and the University of Arizona (37.5%) (33,34). Most infections due to *Nocardia* are sporadic and acquired as outpatients. A few small nosocomial outbreaks have been reported (29,35).

The incidence of nocardial infection in transplant recipients appears to have fallen since the introduction of cyclosporine. Hofflin reported a reduction in the incidence of nocardial infection at Stanford from 13% to 4.2% after the introduction of cyclosporine (12); similarly, the incidence of nocardiosis in the renal transplant population at the University of Texas in Houston declined from 2.6% to 0.7% after the introduction of cyclosporine (36). In this latter study, the authors were able to determine that the decrease in *Nocardia* infection was not due to the introduction of routine pneumocystis prophylaxis with sulfonamides.

Until recently, there were only scattered case reports of nocardial infection occurring after bone marrow transplantation. A 0.3% rate of nocardiosis was reported by van Burik in more than 6,000 marrow recipients at three large marrow transplant centers (37). Cases only occurred in allogeneic marrow recipients, who made up about 80% of the study population. At Vanderbilt University 1.7% of 302 allogeneic marrow recipients developed nocardial infection versus only one of 542 autologous marrow recipients (38). In both series some patients developed nocardial infection despite taking low-dose intermittent TMP-SMX for pneumocystis prophylaxis.

The timing of nocardial infection is similar after solid organ and bone marrow transplantation. In her large review, Wilson has noted that cases of nocardiosis were uncommon in the first 4 weeks after transplantation. The frequency of cases peaked between 1 and 6 months after transplantation and then occurred sporadically at lower rates thereafter (29). Cases of nocardiosis after bone marrow transplantation rarely occur before engraftment. The preponderance of cases occurs in the early postengraftment period (37,38).

The clinical presentation of nocardiosis is similar in solid organ and bone marrow recipients (29,33,37,38). Eighty to ninety percent of patients present with chest symptoms. Usually, these chest symptoms have been present for 1 or more weeks. Typical symptoms are fever, productive cough, pleuritic chest pain, dyspnea, weight loss, and hemoptysis. About one-third of patients have disseminated infection at presentation. The most common sites of dissemination are the CNS (15% to 20%), skin and soft tissues (15% to 20%), and bone or joints (2% to 5%). Occasionally, patients will have disseminated disease at presentation without an identifiable pulmonary focus or have isolated soft-tissue infection arising from a traumatic wound contaminated with soil. Soft-tissue lesions associated with disseminated disease usually present as deep abscesses that are palpable and tender but may not be erythematous. The organism is detected on biopsy or aspiration. *Nocardia* infection in the CNS usually causes brain abscess; meningitis, though reported, is uncommon. The symptoms are those of a space-occupy-ing lesion: focal neurological defects, headache, and seizures (29).

Findings on chest radiographs are variable. Nodules and nodular infiltrates are most common, but alveolar infiltrates are also seen. Cavitation occurs in 20% to 25% of cases and may appear multiloculated. Pleural effusions occur in about 25% of patients (29,33,34,38).

Because prognosis is strongly linked to the presence or absence of CNS disease and brain abscesses may be clinically silent, it may be wise to perform imaging studies of the brain even in patients who are free of neurological symptoms. It is not usually necessary to perform a lumber puncture if meningeal signs are absent.

Confirmation of the diagnosis of *Nocardia* infection is usually straightforward if appropriate steps are taken. The isolation of the organism takes at a minimum 4–5 days and occasional isolates may need 2–3 weeks to grow (31). *Nocardia* species will grow readily on media designed for the isolation of fungi and mycobacteria; thus obtaining these cultures may increase the yield. *Nocardia* is easily visualized on Gram's stain; detection of the delicate beaded and branching Gram-positive rods forms the basis for a presumptive diagnosis. Most strains of *Nocardia* are also weakly acid-fast, a feature that may help identify the organism on smears and differentiate it from *Actinomyces* species.

Sulfonamides have been the drugs of choice for the treatment of nocardiosis. Many clinicians prefer to use TMP-SMX, but excellent results have been achieved with other sulfonamides (29,34,38). Whatever sulfonamide is used, the starting doses should be in the range of 4–8 g daily, depending on renal function and body weight, with the aim of achieving serum levels of 100–150 µg/ml. Other antimicrobials that have good activity against a majority of nocardial strains are minocycline, amikacin, imipenem, cefotaxime, and ceftriaxone (31,39). Selected strains are sensitive to ampicillin, ampicillin/clavulanate, ciprofloxacin, or erythromycin, but use of these is not advised unless there is evidence of susceptibility by *in vitro* testing. Although *in vitro* testing has not been correlated with outcome, it does provide some evidence about relative susceptibility of isolates to different therapies and may be especially useful if therapy has to be changed because of toxicity or inadequate response. A number of recently described strains of *Nocardia*, such as *N. farcinica* or *N. transalvensis*, are resistant to many antimicrobials *in vitro* and may present special problems in treatment (31,39,40). For these strains, sensitivity testing may aid in speciation and help guide initial management.

In animal models of nocardial infection, agents such as imipenem, cefotaxime, or amikacin have killed *Nocardia* more quickly than sulfonamides (41,42). These agents may be excellent alternatives to sulfonamides or may be used as part of a multidrug regimen in patients who are critically ill with disseminated nocardiosis until the patients are stabilized and sensitivity studies are available. Ultimately, almost all patients who have an initial response should be managed on oral monotherapy.

The duration of therapy is generally 3 months or more. Treatment for up to 12 months is preferred in patients with disseminated disease or disease in the CNS. Patients who have a significant exposure to soil or dust, such as daily farming or construction work, may benefit from daily prophylaxis with sulfonamides to prevent reinfection (38).

Lactobacillus

Lactobacilli are non-spore-forming, generally strict or facultatively anaerobic Gram-positive rods that are ubiquitous inhabitants of the human oral cavity, vagina, and gastrointestinal tract. They were previously considered to be relatively innocuous organisms or nonpathogenic contaminants. However, serious infections are being increasingly recognized in transplant recipients and other populations. Bacteremia may follow disturbances of any site along the gastrointestinal tract or vagina. In normal hosts, lactobacilli may cause endocarditis, but this form of infection has only been reported once in a heart transplant recipient (43). Although bacteremia may be the only demonstrable site of infection (44), invasive visceral infections and abscesses have also been reported. Patel and colleagues described lactobacillemia in eight patients who had received liver transplants within the previous 6 months (45). In all but one case, the infections were polymicrobial, together with other enteric flora, and most patients had cholangitis or intra- or perihepatic abscesses. Other serious infections include pneumonia, thought to be transmitted in a transplanted lung (46), and splenic abscess in a renal transplant recipient with concomitant HIV infection (47). Unlike many other Gram-positive organisms, *Lactobacillus* does not appear to be a frequent cause of intravenous catheter infection (48).

Identified risk factors for infections due to *Lactobacillus* are manipulation of the gastrointestinal tract or dental procedures, use of a Roux-en-Y choledochojejunostomy, administration of selective bowel decontamination, and routine use of intravenous vancomycin, to which lactobacilli are uniformly resistant. The diagnosis is made by isolation and identification of the organism from blood or tissue sites. Microbiological data, however, must always be combined with the clinical data to assess their significance.

Definitive therapy should be guided by direct antimicrobial sensitivity testing when possible, but most isolates are sensitive to penicillin. Some investigators have suggested adding an aminoglycoside for the treatment of deep-seated infections on the basis of studies of bactericidal synergy (49). Other antibiotics that have good activity are clindamycin, erythromycin, and imipenem (48).

Rhodococcus equi

Rhodococcus equi is a Gram-positive coccobacillus previously classified as a Corynebacterium. It is a major veterinary pathogen causing chronic suppurative pneumonia in foals and submaxillary lymphadenitis in swine (50). It causes sporadic infections in humans, most of whom have defects in cell-mediated immunity due to AIDS, organ transplantation, cancer, and corticosteroid use (51–56). Herbivores such as horses and cattle are colonized in the gut, and the organism inhabits soil contaminated by their manure. About one-third of those with Rhodococcus infection have regular contact with farms or livestock (50). The infection is rare in organ transplant recipients, but cases have been reported from Australia, New Zealand, the United States, and Europe. No cases have been reported after bone marrow transplantation.

Patients with *Rhodococcus* infection generally present with fever, dyspnea, and nonproductive cough (50,52,57). Other common symptoms are pleuritic chest pain and hemoptysis. Chest radiographs show infiltrates or nodules, which are usually located in the upper lobes. Lung nodules frequently cavitate and develop air fluid levels. Pleural effusions are common and may be infected. In most patients the infection remains confined to the chest cavity, but dissemination to skin, bone, brain, and other organs has been described (50,56,57). The diagnosis is made by isolating the organism from a sterile body site or from pulmonary secretions in the presence of a compatible clinical presentation. In the laboratory, early growth may be seen on agar plates within 24–48 hours, but the mucoid, salmon-colored colonies characteristic of the organism are not apparent until a few days later (50,57). The organism can easily be missed in cultures of nonsterile specimens such as sputum; therefore one should alert the laboratory whenever *R. equi* infection is being considered.

A large number of antibiotics are active against *Rhodococcus*. The most potent agents *in vitro* are vancomycin, imipenem, rifampin, macrolides such as erythromycin and clarithromycin, and ciprofloxacin (50,57–59). Therapy with penicillins and cephalosporins has been unreliable and should be avoided. A regimen of erythromycin and rifampin has had excellent success in treating horses and foals (50). Antibiotic therapy should be prolonged for a number of months. Adjunctive surgical therapy may be useful in selected patients.

Clostridium difficile

Clostridium difficile is a spore-forming, Gram-positive, obligate anaerobic bacillus and is part of the normal intestinal flora in about 3% of healthy adults. Transmission may occur nosocomially, as the organism has been isolated from the hands of hospital personnel caring for colonized patients and the spores of *C. difficile* persist on fomites and surfaces for long periods (60).

Colitis due to *C. difficile* is a common complication of bone marrow and solid organ transplant populations. The frequency of *C. difficile*-mediated colitis in different transplant populations appears to relate to the intensity of their exposure to antibiotics. *C. difficile* has been reported as a very common cause of diarrhea after bone marrow transplantation. Three studies have shown rates of 14% to 18% based on toxin detection (61–63). A fourth and later study detected only six cases in 296 patients (64). Possible reasons for this discrepancy were not discussed. Colitis due to *C. difficile* has been reported in 3% to 6% of liver recipients (65,66) and 1% to 4% of heart and kidney recipients (67,68). Few if any transplant patients develop *C. difficile* disease while taking TMP-SMX for pneumocystis prophylaxis. Presumably, the lack of anaerobic activity in this drug combination causes relatively little perturbation of bowel flora.

Most transplant patients with *C. difficile* colitis present with watery diarrhea and abdominal pain after receiving a course of antibiotics. Fever is a common but not universal finding (69). In symptomatic patients the detection of *C. difficile* cytotoxin in the stool is adequate reason to make a presumptive diagnosis and initiate treatment. In atypical cases, or when another disease is suspected, sigmoidoscopy or colonoscopy may be helpful to establish a definite diagnosis. Culture for *C. difficile* on selective media increases the sensitivity of detection but also requires a laboratory skilled in anaerobic bacteriology. Culture also detects carriers and nontoxigenic strains of bacteria and is therefore somewhat less useful clinically than toxin detection. The latex agglutination assay detects a nontoxigenic protein of the bacteria (70). It suffers from lower sensitivity than other assays and should not be relied upon to exclude the diagnosis.

The usual treatment for *C. difficile* colitis is to stop the offending antibiotic and administer oral metronidazole 500–750 mg TID or oral vancomycin 125 mg QID. Many patients will be cured with 7–10 days of therapy, but longer courses may be necessary in patients who are slow to respond or have suffered relapses. Metronidazole is usually the preferred treatment because of its lower cost (71). It may also be less likely to encourage the emergence of vancomycin-resistant organisms. If only intravenous therapy can be given, metronidazole is the drug of choice because intravenous vancomycin is not thought to enter the bowel in sufficient concentration to be effective (70). Anion exchange resins, such as cholestyramine, have been successfully used to treat *C. difficile* colitis, but they may bind the patient's immunosuppressive medications (70,71). Novel approaches, such as repopulating the bowel with "nonpathogenic" organisms (e.g., lactobacilli), have had anecdotal success but have not been rigorously studied (70). Because commensal organisms in normal hosts may become pathogens in compromised hosts, this approach should only be attempted as a last resort in transplant patients.

GRAM-NEGATIVE ORGANISMS

Legionella

Legionella organisms are fastidious, aerobic, Gram-negative rods that are ubiquitous in nature and have been found in soil and fresh-water lakes and streams (72). There are least 18 separate species of *Legionella*, and several species are further divided into serogroups. Most human illness is caused by *L. pneumophila*, serogroup 1. Other species known to have caused infection in transplant patients include other serogroups of *L. pneumophila*, *L. micdadei*, *L. bozemanii*, and *L. dumoffii* (73–76).

Legionella infection is common among transplant recipients and can be either nosocomial or community-acquired. The exact mode of transmission is unclear, but person-to-person transmission does not occur, and most outbreaks of legionellosis are related to exposure to contaminated water (77) or soil (78). *Legionella* species have a major reservoir in institutional plumbing systems. They enter via contaminated cold water intakes and subsequently colonize hot water heaters. From hot water tanks they are dispersed throughout the water system to contaminate plumbing fixtures and pipes (79,80). Outbreaks have been epidemiologically linked to several sources of aerosolized water, including shower heads, cooling towers, evaporative condensers, humidifiers, and whirlpools (81–85). Health care facilities that experience more than a few cases of nosocomial legionellosis may find it prudent to investigate sources of *Legionella* bacteria in the institutional environment, particularly the hot water system.

The defect in cellular immunity inherent with immunosuppressive therapy makes transplant recipients particularly susceptible to legionellosis. Infection has been frequently reported in patients with renal (75,86,87), cardiac (88–90), bone marrow (91–94), and liver (65,95) transplants. Infection occurs at any time following transplantation, but with greatest frequency within a few weeks of transplantation or when there has been augmentation of immunosuppressive therapy.

The clinical presentation can vary widely. Although there are no pathognomonic findings, some features may suggest legionellosis. Patients often experience a flulike prodrome of high fever, chills, myalgias, and malaise. Antecedent upper respiratory symptoms are usually absent, but the infection then progresses to include dyspnea and a mildly productive cough, often associated with pleuritic chest pain. About one-half of patients develop watery diarrhea. Mild CNS symptoms, such as headache and confusion, are often present. On physical examination, patients often appear quite ill, and some authors have noted the presence of a pulse/temperature disassociation with a relative bradycardia (96). The most common physical findings are those associated with pneumonia, such as tachypnea, pulmonary rales, and, rarely, pleural friction rub or signs of an effusion.

Occasionally, extrapulmonary infection has been observed with or without a primary pneumonia. These complications may result from bacteremic spread of the organism, in the case of pericardial effusion (97) or peritonitis (98), or from direct contamination, in the case of sternal wound infection (99). The mortality of untreated legionellosis in immunocompromised patients has been 80% (96), and even with effective therapy, mortality ranges from 24% to 54% (96,100).

The most common appearance of *Legionella* pneumonia on radiograph is alveolar infiltrates, which are frequently multilobar (101). One-third of patients develop pleural effusions (102), and cavitation occurs in about 20% (87,101,103). The appearance of rapidly expanding pulmonary nodules suggestive of septic emboli is another radiographic pattern noted in transplant patients.

The diagnosis of legionellosis is often difficult and depends on the level of laboratory experience of those working with this organism. *Legionella* organisms have the ultrastructural properties of Gram-negative bacilli, but they are very small, take up stain poorly, and are often not visualized on Gram's stain of clinical specimens. The definitive method to diagnose *Legionella* infection is culture. *Legionella* are very fastidious and their isolation requires the use of specially enriched culture media (buffered charcoal/yeast extract agar, or BCYE) and an environment enriched in CO_2. An average of 3–5 days of incubation is necessary for sufficient growth, and overgrowth by other, less fastidious organisms can mask the presence of the organism, even when media-containing inhibitory antibiotics is used. Cultured organisms are more readily visualized by Gram's staining than organisms in clinical specimens.

Several useful indirect diagnostic methods for legionellosis are available. The most rapid technique is direct fluorescent antibody (DFA) staining of sputum or tissue specimens (104). However, there are several limitations of this procedure: the sensitivity of DFA is only about 50%, and the reagents contain antibodies to only the most common species and serogroups (105). The interpretation of the assay is subjective and therefore requires an experienced technician, and false-positive results can occur because of cross-reactivity with other organisms. Demonstrating the development of a serological response is another indirect method of diagnosis that has been used with some success (106,107). *Legionella* serology is of little value in the acute clinical setting because the diagnosis is made retrospectively. In addition, serology relies on an adequate antibody response, which may be diminished in immunocompromised patients. Also, cross-reactions with other organisms producing false-positive results are a potential problem.

Detection of urinary antigen is a newer assay that has been demonstrated to have a sensitivity of greater than 85% for infections caused by *L. pneumophila* serogroup 1. However, other species and serogroups will not be detected by this technique (106,107).

There are no controlled studies evaluating the treatment for legionellosis, and recommendations are based upon *in vitro* testing, animal studies, and clinical observation. Agents that are known to be the most active include erythromycin, rifampin, tetracyclines, TMP-SMX, and the fluoroquinolones, whereas all β-lactam antibiotics, aminoglycosides, chloramphenicol, vancomycin, and clindamycin are ineffective (96,108). Erythromycin is probably the most commonly used antibiotic, but doses as high as 4 g/day may be required. If the patient does not respond to this regimen, the addition of rifampin may be helpful (109). The use of these two antibiotics can be problematic in the transplant population because of interference with the metabolism of cyclosporine (110,111). Close monitoring of cyclosporine levels is necessary when using either of these agents. For this reason, other active agents—such as TMP-SMX, tetracycline, or the fluoroquinolones—are appealing alternatives, although there is less clinical experience with these drugs. Transplant patients should be treated for at least 3 weeks and until they have had an adequate clinical response to treatment. Prophylaxis with TMP-SMX, erythromycin, or fluoroquinolones may be useful in preventing *Legionella* pneumonia in transplant recipients, particularly in outbreak situations (112–114).

Helicobacter

Helicobacter pylori is a curved, Gram-negative bacillus that infects the stomach in 25% to 50% of adults in developed countries and causes chronic gastritis (115). Infection with this organism has been strongly linked to the occurrence of peptic ulcer disease and is also a risk factor for the development of gastric cancer. The presence of IgG antibodies in serum correlates very well with the presence of chronic infection with *H. pylori* in the stomach, as detected by endoscopic biopsy and culture. A number of studies have looked at *H. pylori* infection in transplant patients. A seroepidemiological study of 202 renal recipients showed a 29% rate of infection, which was similar to rates of infection in healthy blood donors and patients on hemodialysis (116). Seropositive transplant recipients were more likely than seronegative transplant patients to have dyspeptic symptoms. In another study 33 renal recipients underwent upper endoscopy between 2 and 4 months after transplantation. Forty-eight percent had *H. pylori* identified either by histology or by testing for the urease elaborated by the organism; the patients who were infected with *Helicobacter* were more likely to have gastritis, peptic ulcers, or dyspeptic symptoms (117). Somewhat disparate results were seen in a study of 100 heart transplant recipients (115). Thirty-five percent of the patients were seropositive before transplantation. Only one of the 65 seronegative patients seroconverted over a mean follow-up of 3.5 years. Seropositive patients did not have more documented episodes of ulcer disease, gastritis, or gastrointestinal bleeding than seronegative patients. Forty percent of *Helicobacter*-infected patients became seronegative in long-term follow-up, a finding that correlated with more intense use of antibiotics. The patients appeared to have been inadvertently cured of their *Helicobacter* infections while being treated for other infections.

Information on *Helicobacter* infection in patients undergoing bone marrow transplantation is very limited. One study in 276 bone marrow recipients who underwent endoscopy before or after transplantation disclosed only one case of *H. pylori* infection (118). This rate of infection is surprisingly low and should be confirmed by further studies. The result could be explained if *H. pylori* had been eradicated by antibiotic therapy.

Despite the limited scope of the studies, they do show that transplant recipients are no more likely than persons in the general population to be chronically infected with *H. pylori*. They leave unresolved the issue of whether transplant patients with *Helicobacter* are more or less likely than normal hosts to develop gastritis and ulcer disease.

No treatment trials of *Helicobacter* infection have been reported in transplant recipients. Until these are available, treatment regimens devised for normal hosts should be employed. Many regimens have been described. Older regimens combined bismuth salts with one or more antibiotics—such as metronidazole, amoxicillin, or tetracycline—usually for 14–21 days (119). New regimens have employed antisecretory agents, such as omeprazole or ranitidine with these antibiotics or clarithromycin (120). Eradication rates greater than 80% have been achieved with some of these regimens, but failure is not rare. Patients can be monitored for cure with endoscopy, *H. pylori* serology, or a urea breath test.

SPIROCHETES

Treponema pallidum

Treponema pallidum, the causative organism of syphilis, is a motile, slender, tightly coiled, helical organism that cannot be cultivated *in vitro*. Transmission from an infected individual is by sexual or intimate contact, passage through the placenta, transfusion of fresh blood, or accidental direct inoculation. Infection following organ transplantation is rare. Although transmission from contaminated blood products is a theoretical possibility, the risk is currently felt to be negligible (121), particularly because the organism cannot survive longer than 24–48 hours under the conditions of blood bank storage. Indeed, this form of transmission has never been reported in a transplant recipient. The potential risk of transmission from an infected organ is also a concern and underlies the common policy of excluding potential organ donors based upon positive serological tests for syphilis.

This contraindication was questioned by Gibel and colleagues when they reported the successful and safe transplantation of kidneys obtained from donors known to have had syphilis using penicillin prophylaxis in the organ recipients (122).

There have been no reported cases of syphilis in bone marrow transplant recipients. There have been isolated reports of luetic hepatitis in renal and liver transplant recipients (123,124). This is an uncommon manifestation of syphilis in normal hosts. Both patients were homosexual men, and it was postulated that they were predisposed to this form of infection, because of the presence of primary anal lesions that drain spirochetes directly into the liver through the portal venous system.

The diagnosis of syphilis is usually based upon initial serological testing for nontreponemal antibodies (VDRL, RPR) followed by specific treponemal antibodies (FTA). It has been suggested that false-negative tests due to the prozone phenomena may be more common in patients receiving immunosuppressive medication because of dysregulation of the B-cell response (125).

The treatment of choice is parenteral penicillin, but doxycycline or erythromycin may be used if penicillin is absolutely contraindicated.

Borrelia

Lyme disease is a tick-borne infection caused by *Borrelia burgdorferi*, a cultivable spirochete. Animal reservoirs are small mammals (rodents), but large animals, such as deer and cattle, are important in the life cycle of the tick vector, *Ixodes* species. This infection has been reported in a patient 7 years after renal transplantation. Although it is unclear whether transplant recipients are more susceptible to infection, it was felt that this patient's immunocompromised state contributed to unusually severe neurological involvement that began as a painful L4 root radiculoneuritis and progressed to a severe encephalitis. However, the patient recovered completely after a prolonged course of ceftriaxone and doxycycline with no change in immunosuppressive therapy (126).

CHLAMYDIA

Chlamydia species are Gram-negative, obligate intracellular parasites of eukaryotic cells. Chlamydial infections are ubiquitous in birds and mammals, including humans. Transmission of *C. pneumoniae* (TWAR) is thought to be by inhalation of aerosolized organisms. The usual mode of transmission of *C. trachomatis* is by sexual contact or from mother to child during delivery. Pneumonia due to *C. trachomatis* is thought to occur only rarely in nonimmunocompromised adults and the mode of transmission is not known.

C. trachomatis has been described as an occasional cause of pneumonia in transplant patients. It has been reported in 6% of a series of 72 marrow transplant recipients with interstitial pneumonitis (127) and in several case reports of patients after renal transplantation (128,129). Other pathogens, most frequently CMV, are frequently also implicated in these reports, and therefore it is often difficult to determine whether *C. trachomatis* was the primary pathogen.

Although isolation of the organism from lung tissue or pulmonary secretions is the preferred method of diagnosis, the only evidence of infection is often demonstration of serological conversion with or without compatible histologic findings. The diagnosis of *C. trachomatis* infection based on serological conversion alone should be made with caution because some patients may demonstrate a fourfold increase in IgG without clinical disease (130). Recently, the polymerase chain reaction (PCR) has been shown to be a useful adjunct to existing diagnostic tools (131).

In addition to *C. trachomatis*, there have been isolated case reports of other *Chlamydia* infections in renal transplant recipients, such as *C. pneumoniae*/TWAR (74) and feline keratoconjunctivitis agent (132), both based upon serological conversion. *C. pneumoniae*/TWAR infection has been shown to be a common cause of community-acquired pulmonary infections in the general population and is likely more common in transplant recipients than is usually appreciated. It is hoped that newer molecular diagnostic techniques will allow the occurrence of this infection in transplant patients to be studied with greater ease and accuracy than has heretofore been possible.

The therapy of choice of chlamydial infection is either tetracycline or doxycycline, with erythromycin as an alternative.

MYCOPLASMA

The mycoplasmas are distinct from true bacteria in lacking a cell wall and are ubiquitous as saprophytes and/or parasites of the plant and animal kingdom. The mode of transmission varies with each organism. *Mycoplasma pneumonia* is spread by respiratory droplets and *M. hominis* and ureaplasmas are spread during vaginal delivery and sexual contact.

Infections due to *M. pneumoniae* are common in the general population but are rarely reported in transplant recipients, possibly due to failure to perform diagnostic tests or insensitivity of serology in this population (133). In contrast, there are numerous descriptions of infections due to *M. hominis* in transplant recipients (134–137). *M. hominis* is a common commensal of the urinary tract in sexually active men and women (138,139). It is a frequent cause of self-limited postpartum fever, but on occasion it also causes invasive disease such as septic arthritis in new mothers (133,140). Immunosuppressed patients are predisposed to *M. hominis* infection. In a review of invasive *M. hominis* infection occurring outside the genitourinary

tract, 76% of patients had immunosuppressing disorders or were receiving immunosuppressive medication (135).

M. hominis infection has been described in all types of solid organ transplantation (135,136,141), and transmission of *M. hominis* from a lung donor to recipients of both the right and left lung has been reported (142). Commonly, patients have superficial or deep wound infection within a few weeks of a transplant operation. After heart or heart/lung transplantation, patients typically present with fever and have erythema, tenderness, and drainage of purulent secretions along the sternal incision (136). Microscopic examination of a Gram's stain of the wound drainage shows many white cells but few or no organisms. Patients may not appear very ill. Nonetheless, the organism has a destructive effect on sternal bone, and extensive surgical intervention may be required. Single lung recipients usually develop pleural space infection, and renal and liver recipients present with local or diffuse peritoneal infection (143,144). Other well-documented sites of infections are joints, the CNS, and bloodstream (134,135,145). *M. hominis* has occasionally been isolated from the respiratory tract in patients with pneumonia, but its role as a respiratory pathogen is still not well defined (135,137). The only bone marrow recipient reported with *M. hominis* infection had diffuse alveolar hemorrhage in association with isolation of this organism (137).

The clinician should think of *M. hominis* when encountering a pyogenic infection from which cultures are either negative or grow a small amount of normal flora. The organism grows best on specific *Mycoplasma* media such as A8 solid agar but will often grow on routine blood agar, aerobically or anaerobically, if held 4–5 days. Because of this it is important for clinicians to alert their microbiologist that *M. hominis* is suspected (135).

Most *M. hominis* isolates are sensitive to clindamycin, rifampin, fluoroquinolones, and tetracycline (135). The organism is resistant to aminoglycosides, sulfonamides, erythromycin, β-lactams, and other cell wall–active agents. Treatment duration should be at least 2 weeks. A longer duration is indicated when there is severe, deep-seated infection. Bone infection and endocarditis should be treated for a minimum of 6 weeks. Coinfection with *Ureaplasma urealyticum* has been described in a few patients (141,145). Because ureaplasmas are resistant to clindamycin, it may be sensible to avoid the use of clindamycin or employ therapy with more than one active drug pending the results of microbiological studies.

RICKETTSIOSIS

Bartonella

Bartonella (formerly *Rochalimaea*) is a newly recognized fastidious Gram-negative bacillus and has been identified as the etiologic agent of a wide spectrum of clinical illnesses, including cat scratch disease (CSD) in normal hosts and bacillary angiomatosis, bacillary peliosis, and persistent bacteremia with fever in HIV-infected patients. Domestic cats serve as a natural reservoir for *B. henselae*–associated disease in humans. The exact mode of transmission is not known, but a very common epidemiological feature of this infection is recent contact with young cats, usually involving a scratch or bite (146). The clinical syndromes usually associated with HIV infection have also been occasionally reported in immunocompetent hosts and may be caused by *B. quintana*, the etiologic agent of trench fever. Unlike *B. henselae*, humans are the only known reservoir of *B. quintana* and the infection is transmitted by the human body louse (*Pediculus humanus*) (147).

Bartonella infection has been reported in kidney (148–150), liver (151), and heart (152) transplant recipients as early as 11 months and as late as 14 years following transplantation.

The clinical manifestations of *Bartonella* infection in transplant recipients can vary greatly. Patients may present with the typical features of CSD, regional lymphadenopathy, and fever but will usually progress to a more severe, systemic illness if not treated promptly (148,151). Other patients may have no peripheral lymphadenopathy and progress early to visceral involvement (149,150,152). Most transplant patients with *B. henselae* infection will have involvement of the liver, spleen, or visceral lymph nodes detected initially by radiography and confirmed by biopsy and bacteriological studies. The liver and spleen are often studded with small nodules on gross examination and have multiple hypodense lesions (peliosis) either by computerized tomography (CT) scan or ultrasound examination. The histologic appearance of lymph nodes is that of necrotizing granulomas with microabscesses, while visceral organs such as the liver usually have epithelioid hemangiomatous lesions. Although unusual, other organs such as the lungs may also be involved (150). Despite their compromised state, transplant patients have not been reported to develop bacillary angiomatosis, the form of *Bartonella* infection commonly seen in HIV-infected individuals. Patients with bacillary angiomatosis present with fever and highly vascular, friable, red skin tumors. They may also have unusual lytic bone lesions that underlie some skin lesions.

Because the organism is not routinely isolated from blood, the diagnosis can be difficult and frequently requires invasive procedures to obtain tissue. Infection can be confirmed by culture of tissue specimens (such as lymph node, skin, liver, or spleen) using either blood or chocolate agar, but these cultures may require an incubation period of up to 30 days. For this reason PCR of the 16s RNA performed on tissue specimens may be preferable. The diagnosis is also suggested by the appearance of typical coccobacillary organisms with the Warthin-Starry stain and by demonstrating a positive serological response.

Because CSD in normal hosts generally resolves without therapy, reliable information regarding the relative effectiveness of antibiotics is limited. Based upon reports of successful treatment for bacillary angiomatosis, erythromycin or doxycycline should be active (153). Clarithromycin and azithromycin have *in vitro* activity that is superior to erythromycin, and likely will prove to be clinically superior as well (146). There is evidence to suggest that rifampin and aminoglycosides may also be useful (153).

Coxiella burnetti

Coxiella burnetti, the etiologic agent of Q fever, is a pleomorphic coccobacillus with a Gram-negative cell wall. Infection is usually associated with an exposure to infected livestock or unpasteurized milk. The two most common clinical manifestations of disease are an acute febrile illness associated with pneumonia or hepatitis, or a chronic febrile illness associated with endocarditis. Infection has been reported in patients with a variety of immunocompromised conditions, such as leukemia and Hodgkin's disease (154), but there are only two reports of Q fever occurring in transplant recipients. One patient presented with an acute illness characterized by fever and cough 3 months after bone marrow transplantation for acute myeloid leukemia (155). Her symptoms resolved within 7 days without specific therapy, but she was treated with doxycycline for 6 weeks after the serological diagnosis was made. A similar presentation was reported in a young girl who developed acute lymphocytic leukemia 4 years following a fetal liver/thymic transplant (156). The diagnosis was also established retrospectively 6 weeks later by serology, but no treatment was rendered because she was asymptomatic. Nine months later, the patient developed a febrile illness associated with seizures and hemiparesis that was thought to be due to recurrent *C. burnetti* infection based upon a rapid resolution of symptoms after treatment with tetracycline. Based upon these reports it may be prudent to treat patients when a positive serological response is detected to prevent recurrent or chronic infection.

Other rickettsial organisms that have been reported in transplant recipients include Rocky Mountain spotted fever (RMSF) and human monocytic ehrlichiosis (HME). The etiologic agents, *Rickettsia rickettsii* and *Ehrlichia chaffeensis*, respectively, are both fastidious, obligate intracellular bacteria with Gram-negative cell walls transmitted from tick vectors. The single reported patient with RMSF following heart transplantation had a typical illness with a classic petechial rash (157). The patient's course was relatively benign with response to 3 weeks of doxycycline. Although the diagnosis was made by immunofluorescent staining of a skin lesion, the patient had a very delayed antibody response and only demonstrated seroconversion 5 months after the infection. In contrast, the single report of a patient with HME after a liver transplant had a severe illness requiring intensive care monitoring but developed a serological response within 5 days (158). He also made a full recovery after 10 days doxycycline therapy. Both reported patients had a history consistent with potential tick exposure. These reports demonstrate that transplant patients who reenter full lives in the community are at risk for all infections than can afflict normal hosts.

REFERENCES

1. Gellin BG, Broome CV. Listeriosis. *JAMA* 1989;261:1313–1320.
2. Macgowan AP, Marshall RJ, Mackay IM, Reeves DS. *Listeria* faecal carriage by renal transplant recipients, haemodialysis patients and patients in general practice: its relation to season, drug therapy, foreign travel, animal exposure and diet. *Epidemiol Infect* 1991;106: 157–166.
3. Stamm AM, Dismukes WE, Simmons BP, et al. Listeriosis in renal transplant recipients: report of an outbreak and review of 102 cases. *Rev Infect Dis* 1982;4:665–682.
4. Helenglass G, Talbot D, Jameson B, Powles RL. Possible role of person-to-person transmission of *Listeria* infection in immunocompromised patients [Letter]. *Lancet* 1989;1:851.
5. Green HT, Macaulay MB. Hospital outbreak of *Listeria monocytogenes* septicaemia: a problem of cross infection? *Lancet* 1978;2: 1039–1040.
6. Linnan MJ, Mascola L, Xaio DL, et al. Epidemic listeriosis associated with Mexican-style cheese. *N Engl J Med* 1988;319:823–828.
7. Schlech WF, Lavigne PM, Bortolussi RA, et al. Epidemic listeriosis: evidence for transmission by food. *N Engl J Med* 1983;308:203–206.
8. Lorber B. Listeriosis. *Clin Infect Dis* 1997;24:1–11.
9. Hooper DC, Pruitt AA, Rubin RH. Central nervous system infection in the chronically immunosuppressed. *Medicine* 1982;61:166–188.
10. Stamm AM, Smith SH, Kirklin JK, McGiffin DC. Listerial myocarditis in cardiac transplantation. *Rev Infect Dis* 1990;12:820–823.
11. Anonymous. Meningoencephalitis in a heart transplant recipient. *J Tenn Med Assoc* 1987;80:613–614.
12. Hofflin JM, Potasman I, Baldwin JC, Oyer PE, Stinson EB, Remington JS. Infectious complications in heart transplant recipients receiving cyclosporine and corticosteroids. *Ann Intern Med* 1987;106: 209–216.
13. Orenstein R. Relapse of infection or reinfection by *Listeria monocytogenes* in a patient with a heart transplant: usefulness of pulsed-field gel electrophoresis for diagnosis [Letter]. *Clin Infect Dis* 1994;19: 208–209.
14. Zenati M, Milano A, Livi U, Cattelan A, Casarotto D. Successful treatment of disseminated infection with *Listeria monocytogenes* in a heart transplant recipient [Letter]. *J Heart Lung Transplant* 1994;13: 345–346.
15. Bourgeois N, Jacobs F, Tavares ML, et al. *Listeria monocytogenes* hepatitis in a liver transplant recipient: a case report and review of the literature. *J Hepatol* 1993;18:284–289.
16. Peetermans WE, Endtz HP, Janssens AR, van den Broek PJ. Recurrent *Listeria monocytogenes* bacteraemia in a liver transplant patient. *Infection* 1990;18:107–108.
17. Larson CC, Baine WB, Ware AJ, Krejs G. *Listeria* peritonitis diagnosed by laparoscopy. *Gastrointest Endosc* 1988;34:352–354.
18. Chang J, Powles R, Mehta J, Paton N, Treleaven J, Jameson B. Listeriosis in bone marrow transplant recipients: incidence, clinical features, and treatment. *Clin Infect Dis* 1995;21:1289–1290.
19. Long SG, Leyland MJ, Milligan DW. *Listeria* meningitis after bone marrow transplantation. *Bone Marrow Transplant* 1993;12:537–9.
20. Lopez R, Martino R, Brunet S, Altes A, Sureda A, Albos AD. Infection by *Listeria monocytogenes* in the early period post-bone marrow transplantation. *Eur J Haematol* 1994;53:251–252.
21. Martino R, Lopez R, Pericas R, Badell I, Sureda A, Brunet S. Listeriosis in bone marrow transplant recipients [Letter]. *Clin Infect Dis* 1996;23:419–420.
22. Skogberg K, Syrjänen J, Jahkola M, et al. Clinical presentation and outcome of listeriosis in patients with and without immunosuppressive therapy. *Clin Infect Dis* 1992;14:815–821.
23. Abadie SM, Dalovisio JR, Pankey GA, Cortez LM. *Listeria monocytogenes* arthritis in a renal transplant recipient [Letter]. *J Infect Dis* 1987;156:413–414.
24. Algan M, Jonon B, George JL, Lion C, Kessler M, Burdin JC. *Listeria monocytogenes* endophthalmitis in a renal-transplant patient receiving cyclosporine. *Ophthalmologica* 1990;201:23–27.
25. Tuazon CU, Shamsuddin D, Miller H. Antibiotic susceptibility and synergy of clinical isolates of *Listeria monocytogenes*. *Antimicrob Agents Chemother* 1982;21:525–7.
26. Edmiston CE, Gordon RC. Evaluation of gentamicin and penicillin as a synergistic combination in experimental murine listeriosis. *Antimicrob Agents Chemother* 1979;16:862–863.
27. Tappero JW, Schuchat A, Deaver KA, Mascola L, Wenger JD. Reduction in the incidence of human listeriosis in the United States. *JAMA* 1995;273:1118–1122.
28. Watson GW, Fuller TJ, Elms J, Kluge RM. *Listeria* celebritis. Relapse of infection in renal transplant patients. *Arch Intern Med* 1978;138:83–87.
29. Wilson JP, Turner HR, Kirchner KA, Chapman SW. Nocardial infections in renal transplant recipients. *Medicine* 1989;68:38–57.
30. Beaman BL, Burnside J, Edwards B, Causey W. Nocardial infections in the United States, 1972–1974. *J Infect Dis* 1976;134:286–289.
31. Beaman BL, Beaman I. Nocardial species, host-parasite relationship. *Clin Micro Rev* 1994;7:213–264.
32. Forbes GM, Harvey FAH, Philpott-Howard JN, et al. Nocardiosis in liver transplantation: variation in presentation, diagnosis and therapy. *J Infect* 1990;20:11–19.
33. Chapman SW, Wilson JP. Nocardiosis in transplant recipients. *Semin Respir Infect* 1990;5:74–79.
34. Simpson GL, Stinson EB, Egger MJ, Remington JS. Nocardial infections in the immunocompromised host: a detailed study in a defined population. *Rev Infect Dis* 1981;3:492–507.
35. Lovett IS, Houang ET, Burge S, et al. An outbreak of *Nocardia asteroides* infection in a renal transplant unit. *Q J Med* 1981;50:123–135.
36. Arduino RC, Johnson PC, Miranda AG. Nocardiosis in renal transplant recipients undergoing immunosuppression with cyclosporine. *Clin Infect Dis* 1993;16:505–512.
37. van Burik JA, Hackman RC, Nadeem S, et al. Nocardiosis after bone marrow transplantation. *Clin Infect Dis* 1997;24:1154–1160.
38. Choucino C, Goodman SA, Greer JP, Stein RS, Wolff SN, Dummer JS. Nocardial infections in bone marrow transplant recipients. *Clin Infect Dis* 1996;23:1012–1019.
39. McNeil MM, Brown JM, Hutwagner LC, Schiff TA. Evaluation of therapy for *Nocardia asteroides* complex infections. *Infect Dis Clin Pract* 1995;4:287–92.
40. McNeil MM, Brown JM, Magruder CH, et al. Disseminated *Nocardia transvalensis* infection: an unusual opportunistic pathogen in severely immunocompromised patients. *J Infect Dis* 1992;165:175–178.
41. Gombert ME, Berkowitz LB, Aulicino TM, duBouchet L. Therapy of pulmonary nocardiosis in immunocompromised mice. *Antimicrob Agents Chemother* 1990;34:1766–1768.
42. Gombert ME, Aulicino TM, duBouchet L, Silverman GE, Sheinbaum WM. Therapy of experimental cerebral nocardiosis with imipenem, amikacin, trimethoprim-sulfamethoxazole, and minocycline. *Antimicrob Agents Chemother* 1986;30:270–273.
43. Toporoff B, Rosado LJ, Appleton CP, Sethi G, Copeland JG. Successful treatment of early infective endocarditis and mediastinitis in a heart transplant recipient. *J Heart Lung Transplant* 1994;13:546–548.
44. Kalima P, Masterton RG, Roddie PH, Thomas AE. *Lactobacillus rhamnosus* infection in a child following bone marrow transplant. *J Infect* 1996;32:165–167.
45. Patel R, Cockerill FR, Porayko MK, Osmon DR, Ilstrup DM, Keating MR. Lactobacillemia in liver transplant patients. *Clin Infect Dis* 1994;18:207–212.
46. Jones SD, Fullerton DA, Zamora MR, Badesch DB, Campbell DN, Grover FL. Transmission of *Lactobacillus* pneumonia by a transplanted lung. *Ann Thorac Surg* 1994;58:887–9.
47. Sherman ME, Albrecht M, DeGirolami PC, et al. An unusual case of splenic abscess and sepsis in an immunocompromised host. *Am J Clin Path* 1987;88:659–662.
48. Anthony SJ, Stratton CW, Dummer JS. *Lactobacillus* bacteremia: description of the clinical course in adult patients without endocarditis. *Clin Infect Dis* 1996;23:773–778.
49. Bayer AS, Chow AW, Betts D, Guze L. Lactobacillemia: report of nine cases. *Am J Med* 1978;64:808–813.
50. Prescott JF. *Rhodococcus equi*: an animal and human pathogen. *Clin Microbiol Rev* 1991;4:20–34.

51. Harvey RL, Sunstrum JC. *Rhodococcus equi* infection in patients with and without human immunodeficiency virus infection. *Rev Infect Dis* 1991;13:139–145.

52. VanEtta LL, Filice GA, Ferguson RM, Gerding DN. *Corynebacterium equi*: a review of 12 cases of human infection. *Rev Infect Dis* 1983;5:1012–1018.

53. Jones MR, Neale TJ, Say PJ, Horne JG. *Rhodococcus equi*: an emerging opportunistic pathogen? *Aust NZ J Med* 1989;19:103–107.

54. Segovia J, Pulpon LA, Crespo MG, et al. *Rhodococcus equi*: first case in a heart transplant recipient. *J Heart Lung Transplant* 1994;13:332–335.

55. Sabater L, Andreu H, Garcia-Valdecasas JC, et al. *Rhodococcus equi* infection after liver transplantation. *Transplantation* 1996;61:980–982.

56. Novak RM, Polisky EL, Janda WM, Libertin CR. Osteomyelitis caused by *Rhodococcus equi* in a renal transplant recipient. *Infection* 1988;3:186–188.

57. Walsh RD, Schoch PE, Cunha BA. *Rhodococcus*. *Infect Control Hosp Epidemiol* 1993;14:282–207.

58. Nordmann P, Ronco E. *In vitro* antimicrobial susceptibility of *Rhodococcus equi*. *J Antimicrob Chemother* 1992;29:383–393.

59. McNeil MM, Brown JM. Distribution and antimicrobial susceptibility of *Rhodococcus equi* from clinical specimens. *Eur J Epidemiol* 1992;8:437–443.

60. Fekety R, Kim KH, Brown D, Batts D, Cudmore M, Silva J. Epidemiology of antibiotic-associated colitis. Isolation of *Clostridium difficile* from the hospital environment. *Am J Med* 1981;70:906–908.

61. Yolken RH, Bishop CA, Townsend TR, et al. Infectious gastroenteritis in bone-marrow-transplant recipients. *N Engl J Med* 1982;306:1009–1012.

62. Blakey JL, Barnes GL, Bishop RF, Ekert H. Infectious diarrhea in children undergoing bone-marrow transplantation. *Aust NZ J Med* 1989;19:31–36.

63. Aplin MS, Weiner RS, Graham Pole J, Hiemenz J, Elfenbein G, Oblon DJ. Enterocolitis in allogeneic marrow transplant patients (Abstr). *Exp Hematol* 1990;18:696.

64. Cox GJ, Matsui SM, Lo RS, et al. Etiology and outcome of diarrhea after marrow transplantation: a prospective study. *Gastroenterology* 1994;107:1398–1407.

65. Kusne S, Dummer JS, Singh N, et al. Infections after liver transplantation. An analysis of 101 consecutive cases. *Medicine* 1988;67:132–143.

66. George DL, Arnow PM, Fox AS, et al. Bacterial infection as a complication of liver transplantation: epidemiology and risk factors. *Rev Infect Dis* 1991;13:387–396.

67. Lao A, Bach D. Colonic complications in renal transplant recipients. *Dis Colon Rectum* 1988;31:130–133.

68. Kirklin JK, Holm A, Aldrete JS, White C, Bourge RC. Gastrointestinal complications after cardiac transplantation. *Ann Surg* 1990;211:538–541.

69. Green M, Wald ER, Fricker FJ, Griffith BP, Trento A. Infections in pediatric orthotopic heart transplant recipients. *Pediatr Infect Dis J* 1989;8:87–93.

70. Bartlett JG. *Clostridium difficile*: history of its role as an enteric pathogen and the current state of knowledge about the organism. *Clin Infect Dis* 1994;18:S265–S272.

71. Kelly CP, Pothoulakis C, LaMont JT. *Clostridium difficile* colitis. *N Engl J Med* 1994;330:257–330.

72. Fliermans CB, Cherry WB, Orrison LH, et al. Ecological distribution of *Legionella pneumophila*. *Appl Environ Microbiol* 1981;41:9–16.

73. Dowling JN, Pasculle AW, Frola FN, Zaphyr MK, Yee RB. Infections caused by *Legionella micdadei* and *Legionella pneumophila* among renal transplant recipients. *J Infect Dis* 1984;149:703–713.

74. Humphreys H, Marshall RJ, Mackay I, Caul EO. Pneumonia due to *Legionella bozemanii* and *Chlamydia psittaci*/TWAR following renal transplantation. *J Infect* 1992;25:67–71.

75. Jernigan DB, Sanders LI, Waites KB, Brookings ES, Benson RF, Pappas PG. Pulmonary infection due to *Legionella cincinnatiensis* in renal transplant recipients: two cases and implications for laboratory diagnosis. *Clin Infect Dis* 1994;18:385–389.

76. Valantine HA, Hunt SA, Gibbons R, Billingham ME, Stinson EB, Popp RL. Increasing pericardial effusion in cardiac transplant recipients. *Circulation* 1989;79:603–609.

77. Stout J, Yu VL, Vickers RM, et al. Ubiquitousness of *Legionella pneumophila* in the water supply of a hospital with endemic legionnaires' disease. *N Engl J Med* 1982;306:466–468.

78. Redd SC, Lin FYC, Fields BS, et al. A rural outbreak of legionnaires' disease. *Am J Public Health* 1990;80:431–434.

79. Wadowsky RM, Yee RB, Mezmar L, et al. Hot water systems as sources of *Legionella pneumophila* in hospital and nonhospital plumbing fixtures. *Appl Environ Microbiol* 1982;43:1104–1110.

80. Farrell ID, Barker JE, Miles EP, Hutchison JGP. A field study of the survival of *Legionella pneumophila* in a hospital hot-water system. *Epidemiol Infect* 1990;104:381–387.

81. Garbe PL, Davis BJ, Weisfeld JS, et al. Nosocomial legionnaires disease: Epidemiologic demonstration of cooling towers as a source. *JAMA* 1985;254:521–524.

82. Timbury MC, Donaldson JR, McCartney AC, Winter JH, Fallon RJ. How to deal with a hospital outbreak of legionnaires' disease. *J Hosp Infect* 1988;11:S189–S195.

83. Breiman RE, Cozen W, Fields BS, et al. Role of air sampling in investigation of an outbreak of legionnaires' disease associated with exposure to aerosols from an evaporative condenser. *J Infect Dis* 1990;161:1257–1261.

84. Vogt RL, Hudson PJ, Orciari L, Heun EW, Woods TC. Legionnaire's disease and a whirlpool-spa [Letter]. *Ann Intern Med* 1987;107:596.

85. Zuravleff JJ, Yu VL, Shonnard JW, Rihs JD, Best M. *Legionella pneumophila* contamination of a hospital humidifier. Demonstration of aerosol transmission and subsequent subclinical infection in exposed guinea pigs. *Am Rev Respir Dis* 1983;128:657–661.

86. Bock BV, Kirby BD, Edelstein PH, et al. Legionnaires' disease in renal-transplant recipients. *Lancet* 1978;1:410–413.

87. Gombert ME, Josephson A, Goldstein EJC, Smith PR, Butt KM. Cavitary legionnaires' pneumonia: Nosocomial infection in renal transplant recipients. *Am J Surg* 1984;147:402–405.

88. Copeland J, Wieden M, Feinberg W, Salomon N, Hager D, Galgiani J. Legionnaires' disease following cardiac transplantation. *Chest* 1981;79:669–671.

89. Horbach I, Fehrenbach FJ. Legionellosis in heart transplant recipients. *Infection* 1990;18:361–363.

90. Wilkinson HW, Thacker WL, Benson RF, et al. *Legionella birminghamensis* species *novum* isolated from a cardiac transplant recipient. *J Clin Microbiol* 1987;25:2120–2122.

91. Kugler JW, Armitage JO, Helms CM, et al. Nosocomial legionnaires' disease. Occurrence in recipients of bone marrow transplants. *Am J Med* 1983;74:281–288.

92. Benz-Lemoine E, Delwail V, Castel O, et al. Nosocomial legionnaires' disease in a bone marrow transplant unit. *Bone Marrow Transplant* 1991;7:61–63.

93. Schwebke JR, Hackman R, Bowden R. Pneumonia due to *Legionella micdadei* in bone marrow transplant recipients. *Rev Infect Dis* 1990;12:824–828.

94. Harrington RD, Woolfrey AE, Bowden R, McDowell MG, Hackman RC. Legionellosis in bone marrow transplant center. *Bone Marrow Transplant* 1996;18:361–368.

95. Singh N, Gayowski T, Wagener M, Marino IR, Yu VL. Pulmonary infections in liver transplants receiving tacrolimus. Changing pattern of microbial etiologies. *Transplantation* 1996;61:396–401.

96. Kirby BD, Snyder KM, Meyer RD, Finegold SM. Legionnaires' disease: Report of sixty-five nosocomially acquired cases and review of the literature. *Medicine* 1980;59:188–205.

97. Mayock R, Skale B, Kohler RB. *Legionella pneumophila* pericarditis proved by culture of pericardial fluid. *Am J Med* 1983;75:534–536.

98. Arnouts PJ, Ramael MR, Ysebaert DK, et al. *Legionella pneumophila* peritonitis in a kidney transplant patient. *Scand J Infect Dis* 1991;23:119–122.

99. Lowry PW, Blankenship RJ, Gridley W, Troup NJ, Tompkins LS. A cluster of *Legionella* sternal wound infections due to postoperative topical exposure to contaminated tapwater. *N Engl J Med* 1991;324:109–113.

100. Brown A, Yu VL, Elder EM, Magnussen MH, Kroboth F. Nosocomial outbreak of legionnaires' disease at the Pittsburgh Veterans Administration Medical Center. *Trans Assoc Am Physicians* 1980;93:52–59.

101. Rudin JE, Wing EJ. A comparative study of *Legionella micdadei* and other nosocomial acquired pneumonia. *Chest* 1984;86:675–680.

102. Kirby BD, Peck H, Meyer RD. Radiographic features of legionnaires' disease. *Chest* 1979;76:562–565.

103. Bauling PC, Weil RI, Schröter GPJ. *Legionella* lung abscess after renal transplantation. *J Infect* 1985;11:51–55.

104. Broome CV, Cherry WB, Winn WC, MacPherson BR. Rapid diagnosis of legionnaires' disease by direct immunofluorescent staining. *Ann Intern Med* 1979;90:1–4.

105. Edelstein PH, Meyer RD, Finegold SM. Laboratory diagnosis of legionnaires' disease. *Am Rev Respir Dis* 1980;121:317–327.

106. Kohler RB, Winn WC, Wheat LJ. Onset and duration of urinary anti-

gen excretion in legionnaires' disease. *J Clin Microbiol* 1984;20:
605–607.

107. Ruf B, Schürmann D, Horbach I, Fehrenbach FJ, Pohle HD. Prevalence and diagnosis of *Legionella* pneumonia: A 3-year prospective
study with emphasis on application of urinary antigen detection. *J
Infect Dis* 1990;162:1341–1348.

108. Edelstein PH. Antimicrobial chemotherapy for legionnaires' disease:
A review. *Clin Infect Dis* 1995;21:S265–S276.

109. Saravolatz LD, Burch KH, Fisher E, et al. The compromised host and
legionnaires' disease. *Ann Intern Med* 1979;90:533–537.

110. Martell R, Heinrichs D, Stiller C, Jenner M, Keown PA, Dupre J. The
effects of erythromycin in patients treated with cyclosporine. *Ann
Intern Med* 1986;104:660–661.

111. Langhoff E, Madsen S. Rapid metabolism of cyclosporine and prednisone in kidney transplant patient receiving tuberculostatic treatment
[Letter]. *Lancet* 1983;2:1031.

112. LeSaux NM, Sekla L, McLeod J, et al. Epidemic of nosocomial
legionnaires' disease in renal transplant recipients: A case-control and
environmental study. *Can Med Assoc J* 1989;140:1047–1053.

113. Jacobs F, Van de Stadt J, Bourgeois N, et al. Severe infections early
after liver transplantation. *Transplant Proc* 1989;21:2271–2273.

114. Vereerstraeten P, Stolear JC, Schoutens-Serruys E, et al. Erythromycin prophylaxis for legionnaire's disease in immunosuppressed
patients in a contaminated hospital environment. *Transplantation*
1986;41:52–54.

115. Dummer JS, Perez-Perez GI, Breinig MK, et al. Seroepidemiology of
Helicobacter pylori infection in heart transplant recipients. *Clin Infect
Dis* 1995;21:1303–1305.

116. Davenport A, Shallcross TM, Crabtree JE, Davison AM, Will EJ,
Heatley RV. Prevalence of *Helicobacter pylori* in patients with end-
stage renal failure and renal transplant recipients. *Nephron* 1991;59:
597–601.

117. Teenan RP, Burgoyne M, Brown IL, Murray WR. *Helicobacter* pylori
in renal transplant recipients. *Transplantation* 1993;56:100–103.

118. Tobin A, Hackman RC, McDonald GB. *H. pylori* infection in the
immunocompromised host: A prospective study of 276 patients. *Ir J
Med Sci* 1992;161:S64–S65.

119. Graham DY. Treatment of peptic ulcers caused by *Helicobacter pylori*.
N Engl J Med 1993;328:349–350.

120. Unge P. Review of *Helicobacter pylori* eradication regimens. *Scand J
Gastroenterol* 1996;215:74–81.

121. Bove JR. Transfusion-transmitted diseases: Current problems and
challenges. *Prog Hematol* 1986;14:123–147.

122. Gibel LJ, Sterling W, Hoy W, Harford A. Is serological evidence of
infection with syphilis a contraindication to kidney donation? Case
report and review of the literature. *J Urol* 1987;138:1226–1227.

123. Petersen LR, Mead RH, Perlroth MG. Unusual manifestations of secondary syphilis occurring after orthotopic liver transplantation. *Am J
Med* 1983;75:166–170.

124. Johnson PC, Norris SJ, Miller GPG, et al. Early syphilitic hepatitis
after renal transplantation. *J Infect Dis* 1988;158:236–238.

125. Taniguchi S, Osato K, Hamada T. The prozone phenomenon in secondary syphilis. *Acta Derm Venereol* 1995;75:153–154.

126. Chochon F, Kanfer A, Rondeau E, Sraer JD. Lyme disease in a kidney
transplant recipient [Letter]. *Transplantation* 1997;57:1687–1688.

127. Meyers JD, Hackman RC, Stamm WE. *Chlamydia trachomatis* infection as a cause of pneumonia after human marrow transplantation.
Transplantation 1983;36:130–134.

128. Tack KJ, Peterson PK, Rasp FL, et al. Isolation of *Chlamydia trachomatis* from the lower respiratory tract of adults. *Lancet* 1980;1:
116–121.

129. Ito JI, Comess KA, Alexander ER, et al. Pneumonia due to *Chlamydia trachomatis* in an immunocompromised adult. *N Engl J Med*
1982;307:95–97.

130. Wilson DJ, Smith TF, Van Scoy RE, Taswell HF. Prevalence of antibody to *Chlamydia* in renal transplant recipients and other population
groups. *Am J Clin Pathol* 1982;78:228–231.

131. Gaydos CA, Fowler CL, Gill VJ, Eiden JJ, Quinn TC. Detection of
Chlamydia pneumoniae by polymerase chain reaction-enzyme
immunoassay in an immunocompromised population. *Clin Infect Dis*
1993;17:718–723.

132. Griffiths PD, Lechler RI, Treharne JD. Unusual chlamydial infection
in a human renal allograft recipient. *Br Med J* 1978;2:1264–1265.

133. Toomey FB, Bailey LL, Bui RD, et al. Chest radiography in infant cardiac allotransplantation. *Am J Radiol* 1988;150:369–372.

134. Madoff S, Hooper DC. Nongenitourinary infections caused by
Mycoplasma hominis in adults. *Rev Infect Dis* 1988;10:602–613.

135. McMahon DK, Dummer JS, Pasculle AW, Cassell G. Extragenital
Mycoplasma hominis infections in adults. *Am J Med* 1990;89:
275–281.

136. Steffenson DO, Dummer JS, Granick MS, et al. Sternotomy infections
with *Mycoplasma hominis*. *Ann Intern Med* 1987;106:204–208.

137. Kane JR, Shenep JL, Krance RA, Hurwitz CA. Diffuse alveolar hemorrhage associated with *Mycoplasma hominis* respiratory tract infection in a bone marrow transplant recipient. *Chest* 1994;105:
1891–1892.

138. Cassell GH, Cole BC. Mycoplasmas as agents of human disease. *N
Engl J Med* 1981;304:80–89.

139. McCormack WM. Epidemiology of *Mycoplasma hominis*. *Sex Transm
Dis* 1997;10:S261–S262.

140. Platt R, Warren JW, Edelin KC, Lin JS, Rosner B, McCormack WM.
Infection with *Mycoplasma hominis* in postpartum fever. *Lancet* 1980;
2:1217–1221.

141. Haller M, Forst H, Ruckdeschel G, Denecke H, Peter K. Peritonitis
due to *Mycoplasma hominis* and *Ureaplasma urealyticum* in a liver
transplant recipient. *Eur J* Clin Microbiol Infect Dis 1997;10:172.

142. Gass R, Fisher J, Badesch D, et al. Donor-to-host transmission of
Mycoplasma hominis in lung allograft recipients. *Clin Infect Dis*
1996;22:567–568.

143. Jacobs F, Van de Stadt J, Gelin M, et al. *Mycoplasma hominis* infection of perihepatic hematomas in a liver transplant recipient. *Surgery*
1992;111:98–100.

144. Mokhbat JE, Peterson PK, Sabath LD, Robertson JA. Peritonitis due
to *Mycoplasma hominis* in a renal transplant recipient [Letter]. *J Infec
Dis* 1997;146:713.

145. Burdge DR, Reid GD, Reeve CE, Robertson JA, Stemke GW, Bowie
WR. Septic arthritis due to dual infection with *Mycoplasma hominis*
and *Ureaplasma urealyticum*. *J Rheumatol* 1988;15:366–368.

146. Bass JW, Vincent JM, Person DA. The expanding spectrum of *Bartonella* infections: II. Cat-scratch disease. *Pediatr Infect Dis J* 1997;
16:163–179.

147. Bass JW, Vincent JM, Person DA. The expanding spectrum of *Bartonella* infections: I. Bartonellosis and trench fever. *Pediatr Infect Dis
J* 1997;16:2–10.

148. Black JR, Herrington DA, Hadfield TL, Wear DJ, Margileth AM,
Shigekawa B. Life-threatening cat-scratch disease in an immunocompromised host. *Arch Intern Med* 1986;146:394–396.

149. Slater LN, Welch DF, Min KW. *Rochalimaea henselae* causes bacillary angiomatosis and peliosis hepatis. *Arch Intern Med* 1992;
152:602–606.

150. Caniza MA, Granger DL, Wilson KH, et al. *Bartonella henselae*: Etiology of pulmonary nodules in a patient with depressed cell-mediated
immunity. *Clin Infect Dis* 1995;20:1505–1511.

151. Apalsch AM, Nour B, Jaffe R. Systemic cat-scratch disease in a pediatric liver transplant recipient and review of the literature. *Pediatr
Infect Dis J* 1993;12:769–774.

152. Kemper CA, Lombard CM, Deresinski SC, Tompkins LS. Visceral
bacillary epithelioid angiomatosis: Possible manifestations of disseminated cat scratch disease in the immunocompromised host: A report
of two cases. *Am J Med* 1990;89:216–222.

153. Koehler JE, Tappero JW. Bacillary angiomatosis and bacillary peliosis in patients infected with human immunodeficiency virus. *Clin
Infect Dis* 1993;17:612–624.

154. Heard SR, Ronalds CJ, Heath RB. *Coxiella burnetii* infection in
immunocompromised patients. *J Infect* 1985;11:15–18.

155. Kanfer E, Farrag N, Price C, MacDonald D, Coleman J, Barrett AJ. Q
fever following bone marrow transplantation. *Bone Marrow Transplant* 1988;3:165–166.

156. Loudon MM, Thompson EN. Severe combined immunodeficiency
syndrome, tissue transplant, leukaemia, and Q fever. *Arch Dis Child*
1988;63:207–209.

157. Rallis TM, Kriesel JD, Dumler JS, Wagoner LE, Wright ED, Spruance
SL. Rocky Mountain spotted fever following cardiac transplantation.
West J Med 1993;158:625–628.

158. Antony SJ, Dummer JS, Hunter E. Human ehrlichiosis in a liver transplant recipient. *Transplantation* 1995;60:879–881.

Transplant Infections edited by
Raleigh A. Bowden, Per Ljungman, and Carlos V. Paya.
Lippincott–Raven Publishers, Philadelphia © 1998

CHAPTER 16

Cytomegalovirus Infection after BMT

Michael J. Boeckh and Per Ljungman

EPIDEMIOLOGY AND CLINICAL MANIFESTATIONS

Allogeneic Bone Marrow Transplant Recipients

Cytomegalovirus (CMV) has been one of the most feared infectious complications to allogeneic bone marrow transplantation (BMT). Reactivation of CMV occurs in approximately 80% of patients who are seropositive before transplantation; seronegative patients with seropositive marrow donors develop primary CMV infection about one-third of the time (1). Before the introduction of specific prophylaxis, the risk for CMV disease was reported to be 20% to 35% in seropositive recipients (2,3). CMV can cause multiorgan disease after BMT, including pneumonia, gastroenteritis, hepatitis, retinitis, and encephalitis. Pneumonia and gastrointestinal disease are the most common manifestations (4). It is also most likely one important cause of fever early after BMT and has been implicated as a cause of pancytopenia.

Previously, the peak incidence of CMV disease occurred approximately between days 45 and 60 after BMT; however, with current antiviral prophylaxis, CMV disease has been diagnosed more frequently after day 100 (5,6). This appears to be partly because effectively suppressing CMV replication does not allow the mounting of an adequate immune response to CMV (7,8). Incomplete T-cell reconstitution and acute and chronic Graft-versus Host Disease (GvHD), particularly associated with unrelated and mismatched grafts, may be the mechanisms for this phenomenon (6,9). At the Fred Hutchinson Cancer Research Center in Seattle, the incidence of disease before day 100 in CMV-seropositive allogeneic recipients was 35% in 1987 and 6% in 1994. The corresponding figures for disease later than 100 days after BMT were 4%

and 15%, respectively (5). After CD34$^+$-selected allogeneic peripheral blood stem cell (PBSC) transplantation, there appears to be a higher incidence of CMV infection as well as a higher CMV viral load than after marrow transplantation, possibly because of the T-cell depletion that occurs with CD34$^+$ selection (10). CMV infection after unmodified allogeneic PBSC transplantation is not different from that after allogeneic marrow transplantation (10). CMV seropositivity of the recipient was a negative predictor for survival and a risk factor for acute GvHD after umbilical cord blood transplantation in one study (11). Whether there is a different risk of CMV infection and disease in umbilical cord blood transplant recipients has not been reported.

Autologous Stem Cell Transplant Recipients

Several studies show that the incidence of CMV pneumonia after autologous BMT ranges from 1% to 6% (12–16). Furthermore, the outcome of CMV pneumonia after autologous transplantation has been similar to the outcome after allogeneic BMT (13–16). However, these reports included mostly patients with hematologic malignancies, many of whom were treated with Total Body Irradiation (TBI) or toxic combination chemotherapy regimens. CMV disease did not occur in one study of breast cancer patients who were treated with high-dose chemotherapy and autologous PBSC support (17). However, no study has analyzed the impact of the underlying diagnosis on the risk for CMV disease after autologous transplantation. Using the antigenemia assay or polymerase chain reaction (PCR), CMV infection rates of 39% and 42%, respectively, have been reported in seropositive autograft recipients (18,19). There does not seem to be a difference between marrow and PBSC with regard to the incidence of CMV infection (18). CMV disease other than pneumonia has been only rarely reported after autologous marrow and PBSC transplantation. There has been some controversy in the published literature regarding the influence of CMV on marrow engraft-

MB: From the Program in Infectious Diseases, Fred Hutchinson Cancer Research Center, Seattle, WA 98109. PL: From the Department of Hematology, Huddinge University Hospital, Karolinska Institutet, S-14186 Huddinge, Sweden.

ment (12,13). No data exist regarding CMV and engraftment after autologous PBSC transplantation.

PATHOGENESIS

The pathogenesis of CMV infection and disease after hematopoietic stem cell transplantation is complex, and substantial data have been accumulated with regard to viral factors and the interactions between CMV and the immune system. In seropositive recipients, reactivation of latent endogenous virus appears to be the most likely cause of infection. The role of exogenous virus in seropositive patients is not well defined, but co-infection with different strains can occur (20). Whether infection with multiple CMV strains results in a higher overall incidence or severity of CMV disease or higher systematic viral load is not known. In seronegative individuals, CMV is acquired from blood products or from transplanted organs (21). Both host and viral factors appear to be responsible for the progression from infection to disease. Host factors that have been associated with the CMV disease after transplant include CMV serostatus before transplant, patient's age, post-transplant immunosuppression, development of acute graft-versus-host disease (GvHD) and its treatment, and total body irradiation (4,22). Dissemination of CMV in the blood is an important factor in the pathogenesis of disease. Earlier studies have established that culture-proven viremia is highly predictive for CMV disease, but simultaneous detection of viremia and development of disease occur in more than 50% of patients (3,16,23). Using more sensitive techniques for detection of CMV in blood such as the antigenemia assay or PCR for CMV DNA, CMV can be detected in almost all patients with CMV disease. Because of the high sensitivity of these assays, CMV is also detectable in a substantial number of patients with asymptomatic infection who never progress to disease, resulting in a low positive predictive value (24,25). However, patients with disease often have higher viral loads than those who remain asymptomatic (26,27). Patients with higher viral load are also more likely to develop CMV disease both early and late (after day 100) after transplant (28,29).

There is increasing evidence that strain differences play an important role in the pathogenesis of CMV disease. Recent studies suggest that strain differences based on the CMV gB envelope protein (30) may contribute to the tropism and pathogenicity of CMV both in marrow transplant and in AIDS patients. In one study of allogeneic marrow transplant recipients, CMV gB type I was associated with favorable outcome of CMV infection (20). An association between gB types 3 and 4 and death due to secondary marrow graft failure after marrow transplantation has been reported (31).

Studies in the murine model and in human transplant recipients suggest that HLA-restricted CMV-specific cytotoxic T-cell responses (CTL) responses play an important role in the elimination of active infection and protective immunity (32,33). The virus/T-cell interaction is mediated through several mechanisms, including the virus effects on HLA expression, cytokine production, and adherence molecules. In allogeneic marrow transplant recipients who develop CMV disease, both CMV-specific CD8[+] CTL and CD4[+] Th responses are usually undetectable, although in an occasional patient, weak CD4[+] Th reactivity is observed (34,35). There is also a direct correlation between absence of CMV-specific CTL and Th responses and high CMV viral load in allogeneic marrow transplant recipients (5). In autologous peripheral blood and marrow transplant recipients, recovery of CD8[+] CTL responses is associated with subsequent protection from CMV infection (36).

Another effect of the interaction of CMV with the immune system is the association between CMV and acute and chronic GvHD. It has been clearly documented that patients with acute GvHD are at an increased risk for CMV disease (3,4). Studies in animal models have suggested that CMV increases the risk for acute GvHD (37–39). However, this has not been conclusively shown in humans (40). Seroepidemiological studies have shown an association between CMV infection and chronic GvHD (41–43). Recently, Söderberg and colleagues found that patients with chronic GvHD who had experienced CMV disease in a very high frequency had cytotoxic antibodies to CD13, an antigen that is expressed on many target cells for chronic GvHD (44,45).

PROPHYLAXIS

Prevention of Primary CMV Infection

Patients who are CMV seronegative before transplantation should, if possible, be transplanted from a CMV negative donor. This is, of course, often not possible because only a limited number of donors are available and time to find a donor is frequently critical. The risk for CMV transmission in CMV seronegative patients with seronegative marrow donors is mainly through blood products (21). Today two options exist for reducing this risk of CMV transmission: the use of blood products from CMV seronegative donors or the use of leukocyte-filtered blood products. These two options were tested in a randomized trial and shown to be comparable (46). If only a CMV-seropositive donor is available, the risk for transmission of CMV by the marrow product to the recipient is approximately 30% (1). Thus, these patients should be considered at risk for CMV disease and preventive strategies similar to those used in CMV-seropositive patients (i.e., antigenemia- or PCR-guided antiviral therapy) should be used. Two studies have been performed with intravenous immune globulin (IVIG) as prophylaxis. Bowden and colleagues showed a reduction in the rate of CMV infection but no reduction in CMV disease (47). In a similarly designed study performed by the Nordic BMT group, there was no reduction in CMV infection (48).

Antiviral Chemotherapy in Allogeneic Stem Cell Transplant

Acyclovir

The first study to demonstrate a reduction in reactivation of CMV in seropositive allogeneic recipients was the nonrandomized prospective study by Meyers and colleagues (49). In this study, patients seropositive for CMV and HSV received acyclovir (500 mg/m^2 IV every 8 hours from day −5 until day +30); patients seropositive for CMV only served as controls. CMV infection, CMV disease, and transplant survival were significantly improved in high-dose acyclovir recipients. In a prospective double-blind study performed by the European Acyclovir for CMV Study Group, patients received either high-dose IV acyclovir as used by Meyers and colleagues followed by oral acyclovir (3,200 mg/day) until day 210 after transplant, high-dose acyclovir from day −5 until day +30 followed by placebo, or HSV doses of acyclovir (1,600 mg/day p.o.) followed by placebo (50). Acyclovir significantly reduced the probability of and delayed the onset of CMV infection. There was no difference in the incidence of CMV pneumonia and all CMV diseases between the groups. Survival was improved among patients who received IV acyclovir followed by oral acyclovir when compared with patients who received low-dose acyclovir followed by placebo. The role of high-dose acyclovir in current prevention strategies consisting of prophylactic or preemptive use of ganciclovir cannot be determined from these studies. A recent retrospective analysis suggests that there is no additional survival benefit of giving high-dose acyclovir when ganciclovir was given either for prophylaxis or for antigenemia (51).

Ganciclovir

There are two strategies for antiviral prophylaxis with ganciclovir. First, ganciclovir can be given to patients who have evidence of CMV infection after marrow transplant, as indicated by a positive culture from blood, urine, throat, or bronchoalveolar lavage (BAL) fluid; CMV antigenemia; or PCR positivity (i.e., "early treatment" or "preemptive therapy"). The second strategy is the prophylactic administration of ganciclovir to all patients at risk based on the pretransplant serological status regardless of post-transplant excretion, antigenemia, or PCR positivity (i.e., "early prophylaxis" or "universal prophylaxis").

Three randomized double-blind studies have been published using an early prophylaxis strategy (52–54). Winston and colleagues randomized patients before transplant to either ganciclovir or placebo, whereas Goodrich and colleagues, and Boeckh and colleagues started pro-

phylaxis at engraftment. Goodrich and colleagues compared prophylaxis with ganciclovir given for CMV excretion from blood, urine, or throat, whereas Boeckh and colleagues compared prophylaxis with strategy based on quantitative antigenemia (see later). All three studies showed a significant reduction of infection and/or disease. Indeed, two studies showed an almost complete elimination of CMV disease while ganciclovir was given (52,54). However, severe neutropenia was a limiting factor in all three studies. There was no benefit in overall survival in any of the studies. Salzberger and colleagues analyzed risk factors for neutropenia in 278 patients who received ganciclovir at engraftment and found that early liver failure, renal insufficiency after engraftment, and a low marrow cellularity at day 28 are significantly associated with the development of neutropenia (55).

Five nonrandomized studies have been reported using a pretransplant induction course of ganciclovir from day -8 to -1 followed by lower maintenance doses of ganciclovir (i.e., 5 mg/kg, three times a week) starting at engraftment (56–60). Two of these studies, which were performed in unrelated marrow transplant recipients and recipients of T-cell-depleted marrow, respectively, showed unacceptably high rates of CMV disease (57,58). Thus this strategy may be unsafe in high-risk patients.

Although early ganciclovir prophylaxis appears to be highly effective in preventing CMV disease, significant disadvantages are associated with this strategy. Ganciclovir given at engraftment causes prolonged neutropenia, leading to more invasive bacterial and fungal infections (52,54,55). In addition, a substantial number of patients not at risk for disease (i.e., 60% to 65%) will unnecessarily receive a potentially marrow-toxic drug. Both factors may contribute substantially to morbidity and financial cost. An interference of ganciclovir with the recovery of CMV-specific immune responses has been described (8). Finally, there appears to be an increased risk of late-onset CMV disease (i.e., after day 100) when ganciclovir is given at engraftment that may be as high as 17% (54).

Foscarnet

The role of foscarnet for prevention of CMV disease remains undefined because no controlled studies have been published. Two uncontrolled studies have been reported (61,62). Reusser and colleagues reported breakthrough CMV infection in four of 12 allograft recipients and none of the seven autograft recipients but no CMV disease, and renal toxicity occurred in 11 of 19 patients who received relatively low doses of foscarnet (40 mg/kg three times daily from day -7 to day 30 followed by 60 mg/kg/day (-1 until day 75) (61). Bacigalupo and colleagues treated 11 allograft recipients (60 mg/kg three times daily from day 10 until day 15 followed by 90 mg/kg three times per week until day 100), five of whom developed CMV antigenemia and one of whom progressed to CMV disease (62).

Intravenous Immunoglobulin

The use of intravenous immunoglobulin (IVIG) or hyperimmune globulin for the prophylaxis of CMV infection and disease after allogeneic transplants remains controversial. Although the prophylactic use of IVIG is associated with virtually no toxicity, the regimens proposed are costly, and controlled studies assessing the effect in preventing CMV disease show conflicting results with regard to the prevention of CMV disease (21,47,48,63–67). In addition, some studies showed a reduction of bacteremia, non-CMV interstitial pneumonia, and/or acute GVHD, whereas other studies did not report such a difference. An improvement of survival has not been reported in any of the studies.

Critique of Prophylaxis Strategies

An attractive feature of any effective prophylaxis strategy is that it is simple and does not require virologic monitoring. Presently, intravenous ganciclovir prophylaxis appears to be the most effective way of preventing CMV disease. This strategy should be used in CMV-seropositive allograft recipients when no virologic monitoring by PCR or the antigenemia assay is available. However, ganciclovir prophylaxis has significant disadvantages (Table 1) that can be overcome, in part, by PCR- or antigenemia-guided preemptive treatment strategies. Whether empiric reduction of the maintenance dose can reduce neutropenia has not been studied in a controlled fashion. There is, however, good evidence that such a strategy is not safe in high-risk patients, including those with severe GvHD or after T-cell depletion (57,58). High-dose acyclovir prophylaxis, although it has only a limited effect on CMV disease, is associated with a survival benefit in low-risk patients (i.e., those with a low risk of acute GvHD) when no ganciclovir prophylaxis or antigenemia- or PCR-guided therapy is given (49,50,68). However, there does not seem to be a survival advantage when either of these ganciclovir strategies is used (51). Because of the high cost, the only moderate effect on CMV, and the lack of data demonstrating that high-dose acyclovir adds additional benefit when ganciclovir is given as prophylaxis at engraftment or for antigenemia or PCR positivity, most centers do not use acyclovir for prophylaxis of CMV disease. The reason that acyclovir and not ganciclovir prophylaxis has been associated with a survival benefit in randomized trials is difficult to determine because no comparative study has been done. There are several possible explanations: first, the toxic side effects of ganciclovir may lead to more fatal fungal infections that outweigh the reduction in CMV-related mortality (54). Second, the risk profile of the patient population may be important. Acyclovir studies have been performed in patients with a low incidence of severe acute GvHD (49,50,68). In these patients the protection from fatal CMV disease provided by acyclovir may be sufficient, possibly because of better CMV-specific immune reconstitution resulting from the only moderate inhibition of CMV reactivation by acyclovir and reduced use of high-

TABLE 1. *Options for prevention of CMV diseases in allogeneic BMT recipients*

Strategy	Advantages	Disadvantages	References
Prophylaxis			
Intravenous immunoglobulin	Low risk for side effects	Low efficacy High cost Overtreatment	(21,47,48,63–67)
High-dose acyclovir	Low risk for side effects	Low effectiveness for prevention of CMV disease	(49,50)
	Survival benefit in patients not receiving ganciclovir prophylaxis or preemptive therapy	High cost Overtreatment	
Ganciclovir at engraftment	Highly effective	High risk of neutropenia High risk of invasive fungal infections High risk of late CMV disease Delay of recovery of CMV-specific T-cell function Overtreatment	(5,8,52,53,55)
Preemptive therapy			
Based on PCR for CMV-DNA	Effective Targeted treatment	Requirement for close monitoring Occasionally missed cases of CMV disease	(74)
Based on pp65 antigenemia	Effective Targeted treatment Less invasive fungal infections (compared with ganciclovir at engraftment)	Requirement for close monitoring Increased risk of CMV disease (compared with ganciclovir at engraftment) when ganciclovir is delayed until ≥2 positive cells per slide and discontinued based on a negative test	(54)

dose corticosteroids. Third, the survival benefit in acyclovir studies may have been due to a significant reduction of other herpesviruses, such as HHV-6 during the preengraftment period (40). Finally, both design and sample size of the studies may explain results. In two of three ganciclovir studies, patients in the control group also received some ganciclovir, and the sample size in all studies was calculated to detect differences in the incidence of CMV disease rather than survival (52–54). Study design plays an important role, as is illustrated by the fact that ganciclovir did show a survival benefit when only high-risk patients (i.e., isolation from blood, urine, throat) were studied (69). In this group of patients, the anti-CMV effect probably outweighed the neutropenia-associated deaths.

With regard to the use of IVIG, there are several factors that may explain the inconsistency of the results, including (a) use of nonspecific IVIG versus hyperimmune globulin; (b) differing doses, dose schedules, duration of administration after transplant, and preparation of the product; (c) mixed patient populations with different risk for CMV disease (i.e., inclusion of autologous and allogeneic patients with different CMV serostatus); (d) varying supportive care techniques; and (e) different GvHD prophylaxis regimens. Recently, the available studies have been analyzed in three reviews that result in conflicting conclusions (70–72). Furthermore, there is no randomized trial that evaluates IVIG when ganciclovir prophylaxis or preemptive treatment is given. Therefore most transplant centers do not use IVIG for prevention of CMV disease after allogeneic transplant.

Autologous Stem Cell Transplant

There was no evidence that high-dose acyclovir had any impact on the incidence of disease in the study by Boeckh and colleagues (15). There is also no evidence that IVIG is effective for prevention of CMV disease in autologous transplant recipients (73).

PREEMPTIVE THERAPY

Allogeneic Stem Cell Transplant Patients

A disadvantage with prophylaxis given at engraftment is that all patients with varying risks for CMV disease will receive the antiviral drug and will thereby be at risk for drug-related side effects. It would therefore be of value to identify the patients who have the highest risk for development of CMV disease. The preemptive therapy strategy is based on detection of CMV reactivation with a rapid diagnostic technique and then initiation of antiviral therapy. One advantage of this strategy is that only those patients who are judged to be at high risk for CMV disease will get treatment that would reduce the risk of side effects and, potentially, the cost. The disadvantages with this strategy are the requirement to monitor patients and

the possibility that some patients might develop CMV disease before the indicator test becomes positive.

Thus the requirements for use of a preemptive strategy are (a) availability of a reliable and rapid early diagnostic technique; (b) close surveillance (e.g., weekly) with the selected technique; (c) selection of the adequate samples for detection of virus. Several studies have shown that CMV viremia is predictive for the development of CMV disease (3,9,23). However, the rapid or standard isolation techniques used in the early studies were not sensitive enough to allow initiation of antiviral therapy before CMV disease had developed in a significant proportion of the patients. This was shown in a study by Goodrich and colleagues in which, although the risk for CMV disease was significantly reduced in the preemptive therapy group, 12% of the patients developed CMV disease before antiviral therapy had been initiated (70). Schmidt and colleagues used BAL fluid obtained from asymptomatic patients at day 35 after transplantation that was analyzed by rapid isolation and showed that preemptive therapy reduced the risk for progression to CMV pneumonia (23). However, this technique also failed to identify 13% of the patients who developed CMV pneumonia. More recent studies that included a high number of seropositive unrelated and HLA-mismatched recipients showed disease rates of up to 30% with shell vial-guided early treatment (52,74). Today more sensitive techniques are available, such as the antigenemia assay and PCR (see later).

PCR for CMV DNA

PCR for detection of CMV DNA has been evaluated in several studies. Einsele and colleagues showed that PCR on leukocytes can detect CMV infection earlier than rapid isolation (75). Similar data were presented by Wolf and colleagues, who used plasma for detection of CMV DNA (76). A direct comparison between PCR in leukocytes and plasma suggests that PCR in plasma is less sensitive (25,77). Several laboratories are now evaluating quantitative PCR and also PCR for CMV RNA (78–80). Recently, Einsele and colleagues showed in a randomized trial that the use of PCR-based ganciclovir treatment reduced the incidence of CMV disease and CMV-associated mortality compared with ganciclovir based on rapid isolation (74) (Table 2). Ljungman and colleagues showed, in a trial that compared PCR-based diagnosis with historical control patients monitored with rapid isolation techniques, that PCR allowed significantly earlier initiation of therapy and led to a reduced risk for CMV disease (81). Furthermore, when the samples that were positive by PCR were analyzed in a semi-quantitative fashion, a higher amount of CMV DNA was associated with an increased risk for CMV disease (81). This finding indicates that the preemptive therapy strategy could be developed even further and that the proportion of patients requiring antiviral therapy might be reduced

TABLE 2. *Design and results of randomized studies using PCR- or antigenemia-guided early treatment*

Characteristic/end point	Einsele et al. (71)		Boeckh et al. (7)
Recipient pretransplant CMV serostatus	Seropositive or seronegative[a]		Seropositive
Treatment study group	• Ganciclovir and CMV-Ig for two consecutive positive PCR results • Discontinuation after 2 weeks or when PCR negative • Repeated treatment if PCR positivity recurred		• Ganciclovir for antigenemia (≥2 positive cells/slide) • Discontinuation after 3 weeks or 6 days after negative antigenemia assay • Repeated treatment at same level when of antigenemia if antigenemia recurred
Treatment control group	• Ganciclovir for 2 weeks detection of CMV by shell vial cultures from blood, urine, or throat wash • Thereafter same PCR-guided ganciclovir as above		• Ganciclovir from engraftment until day 100
Design	Randomized, open-label		Randomized, double-blind
Time of randomization	Before transplant		At engraftment
Primary end points	CMV disease, CMV-related mortality, survival		CMV disease, neutropenia
Sample size	71[a]		226
Incidence of CMV disease[b]	All randomized patients	High-risk engrafted patient[d]	
Day 100	5.4% vs. 23.5%, $p=0.004$	7.7% vs. 32%, $p=0.03$	14.1% vs. 2.7%, $p=0.002$[e]
Day 180	8.1% vs. 32.4%, $p=$NR	11.5% vs. 44%, $p=$NR	15.8% vs. 9.8%, $p=0.17$
Day 400	13.5% vs. 38.2%, $p=$NR	19.2% vs. 52%, $p=$NR	20.2% vs. 16.1%, $p=0.42$
CMV-related mortality[b,c]			
Day 100	0% vs. 14.7%, $p=0.02$	NR	6.1% vs. 0.9%, $p=0.07$
Day 180	NR	NR	7.0% vs. 3.6%, $p=0.21$
Day 400	NR	NR	11.4% vs. 11.6%, $p=1.0$
Neutropenia[a] <500/mm³	5.4% vs. 23.5%, $p=0.02$	NR	26% vs. 20%, $p=0.27$
Invasive infections[b]			
Fungal	2.7% vs. 17.6%, $p=0.03$	NR	6% vs. 16%, $p=0.03$
Transplant survival[b]			
Day 100	87% vs. 67%, $p=0.05$	92% vs. 72%, $p=0.05$	84% vs. 87%, $p=0.51$
Day 180	84% vs. 59%, $p=0.02$	88% vs. 60%, $p=0.02$	73% vs. 71%, $p=0.91$
Day 400	NR	NR	61% vs. 59%, $p=0.80$

NR, not reported.

[a]Study included 14 seronegative recipients with seronegative donors and 18 seronegative recipients with seropositive donors.

[b]Results show study group versus control group.

[c]Defined as histopathologic evidence at autopsy (Einsele et al.) or death within 6 weeks after diagnosis of CMV disease (Boeckh et al.).

[d]To compare both studies, results from high-risk patients who have engrafted are presented (excluding serenegative recipients of seropositive marrow).

[e]Disease before or following antigenemia of ≥2 positive cells per slide 8.8%; disease shortly after discontinuation of ganciclovir based on a negative test 5.3%.

without increasing the risk for breakthrough CMV disease. However, because even patients with low systemic CMV viral load can develop CMV disease after allogeneic BMT, this strategy might fail in patients who progress rapidly from low viral load to overt disease, such as those with severe acute GvHD (54).

Antigenemia

The antigenemia assay is based on the detection of the CMV lower matrix protein pp65 in polymorphonuclear leukocytes by immunostaining with monoclonal antibodies (28,82,83). Results are available within 5 hours, and the technique is more sensitive than rapid isolation. Furthermore, it is quantitative so that patients who have a high number of antigenemia-positive leukocytes are at a higher risk for developing CMV disease (28). Boeckh and colleagues, in a randomized, double-blind study, evaluated a preemptive therapy strategy based on CMV viral load measured by quantitative antigenemia (see Table 2). The study indicated that antigenemia-guided early treatment based on a certain level of antigenemia could be used with similar efficacy in preventing CMV disease by 1 year as ganciclovir prophylaxis (54). However, ganciclovir prophylaxis was more effective in preventing CMV disease during the time it was given (the first 100 days after BMT), but the risk for late CMV disease was higher in the ganciclovir prophylaxis group, equalizing the risk for CMV disease at 180 days after transplantation. Survival was similar at any time during the first 400 days after transplant. The higher incidence of CMV disease before day 100 was likely due to the delay of ganciclovir until levels of antigenemia of ≥2 positive cells per slide and discontinuation based on a negative test in patients with severe GvHD.

Another risk-adapted strategy that combines both immunologic and virologic risk factors is to give a short course of ganciclovir to patients who receive high-dose steroids for treatment of acute GvHD or for CMV antigenemia (84). In an uncontrolled trial that included HLA-matched related allogeneic transplant recipients, there was no case of CMV disease within the first 180 days after transplant using such an approach (84). Whether this approach is useful in unrelated and HLA-mismatched patients and whether it is superior to early treatment strategies based on virologic marker only has not been studied in a randomized fashion.

Either of two antiviral drugs can be used for preemptive therapy, ganciclovir and foscarnet. Ganciclovir has been used in most published studies. Foscarnet has been studied in two small uncontrolled studies that showed rates of effectiveness similar to that of ganciclovir (85,86). A randomized trial comparing ganciclovir and foscarnet has just been performed within the European Group for Blood and Marrow Transplantation. In a retrospective comparison of patients who presented with antigenemia of more than four positive cells per slide, patients who received both ganciclovir and foscarnet had a reduced transplant-related mortality compared with those treated with either ganciclovir or foscarnet as a single agent (87). This result requires confirmation in a randomized trial. Until now, there are no data regarding oral ganciclovir as preemptive therapy.

The duration of preemptive therapy has varied greatly in published studies. In the early studies ganciclovir therapy, once started, continued until day 100 after transplantation, which gives a therapy duration of 6–8 weeks in most patients (23,70). More recently, shorter periods of therapy have been used. For example, Einsele and colleagues (74) gave ganciclovir for a mean of 3 weeks and Ljungman and colleagues gave a mean of 2 weeks of therapy (81). Drawbacks with shorter courses of therapy are that treatment might have to be reinstituted in up to 30% of patients and occasional cases of CMV disease shortly after discontinuation of ganciclovir (24,54). However, the advantages are lower cost, lower risk for side effects, and the possibility that short duration of therapy might allow a better reconstitution of the specific immune response to CMV, thereby reducing the risk of late CMV disease (54).

Critique of Preemptive Strategies

Recent studies suggest that preemptive treatment strategies based on rapid culture techniques cannot be considered optimal for prevention of CMV disease (52,74). Based on data from two randomized trials, both antigenemia- and PCR-guided strategies currently provide the best results using this strategy. There are important differences in the design and outcome of these two trials. Whereas Einsele and colleagues performed a superiority trial that was designed to show an advantage of PCR-guided therapy compared with the less effective rapid culture-guided treatment, Boeckh and colleagues performed a larger equivalence trial comparing short-term ganciclovir based on quantitative antigenemia with ganciclovir at engraftment, presently the most effective way of preventing CMV disease. The shell vial culture–based strategy used in the control group of the study by Einsele and colleagues showed particularly poor results, with an incidence of CMV disease of 32% by day 100 in high-risk patients (i.e., seropositive patients or donors, engrafted) (74). Consequently, the results of both trials are different. Einsele and colleagues found a significant reduction of CMV disease and improved survival with PCR-guided ganciclovir, whereas the antigenemia-guided treatment as used by Boeckh and colleagues was associated with more CMV disease by day 100. However, the actual incidence of CMV disease before day 100 is quite similar, especially if one considers that in the Seattle study only seropositive individuals were included. Because the control group in the Seattle study had received the best available prophylaxis for CMV disease, there was no apparent difference in survival. Although both studies used a short-term treatment regimen for ganciclovir, the incidence of severe neutropenia seemed lower in patients who received PCR-guided treated (74) when compared with patients treated based on antigenemia (54) (see Table 2). However, Einsele and colleagues did not report the incidence of neutropenia in high-risk patients (i.e., seropositive recipients), and the use of hematopoietic growth factors was not standardized in either study. Also, patients in the Seattle study may have included a population at higher risk for ganciclovir-related neutropenia (55). The Seattle study also provided important insight regarding the use of systemic viral load to direct antiviral treatment. The results suggest that measuring systemic viral load is of limited value in patients with severe GvHD because of the rapid tempo of progression. Thus using viral load measured by antigenemia to limit the amount of antiviral drug treatment does not appear to be safe in these patients, and even low levels of antigenemia should be treated. Whether viral load measurement by a highly sensitive quantitative PCR assay can overcome these problems has not been studied. In patients without or with mild GvHD, CMV viral load measurement appears to be a useful strategy to target antiviral drug treatment (54).

Autologous Stem Cell Transplant Patients

Autologous stem cell transplant patients have a lower risk for development of CMV, and few studies have studied preemptive therapy after autologous transplantation. Boeckh and colleagues investigated the use of antigenemia in surveillance of autologous stem cell transplant patients and found that it is more sensitive than viremia and that the technique's ability to quantify viral load might be useful (18). Hebart and colleagues, using semi-quantitative PCR for CMV DNA in whole blood, reported similar findings (19). However, because CMV disease after autologous transplantation is rare, the cost of monitoring for CMV with any technique is unlikely to be cost-effective in all seropositive patients. A high-risk group for CMV disease after autologous transplant that might benefit most from virologic monitoring has not been defined.

DIAGNOSIS AND THERAPY OF ESTABLISHED CMV DISEASE

Today the need to treat established disease has to be regarded as a failure of the preventive strategy used. However, in some high-risk patient populations the incidence of the disease is still substantial, especially CMV disease of delayed onset. Although the risk for CMV disease occurring before day 100 has decreased, in most centers the risk for late CMV disease has increased. It is important in assessing different centers' experiences that the same definitions of CMV disease are used. Therefore the fourth and fifth International CMV conferences produced a set of definitions for use in clinical studies of CMV infection and disease in immunocompromised patients (88,89). These definitions are used in the remainder of this chapter.

CMV Pneumonia in Allogeneic Bone Marrow Transplant Recipients

CMV pneumonia continues to be associated with a high mortality. The symptoms of pneumonia are initially nonspecific, with dry cough, hypoxemia, and low-degree fever, but it can progress rapidly to respiratory failure. The radiograph often shows an interstitial pattern, but other patterns, including alveolar changes or diffuse nodular changes, can be seen. Severe hypoxemia at presentation is a poor prognostic sign, and most patients who require ventilator assistance will succumb to the disease (16).

Diagnosis of CMV Pneumonia

No clinical or radiologic features distinguish CMV pneumonia from pneumonia caused by other opportunistic pathogens. Thus the diagnosis has to rely on pneumonia in the appropriate clinical setting combined with identification of CMV from the lower respiratory tract, such as bronchoalveolar lavage (BAL), transbronchial biopsy, or open lung biopsy. Open lung biopsy was previously the

gold standard for diagnosis of CMV infection in the immunocompromised host. This procedure was associated with significant morbidity and has today been replaced by BAL in most centers based on a comparative trial that showed equivalence of diagnosis by BAL and biopsy (90). The problem with the use of BAL is the risk of overdiagnosis. It has been shown that CMV can be isolated from BAL in patients without any signs or symptoms of respiratory disease (23,91). In BMT recipients, Schmidt and colleagues showed in a randomized trial that CMV detection in BAL from asymptomatic patients at day 35 after transplant was highly predictive for later development of CMV pneumonia (23). However, approximately one-third of asymptomatic patients who had CMV detected in BAL fluid did not go on to develop CMV pneumonia. Thus the finding of CMV in BAL in asymptomatic patients must be interpreted with caution. During the last few years, even more sensitive techniques such as PCR have been introduced for the detection of CMV DNA from BAL but have the same or greater problem as shell vial cultures or direct fluorescent antibody tests (i.e., overdiagnosis). In a study by Cathomas and colleagues, PCR of BAL had a very high negative predictive value; however, the positive predictive value of a positive PCR was low because of the high sensitivity of PCR assay (92). It was suggested that the combination of such techniques as PCR and immune-staining of alveolar cells can improve the specificity and positive predictive value (92). Thus qualitative PCR of BAL can be used to rule out CMV as a cause of pneumonia in BMT recipients.

Quantitation of CMV from the lung or BAL specimens has been explored as a way of differentiating asymptomatic virus shedding from CMV pneumonia. In BMT recipients there was no relation between the virus load in centrifugation culture and asymptomatic CMV excretion or CMV pneumonia (93). More recently, Boivin and colleagues measured CMV viral load by quantitative PCR and CMV gene expression in 18 patients with asymptomatic pulmonary shedding and 19 patients with definite or probable CMV pneumonitis (94). There was >2 $\log_{10}$ difference in the amount of DNA between patients with asymptomatic shedding and definite or probable CMV pneumonia. In addition, all patients with definite or probable CMV pneumonitis had detectable CMV glycoprotein H mRNA compared with none of the asymptomatic shedders (94). These data suggest that CMV viral load in the lung plays an important role in the pathogenesis of CMV pneumonia.

One important challenge is what to do when CMV is found in BAL fluid together with another opportunistic organism. The interpretation of the results of the diagnostic procedures must depend on the risk for severe CMV disease occurring in the individual patient under consideration. Currently, no test can differentiate between CMV pneumonia and asymptomatic pulmonary shedding. Presence of CMV-infected endothelial cells in the peripheral blood, previously associated with organ site disease in solid organ and AIDS patients, was of only limited value in making that distinction after BMT (95).

Treatment of CMV Pneumonia

The earliest treatment studies used agents with limited effectiveness against CMV such as vidarabine, alpha-interferon, acyclovir, and combinations of alpha-interferon with acyclovir or vidarabine. Patient survival in these studies ranged from 0 to 20%. Early experience with ganciclovir or foscarnet used as single agents in BMT patients did not improve survival despite the fact that these agents are effective against CMV (96,97). Treatment with CMV hyperimmune globulin alone gave conflicting results (98,99). The concept of combining antiviral treatment with IVIG came from animal studies that had shown that the course of CMV pneumonia can be modified by a combination of ganciclovir and anti-CMV antiserum, whereas ganciclovir alone was not successful (100,101). In 1988, this hypothesis was tested in noncontrolled studies performed by three different transplant groups. In these studies, a short-term survival of 50% to 70% was found, indicating an improvement compared with previous results with single-agent therapy (102–104). Similar results were reported recently from the University of Minnesota, although patients who were ventilator dependent at the time of diagnosis seemed to have an extremely poor prognosis (16). However, in a survey of patients treated in different centers belonging to the European Group for Blood and Marrow Transplantation (EBMT), the survival at 30 days after start of treatment was only 31% (105). In the EBMT study two potential prognostic factors were suggested—namely, a negative effect of conditioning regimens that included TBI and a positive effect of BAL as the used diagnostic procedure, rather than open lung biopsy or transbronchial biopsy. The survival in the European survey increased to 53% when only patients who had CMV pneumonia diagnosed by BAL were included.

Based on these studies, most transplant centers today use a combined treatment regimen consisting of ganciclovir 5 mg/kg BID for 14–21 days followed by maintenance therapy with a lower dosage for at least 2 weeks and IVIG. Many different dosages of IVIG were used in the early reports, and none was clearly superior to any other. There has been no advantage for using CMV hyperimmune globulin rather than standard IVIG. A dosage frequently used today is 0.5 g/kg body weight of standard intravenous immune globulin given every other day during the first 2 weeks of ganciclovir therapy.

Although the efficacy of foscarnet *in vitro* is similar to that of ganciclovir in the treatment of CMV retinitis in HIV-infected patients (106), only anecdotal cases have been reported concerning the use of foscarnet combined with immune globulin for therapy for CMV pneumonia

in allogeneic BMT recipients. Combination antiviral therapy has not been evaluated in BMT recipients with CMV disease.

Based on the early promising results with the combination of ganciclovir and intravenous immune globulin and the good results of preventing CMV disease with prophylaxis and preemptive therapy, there has been limited interest in and opportunities for performing treatment studies for established CMV pneumonia. Boeckh and colleagues recently reported results of treatment collected during the last decade, and the mortality in established CMV pneumonia remains more than 50% (5). Furthermore, they could find no difference in outcome of therapy in early (before day 100) and late (after day 100) CMV pneumonia.

Thus the results of treatment of established CMV pneumonia are clearly unsatisfactory, and the increased risk for late CMV disease in unrelated and HLA mismatched transplant recipients, despite good preventive strategies during the early phase after BMT, underscores the need for more effective treatment of established CMV pneumonia.

CMV Pneumonia in Autologous Bone Marrow Transplant Recipients

Less information is available concerning therapy for CMV pneumonia in autologous BMT recipients. In a survey from the EBMT the survival at 30 days from diagnosis was only 43% (14). Similar survival data were published from the Minnesota group and from Seattle (13,15,16). Thus although CMV pneumonia is rare after autologous BMT, survival does not seem to be better than in allogeneic BMT recipients. It is not possible from the published data to draw any conclusion about the best treatment regimen or if addition of high dosage of immune globulin to antiviral therapy would be of value in autologous BMT recipients.

CMV Gastrointestinal Disease

CMV gastrointestinal disease can occur all the way from the esophagus to the colon. Thus the symptoms vary, depending on the location of the disease, including epigastric pains, vomiting, abdominal cramps, and diarrhea. At endoscopy, ulcerations are frequently seen, but macroscopic appearance cannot differentiate from other causes such as GvHD and HSV infection. Furthermore, CMV gastrointestinal disease can occur together with acute GvHD of the gut, which makes each factor's contribution to the symptoms of the patient difficult to assess. This makes specific diagnosis crucial. Therefore this diagnosis should be based on biopsy material analyzed by appropriate histopathological and virologic techniques (88,107).

There is no established therapy for CMV gastrointestinal disease. Reed and colleagues performed a double-blind, placebo-controlled, randomized study of 2 weeks of therapy with ganciclovir and could not show any difference in symptoms, progression to CMV pneumonia, or survival (108). Possible reasons for the failure to show a benefit of ganciclovir therapy include the short duration or inadequate dose of ganciclovir (7.5 mg/kg/day for 14 days) and other concomitant causes of gastrointestinal symptoms, such as GvHD, or ineffectiveness of ganciclovir alone. Because of the latter hypothesis many centers have added IVIG to ganciclovir, similar to the treatment regimen for CMV pneumonia. Recently, the Infectious Diseases Working Party of the EBMT performed a retrospective study showing no advantage with the addition of immune globulin (109). Aschan and colleagues published data supporting the use of foscarnet as alternative therapy of CMV gastrointestinal disease (97). No controlled studies of therapy duration have been performed. Because of the unsatisfactory experience with using 2 weeks of antiviral therapy in the study by Reed and colleagues, many centers now give longer courses of therapy. These courses usually include at least 2 weeks of induction therapy (5 mg/kg twice daily) followed by 2–4 weeks maintenance. If CMV ulcers are significant in size on endoscopic examination or if symptoms persist, longer maintenance courses may be required.

Other CMV-Associated Diseases

CMV hepatitis occurs in BMT recipients but is difficult to document and appears to be rarely severe. To differentiate from other causes of liver function abnormalities, biopsy material is needed, and documentation of CMV by culture or histopathology and histologic evidence of hepatitis is required. Encephalitis and retinitis have been rare complications, but recent reports indicate that these manifestations might become more common in unrelated transplant recipients developing CMV disease late after transplantation. Symptoms of encephalitis are frequently nonspecific, with headache, confusion, and fatigue, and the diagnosis must therefore rely on detection of CMV in the cerebrospinal fluid. Recent data support that PCR for CMV DNA is both sensitive and highly specific for the diagnosis of CMV CNS disease (110). The diagnosis of retinitis is based on typical retinal lesions. The so-called CMV syndrome with fever and bone marrow suppression is difficult to differentiate from several other etiologies, such as other viral infections, drug toxicity, and marrow rejection; therefore it is currently not accepted as a separate disease entity in the definitions adopted by the CMV conferences. However, *in vitro* studies support that CMV has an inhibitory effect on hematopoiesis, and there are well-documented cases of late marrow failures after BMT that can also occur with low or undetectable systemic viral load (111).

There have been no controlled treatment trials in any of these more rare CMV-associated diseases in BMT recipients. The experience of many centers, however, supports the idea that either ganciclovir or foscarnet can be used for therapy. This is consistent with studies in HIV-infected patients that show that both agents are effective in the treatment of CMV retinitis (106). Resistance to ganciclovir or foscarnet is common in HIV-infected patients but has been rare in BMT patients. However, with the increased use of repeated courses of therapy needed for controlling CMV in patients with severe acute and chronic GvHD, it is likely that more resistant CMV mutants will also be found in BMT recipients.

NEW IMMUNOLOGIC STRATEGIES

Because the principal immunologic defect in the host defense against CMV seems to be a delayed recovery of HLA-restricted CMV-specific CD8$^+$ cytotoxic T-lymphocyte (CTL) function, studies are currently being conducted to adoptively transfer donor-derived CTL after transplant. In a pioneering study, Riddell and co-workers demonstrated that donor CMV-specific CTL can be expanded *in vitro* and can be safely infused after transplant. The clones were detectable for up to 12 weeks (112). A phase II study is currently under way. Another approach that might be useful in the future is to augment the donor immunity before transplant by donor vaccination, possibly combined with recipient vaccination. The most promising candidate antigen for vaccine development is pp65 (UL83), which has been shown to be a target antigen for CMV-specific CTL (113).

NEW CHEMOTHERAPEUTIC APPROACHES

Several new anti-CMV drugs are currently in various stages of clinical evaluation. Oral ganciclovir has been evaluated in a phase I/II study and has shown an absorption rate similar to that reported in other settings (114). However, gastrointestinal intolerance seems to be a limiting factor in the early post-transplant period with the current formulation (114). Whether oral ganciclovir can prevent CMV disease, especially in patients with acute GvHD, has not been studied. An oral pro-drug of ganciclovir that has a higher bioavailability is currently under study in HIV-infected patients. A randomized phase II trial of a human monoclonal antibody specific to the glycoprotein gH (MSL-109) has been completed in allogeneic marrow transplant recipients and results are forthcoming. Valaciclovir, the pro-drug of acyclovir, is currently being tested in two different phase III trials. Cidofovir (HPMPC) has been used successfully for treatment of CMV retinitis in AIDS patients. Its principal toxicity, renal insufficiency, can be ameliorated by concomitant use of probenecid (115). Whether cidofovir is safe and effective after BMT has not been studied. Lobucavir, a cyclobutyl analog of guanine with broad *in vitro* activity against most herpesviruses, and 1263W94, a benzimidazole riboside with potent anti-CMV activity, have entered clinical trials in HIV-infected patients. Both compounds are promising and may be evaluated in hematopoietic stem cell transplant recipients in the future.

ACKNOWLEDGMENTS

Grant support: Michael Boeckh was supported in part by the National Institutes of Health (CA 18029).

REFERENCES

1. Boeckh M, Riddell SR, Woogerd P, Cunningham T, White K, Bowden RA. Primary CMV infection via marrow: incidence, response to early treatment, CMV-specific immune response, and risk of late CMV disease. In: 9th International Symposium on Infections in the Immunocompromised Host. Assisi, Italy, 1996.
2. Meyers JD, Flournoy N, Thomas ED. Nonbacterial pneumonia after allogeneic marrow transplantation: a review of ten years' experience. *Rev Infect Dis* 1982;4:1119–1132.
3. Meyers JD, Ljungman P, Fisher LD. Cytomegalovirus excretion as a predictor of cytomegalovirus disease after marrow transplantation: importance of cytomegalovirus viremia. *J Infect Dis* 1990;162:373–380.
4. Meyers JD, Flournoy N, Thomas ED. Risk factors for cytomegalovirus infection after human marrow transplantation. *J Infect Dis* 1986;153:478–488.
5. Boeckh M, Riddell SR, Cunningham T, Myerson D, Flowers M, Bowden PA. Increased incidence of late CMV disease in allogeneic marrow transplant recipients after ganciclovir prophylaxis is due to a lack of CMV-specific T cell responses. *Blood* 1996;88[Supplement 1]:302a.
6. Krause H, Hebart H, Jahn G, Müller CA, Einsele H. Screening for CMV-specific T cell proliferation to identify patients at risk of developing late onset CMV disease. *Bone Marrow Transplant* 1997;19:1111–1116.
7. Bowden RA, Digel J, Reed EC, Meyers JD. Immunosuppressive effects of ganciclovir on *in vitro* lymphocyte responses. *J Infect Dis* 1987;156:899–903.
8. Li CR, Greenberg PD, Gilbert MJ, Goodrich JM, Riddell SR. Recovery of HLA-restricted cytomegalovirus (CMV)-specific T-cell responses after allogeneic bone marrow transplant: correlation with CMV disease and effect of ganciclovir prophylaxis. *Blood* 1994;83:1971–1979.
9. Ljungman P, Aschan J, Azinge JN, et al. Cytomegalovirus viraemia and specific T-helper cell responses as predictors of disease after allogeneic marrow transplantation. *Br J Haematol* 1993;83:118–124.
10. Boeckh M, Gooley T, Bowden RA. CMV infection and viral load after peripheral blood stem cell transplant versus marrow transplant. In: 6th International Cytomegalovirus Workshop. Perdido Beach, AL, 1997.
11. Gluckman E, Rocha V, Boyer-Chammard A, et al. Outcome of cord-blood transplantation from related and unrelated donors. *N Engl J Med* 1997;337:373–381.
12. Wingard JR, Chen DY, Burns WH, et al. Cytomegalovirus infection after autologous bone marrow transplantation with comparison to infection after allogeneic bone marrow transplantation. *Blood* 1988;71:1432–1437.
13. Reusser P, Fisher LD, Buckner CD, Thomas ED, Meyers JD. Cytomegalovirus infection after autologous bone marrow transplantation: occurrence of cytomegalovirus disease and effect on engraftment. *Blood* 1990;75:1888–1894.
14. Ljungman P, Biron P, Bosi A, et al. Cytomegalovirus interstitial pneumonia in autologous bone marrow transplant recipients. Infectious Disease Working Party of the European Group for Bone Marrow Transplantation. *Bone Marrow Transplant* 1994;13:209–212.
15. Boeckh M, Gooley TA, Reusser P, Buckner CD, Bowden RA. Failure of high-dose acyclovir to prevent cytomegalovirus disease after autologous marrow transplantation. *J Infect Dis* 1995;172:939–943.
16. Enright H, Haake R, Weisdorf D, et al. Cytomegalovirus pneumonia after bone marrow transplantation. Risk factors and response to therapy. *Transplantation* 1993;55:1339–1346.
17. Holland HK, Dix SP, Geller RB, et al. Minimal toxicity and mortality in high-risk breast cancer patients receiving high-dose cyclophosphamide, thiotepa, and carboplatin plus autologous marrow/stem-cell transplantation and comprehensive supportive care. *J Clin Oncol* 1996;14:1156–1164.
18. Boeckh M, Stevens-Ayers T, Bowden RA. Cytomegalovirus pp65 antigenemia after autologous marrow and peripheral blood stem cell transplantation. *J Infect Dis* 1996;174:907–912.
19. Hebart H, Schröder A, Löffler J, et al. Cytomegalovirus monitoring by polymerase chain reaction of whole blood samples from patients undergoing autologous bone marrow or peripheral blood progenitor cell transplantation. *J Infect Dis* 1997;175:1490–1493.
20. Fries BC, Chou S, Boeckh M, Torok-Storb B. Frequency distribution of cytomegalovirus envelope glycoprotein genotype in bone marrow transplant recipients. *J Infect Dis* 1994;169:769–774.
21. Bowden RA, Sayers M, Flournoy N, et al. Cytomegalovirus immune globulin a seronegative blood products to prevent primary cytomegalovirus infection after marrow transplantation. *N Engl J Med* 1986;314:1006–1010.
22. Miller W, Flynn P, McCullough J, et al. Cytomegalovirus infection after bone marrow transplantation: an association with acute graft-vs-host disease. *Blood* 1986;67:1162–1167.
23. Schmidt GM, Horak DA, Nlland JC, Duncan SR, Forman SJ, Zaia JA. A randomized, controlled trial of prophylactic ganciclovir for cytomegalovirus pulmonary infection in recipients of allogeneic bone marrow transplants. The City of Hope-Stanford-Syntex CMV Study Group. *N Engl J Med* 1991;324:1005–1011.
24. Vlieger AM, Boland GJ, Jiwa NM, et al. Cytomegalovirus antigenemia assay or PCR can be used to monitor ganciclovir treatment in bone marrow transplant recipients. *Bone Marrow Transplant* 1992;9:247–253.
25. Boeckh M, Hawkins G, Myerson D, Zaia J, Bowden RA. Plasma PCR for cytomegalovirus DNA after allogeneic marrow transplantation: comparison with PCR using peripheral blood leukocytes, pp65 antigenemia, and viral culture. *Transplantation* 1997;64:108–113.
26. The TH, van der Ploeg M, van den Berg AP, Vlleger AM, van der Giessen M, van Son WJ. Direct detection of cytomegalovirus in peripheral blood leukocytes—a review of the antigenemia assay and polymerase chain reaction. *Transplantation* 1992;54:193–198.
27. Gerna G, Furione M, Baldanti F, Sarasini A. Comparative quantitation of human cytomegalovirus DNA in blood leukocytes and plasma of transplant and AIDS patients. *J Clin Microbiol* 1994;32:2709–2717.
28. Boeckh M, Bowden RA, Goodrich JM, Pettinger M, Meyers JD. Cytomegalovirus antigen detection in peripheral blood leukocytes after allogeneic marrow transplantation. *Blood* 1992;80:1358–1364.
29. Zaia A, Gallez-Hawkins GM, Tegtmeier BR, et al. Late cytomegalovirus disease in marrow transplantation is predicted by virus load in plasma. *J Infect Dis* 1997;176:782–785.
30. Chou SW. Differentiation of cytomegalovirus strains by restriction analysis of DNA sequences amplified from clinical specimens. *J Infect Dis* 1990;162:738–742.
31. Torok-Storb B, Boeckh M, Hoy C, Leisenring W, Myerson D, Gooley T. Association of specific cytomegalovirus genotypes with death from myelosuppression after marrow transplantation. *Blood* 1997;90:2097–2102.
32. Quinnan GV Jr, Kirmani N, Rook AH, et al. Cytotoxic T cells in cytomegalovirus infection: HLA-restricted T-lymphocyte and non-T-lymphocyte cytotoxic responses correlate with recovery from cytomegalovirus infection in bone-marrow-transplant recipients. *N Engl J Med* 1982;307:7–13.
33. Reddehase MJ, Mutter W, Munch K, Buhring HJ, Koszinowski UH. CD8-positive T lymphocytes specific for murine cytomegalovirus immediate-early antigens mediate protective immunity. *J Virol* 1987;61:3102–3108.
34. Reusser P, Riddell SR, Meyers JD, Greenberg PD. Cytotoxic T-lymphocyte response to cytomegalovirus after human allogeneic bone marrow transplantation: pattern of recovery and correlation with cytomegalovirus infection and disease. *Blood* 1991;78:1373–1380.
35. Riddell SR. Pathogenesis of cytomegalovirus pneumonia in immunocompromised hosts. *Semin Respir Infect* 1995;10:199–208.

36. Reusser P, Attenhofer R, Hebart H, Helg C, Chapuis B, Einsele H. Cytomegalovirus-specific T-cell immunity in recipient of autologous peripheral blood stem cell or bone marrow transplant. *Blood* 1997;89: 3873–3879.

37. Cray C, Levy RB. CD8+ and CD4+ T cells contribute to the exacerbation of class I MHC disparate graft-vs-host reaction by concurrent murine cytomegalovirus infection. *Clin Immunol Immunopathol* 1993;67:84–90.

38. Via CS, Shanley JD, Shearer GM. Synergistic effect of murine cytomegalovirus on the induction of acute graft-vs-host disease involving MHC class I differences only. Analysis of *in vitro* T cell function. *J Immunol* 1990;145:328–334.

39. Jones M, Cray C, Levy RB. Concurrent MCMV infection augments donor antihost-specific activity and alters clinical outcome following experimental allogenic bone marrow transplantation. *Transplantation* 1996;61:856–861.

40. Wang FZ, Dahl H, Linde A, Brytting M, Ehrnst A, Ljungman P. Lymphotropic herpesviruses in allogeneic bone marrow transplantation. *Blood* 1996;88:3615–3620.

41. Boström L, Ringdén O, Sundberg B, Ljungman P, Linde A, Nilsson B. Pretransplant herpes virus serology and chronic graft-versus-host disease. *Bone Marrow Transplant* 1989;4:547–552.

42. Lönnqvist B, Ringdén O, Wahren B, Gahrton G, Lundgren G. Cytomegalovirus infection associated with and preceding chronic graft-versus-host disease. *Transplantation* 1984;38:465–468.

43. Jacobsen N, Andersen HK, Skinhøj P, et al. Correlation between donor cytomegalovirus immunity and chronic graft-versus-host disease after allogeneic bone marrow transplantation. *Scand J Haematol* 1986;36: 499–506.

44. Söderberg C, Larsson S, Rozell BL, Sumitran-Karuppan S, Ljungman P, Möller E. Cytomegalovirus-induced CD13-specific autoimmunity—a possible cause of chronic graft-vs-host disease. *Transplantation* 1996;61:600–609.

45. Söderberg C, Sumitran-Karuppan S, Ljungman P, Möller E. CD13-specific autoimmunity in cytomegalovirus-infected immunocompromised patients. *Transplantation* 1996;61:594–600.

46. Bowden RA, Slichter SJ, Sayers M, et al. A comparison of filtered leukocyte-reduced and cytomegalovirus (CMV) seronegative blood products for the prevention of transfusion-associated CMV infection after marrow transplant. *Blood* 1995;86:3598–3603.

47. Bowden RA, Fisher LD, Rogers K, Cays M, Meyers JD. Cytomegalovirus (CMV)-specific intravenous immunoglobulin for the prevention of primary CMV infection and disease after marrow transplant. *J Infect Dis* 1991;164:483–487.

48. Ruutu T, Ljungman P, Brinch L, et al. No prevention of cytomegalovirus infection by anti-cytomegalovirus hyperimmune globulin in seronegative bone marrow transplant recipients. The Nordic BMT Group. *Bone Marrow Transplant* 1997;19:233–236.

49. Meyers JD, Reed EC, Shepp DH, et al. Acyclovir for prevention of cytomegalovirus infection and disease after allogeneic marrow transplantation. *N Engl J Med* 1988;318:70–75.

50. Prentice HG, Gluckman E, Powles RL, et al. Impact of long-term acyclovir on cytomegalovirus infection and survival after allogeneic bone marrow transplantation. European Acyclovir for CMV Prophylaxis Study Group. *Lancet* 1994;343:749–753.

51. Boeckh M, Gooley T, Bowden R. Effect on survival of high-dose acyclovir in patients who receive ganciclovir prophylaxis at engraftment or for pp65 antigenemia after allogeneic marrow transplantation *J Infect Dis (in press)*.

52. Goodrich JM, Bowden RA, Fisher L, Keller C, Schoch G, Meyers JD. Ganciclovir prophylaxis to prevent cytomegalovirus disease after allogeneic marrow transplant. *Ann Intern Med* 1993;118:173–178.

53. Winston DJ, Ho WG, Bartoni K, et al. Ganciclovir prophylaxis of cytomegalovirus infection and disease in allogeneic bone marrow transplant recipients. Results of a placebo-controlled, double-blind trial. *Ann Intern Med* 1993;118:179–184.

54. Boeckh M, Gooley TA, Myerson D, Cunningham T, Schoch G, Bowden RA. Cytomegalovirus pp65 antigenemia-guided early treatment with ganciclovir versus ganciclovir at engraftment after allogeneic marrow transplantation: a randomized double-blind study. *Blood* 1996;88:4063–4071.

55. Salzberger B, Bowden RA, Hackman R, Davis C, Boeckh M. Neutropenia in allogeneic marrow transplant recipients receiving ganciclovir for prevention of CMV disease: risk factors and outcome. *Blood* 1997;90:2502–2508.

56. Atkinson K, Downs K, Golenia M, et al. Prophylactic use of ganciclovir in allogeneic bone marrow transplantation: absence of clinical cytomegalovirus infection. *Br J Haematol* 1991;79:57–62.

57. Atkinson K, Arthur C, Bradstock K, et al. Prophylactic ganciclovir is more effective in HLA-identical family member marrow transplant recipients than in more heavily immune-suppressed HLA-identical unrelated donor marrow transplant recipients. Australasian Bone Marrow Transplant Study Group. *Bone Marrow Transplant* 1995;16: 401–405.

58. Przepiorka D, Ippolitl C, Panina A, et al. Ganciclovir three times per week is not adequate to prevent cytomegalovirus reactivation after T cell-depleted marrow transplantation. *Bone Marrow Transplant* 1994; 13:461–464.

59. Von Bueltzingsloewen A, Bordigoni P, Witz F, et al. Prophylactic use of ganciclovir for allogeneic bone marrow transplant recipients. *Bone Marrow Transplant* 1993;12:197–202.

60. Yau JC, Dimopoulos MA, Huan SD, et al. Prophylaxis of cytomegalovirus infection with ganciclovir in allogeneic marrow transplantation. *Eur J Haematol* 1991;47:371–376.

61. Reusser P, Gambertoglio JG, Lilleby K, Meyers JD. Phase I–II trial of foscarnet for prevention of cytomegalovirus infection in autologous and allogeneic marrow transplant recipients. *J Infect Dis* 1992;166: 473–479.

62. Bacigalupo A, Tedone E, Van Lint MT, et al. CMV prophylaxis with foscarnet in allogeneic bone marrow transplant recipients at high risk of developing CMV infections. *Bone Marrow Transplant* 1994;13: 783–788.

63. Meyers JD, Leszczynski J, Zaia JA, et al. Prevention of cytomegalovirus infection by cytomegalovirus immune globulin after marrow transplantation. *Ann Intern Med* 1983;98:442–446.

64. Winston DJ, Ho WG, Lin CH, Budinger MD, Champlin RE, Gale RP. Intravenous immunoglobulin for modification of cytomegalovirus infections associated with bone marrow transplantation. Preliminary results of a controlled trial. *Am J Med* 1984;76:128–133.

65. Winston DJ, Ho WG, Lin CH, et al. Intravenous immune globulin for prevention of cytomegalovirus infection and interstitial pneumonia after bone marrow transplantation. *Ann Intern Med* 1987;106:12–18.

66. Ringdén O, Pihlstedt P, Volin L, et al. Failure to prevent cytomegalovirus infection by cytomegalovirus hyperimmune plasma: a randomized trial by the Nordic Bone Marrow Transplantation Group. *Bone Marrow Transplant* 1987;2:299–305.

67. Sullivan KM, Kopecky KJ, Jocom J, et al. Immunomodulatory and antimicrobial efficacy of intravenous immunoglobulin in bone marrow transplantation. *N Engl J Med* 1990;323:705–712.

68. Prentice HG, Gluckman E, Powles RL, et al. Long-term survival in allogeneic bone marrow transplant recipients following acyclovir prophylaxis for CMV infection. *Bone Marrow Transplant* 1997;19: 129–133.

69. Goodrich JM, Mori M, Gleaves CA, et al. Early treatment with ganciclovir to prevent cytomegalovirus disease after allogeneic bone marrow transplantation. *N Engl J Med* 1991;325:1601–1607.

70. Bass EB, Powe NR, Goodman SN, et al. Efficacy of immune globulin in preventing complications of bone marrow transplantation: a meta-analysis. *Bone Marrow Transplant* 1993;12:273–282.

71. Guglielmo BJ, Wong-Beringer A, Linker CA. Immune globulin therapy in allogeneic bone marrow transplant: a critical review. *Bone Marrow Transplant* 1994;13:499–510.

72. Messori A, Rampazzo R, Scroccaro G, Martini N. Efficacy of hyperimmune anti-cytomegalovirus immunoglobulins for the prevention of cytomegalovirus infection in recipients of allogeneic bone marrow transplantation: a meta-analysis. *Bone Marrow Transplant* 1994;13: 163–167.

73. Wolff SN, Fay JW, Herzig RH, et al. High-dose weekly intravenous immunoglobulin to prevent infections in patients undergoing autologous bone marrow transplantation or severe myelosuppressive therapy. A study of the American Bone Marrow Transplant Group. *Ann Intern Med* 1993;118:937–942.

74. Einsele H, Ehninger G, Hebart H, et al. Polymerase chain reaction monitoring reduces the incidence of cytomegalovirus disease and the duration and side effects of antiviral therapy after bone marrow transplantation. *Blood* 1995;86:2815–2820.

75. Einsele H, Ehninger G, Steidle M, et al. Polymerase chain reaction to evaluate antiviral therapy for cytomegalovirus disease. *Lancet* 1991;338:1170–1172.

76. Wolf DG, Spector SA. Early diagnosis of human cytomegalovirus dis-

ease in transplant recipients by DNA amplification in plasma. *Transplantation* 1993;56:330–334.

77. Brytting M, Mousavi-Jazi M, Boström L, et al. Cytomegalovirus DNA in peripheral blood leukocytes and plasma from bone marrow transplant recipients. *Transplantation* 1995;60:961–965.

78. Gerna G, Furione M, Baldanti F, Percivalle E, Comoli P, Locatelli F. Quantitation of human cytomegalovirus DNA in bone marrow transplant recipients. *Br J Haematol* 1995;91:674–683.

79. Boivin G, Handfield J, Murray G, et al. Quantitation of cytomegalovirus (CMV) DNA in leukocytes of human immunodeficiency virus-infected subjects with and without CMV disease by using PCR and the Sharp Signal Detection System. *J Clin Microbiol* 1997;35:525–526.

80. Bitsch A, Kirchner H, Dupke R, Bein G. Cytomegalovirus transcripts in peripheral blood leukocytes of actively infected transplant patients detected by reverse transcription-polymerase chain reaction. *J Infect Dis* 1993;167:740–743.

81. Ljungman P, Loré K, Aschan J, et al. Use of semi-quantitative PCR for cytomegalovirus DNA as a basis for pre-emptive antiviral therapy in allogeneic bone marrow transplant patients. *Bone Marrow Transplant* 1996;17:583–587.

82. Van der Bij W, Torensma R, van Son WJ, et al. Rapid immunodiagnosis of active cytomegalovirus infection by monoclonal antibody staining of blood leucocytes. *J Med Virol* 1988;25:17,88.

83. Van der Bij W, van Son WJ, van der Berg AP, Tegzess AM, Torensma R, The TH. Cytomegalovirus (CMV) antigenemia rapid diagnosis and relationship with CMV-associated clinical syndromes in renal allograft recipients. *Transplant Proc* 1989;21:2061–2064.

84. Verdonck LF, Dekker AW, Rozenbergarska M, Vandenhoek MR. A risk-adapted approach with a short course of ganciclovir to prevent cytomegalovirus (CMV) pneumonia in CMV-seropositive recipients of allogeneic bone marrow transplants. *Clin Infect Dis* 1997;24:901–907.

85. Bacigalupo A, van Lint MT, Tedone E, et al. Early treatment of CMV infections in allogeneic bone marrow transplant recipients with foscarnet or ganciclovir. *Bone Marrow Transplant* 1994;13:753–758.

86. Ljungman P, Öberg G, Aschan J, et al. Foscarnet for pre-emptive therapy of CM infection detected by a leukocyte-based nested PCR in allogeneic bone marrow transplant patients. *Bone Marrow Transplant* 1996;18:565–568.

87. Bacigalupo A, Bregante S, Tedone E, et al. Combined foscarnet-ganciclovir treatment for cytomegalovirus infections after allogeneic hemopoietic stem cell transplantation. *Transplantation* 1996;62:376–380.

88. Ljungman P, Griffiths P. Definitions of cytomegalovirus infection and disease. In: *Multidisciplinary approach to understanding cytomegalovirus disease.* Amsterdam: Exerpta Medica; 1993.

89. Ljungman P, Plotkin SA. Workshop on CMV disease: definitions, clinical severity scores, and new syndromes. *Scand J Infect Dis* 1995;99:S87–S88.

90. Crawford SW, Bowden RA, Hackman RC, Gleaves CA, Meyers JD, Clark JG. Rapid detection of cytomegalovirus pulmonary infection by bronchoalveolar lavage and centrifugation culture. *Ann Intern Med* 1988;108:180–185.

91. Ruutu P, Ruutu T, Volin L, Tukiainen P, Ukkonen P, Hovi T. Cytomegalovirus is frequently isolated in bronchoalveolar lavage fluid of bone marrow transplant recipients without pneumonia. *Ann Intern Med* 1990;112:913–916.

92. Cathomas G, Morris P, Pekle K, Cunningham I, Emanuel D. Rapid diagnosis of cytomegalovirus pneumonia in marrow transplant recipients by bronchoalveolar lavage using the polymerase chain reaction, virus culture, and the direct immunostaining of alveolar cells. *Blood* 1993;81:1909–1914.

93. Slavin MA, Gleaves CA, Schoch HG, Bowden RA. Quantification of cytomegalovirus in bronchoalveolar lavage fluid after allogeneic marrow transplantation by centrifugation culture. *J Clin Microbiol* 1992;30:2776–2779.

94. Bolvin G, Olson CA, Quirk MR, Kringstad B, Hertz MI, Jordan MC. Quantitation of cytomegalovirus DNA and characterization of viral gene expression in bronchoalveolar cells of infected patients with and without pneumonitis. *J Infect Dis* 1996;173:1304–1312.

95. Salzberger B, Myerson D, Boeckh M. Circulating CMV-infected endothelial cells in marrow transplant patients with CMV disease and CMV infection. *J Infect Dis* 1997;176:778–781.

96. Shepp DH, Dandliker PS, de Miranda P, et al. Activity of 9-[2-

hydroxy-1-(hydroxymethyl)ethoxymethyl]guanine in the treatment of cytomegalovirus pneumonia. *Ann Intern Med* 1985;103:368–373.

97. Aschan J, Ringdén O, Ljungman P, Lönnqvist B, Ohlman S. Foscarnet for treatment of cytomegalovirus infections in bone marrow transplant recipients. *Scand J Infect Dis* 1992;24:143–150.

98. Blacklock HA, Griffiths P, Stirk P, Prentice HG. Specific hyperimmune globulin for cytomegalovirus pneumonitis [letter]. *Lancet* 1985;2:152–153.

99. Reed EC, Bowden RA, Dandliker PS, Gleaves CA, Meyers JD. Efficacy of cytomegalovirus immunoglobulin in marrow transplant recipients with cytomegalovirus pneumonia. *J Infect Dis* 1987;156:641–645.

100. Wilson EJ, Medearis DN Jr, Hansen LA, Rubin RH. 9-(1-3-Dihydroxy-2-propoxymethyl)guanine prevents death but not immunity in murine cytomegalovirus-infected normal and immunosuppressed BALB/c mice. *Antimicrob Agents Chemother* 1987;31:101–120.

101. Shanley JD, Pesanti EL. The relation of viral replication to interstitial pneumonitis in murine cytomegalovirus lung infection. *J Infect Dis* 1985;151:454–458.

102. Emanuel D, Cunningham I, Jules-Elysee K, et al. Cytomegalovirus pneumonia after bone marrow transplantation successfully treated with the combination of ganciclovir and high-dose intravenous immune globulin. *Ann Intern Med* 1988;109:777–782.

103. Reed EC, Bowden RA, Dandliker PS, Lilleby KE, Meyers JD. Treatment of cytomegalovirus pneumonia with ganciclovir and intravenous cytomegalovirus immunoglobulin in patients with bone marrow transplants. *Ann Intern Med* 1988;109:783–788.

104. Schmidt GM, Kovacs A, Zaia JA, et al. Ganciclovir/immunoglobulin combination therapy for the treatment of human cytomegalovirus-associated interstitial pneumonia in bone marrow allograft recipients. *Transplantation* 1988;46:905–907.

105. Ljungman P, Engelhard D, Link H, et al. Treatment of interstitial pneumonitis due to cytomegalovirus with ganciclovir and intravenous immune globulin: experience of European Bone Marrow Transplant Group. *Clin Infect Dis* 1992;14:831–835.

106. Anonymous. Mortality in patients with the acquired immunodeficiency syndrome treated with either foscarnet or ganciclovir for cytomegalovirus retinitis. Studies of Ocular Complications of AIDS Research Group, in collaboration with the AIDS Clinical Trials Group. *N Engl J Med* 1992;326:213–220.

107. Hackman RC, Wolford JL, Gleaves CA, et al. Recognition and rapid diagnosis of upper gastrointestinal cytomegalovirus infection in marrow transplant recipients. A comparison of seven virologic methods. *Transplantation* 1994;57:231–237.

108. Reed EC, Wolford JL, Kopecky KJ, et al. Ganciclovir for the treatment of cytomegalovirus gastroenteritis in bone marrow transplant patients. A randomized, placebo-controlled trial. *Ann Intern Med* 1990;112:505–510.

109. Ljungman P, Cordonnier C, Einsele H, et al. Use of intravenous immune globulin in addition to antiviral therapy in the treatment of CMV gastrointestinal disease in allogeneic bone marrow transplant patients. A report from the European Group for Blood and Marrow Transplantation (EBMT). *Bone Marrow Transplant* 1998;21:473–76.

110. Cinque P, Vago L, Dahl H, et al. Polymerase chain reaction on cerebrospinal fluid for diagnosis of virus-associated opportunistic diseases of the central nervous system in HIV-infected patients. *AIDS* 1996;10:951–958.

111. Boeckh M, Hoy C, Torok-Storb B. Occult cytomegalovirus infection of marrow stroma. *Clin Infect Dis* 1998;26:209–10.

112. Walter EA, Greenberg PD, Gilbert MJ, et al. Reconstitution of cellular immunity against cytomegalovirus in recipients of allogeneic bone marrow by transfer of T-cell clones from the donor. *N Engl J Med* 1995;333:1038–1044.

113. McLaughlin-Taylor E, Pande H, Forman SJ, et al. Identification of the major late human cytomegalovirus matrix protein pp65 as a target antigen for CD8+ virus-specific cytotoxic T lymphocytes. *J Med Virol* 1994;43:103–110.

114. Boeckh M, Zaia J, Jung D, Skettino S, Chauncey T, Bowden RA. Phase I/II Study of the pharmacokinetics, antiviral activity and tolerability of oral ganciclovir for CMV prophylaxis in marrow transplantation. *Biology of Blood and Marrow Transplant* 1998;4:13–19.

115. Lewis RA, Carr LM, Doyle K, et al. Parenteral cidofovir for cytomegalovirus retinitis in patients with AIDS—the HPMPC peripheral cytomegalovirus retinitis trial—a randomized, controlled trial. *Ann Intern Med* 1997;126:267ff.

Transplant Infections edited by
Raleigh A. Bowden, Per Ljungman, and Carlos V. Paya.
Lippincott–Raven Publishers, Philadelphia © 1998

CHAPTER 17

Cytomegalovirus Infection and Disease in Solid Organ Transplant Recipients

Robin Patel and Carlos V. Paya

PATHOGENESIS

Cytomegalovirus (CMV) is a widely distributed human pathogen with the prevalence of anti-CMV IgG antibodies in adults in the general population ranging from 30% to 97% (1). CMV is a member of the herpesvirus family and shares with other herpesviruses the capacity to remain latent after recovery from an acute infection. Although the exact site of latency remains to be elucidated, monocytes/macrophages (2), neutrophils (3), lymphocytes (4), and endothelial cells (5) have been shown to harbor CMV genome. The replication of CMV is initially regulated through the promoter of the immediate early (IE) genes. Cell activation and certain drugs used in transplantation have been shown to reactivate and increase CMV replication. In addition, a low degree of viral persistence may be present in infected cells that is tightly controlled by immune surveillance. Hence conditions that decrease functional immune surveillance such as exogenous immunosuppression following transplantation will result in enhanced viral replication. Therefore these two mechanisms (latency and persistence) are functional following transplantation.

CMV infection occurs in the majority of solid organ transplant (SOT) recipients (6), primarily in the first 3 post-transplant months, when immunosuppression is most intense. CMV disease incidence ranges from 8% to 55%, depending on the type of transplanted organ. The reasons for this wide range depend on specific risk factors that will be discussed later (7–9) (Table 1). CMV is transmitted to transplant recipients mainly by the donor organ and to a lesser degree by blood products (10). Three major patterns of CMV transmission are observed in SOT

recipients. Primary infection occurs when a CMV-seronegative individual receives cells latently infected with the virus from a seropositive donor followed by viral reactivation. Secondary infection or reactivation infection occurs when endogenous latent virus is reactivated in a CMV-seropositive individual following transplantation. Superinfection or reinfection occurs when a seropositive recipient receives latently infected cells from a seropositive donor and the virus that reactivates after transplantation is of donor origin (11).

Following primary infection with CMV in the normal host, long-term cellular and humoral immunity develop, thus controlling viral persistence, a situation that is lacking following solid organ transplantation and that leads to uncontrolled viral replication and consequently symptomatic CMV infection. The level of immunosuppression in any given patient is determined by the dose, duration, and temporal sequence in which immunosuppressive medications are administered. Most immunosuppressive agents used in solid organ transplantation depress cell-mediated immunity; however, blunted antibody responses and leukopenia may also result from the use of these agents. The resultant depressed cell-mediated immunity leads to increased susceptibility to infections caused by intracellular pathogens. The upcoming availability of more potent immunosuppressive agents may thus change the incidence and severity of CMV infection.

Epidemiologic studies of risk factors have provided important clues to identify those patients at high risk for symptomatic CMV infection, reflecting in part the pathogenesis of CMV infection following solid organ transplantation. A lack of cellular and humoral immunity, as defined by the absence of anti-CMV antibodies, places the recipient in the high-risk category upon receiving a CMV seropositive donor's organ or other exogenous source of CMV (e.g., blood transfusion). This situation

---

From the Division of Infectious Diseases, Mayo Clinic and Foundation, Rochester, MN 55905.

TABLE 1. *CMV disease in solid organ transplant recipients*

	Frequency of CMV disease (7–9)	Organ predisposed to CMV disease
Kidney transplant recipients	8%	Kidney
Liver transplant recipients	29%	Liver
Heart transplant recipients	25%	Heart
Kidney–Pancreas transplant recipients	50%	Pancreas
Human small bowel transplant recipients	22%	Intestine
Heart–Lung transplant recipients	39%	Lung

reflects the lack of preexisting immune surveillance, which allows viral persistence in the transplanted graft to remain unchecked. Compounds such as antilymphocyte immunoglobulins (antithymocyte or antilymphocyte globulins, and OKT3 monoclonal antibodies), employed either as induction therapy or for allograft rejection treatment, enhance the rate of symptomatic CMV infection, especially in CMV-seropositive individuals (12,13). These compounds may not only further diminish the immune surveillance but reactivate latent CMV from infected cells by means of the induction of cytokines such as Tumor Necrosis Factor (TNF) (14). In addition to pharmacologic agents, pre- and post-transplant events that contribute to further immunosuppressing the transplant recipient and/or reactivating latent CMV have been identified as risk factors for symptomatic CMV infection in additional epidemiologic studies. These include fulminant hepatitis before liver transplantation, occurrence of bacterial infection following transplantation, and intercurrent infection with other viruses of the herpes family (human herpesvirus 6 and 7) (15). The viral load present in the transplanted graft may impact the frequency and severity of CMV infections following transplantation. Although this postulate remains to be proven, it could explain the high rate of symptomatic CMV infection observed in lung and gastrointestinal transplant recipients, reflecting the transplantation of a higher latent CMV load contained in a larger amount of tissue with an increased endothelial and lymphoid compartment. As mentioned earlier, the severity would be proportional to the presence or absence of specific CMV immunity in the recipient patient. Thus prophylactic measures found to be effective for renal transplant recipients may not apply to lung or gastrointestinal transplant recipients. Likewise, lessons learned from CMV infection in bone marrow transplantation (BMT) can be only partially extrapolated to the nonhomogeneous field of solid organ transplantation because of potential differences in pathogenesis.

CLINICAL MANIFESTATIONS

In the immunosuppressed SOT recipient, CMV has four major effects. It (a) causes characteristic infectious diseases syndromes (see later); (b) has been implicated in causing increased immunosuppression, which may explain the frequent association of CMV with other infections, such as bacterial, fungal, and pneumocystis infections as well as Epstein-Barr virus–induced post-transplant lymphoproliferative disorder (16–18); (c) has been associated with allograft rejection (e.g., early-onset allograft rejection in renal transplant recipients [19] and allograft atherosclerosis in cardiac transplant recipients (in some but not all studies) [20–23]); and (d) has been associated with a deleterious effect on the outcome and survival of the transplant recipient, as recently demonstrated in epidemiologic studies. CMV infection therefore has a potential impact on both patient and graft outcome.

CMV infection in SOT recipients exhibits a wide range of clinical manifestations, from asymptomatic infection to severe, lethal CMV disease (24). The wide range of the incidence of CMV infection and its clinical forms and manifestations reported in the SOT literature is in part due to differences in the use of diagnostic techniques and clinical definitions, as well as to differences inherent in each type of transplant and transplant program. In general, CMV infection is defined as the documentation of CMV by culture of body fluids and tissues, by immunostaining of CMV antigens in peripheral blood leukocytes (e.g., antigenemia) or by histopathology, including immunostaining and/or *in vitro* hybridization of tissues. In addition, seroconversion to CMV has been used to define CMV infection. The recent availability of more sensitive techniques such as polymerase chain reaction (PCR)–based techniques resulted in an increase in the number of patients with evidence of CMV infection within a defined cohort of transplant patients. Clinically, CMV infection can be defined as asymptomatic or symptomatic; the latter is also defined as disease. Symptomatic CMV infection or disease is applied to those patients with symptomatology specific to CMV, together with concomitant evidence of CMV infection (as described earlier). This group of patients can be further subdivided into those with and those without organ involvement. Symptomatic infection (disease) without documentation of organ involvement is usually reserved for patients with a viral syndrome (fever, leukopenia, thrombocytopenia, and other constitutional symptoms such as malaise and arthralgia). The presence of CMV viremia (detection of CMV by culture and/or antigenemia) in a SOT recipient can fall into the asymptomatic

TABLE 2. *Summary of randomized passive immunoprophylaxis trials in solid organ transplant recipients*

Type of transplant	Reference	Type of study	Number of patients studied (# of D⁺/R⁻ Patient[a])	Prophylactic regimen	Outcome	CMV Disease[b]	Mortality[b]
Kidney	(119)	Primary and secondary prophylaxis, randomized, nonplacebo controlled	24	Hyperimmune serum 0.1 g/kg biweekly day 0, 1 and q 3 weeks for 6 months vs. no treatment	Beneficial effect on CMV illness but not infection in patients on cyclosporin but not those on azathioprine/ATG	0% vs. 17% (cyclosporine); 58%vs. 37% (azathioprine/ATG)	none reported
	(121)	Primary and secondary prophylaxis, randomized	24 42 34	Cytotect 10 g days 0, 18, 38, intraglobulin 10 g (same regimen) 58, 78 vs. (same regimen) intraglobulin 10 g	No change in CMV infections; decrease in severity of symptom of primary infection in Cytotect group	Disease rates not shown	0% vs. 0%
	(120)	Primary prophylaxis (D⁺/R⁻), randomized nonplacebo controlled	24(24)	CMV immune globulin (MA Public Health Biological Laboratories) 150 mg/kg for 72 hours; 100 mg/kg at weeks 2 and 4; 50 mg/kg at weeks 6, 8, 12, 16 vs. no treatment	Reduced CMV-associated syndromes fungal and parasitic superinfections	21% vs. 60%	4% vs. 14%
	(129)	Primary prophylaxis (D⁺/R⁻), randomized, nonplacebo controlled	35(35) 27(27) 24(24)	Unselected immune globulin 500 mg/kg within 48 hr, and week 1; 250 mg/kg q week × 5 vs. ganciclovir 2.5 mg/kg/iv/day × 21 days	Both regimens reduced CMV syndrome invasive CMV infection (compared to historical controls); ganciclovir was much cheaper	22% vs. 21%	0% vs. 0%
	(122)	Primary and secondary prophylaxis, randomized, nonplacebo controlled	15(1)	Gamimmune-N 500 mg/kg within 48 hr post-transplant; then weekly for 23 wks vs. no treatment	No benefit	53% vs. 77%	Not reported
Liver	(123)	Primary and secondary prophylaxis, randomized, prospective, placebo controlled	13(1) 25(0) 25(4)	Sandoglobulin 500 mg/kg days 1, 7, 14, 21, 28, 42, 56, 70, 84 vs. albumin in a similar concentration on same days	No benefit	32% vs. 20%	None reported
	(125)	Primary prophylaxis of R, randomized, controlled, prospective	22(15) 12(7)	CMV immunoglobulin 250 mg/kg day 0; then 125 mg/kg q 10 days × 3 months vs. no prophylaxis	Decreased rate of disease in D⁺/R⁻	27% vs. 86% (D⁺/R⁻) 14% vs. 0% (D⁻/R⁻)	Not
	(124)	Primary and secondary prophylaxis, randomized, double-blind	69(19)	CMV immune globulin (Massachusetts Public Health Biological Laboratories) 150 mg/kg within 72 hours of transplant and at weeks 2, 4, 6, 8 8, 100 mg/kg at weeks 12 and 16 vs. placebo (1% serum albumin)	Reduction in several CMV disease; no effect in D⁺/R⁻	19% vs. 31%	17 vs. 25%
	(126)	Primary prophylaxis (R⁻); compared with CMV seronegative recipients receiving placebo in above random-assignment trial	72(19) 21(9) 44(19)	CMV immune globulin (Massachusetts Public Health Biological Laboratories) 150 mg/kg within 72 hours of transplant and at weeks 2, 4, 6, 8; 100 mg/kg at weeks 12 and 16 vs. patients previously randomized to placebo	Reduction in severe CMV disease in the D⁺/R⁻ group	14% vs. 32%	Not reported
Heart, lung, and kidney	(127)	Primary prophylaxis (D⁺/R⁻), randomized, prospective, stratified (type of transplant and prophylactic immunosuppression)	11(11) 10(10)	Acyclovir 800 mg po 4/day × 12 weeks vs. acyclovir 800 mg po 4/day × 12 weeks with IV immune globulin 300 mg/kg q 2 weeks × 6 doses	Acyclovir with or without immune globulin did not prevent primary infection or disease	64% vs. 80%	9% vs. 0%

[a]If known, the number of patients who were D⁺/R⁻ is given in parentheses.

[b]Among patients given, first listed vs. second listed regimen.

CMV infection category, or alternatively, into the symptomatic (disease) category if the mentioned clinical symptomatology and/or documentation of CMV organ involvement are present (25,26).

Organ involvement with CMV correlates with the organ transplanted as follows: CMV hepatitis occurs most frequently in liver transplant recipients, CMV pancreatitis occurs most frequently in pancreas transplant recipients, and CMV pneumonitis occurs most frequently in lung and heart-lung transplant recipients, especially CMV-seronegative recipients of the corresponding organ from CMV-seropositive donors (Table 1). This may relate to the yet to be proven hypothesis raised earlier regarding the issue of the viral load inherent to each organ. In addition, CMV myocarditis, although rare, typically presents in heart transplant recipients (27). Moreover, it remains unknown, but possible, that the apparent predisposition of CMV to cause disease in the allograft is secondary to increased surveillance of the transplanted graft for diagnosing rejection. Other sites of involvement of CMV include the gastrointestinal tract, gallbladder, pancreas, epididymis, biliary tree, retina, skin, endometrium, and central nervous system (28–36). CMV in renal transplant recipients has also been associated with a glomerulopathy characterized by enlargement or necrosis of endothelial cells and accumulation of mononuclear cells and fibrillar material in glomerular capillaries (37). CMV has been associated with left ventricular dysfunction in heart transplant recipients (36). Congenital CMV infection has been reported in the offspring of female liver transplant recipients (39).

CMV hepatitis typically manifests as elevated concentrations of gamma-glutamyltransferase and alkaline phosphatase, peaking 2–4 days later than aminotransferase elevations with only minimally increased bilirubin levels (40). CMV pneumonitis results in fever, dyspnea, and cough with findings of hypoxemia and pulmonary infiltrates (41). Roentgenographic appearances include bilateral interstitial, unilateral lobar, and nodular infiltrates. As suggested earlier, recipients of lung allografts are particularly prone to CMV pneumonitis, which may be severe in this population. CMV can affect any segment of the gastrointestinal tract, including the esophagus, stomach, and small and large intestines. Symptoms include dysphagia, odynophagia, nausea, vomiting, delayed gastric emptying, abdominal pain, gastrointestinal hemorrhage, and diarrhea (42,43). Endoscopic findings include erythema and diffuse, shallow erosions or localized ulcerations, but endoscopic findings are not specific, so biopsy is essential (44). Intestinal perforation may ensue. CMV inclusion bodies or positive CMV cultures may be found from tissue obtained at endoscopy in the absence of endoscopic findings; the significance and relevance of this finding are unclear (42). A high index of suspicion for CMV colitis should be maintained in any transplant recipient who presents with lower gastrointestinal bleeding in the first 4 months following transplantation. CMV has also been associated with biliary disease in SOT recipients (45). CMV may also cause vasculitis, resulting in ischemic colitis (46). CMV retinitis is distinctive in that it usually presents more than 6 months following transplantation. Patients may be asymptomatic or may experience blurring of vision, scotomata, or decreased visual acuity. The diagnosis is made funduscopically. Because many of these manifestations of CMV organ involvement may be difficult to differentiate from allograft rejection, it is imperative that tissue biopsy be performed to document the presence or absence of CMV.

TREATMENT

Effective, currently available antiviral agents for the treatment of CMV include ganciclovir, foscarnet, and cidofovir. Ganciclovir {9-[2-hydroxy-1-(hydroxymethyl)-ethoxymethyl]guanine} has excellent activity against all members of the herpes family of viruses. It is a pro-drug that is phosphorylated to ganciclovir 5′-monophosphate by a protein encoded by the UL97 open reading frame of human CMV, and then to the di- and triphosphate form by host cellular kinases (47,48). The active drug inhibits DNA polymerase and competes with deoxyguanosine triphosphate to act as a terminator of biosynthesis of the viral strand (49).

Intravenous ganciclovir has been successfully used in uncontrolled, nonrandomized therapeutic trials to treat SOT recipients with CMV disease (50–82). As an example, of 81 liver transplant recipients with CMV disease treated with ganciclovir, 74% responded to treatment and 21% developed recurrent CMV disease after stopping treatment (of these, 65% were successfully retreated) (82). One caveat is that treatment of CMV may not reduce disease if the pathogenesis of the disease is immune mediated, as exemplified by the only randomized, placebo-controlled trial of ganciclovir for the treatment of gastrointestinal CMV infection in BMT recipients (83).

The usual dose of intravenous ganciclovir is 5 mg/kg every 12 hours, administered as a 1-hour infusion, and because of its predominantly renal excretion, the dosage should be decreased in patients with renal impairment. Concentrations of ganciclovir in the blood are decreased by 50% after 4 hours of hemodialysis; thus ganciclovir must be readministered shortly after dialysis (84). CMV disease is typically treated with 2 weeks of intravenous ganciclovir, although it has been suggested that a longer duration of treatment may be required for gastrointestinal CMV disease (85). Unlike treatment of CMV in patients with human immunodeficiency virus infection, long-term maintenance is seldom required in recipients of solid organs. CMV retinitis and pneumonitis, the latter in lung transplant recipients, are possible exceptions. The optimal duration of antiviral therapy in an individual patient remains unknown. In studies of BMT recipients, a negative result of a PCR assay in either blood or urine at the conclusion of antiviral therapy seemed to be a better marker for effective antiviral treatment than did clinical improvement or negative blood cultures (86). In SOT recipients, a similar approach might indicate that ganciclovir therapy should be continued or discontinued. Quantitative antigenemia and CD8$^+$ bright T-lymphocytes in peripheral blood are other potential markers that indicate appropriate times to discontinue antiviral therapy (87). Recurrent tissue-invasive CMV disease has been reported in 25% of SOT patients in whom an initial episode of tissue-invasive CMV disease occurs. Recurrent CMV disease appears to respond to ganciclovir as well as initial CMV disease (88). As with recent advances in the management of human immunodeficiency virus infection, the value of quantifying CMV viral load for response to specific antiviral therapy remains to be elucidated.

Oral ganciclovir has recently been approved for use in human immunodeficiency virus–infected patients, as maintenance therapy to prevent the relapse of CMV retinitis. The absorption of ganciclovir following oral administration is low and its role in the treatment of CMV infection and disease following solid organ transplantation is under study. Oral ganciclovir may be useful as maintenance therapy in those patients treated with intravenous ganciclovir with identified risk factors for relapse; however, this also remains to be studied, as the current knowledge of the use of oral ganciclovir in solid organ transplantation is limited to its use as a prophylactic agent (see the section on prophylaxis).

Side effects of ganciclovir in SOT patients are less frequent than in human immunodeficiency virus–infected patients and in BMT recipients, and include leukopenia, thrombocytopenia, anemia, eosinophilia, bone marrow hypoplasia, hemolysis, nausea, infusion site reactions, diarrhea, renal toxicity, seizures, mental status changes, fever, rash, and abnormal liver function tests (28,56,89–91). Hematologic and renal function should be monitored while the patient is on ganciclovir. Renal toxicity may occur when ganciclovir is used in conjunction with other nephrotoxic agents such as amphotericin B, azathioprine, and cyclosporine A, and when used in children. The long-term safety of ganciclovir in adult and especially pediatric transplant recipients remains to be established (92).

The possibility of viral resistance should be considered in patients with poor clinical response or persistent viral excretion during ganciclovir therapy. Mutations in viral thymidine kinase and/or DNA polymerase genes appear to mediate resistance (91). Although an early study showed that ganciclovir prophylaxis in SOT recipients did not select ganciclovir-resistant isolates of CMV (93), a more recent study indicates that the use of ganciclovir

prophylaxis and treatment may select for ganciclovir-resistant CMV (94).

There is less experience with the use of foscarnet (trisodium phosphonoformate hexahydrate) for the treatment of CMV disease in SOT recipients (95–98). Until more data are available, foscarnet should be reserved for patients who are intolerant of ganciclovir or who have failed ganciclovir therapy. Foscarnet inhibits viral DNA polymerase. Its main side effects are nephrotoxicity, anemia, hyperphosphatemia, hypophosphatemia, hypercalcemia, hypocalcemia, nausea, vomiting, and seizures. Foscarnet is administered intravenously at a dosage of 60 mg/kg thrice daily. The dosage must be adjusted in renal failure. It has been suggested that combination antiviral therapy with ganciclovir and foscarnet should be investigated, because *in vitro* these agents are synergistic for antiviral activity (99). Studies done in BMT recipients suggest that the combination of ganciclovir and foscarnet may provide effective therapy for CMV infection (100,101).

Although high concentrations of acyclovir inhibit CMV *in vitro*, clinical trials have demonstrated no benefit in the treatment of CMV infection (102).

CMV hyperimmune globulin has been found by some investigators to be ineffective in the treatment of CMV disease in SOT recipients (103) and by others to possibly be an effective therapeutic agent (104,105). Although the combination of CMV immune globulin and ganciclovir has been suggested to be efficacious in the treatment of CMV disease in some studies (53), a lack of large randomized studies addressing its value, and the expense of immune globulin needs to be considered before becoming a valuable therapeutical tool. Combination therapy may be useful in specific subsets of patients (e.g., those with severe CMV pneumonia). Cidofovir has recently been found to be effective for the treatment of CMV infection in human immunodeficiency virus–infected patients. A newer pro-drug of cidofovir may be less nephrotoxic than the parent compound. This may prove to be an ideal agent to use in transplantation because it needs only infrequent administration. Phase II and III trials are in progress to address this issue. In summary, intravenous ganciclovir remains the drug of choice for the treatment of CMV disease in SOT recipients.

PROPHYLAXIS

To date, a number of prophylactic measures have been evaluated in an attempt to prevent the occurrence of CMV infection and disease in SOT recipients. These include (a) use of CMV-seronegative, filtered, or leukocyte-poor blood products; (b) active immunization with a vaccine; (c) passive immunization with immune globulins; (d) prophylaxis with antiviral agents; and (e) preemptive therapy. In that which follows we outline what is known and recommended as concerns each of these approaches.

CMV Seronegative Blood Products and Protective Matching

The use of CMV seronegative blood products, previously shown to be effective in preventing CMV infection in CMV-seronegative BMT recipients (106), has been later shown to be of value in SOT recipients (107). A disadvantage of CMV-seronegative blood products is their scarcity in areas with a high prevalence of CMV seropositivity. In this situation, filtered or leukocyte-poor products, which are associated with a very low risk of CMV transmission, are useful (107). CMV-seronegative, filtered blood products, or leukocyte-poor blood should be used for all transfusions given to seronegative recipients (107).

Knowledge of CMV serostatus of the donor and recipient before transplantation will predict which patients will develop CMV disease. Although the patient at highest risk for CMV infection is the seronegative recipient of a seropositive allograft, protective matching of seronegative donors and seronegative recipients is not practical because of the scarcity of donor organs.

Vaccination

In theory, one of the simplest interventions to prevent CMV infection and disease after solid organ transplantation would be immunization of seronegative recipients with a vaccine given once in anticipation of future viral challenge.

A candidate live attenuated CMV vaccine, which used the Towne strain of virus, was developed and extensively tested. The first trials of the Towne vaccine were conducted in the mid-1970s in normal volunteers, and randomized, placebo-controlled, double-blind trials of the Towne vaccine in renal transplant recipients were subsequently carried out demonstrating that the vaccine was both safe and immunogenic. At the University of Minnesota, 236 subjects (117 vaccine and 119 placebo recipients) were enrolled from 1979 through 1984. Unfortunately, there was no significant decrease in the incidence or severity of CMV disease in vaccinated patients. In the donor CMV-seropositive pretransplant (D^+)/recipient CMV seronegative pretransplant (R^-) subgroup, the proportions infected and the number of patients with disease did not differ between vaccine and placebo recipients, but the vaccinees tended to have a less severe form of CMV disease than the placebo recipients, although this difference was not statistically significant (108–110).

At the University of Pennsylvania, 237 subjects (124 vaccine and 113 placebo recipients) were enrolled from 1979 through 1989. As in the Minnesota study, the Towne live attenuated CMV vaccine did not alter the incidence of CMV infection or disease; however, there was a statistically significant decrease in the severity of CMV disease in the D^+/R^- subgroup (111–115). In 1983 Merck Sharp and Dohme Research Laboratories (West Point, PA), discontinued support for clinical trials of the Towne live attenuated CMV vaccine.

The future of the CMV vaccine will likely be a subunit product, lacking any potential for latency. Renewed efforts are under way by several biotechnology companies to evaluate subunit vaccines containing recombinant glycoproteins (B, H) (116). Although complete protection against CMV may not be achieved by a vaccine, partial protection against the serious manifestations of CMV infection and disease could be possible. Moreover, a suboptimal vaccine could suffice when considered in combination with other current regimens, such as antiviral agents and/or immunoglobulin.

Passive Immunoprophylaxis

Because immunity to CMV prior to transplantation decreases the incidence of CMV disease following transplantation, boosting the immune system after transplantation should have a beneficial effect in decreasing CMV disease. Expanding the number and function of virus-specific cytotoxic T-lymphocytes to reduce the incidence of CMV disease following BMT is now a reality (117), although its role in solid organ transplantation remains to be studied. In addition, the humoral CMV immune response can theoretically be boosted with specific CMV immunoglobulin. Passive immunization with intravenous immunoglobulin has been used in an attempt to prevent CMV infection and disease in SOT recipients. Both unscreened (unselected) and hyperimmune globulin preparations have been studied.

CMV hyperimmune globulin is obtained from CMV-seropositive donors and standardized for a high titer of CMV antibody content; it is enriched four- to eightfold in anti-CMV titer as compared with unselected immune globulin. The currently approved unselected polyclonal immune globulin preparations are difficult to compare because of differences in the process of manufacturing, donor pool sources, and IgG compositions even among lots of the same preparation. Furthermore, there are no standardized laboratory assays for evaluating their efficacy.

The incidence of adverse effects related to immune globulin administration is usually less than 5% and manifestations are typically mild and self-limited. Headaches, back or abdominal pain, nausea, vomiting, shortness of breath, fever, chills, and myalgias are the most common adverse effects. Anaphylactic reactions have been described in patients with IgA deficiency given preparations that contain IgA. Contamination of some immune globulin preparations with hepatitis C virus has been demonstrated (118). However, all currently manufactured preparations require both screening of plasma pools for anti-hepatitis C virus antibody and removal of such pools from the immune globulin, as well as a specific additional viral inactivation step. Whether there is the potential for transmission of other yet unidentified pathogens is unknown.

Critique of Passive Immunoprophylaxis Studies

Results from randomized controlled trials in renal transplant recipients indicate that immune globulins (both unscreened and hyperimmune globulin) prevent CMV disease in some (119–121) but not all (122) trials (see Table 2). There are several factors that may explain the inconsistency of the results, including (a) use of both unscreened and hyperimmune globulin; (b) differing doses, dose schedules, duration of administration after transplant and preparation of the product; and (c) varying immunosuppressive regimens and supportive care techniques. CMV immune globulin is licensed by the U.S. Food and Drug Administration for use in renal transplantation. In liver transplantation, unselected immune globulin does not reduce CMV disease (123), whereas use of CMV hyperimmune globulin prevents CMV disease in non-D$^+$/R$^-$ liver transplant recipients (124). A subsequent analysis of the latter study, however, and one additional study demonstrated a reduction in CMV disease in D$^+$/R$^-$ liver transplant recipients given CMV hyperimmune globulin (125,126). A randomized trial in heart, lung, and kidney transplant recipients showed no difference when acyclovir was used with or without unselected immune globulin (127). A secondary beneficial effect of CMV hyperimmune globulin is that it reduces other opportunistic infections following transplantation (124). A recent meta-analysis of the use of immune globulin to prevent symptomatic CMV disease in transplant recipients showed a beneficial effect (common odds ratio, 0.59 [95% confidence interval, 0.39–0.86]) of immune globulin as compared with no treatment (128). Although in this analysis no apparent advantage was provided by the use of hyperimmune globulin over unselected immune globulin, bone marrow and SOT recipients were pooled together; thus two separate pathogenic processes were combined. When the solid organ transplantation data are analyzed in isolation, there is evidence that hyperimmune globulin is superior to unselected immune globulin in preventing CMV disease.

Together, results from randomized trials in SOT indicate the following:

1. Immune globulin confers some degree of efficacy in preventing CMV disease, being more consistent with CMV hyperimmune globulin preparations.
2. These benefits are attenuated when antilymphocyte antibody therapy is used.

3. Renal transplant recipients are more likely to have a beneficial effect from CMV hyperimmune globulin than are extrarenal (e.g., liver) transplant recipients, especially within the high-risk (D$^+$/R$^-$) group.
4. Advantages include relatively infrequent administration (weekly intervals) and no need for continuous intravenous access.
5. The main disadvantage is cost. Formal comparisons between effective antiviral agents and CMV hyperimmune globulin will need to be performed to address cost and side effects (129). Such pharmacoeconomic studies, which apply to any other antiviral agents, need to clearly establish not only the cost of the prophylactic agent, but also the cost of direct and indirect effects of CMV infection previously outlined. In liver and perhaps in heart and pancreas transplant recipients, the high-risk (D$^+$/R$^-$) group requires enhanced prophylaxis, which may be achieved by combining CMV hyperimmune globulin with antiviral agents.

Antiviral Agents

The ideal CMV prophylactic regimen would be characterized as (a) effective in an oral formulation if frequent administration is required or in an intravenous formulation that can be given at infrequent intervals (i.e., weekly); (b) safe, thus requiring minimal laboratory evaluations and having a wide therapeutic range to avoid monitoring of levels; (c) having minimal interactions with conventional "transplantation" medications; (d) pan virostatic/cidal to cover not only CMV but other herpesviruses (herpes simplex virus, varicella-zoster virus, Epstein-Barr virus, human herpesvirus 6, 7 and 8), with a low chance of inducing antiviral resistance; (e) administered only to patients at risk for symptomatic CMV infection; (f) cost-effective; and (g) not requiring virologic monitoring (Table 3).

Based on the current state-of-the-art CMV prophylaxis and treatment, significant advances need to be made to achieve the preceding goals. Current prophylactic approaches vary widely among different transplant programs. Reasons for the discrepancies reflect the absence of large, multicentered, randomized trials. In addition, results of small single-center studies are frequently difficult to reproduce, as differences in endpoints, definitions, viral surveillance (frequency, methodology), type of immunosuppressive regimen, patient populations, and frequency of antilymphocyte antibody treatment are common. More important, inherent differences among the type of solid organ transplanted need to be considered. This results in a myriad of prophylactic regimens, many of which may be insufficient or even excessive, from both effectiveness and cost perspectives.

TABLE 3. *Summary of Randomized Antiviral Medication Prophylaxis Trials in Solid Organ Transplant Recipients*

Type of transplant	Reference	Type of study	Number of patients studied (# of D+/R− patients[a])	Prophylactic Regimen	Outcome	CMV Disease[b]	Mortality[b]
Acyclovir							
Kidney	(131)	Primary and secondary prophylaxis, randomized, double-blind, placebo-controlled	53 (6) / 51 (7)	Acyclovir 800 mg po 4/day × 12 weeks beginning before transplant vs. placebo	Decreased CMV infection and disease, especially in the D+/R− subgroup	8% vs. 29%	4% vs. 6%
	(134)	Primary prophylaxis, prospective, randomized	22 (22) / 10 (10)	Acyclovir 800–3,200 mg/day × 12 weeks vs. no prophylaxis	No difference	40% vs. 40%	not reported
Liver	(133)	Primary and secondary prophylaxis, randomized, pediatric	10 (1) / 19 (3)	Ganciclovir 5 mg/kg IV 2/day × 2 weeks; then acyclovir 800 mg/m² po 4/day × 1 year vs. ganciclovir 5 mg/kg IV 2/day × 2 weeks	No difference	20% vs. 5%	
	(132)	Secondary prophylaxis, randomized, controlled, prospective	60 (0) / 60 (0)	Acyclovir 500 mg/m² IV 3/day × 10 days, then acyclovir 3200 mg/day po through 3 months vs. no prophylaxis	Decreased CMV infection and disease	7% vs. 23%	"no effect on survival"
Ganciclovir							
Kidney–cadaver	(138)	Primary prophylaxis (D+/R−), randomized	17 (17) / 17 (17)	Ganciclovir 5 mg/kg IV 2/day × 14 days (days 14–28) vs. no ganciclovir	Delayed onset CMV infection; reduce severity of CMV disease; no change in incidence of CMV infection or disease	47% vs. 73%	0% vs. 0%
Kidney, kidney–pancreas, kidney–islet cell, pancreas, liver	(139)	Primary and secondary prophylaxis, randomized, prospective, nonplacebo controlled	133 (32) / 133 (31)	Acyclovir 800 mg po or 400 mg IV 4/day × 12 weeks or 6 weeks after any antirejection therapy vs. Ganciclovir 5 mg/kg IV 2/day × 7 days plus Sandoglobulin or Minnesota CMV immune globulin 100 mg/kg IV days 1, 4, 7	Decreased CMV disease in the acyclovir group	21% vs. 32%	10% vs. 14%
Heart	(136)	Primary and secondary prophylaxis (stratified (D+ vs. D+/R+), prospective, randomized, double-blind, placebo controlled	76 (19) / 73 (16)	Ganciclovir 5 mg/kg IV 2/day × 14 days, then 6 mg/kg 5/week × 14 days vs. placebo	Reduced incidence of CMV illness in R+ subgroup, decreased incidence of CMV shedding	16% vs. 43%	4% vs. 1%
	(165)	Secondary prophylaxis, prospective, randomized, nonplacebo controlled	16 (0) / 15 (0)	Ganciclovir 5 mg/kg IV 2/day × 14 days vs. Cytotect 100 mg/kg within 24 hr of transplant and at weeks 2, 4, 6, 8, 10	Higher incidence of CMV disease in the immunoglobulin group	6% vs. 40%	6% vs. 13%

236

TABLE 3. *(Continued)*

Type of transplant	Reference	Type of study	Number of patients studied (# of D+/R− patients[a])	Prophylatic Regimen	Outcome	CMV Disease[b]	Mortality[b]
Lung	(143)	Primary and secondary prophylaxis (excluding (D⁻/R⁻), randomized	13 (3)	Ganciclovir 5 mg/kg IV 4/day × 2 weeks, starting day 7; then 5 mg/kg/day × 1 week; then 5 mg/kg/day 5 days/week through 90 days vs.	Decreased CMV infection and disease, increased median infection-free duration	0% vs. 25%	15% vs. 25%
			12 (3)	ganciclovir 5 mg/kg IV 4/day × 2 weeks, starting day 7; then 5 mg/kg/day × 1 week; then acyclovir 800 mg po 4/day through 90 days			
Liver	(141)	Primary and secondary prophylaxis, randomized, prospective	52 (9)	Sandoglobulin 200 mg/kg IV 2/week with acyclovir 5 mg/kg/day IV until discharge, then acyclovir 5 mg/kg/day po vs.	Decreased CMV disease in ganciclovir group	15% vs. 4%	14% vs. 13%
			52 (7)	Sandoglobulin 200 mg/kg IV 2/week with ganciclovir 5 mg/kg/day IV until discharge, then acyclovir 5 mg/kg/day po			
	(142)	Primary and secondary prophylaxis, randomized, prospective	71 (11)	Acyclovir 800 mg po 4/day . × 3 months vs.	Decreased CMV infection and disease and delayed onset of CMV infection in ganciclovir group; no decrease in primary CMV infection	28% vs. 9%	7% vs. 12%
			68 (7)	ganciclovir 5 mg/kg/day IV × 2 weeks, then acyclovir 800 mg po 4/day × 2.5 months			
	(140)	Primary and secondary prophylaxis (excluding D⁻/R⁻), randomized, prospective	33 (3)	Ganciclovir 5 mg/kg IV 2/day × 14 days during 3rd and 4th post-transplant weeks vs.	No difference in clinical infections; lower incidence of serologically diagnosed infection in ganciclovir group	27% vs. 34%	3% vs. 19%
			32 (7)	no prophylaxis			
	(144)	Primary and secondary prophylaxis, randomized, prospective, nonplacebo controlled	124 (10)	Ganciclovir 6 mg/kg IV/day days 1–30; then Monday–Friday through day 100 vs.	Decreased CMV infection and disease in ganciclovir group	0.8% vs. 10%	15% vs. 14%
			126 (11)	acyclovir 10 mg/kg IV 3/day through discharge; then 800 mg 4/day through day 100			
	(46)	Primary and secondary prophylaxis, randomized, prospective, placebo controlled	150 (21)	Ganciclovir 1000 mg po 3/day × 98 days vs.	Decreased CMV disease in ganciclovir group including among D⁺/R⁻ patients	4.8% vs. 18.9%	6.7% vs. 10.4%
			154 (25)	Placebo			

[a]If known, the number of patients who were D⁺/R⁻ is given in parentheses.
[b]Among patients given, first listed vs. second listed regimen.

237

Critique of Antiviral Prophylaxis Studies

Acyclovir

Acyclovir, in its phosphorylated form, acts as a competitive inhibitor of viral DNA polymerase. It should be an ideal prophylactic agent for CMV for several reasons. First, it can be given orally; second, it is relatively inexpensive; and third, it has minimal adverse effects at low doses. However, it possesses little *in vitro* activity against CMV at clinically achievable levels. In spite of this, in the past, acyclovir has been the only available potential oral anti-CMV agent and has been successfully used to prevent CMV infection and disease in BMT populations (130). For these reasons, many investigators have studied the role of acyclovir in CMV prophylaxis following solid organ transplantation. One prospective, randomized, placebo-controlled study has shown acyclovir to be effective in preventing CMV infection and disease following renal transplantation (131), and a randomized, but non-placebo-controlled study has shown acyclovir to be effective in preventing CMV infection and disease following liver transplantation (132). However, these results have not been confirmed by other studies (133,134), and further analysis from the same institution that demonstrated the prophylactic efficacy of acyclovir in renal transplant recipients (including some of the patients in the original study) showed, as part of a study of rejection prophylaxis regimens, no difference in the incidence of CMV disease in D+/R− patients (a subgroup of patients who were particularly benefited in the original study) (135). Side effects of acyclovir include phlebitis after intravenous infusion, renal toxicity, confusion, delirium, lethargy, lightheadedness, tremors, seizures, nausea, vomiting, and rash.

Although acyclovir meets many of the criteria of an ideal prophylactic drug, its efficacy as an anti-CMV compound is suboptimal and based on the current data, it can only be indicated as a primary agent for non-high-risk renal transplant recipients.

Ganciclovir

As with acyclovir, most studies of intravenous ganciclovir prophylaxis are difficult to interpret because they lack control groups receiving placebo and instead compare ganciclovir with acyclovir or different preparations of immune globulins. In general, the idea of intravenous antiviral prophylaxis is to administer medication during the initial period following transplantation (first 2–4 weeks), when patients are usually hospitalized and intravenous access is feasible. In heart transplant recipients, intravenous ganciclovir administered for 2–4 weeks after transplantation reduces CMV disease in CMV-seropositive recipients (136,137) but not in the high-risk (D+/R−) group (136). Similarly, in the D+/R− renal transplant recipients, intravenous ganciclovir administered from days 14 to 28 after transplantation is of little use in reducing CMV disease (138). Additional studies in mixed SOT populations (139) and liver recipients (140) show contradictory results. Although some indicate a lack of effectiveness of ganciclovir alone or when combined sequentially with high-dose acyclovir (139,140), others indicate its effectiveness (141,142). Consistently, the high-risk patient group (D+/R−) is seldom benefited by short-term (2–4 weeks) intravenous ganciclovir administration. In lung transplantation recipients, the rate of CMV infection and disease is higher than in other SOTs, and thus prolonging the administration of ganciclovir could theoretically reduce this rate. Within this context, ganciclovir administration beginning 1 week after lung transplantation and continued until day 90 was slightly more effective than a 3-week course of ganciclovir followed by high-dose oral acyclovir in terms of reducing CMV infection, although this effect was not maintained as the follow-up period increased (143). A similar approach of using prolonged (100 days) intravenous ganciclovir administration has been shown to be beneficial in reducing CMV disease in liver transplantation, including in the D+/R− group (144). It is possible that lung and gastrointestinal transplant recipients, and high-risk recipients of other types of organs may require more prolonged prophylaxis. Prophylaxis against CMV may have the added benefit of preventing other infections, especially those for which CMV infection is itself a risk factor. For example, it has been shown that prophylactic ganciclovir reduces fungal as well as CMV infections in heart transplant recipients (145).

Recently, oral ganciclovir has been shown to be an effective agent for CMV prophylaxis when administered for 4 months following transplantation, even in D+/R− individuals (146). Although ganciclovir levels in serum following oral administration are, in general, lower than those achieved following parenteral administration, they may be sufficient to inhibit viral replication following transplantation. Studies are under way to confirm the efficacy of oral ganciclovir in other types of SOT recipients.

Prolonged ganciclovir prophylaxis may affect the emergence of resistant viral strains. Although an early study showed that ganciclovir prophylaxis in SOT recipients does not select ganciclovir-resistant isolates of CMV (93), a more recent study indicates that ganciclovir prophylaxis and treatment may select for ganciclovir-resistant CMV (94). As with any agent, the cost of ganciclovir needs to be considered, especially of the intravenous formulation, because of the need for prolonged intravenous access, which usually implies placing central intravenous lines and the consequent risk of line infections.

New Antiviral Agents

Several drugs are under investigation as possible agents for CMV prophylaxis in solid organ transplantation. No randomized studies of foscarnet prophylaxis have been performed in SOT recipients. This medication must be administered intravenously and is not an ideal candidate, especially in renal transplant recipients, because of its nephrotoxicity. CMV-monoclonal antibody is being developed but is likely to be expensive; unless it proves to be highly efficacious, it seems unlikely to be cost-effective. Valaciclovir, a valine ester of acyclovir that is more readily absorbed than its parent drug and that is subsequently metabolized to acyclovir, is being studied for CMV prophylaxis in kidney transplant recipients in a blinded, placebo-controlled, randomized fashion. Cido-fovir has strong activity against CMV, including ganci-clovir-resistant strains, and is also under evaluation. Its long half-life may allow once weekly or even less frequent dosing, albeit by parenteral administration, which would make it an attractive candidate for CMV prophylaxis. A major drawback is its nephrotoxicity, which can be decreased when coadministered with probenecid (147). In addition, a new pro-drug of cidofovir may be less nephrotoxic. Lobucavir (Bristol Myers-Squibb, Princeton, NJ) is an active oral anti-CMV agent (148) whose clinical efficacy in terms of CMV prophylaxis remains unknown. Oral agents for CMV prophylaxis are an important advance because they avoid the need for intravenous access.

PREEMPTIVE THERAPY

Preemptive therapy of CMV infection involves the administration of antiviral agents to a subgroup of patients prior to the appearance of disease. This depends on a laboratory marker or a patient's characteristic that identifies a subgroup of individuals with a high risk of disease at a time when antimicrobial intervention would be maximally effective in aborting the impending disease process (149). Compared with a prophylactic approach of administering antiviral agents to all patients, only patients at risk of developing symptomatic CMV infection would receive specific antiviral therapy. Therefore fewer patients would receive an antiviral agent, and probably for a shorter period of time, which brings advantages in terms of cost, emergence of resistant viral strains, and medication side effects.

Critique of Preemptive Therapy

Candidate laboratory tests for this therapeutic mode include PCR to detect CMV DNA or CMV RNA, anti-genemia tests, and viral culture, among others (Table 4). A study in liver transplant recipients demonstrated that a 7-day course of ganciclovir given when CMV was identified by surveillance blood or urine cultures provided effective prophylaxis against CMV disease (150). However, CMV disease developed in 63% of patients in this study without prior positive surveillance cultures. Other

TABLE 4. *Prognostic values of methods for CMV detection in blood*

Method	Sensitivity[a]	Specificity[a]
Shell Vial Assay (164)	63%	88%
Polymerase chain reaction		
Serum (151)	83%	57%
Peripheral blood leukocytes cells (166)	57%	35%
Antigenemia (157)	83%	71%

[a]Sensitivity and specificity as a marker of future CMV disease.

methods of surveillance, including molecular biological methods and antigenemia tests, are also being studied in this mode. We have shown that PCR can detect CMV DNA in the sera of 83% of liver transplant recipients prior to the onset of symptomatic CMV infection and could be a useful marker for preemptive therapy (151). Importantly, PCR serum was positive a mean of 13 days prior to the onset of symptomatic CMV infection. Quantitation of PCR-amplified CMV in bronchoalveolar lavage specimens has been successfully used to predict the development of CMV pneumonitis in lung and heart/lung transplant patients, and has been proposed as a marker for preemptive therapy (152). Quantitation of CMV DNA in blood and in urine using PCR has also been studied; high levels of CMV DNA correlate with the presence of CMV disease (153,154). Antigenemia is another promising marker for preemptive therapy (155,156) and has been shown, in heart transplant recipients, to have an 83% sensitivity as a marker for the future development of symptomatic CMV infection, but preceding its onset by only 5 days (157). In one study, PCR performed on peripheral blood leukocytes was the earliest signal of CMV replication, followed by PCR performed on plasma and then by antigenemia (158). In another study, detection of CMV mRNA by PCR was inferior to antigenemia with respect to the early diagnosis of CMV disease (159).

The usefulness of any of these markers will be established only when evaluated in the context of an effective antiviral agent. The ideal scenario would consist of performing a relatively inexpensive surveillance of CMV disease markers at the time of highest risk following transplantation (i.e., 2–6 weeks) and treating those patients with positive markers with a highly effective anti-CMV oral agent.

Identifying patient characteristics that place transplant recipients at risk for CMV infection is another aspect of preemptive therapy. This requires the active investigation of risk factors for CMV infection following solid organ transplantation. Such risk factors include the use of anti-lymphocyte antibodies after transplantation (12,160). The principle is that the intensity of antiviral strategies needs to be linked to the intensity of the antirejection program.

TABLE 5. *Preemptive therapy in solid organ transplant recipients*

Type of transplant	Reference	Type of study	Number of patients studied (# of D+/R− Patients)[a]	Prophylactic regimen	Outcome	CMV Disease[b]	Mortality[b]
Kidney	(163)	Secondary prophylaxis, randomized, >6 days of prophylactic treatment post-transplant with ALG or OKT3 or treatment within the first 2 weeks for acute rejection	16 (0)[a]	Sandoglobulin 500 mg/kg day 0 and weeks 2 and 4; 250 mg/kg weeks 6 and 8 vs. untreated controls	Reduction in severity of symptomatic CMV illness and incidence of CMV complications	13% vs. 39%	not reported
			18 (0)				
	(167)	Primary and secondary prophylaxis of patients receiving ATG for rejection, randomized, double-blind, placebo controlled	19 (5)	Cytotect 100 mg/kg/day of ATG therapy and day 7, 14, 35, 56, and 77; thereafter vs. placebo (albumin)	Prevented fatal CMV disease; should be targeted to D+/R−	37% vs. 30%	0% vs. 20%
			20 (4)				
	(13)	Secondary prophylaxis of patients receiving OKT3 or ALG, randomized, non–placebo controlled, prospective	64 (0)	Ganciclovir 2.5 mg/kg 2/day until termination of antilymphocyte therapy vs. untreated controls	Preemptive therapy with ganciclovir reduced the excessive occurrence of CMV disease	14% vs. 33%	2% vs. 4%
			49 (0)				
	(161)	Primary and secondary prophylaxis patients on OKT3, randomized, controlled, prospective, non–placebo controlled	22 (0)	Ganciclovir 2.5 mg/kg/IV q day that antilymphocyte antibody therapy was given vs. no prophylaxis	0% vs. 17% Reduction in CMV disease	100% vs. 100%	
			18 (0)				
Liver	(162)	Secondary prophylaxis patients on antilymphocyte antibody preparations, randomized, prospective, non–placebo controlled	50 (14)	Gammagard 0.5 g/kg IV days 1, 3, 5, then q week × 3 weeks 3 weeks with acyclovir 400 mg po 5 × q day × 3 months vs. no prophylaxis	No benefit	not shown	10% vs. 22%
			50 (3)				
	(150)	Primary and secondary prophylaxis; randomized; stratified by CMV serostatus of donor and recipient	24 (2)	Acyclovir 800 mg po 4/day × 24 weeks vs. ganciclovir 5 mg/kg IV 2/day × 7 days if surveillance cultures (buffy coat, urine) yielded CMV	Preemptive therapy with ganciclovir provided effective prophylaxis against CMV disease	29% vs. 4%	13% vs. 13%
			23 (2)				

[a]If known, the number of patients who were D+/R− is given in parentheses.
[b]Among patients given, first listed vs. second listed regimen.
Abbreviations used. ALG-antilymphocyte globulin; ATG-antithymocyte globulin.

In particular, antilymphocyte antibody therapy was recently demonstrated to be a risk factor for CMV disease in renal transplant recipients, and intravenous ganciclovir, when administered concomitantly with antilymphocyte antibodies, decreased the incidence of CMV disease (13,161) (Table 5). In liver transplant recipients, immune globulin with acyclovir administered with antilymphocyte therapy did not reduce the rate of CMV disease (162). In contrast, in renal transplant recipients, immune globulin alone did reduce the severity of CMV disease associated with antilymphocyte globulin or OKT3 use (163,164).

Overall, preemptive therapy is a promising approach, whether based on the early detection of CMV or targeting of patients with risk factors for CMV. These areas need further investigation needs. We are currently performing a trial of preemptive ganciclovir in liver transplantation recipients based on the detection of CMV DNA in peripheral blood leukocytes.

CONCLUSIONS

In conclusion, over the last decade we have made significant strides in diagnosing and treating CMV infection in SOT recipients. What remains to be determined is the optimal preventive measure(s). Certainly, an effective, safe, inexpensive oral antiviral agent, akin to the use of trimethoprim-sulfamethoxazole to prevent *Pneumocystis carinii* infection, would be one option, if feasible. Another option would be an effective vaccine. A third solution lies in preemptive therapy. We need to continue to identify risk factors for CMV infection and to study new technologies for early CMV detection as markers for preemptive therapy. Then we need to use these methodologies to study preemptive therapy and assess its benefits in terms of decreasing CMV infection and disease, morbidity, and mortality and in terms of cost-effectiveness.

REFERENCES

1. Alexander JA, Cuellar RE, Fadden RJ, Genovese JJ, Gavaler JS, Van Thiel DH. Cytomegalovirus infections of the upper gastrointestinal tract before and after liver transplantation. *Transplantation* 1988;46:378–382.
2. Soderberg C, Larsson S, Bergstedt-Lindqvist, Moller E. Definition of a subset of human peripheral blood mononuclear cells that are permissive to human cytomegalovirus infection. *J Virol* 1993;67:3166–3175.
3. Gerna G, Zipeto D, Percivalle E, et al. Human cytomegalovirus infection of the major leukocyte subpopulations and evidence for initial viral replication in polymorphonuclear leukocytes from viremic patients. *J Infect Dis* 1992;166:1236–1244.
4. Schrier RD, Nelson JA, Oldstone MBA. Detection of human cytomegalovirus in peripheral blood lymphocytes in a natural infection. *Science* 1985;230:1048–1051.
5. Grefte A, Van der Giessen M, Van Son W, The TH. Circulating cytomegalovirus (CMV)-infected endothelial cells in patients with an active CMV infection. *J Infect Dis* 1993;167:270–277.
6. Dummer JS, Hardy A, Poorsattar A, Ho M. Early infections in kidney, heart, and liver transplant recipients on cyclosporine. *Transplantation* 1983;36:259–267.
7. Ho M. Advances in understanding cytomegalovirus infection after transplantation. *Transplant Proc* 1994;26:7–11.
8. Lumbreras C, Fernandez I, Velosa JA, Munn SR, Paya CV. High incidence of CMV infection following pancreas transplantation. In: Michelson S, Plotkin SA, eds. *Multidisciplinary approach to understanding cytomegalovirus disease.* New York: Elsevier Science Publishers; 1993:165–167.
9. Reyes J, Abu-Elmagd K, Tzakis A, et al. Infectious complications after human small bowel transplantation. *Transplant Proc* 1992;24:1249–1250.
10. Stratta RJ. Clinical patterns and treatment of cytomegalovirus infection after solid-organ transplantation. *Transplant Proc* 1993;25:15–21.
11. Chou S. Cytomegalovirus infection and reinfection transmitted by heart transplantation. *J Infect Dis* 1987;155:1054–1056.
12. Portela D, Patel R, Larson-Keller J, et al. OKT3 treatment for allograft rejection is a risk factor for cytomegalovirus disease in liver transplantation. *J Infect Dis* 1995;171:1014–1018.
13. Hibberd PL, Tolkoff-Rubin NE, Conti D, et al. Preemptive ganciclovir therapy to prevent cytomegalovirus disease in cytomegalovirus antibody-positive renal transplant recipients. A randomized controlled trial. *Ann Intern Med* 1995;123:18–26.
14. Fietze E, Prosch S, Reinke P, et al. Cytomegalovirus infection in transplant recipients. The role of tumor necrosis factor. *Transplantation* 1994;58(6):675–680.
15. Osman HK, Peiris JS, Taylor CE, Warwicker P, Jarrett RF, Madeley CR. "Cytomegalovirus disease" in renal allograft recipients: is human herpesvirus 7 a co-factor for disease progression? *J Med Virol* 1996;48(4):295–301.
16. Rook A. Interactions of cytomegalovirus with the human immune system. *Rev Infect Dis* 1988;10[Suppl. 3]:S460–S467.
17. Falagas ME, Snydman DR, Griffith J, et al. Exposure to cytomegalovirus from the donated organ is a risk factor for bacteremia in orthotopic liver transplant recipients. *Clin Infect Dis* 1996;23(3):468–474.
18. van den Berg AP, Klompmakre IJ, Haagsma EB, et al. Evidence for an increased rate of bacterial infections in lier transplant patients with cytomegalovirus infection. *Clin Transplant* 1996;10:224–231.
19. Fox AS, Tolpin MD, Baker AL, et al. Seropositivity in liver transplantation recipients as a predictor of cytomegalovirus disease. *J Infect Dis* 1988;157:383–384.
20. Grattan MT, Moreno-Cabral CE, Starnes VA, Oyer PE, Stinson EB, Shumway NE. Cytomegalovirus infection is associated with cardiac allograft rejection and atherosclerosis. *JAMA* 1989;261:3561–3566.
21. Kendall TJ, Wilson JE, Radio SJ, et al. Cytomegalovirus and other herpesvirus: do they have a role in the development of accelerated coronary arterial disease in human heart allografts. *J Heart Lung Transplant* 1992;11:S14–S20.
22. Sharples LD, Caine N, Mullins P, et al. Risk factor analysis for the major hazards following heart transplantation-rejection, infection, and coronary occlusive disease. *Transplantation* 1991;52:244–252.
23. Gao SZ, Hunt SA, Schroeder JS, Alderman EL, Hill IR, Stinson EB. Early development of accelerated graft coronary artery disease: risk factors and course. *J Am Coll Cardiol* 1996;28(3):673–679.
24. Simmons RL, Matas AJ, Rattassi LC, Balfour HH, Howard RJ, Najarian JS. Clinical characteristics of the lethal cytomegalovirus infection following renal transplantation. *Surgery* 1977;82:537–546.
25. Paya CV, Wiesner RH, Herman PE, et al. Risk factors for cytomegalovirus and severe bacterial infections following liver transplantation: a prospective multivariate time-dependent analysis. *J Hepatol* 1993;18:185–195.
26. Paya CV, Marin E, Keating M, Dickson R, Porayko M, Wiesner R. Solid organ transplantation: results and implications of acyclovir use in liver transplants. *J Med Virol* 1993;1:123–127.
27. Grossi P, Revello G, Minoli L, et al. Three-year experience with human cytomegalovirus infections in heart transplant recipients. *J Heart Transplant* 1990;9:712–719.
28. Sayage LH, Gonwa TA, Goldstein RM, Husberg BS, Klintmalm GB. Cytomegalovirus infection in orthotopic liver transplantation. *Transplant Int* 1989;2:96–101.
29. Stratta RJ, Shaefer MS, Markin RS, et al. Cytomegalovirus infection and disease after liver transplantation. An overview. *Dig Dis Sci* 1992;37:673–688.
30. Pehlivanoglu E, Amant ME, Jenkins RL, et al. Severe cytomegalovirus

infection and immunosuppressive therapy in pediatric liver transplantation. *Turk J Pediatr* 1990;32:3–11.

31. Starzl T, Porter KA, Schroter G, Corman J, Groth C, Sharp HL. Autopsy findings in a long-surviving liver recipient. *N Engl J Med* 1973;289:82–84.

32. Palestine AG. Clinical aspects of cytomegalovirus retinitis. *Rev Infect Dis* 1988;10:S515–S521.

33. Patterson JW, Broeker AH, Kornstein MJ, Mills AS. Cutaneous cytomegalovirus infection in a liver transplant recipient. *Am J Dermatopathol* 1988;10:524–530.

34. Lee JY. Cytomegalovirus infection involving the skin in immunocompromised hosts. *Am J Clin Pathol* 1989;92:96–100.

35. Power C, Poland SD, Kassim KH, Kaufman JCE, Rice GPA. Encephalopathy in liver transplantation: neuropathology and CMV infection. *Can J Neurol Sci* 1990;17:378–381.

36. McCarthy JM, McLoughlin MG, Shackleton CR, et al. Cytomegalovirus epididymitis following renal transplantation. *J Urol* 1991;146:417–419.

37. Richardson W, Colvin RB, Cheeseman SH, et al. Glomerulopathy associated with cytomegalovirus viremia in renal allografts. *N Engl J Med* 1981;305:57–63.

38. McNamara D, Di Salvo T, Mathier M, Keck S, Semigran M, Dec GW. Left ventricular dysfunction after heart transplantation: incidence and role of enhanced immunosuppression. *J Heart Lung Transplant* 1996;15(5):506–515.

39. Laifer SA, Ehrlich GD, Huff DS, Balsan MJ, Scantlebury VP. Congenital cytomegalovirus infection in offspring of liver transplant recipients. *Clin Infect Dis* 1995;20:52–55.

40. Paya CV, Hermans PE, Wiesner RH, et al. Cytomegalovirus hepatitis in liver transplantation: prospective analysis of 93 consecutive orthotopic liver transplantations. *J Infect Dis* 1989;160:752–758.

41. Jensen WA, Rose RM, Hammer SM, et al. Pulmonary complications of orthotopic liver transplantation. *Transplantation* 1986;42:484–490.

42. Spencer GD, Hackman RC, McDonald GB, et al. A prospective study of unexplained nausea and vomiting after marrow transplantation. *Transplantation* 1986;42:602–607.

43. Van Thiel DH, Gavaler JS, Schade RR, Clien M-C, Starzl TE. Cytomegalovirus infection and gastric emptying. *Transplantation* 1992;54:70–73.

44. Sutherland DER, Chan FY, Foucar E. The bleeding cecal ulcer in transplant patients. *Surgery* 1979;86:386–398.

45. Kowdley KV, Fawaz KA, Kaplan MM. Extrahepatic biliary stricture associated with cytomegalovirus in a liver transplant recipient. *Transplant Int* 1996;9(2):161–163.

46. Muldoon J, O'Riordan K, Rao S, Abecassis M. Ischemic colitis secondary to venous thrombosis. A rare presentation of cytomegalovirus vasculitis following renal transplantation. *Transplantation* 1996;61(11):1651–1653.

47. Littler E, Stuart A, Cree M. Human cytomegalovirus UL97 open reading frame encodes a protein that phosphorylates the antiviral analogue ganciclovir. *Nature* 1992;358:160–162.

48. Sullivan V, Talarico C, Stanat S, al. e. A protein kinase homologue controls phosphorylation of ganciclovir in human cytomegalovirus-infected cells. *Nature* 1992;358:162–164.

49. Keating M. Antiviral agents. *Mayo Clin Proc* 1992;67:160–178.

50. Stratta RJ, Shaefer MS, Markin RS, et al. Clinical patterns of cytomegalovirus disease after liver transplantation. *Arch Surg* 1989;124:1443–1450.

51. Gudnason T, Belani KK, Balfour HH. Ganciclovir treatment of cytomegalovirus disease in immunocompromised children. *Pediatr Infect Dis* 1989;8:436–440.

52. Mai M, Nery J, Sutker W, Husberg B, Klintmalm G, Gonwa T. DHPG (ganciclovir) improves survival in CMV pneumonia. *Transplant Proc* 1989;21:2263–2265.

53. D'Allesandro AM, Pirsch JD, Stratta RJ, Sollinger HW, Kalayoglu M, Belzer FO. Successful treatment of severe cytomegalovirus infections with ganciclovir and CMV hyperimmune globulin in liver transplant recipients. *Transplant Proc* 1989;21:3560–3561.

54. Salmela K, Hockerstedt K, Lautenschlager I, et al. Ganciclovir in the treatment of severe cytomegalovirus disease in liver transplant patients. *Transplant Proc* 1990;22:238–240.

55. De Hemptinne B, Lamy ME, Salizzoni M, et al. Successful treatment of cytomegalovirus disease with 9-(1,3-dihydroxy-2-propoxymethyl guanine). *Transplant Proc* 1988;20:652–655.

56. Buhles WC, Mastre BJ, Tinker AJ, Strand V, Koretz SH, Group SCGTS. Ganciclovir treatment of life- or sight-threatening cytomegalovirus infection: experience in 314 immunocompromised patients. *Rev Infect Dis* 1988;106:S495–S506.

57. De Koning J, van Dorp WT, van Es LA, van't Wout JW, van der Woude FJ. Ganciclovir effectively treats cytomegalovirus disease after solid-organ transplantation, even during rejection treatment. *Nephrol Dial Transplant* 1992;7:350–356.

58. Lang P, Buisso C, Rostoker G, et al. DHPG treatment of kidney transplant recipients with severe CMV infection. *Transplant Proc* 1989;21:20842–2086.

59. Guerin C, Pozzetto B, Broyet C, Gaudin O, Berthoux F. Ganciclovir therapy of symptomatic cytomegalovirus infection in renal transplant recipients. *Nephrol Dial Transplant* 1989;4:906–910.

60. Jordan ML, Hrebinko RLJ, Dummer JS, et al. Therapeutic use of ganciclovir for invasive cytomegalovirus infection in cadaveric renal allograft recipients. *J Urol* 1992;148:1388–1392.

61. Nicholson ML, Veitch PS, Donnelly PK, Flower AJE, Bell PRF. Treatment of renal transplant-associated cytomegalovirus infection with ganciclovir. *Transplant Proc* 1990;22:1811–1812.

62. Cerrina J, Bavoux E, Le Roy Ladurie F, et al. Ganciclovir treatment of cytomegalovirus infection in heart-lung and double-lung transplant recipients. *Transplant Proc* 1991;23:1174–1175.

63. Cooper DKC, Novitzky D, Schlegel V, Muchmore JS, Cucchiara A, Zudhi N. Successful management of symptomatic cytomegalovirus disease with ganciclovir after heart transplantation. *J Heart Lung Transplant* 1991;10:656–663.

64. Icenogle TB, Peterson E, Ray G, Minnich L, Copeland JG. DHPG effectively treats CMV infection in heart and heart-lung transplant patients: a preliminary report. *J Heart Transplant* 1987;6:199–203.

65. Keay S, Petersen E, Icenogle T, et al. Ganciclovir treatment of serious cytomegalovirus infection in heart and heart-lung transplant recipients. *Rev Infect Dis* 1988;10:S563–S572.

66. Stein DS, Verano AS, Levandowski RA. Successful treatment with ganciclovir of disseminated cytomegalovirus infection after liver transplantation. *Am J Gastroenterol* 1988;83:684–686.

67. Snydman DR. Ganciclovir therapy for cytomegalovirus disease associated with renal transplants. *Rev Infect Dis* 1988;10:S554–S562.

68. Rondeau E, Farquet C, Ruedin P, Fries D, Sraer JD. Efficacy of early treatment of cytomegalovirus infection by ganciclovir in renal transplant recipients. *Transplant Proc* 1990;22:1813–1814.

69. Hrebinko R, Jordan ML, Dummer JS, et al. Ganciclovir for invasive cytomegalovirus infection in renal allograft recipients. *Transplant Proc* 1991;23:1346–1347.

70. Watson FS, O'Connell JB, Amber IJ, et al. Treatment of cytomegalovirus pneumonia in heart transplant recipients with 9(1,3-dihydroxy-2-propoxymethyl)-guanine (DHPG). *J Heart Transplant* 1988;7:102–105.

71. Smyth RL, Scott JP, Borysiewicz LK, et al. Cytomegalovirus infection in heart-lung transplant recipients: risk factors, clinical associations, and response to treatment. *J Infect Dis* 1991;164:1045–1050.

72. Steinhoff G, Behrend M, Wagner TOF, Hoper MH, Haverich A. Early diagnosis and effective treatment of pulmonary CMV infection after lung transplantation. *J Heart Lung Transplant* 1991;10:9–14.

73. Dunn DL, Mayoral JL, Gillingham KJ, et al. Treatment of invasive cytomegalovirus disease in solid organ transplant patients with ganciclovir. *Transplantation* 1991;51:98–106.

74. Megison SM, Andrews WS. Combination therapy with ganciclovir and intravenous IgG for cytomegalovirus infections in pediatric liver transplant recipients. *Transplantation* 1991;52:151–154.

75. Paya CV, Hermans PE, Smith TF, et al. Efficacy of ganciclovir in liver and kidney transplant recipients with severe cytomegalovirus infection. *Transplantation* 1988;46:229–234.

76. Markin RS, Langnas AN, Donovan JP, Zetterman RK, Stratta RJ. Opportunistic viral hepatitis in liver transplant recipients. *Transplant Proc* 1991;23:1520–1521.

77. Winston DJ, Ho WG, Bartomi K, et al. Ganciclovir therapy for cytomegalovirus infections in recipients of bone marrow transplants and other immunosuppressed patients. *Rev Infect Dis* 1988;10:S547–S553.

78. Erice A, Jordan MC, Chace BA, Fletcher C, Chinnock BJ, Balfour HH. Ganciclovir treatment of cytomegalovirus disease in transplant recipients and other immunocompromised hosts. *J Am Med Assoc* 1987;257:3082–3087.

79. Harbison MA, De-Girolami PC, Jenkins RL, Hammer SM. Ganciclovir therapy of severe cytomegalovirus infections in solid-organ transplant recipients. *Transplantation* 1988;46:82–88.

80. O'Hair DP, Johnson CP, Roza AM, Adams MB. Treatment of transplant rejection in the presence of cytomegalovirus viremia. *Transplant Proc* 1990;22:1815–1817.

81. Ross C, Reynon H, Savill J, et al. Ganciclovir treatment for cytomegalovirus infection in immunocompromised patients with renal disease. *Q J Med* 1991;81:929–936.

82. Stratta R, Shaefer M, Markin R, et al. Ganciclovir therapy for viral disease in liver transplant recipients. *Transplant Proc* 1991;23:1968.

83. Reed EC, Wolford JL, Kopecky KJ, et al. Ganciclovir for the treatment of cytomegalovirus gastroenteritis in bone marrow transplant patients. *Ann Intern Med* 1990;112:505–510.

84. Swan S, Munar M, Wigger M, et al. Pharmacokinetics of ganciclovir in a patient undergoing hemodialysis. *Am J Kidney Dis* 1991;17:69–72.

85. Shrestha BM, Parton D, Gray A, et al. Cytomegalovirus involving gastrointestinal tract in renal transplant recipients. *Clin Transplant* 1996;10(2):170–175.

86. Einsele H, Ehninger G, Steidle M, et al. Polymerase chain reaction to evaluate antiviral therapy for cytomegalovirus disease. *Lancet* 1991;338:1170–1172.

87. Van den Berg AP, van Son WJ, Haagsma EB, et al. Prediction of recurrent cytomegalovirus disease after treatment with ganciclovir in solid-organ transplant recipients. *Transplantation* 1993;55:847–851.

88. Sawyer MD, Mayoral JL, Gillingham KJ, KrAm MA, Dunn DL. Treatment of recurrent cytomegalovirus disease in patients receiving solid organ transplants. *Arch Surg* 1993;128:165–170.

89. Davis C, Springmeyer S, Gmerek B. Central nervous system side effects of ganciclovir. *N Engl J Med* 1990;322:933–934.

90. Shea BF, Hoffman S, Sesin GP, Hammer SM. Ganciclovir hepatotoxicity. *Pharmacotherapy* 1987;7:223–226.

91. Faulds D, Heel R. Ganciclovir. A review of its antiviral activity, pharmacokinetic properties and therapeutic efficacy in cytomegalovirus infections. *Drugs* 1990;39:597–638.

92. De Armond B. Safety considerations in the use of ganciclovir in immunocompromised patients. *Transplant Proc* 1991;23[Suppl. 1]:26–29.

93. Boivin G, Erice A, Crane DD, Dunn DL, Balfour HH. Ganciclovir susceptibilities of cytomegalovirus (CMV) isolates from solid organ transplant recipients with CMV viremia after antiviral prophylaxis. *J Infect Dis* 1993;168:322–325.

94. Lurain NS, Ammons HC, Kapell KS, Yeldandi W, Garrity ER, O'Keefe JP. Molecular analysis of human cytomegalovirus strains from two lung transplant recipients with the same donor. *Transplantation* 1996;62(4):497–502.

95. Klintmalm G, Lonnqvist B, Oberg B, et al. Intravenous foscarnet for the treatment of severe cytomegalovirus infection in allograft recipients. *Scand J Infect Dis* 1985;17:157–163.

96. Barkholt LM, Ericzon BG, Ehrnst A, Forsgren M, Andersson JP. Cytomegalovirus infections in liver transplant patients: incidence and outcome. *Transplant Proc* 1990;22:235–237.

97. Ringdén O, Lönnqvist B, Paulin T, et al. Pharmacokinetics, safety and preliminary clinical experiences using foscarnet in the treatment of cytomegalovirus infections in bone marrow and renal transplant recipients. *J Antimicrob Chemother* 1986;17:373–387.

98. Locke TJ, Odom NJ, Tapson JS, Freeman R, McGregor CGA. Successful treatment with trisodium phosphonoformate for primary cytomegalovirus infection after heart transplantation. *J Heart Transplant* 1987;6:120–122.

99. Manischewits J, Guinnan G, Lane H, et al. Synergistic effect of ganciclovir and foscarnet on cytomegalovirus replication *in vitro*. *Antimicrob Agents Chemother* 1990;34:373–375.

100. Bacigalupo A, Bregante S, Tedone E, et al. Combined foscarnet–ganciclovir treatment for cytomegalovirus infections after allogeneic hemopoietic stem cell transplantation (Hsct). *Bone Marrow Transplant* 1996;2:110–114.

101. Bacigalupo A, Bregante S, Tedone E, et al. Combined foscarnet-ganciclovir treatment for cytomegalovirus infections after allogeneic hemopoietic stem cell transplantation. *Transplantation* 1996;62(3):376–380.

102. Wade JC, Hintz M, McGuffin RW, Springmeyer SC, Connor JD, Meyers JD. Treatment of cytomegalovirus pneumonia with high dose acyclovir. *Am J Med* 1982;73:249–256.

103. Burdelski M, Schmidt K, Hoyer PF, et al. Liver transplantation in children: the Hanover experience. *Transplant Proc* 1987;19:3277–3281.

104. Lautenschlager I, Ahonen J, Eklund B, et al. Hyperimmune globulin therapy of clinical CMV disease in renal allograft recipients. *Transplant Proc* 1989;21:2087–2088.

105. Rancewicz Z, Halama G, Smogorzewski M, et al. The usefulness of hyperimmune globulin for treatment of overt cytomegalovirus infection in allograft recipients. *Transplant Proc* 1990;22:1818–1819.

106. Bowden R, Sayers M, Flournoy N, et al. Cytomegalovirus immune globulin and seronegative blood products to prevent primary cytomegalovirus infection after marrow transplantation. *N Engl J Med* 1986;314(16):1006–1010.

107. Sayers MH, Anderson KC, Goodnough LT, et al. Reducing the risk for transfusion-transmitted cytomegalovirus infection. *Ann Intern Med* 1992;116:55–62.

108. Marker SC, Simmons RL, Balfour HHJ. Cytomegalovirus vaccine in renal allograft recipients. *Transplant Proc* 1981;13:117–119.

109. Balfour BHJ, Sachs GW, Welo P, Gerhz RC, Simmons RL, Najarian JS. Cytomegalovirus vaccine in renal transplant candidates: progress report of a randomized, placebo-controlled, double-blind trial. *Birth Defects* 1984;20:289–304.

110. Balfour HHJ, Welo PK, Sachs GW. Cytomegalovirus vaccine trial in 400 renal transplant candidates. *Transplant Proc* 1985;17:81–83.

111. Brayman KL, Dafoe DC, Smythe WR, et al. Prophylaxis of serious cytomegalovirus infection in renal transplant candidates using live human cytomegalovirus vaccine. *Arch Surg* 1988;123:1502–1508.

112. Glazer JP, Friedman HM, Grossman RA, et al. Live cytomegalovirus vaccination of renal transplant candidates. A preliminary trial. *Ann Intern Med* 1979;91:676–683.

113. Plotkin SA, Friedman HM, Fleisher GR, et al. Towne-vaccine-induced prevention of cytomegalovirus disease after renal transplants. *Lancet* 1984;1:528–530.

114. Plotkin SA, Starr SE, Friedman HM, et al. Effect of Towne live virus vaccine on cytomegalovirus disease after renal transplant. *Ann Intern Med* 1991;114:525–531.

115. Plotkin SA, Huang E-S. Cytomegalovirus vaccine virus (Towne strain) does not induce latency. *J Infect Dis* 1985;152:395–397.

116. Britt W, Fay J, Seals J, Kensil C. Formulation of an immunogenic human cytomegalovirus vaccine: responses in mice. *J Infect Dis* 1995;171:18–25.

117. Riddell SR, Greenberg PD. Therapeutic reconstitution of human viral immunity by adoptive transfer of cytotoxic T lymphocyte clones. *Curr Top Microbiol Immunol* 1994;198:9.

118. Bjøro K, Frøland S, Yun Z, et al. Hepatitis C infection in patients with hypogammaglobulinemia after treatment with contaminated immune globulin. *N Engl J Med* 1994;331:1607–1611.

119. Greger B, Vallbracht A, Kurth J, et al. The clinical value of CMV prophylaxis by CMV hyperimmune serum in the kidney transplant patient. *Transplant Proc* 1986;18:1387–1389.

120. Snydman DR, Werner BG, Heinze-Lacey B, et al. Use of cytomegalovirus immune globulin to prevent cytomegalovirus disease in renal-transplant recipients. *N Engl J Med* 1987;317:1049–1054.

121. Fassbinder W, Ernst W, Hanke P, Bechstein PB, Scheuermann EH, Schoeppe W. Cytomegalovirus infections after renal transplantation: effect of prophylactic hyperimmunoglobulin. *Transplant Proc* 1986;18:1393–1396.

122. Kasiske BL, Heim-Duthoy KL, Tortorice KL, Ney AL, Odlanc MD, Venkateswara Rao K. Polyvalent immune globulin and cytomegalovirus infection after renal transplantation. *Arch Intern Med* 1989;149:2733–2736.

123. Cofer JB, Morris CA, Sutker WL, et al. A randomized double-blind study of the effect of prophylactic immune globulin on the incidence and severity of CMV infection in the liver transplant recipient. *Transplant Proc* 1991;23:1525–1527.

124. Snydman DR, Werner BG, Dougherty NN, et al. Cytomegalovirus immune globulin prophylaxis in liver transplantation. A randomized, double blind, placebo-controlled trial. The Boston Center for Liver Transplantation CMVIG Study Group. *Ann Intern Med* 1993;10:984–991.

125. Saliba F, Arulnaden JL, Gugenheim J, et al. CMV hyperimmune globulin prophylaxis after liver transplantation: a prospective randomized controlled study. *Transplant Proc* 1989;21:2260–2262.

126. Snydman DR, Werner BG, Dougherty NN, et al. A further analysis of the use of cytomegalovirus immune globulin in orthotopic liver trans-

plant recipients at risk for primary infection. *Transplant Proc* 1994; 26:23–27.

127. Bailey TC, Ettinger NA, Trulock EP, Storch GA, Cooper JD, Powderly WG. Failure of high-dose oral acyclovir with or without globulin to prevent primary cytomegalovirus disease in recipients of solid organ transplants. *Am J Med* 1993;95:273–278.

128. Glowacki LS, Smaill FM. Use of immune globulin to prevent symptomatic cytomegalovirus disease in transplant recipients—a metaanalysis. *Clin Transplant* 1994;8:10–18.

129. Conti DJ, Freed BM, Gruber SA, Lempert N. Prophylaxis of primary cytomegalovirus disease in renal transplant patients. A trial of ganciclovir vs. immunoglobulin. *Arch Surg* 1994;129:443–447.

130. Meyers JD, Reed EC, Shepp DH, et al. Acyclovir for prevention of cytomegalovirus infection and disease after allogeneic marrow transplantation. *N Engl J Med* 1988;318(2):70–75.

131. Balfour HH, Chace BA, Stapleton JT, Simmons RL, Fryd DS. A randomized placebo-controlled trial of oral acyclovir for the prevention of cytomegalovirus disease in recipients of renal allografts. *N Engl J Med* 1989;320:1381–1387.

132. Saliba F, Eyraud D, Samuel D, et al. Randomized controlled trial of acyclovir for the prevention of cytomegalovirus infection and disease in liver transplant recipients. *Transplant Proc* 1993;25:1444–1445.

133. Green M, Reyes J, Nour B, et al. Randomized trial of ganciclovir followed by high dose oral acyclovir vs. ganciclovir alone in the prevention of cytomegalovirus disease in pediatric liver transplant recipients: preliminary analysis. *Transplant Proc* 1994;26:173–174.

134. Kletzmayr J, Kotzmann H, Popow-Kraupp T, Kovarik J, Klauser R. Impact of high-dose oral acyclovir prophylaxis on cytomegalovirus (CMV) disease in CMV high-risk renal transplant recipients. *J Am Soc Nephrol* 1996;7(2):325–330.

135. Frey DJ, Matas AJ, Gillingham KJ, et al. Sequential therapy—a prospective randomized trial of MALG versus OKT3 for prophylactic immunosuppression in cadaver renal allograft recipients. *Transplantation* 1992;54:50–56.

136. Merigan TC, Renlund DG, Keay S, et al. A controlled trial of ganciclovir to prevent cytomegalovirus disease after heart transplantation. *N Engl J Med* 1992;326:1182–1186.

137. Aguado JM, Gomez-Sanchez MA, Lumbreras C, et al. Prospective randomized trial of efficacy of ganciclovir versus that of anticytomegalovirus (CMV) immunoglobulin to prevent CMV disease in CMV-seropositive heart transplant recipients treated with OKT3. *Antimicrob Agents Chemother* 1995;39:1643–1645.

138. Rondeau E, Bourgeon B, Peraldi MN, et al. Effect of prophylactic ganciclovir on cytomegalovirus infection in renal transplant recipients. *Nephrol Dial Transplant* 1993;8:858–862.

139. Dunn DL, Gillingham KJ, Kramer MA, et al. A prospective randomized study of acyclovir versus ganciclovir plus human immune globulin prophylaxis of cytomegalovirus infection after solid organ transplantation. *Transplantation* 1994;57:876–884.

140. Cohen AT, O'Grady JG, Sutherland S, Sallie R, Tan K-C, Williams R. Controlled trial of prophylactic versus therapeutic use of ganciclovir in liver transplantation in adults. *J Med Virol* 1993;40:5–9.

141. Nakazato PZ, Burns W, Moore P, Garcia-Kennecy R, Cox K, Esquivel C. Viral prophylaxis in hepatic transplantation: preliminary report of a randomized trial of acyclovir and ganciclovir. *Transplant Proc* 1993;25:1935–1937.

142. Martin FM, Mañez R, Linden P, et al. A prospective randomized trial comparing sequential ganciclovir—high dose acyclovir to high dose acyclovir for prevention of cytomegalovirus disease in adult liver transplant recipients. *Transplantation* 1994;58:779–785.

143. Duncan SR, Grgurich WF, Iacono AT, et al. A comparison of ganciclovir and acyclovir to prevent cytomegalovirus after lung transplantation. *Am J Respir Crit Care Med* 1994;150:146–152.

144. Winston DJ, Wirin D, Shaked A, Busuttil RW. Randomised comparison of ganciclovir and high-dose acyclovir for long-term cytomegalovirus prophylaxis in liver-transplant recipients. *Lancet* 1995;346:69–74.

145. Wagner JA, Ross H, Hunt S, et al. Prophylactic ganciclovir treatment reduces fungal as well as cytomegalovirus infections after heart transplantation. *Transplantation* 1995;60(12):1473–1477.

146. Gane E, Saliba F, Valdecasas GJ, et al. Randomised trial of efficacy and safety of oral ganciclovir in the prevention of cytomegalovirus disease in liver transplant recipients. The Oral Ganciclovir International Transplantation Study Group. *Lancet* 1997;350:1729–1733.

147. Bailey TC. Prevention of cytomegalovirus disease. *Semin Respir Infect* 1993;8:225–232.

148. Braitman A, Suerdel MR, Olsen SJ, et al. Evaluation of SQ 34,514L pharmacokinetics and efficacy in experimental herpesvirus infections in mice. *Antimicrob Agents Chemother* 1991;35:1464–1468.

149. Rubin RH, Tolkoff-Rubin NE. Antimicrobial strategies in the care of organ transplant recipients. *Antimicrob Agents Chemother* 1993;37:619–624.

150. Singh N, Yu VL, Mietes L, Wagener MW, Miner RC, Gayoski T. High-dose acyclovir compared with short-course preemptive therapy to prevent cytomegalovirus disease in liver transplant recipients. A randomized trial. *Ann Intern Med* 1994;120:375–381.

151. Patel R, Smith TF, Espy MJ, et al. Detection of Cytomegalovirus DNA in sera of liver transplant recipients. *J Clin Microbiol* 1994;32:1431–1434.

152. Cagle PT, Buttone G, Holland VA, et al. Semiquantitative measurement of cytomegalovirus DNA in lung and heart-lung transplant patients by *in vitro* DNA amplification. *Chest* 1992;101:93–96.

153. Drouet E, Colimon R, Michelson S, et al. Monitoring levels of human cytomegalovirus DNA in blood after liver transplantation. *J Clin Microbiol* 1995;33(2):389–394.

154. Fox JC, Kidd IM, Griffiths PD, Sweny P, Emery VC. Longitudinal analysis of cytomegalovirus load in renal transplant recipients using a quantitative polymerase chain reaction: correlation with disease. *J Gen Virol* 1995;76(Pt 2):309–319.

155. Iberer F, Tscheliessnigg K, Halwachs G, et al. Definitions of cytomegalovirus disease after heart transplantation: antigenemia as a marker for antiviral therapy. *Transplant Int* 1996;9(3):236–242.

156. Egan JJ, Barber L, Lomax J, et al. Detection of human cytomegalovirus antigenaemia: a rapid diagnostic technique for predicting cytomegalovirus infection/pneumonitis in lung and heart transplant recipients. *Thorax* 1995;50(1):9–13.

157. Koskinen PK, Nieminen MS, Marrila SP, Hayry PJ, Lautenschlager IT. The correlation between symptomatic CMV infection and CMV antigenemia in heart allograft recipients. *Transplantation* 1993;55:547–551.

158. Wolff C, Skourtopoulos M, Hornschemeyer D, et al. Significance of human cytomegalovirus DNA detection in immunocompromised heart transplant patients. *Transplantation* 1996;61(5):750–757.

159. Meyer-Konig U, Serr, A, von Laer D, et al. Human cytomegalovirus immediate early and late transcripts in peripheral blood leukocytes: diagnostic value in renal transplant recipients. *J Infect Dis* 1995;171(3):705–709.

160. Krogsgaard K, Boesgaard S, Aldershvile J, Arendrup H, Mortensen SA, Petterson G. Cytomegalovirus infection rate among heart transplant patients in relation to anti-thymocyte immunoglobulin induction therapy. Copenhagen Heart Transplant Group. *Scand J Infect Dis* 1994;26(3):239–247.

161. Conti DJ, Freed BM, Singh TP, Gallichio M, Gruber SA, Lempert N. Preemptive ganciclovir therapy in cytomegalovirus-seropositive renal transplants recipients. *Arch Surg* 1995;130(11):1217–1221.

162. Stratta RJ, Shaefer MS, Cushing KA, et al. A randomized prospective trial of acyclovir and immune globulin prophylaxis in liver transplant recipients receiving OKT3 therapy. *Arch Surg* 1992;127:55–64.

163. Steinmuller DR, Novick AC, Streen SB, Graneto D, Swift C. Intravenous immunoglobulin infusions for the prophylaxis of secondary cytomegalovirus infection. *Transplantation* 1990;49:68–70.

164. Pillay D, Ali AA, Liu SF, Kops E, Sweny P, Griffiths PD. The prognostic significance of positive CMV cultures during surveillance of renal transplant recipients. *Transplantation* 1993;56:103–108.

165. Aguado JM, Gomez-Sanchez MA, Lumbreras C, et al. Prospective randomized trial of efficacy of ganciclovir versus that of anticytomegalovirus (CMV) immunoglobulin to prevent CMV disease in CMV-seropositive heart transplant recipients treated with OKT3. *Antimicrob Agents Chemother* 1995;39(7):1643–1645.

166. Delgado R, Lumbreras C, Alba C, et al. Low predictive value of polymerase chain reaction for diagnosis of CMV disease in liver transplant recipients. *J Clin Microbiol* 1992;30:1876–1878.

167. Metselaar HJ, Rothbarth PH, Brouwer RM, Wentimg GJ, Jeekel J, Weimar W. Prevention of cytomegalovirus-related death by passive immunization. A double-blind placebo-controlled study in kidney transplant recipients treated by rejection. *Transplantation* 1989;48:264–266.

Transplant Infections edited by
Raleigh A. Bowden, Per Ljungman, and Carlos V. Paya.
Lippincott–Raven Publishers, Philadelphia © 1998

CHAPTER 18

Epstein-Barr Virus and Lymphoproliferative Disorders after Transplantation

Jutta K. Preiksaitis and Sandra M. Cockfield

In 1964, Epstein, Achong, and Barr described a new herpesvirus in lymphoblastoid cell lines derived from a Burkitt's lymphoma tumor biopsy. This virus was later named Epstein-Barr virus (EBV). The preeminent example of a human tumor virus, EBV is strongly associated with the development of Burkitt's lymphoma, nasopharyngeal carcinoma, and Hodgkin's disease. In immunodeficient or immunosuppressed individuals, it plays a critical pathogenic role in lymphoproliferative disorders and immunoblastic lymphoma (1). Other clinical syndromes such as multiple myeloma, smooth muscle tumors, and oral hairy leukoplakia have been associated with EBV in the setting of post-transplant immunosuppression.

Like other herpesviruses, EBV is characterized by lifelong persistence arising from the establishment and maintenance of a state of equilibrium between the virus and the host immune response. In recipients of bone marrow and solid organ transplants, this balance is disrupted in favor of the virus. The uncontrolled proliferation of EBV-infected B cells that may occur in this setting results in a spectrum of post-transplant lymphoproliferative disorders (PTLD). The use of the term *PTLD* is not consistent in the literature; we use this term to include all clinical syndromes associated with EBV-driven lymphoproliferation ranging from a benign self-limited form of polyclonal proliferation to true malignancies containing clonal chromosomal abnormalities. Although PTLD occurs relatively infrequently, it is associated with significant morbidity and mortality. This chapter will review the pathogenesis of EBV-associated PTLD, risk factors for its development, and strategies that may permit early diagnosis, management, and prevention of this disorder.

THE BIOLOGY OF EPSTEIN-BARR VIRUS INFECTION

EBV, a member of the gamma-herpesvirus subfamily, is an enveloped icosahedral virus whose genome is encoded by a 172-kb linear double-stranded DNA (reviewed in reference 2). It is ubiquitous and has a narrow host range. EBV infection is transmitted by exchange of saliva. In lower socioeconomic strata and developing nations, infection is almost universally acquired in early childhood and is usually subclinical. In industrialized nations, particularly among upper socioeconomic strata, subjects are often infected in adolescence and early adult life. Infection at this time frequently results in the infectious mononucleosis syndrome, the symptoms of which are the result of an exaggerated T-cell response to a self-limited lymphoproliferative process. However, even in Western industrialized societies, more than 90% of the population has immunity to EBV by the age of 40.

EBV isolates have been classified into two strains, EBV-1 and EBV-2, based on the allelic polymorphism of genes encoding the nuclear antigens, EBNA-2, -3A, -3B, and -3C. EBV-1 transforms B cells more efficiently than EBV-2. The two types of EBV differ in their geographic distribution, with EBV-1 being ubiquitous and predominating in Western societies, whereas EBV-2 is prevalent in Africa and New Guinea (3). Although single predominant strains of EBV are detected in most healthy virus carriers, infection with multiple strains has been described in the oropharynx and peripheral blood of cardiac (4) and bone marrow transplant (BMT) recipients (5).

EBV is characterized by its ability to persist for the lifetime of the host despite the presence of a strong humoral and cell-mediated immune response to the virus. Ongoing low-grade replication in the oropharynx occurs simultaneously with a predominantly latent infection of B cells in the peripheral blood and lymphoid tissues.

From the Department of Medicine, University of Alberta, Edmonton, Alberta, Canada T6G 2B7.

Although the epithelial cell of the oropharynx was believed to be the major site of lytic EBV infection, recent data suggest that, in the normal host, infection of epithelial cells by EBV occurs only rarely. Using sensitive *in situ* hybridization techniques, EBV has not been detected in the tonsillar epithelium or exfoliated oropharyngeal epithelial cells of acutely infected patients (6–8). Instead, B cells, particularly those demonstrating features of plasmacytoid differentiation, have been identified as the predominant site of EBV replication in the oropharynx. It has been suggested that latently infected B cells home to the mucosal epithelium when activated. Here the lytic EBV cycle may be reactivated as these B cells terminally differentiate or undergo apoptosis (6). During its lytic cycle EBV expresses more than 80 genes several of which display distant but functional homology to the cellular genes *jun/fos*, *Bcl-2*, and IL-10. The biological consequences of expression of these genes *in vivo* are unclear, although they may influence the survival of EBV-infected cells, permitting replication of the virus prior to cell death.

Infection of susceptible B-lymphocytes is initiated by the binding of the major EBV outer envelope glycoprotein gp 350/220 with the cellular complement receptor C3d, also known as CD21. Infection results in cellular activation and immortalization. In addition to up-regulating expression of certain B-cell activation markers and adhesion molecules, infected B cells express a limited subset of latent viral proteins (reviewed in reference 6). During primary infection, as in infectious mononucleosis, the viral antigens expressed by peripheral blood B cells include six nuclear antigens (EBNA-1, -2, -3A, -3B, -3C, and -LP) and three integral membrane proteins (LMP-1, -2A, and -2B). Two small EBV-encoded nonpolyadenylated RNAs (EBER-1 and EBER-2) are also found in very high copy numbers in the nuclei of latently infected cells, a feature that has facilitated detection of EBV in the clinical setting. This expression pattern, known as latency III or the "growth program," appears to drive limited proliferation of B cells prior to differentiation and the establishment of persistent infection. At least 5 of the viral proteins expressed during the "growth program" (EBNA-1, -2, -3A, -3C and LMP-1) are essential for the transformation or immortalization process of B cells (reviewed in references 2 and 9). How these proteins interact with the host cell machinery to induce B cell transformation has been most clearly elucidated for LMP-1, a viral analogue of the family of tumor necrosis factor (TNF) receptors in human cells. LMP-1 binds to intracellular signal transducing proteins known as TNF-receptor associated factors (TRAFs), thereby activating 2 families of broad-spectrum transcriptional activators, nuclear factor-κB (NF-κB) and, through the activation of c-jun kinase, activator protein-1. This causes the B cell to proliferate.

Cells expressing the "growth pattern" of viral proteins are not found in peripheral blood of healthy EBV carriers, as these cells are rapidly eliminated by host cytotoxic T-lymphocytes (CTLs). However, in the post-transplant setting, suppression of the CTL response permits the survival of cells expressing this growth program, resulting in expansion of the infected cell population and increased viral shedding. This expression pattern is characteristic of both lymphoblastoid cell lines *in vitro* and many lymphomas arising in immunodeficient individuals.

With recovery from the primary infection, long-term viral persistence occurs. During infectious mononucleosis as many as 10% (more commonly, 0.1% to 1%) of circulating B cells are infected (10). In contrast, only 1-60 per 10^6 B cells are infected in the peripheral blood of healthy seropositive subjects. These immortalized B cells carry intact episomal viral genomes in low copy number. However, unlike B-cell infection in the oropharynx, EBV is actually replicating in fewer than one in 40 of the EBV-infected B cells in peripheral blood of healthy carriers (11). This results in intermittent shedding of virus at a low level. The observation that total lymphoid irradiation prior to bone marrow transplantation results in elimination of the resident EBV carrier state supports the role of the B cell, not the oropharyngeal epithelium, as the true site of viral persistence (12). Recent data suggest that the major site of long-term viral persistence is a resting, nonproliferating CD23⁻ B-cell population in peripheral blood (13). Phenotyping of these cells has revealed that they express only the viral gene LMP-2A, the product of which is a known target for CTLs. However, these B cells also lack expression of the costimulatory molecule B7, which is necessary to reactivate a memory T-cell response. Thus these latently infected resting B cells may escape detection by the host immune response. The term "latency program" has been proposed to describe this pattern of gene expression. Certain physiologic signals may be capable of reactivating viral replication in these latently infected cells *in vivo*.

In contrast, certain EBV-associated tumors are characterized by other patterns of viral gene expression not thought to have normal cellular counterparts (reviewed in reference 6). Burkitt's lymphoma cells express only EBNA-1, a viral product required for replication of the EBV episome in proliferating cells. It has been hypothesized that B cells expressing the latency program switch to EBNA-1-only expression (latency I) in response to physiological signals driving B-cell activation and proliferation. Interestingly, EBNA-1 contains a 200-residue glycine/alanine repeat domain that protects the protein from the HLA class I processing pathway, preventing it from being presented to CD8⁺ CTLs. This would limit the cytotoxic immune response to Burkitt's lymphoma cells. A further pattern, latency II (EBNA-1 and LMP-1 and/or LMP-2A and/or LMP-2B) has been associated with nasopharyngeal carcinoma, T/NK cell lymphomas, and Hodgkin's disease. This may represent deviation of the latency program with aberrant expression of the oncogenic LMP-1 protein.

The Normal Immune Response to EBV Infection

The immune response to EBV infection is the result of a complex interaction between humoral and cell-mediated responses (reviewed in references 10 and 14). The production of alpha and gamma interferon appears to be important in the early response to EBV infection. Subsequently, both neutralizing and nonneutralizing antibodies directed against a variety of virally encoded products are generated (Table 1). Many of these persist throughout the lifetime of the host. Neutralizing antibody may function by limiting the spread of cell-free virus, preventing superinfection with other virus strains and rendering lytically infected cells susceptible to antibody-dependent cell-mediated cytotoxicity. However, despite the presence of such antibodies, viral replication continues in the oropharynx.

Initial cell-mediated defense consists of direct cytolysis by early nonspecific T-cell or natural killer responses. These are followed by the development of virus-specific CD4+ or CD8+ T-cell responses. *In vitro* and *in vivo* evidence suggest that HLA-restricted, EBV-specific CD8+ CTLs play a particularly crucial role in controlling the outgrowth of EBV-infected B-lymphocytes during both primary and persistent infection (15). These CTLs recognize epitopes from the EBNA-3A, -3B, and -3C family of latent proteins, although less common reactivities against EBNA-2, EBNA-LP, LMP-1, and LMP-2 have been described. In the peripheral blood of healthy EBV-seropositive subjects the frequency of EBV-specific memory CTLs is high, ranging from 1/540 to 1/8,300 T cells (16). After transplantation this CTL response is impaired or ablated. This is particularly true in recipients of allogeneic bone marrow; most demonstrate a significant reduction in anti-EBV CTL precursor frequency when studied at 3 months following transplant (17). The use of T-cell-depleted donor marrow results in a greater delay in reconstitution of the T-cell population (18). However, these responses recover in most patients by 6 months after transplant. This interval of deficient CTL activity corresponds to the period of greatest risk for the development of PTLD in BMT recipients. Detailed kinetics of the EBV-specific CTL response in solid organ transplant (SOT) recipients receiving current immunosuppressive regimens has not been reported.

EBV Infection After Organ and Bone Marrow Transplantation

Primary EBV infection is almost universal in the EBV seronegative transplant recipient who receives a seropositve donor organ or bone marrow. Transmission of the donor EBV isolate to the recipient has been clearly documented in this setting (20,23). Although a case of primary EBV infection leading to PTLD acquired from a recently EBV-infected blood donor has been described in a liver transplant recipient (21), the importance of transfusion as a source of EBV infection after transplantation is uncertain. The median time to onset of oropharyngeal EBV shedding in patients experiencing primary infection after solid organ transplantation is 6 weeks, an interval identical to the incubation period documented in the transmission of EBV mononucleosis (22). Reinfection with a second EBV strain transmitted from the donor to EBV-seropositive bone marrow (5) and SOT (23) recipients has also been reported.

With immunosuppressive therapy, solid organ and bone marrow allograft recipients demonstrate both increased oropharyngeal EBV excretion and increased numbers of circulating EBV-infected B cells. Among SOT recipients, higher levels of oropharyngeal EBV shedding are observed in patients experiencing primary infection compared with those who are seropositive prior to transplantation, and shedding increases with courses of antilymphocyte antibodies or multiple doses of methylprednisolone (22).

Several groups have recently reported the results of prospective monitoring of EBV viral load in peripheral blood lymphocytes (PBLs) of bone marrow and SOT recipients (24–27). Increases in EBV viral load, even in the presence of acyclovir or ganciclovir prophylaxis, are consistently seen following transplant. Among SOT recipients, patients undergoing a primary EBV infection experience significantly higher viral loads than those recipients who are seropositive before transplant. Moreover, in the setting of both bone marrow and solid organ transplantation,

TABLE 1. *Antibody responses to EBV infections*

EBV status	VCA		EA	EBNA	
	IgM	IgG	IgG	IgG	IgM
Susceptible	–	–	–	–	–
Postinfection	–	+	–	+	–
Primary infection	+	+	+/–	–	+/–
Normal host	+/–	++/–	?	–	?
Transplant recipient					
Reactivated infection					
Normal host	+/–	++	+/––	++	+/–
Transplant recipient	+/–	+++	?	++/+	?

VCA, viral capsid antigen; EA, early antigen; EBNA, EBV nuclear antigen.

patients developing PTLD have greater viral loads than those without PTLD, suggesting that quantitative surveillance of EBV viral load in the peripheral blood may identify transplant recipients at high risk for this complication.

Early studies of EBV infection in SOT recipients used serological responses to EBV as a measure of infection. High levels of antibody to viral proteins expressed in the lytic EBV cycle (anti-VCA IgG) are often seen in seropositive recipients of solid organ and bone marrow transplants. However, our studies of oropharyngeal shedding of EBV by immunosuppressed kidney and heart transplant recipients suggest that serological responses seriously underestimate EBV infection (22). Patients shedding the highest levels of EBV have the poorest serological responses. Cen and colleagues also demonstrated that SOT recipients experiencing a primary EBV infection produce low to undetectable levels of anti-EBNA antibodies (28). Moreover, in seropositive individuals, the titer of anti-EBNA antibodies may actually decrease from pretransplant levels. The absence or decrease in EBNA antibody after solid organ transplantation appears to correlate with high EBV viral loads and an increased risk of developing PTLD (24). Furthermore, the presence of passive antibody from blood products and intravenous immunoglobulin preparations complicates the interpretation of humoral immune responses to EBV after transplantation, particularly in the setting of bone marrow transplantation.

PATHOGENESIS OF LYMPHOPROLIFERATIVE LESIONS IN THE IMMUNOSUPPRESSED HOST

The evidence currently suggests that early EBV-induced lymphoproliferative disorders result from an uncontrolled proliferation of EBV-infected B cells (Fig. 1). Although this proliferation is initially polyclonal in nature, it is evident that most phenotypically polyclonal lesions contain oligoclonal or monoclonal elements. Certain clones may experience a selective growth advantage, transforming the polyclonal lesion into an oligoclonal or monoclonal one. Ongoing proliferation may predispose to the development of cytogenetic abnormalities, completing the transformation into a truly malignant state. This theory has received validation from a murine model of early EBV-induced lymphoproliferation in which severe combined immunodeficiency (SCID) mice are engrafted with human hemopoietic cells (29). When PBLs from EBV-seropositive individuals, particularly those infected with EBV-1 isolates, are used as a source of the human cells, human B-cell lymphomas containing EBV DNA consistently develop 2–4 months after engraftment. There are often multiple discrete tumors with each focus usually derived from a single B-cell clone. These lymphoproliferative lesions bear remarkable similarity to those developing in the early post-transplant period in man.

In both the murine model and PTLD lesions in man, there is significant heterogeneity in the latency phenotype of the EBV-infected B cells comprising the tumor

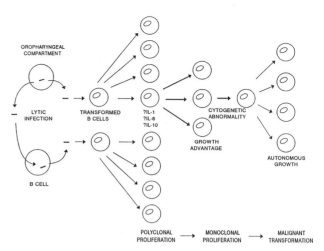

Figure 1. The pathogenesis of EBV-associated PTLD. Infectious virus released from either oropharyngeal or peripheral blood B cells infects resting B cells resulting in B cell transformation and polyclonal proliferation. Certain transformed B cells may have a selective growth advantage leading to clonal components of the lymphoproliferative process. Malignant transformation may occur as a consequence of the development of cytogenetic abnormalities. (–) represents linear viral genome in lytic cycle. (0) represents circular episomal virus in latently infected B cell.

(30–32). Because certain of these proteins are important target antigens for CTLs, B-cell clones expressing latency phenotype I or II may have a growth advantage in patients with a functional but impaired CTL response. These cells may have the ability to evade cell-mediated immunity due to their restricted display of viral antigens. It has been suggested that, in patients lacking a competent EBV-specific CTL response, B cells expressing a greater number of viral proteins (latency III phenotype or "growth program") would also have a distinct growth advantage. This heterogeneity in the latency phenotype of the B cells within lymphoproliferative lesions also results in substantial variation in the density of expression of host genes transactivated by EBV latent proteins, including B-cell activation markers, adhesion molecules, and IL-10 or bcl-2 (30–33). These features may also influence the proliferative capacity of specific clones.

In the murine model two cell populations have been identified in lymphoproliferative lesions: a lymphoblastoid population expressing EBV latent genes and a plasmacytoid population expressing EBV lytic cycle genes (32,34). In man, studies have demonstrated that tissue from approximately 40% of cases of PTLD contain linear replicative forms in addition to the latent episomal forms of EBV (35,36). When examined at the single-cell level, most PTLD lesions contain replicative EBV (30). However, only a small minority (usually less than 5%) of cells in most PTLD lesions demonstrate progression through the lytic cycle. This observation has important implications for the potential efficacy of antiviral agents that are directed against the replicative viral cycle. Because the major pathology in lymphoproliferative disorders is a failure to control the proliferation of latently infected B cells, antiviral drugs would, at best, only prevent recruitment of newly infected B cells.

With enhanced proliferation, these expanding clones of cells are susceptible to developing cytogenetic alterations. This may result in the activation of proto-oncogenes or the inactivation of tumor suppressor genes, thus increasing the risk of malignant transformation to a monoclonal tumor mass that satisfies the criteria for the diagnosis of lymphoma or myeloma. This hypothesis is compatible with reports in the literature that emphasize the ability of lymphoproliferative lesions to evolve with time toward monoclonal populations and the presence of multifocal lesions with apparently different clonal origins (37,38). The role of EBV in driving lymphoproliferation or maintaining susceptibility to immune regulation in these lesions is unclear. Recent data suggest that an intermediate stage in malignant transformation can be observed in PTLD lesions *in vivo* where oncogene expression exists simultaneously with LMP-1 expression and function suggesting that cytogenetic events do not necessarily render B cell growth independent of the EBV genome (38b).

This murine model of EBV-induced lymphomagenesis is a potentially important tool for understanding the pathogenesis of early polyclonal and oligoclonal phases of EBV-induced PTLD in immunosuppressed transplant recipients, and for testing strategies for the prevention and treatment of this clinical problem.

RISK FACTORS FOR THE DEVELOPMENT OF PTLD

Certain risk factors have been identified in the development of PTLD.

1. *The development of PTLD is strongly linked to infection with Epstein-Barr virus.* On the basis of both histologic and epidemiological studies, there is strong evidence that EBV plays a major pathophysiologic role in the development of the great majority of cases of PTLD. EBV DNA has been found in PTLD tumor tissue by *in situ* hybridization (30,31,35,39,40), Southern (31,36,40–42), and Western blotting (28). EBV-specific proteins have also been detected by immunohistochemistry (30,31,40, 43,44). However, not all lesions occurring after solid organ transplantation are clearly linked to EBV; approximately 13% to 21% of PTLD lesions are negative when assessed by these various techniques. The role of EBV in the pathogenesis of these lesions is uncertain.

Most PTLD lesions have been found to contain EBV-1 (45). Knecht and colleagues reported that EBV strains derived from some PTLD lesions were characterized by a series of mutations in the carboxy terminal region of LMP-1 (46); these mutations could render the LMP-1 protein nonimmunogenic or affect critical aspects of its function. Others, however, have been unable to confirm

an increased incidence of these mutations in patients with PTLD (47). At present it is not clear whether some EBV isolates are more virulent than others with respect to the development of PTLD.

Ho and colleagues first reported that recipients of solid organ allografts who are EBV seropositive before transplant are at substantially lower risk of developing PTLD than their seronegative counterparts (41). The profound impact of pretransplant EBV seronegativity on the risk of PTLD has been emphasized in recent single-center analyses (48–51), where a 24- to 33-fold greater incidence of PTLD has been reported in patients at risk for a primary EBV infection compared with those who were seropositive before transplant. The relative risk of PTLD in seropositive individuals experiencing EBV reactivation versus reinfection with a second strain is unknown. Data on the relationship of pretransplant EBV serology to PTLD risk after bone marrow transplantation are limited. In a study of children who received non-HLA-identical bone marrow transplants the pretransplant EBV serostatus of the donor and recipient did not influence the risk of developing PTLD (18).

2. *The risk of PTLD is related to the type of organ allografted.* The incidence of PTLD is correlated with the type of organ transplant. Although this may be partially due to the relative potencies of the immunosuppressive protocols used in recipients of these different organs, characteristics peculiar to the allografted organ may also predispose to the development of PTLD. Recipients of renal allografts are at the lowest risk of developing PTLD, with an incidence of approximately 1%. Recipients of nonrenal organs are at greater risk, with rates of 2.2% reported for liver allograft recipients, 3.5% for recipients of cardiac allografts, 7.9% for recipients of lung allografts, and up to 9.4% for recipients of heart/lung allografts (52–54). The Collaborative Transplant Study, involving more that 50,000 patients transplanted between January 1983 and June 1991, reported a three-fold greater risk of PTLD occurring in the first post-transplant year in heart allograft recipients when compared with kidney transplant recipients (55). Although the incidence of PTLD declined substantially beyond the first post-transplant year, recipients of cardiac transplants continued to experience a relative risk that was 7.7 times greater than that of renal allograft recipients. The incidence of PTLD is particularly high in recipients of intestinal transplants, where it has been reported to occur in 28.5% of patients (56).

In allogeneic bone marrow transplantation PTLD is uncommon (less than 1%) despite intensive immunosuppression (57). However, strategies employed when the donor matching is not optimal may significantly increase the risk of PTLD. The potent combination of T-cell depletion by E-rosetting, the use of myeloablative conditioning regimes, and the *in vivo* administration of monoclonal or polyclonal antibody preparations to promote engraftment is associated with an increased incidence of EBV-associated PTLD of 18% (18). An analysis of secondary malignancies following bone marrow transplant revealed that the factors associated with the development of non-Hodgkin's lymphomas included treatment with an anti-CD3 monoclonal antibody (relative risk 15.6) or antithymocyte globulin (ATG) (relative risk 4.9), T-cell depletion of the donor marrow (relative risk 12.4), and HLA mismatch (relative risk 4.3) (58). Others have also emphasized the potent combination of HLA mismatching and T-cell-depleted marrow where the risk of PTLD rose from 12–14% with the use of T-cell-depleted marrow alone to 24% with HLA mismatching of the donor and recipient (59).

3. *Chronic antigenic stimulation may increase the risk of PTLD.* Antigenic differences between the donor/recipient pair may induce polyclonal B-cell proliferation, predisposing to the development of PTLD. The most convincing clinical data to support this hypothesis are derived from recipients of mismatched, T-cell-depleted bone marrow where the degree of HLA mismatching with its risk of graft-versus-host disease (GVHD) is a significant risk factor for the development of PTLD (18,58,59). Whether cytokines produced in the setting of GVHD promote EBV-driven lymphoproliferation remains speculative. In contrast, the degree of HLA mismatching does not appear to influence the risk of PTLD in recipients of solid organ transplants.

In solid organ transplantation, PTLD has a tendency to involve the allograft. Although it is possible that EBV-transformed donor B cells transmitted with the allograft undergo local proliferation, the proliferating cells of PTLD are usually of recipient origin (19,60,61). This would suggest that transmission from EBV-infected donor cells to recipient B cells occurs initially in the allograft, resulting in local lymphoproliferation. Since several cytokines may act as autocrine growth factors for EBV-transformed B cells *in vitro*—including IL-1-like activity (62), IL-6 (63,64), lymphotoxin (65), and IL-10 (33)—the cytokine milieu within the allograft, particularly during rejection episodes, may promote local lymphoproliferation (reviewed in reference 66). We and others have observed extremely high serum IL-6 levels in several patients with PTLD, suggesting that this cytokine may act as an autocrine growth factor *in vivo* (67). In addition to direct promotion of cellular proliferation, cytokines may facilitate homing of EBV-transformed cells to the allograft.

4. *PTLD is strongly associated with the presence and intensity of the immunosuppressed state.* Any immunosuppressive that blunts cellular immunity to EBV constitutes a risk factor for the development of PTLD. However, the development of increasingly complex and targeted immunosuppressive protocols in solid organ transplantation invites the possibility of increased incidence of this complication. Indeed, there is now abundant evidence that current protocols favor EBV-driven lymphoproliferation, thus requiring great vigilance by transplant programs to identify patients at high risk and appropriately reduce immunosuppression.

Experimental data would support a role for both cyclosporine (CsA) and tacrolimus (FK506) in permitting the development of PTLD. These agents inhibit the maturation of T-cell-dependent immune responses, including the generation of CTLs. Because EBV-specific CTLs are critical in limiting the proliferation of EBV-infected B cells, it is not surprising that CsA and FK506 facilitate the outgrowth of EBV-transformed lymphoblastoid cells *in vitro* (68–70) and *in vivo* (71). CsA has also been reported to induce IL-6 gene transcription (72) and the release of soluble CD23 (73). The former supports B-cell activation and growth of EBV-transformed B cells, and the latter influences B-cell proliferation and differentiation. Thus there may be several mechanisms by which this class of immunosuppressive may potentiate the development of PTLD.

The initial experience with high-dose CsA in solid organ transplantation suggested that its use was associated with an increased incidence of PTLD (74,75). Although the risk of PTLD has diminished with lowering of the CsA dose, PTLD tends to appear earlier with CsA therapy, shifting the mean time to presentation from 48 months after transplantation to 15 months with CsA treatment; 32% of lesions appear within 4 months (76). There is a greater tendency to involve the gastrointestinal tract and lymph nodes, with less central nervous system involvement. Lesions in CsA-treated patients more commonly regress with a reduction in immunosuppression or antiviral therapy. Because many CsA-treated patients also receive azathioprine and/or antilymphocyte antibody therapy, it is difficult to conclude that the increased incidence of PTLD is due solely to CsA. Although the data are limited, the use of CsA, methotrexate, or methylprednisolone was not associated with an increased risk of PTLD in children receiving HLA-mismatched bone marrow transplants (18).

PTLD has also been observed in SOT patients treated with FK506. Several groups have reported a several-fold increase in the incidence of PTLD in young pediatric recipients of liver (77,78) and renal (79,80) allografts with FK506-based immunosuppression. This suggests that FK506 may permit greater lymphoproliferation relative to CsA, at least in the setting of primary EBV infection. In some of these patients, FK506 was initiated as salvage therapy; these individuals may have received more aggressive immunosuppression for refractory acute rejection prior to the conversion to FK506. Thus it is difficult to determine whether this trend is the result of greater immunosuppression with FK506 or of the selection of a high-risk population.

The addition of CsA to steroid and azathioprine (triple therapy) has been variably associated with an increased appearance of PTLD in SOT recipients (81–83). Multivariate analysis of the Collaborative Transplant Study database suggests that triple therapy is associated with a 1.5-fold relative risk of PTLD in the first post-transplant year when compared with either azathioprine and steroid or

CsA alone or in combination with steroid (55). There was no influence of maintenance immunosuppression on the incidence of PTLD occurring beyond the first post-transplant year. Pooled data from the multicenter trials evaluating mycophenolate mofetil (MMF) in renal allograft recipients did not reveal a statistically significant increase in the incidence of PTLD when MMF was used with CsA (0.8%) when compared with the azathioprine/CsA combination (0.3%) or CsA alone (0.0%) (84–86).

Substantial evidence supports the conclusion that the use of potent antilymphocyte antibodies for induction or the treatment of acute rejection after solid organ transplantation is associated with an increased incidence of early PTLD (76,87–90). Increased dose, duration, or repeated courses of antilymphocyte therapy within short time intervals substantially increase the risk, particularly in that subgroup undergoing a primary EBV infection (48,51,91). The Collaborative Transplant Study reported a relative risk of PTLD of 1.80-fold when antilymphocyte antibodies (ALG/ATG or OKT3) were employed as induction agents (55). Univariate analysis of the nonrenal transplant programs at the Mayo Clinic revealed that antirejection therapy with OKT3 alone or following induction with ALG/ATG resulted in a four- to six-fold increase in the incidence of PTLD (51). Similarly, Swinnen and colleagues reported that OKT3 was the predominant variable associated with the increase in incidence of PTLD from 1.3% to 11.4% in a group of cardiac allograft recipients (92). Our experience in renal transplantation suggests that sequential courses of ALG and OKT3, particularly in the setting of primary EBV infection, are a highly significant risk factor (48,91). Those patients who received ALG induction followed by OKT3 treatment for an episode of steroid-resistant rejection had an incidence of PTLD of 12.5%. This was significantly greater than the 0.6% incidence in patients receiving other immunosuppressive protocols.

OKT3 induces a state of virtual paralysis of T-cell effector function. Thus both the helper function required for the development of cytotoxic T cells and the activity of the CTLs themselves may be affected. OKT3 permits the outgrowth of EBV-transformed B cells *in vitro* (93,94). The particular predisposition of OKT3 to promote the development of PTLD may also be linked to its mitogenic activity or the cytokine release syndrome seen with the first or second dose of the drug. It is possible that the cytokine milieu generated by OKT3, especially the secretion of B-cell growth factors such as interleukin-6 or -10, directly promotes proliferation of EBV-infected B cells (66,95). The relative importance of these mechanisms with polyclonal preparations is uncertain.

In the setting of bone marrow transplantation, the delay in reconstitution of the T-cell compartment is largely responsible for the profound early immunodeficiency. Factors that delay recovery of EBV-specific T-cell function—such as HLA mismatching, acute GVHD, and the use of T-cell-depleted marrow or certain T-cell-spe-

cific antibody preparations—greatly escalate the risk of PTLD by turning the balance in favor of EBV. The administration of certain monoclonal antibodies (Campath IG and antileukocyte functional antigen [LFA]-1) to enhance engraftment is also associated with an increased risk of developing PTLD (18). This was particularly evident in children who had received a T-cell-depleted marrow graft in the setting of less than optimal donor matching and who were conditioned with Ara-C, cyclophosphamide and total body irradiation. The use of ATG and anti-CD3 mAb to treat GVHD is also associated with a several-fold increased risk of PTLD (58).

In summary, it is probably not a single immunosuppressive agent, but rather the cumulative intensity of immunosuppression that poses the greatest risk. The specificity of agents such as CsA, FK506, ALG/ATG, and OKT3 for the T-cell limb of the immune response probably accounts for the recent surge in the incidence of PTLD in solid organ transplantation. Repeated or prolonged courses of antilymphocyte therapy may inhibit the ability of the immune system to control virally driven lymphoproliferation. In addition, the use of multiple agents in complex protocols may result in more global immunosuppression by attacking multiple points of the immune response.

5. The risk of PTLD is increased in the setting of cytomegalovirus infection. Although the pathogenesis of PTLD is not directly related to cytomegalovirus (CMV), recent data from the nonrenal SOT programs at the Mayo Clinic suggest that mismatching for CMV, such that a seronegative recipient receives a donor organ from a seropositive individual, amplifies the risk of PTLD several-fold (51). The magnitude of this effect was similar to that seen with the risk attributed to the use of OKT3 for rejection. Importantly, the three identified risk factors (pretransplant seronegativity for EBV, CMV mismatch, and OKT3 treatment for rejection) acted synergistically to increase the risk of PTLD more than 500-fold compared with the lowest-risk patients who lacked all these parameters. The development of CMV disease in patients with a primary EBV infection also increased the risk of PTLD by 7.8-fold in a second series of 40 adult liver transplant recipients (95b). There have been no published reports examining CMV infection as a risk factor for PTLD development after bone marrow transplantation.

The observation that CMV is an additional risk factor for the development of PTLD is not surprising. CMV increases the incidence of other opportunistic infections (96) and is itself immunosuppressive (97). Infection with other members of the herpesvirus family may also facilitate the development of PTLD through similar mechanisms.

CLINICAL PRESENTATION

Patients should be considered to have PTLD if a lymphoproliferative lesion is observed histologically in association with one of several clinical syndromes. The spectrum of disease ranges from an indolent self-limited form of lymphoproliferation to fulminant disease and from localized nodular lesions to widely disseminated disease (52,98–100). Although the pathogenic mechanisms may be similar, the clinical features, response to reduction in immunosuppression, and prognosis differ substantially.

A common presentation, particularly among younger patients in the first year after transplantation, is an infectious mononucleosis-like illness. Fever, sore throat, myalgia, and lymphadenopathy are typical features. Cervical adenopathy and tonsillar hypertrophy may be prominent. The diagnosis may be suspected on the basis of the characteristic clinical presentation and confirmed on histologic evaluation. Patients with disease limited to the lymph nodes, tonsils, or a single organ frequently respond to a reduction in immunosuppression or antiviral therapy. Unfortunately, dissemination may occur, and once widespread, the course is rapidly progressive and fatal in more than 75% of cases.

PTLD limited to the allograft is a common manifestation of early PTLD in SOT recipients. Certain allografts may have a particular predisposition for involvement with PTLD, suggesting organ-specific features that promote lymphoproliferation (52,53,76). Primary presentation in the allograft has been reported in 17% of cases in renal allograft recipients, 8.6% of cases in liver allograft recipients, and up to 60%–80% of cases in recipients of lung or intestinal allografts. Our experience in renal allograft recipients who develop early PTLD suggests that renal allograft involvement is extremely common (48,91); others have reported involvement in 36% to 100% of cases (101,102). In contrast, the cardiac allograft appears to be relatively spared from clinically relevant disease (55), although investigators have identified an increased number of EBV-positive lymphocytes in cardiac biopsies of patients with PTLD (103). Because of the tendency for early allograft involvement with PTLD, a high index of suspicion must exist for patients presenting with allograft dysfunction, particularly in the presence of known risk factors for PTLD. One of the challenges for the pathologist is to differentiate the infiltrate of PTLD from that seen in acute rejection (101,104). An incorrect diagnosis of acute rejection can easily lead to inappropriate or prolonged treatment for rejection, resulting in overimmunosuppression and PTLD.

Central nervous system involvement occurs in fewer than 10% of patients with PTLD using current immunosuppressive protocols. Disseminated multiorgan disease may be associated with CNS involvement isolated to the leptomeninges or CSF without overt lesions in the brain or spinal cord parenchyma. In an analysis of the Cincinnati Transplant Tumor Registry, the average time of appearance of CNS involvement was 33 months with 48% of tumors appearing within the first post-transplant year (105). In 55% of patients, disease was confined to the CNS, a feature that is uncommon in the untransplanted population. Patients typically present with an altered mental status or focal neurologic findings. Lesions usually appear isodense or hypodense radiologically and enhance when contrast is administered. Cerebrospinal fluid is diagnostic in approximately 50% of cases; the diagnosis is confirmed by stereotactic biopsy. The prognosis of patients with CNS involvement is poor, although certain patients have survived in excess of ten years after diagnosis.

Gastrointestinal involvement occurs in approximately 25% of cases in the CsA era (106) and tends to be aggressive, with rapid growth of multiple tumors. Local invasion results in tissue necrosis, bleeding, and perforation. The diagnosis is usually made on exploratory laparotomy. Because disease is frequently restricted to the bowel, definitive treatment with resection of the affected areas permits a good prognosis in this group of patients, with 80% surviving more than a year after diagnosis.

Involvement of the lungs is particularly common in recipients of cardiac, lung, or heart/lung allografts. Patients typically present with deteriorating blood gases and the radiologic appearance of multiple pulmonary nodules. The lymphoproliferative process may extend through the visceral pleura. Cell necrosis with necrotizing vasculitis resulting in destruction of the terminal and respiratory bronchioles is consistently seen on pathological examination. The lesions may be indistinguishable from a primary pulmonary lymphoma. The distinction between acute rejection and PTLD is particularly difficult, given the small size of transbronchial biopsies; stains for EBV-associated proteins or EBER RNA may be useful (Fig. 2) (104). Frequently, consideration must be given to open lung biopsy to ensure a definitive diagnosis. Pulmonary disease is frequently associated with

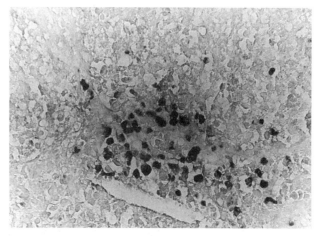

Figure 2. *In situ* hybridization with digoxigenin-labeled EBER-1 probe. Large lymphoid cells seen in this section of a mass lesion taken from the native lung of a lung transplant recipient demonstrate focal positively for EBER-1 mRNA.

either CMV or *Pneumocystis carinii* pneumonia. PTLD can also present as a necrotizing ulcerative bronchitis in heart/lung transplant recipients (107).

Multisystem involvement with lymphoproliferation is said to be relatively rare in recipients of solid organ allografts. However, data suggest that an increasing percentage of patients have multisystem disease that follows a fulminant clinical course (76,90–92). Recipients of bone marrow transplants are at particular risk of developing disseminated disease (18). Such patients usually develop PTLD within the early post-transplant period and have recently received antilymphocyte antibody preparations for the treatment of GVHD. They present with widespread lymphoproliferation and multiorgan failure complicated by concomitant viral infections or systemic sepsis. The CNS is frequently involved with the lymphoproliferative process. Polyclonal and monoclonal disease have a similarly poor prognosis. In contrast to that seen in solid organ transplantation, proliferating cells are frequently of donor origin. In a series of 12 cases tested, the lymphoproliferative lesion was of host origin in two cases and donor origin in ten cases (57). Presumably, this aggressive form of PTLD is a reflection of the greater global immunosuppression produced by protocols used in the setting of less optimally matched marrow donors. The resulting delay in reconstitution of the T-cell immune response constitutes a period of high risk for uncontrolled EBV-driven lymphoproliferation. If engraftment is delayed and disease is disseminated, approximately 90% of such patients succumb despite aggressive management (107b). Even if disease is localized, mortality approaches 30%.

Patients may also present with PTLD several years after transplantation. These patients tend to be older and are more likely to develop mass lesions in the CNS, head and neck, or bowel. Disease is primarily extranodal and the pathology is more typical of that of a large cell or immunoblastic non-Hodgkin's lymphoma. Evidence of active EBV infection is usually absent, although sensitive studies of expression of viral proteins, EBER RNA or EBV genome have not often been done in this setting. In this group, there is less evidence that differences in maintenance immunosuppression or prior use of antilymphocyte antibody therapy identify patients at particular risk. Although their course may not be as fulminant, the disease is fatal in more than 70% of patients. It is unusual for these tumors to respond to a reduction in immunosuppression or antiviral agents. However, traditional chemotherapeutic approaches may induce complete remissions in selected patients.

Recently, it has been appreciated that PTLD may rarely present as a plasma cell dyscrasia with extramedullary plasmacytomas and a circulating paraprotein (108). It should be noted that the presence of a monoclonal paraprotein does not necessarily indicate a plasma cell dyscrasia. Immunosuppressed patients have been reported to have a 30% incidence of monoclonal gammopathy of uncertain significance. Although the extramedullary plasmacytomas may resolve with a reduction in immunosuppression alone or in combination with radiotherapy, the development of clinical multiple myeloma is best managed with chemotherapy.

OTHER EBV CLINICAL SYNDROMES

An increase in EBV viral load is an inevitable consequence of both solid organ and bone marrow transplantation. However, other than PTLD, clinical syndromes associated with this increased viral load have not been definitively identified. It has been our impression that a large number of lymphoproliferative processes related to EBV infection and immunosuppression after solid organ transplantation are subclinical. Patients may present with a nonspecific viral syndrome of fever and leukopenia. This may be interpreted as clinical evidence of a CMV infection and managed with a reduction in immunosuppression and antiviral therapy. As resolution in limited forms of PTLD after solid organ transplantation usually occurs with this therapeutic strategy, the association of these syndromes with EBV may remain unrecognized.

In the setting of bone marrow transplantation, case reports of fatal aplastic anemia (109) and meningoencephalitis (110) attributed to EBV infection have been described. Oral hairy leukoplakia, a nonmalignant lesion of the lateral borders of the tongue, is uncommon after solid organ transplantation. However, spontaneously reversible hairy leukoplakia has been reported in patients early after bone marrow transplantation (111). In a series of 10 patients reported by Epstein and colleagues, three lesions were positive for EBV genome by *in situ* hybridization. It is unclear whether EBV infection of the epithelial cells is pathogenic or simply an epiphenomenon.

EBV is also believed to play a pathophysiologic role in the development of smooth-muscle tumors reported in children after solid organ transplantation (112). It is not clear whether other EBV-associated malignancies such as Hodgkin's disease (113,114) and Burkitt's lymphoma (115) occur more frequently in transplant recipients than in immunocompetent patients. Although the role of EBV is firmly established in the development of B cell lymphoproliferative disease, there is increasing recognition that EBV may also be pathogenic in a subset of T cell lymphomas occurring after solid organ transplantation (116–118,121). EBV may infect T cells; the presence of EBV episomal monoclonality suggests that this is not simply due to bystander infection (119,120). T cell lymphomas currently account for 14% of post-transplant lymphomas (76). They tend to occur late after transplant with a mean time to presentation of more than 10 years.

The lesions are frequently in extra-nodal sites, including the spleen, liver, and gastrointestinal tract. Bone marrow involvement with a leukoerythroblastic blood picture is frequent at the time of presentation. The allograft is rarely affected. The lesions are usually monoclonal as demonstrated by the presence of clonal T cell receptor gene rearrangements. Immunophenotyping reveals positivity for CD2, CD3 and CD8 with variable expression of other T cell markers. Disease is often aggressive and refractory to therapy; those that survive often have only limited disease.

Although EBV-associated PTLD is a known complication of bone marrow transplantation, this therapy has been used to successfully treat patients with X-linked lymphoproliferative disease, an inherited lack of immune response of EBV, even during fulminant infection (122). This approach has also been advocated for the management of severe EBV-associated hemophagocytic syndrome, a multisystem disease arising from active EBV infection of T cells in young children or as a complication of EBV-associated T cell lymphoma in adults (123).

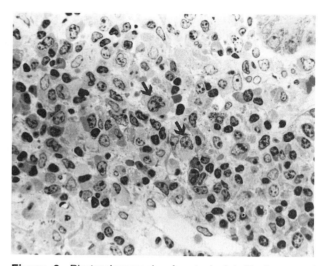

Figure 3. Photomicrograph of a typical infiltrate seen in PTLD. Representative sections from a case of PTLD involving the renal allograft. The expansile interstitial infiltrate is polymorphic, containing a large number of plasmacytoid cells and atypical immunoblasts (*arrows*) (×700).

DIAGNOSIS

The diagnosis of PTLD relies on the presence of an abnormal lymphoid proliferation that may be either polymorphic or monomorphic in nature. Biopsy material is essential, although cytologic analysis of urine, bronchoalveolar washings, or cerebrospinal fluid can support the diagnosis of PTLD (123b). The appearance of PTLD in various organs has been recently reviewed (101,104, 124,125). The lesions characteristically contain B cells in all stages of maturation, resulting in an extremely polymorphic appearance (Fig. 3). Varying proportions of small lymphocytes, small and large cleaved and non-cleaved cells, immunoblasts, plasmacytoid cells, and mature plasma cells may be found. Plasmacytoid features include an eccentric round or oval nucleus with peripheralization of chromatin. Atypical immunoblasts appear as large mononuclear cells with abundant eosinophilic cytoplasm and irregular nuclei that may be bi- or multilobed, and contain vesicular chromatin and prominent central nucleoli. Particular attention should be paid to the degree of pleomorphism of the infiltrating cells, the extent of plasmacytic differentiation, and the presence of atypical immunoblasts, as these features often permit one to distinguish PTLD from acute rejection in the SOT setting.

Attempts have been made to define the "malignant" nature of PTLD by assessing its clonality (monoclonal vs. oligoclonal vs. polyclonal). A variety of parameters have been studied, including cellular morphology, histologic immunophenotyping, expression of virally determined markers, presence of immunoglobulin gene rearrangements, and cytogenetic analysis. In 1984, Cleary and colleagues pointed out a potential sampling

error in assessing the clonality of PTLD (126). Patients presenting with multicentric disease frequently have lesions with quite different histologic appearance in separate locations. In addition, analysis of tissues from several sites or at various times in patients developing PTLD may reveal different clonal immunoglobulin gene rearrangements and contain different clonal EBV infections (38). Thus sampling at any single site in a patient may not accurately reflect the systemic clonality of the lesion. Determining the cellular origin as B cell, T cell, or null cell may be improtant in considering therapy or prognosis.

A systematic approach to the pathology of PTLD was reported by Frizzera (127) and subsequently modified by Nalesnik (52). They recognized that the lesions represent a continuum of disease (Table 2) (reviewed in reference 128). At one end of the spectrum are lesions usually arising in the oropharynx or lymph nodes that are consistent with a benign plasmacytic hyperplasia similar to that seen in infectious mononucleosis. Underlying architecture of the lymph node or tissue is preserved. These are almost always polyclonal, contain evidence for multiple EBV infection events, and lack oncogene or tumor suppressor gene alterations (129). They tend to develop shortly after transplant and regression is common, with a reduction in immunosuppression. At the other end of the spectrum are tumor masses with features consistent with true monoclonal non-Hodgkin's lymphoma. These lesions appear monomorphic (monomorphic PTLD) with little or no differentiation to mature plasma cells and are indistinguishable from those found in a nontransplant non-Hodgkin's lymphoma. They have been designated as immunoblastic lymphomas in Frizzera's classification. These lesions usually contain an overwhelming monoclonal population

TABLE 2. *Classification of the histologic lesions found in PTLD*

Category		Plasmacytic differentiation	Immunoblasts	Cytologic atypia	Necrosis	Clonality	Activation of oncognes/ tumor suppressor genes
Polymorphic I	Plasmacytic hyperplasia	++	+/++	–	–	Polyclonal	No
II	Polymorphic B cell hyperplasia	++	++/+++	–	–	Usually Monoclonal	No
	Polymorphic B cell lymphoma	+	++/+++	+/+++	+++	Monoclonal	No
Monomorphic III	Immunoblastic lymphoma	+	+++	+/+++	+	Monoclonal	Yes
IV	Multiple myeloma	+	–	+++	+	Monoclonal	Yes

Adapted from references 52, 127, and 129.

of small or large noncleaved lymphocytes, are infected with one form of EBV, and frequently have cytogenetic abnormalities resulting in activation of one or more proto-oncogenes (*c-myc*, N-*ras*) or mutations involving the p53 tumor suppressor gene, *bcl-2* or *bcl-6* (128–133). The presence of cytogenetic abnormalities may identify lesions that are likely to progress despite a reduction of immunosuppression and should be considered for chemotherapy.

Unfortunately, the malignant potential of lesions intermediate to these two forms is frequently difficult to determine. Morphological features suggesting a clonal malignancy (cellular atypia, necrosis, and obliteration of the underlying architecture) can exist despite the polymorphous nature of the infiltrating cell population. Initially, this dilemma was resolved by designating this lesion a polymorphic B-cell lymphoma. Lesions with a similar degree of polymorphism but exhibiting marked plasmacytoid differentiation and relatively little necrosis or cellular atypia were designated as polymorphic B-cell hyperplasia.

Unfortunately, the predictive value of the presence of the classic pathological features of malignancy—namely, cellular atypia, necrosis, and invasiveness—has not been substantiated in the clinical setting. Even nonimmunosuppressed patients with acute infectious mononucleosis may have lymph node biopsies that reveal atypical immunoblasts, necrosis, distortion of the normal architecture, and Reed Sternberg cells, features that could suggest a clonal malignancy (134,135). The distinction between polymorphic hyperplasia and polymorphic lymphoma has proved artificial; it fails to predict either the clinical course or response to a reduction in immunosuppressive therapy or antiviral therapy. Both lesions frequently have monoclonal or oligoclonal components, contain a single form of EBV, and do not have oncogene or tumor suppressor gene alterations. Thus it has been

suggested that these terms be avoided and that these lesions be combined under the designation of polymorphic PTLD (52,128,129). The clinical course of these patients is variable and cannot be predicted at diagnosis. Most patients should be allowed a short trial of reduced immunosuppression before initiating cheomotherapy or radiation.

Disease in all patients should be viewed as potentially curable. It may be more appropriate to think of early PTLD as an infectious complication rather than as a malignant process. Differentiating between these two possibilities is important, not only to understand the pathogenesis of PTLD, but also to determine whether optimal therapy in patients should include antiviral agents or the use of cytotoxic therapy.

TREATMENT OF PTLD

Regimens for the management of patients with PTLD have often been based on clinical outcomes described in case reports or limited series of patients. No controlled trials of therapeutic intervention have been performed. Furthermore, spontaneous regression of PTLD after solid organ transplantation occurs in many patients following a reduction in immunosuppression. As most patients receive other therapy concomitant with a reduction in immunosuppression, it is difficult to evaluate the true efficacy of these therapeutic approaches. Agreement regarding standardized therapeutic protocols that can be tested in a multicenter controlled trial format would be an important first step to improving the therapeutic approach to PTLD.

The following discussion will focus largely on the management of early EBV-associated PTLD, which usually occurs within the first six months following transplantation (Table 3). These strategies may have limited application in the setting of PTLD occurring after the first posttransplant year.

TABLE 3. *Options for the treatment of PTLD*

Reduction of immunosuppression
Surgical resection/local irradiation
Adoptive immunotherapy
Passive antibody (IVIG)
Alpha-interferon
Monoclonal B cell antibody therapy (CD21 and CD24)
Antiviral agents (acyclovir, ganciclovir)
Cytotoxic chemotherapy

In 1984, Starzl and colleagues first reported that a reduction of immunosuppression led to complete regression of PTLD after solid organ transplantation in some cases (136); this has been confirmed by others (48,52,98). Thus the most important initial strategy in the management of early PTLD after solid organ transplantation is to reduce and even discontinue the immunosuppressive therapy. Although the risk of precipitating rejection by reducing immunosuppression is of particular concern in heart, lung, and liver transplant recipients, patients with PTLD are already profoundly immunosuppressed, as illustrated by the high frequency of opportunistic infections. It has been our experience that immunosuppression can be significantly reduced and even withdrawn for periods of weeks with a relatively low risk of rejection. In contrast, a reduction in immunosuppression is unlikely to have a significant impact on the course of disease that appears truly malignant, such as late-occurring cases of non-Hodgkin's lymphoma or multiple myeloma.

In some settings, reduction of immunosuppression is not possible. In recipients of T-cell-depleted donor bone marrow, the development of PTLD has been clearly linked to persistently low T-cell numbers (18). To facilitate the restoration of EBV-specific cytotoxic T-cell responses, adoptive transfer of T-cell immunity has been used to treat these patients. Papadopoulos and colleagues initially described dramatic responses to infusions of unfractionated donor leukocytes in patients with PTLD, although their subsequent course was complicated by the development of GVHD (137). A refinement of this approach includes the infusion of polyclonal EBV-specific CTL cell lines prepared from donor leukocytes (138). This approach has been shown to be safe and effective, with functional EBV-specific CTL responses persisting for as long as 18 months in the recipient (139). Although this represents an elegant example of specific reconstitution of the most significant immunologic defect contributing to the development of PTLD, this treatment is likely to be of limited value in solid organ transplantation, where PTLD lesions are usually of recipient origin (140). Preliminary data evaluating the use of autologous lymphokine-activated killer (LAK) cells for the treatment of refractory PTLD in solid organ transplantation has proven disappointing (141).

In many cases reduction of immunosuppression has been combined with surgical resection for tumor debulking or as management of local complications such as gastrointestinal hemorrhage or perforation (52). Local radiotherapy has also been used. The role of surgical intervention and radiotherapy in these cures is uncertain. Because CNS lesions tend to relapse or fail to regress despite remission of disease elsewhere (48,142), the CNS may be an immunologically privileged site. Special intervention, perhaps in the form of local radiotherapy, may be indicated when CNS involvement is documented. An alternative approach is suggested by a report that describes the successful treatment of CNS PTLD using intrathecal administration of an anti-B-cell antibody directed against the CD21 molecule (143).

It is not clear that a standard cytotoxic chemotherapeutic approach, as would be used in a truly "malignant" lymphoproliferative process, is ever indicated as the first-line therapy in the setting of early PTLD. Although responses to cytotoxic chemotherapy have been described, a significant number of patients succumb to septic complications (52,144,145). Prophylactic regimens for the prevention of *Pneumocystis carinii* pneumonia and gram-negative pathogens should be considered whenever this approach is attempted. Unfortunately, the relationship between clonality or cytogenetic abnormalities and prognosis is not clear enough at the present time to accurately select the subset of patients who may benefit from a chemotherapeutic approach. Its use is less controversial in the setting of monomorphic PTLD occurring late in the post-transplant course.

Hanto and colleagues were the first to suggest the potential efficacy of the antiviral acyclovir in the management of the early polyclonal phase of PTLD (37). Patients with PTLD who responded to ganciclovir therapy after an initial poor response to acyclovir have also been reported (146). Because CMV is an extremely common co-infection in transplant recipients and is a risk factor for PTLD, the use of ganciclovir therapy may be theoretically more effective than that of acyclovir. We have demonstrated that EBV shedding from the oropharynx is eliminated in transplant recipients receiving ganciclovir in doses used for the treatment of CMV infections; however, rapid rebound of EBV shedding occurs after therapy is withdrawn (22,48). Because both acyclovir and ganciclovir block EBV DNA replication by interfering with EBV-associated DNA polymerase, they are only effective in the lytic phase of EBV infection. Unfortunately, the importance of the replicative EBV infection in B cells in the oropharynx or peripheral blood in maintaining or expanding the EBV-transformed B-cell population in patients with PTLD is unknown. Of note, PTLD has developed in patients receiving both acyclovir and ganciclovir prophylaxis (147). Antiviral agents may be useful to prevent infection of resting B cells, thereby limiting the numbers of EBV-infected cells until control of B-cell proliferation by the host immune response is reestablished. Antiviral therapy may be less effective when the numbers of latently infected circulating or tissue-invasive B cells are already extremely high, as in the setting of profound immunosuppression.

Alpha interferon (IFN-α) has not only antiviral and antiproliferative actions but also an effect on the host immune response. Rapid resolution of PTLD with IFN-α has been reported in some patients who received mismatched T-cell-depleted bone marrow transplants or had underlying immunodeficiency states (59). A similar response was seen in a case report of a pediatric recipient of a double lung transplant (148). The authors were able to document a reduction in IL-4 and IL-10 mRNA levels in bronchoalveolar washings with the IFN-α therapy, leading them to speculate that the IFN-α led to a down-regulation of Th2 cytokines that could serve as growth factors for the proliferating B-cell population. Interferon therapy is associated with a theoretical risk of precipitating rejection because of its ability to up-regulate HLA expression in the allograft. Whether this has any clinical relevance in the setting of the profound immunosuppression present in patients with PTLD is uncertain.

Monoclonal antibodies directed against CD21 and CD24 expressed on B bells have also been used for the treatment of PTLD (142,149,150). However, many of these patients also received concomitant therapy with acyclovir, ganciclovir, or steroids in association with a reduction in immunosuppression. Nonetheless, regression of disease has occurred after treatment of patients who would normally be considered to have a poor prognosis, such as those developing PTLD in the setting of a bone marrow transplant. This suggests that these antibodies have some efficacy as a treatment modality. Failure of treatment associated with defective expression of both CD21 and CD24 on the surface of the proliferating B lymphoblasts has been reported (149). Unfortunately, these antibodies are no longer commercially available.

Successful retransplantation of kidney (151) and liver (152) has been reported, as have cardiac (22) allograft recipients who recovered from PTLD. It is reasonable to assume that patients in whom PTLD was clearly associated with primary EBV infection would be at significantly lower risk of recurrent EBV-associated PTLD, assuming they remained disease-free for a significant interval and an immune response to the initial EBV infection occurred. Retransplantation in patients who developed PTLD associated with a remote EBV infection is more problematic. They should probably be viewed as patients who obtain a greater immunosuppressive effect than average from standard protocols; aggressive immunosuppression should therefore be avoided.

STRATEGIES FOR THE PREVENTION OF PTLD

From this discussion it is apparent that maintaining a careful balance between sufficient immunosuppression to prevent rejection and overimmunosuppression resulting in PTLD is critical in solid organ transplantation. Aggressive immunosuppression should only be employed in the presence of biopsy-proven acute rejection. Because PTLD frequently presents with allograft dysfunction, it is important to make a pathological diagnosis of rejection using standardized criteria and to clearly distinguish early PTLD from rejection prior to the use of more potent antirejection therapy. Recognition of limited forms of PTLD permits intervention with a reduction in immunosuppression and institution of adjunctive therapy. This offers the best opportunity to prevent dissemination or progression of early disease to an unresponsive state. (Table 4).

If uncontrolled EBV-induced lymphoproliferation is central to the pathogenesis of most cases of PTLD, it is important to determine which immunosuppressive drugs have the greatest impact on EBV activity. Our studies suggest that the timing of rejection therapy, particularly antilymphocyte antibodies, after solid organ transplantation may be important in permitting PTLD. If steroid-resistant rejection occurs, it is frequently between 4 and 12 weeks following transplant. Over the same interval, EBV viral load in the blood (24–26,147) and oropharyngeal shedding increase in both EBV-seropositive patients and those experiencing primary infection (22). Thus the most potent immunosuppression may be administered at a time when the immune system is required to control virally driven lymphoproliferation. The risk/benefit ratio associated with the use of second or prolonged courses of antilymphocyte antibodies in the first 3 post-transplant months should therefore be carefully assessed in each patient.

Reconstitution of the EBV-specific cytotoxic T-cell responses by infusion of cloned donor T-cell lines has been used prophylactically for the prevention of PTLD in the setting of high-risk BMT recipients receiving T-cell-depleted bone marrow (138). Preliminary observations are promising, but the efficacy of this approach requires

TABLE 4. *Options for the prevention of PTLD*

Differentiate early PTLD from rejection in the setting of allograft dysfunction after solid organ transplantation
EBV viral load surveillance in peripheral blood and allograft biopsies
Prophylactic adoptive immunotherapy (cloned T-cell lines)
Identify the patient at risk (primary EBV infection, primary CMV infection, prolonged or repetitive courses of ALG after solid organ transplantation, non-HLA identical, T-cell-depleted bone marrow transplant recipients)
Prophylactic antiviral drugs +/– passive antibody
Vaccine

further validation. This approach would be less applicable in the setting of solid organ transplantation. In the patient who is EBV seropositive before transplant, the low incidence of PTLD would make it costly and impractical to routinely produce cloned T-cell lines from pretransplant blood for use as prophylaxis. In the patient group at greatest risk, those experiencing primary infection, this approach using current protocols for cytotoxic T-cell cloning is not possible. The use of autologous dendritic cells genetically modified to express EBV antigens may overcome this problem (166).

An important strategy for the prevention of PTLD is to identify high risk patients prior to transplantation. Although patients who are EBV seronegative before transplant represent a small group of patients in adult SOT programs, these patients are at particularly high risk of developing PTLD. Identification of patients who are also at risk of primary CMV infection would select a particularly vulnerable subgroup of recipients. Such patients should be monitored carefully for evidence of EBV infection including careful review of their allograft biopsies for evidence of early PTLD. If seroconversion or EBV activity is documented in the oropharynx or peripheral blood of these patients, the use of antilymphocyte antibodies for rejection therapy should be avoided if possible and, if they are necessary, consideration should be given to preemptive antiviral therapy. EBV seronegative patients also represent a particularly important subgroup for the study of the potential efficacy of antiviral and vaccine prophylaxis for the prevention of EBV infection. In the setting of bone marrow transplantation the patient receiving a T-cell-depleted non-HLA-identical or mismatched bone marrow has been clearly at highest risk of PTLD development.

Both acyclovir and ganciclovir may be of benefit as prophylactic antiviral agents for the prevention of PTLD (153,154). By limiting recruitment of newly infected B cell clones or reducing the impact of other viruses on EBV-driven lymphoproliferation, prophylaxis initiated at the time of transplantation might be more efficacious than adding antiviral agents at the time of rejection therapy, when levels of shedding and the number of EBV-transformed B cells may already be high. Antiviral drugs which could be administered orally and achieve serum levels that would block EBV replication would be preferable to existing agents for prophylactic use. The role of prophylactically administered neurtralizing antibodies to EBV has also not been fully explored although preliminary results in the SCID mouse model of PTLD are promising (155). Efficacy of this approach appears to be related to the titer of EBV-specific antibodies rather than the immunomodulatory effects of intravenous immunoglobulin.

Research in vaccine development has recently focused on strategies that would impact EBV-associated disorders such as PTLD, Burkitt's lymphoma, and nasopharyngeal carcinoma. Of particular interest is work aimed at the generation of a cytotoxic T-cell response by using formulations of synthetic EBV peptides derived from certain latent EBV antigens (e.g., EBNA-3) that mimic immunodominant epitopes recognized by EBV-induced cytotoxic T cells *in vivo* (14). This strategy would specifically aim at generating an immune response targeting latently infected B cells. If administered before transplant to the EBV seronegative individual, it may not protect against the acquisition of EBV infection; instead it could circumvent the need for an intact T-cell response to generate cellular immunity to EBV during the early post-transplant period. This type of vaccine approach has yet to enter clinical trials.

It may also be possible to standardize techniques to quantify and prospectively monitor EBV activity and determine "safe" levels in transplant recipients. In general, serological responses to EBV are not useful predictors of PTLD, although the observation of Riddler and colleagues (24) that poor anti-EBNA serological responses may identify patients at risk of PTLD is interesting. Several alternative laboratory surveillance methods have been examined in SOT recipients, including monitoring of soluble CD23 in plasma (156), quantifying $CD19^+$ cells by flow cytometry (157), and quantifying EBV-infected cells in peripheral blood by immunohistochemistry (158). In children receiving non-HLA-identical bone marrow transplants, it has been suggested that T-cell numbers below $50/\mu l$ of peripheral blood at 1 month and $100/\mu l$ at 2 months following transplant were associated with an increased risk of PTLD (18). Attempts to determine EBV viral load have also been made, both in oropharyngeal secretions by dot-blot hybridization (22) and in peripheral blood using PCR technology (24–27,147,159). The measurement of EBV viral load in peripheral blood appears to be the most promising of these techniques. Several groups have demonstrated that a high EBV load can be detected prior to the development of clinical PTLD. In a BMT population, Rooney and colleagues (159) found a correlation between EBV viral load of more than 20,000 EBV genome copies/μg of DNA extracted from peripheral blood mononuclear cells and the development of PTLD. Riddler and colleagues (24) have suggested that SOT recipients who exhibit greater than 500 genome equivalents per 10^5 PBLs be considered at increased risk for PTLD. In a group of 26 pediatric recipients of solid organ allografts, Rowe and colleagues used quantitative competetive PCR to assess viral load in PBLs. Using a value of more than 200 EBV genomes/10^5 PBLs as a positive test predictive of PTLD, they found that the assay had a sensitivity and specificity of 92.8% and 100%, respectively. In contrast, 10 healthy seropositive individuals had 0.1–2 copies/10^5 PBLs. There is a need to standardize these surveillance methods and validate the level at which EBV viral load is predictive of PTLD in multicenter trials. This may permit a targeted preemptive approach to intervention. The potential efficacy of this approach is illustrated by preliminary data from Green and colleagues, who preemptively administered ganciclovir and immunoglobulin to pediatric intestinal transplant recipients when their EBV viral load exceeded 500 genome equivalents/10^5 PBLs (160). This laboratory technique is also an important tool for monitoring the response to therapeutic intervention in patients with high EBV viral load.

Because PTLD frequently affects the allografted organ, an alternative approach might consist of identifying and quantifying EBV-transformed B cells in transplant biopsies performed for any reason. Using *in situ* hybridization directed at EBER-1 RNA, which is present in high copy number in latently infected B cells, EBER-positive cells have been found in transplant biopsies from liver allograft recipients prior to the development of PTLD (161). Although small numbers of these cells have also been described in non-PTLD inflammatory diseases of the liver (162), the presence of significant or increasing numbers of EBER-positive cells may be useful for identifying patients at risk for PTLD. Further prospective studies to evaluate this conclusion and determine safe levels of EBER-positive cells are warranted.

POTENTIAL FUTURE TREATMENT OPTIONS

Over the past decade there has been a significant increase in our understanding of mechanisms underlying EBV latency and B-cell transformation. In the past, antiviral drug therapy has targeted the replicative phase of EBV infection. Because the proliferation of latently infected B cells is instrumental in the pathogenesis of EBV, antiviral therapy targeting latent infection is likely to be more effective. A clinical trial evaluating the efficacy of hydoxyurea for disruption of viral latency is underway (162b). Alternatively, strategies to disrupt the expression of essential viral proteins may be developed. The potential clinical use of an EBNA-1 antisense oligodeoxynucleotide that has demonstrated efficacy in inhibiting maintenance replication of the EBV genome *in vitro* is being evaluated (163). The recent report of the crystal structure of the EBNA-1 DNA-binding site may allow the design of antiviral drugs that disrupt this binding and clear viral episomes (164).

Future strategies could also use immunomodulation, which exploits our understanding of the immune response to EBV infection in the immunocompromised host, including factors influencing the proliferation of EBV-infected B cells. Preliminary evidence from the murine model of EBV-induced lymphomagenesis suggest that anti-IL-6 antibodies may be effective in the prevention and treatment of PTLD (Durandy, personal communication). CD40, a cell surface antigen expressed on B cells, plays an important role in the expansion and differentiation of normal B cells. However, in EBV-transformed cells, signalling through CD40 exerts an inhibitory effect. In the SCID mouse model, CD40 stim-

ulation was found to prevent the development of lymphomas (165). This approach may be useful for the treatment or prevention of PTLD in transplant reipients.

SUMMARY

PTLD is one of the consequences of immunosuppression associated with organ and bone marrow transplantation. It results from the imbalance created when virally driven lymphoproliferation, usually restrained by EBV-specific cytotoxic T cells, proceeds unchecked in the presence of procedures and immunosuppressive agents that inhibit or ablate T-cell function. With the current multipronged approach to immunosuppression in solid organ transplantation and the increased use of non-HLA-identical bone marrow donors, PTLD appears to be occurring more frequently and earlier in the post-transplant course. In solid organ transplantation much of the disorder is probably subclinical, and there is a particular predilection to involve the allograft early in the course of disease. If limited forms of the disorder go unrecognized, widespread dissemination may occur, particularly in the setting of aggressive immunosuppression. For PTLD occurring in the early post-transplant period, the distinction between infection and malignancy is blurred. Thus all lesions should be viewed as potentially curable. In the setting of solid organ transplantation reduction in immunosuppression remains the mainstay of therapy, although antiviral agents and other adjunctive treatment may also be useful. For monoclonal lesions with evidence of activation of proto-oncogenes or alterations of tumor suppressor genes, a conventional chemotherapeutic approach may be warranted. In BMT recipients, adoptive immunotherapy using EBV-specific cloned cytotoxic T cells as prophylaxis and therapy for PTLD has produced the most consistently positive results.

The best strategy for the management of PTLD is prevention. Identification of patients at particular risk for the development of PTLD by virtue of their EBV status or immunosuppressive regimen is critical. The introduction of a new agent into an established protocol must always balance the advantages of greater immunosuppression, resulting in improved graft survival and the consequences of overimmunosuppression, namely, infection and malignancy. New techniques for monitoring EBV viral load or demonstrating evidence of virally driven lymphoproliferation in tissues hold promise but suffer from a lack of standardization. Resolving these difficulties would offer the opportunity to design rational programs for the prevention and treatment of this potentially fatal consequence of immunosuppression.

REFERENCES

1. Anagnostopoulos I, Hummel M. Epstein-Barr virus in tumours. *Histopathol* 1996;29:297–315.
2. Kieff E. Epstein-Barr virus and its replication. In: Fields BN, Howley

PM, Knipe DM, eds. *Fields Virology*, 3rd ed. Philadelphia: Lippincott-Raven; 1995:2343–2396.

3. Sixbey JW, Shirley P, Chesney PJ, Buntin D, Resnik L. Detection of a second widespread strain of Epstein-Barr virus. *Lancet* 1989;2: 761–765.

4. Kyaw-Tanner MT, Esmore D, Burrows SR, Benson EM, Sculley TB. Epstein-Barr virus-specific cytotoxic T cell response in cardiac transplant recipients. *Transplantation* 1994;57:1611–1617.

5. Gratama JW, Oosterveer MAP, Weimar W, Sintnicolaas K, Sizoo W, Bolhuis RL, Ernberg I. Detection of multiple "Ebnotypes" in individual Epstein-Barr virus carriers following lymphocyte transformation by virus derived from peripheral blood and oropharynx. *J Gen Virol* 1994;75(1):85–94.

6. Thorley-Lawson DA, Miyashita EM, Khan G. Epstein-Barr virus and the B cell: that's all it takes. *Trends Microbiol* 1996;4(5):204–208.

7. Niedobitek G, Agathanggelou A, Herbst H, Whitehead L, Wright DH, Young LS. Epstein-Barr virus infection in infectious mononucleosis: virus latency, replication and phenotype of EBV-infected cells. *J Pathol* 1997;182:151–159.

8. Anagnostopoulos I, Hummel M, Kreschel C, Stein H. Morphology, immunophenotype, and distribution of latently and/or productively Epstein-Barr virus-infected cells in acute infectious mononucleosis: implications for the interindividual infection route of Epstein-Barr virus. *Blood* 1995;85(3):744–750.

9. Rickinson AB. Epstein-Barr virus in action *in vivo. N Engl J Med* 1998;338:1461–1463.

10. Rickinson AB, Kieff E.; Fields BN, Howley PM, Knyse DM, eds. Epstein-Barr virus. *Fields Virology*, 3rd ed. Philadelphia: Lippincott-Raven; 1995:2397–2446.

11. Decker LL, Klaman LD, Thorley-Lawson DA. Detection of the latent form of Epstein-Barr virus DNA in the peripheral blood of healthy individuals. *J Virol* 1996;70(5):3286–3289.

12. Gratama JW, Oosterveer MAP, Zwaan FE, Lepoutre J, Klein G, Ernberg I. Eradication of Epstein-Barr virus by allogeneic bone marrow transplantation: implications for sites of viral latency. *Proc Natl Acad Sci USA* 1988;85:8693–8696.

13. Miyashita EM, Yang B, Babcock GJ, Thorley-Lawson DA. Identification of the site of Epstein-Barr virus persistence *in vivo* as a resting B cell. *J Virol* 1997;71(7):4882–4891.

14. Khanna R, Burrows SR, Moss DJ. Immune regulation in Epstein-Barr virus-associated diseases. *Microbiol Rev* 1995;59(3):387–405.

15. Rickinson AB, Lee SP, Steven NM. Cytotoxic T lymphocyte responses to Epstein-Barr virus. *Curr Opin Immunol* 1996;8:492–497.

16. Bourgault I, Gomez A, Gomard E, Levy JP. Limiting dilution analysis of the HLA restriction of anti-Epstein-Barr virus specific cytolytic T lymphocytes. *Clin Exp Immunol* 1991;84:501–507.

17. Lucas KG, Small TN, Heller G, Dupont B, O'Reilly RJ. The development of cellular immunity to Epstein-Barr virus after allogeneic bone marrow transplantation. *Blood* 1996;87(6):2594–2603.

18. Gerritsen EJA, Stam ED, Hermans J, et al. Risk factors for developing EBV-related B cell lymphoproliferative disorders (BLPD) after non-HLA-identical BMT in children. *Bone Marrow Transplant* 1996;18: 377–382.

19. Randhawa PS, Yousem SA. Epstein-Barr virus-associated lymphoproliferative disease in a heart-lung allograft. Demonstration of host origin by restriction fragment-length polymorphism analysis. *Transplantation* 1990;49:126–130.

20. Haque T, Thomas JA, Falk KI, et al. Transmission of donor Epstein-Barr virus (EBV) in transplanted organs causes lymphoproliferative disease in EBV-seronegative recipients. *J Gen Virol* 1996;77:1169–1172.

21. Alfieri C, Tanner J, Carpentier L, et al. Epstein-Barr virus transmission from a blood donor to an organ transplant recipient with recovery of the same virus strain from the recipient's blood and oropharynx. *Blood* 1996;87(2):812–817.

22. Preiksaitis J, Diaz-Mitoma F, Mirzayans F, Roberts S, Tyrrell DLJ. Quantitative oropharyngeal Epstein-Barr virus shedding in renal and cardiac transplant recipients: relationship to immunosuppressive therapy, serological responses and the risk of post-transplant lymphoproliferative disorder. *J Infect Dis* 1992;166:986–994.

23. Cen H, Breinig MC, Atchison RW, Ho M, McKnight JLC. Epstein-Barr virus transmission via the donor organs in solid organ transplantation: polymerase chain reaction and restriction fragment length polymorphism analysis of IR2, IR3, and IR4. *J Virol* 1991;65:976–980.

24. Riddler SA, Breinig MC, McKnight JLC. Increased levels of circulat-ing Epstein-Barr virus (EBV)-infected lymphocytes and decreased EBV nuclear antigen antibody responses are associated with the development of posttransplant lymphoproliferative disease in solid-organ transplant recipients. *Blood* 1994;84(3):972–984.

25. Savoie A, Perpete C, Carpentier L, Joncas J, Alfieri C. Direct correlation between the load of Epstein-Barr virus-infected lymphocytes in the peripheral blood of pediatric transplant patients and risk of lymphoproliferative disease. *Blood* 1994;83(9):2715–2722.

26. Crompton CH, Cheung RK, Donjon C, et al. Epstein-Barr virus surveillance after renal transplantation. *Transplantation* 1994;57(8): 1182–1189.

27. Rowe DT, Qu L, Reyes J, et al. Use of quantitative competitive PCR to measure Epstein-Barr virus genome load in the peripheral blood of pediatric transplant patients with lymphoproliferative disorders. *J Clin Microbiol* 1997;35(6):1612–1615.

28. Cen H, Williams PA, McWilliams HP, Breinig MC, Ho M, McKnight JLC. Evidence for restricted Epstein-Barr virus latent gene expression and anti-EBNA antibody response in solid organ transplant recipients with posttransplant lymphoproliferative disorders. *Blood* 1993;81: 1393–1403.

29. Mosier DE, Gulizia RJ, Baird SM, Wilson DB. Transfer of a functional human immune system to mice with severe combined immunodeficiency. *Nature* 1988;335:256–259.

30. Oudejans JJ, Jiwa M, van den Brule AJC, et al. Detection of heterogeneous Epstein-Barr virus gene expression patterns within individual post-transplantation lymphoproliferative disorders. *Am J Pathol* 1995; 147(4):923–933.

31. Rea D, Fourcade C, Leblond V, et al. Patterns of Epstein-Barr virus latent and replicative gene expression in Epstein-Barr virus B cell lymphoproliferative disorders after organ transplantation. *Transplantation* 1994;58(3):317–324.

32. Rochford R, Mosier DE. Differential Epstein-Barr virus gene expression in B-cell subsets recovered from lymphomas in SCID mice after transplantation of human peripheral blood lymphocytes. *J Virol* 1995; 69(1):150–155.

33. Baiocchi RA, Ross ME, Tan JC, et al. Lymphomagenesis in the SCID-hu mouse involves abundant production of human interleukin-10. *Blood* 1995;85(4):1063–1074.

34. Rowe M, Young LS, Crocker J, Stokes H, Henderson S, Rickinson AB. Epstein-Barr virus (EBV)-associated lymphoproliferative disease in the SCID mouse model: implications for the pathogenesis of EBV-positive lymphomas in man. *J Exp Med* 1991;173:147–158.

35. Katz BZ, Raab-Traub N, Miller G. Latent and replicating forms of Epstein-Barr virus DNA in lymphomas and lymphoproliferative diseases. *J Infect Dis* 1989;160:589–598.

36. Patton DF, Wilkowski CW, Hanson CA, et al. Epstein-Barr virus-determined clonality in posttransplant lymphoproliferative disease. *Transplantation* 1990;49:1080–1084.

37. Hanto DW, Frizzera G, Gajl-Peczalska KJ, et al. Epstein-Barr virus-induced B-cell lymphoma after renal transplantation. Acyclovir therapy and transition from polyclonal to monoclonal B-cell proliferation. *N Engl J Med* 1982;306:913–918.

38. Chadburn A, Cesarman E, Liu YF, et al. Molecular genetic analysis demonstrates that multiple posttransplant lymphoproliferative disorders occurring in one anatomic site in a single patient represent distinct primary lymphoid neoplasms. *Cancer* 1995;75(11) 2747–2756.

38b. Liebowitz D. Epstein-Barr virus and a cellular signaling pathway in lymphomas from immunosuppressed patients. *N Engl J Med* 1998;338: 1413–1421.

39. Berg LC, Copenhaver CM, Morrison VA, et al. B cell lymphoproliferative disorder in solid organ transplant patients: detection of EB virus by *in situ* hybridization. *Hum Pathol* 1992;23:159–163.

40. Ambinder RF, Mann RB. Detection and characterization of Epstein-Barr virus in clinical specimens. *Am J Pathol* 1994;145(2):239–252.

41. Ho M, Miller G, Atchison RW. Epstein-Barr virus infections and DNA hybridization studies in posttransplantation lymphoma and lymphoproliferative lesions: the role of primary infection. *J Infect Dis* 1985; 152:876–886.

42. Ho M, Jaffe R, Miller G, et al. The frequency of Epstein-Barr virus infection and associated lymphoproliferative syndrome after transplantation and its manifestations in children. *Transplantation* 1988;45:719–727.

43. Young L, Alfieri C, Hennessy K, et al. Expression of Epstein-Barr virus transformation-associated genes in tissues of patients with EBV lymphoproliferative disease. *N Engl J Med* 1989;321:1080–1085.

44. Delecluse H, Kremmer E, Rouault J, Cour C, Bornkamm G, Berger F. The expression of Epstein-Barr virus latent proteins is related to the pathological features of post-transplant lymphoproliferative disorders. *Am J Pathol* 1995;146(5):1113–1120.

45. Frank D, Cesarman E, Liu YF, Michler RE, Knowles DM. Posttransplantation lymphoproliferative disorders frequently contain type A and not type B Epstein-Barr virus. *Blood* 1995;85(5):1396–1403.

46. Knecht H, Bachmann E, Brousset P, et al. Mutational hot spots within the carboxy terminal region of the LMP1 oncogene of Epstein-Barr virus are frequent in lymphoproliferative disorders. *Oncogene* 1995;10:523–528.

47. Smir BN, Hauke RJ, Bierman PJ, et al. Molecular epidemiology of deletions and mutations of the latent membrane protein 1 oncogene of the Epstein-Barr virus in post-transplant lymphoproliferative disorders. *Lab Invest* 1996;75:575–588.

48. Cockfield SM, Preiksaitis JK, Jewell LD, Parfrey NA. Post-transplant lymphoproliferative disorder in renal allograft recipients: clinical experience and risk factor analysis in a single center. *Transplantation* 1993;56:88–96.

49. Renard TH, Andrews WS, Foster ME. Relationship between OKT3 administration, EBV seroconversion, and the lymphoproliferative syndrome in pediatric liver transplant recipients. *Transplant Proc* 1991;23:1473–1476.

50. Walker RC, Paya CV, Marshall WF, et al. Pretransplantation seronegative Epstein-Barr virus status is the primary risk factor for post-transplantation lymphoproliferative disorder in adult heart, lung, and other solid organ transplantations. *J Heart Lung Transplant* 1995;14:214–221.

51. Walker RC, Marshall WF, Strickler JG, et al. Pretransplantation assessment of the risk of lymphoproliferative disorder. *Clin Infect Dis* 1995;20:1346–1353.

52. Nalesnik MA, Jaffe R, Starzl TE, et al. The pathology of posttransplant lymphoproliferative disorders occurring in the setting of cyclosporine A-prednisone immunosuppression. *Am J Pathol* 1988; 133:173–192.

53. Randhawa P, Yousem SA, Paradis IL, et al. The clinical spectrum, pathology, and clonal analysis of Epstein-Barr virus-associated lymphoproliferative disorders in heart-lung transplant recipients. *Am J Clin Pathol* 1989;92:177–185.

54. Armitage JM, Kormos RL, Stuart RS, et al. Posttransplant lymphoproliferative disease in thoracic organ transplant patients: ten years of cyclosporine-based immunosuppression. *J Heart Lung Transplant* 1991;10:877–887.

55. Opelz G, Henderson R. Incidence of non-Hodgkin lymphoma in kidney and heart transplant recipients. *Lancet* 1993;342:1514–1516.

56. Reyes J, Green M, Rowe D, et al. Spectrum of Epstein Barr virus disease after intestinal transplantation in humans. International Congress of the Transplantation Society 1996; Abstract 21.

57. Zutter MM, Martin PJ, Sale GE, et al. Epstein-Barr virus lymphoproliferation after bone marrow transplantation. *Blood* 1988;72(2):520–529.

58. Witherspoon RP, Fisher LD, Schoch G, et al. Secondary cancers after bone marrow transplantation for leukemia or aplastic anemia. *N Engl J Med* 1989;321:784–789.

59. Shapiro RS, McClain K, Frizzera G, et al. Epstein-Barr virus associated B cell lymphoproliferative disorders following bone marrow transplantation. *Blood* 1988;71:1234–1243.

60. Weissmann DJ, Ferry JA, Harris NL, Louis DN, Delmonico F, Spiro I. Posttransplantation lymphoproliferative disorders in solid organ recipients are predominantly aggressive tumors of host origin. *Am J Clin Pathol* 1995;103(6):748–755.

61. Chadburn A, Suciu-Foca N, Cesarman E, Reed E, Michler RE, Knowles DM. Post-transplantation lymphoproliferative disorders arising in solid organ transplant recipients are usually of recipient origin. *Am J Pathol* 1995;147(6):1862–1870.

62. Wakasugi H, Rimsky L, Mahe Y, et al. Epstein-Barr virus-containing B-cell line produces an interleukin 1 that it uses as a growth factor. *Proc Natl Acad Sci USA* 1987;84:804–808.

63. Tosato G, Tanner J, Jones KD, Revel M, Pike SE. Identification of interleukin-6 as an autocrine growth factor for Epstein-Barr virus-immortalized B cells. *J Virol* 1990;64:3033–3041.

64. Yokoi T, Miyawaki T, Yachie A, Kato K, Kasahara Y, Taniguchi N. Epstein-Barr virus-immortalized B cells produce IL-6 as an autocrine growth factor. *Immunology* 1990;70:100–105.

65. Estrov Z, Kurzrock R, Pocski E, et al. Lymphotoxin is an autocrine growth factor for Epstein-Barr virus-infected B cell lines. *J Exp Med* 1993;177:763–774.

66. Randhawa PS, Demetris AJ, Nalesnik MA. The potential role of cytokines in the pathogenesis of Epstein-Barr virus associated post-transplant lymphoproliferative disorder. *Leuk Lymphoma* 1994;15: 383–387.

67. Tosato G, Jones K, Breinig MK, McWilliams HP, McKnight JLC. Interleukin-6 production in posttransplant lymphoproliferative disease. *J Clin Invest* 1993;91:2806–2814.

68. Beatty PR, Krams SM, Esquivel CO, Martinez OM. Effect of cyclosporine and tacrolimus on the growth of Epstein-Barr virus-transformed B-cell lines. *Transplantation* 1998;65:1248–1255.

69. Bird AG, McLachlan SM, Britton S. Cyclosporin A promotes spontaneous outgrowth *in vitro* of Epstein-Barr virus-induced B-cell lines. *Nature* 1981;289:300–301.

70. Burman K, Crawford DH. Effect of FK506 on Epstein-Barr virus specific cytotoxic T cells. *Lancet* 1991;337:297–298.

71. Crawford DH, Edwards JMB, Sweny P, Hoffbrand AV, Janossy G. Studies on long-term T-cell-mediated immunity to Epstein-Barr virus in immunosuppressed renal allograft recipients. *Int J Cancer* 1981;28: 705–709.

72. Walz G, Zanker B, Melton LB, Suthanthiran M, Strom TB. Possible association of the immunosuppressive and B cell lymphoma-promoting properties of cyclosporine. *Transplantation* 1990;49:191–194.

73. Hornung N, Degiannis D. Up-regulation by cyclosporine (CsA) of the *in vitro* release of soluble CD23 (sCD23) and of the *in vitro* production of IL-6 and IgM. *Scand J Immunol* 1993;38:287–292.

74. Calne RY, Rolles S, Thiru S, et al. Cyclosporin A initially as the only immunosuppressant in 34 recipients of cadaveric organs: 32 kidneys, 2 pancreases, and 2 livers. *Lancet* 1979;2:1033–1036.

75. Bieber CP, Heberling RL, Jamieson SW, et al. Lymphoma in cardiac transplant recipients associated with cyclosporin A, prednisone and anti-thymocyte globulin (ATG). In: Purtillo DI, ed. *Immune deficiency and cancer.* New York: Plenum; 1984:309–320.

76. Penn I. The changing pattern of posttransplant malignancies. *Transplant Proc* 1991;23:1101–1103.

77. Cox KL, Lawrence-Miyasaki LS, Garcia-Kennedy R, et al. An increased incidence of Epstein-Barr virus infection and lymphoproliferative disorder in young children on FK506 after liver transplantation. *Transplantation* 1995;59(4):524–529.

78. Reding R, Wallemacq PE, Lamy ME, et al. Conversion from cyclosporine to FK506 for salvage of immunocompromised pediatric liver allografts. *Transplantation* 1994;57(1):93–100.

79. Scantlebury VP, Shapiro R, Tzakis A, et al. Pediatric kidney transplantation at the University of Pittsburgh. *Transplant Proc* 1994;26 (1):46–47.

80. Ellis D. Clinical use of tacrolimus (FK506) in infants and children with renal transplants. *Pediatric Nephrol* 1995;9:487–494.

81. Wilkinson AH, Smith JL, Hunsicker LG, et al. Increased frequency of posttransplant lymphomas in patients treated with cyclosporine, azathioprine, and prednisone. *Transplantation* 1989;47:293–296.

82. Lopatin WB, Hickey DP, Nalesnik MA, et al. Post-transplant lymphoproliferative disease and triple therapy. *Clin Transplant* 1990;4:47–50.

83. Stephanian E, Gruber SA, Dunn DL, Matas AJ. Posttransplant lymphoproliferative disorders. *Transplant Reviews* 1991;5:120–129.

84. Sollinger HW. Mycophenolate mofetil for the prevention of acute rejection in primary cadaveric renal allograft recipients. *Transplantation* 1995;60(3):225–232.

85. European Mycophenolate Mofetil Cooperative Study Group. Placebo-controlled study of mycophenolate mofetil combined with cyclosporin and corticosteroids for prevention of acute rejection. *Lancet* 1995; 345:1321–1325.

86. The Tricontinental Mycophenolate Mofetil Renal Transplantation Study Group. A blinded, randomized clinical trial of mycophenolate mofetil for the prevention of acute rejection in cadaveric renal transplantation. *Transplantation* 1996;61(7):1029–1037.

87. Touraine JL, Bosi E, El Yafi MS, et al. The infectious lymphoproliferative syndrome in transplant patients under immunosuppressive treatment. *Transplant Proc* 1985;17:96–98.

88. Iwatsuki S, Geis WP, Molnar Z, Giacchino JL, Ing TS, Hano JE. Systemic lymphoblastic response to antithymocyte globulin in renal allograft recipients: an initial report. *J Surg Res* 1978;24:428–434.

89. Brumbaugh J, Baldwin JC, Stinson EB. Quantitative analysis of immunosuppression in cyclosporine treated heart transplant patients with lymphoma. *Heart Transplant* 1985;4:307–311.

90. Canfield CW, Hudnall SD, Colonna JO, et al. Fulminant Epstein-Barr

virus–associated post-transplant lymphoproliferative disorders following OKT3 therapy. *Clin Transplant* 1992;6:1–9.

91. Cockfield SM, Preiksaitis J, Harvey E, et al. Is sequential use of ALG and OKT3 in renal transplants associated with an increased incidence of fulminant post-transplant lymphoproliferative disorder? *Transplant Proc* 1991;23:1106–1107.

92. Swinnen LJ, Costanzo-Nordin MR, Fisher SG, et al. Increased incidence of lymphoproliferative disorder after immunosuppression with the monoclonal antibody OKT3 in cardiac-transplant recipients. *N Engl J Med* 1990;323:1723–1728.

93. Tsoukas CD, Carson DA, Fong S, Vaughan JH. Molecular interactions in human T cell-mediated cytotoxicity to EBV. II. Monoclonal antibody OKT3 inhibits a post-killer-target recognition/adhesion step. *J Immunol* 1982;129:1421–1425.

94. Ren EC, Chan SH. Possible enhancement of Epstein-Barr virus infections by the use of OKT3 in transplant recipients. *Transplantation* 1988;45:988–989.

95. Swinnen LJ, Fisher RI. OKT3 monoclonal antibodies induce interleukin-6 and interleukin-10: possible cause of lymphoproliferative disorders associated with transplantation. *Curr Opin Nephrol Hyperten* 1993;2:670–678.

95b. Manez R, Breinig MC, Linden P, et al. Posttransplant lymphoproliferative disease in primary Epstein-Barr virus infection after liver transplantation: the role of CMV disease. *J Infect Dis* 1997;176:1462–1467.

96. Rand KH, Pollard RB, Merigan TC. Increased pulmonary superinfections in cardiac transplant patients undergoing primary cytomegalovirus infection. *N Engl J Med* 1978;298:951–953.

97. Grundy JE. Virologic and pathogenetic aspects of cytomegalovirus infection. *Rev Infect Dis* 1990;12:[Suppl 7]:S711–S719.

98. Hanto DW, Frizzera G, Gajl-Peczalska KJ, Simmons RL. Epstein-Barr virus, immunodeficiency, and B cell lymphoproliferation. *Transplantation* 1985;39:461–472.

99. Garnier JL, Berger F, Betuel H, et al. Epstein-Barr virus associated lymphoproliferative diseases (B cell lymphoma) after transplantation. *Nephrol Dial Transplant* 1989;4:818–823.

100. Nalesnik MA, Starzl TE. Epstein-Barr virus, infectious mononucleosis, and post-transplant lymphoproliferative disorders. *Transplant Sci* 1994;4(1):61–79.

101. Randhawa PS, Magnone M, Jordan M, Shapiro R, Demetris AJ, Nalesnik MA. Renal allograft involvement by Epstein-Barr virus associated post-transplant lymphoproliferative disease. *Am J Surg Pathol* 1996;20(5):563–571.

102. Houle AM, McLorie GA, Churchill BM, Khoury AE, Harvey E, Hebert D. Rapid development of an immunoblastic lymphoma and death in children following cadaveric renal transplantation. *J Pediatr Surg* 1992;27:626–628.

103. Hanasono MM, Kamel OW, Chang PP, Riseq MN, Billingham ME, van de Rijn M. Detection of Epstein-Barr virus in cardiac biopsies of heart transplant patients with lymphoproliferative disorders. *Transplantation* 1995;60(5):471–473.

104. Rosendale B, Yousem SA. Discrimination of Epstein-Barr virus-related posttransplant lymphoproliferations from acute rejection in lung allograft recipients. *Arch Pathol Lab Med* 1995;119:418–423.

105. Penn I, Porat G. Central nervous system lymphomas in organ allograft recipients. *Transplantation* 1995;59(2):240–244.

106. Nalesnik MA, Makowka L, Starzl TE. The diagnosis and treatment of post-transplant lymphoproliferative disorders. *Curr Prob Surg* 1988;25:371.

107. Egan JJ, Hasleton PS, Yonan N, et al. Necrotic, ulcerative bronchitis, the presenting feature of lymphoproliferative disease following heart-lung transplantation. *Thorax* 1995;50:205–207.

107b. Orazi A, Hromas RA, Neiman RS, et al. Posttransplantation lymphoproliferative disorders in bone marrow transplant recipients are aggressive diseases with a high incidence of adverse histologic and immunobiologic features. *Am J Clin Pathol* 1997;107:419–429.

108. Joseph G, Barker RL, Yuan B, Martin A, Medeiros J, Peiper SC. Post-transplantation plasma cell dyscrasias. *Cancer* 1994;74(7):1959–1964.

109. Inoue H, Shinohara K, Nomiyama J, Oeda E. Fatal aplastic anemia caused by Epstein-Barr virus infection after autologous bone marrow transplantation for non-Hodgkin malignant lymphoma. *Intern Med* 1994;33(5):303–307.

110. Dellemijn PLI, Brandenburg A, Niesters HGM, van den Bent MJ, Rothbarth PH, Vlasveld LT. Successful treatment with ganciclovir of

111. presumed Epstein-Barr meningo-encephalitis following bone marrow transplant. *Bone Marrow Transplant* 1995;16:311–312.

111. Epstein JB, Sherlock CH, Wolber RA. Hairy leukoplakia after bone marrow transplantation. *Oral Surg Oral Med Oral Pathol* 1993;75:690–695.

112. Lee ES, Locker J, Nalesnik MA, et al. The association of Epstein-Barr virus with smooth muscle tumors occurring after organ transplantation. *N Engl J Med* 1995;332(1):19–25.

113. Garnier J-L, Lebranchu Y, Dantal J, et al. Hodgkin's disease after transplantation. *Transplantation* 1996;61(1):71–76.

114. Bierman PJ, Vose JM, Langnas AN, et al. Hodgkin's disease following solid organ transplantation. *Ann Oncol* 1996;7(3):265–270.

115. Hunt BJ, Thomas JA, Burke M, Walker H, Yacoub M, Crawford DH. Epstein-Barr virus associated Burkitt lymphoma in a heart transplant recipient. *Transplantation* 1996;62(6):869–872.

116. Hanson MN, Morrison VA, Peterson BA, et al. Posttransplant T-cell lymphoproliferative disorders—an aggressive, late complication of solid-organ transplantation. *Blood* 1996;9:3626–3633.

117. Leblond V, Sutton L, Dorent R, et al. Lymphoproliferative disorders after organ transplantation: a report of 24 cases observed in a single centre. *J Clin Oncol* 1995;13(4):961–968.

118. Macon WR, Williams ME, Greer JP, et al. Natural killer-like T-cell lymphomas: aggressive lymphomas of T-large granular lymphocytes. *Blood* 1996;87:1474–1483.

119. Su I-J, Hsieh H-C, Lin K-H, et al. Aggressive peripheral T-cell lymphomas containing Epstein-Barr vial DNAs: a clinicopathologic and molecular analysis. *Blood* 1991;77(4):799–808.

120. Kumar S, Kumar D, Kingma DW, Jaffe ES. Epstein-Barr virus-associated T-cell lymphoma in a renal transplant patient. *Am J Surg Pathol* 1993;17(10):1046–1053.

121. Van Gorp J, Doornewaard H, Verdonck LF, Klopping C, Vos PF, van den Tweel JG. Posttransplant T-cell lymphoma: a report of three cases and a review of the literature. *Cancer* 1994;73:3064–3072.

122. Pracher E, Grumayer-Panzer ER, Zoubek A, Peters C, Gadner H. Bone marrow transplantation during fulminant EBV-infection in Duncan's syndrome. *Lancet* 1993;342:1362.

123. Su IJ, Wang CH, Cheng AL, Chen RL. Hemophagocytic syndrome in Epstein-Barr virus-associated T-lymphoproliferative disorders: disease spectrum, pathogenesis, and management. *Leuk Lymphoma* 1995;19:401–406.

123b. Davey DD, Gulley ML, Walker WP, Zaleski S. Cytologic findings in posttransplant lymphoproliferative disease. *Acta Cytol* 1990;34:304–310.

124. Randhawa PS, Markin RS, Starzl TE, Demetris AJ. Epstein-Barr virus-associated syndromes in immunosuppressed liver transplant recipients. Clinical profile and recognition on routine allograft biopsy. *Am J Surg Pathol* 1990;14:538–547.

125. Markin RS, Wood RP, Shaw BWJ, Brichacek B, Purtilo DT. Immunohistologic identification of Epstein-Barr virus-induced hepatitis reactivation after OKT-3 therapy following orthotopic liver transplant. *Am J Gastroenterol* 1990;85:1014–1018.

126. Cleary ML, Sklar J. Lymphoproliferative disorders in cardiac transplant recipients are multiclonal lymphomas. *Lancet* 1984;2:489–93.

127. Frizzera G, Hanto DW, Gajl-Peczalska KJ, et al. Polymorphic diffuse B-cell hyperplasias and lymphomas in renal transplant recipients. *Cancer Res* 1981;41:4262–4269.

128. Chadburn A, Cesarman E, Knowles DM. Molecular pathology of post-transplant lymphoproliferative disorders. *Semin Diag Pathol* 1997;14(1):15–26.

129. Knowles DM, Cesarman E, Chadburn A, et al. Correlative morphologic and molecular genetic analysis demonstrates three distinct categories of posttransplantation lymphoproliferative disorders. *Blood* 1995;85(2):552–565.

130. Delecluse H, Rouault JP, Ffrench M, Dureau G, Magaud JP, Berger F. Post-transplant lymphoproliferative disorders with genetic abnormalities commonly found in malignant tumours. *Br J Hematol* 1995;89(1):90–97.

131. Delecluse H, Rouault J, Jeammot B, Kremmer E, Bastard C, Berger F. Bcl6/Laz3 rearrangements in post-transplant lymphoproliferative disorders. *Br J Hematol* 1995;91(1):101–103.

132. Seiden MV, Sklar J. Molecular genetic analysis of post-transplant lymphoproliferative disorders. *Hematol Oncol Clin North Am* 1993;7:447–465.

133. Gaulard P, d'Agay MF, Peuchmaur M, et al. Expression of the bcl-2

gene product in follicular lymphoma. *Am J Pathol* 1992;140(5): 1089–1095.

134. Gall EA, Stout HA. The histological lesion in lymph nodes in infectious mononucleosis. *Am J Pathol* 1940;16:4433–4481.

135. Tindle BH, Parker JW, Lukes RJ. "Reed-Sternberg cells" in infectious mononucleosis. *Am J Clin Pathol* 1972;58:607–617.

136. Starzl TE, Porter KA, Iwatsuki S, et al. Reversibility of lymphomas and lymphoproliferative lesions developing under cyclosporine-steroid therapy. *Lancet* 1984;1:583–587.

137. Papadopoulos EB, Ladanyi M, Emanuel D, et al. Infusions of donor leukocytes to treat Epstein-Barr virus-associated lymphoproliferative disorders after allogeneic bone marrow transplantation. *N Engl J Med* 1994;330(17):1185–1191.

138. Rooney CM, Smith CA, Ng CYC, et al. Use of gene-modified virus-specific T lymphocytes to control Epstein-Barr-virus-related lymphoproliferation. *Lancet* 1995;345(1):9–13.

139. Heslop HE, Ng CYC, Li C, et al. Long-term restoration of immunity against Epstein-Barr virus infection by adoptive transfer of gene-modified virus-specific T lymphocytes. *Nature Med* 1996;2(5):551–555.

140. Emanuel DJ, Lucas KG, Mallory GB, et al. Treatment of posttransplant lymphoproliferative disease in the central nervous system of a lung transplant recipient using allogeneic leukocytes. *Transplantation* 1997;63(11):1691–1694.

141. Minervini MI, Pavlick M, Zeevi A, et al. Cytotoxicity of LAK cell and EBV-specific T cells against lymphoblastoid EBV-positive B cells: a model for cellular therapy of PTLD. *Transplantation* 1998;65:5176.

142. Fischer A, Blanche S, LeBidois J, et al. Anti-B-cell monoclonal antibodies in the treatment of severe B-cell lymphoproliferative syndrome following bone marrow and organ transplantation. *N Engl J Med* 1991;324:1451–1456.

143. Stephan JL, Le Deist F, Blanche S, et al. Treatment of central nervous system B lymphoproliferative syndrome by local infusion of a B cell-specific monoclonal antibody. *Transplantation* 1992;54:246–249.

144. Garrett TJ, Chadburn A, Barr ML, et al. Posttransplantation lymphoproliferative disorders treated with cyclophosphamide-doxorubicin-vincristine-prednisone chemotherapy. *Cancer* 1993;72(9):2782–2785.

145. Swinnen LJ, Mullen GM, Carr TJ, Costanzo MR, Fisher RI. Aggressive treatment for post-cardiac transplant lymphoproliferation. *Blood* 1995;86(9):3333–3340.

146. Pirsch JD, Stratta RJ, Sollinger HW, et al. Treatment of severe Epstein-Barr virus-induced lymphoproliferative syndrome with ganciclovir: two cases after solid organ transplantation. *Am J Med* 1989;86:241–244.

147. Kenagy DN, Schlesinger Y, Weck K, Ritter JH, Gaudreault-Keener MM, Storch GA. Epstein-Barr virus DNA in peripheral blood leukocytes of patients with posttransplant lymphoproliferative disease. *Transplantation* 1995;60(6):547–554.

148. Faro A, Kurland G, Michaels MG, et al. Interferon-alpha affects the immune response in post-transplant lymphoproliferative disorder. *Am J Respir Crit Care Med* 1996;153:1442–1447.

149. Benkerrou M, Durandy A, Fischer A. Therapy for transplant-related lymphoproliferative diseases. *Hematol Oncol Clin North Am* 1993; 7:467–475.

150. Lazarovits AI, Tibbles LA, Grant DR, Ghent CN, Wall WJ, White MJ. Anti-B cell antibodies for the treatment of monoclonal Epstein-Barr virus-induced lymphoproliferative syndrome after multivisceral transplantation. *Clin Invest Med* 1994;17(6):621–625.

151. Hickey DP, Nalesnik MA, Vivas CA, et al. Renal retransplantation in patients who lost their allografts during management of previous posttransplant lymphoproliferative disease. *Clin Transplant* 1990;4:187–190.

152. Chachap P, Filho EC, Porta G, et al. Posttransplant lymphoproliferative disease of the liver successfully treated by retransplantation. *Transplantation* 1991;52:736–737.

153. Davis CL, Harrison KL, McVicar JP, Forg P, Bronner M, Marsh CL. Antiviral prophylaxis and the Epstein-Barr virus-related post-transplant lymphoproliferative disorder. *Clin Transplant* 1995;9:53–59.

154. Darenkov IA, Marcarelli MA, Basadonna GP, et al. Reduced incidence of Epstein-Barr virus-associated post-transplant lymphoproliferative disorder using preemptive antiviral therapy. *Transplantation* 1997;64:848–852.

155. Abedi MR, Linde A, Christensson B, Mackett M, Hammarstrom L, Smith CIE. Preventative effects of IgG from EBV-seropositive donors on the development of human lymphoproliferative disease in SCID mice. *Int J Cancer* 1997;71:624–629.

156. Kato H, Inamoto T, Nakamura H, et al. Soluble CD23 as a sensitive marker for Epstein-Barr virus-related disorders after liver transplantation. *Transplantation* 1993;56:1109–1113.

157. Morrissey PE, Lorber KM, Marcarelli M, Bia MJ, Kliger AS, Lorber MI. Posttransplant Epstein-Barr virus infection is associated with elevated levels of CD19+ B lymphocytes. *Transplantation* 1995;59(4):637–640.

158. Hornef MW, Wagner H, Fricke L, Bein G, Kirchner H. Immunocytochemical detection of Epstein-Barr virus antigens in peripheral B lymphocytes after renal transplantation. *Transplantation* 1995;59(1): 138–140.

159. Rooney CM, Loftin SK, Holladay MS, Brenner MK, Krance RA, Heslop HE. Early identification of Epstein-Barr virus-associated posttransplantation lymphoproliferative disease. *Br J Hematol* 1995;89: 98–103.

160. Green M. Preemptive therapy: Epstein Barr virus. *Transplant Proc* 1996;28:(6)[Suppl 2]:5–6.

161. Randhawa PS, Jaffe R, Demetris AJ, et al. Expression of Epstein-Barr virus-encoded small RNA (by the EBER-1 gene) in liver specimens from transplant recipients with post-transplantation lymphoproliferative disease. *N Engl J Med* 1992;327:1710–1714.

162. Hubscher SG, Williams A, Davison SM, Young LS, Niedobitek G. Epstein-Barr virus in inflammatory diseases of the liver and liver allografts: an *in situ* hybridization study. *Hepatology* 1994;20(4):899–907.

162b. Chodosh J, Holder VP, Gan Y, Belgaumi A, Sample J, Sixbey JW. Eradication of latent Epstein-Barr virus by hydroxyurea alters the growth-transformed cell phenotype. *J Infect Dis* 1998;177:1194–1201.

163. Roth G, Curiel T, Lacy J. Epstein-Barr viral nuclear antigen-1 antisense oligodeoxynucleotide inhibits proliferation of Epstein-Barr virus-immortalized B cells. *Blood* 1994;84:582–587.

164. Bochkarev A, Barwell J, Pfuetzner R, Bochkareva E, Frappier L, Edwards AM. Crystal structure of the DNA-binding domain of the Epstein-Barr virus origin binding protein EBNA-1 bound to DNA. *Cell* 1996;84:791–800.

165. Funakoshi S, Taub DD, Asai O, et al. Effects of CD40 stimulation in the prevention of human EBV-lymphomagenesis. *Leuk Lymphoma* 1997;24:187–99.

166. Rooney CM, Smith CA, Heslop HE. Control of virus-induced lymphoproliferation: Epstein-Barr virus-induced lymphoproliferation and host immunity. *Mol Med Today* 1997;24–30.

Transplant Infections edited by
Raleigh A. Bowden, Per Ljungman, and Carlos V. Paya.
Lippincott–Raven Publishers, Philadelphia © 1998

CHAPTER 19

Other Herpesviruses: Herpes Simplex Virus, Varicella-Zoster Virus, Human Herpesvirus Types 6, 7, and 8

John W. Gnann, Jr.

The human herpesvirus family currently includes eight viruses. All human herpesviruses (with the possible exception of human herpesvirus-8 (HHV8)) commonly cause infection in immunocompetent individuals but rarely cause severe or life-threatening disease. In immunocompromised patients, however, human herpesviruses are important causes of morbidity and mortality. As a consequence of the impairment of cell-mediated immunity that accompanies organ transplantation and antirejection therapy, clinical manifestations of herpesvirus diseases occurring in transplant recipients tend to be more frequent, severe, and prolonged than those seen in healthy individuals.

A key characteristic of all herpesviruses is the ability to establish latent infections. Following primary infection, latent infection of specific tissues (e.g., neural ganglia cells for varicella-zoster virus (VZV); lymphocytes for Epstein-Barr virus (EBV)) occurs and persists for life. The viral genome is present within latently infected cells but does not undergo full replication cycles and does not produce infectious progeny virus. The latent infection establishes an equilibrium with the immune response in which viral replication is restricted, but immune-mediated eradication of the infection does not occur. Periodically, the latent virus will undergo a replication cycle that temporarily overwhelms the immune response, resulting in symptomatic, recurrent herpesvirus disease (e.g., herpes labialis or herpes zoster). Impairment of cell-mediated immune responses by disease (e.g., Hodgkin's disease or acquired immunodeficiency syndrome [AIDS]) or by medical interventions (e.g., antirejection drug therapy)

strongly predisposes to symptomatic reactivation of herpesvirus infections.

Human infections with herpes simplex virus (HSV), cytomegalovirus (CMV), and EBV are very common (well over 50% seroprevalence in most populations) and infections with VZV, human herpesvirus-6, and human herpesvirus-7 are virtually universal. Diagnosis of latent infection is readily established by serological testing. Most primary herpesvirus infections occur during childhood, meaning that diseases in adult transplant patients are usually due to viral reactivation (1). However, when primary infection does occur in the transplant setting, the disease manifestations are frequently severe and prolonged. Because latent infections with HSV, VZV, and EBV are ubiquitous, serological matching of recipients with donors is generally not feasible.

Viruses cause 25% to 30% of all post-transplant infections, with herpesviruses accounting for the preponderance of viral opportunistic infections. More than half of the viral infections in transplant patients are caused by CMV, followed by HSV, VZV, and EBV (2). A direct association exists between the intensity of immunologic suppression and the frequency and severity of reactivated herpesvirus diseases. For example, the attack rate for herpes zoster is about five times higher after bone marrow transplantation than after renal transplantation. In some circumstances, reduction in immunosuppressive therapy may be necessary to achieve control of serious or life-threatening herpesvirus infections. Although prophylactic antiviral drugs have significantly reduced the risk of herpesvirus disease in transplant patients, the ultimate goal is to develop more selective immunosuppression that will effectively prevent graft rejection without simultaneously suppressing antiviral cellular immune responses.

From the Department of Medicine, University of Alabama at Birmingham, Birmingham, AL 35294-2170.

DESCRIPTION OF THE PATHOGENS

The eight human pathogens in the family Herpesviridae can be classified into three subfamilies (3). Herpes simplex viruses type 1 and type 2 (HSV-1, HSV-2) (4) and VZV are alpha herpesviruses, characterized by short replication cycles, rapid spread in culture, destruction of host cells during replication, and latency in sensory ganglia. The beta herpesviruses—including human CMV, human herpesvirus-6 (HHV-6), and human herpesvirus-7 (HHV-7)—exhibit a more restricted host range, long replication cycle, slow progression in culture, and latency in hematologic and epithelial cells. EBV is a gamma herpesvirus and exhibits a restricted host range, replication in lymphoblastoid cells, and latency in lymphoid tissue. The recently described HHV-8 is probably also a gamma herpesvirus.

All members of the family Herpesviridae share many features of structure and genomic organization. A complete virion is approximately 100–200 nm in diameter. The nucleocapsid measures about 100 nm in diameter and is composed of 162 capsomeres arranged in icosahedral symmetry. An amorphous tegument layer surrounds the capsid. The entire virion is enclosed in a lipid-containing laminated envelope with external glycoproteins, which are key antigenic determinants. The herpesvirus genome consists of a linear, double-stranded DNA molecule (120–230 kb) with unique regions flanked by terminal repeating sequences (3).

Herpesviruses specify a variety of enzymes to catalyze steps in the replication cycle, including nucleic acid metabolism (e.g., thymidine kinase), DNA synthesis (e.g., DNA polymerase), and protein processing (e.g., protein kinase). Synthesis of viral DNA and assembly of capsids occurs in the nucleus of the host cell and the envelope is acquired as the capsid passes through the nuclear membrane. Productive infection with release of progeny virus results in host cell death. In terms of disease pathogenesis, the most critical feature of the herpesvirus replication cycle is the ability to establish latent infections that persist for the life of the host (3).

HERPES SIMPLEX VIRUS

Epidemiology of HSV Infections

There is extensive sequence homology between HSV-1 and HSV-2; consequently, corresponding polypeptides from the two virus types are highly antigenically cross-reactive. HSV-1 is transmitted by oral secretions and predominantly causes orolabial infections. HSV-2 is sexually transmitted and most often causes genital infections, but there is considerable overlap, and either virus can cause disease at either location.

Both HSV-1 and HSV-2 are extremely common causes of infection, although exact seroprevalence rates vary somewhat among different populations (5). HSV-1 is most often acquired during childhood and causes gingivostomatitis, although the primary infection is frequently asymptomatic. Viral reactivation causes herpes labialis (cold sores or fever blisters) (6,7). Seroprevalence rates for HSV-2, in contrast, remain low until puberty and the onset of sexual activity (8). Primary and recurrent genital HSV infections are characterized by clusters of painful vesicles and ulcers. Asymptomatic shedding of HSV in genital secretions from infected individuals is common and a major source of disease transmission (9). In the United States, overall seroprevalence rates for HSV-1 and HSV-2 is estimated to be 62% and 22%, respectively, although rates vary significantly among age and socioeconomic groups (10,11).

Pathogenesis of HSV Infections

HSV is transmitted by direct contact with the skin or mucosal surfaces of a person actively shedding virus. In the newly infected individual, an initial round of viral replication takes place on the mucocutaneous surface, followed by transport of the virus via cutaneous neurons to nerve cell bodies in ganglia where latency is established. When latent HSV is subsequently reactivated, virus travels by way of peripheral sensory nerves back to the skin, where replication occurs in dermal and epidermal layers, producing the characteristic cluster of painful vesicles (5).

Almost all the HSV infections that occur following bone marrow (BMT) or solid organ transplantation (SOT) result from reactivation of endogenous latent virus, rather than from primary infection acquired from an exogenous source. Primary infections account for only about 2% of HSV disease occurring in BMT recipients (12). HSV can be cultured from oropharyngeal secretions in 70% to 80% of seropositive transplant patients not receiving antiviral prophylaxis (13). About two-thirds of these patients will develop clinically apparent lesions. Patients occasionally transmit virus to distant sites via autoinoculation, resulting in syndromes such as herpes keratitis or herpetic whitlow (14).

Herpesviruses can be transmitted via the graft from a seropositive donor to a seronegative recipient. For HSV, this has been most clearly described in the setting of renal transplantation (15–19). If the recipient is seronegative, primary infection occasionally results in viremia, a rare but frequently lethal event resulting in widespread visceral organ involvement. In one well-documented instance, two patients received kidneys from the same donor. Both recipients developed fulminant HSV-2 hepatitis and died. HSV isolates obtained from both recipients had identical restriction endonuclease patterns, strongly suggesting that infection was transmitted via the donor organs (16).

Most HSV infections occur within the first 30 days after transplantation (20). HSV reactivates rapidly after initiation of immunosuppressive therapy, which coincides with the time of maximal suppression of lymphocyte responsiveness to HSV antigens (21–23). Donor immunity does not prevent reactivation of HSV in the graft recipient. Following SOT, lymphocyte responsiveness to HSV antigens returns to normal within 6 months, and the frequency of HSV recurrences also declines (23). In BMT recipients, reestablishment of specific lymphocyte reactivity is dependent on reexposure to HSV antigens via HSV infection (symptomatic or asymptomatic) (21,24). Those patients who fail to develop a positive lymphocyte response to HSV antigens after the first post-transplantation HSV recurrence tend to maintain a higher frequency of subsequent HSV recurrences (21). No clear detrimental effect of HSV infection on graft survival has been demonstrated.

Clinical Presentation and Natural History of HSV Disease

In patients who do not receive antiviral prophylaxis, HSV disease occurs within 2–3 weeks of BMT or SOT (22,25–27). In BMT patients, the median time to onset of HSV disease is 17 days (22,25). Following liver transplantation, 50% of all symptomatic HSV disease occurs within 3 weeks of transplantation (26–28). Significant disease caused by HSV is uncommon beyond post-transplant day 60.

Overall, at least 50% of transplant patients will have serological evidence of prior HSV infection at the time of transplantation and at least 40% will subsequently develop HSV disease, which means that HSV reactivation occurs in 70% to 80% of seropositive patients (21,28–31). In a study of 107 BMT recipients, HSV lesions developed in 37 of 51 seropositive patients and in six of 42 seronegative patients with a median time to onset of 8 days following transplantation (13). Similarly, culture-proven HSV disease occurred in 15 of 18 (83%) seropositive cardiac transplant patients during the early post-transplant period (30). These high attack rates provide rationale for antiviral prophylaxis to prevent HSV disease during the first few weeks after transplantation.

In many instances, the initial presentation of mucocutaneous HSV disease in transplant patients does not differ much from that seen in the immunocompetent host. However, as a consequence of the impaired immune responses, herpetic lesions in immunocompromised patients exhibit prolonged viral shedding, are more invasive, heal more slowly, and have the potential to disseminate (30,32). A review of 101 liver transplant patients at the University of Pittsburgh revealed 35 cases of HSV disease. Thirty-two of the HSV cases (91%) were limited to mucocutaneous disease and were considered nonsevere (28). However, the other three had fatal disseminated HSV infection with hepatic or gastrointestinal involve-

ment, demonstrating the lethal potential of HSV infections in transplant populations.

On intact skin, herpetic lesions begin as painful erythematous papules that rapidly develop into clusters of vesicles. If the vesicles remain intact, they evolve into pustules with the influx of inflammatory cells. The vesicles are fragile and soon rupture, resulting in shallow ulcerations on an erythematous base that eventually form crusts. Although healing takes places over 5–10 days in the normal host, healing (without antiviral therapy) may be delayed for 4–6 weeks in the immunocompromised host (30,32). In some patients, large, chronic, mucocutaneous ulcerations may develop that are very atypical in appearance and require biopsy or viral culture for accurate diagnosis (33,34).

The most common presentation of HSV in transplant patients is orolabial disease, which accounts for 85% of all HSV disease in the early post-transplant period (12,35). HSV causes about half of all oral lesions in the first month following transplantation (35). Herpetic lesions may involve the lips, oral mucosa (including the gingiva, tongue, and posterior pharynx), and the perioral facial skin. In bone marrow transplant patients, intraoral HSV infections occurring during the granulocytopenic period may be difficult to distinguish from mucositis resulting from other etiologies. If typical herpetic labial or perioral lesions are present, the diagnosis of HSV gingivostomatitis is strongly suggested. If the process is limited to nonspecific intraoral erosions and ulcerations, a viral culture will be necessary to detect the presence of HSV. Herpetic gingivostomatitis can cause severe mouth pain and result in diminished nutritional intake and may predispose the patient to bacterial superinfections of the oral cavity as well as to HSV esophagitis and pneumonitis.

The next most common presentation is genital or perianal HSV disease. Anogenital herpes is most commonly due to HSV-2 and results from reactivation of virus in sacral ganglia. HSV-2 accounts for 10% to 15% of all HSV infections in BMT patients (36). As with orolabial disease, anogenital herpes can range from self-limited lesions similar to those seen in the normal host to extensive chronic ulcerations that may persist for weeks or months (34,37). Anogenital reactivations of HSV-2 may be complicated by lymphocytic meningitis, which is usually self-limited and does not progress to HSV encephalitis (38).

Mucocutaneous HSV infections can cause serious morbidity but are usually self-limited and rarely fatal. However, dissemination of virus can result in visceral organ infections that are difficult to diagnose and frequently lethal. HSV can spread by direct extension from the oropharynx to the gastrointestinal or respiratory tracts, causing herpetic esophagitis or pneumonia. Viremic dissemination with widespread involvement of multiple visceral organs is associated with an extremely high mortality rate, but fortunately is rare. Herpes simplex encephalitis does not occur with increased frequency in immunocompromised patients and is rarely observed as a post-transplant complication (39,40).

Patients with HSV esophagitis present with symptoms of dysphagia and odynophagia that may be clinically indistinguishable from syndromes caused by candida or CMV. In BMT patients, CMV and HSV esophagitis occur with approximately equal frequency (41). In most cases, HSV esophagitis is thought to result from direct extension from herpes gingivostomatitis. An alternative hypothesis suggests that HSV esophagitis could result from reactivation of virus from the vagus ganglia (42). The presence of a nasogastric tube may increase the risk of esophagitis in a transplant patient with HSV oral infection. Because clinical and radiographic findings cannot reliably distinguish among the infectious etiologies of esophagitis, endoscopy for biopsy and cultures is usually required. In cases of HSV esophagitis, endoscopic examination will reveal superficial erosions and punched- out ulcerations that, in severe cases, become almost confluent (41,43). Colitis in transplant patients is more commonly caused by CMV than by HSV, but cases of HSV colitis have been reported (44).

HSV pneumonia is diagnosed most frequently in bone marrow, lung, and heart/lung transplant recipients, and less frequently in other SOT patients (45–50). Lung allografts are highly susceptible to HSV, especially in the early post-transplant period (46,48). Pulmonary involvement with HSV may result either from aspiration or local extension from the upper airway (which is most common) or as a result of viremia (which is infrequent). In a study of HSV pneumonia in BMT patients, 17 of 20 patients (85%) had prior evidence of mucocutaneous HSV disease, providing a clue to the pulmonary diagnosis (45). HSV pneumonia resulting from contiguous spread of virus from the oropharynx via the trachea is usually caused by HSV-1 and is characterized radiographically by focal or multifocal infiltrates on the chest radiograph (45). Bronchoscopic findings will include extensive erosive tracheobronchitis. The presence of an endotracheal tube appears to significantly increase the risk of direct extension of HSV to the tracheobronchial tree. In contrast, HSV pneumonia resulting from viremia may be due to either HSV-1 or HSV-2, presents radiographically with diffuse infiltrates on the chest film, and is usually accompanied by HSV disease affecting other organs (45).

Transplant patients with HSV pneumonia will present with fever, cough, dyspnea, hypoxemia, and abnormalities on the chest radiograph that may be indistinguishable from bacterial pneumonia. Bronchoscopy to examine the airways and obtain biopsies and cultures is necessary to establish a diagnosis of HSV pneumonia. Since HSV is frequently present in oral secretions, positive viral cultures from expectorated sputum can be misleading. A definitive diagnosis of HSV pneumonia is based on positive cultures of deep lung specimens obtained by bronchoscopy, coupled with histopathologic evidence of HSV infection on lung biopsy (45). A diagnosis of HSV pneumonia should be entertained in any transplant patient with known HSV disease who develops pulmonary infiltrates, particularly if the patient has clinical findings suggestive of esophagitis, tracheitis, or HSV dissemination to other visceral organs (45).

Viremic dissemination of HSV can result in infection of multiple organs, most notably the liver, but also lungs, adrenal glands, gastrointestinal tract, and skin. This syndrome has been described most frequently in renal and liver transplant patients but occurs in BMT recipients as well (14,16,19,51–57). The mortality rate for disseminated HSV disease is very high; rapid diagnosis and initiation of aggressive antiviral therapy and supportive care are essential for patient survival. The systemic HSV syndrome usually occurs within 1 month of organ transplantation. Patients may present with signs of hepatitis, including fever and abnormal liver function tests. In some cases, primary HSV infection with dissemination has occurred when an organ is transplanted from a seropositive donor to a seronegative recipient (16,19). In other cases, dissemination has occurred in seropositive transplant patients who develop reactivated HSV disease. Twelve patients with HSV hepatitis were identified in a population of 3,536 SOT recipients, yielding an incidence of 0.3% (17). The median time to onset of hepatitis was 18 days following transplantation. Clinical findings included abdominal pain and tenderness, fever, and abnormal liver function tests. Some, but not all, patients had HSV skin lesions. Eight of the 12 patients (67%) died, and the diagnosis was often made post mortem. Presence of disseminated intravascular coagulopathy in the setting of HSV hepatitis is associated with 100% mortality (17). Liver biopsy for HSV cultures and histopathology is the diagnostic method of choice (17,58).

CMV can also cause hepatitis in this population, but the presentations differ. HSV hepatitis tends to occur within 5–25 days of transplantation, is fulminant and rapidly progressive, and is associated with an increased percentage of band forms on the white blood cell differential. CMV hepatitis usually occurs at least 20–50 days after transplantation, has a subacute and smoldering course, and is associated with leukopenia and atypical lymphocytes on the white blood cell differential (17). A liver biopsy is essential to provide an accurate diagnosis, especially in liver transplant recipients when the differential diagnosis also includes hepatitis B or graft rejection (58).

Diagnosis of HSV Infections

Although typical mucocutaneous herpetic lesions can be accurately identified by experienced clinicians, atypical lesions or visceral organ involvement will require laboratory confirmation. Viral culture remains the preferred method for diagnosis of HSV infections (59). When performed early in the course of infection (during the vesicle or ulcer stage), culture is a sensitive diagnostic technique. For mucocutaneous lesions, vesicle fluid or ulcer exudate is collected on a swab and placed in appropriate viral transport media. Tissue specimens from biopsies can be minced and extracted for viral culturing. The specimen should be inoculated onto tissue culture cells as soon as possible. If necessary, the specimen can be stored at 4°C for up to 48 hours, although some reduction in yield may result. HSV grows readily on a variety of mammalian cell lines, including primary rabbit kidney, human fibroblasts, and Vero cells. Characteristic cytopathic changes can be observed within 24–48 hours, although viral growth occasionally takes as long as a week. Definitive identification and typing of the virus can be performed by staining cells from the tissue culture monolayer with fluorescein-labeled HSV-1 and HSV-2–specific monoclonal antibodies.

The direct fluorescent antigen (DFA) assay can be used for rapid diagnosis of mucocutaneous lesions (60). Cells scraped from the base of a vesicular or ulcerative lesion are fixed on a glass slide and stained with fluorescein-labeled monoclonal antibodies specific for HSV-1, HSV-2, or VZV and examined under a fluorescent microscope. This method is more sensitive than the Tzanck smear and provides a virus-specific diagnosis in as little as an hour.

A variety of rapid diagnostic assays to detect HSV antigens or nucleic acids are currently under development and may eventually replace virus culture. One promising technique for diagnosis of HSV infections employs the polymerase chain reaction (PCR) (40,61). PCR is now the method of choice for diagnosing CNS infections due to HSV and may eventually be adapted for diagnosis of HSV infections in other tissues (62).

Because most HSV infections are due to reactivation in patients with preexisting antibody, serology is generally not helpful. Except in the case of seroconversion, serological testing is useful to define susceptibility, but not to diagnose active disease. A negative assay for anti-HSV antibodies may help exclude HSV from the differential diagnosis. Most laboratories currently use an enzyme-linked immunosorbent assay (ELISA), although a variety of other serological tests are available (including complement fixation, passive hemagglutination, neutralization, and immunofluorescence tests) (59). The ELISA is simple and sensitive but cannot distinguish between antibodies directed against HSV-1 or HSV-2. If type-specific HSV serological testing is required, Western blotting is available at reference laboratories. A variety of simpler serological assays that distinguish between HSV-1 and HSV-2 antibodies are under development.

Therapy of HSV Infections

Prior to about 1980, no effective systemic therapy for herpesvirus infections was available. Administration of interferon in immunocompromised patients with HSV infections produced some clinical benefit but was associated with multiple adverse effects (63). Vidarabine was the first systemically administered antiviral drug to have both significant clinical benefit and an acceptable toxicity profile (64). The release of acyclovir in the early 1980s revolutionized the treatment and prophylaxis of HSV infection. Small trials of intravenous acyclovir therapy of mucocutaneous HSV infections in immunocompromised patients clearly demonstrated the efficacy and safety of the drug (65,66). These were followed by large, randomized, placebo-controlled trials of intravenous acyclovir (5 mg/kg or 250 mg/m^2 IV every 8 hours) in BMT and SOT populations (67). In a study of 97 immunocompromised patients with mucocutaneous HSV infections (85% orolabial infections), intravenous acyclovir reduced the duration of viral shedding (median 2.8 versus 16.8 days), accelerated resolution of pain (median 8.9 versus 13.1 days), and accelerated lesion healing (median 13.7 versus 20.1 days), compared with placebo (67).

Orally administered acyclovir is also highly effective for HSV infections. Although intravenous acyclovir is preferred for patients with severe or potentially life-threatening infections, oral acyclovir is more convenient for patients with less serious HSV infections. Orally administered acyclovir is extremely safe and well tolerated. In a study of mucocutaneous HSV infections in 21 BMT recipients, oral acyclovir reduced the duration of virus shedding (median 2 versus 9 days), hastened pain resolution (median 6 versus 16 days), and accelerated total lesion healing (median 8 versus 21 days), compared with placebo (Fig. 1) (68). Newer oral antiherpesvirus drugs with improved pharmacokinetic properties may replace oral acyclovir for this indication. Valacyclovir (a pro-drug of acyclovir) and famciclovir (a pro-drug of penciclovir) have antiviral activity similar to that of acy-

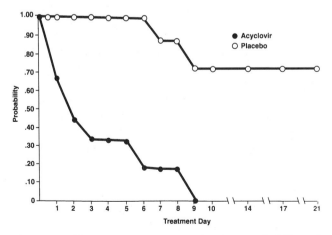

Figure 1. Time-to-event curves showing probability of remaining culture-positive for HSV, from a study of BMT patients with mucocutaneous HSV disease treated with oral acyclovir (*closed circles*) or placebo (*open circles*) for 10 days (*p* = 0.0008). Modified from Shepp et al. (68), with permission.

clovir, but produce higher serum drug levels and have simpler dosing schedules (69,70). Preliminary indications suggest that valacyclovir and famciclovir will be highly effective for HSV infections in transplant patients, but published experience with these drugs in immunocompromised patients is currently limited.

A topical preparation of acyclovir is available and was proven to be beneficial for treatment of mucocutaneous HSV infections in immunocompromised patients (32). However, topically applied acyclovir is clearly not as effective as systemically administered drug. In view of the safety and efficacy of the orally administered anti-HSV drugs, there is probably no role for topical acyclovir or penciclovir for HSV infections in transplant patients.

No prospective, controlled studies have been performed to evaluated the efficacy of acyclovir in transplant patients with disseminated or visceral HSV infections. However, clinical experience and anecdotal reports clearly support the value of intravenous acyclovir in this setting (28,58,71). High-dose intravenous acyclovir (10 mg/kg IV every 8 hours) should be considered the treatment of choice for any immunocompromised patient with known or suspected HSV infection of visceral organs.

Antiviral therapy of mucocutaneous HSV disease should be continued until the lesions are completely healed, which will be at least 10 days in most cases. Premature discontinuation of antiviral therapy can result in relapsing infection and set the stage for emergence of acyclovir-resistant HSV. Ganciclovir, foscarnet, and cidofovir are antiviral drugs primarily used to treat CMV diseases, but have excellent activity against HSV as well. Acyclovir, conversely, has essentially no useful therapeutic activity against CMV. In transplant patients who have infections caused by both CMV and HSV, ganciclovir, foscarnet, or cidofovir will provide effective treatment for both viral pathogens.

Infections caused by HSV isolates resistant to acyclovir are occasionally encountered in bone marrow transplant patients, but rarely in SOT patients (72–75). In one study, the frequency of acyclovir-resistant HSV isolates in BMT patients was estimated to be 2% (72). The most common manifestation of acyclovir-resistant HSV is extensive and chronic mucocutaneous disease. Although acyclovir-resistant HSV strains appear to be less virulent in animal models, instances of serious visceral infection due to acyclovir-resistant HSV have been reported (73,76). Immunocompromised patients with HSV lesions that fail to heal or that progress despite acyclovir therapy should be recultured and isolates submitted for antiviral susceptibility testing.

The hypothesis that appropriate use of acyclovir prophylaxis will suppress viral replication and reduce the probability of mutations leading to resistance appears to be supported by clinical experience (77). In BMT patients, acyclovir resistance develops more frequently in patients repeatedly treated for recurrent HSV disease than in patients maintained on long-term prophylaxis

(13,72,78). The initial phosphorylation step in activation of acyclovir is catalyzed by virally encoded thymidine kinase. HSV isolates with mutations that result in quantitatively or qualitatively altered thymidine kinase will be resistant to acyclovir (74,79). Since famciclovir/penciclovir and ganciclovir are also dependent upon thymidine kinase for activation, these drugs will also be ineffective against acyclovir-resistant HSV strains. Foscarnet and cidofovir, which are not dependent upon thymidine kinase, can be used to treat disease caused by acyclovir-resistant HSV (44,75,80,81).

Prophylaxis of HSV Disease

The widespread adoption of antiviral prophylactic therapy has dramatically altered the natural history of HSV infections in transplant patients. Prophylaxis minimizes the risks of HSV-associated morbidity and mortality in the post-transplant period and reduces the risks of emergence of acyclovir-resistant HSV strains (77,82). Clinical trials using intravenous acyclovir prophylaxis in BMT patients documented reduction in the incidence of HSV infection from 70% to 5% or less (83–85). These studies demonstrated that intravenous acyclovir given at a dose of 5 mg/kg (or 250 mg/m^2) every 8–12 hours during the neutropenic phase following bone marrow transplantation could essentially eliminate the occurrence of HSV disease. Prophylaxis using oral acyclovir was nearly as effective as intravenous administration (Fig. 2), although some patients in the immediate post-transplant period had difficulty taking oral medications due to stomatitis or nausea (85,86). However, these investigators noted an increased frequency of HSV disease beginning very shortly after acyclovir prophylaxis was discontinued (13,85,86). This led to a strategy of initiating prophylaxis

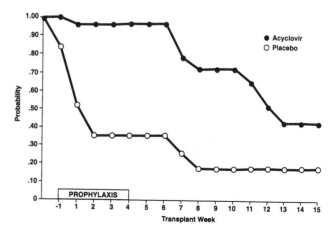

Figure 2. Time-to-event curves showing probability of remaining culture-negative for HSV, from a study of BMT patients receiving prophylaxis with acyclovir (*closed circles*) or placebo (*open circles*) for 5 weeks (*p* = 0.0002). Modified from Wade et al. (86), with permission.

with intravenous acyclovir during the immediate post-transplant period and then switching to long-term prophylaxis with oral acyclovir (84,87). In a placebo-controlled study, 42 BMT recipients were treated with intravenous acyclovir from 5 days prior to transplant until 5 weeks following transplant. At that point, they were switched to oral acyclovir and therapy was continued until 6 months following transplant, a regimen that proved to be highly effective for preventing HSV disease (84). Sequential therapy with intravenous and oral acyclovir has the advantages of avoiding frequent oral dosing during the immediate post-transplant phase (when compliance may be problematic) while permitting a longer duration of effective prophylaxis than would be feasible with intravenous acyclovir (87). A simplified oral acyclovir regimen of 800 mg b.i.d. provides greater than 90% virologic efficacy with reduced costs and improved patient compliance (88). Acyclovir prophylaxis is well tolerated in BMT patients. Some initial reports indicated that marrow engraftment might actually be faster in groups treated with acyclovir (85,86), but these findings were not confirmed by other investigators (84,89).

Few controlled trials have been performed in other organ transplant populations, although clinical experience suggests that acyclovir prophylaxis is safe and effective in these groups (88,90). A study of 35 renal transplant patients documented no HSV recurrences in 18 acyclovir recipients, compared with 9 recurrences in 17 placebo patients (91). In one study of liver transplant recipients, the incidence of HSV in patients receiving acyclovir prophylaxis was 4% (92), whereas the incidence of HSV disease in historical control groups where prophylaxis was not used was 53% (31). In all transplant populations, prophylaxis appears to be a superior strategy to repeated therapeutic administration of antiviral drugs for management of recurrent HSV disease.

Immunoprophylaxis of HSV Infections

Vaccinating HSV-seronegative transplant candidates is theoretically attractive, but an effective HSV vaccine has proven very difficult to devise (93). Clinical trials are ongoing with vaccines containing a variety of attenuated, inactivated, subunit, and genetically engineered HSV preparations. Furthermore, passive immunotherapy with polyclonal immunoglobulin preparations has not proven beneficial for management of HSV disease in immunocompromised patients. High-titered preparations of anti-HSV monoclonal antibodies in combination with antiviral drugs are being evaluated.

VARICELLA-ZOSTER VIRUS

Epidemiology of VZV Infections

Humans are the only known reservoir for VZV. In temperate regions, epidemics of varicella (or chickenpox) occur annually in the late winter and early spring (94). About 3.8 million cases of varicella occur each year in the United States (15 cases per 100,000 population), which approximately equals the annual birth cohort (95). About 60% of varicella cases occur in children between 5 and 9 years of age, and 90% of cases occur in patients under 15 years of age. More than 90% of the U.S. population is VZV seropositive by age 20 (96). Herpes zoster (or shingles) results from reactivation of latent VZV. The annual incidence rate for herpes zoster is 1.5–3.0 cases per 1,000 population, predicting about 500,000 cases of herpes zoster cases annually in the United States (97). The incidence of zoster is clearly age related, reaching 10 cases per 1,000 patient-years in individuals more than 75 years of age (97). Individuals with impaired cell-mediated immunity (including patients with lymphoproliferative malignancies, AIDS, and organ transplantation) are at very high risk for development of herpes zoster (98).

Pathogenesis of VZV Infections

Primary varicella infection occurs when a susceptible individual is exposed to airborne virus via the respiratory route (99). Patients with chickenpox are infectious for about 48 hours prior to rash onset and for 4–5 days after. Varicella is most often acquired from exposure to another individual with chickenpox, but infection can also occur from exposure to a patient with herpes zoster. Varicella is highly infectious; following household exposure, attack rates are more than 70% (94,100). After entry through mucosal surfaces of the upper respiratory tract, VZV undergoes an initial round of replication, probably in cervical lymph nodes. A primary viremia follows, with widespread dissemination of VZV to the reticuloendothelial system. Following additional rounds of replication, a second viremic phase occurs about 1 week after the initial viremia. This second viremic phase heralds the onset of clinical symptoms and the characteristic cutaneous vesicles (101).

As VZV replicates in the skin during acute varicella, some virions are transported via sensory nerves to the corresponding dorsal root ganglia, where latent infection is established (102). The specific immune responses that limit reactivation of VZV from the sensory ganglia are poorly understood. The most important factor predisposing to the development of herpes zoster is declining VZV-specific cellular immunity, resulting from natural aging or from immunosuppressive illness or therapy. Following VZV reactivation and replication in the ganglion, virus travels along the sensory nerve to the skin, where it replicates in epithelial cells, producing the characteristic vesicular eruption of herpes zoster (Fig. 3).

Several factors have been identified that predispose organ transplant recipients to develop herpes zoster. Among autologous bone marrow transplant patients, the underlying disease is clearly associated with the likelihood of develop-

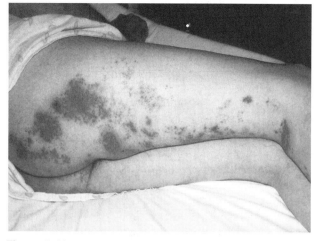

Figure 3. Herpes zoster in a heart transplant patient involving the right S2 dermatome.

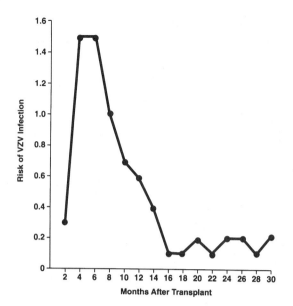

Figure 4. Risk of herpes zoster by month after BMT expressed as incidence per patient-day (%). Modified from Locksley et al. (105), with permission.

ing herpes zoster (103). The risk is 46% among patients transplanted for Hodgkin's disease or lymphoma, 23% for leukemia, and 9% for solid tumors. Furthermore, patients who have an episode of herpes zoster after the diagnosis of Hodgkin's disease but prior to marrow transplantation are at especially high risk for shingles after transplantation (104). The importance of graft-versus-host-disease (GVHD) as a risk factor for zoster has been debated. Among allogeneic marrow transplant patients, GVHD probably increases the incidence of herpes zoster and the risk of VZV dissemination once zoster occurs (105). Other investigators find no association between acute or chronic GVHD and reactivation of VZV (106). Overall, the incidence of herpes zoster is approximately equal in autologous and allogeneic BMT populations (103).

No correlation exists between titers of IgG antibody against VZV measured close to the time of transplantation and subsequent risk of zoster (107). Instead the zoster risk appears to correlate with the level of VZV-specific cell-mediated immune responses, which are suppressed in the post-transplant period (23,108). Following BMT, VZV-specific immune responses may be lost, although both the donor and the recipient were initially seropositive (109,110). Lymphocyte responsiveness to VZV antigens is slowly recovered after bone marrow transplantation (110,111). As previously described with HSV, T-cell recognition of VZV proteins may not be fully reconstituted until the patient experiences a reexposure to VZV antigens via clinical disease or possibly through subclinical reactivation (105,110–112). However, most patients develop durable immunity, as evidenced by the fact that few transplant patients experience more than one episode of herpes zoster (106,108).

Unlike HSV infections that occur in the immediate post-transplant period, VZV reactivation usually occurs after day 100 in BMT and SOT patients (Fig. 4) (25,104,113,114). Following BMT, the median time to onset of herpes zoster is 5 months, with 78% to 85% of

cases occurring in the first year after transplantation (104,105,115).

Herpes zoster in transplant patients can follow one of three clinical patterns. In most instances, the patient will develop a dermatomal skin eruption similar to that seen in immunocompetent patients, although the risk of dissemination is higher. Less commonly, immunocompromised patients can develop varicella-like skin lesions with no primary dermatomal eruption, a syndrome termed *atypical generalized zoster* (106,116). This probably represents reactivation of endogenous virus with cutaneous dissemination, but no clinically apparent dermatomal rash, although a second primary infection following reexposure to exogenous VZV may occasionally occur (106). Lastly, patients may develop subclinical reactivation of latent VZV as evidenced by boosted humoral and cellular immune responses with no evidence of cutaneous VZV lesions (111,112). In some BMT patients, subclinical VZV reactivation has been documented by PCR detection of VZV DNA in circulating mononuclear cells, accompanied by restoration of lymphocyte proliferation responses to VZV antigens (111). Patients with subclinical reactivation are at very low risk for subsequent herpes zoster (112). A related group of patients has been described who developed neuralgic pain typical of herpes zoster but no cutaneous lesions, followed by a boost in VZV-specific humeral and cellular immune responses (102).

Clinical Presentation and Natural History of VZV Disease

Because more than 90% of adults are latently infected with VZV, true primary infection in transplant recipients occurs chiefly in pediatric patients. Chickenpox in children (or adults) with bone marrow or solid organ transplantation is associated with high rates of morbidity and mortality (117–119). Skin lesions may be unusually numerous and severe, with ongoing new lesion formation for up to a week. Cutaneous complications in immunocompromised children include bullous or hemorrhagic varicella lesions, necrotizing fasciitis, purpura fulminans, and bacterial superinfections. Prior to the availability of antiviral therapy, visceral involvement (especially pneumonitis and hepatitis) developed in nearly half of immunocompromised children with chickenpox, resulting in 10% to 20% mortality (118,120). VZV pneumonia occurred in 25% to 30% of these children, presenting with fever, cough, and dyspnea usually within 3–5 days after the onset of the skin lesions. Aggressive antirejection therapy and absolute lymphopenia (less than 500/mm^3) are risk factors for VZV dissemination and death (120,121).

The frequency of herpes zoster in transplant populations correlates with the intensity of immune suppression. During the 12 months following transplantation, the incidence of herpes zoster is 28% to 40% for BMT, about 20% for cardiac transplant, and 3% to 10% for renal or liver transplant (28,103–106,112–114,122–124). Second episodes of herpes zoster are seen in fewer than 5% of transplant patients (106). The initial presentation of herpes zoster in transplant patients is usually similar to that seen in the normal host. Malaise and neuralgic pain in the involved dermatome may precede the onset of the rash by hours to a few days. About 10% of patients present with a syndrome of fever, abdominal pain, nausea, and vomiting, which precedes the appearance of the rash by 1–4 days (105,125). In a population of 195 BMT patients with herpes zoster, the rash involved the following dermatomes: cranial, 16%; cervical, 17%; thoracic, 47%; lumbar, 21%; and sacral, 12% (105). Multiple or noncontiguous dermatomes are involved more frequently in transplant recipients than in immunocompetent hosts (106). Without antiviral therapy, the events of cutaneous healing are also more prolonged in immunocompromised patients (126). In the normal host, cessation of new vesicle formation occurs in about 3–5 days and compete lesion healing requires 2–3 weeks; in immunocompromised patients, the intervals are 8 days and 3–4 weeks, respectively. Prior to the availability of antiviral therapy, transplant patients sometimes developed indolent zoster lesions that persisted for weeks or months and only resolved when immunosuppression therapy was reduced (126). Complications related to herpes zoster may include postherpetic neuralgia (25%), cutaneous scarring (19%), and bacterial superinfection of skin lesions (17%) (105). Dissemination of VZV to the eye can cause acute retinal necrosis and blindness (127).

Fifteen to twenty percent of the reactivation VZV episodes in BMT patients will present as atypical generalized zoster. This syndrome resembles varicella, with widely disseminated cutaneous lesions, no clinically apparent dermatomal localization, and a high risk of visceral involvement (105,106). Although this syndrome resembles primary VZV infection, it is thought to represent reactivation and dissemination of latent VZV in a patient with no effective immune responses.

Cutaneous dissemination of VZV will occur in 20% to 30% of transplant patients who initially present with dermatomal herpes zoster (103,105,106). Rates of dissemination appear to be significantly higher among BMT patients undergoing allogeneic transplantation (45%) compared with autologous transplantation (26%) (103). Cutaneous dissemination alone does not significantly increase the mortality rate associated with herpes zoster. However, cutaneous dissemination is a clinical predictor of the subsequent development of a visceral infection, such as VZV pneumonitis, hepatitis, or encephalitis. Approximately one-third of BMT patients with dermatomal zoster and cutaneous dissemination will subsequently develop visceral complications (103,105,106). Among patients with the varicella-like syndrome, the risk of visceral involvement is 40% to 50% (103,105,106).

Visceral VZV disease without cutaneous involvement is very uncommon and may be difficult to diagnose. A small number of BMT patients have been described who present with a syndrome of fever, severe abdominal pain, and gastrointestinal bleeding but no apparent cutaneous lesions (125,128,129). At autopsy, these patients were found to have ulcerations in the gastrointestinal tract and hemorrhage necrosis in the liver, pancreas, and kidneys. Cultures from the involved organs were positive for VZV (105,125,128).

Prior to the availability of specific antiviral therapy, the mortality rate for herpes zoster in transplant populations was about 10%, with deaths due to visceral dissemination, especially VZV pneumonitis (105,106). In a review of 195 BMT patients with dermatomal zoster, 26 (13%) developed visceral dissemination and 13 (6.7%) died (105). In the same study, 36 patients presented with the varicella-like syndrome and 10 (28%) of those patients died (105). In a more recent study of 43 episodes of zoster occurring in autologous BMT patients, all patients were treated with acyclovir and all patients survived, including 10 patients with varicella-like syndrome (103).

Diagnosis of VZV Infections

The appearances of varicella and herpes zoster are quite distinctive, and in most cases, a clinical diagnosis is accurate and reliable. The presentation of a child with fever, a diffuse vesicular rash, and no prior history of chickenpox is strongly suggestive of the diagnosis, particularly if there has been a known exposure to VZV in the previous 10–14 days. Herpes zoster, with its characteristic neuralgic pain and dermatomal vesicular rash, is also readily diagnosed on the basis of clinical appearance. In transplant patients, however, distinguishing between VZV and HSV disease on clinical grounds can sometimes be difficult. Zoster presenting with localized vesicles on the face or genital area may be confused with HSV. Conversely, HSV presenting in a zosteriform or pseudodermatomal pattern, especially in the sacral area, may closely resemble herpes zoster. In these settings or when visceral disease is suspected, laboratory confirmation of the diagnosis should be pursued.

Unlike HSV or CMV, VZV is not shed asymptomatically. Therefore identification of VZV virions, antigens, or nucleic acids from cutaneous lesions or tissue biopsies is diagnostic of active infection. VZV can be cultured by inoculation of vesicular fluid or tissue extracts into monolayers of human fetal diploid kidney or lung cells (130). Unlike HSV, VZV is very labile and every effort should be made to minimize time spent in specimen transport or storage. Characteristic cytopathic effects are seen in tissue culture within 3–7 days, and identification of the isolate can be confirmed by direct immunofluorescent staining of infected cells using VZV-specific monoclonal antibodies (131). A more rapid diagnosis can be made by using fluorescein-conjugated monoclonal antibodies to detect VZV glycoprotein antigens in cellular scrapings obtained from the base of a fresh vesicle (132). This DFA assay is especially helpful for making a rapid diagnosis when the clinical presentation is atypical (133,134). PCR is a very promising technique for detecting VZV DNA in tissues or fluids (e.g., CSF) when viral culture may be insensitive, but the procedure is not yet widely available (129,135–137).

Serological techniques are helpful for determining patient susceptibility to VZV but not generally useful for diagnosing acute infections. Most laboratories use an ELISA method that can detect either IgG or IgM responses (138). Serum antibodies appear several days after the onset of varicella and peak at 2–3 weeks. Patients with herpes zoster are usually VZV seropositive at the time of disease onset, but most show a significant rise in titer during the convalescent phase. In either event, the serological result only provides retrospective confirmation of the diagnosis.

Therapy of VZV Infections

The availability of safe and effective antiviral drugs has greatly reduced the high mortality rate associated with VZV infections in transplant patients. Nonetheless, occasional deaths from disseminated VZV still occur despite appropriate antiviral therapy. In addition, complications such as cutaneous scarring and postherpetic neuralgia are not reliably prevented by antiviral therapy. Interferon and vidarabine were both shown to provide therapeutic benefit in immunocompromised patients with VZV infections, but these drugs have now been replaced by antiviral compounds such as acyclovir that offer more potent antiviral effect and less toxicity (139,140).

Because of the high frequency of visceral involvement in immunocompromised children (or adults) with chickenpox, aggressive antiviral therapy is warranted. Controlled trials of intravenous acyclovir in immunocompromised patients with varicella clearly demonstrated a significant reduction in the frequency of VZV pneumonitis (119,141,142). Therapy should be initiated as soon as possible with intravenous acyclovir (10 mg/kg or 500 mg/m² for 7–10 days). A switch to oral acyclovir can be considered when the patient is afebrile and new lesion formation has terminated. If the patient is hospitalized, isolation procedures are essential to prevent nosocomial transmission of VZV.

Initial clinical trials with intravenous acyclovir for localized or disseminated herpes zoster in immunocompromised patients clearly demonstrated that treatment achieved more rapid virus clearance and halted disease progression (143,144). Subsequent studies in BMT patients proved that acyclovir, in addition to promoting faster disease resolution, was highly effective at preventing VZV dissemination (139,145). Since most VZV-related fatalities result from disseminated infection, the ability to prevent dissemination has dramatically reduced the herpes zoster mortality rate in transplant patients. In addition, intravenous acyclovir is effective for treating dissemination if it occurs and is considered the drug of choice for that indication (140,143).

Since herpes zoster tends to occur late after transplantation, most patients have been discharged from the hospital when herpes zoster develops. Treating zoster on an outpatient basis with oral antiviral drugs is an attractive approach, although data are currently limited. In one small study, 27 allogeneic BMT patients with zoster were randomized to receive oral or intravenous acyclovir (146). No VZV dissemination occurred in either group and no differences in healing or clinical outcome were apparent. Recent clinical trials with oral acyclovir and famciclovir have demonstrated that outpatient therapy for herpes zoster is appropriate in selected immunocompromised patients (147,148). Published data from clinical trials with famciclovir and valacyclovir for herpes zoster in immunocompromised patients remain limited, but a growing body of clinical experience suggests that these drugs are safe and effective in this setting and will likely replace oral acyclovir (69,70).

Intravenous acyclovir remains the therapy of choice for VZV disease in severely immunocompromised patients, including allogeneic BMT patients within 4 months of transplantation, BMT patients with moderate to severe acute or chronic GVHD, or any transplant patient requiring aggressive antirejection therapy. In addition, any transplant patient with suspected visceral dissemination should receive intravenous acyclovir. The recommended dose is 10 mg/kg (or 500 mg/m²) every 8 hours. For less severely immunosuppressed patients, including most SOT and autologous BMT patients, oral therapy with acyclovir (800 mg p.o. 5 times daily), valacyclovir (1,000 mg p.o. t.i.d.), or famciclovir (500 mg p.o. t.i.d.), coupled with close clinical observation, is a reasonable option. Patients should be treated until healing is complete (or a minimum of 10–14 days) to reduce the risk of relapsing disease. When the infection is under control, the patient can be switched from intravenous to oral drug to complete the course of therapy.

Resistance to acyclovir is not seen nearly as often with VZV as it is with HSV (75). Acyclovir-resistant VZV isolates have been identified much more frequently in AIDS patients than in transplant populations (149). On the basis of anecdotal experience, foscarnet is recommended for therapy of disease due to acyclovir-resistant VZV (150).

Prophylaxis of VZV Disease

Drug regimens designed to prevent HSV recurrences in transplant patients will also effectively prevent herpes zoster. Combined results from two placebo-controlled trials of long-term (6 months) acyclovir prophylaxis in BMT patients showed herpes zoster in 11 of 62 placebo recipients (18%) and in none of 62 acyclovir-treated patients (84,89). These studies revealed no negative impact of acyclovir therapy on marrow engraftment or organ rejection. Interestingly, the incidence of zoster increased dramatically after the prophylaxis was discontinued, so that 12 months following transplant the cumulative number of herpes zoster cases was virtually identical between the acyclovir and placebo groups (Fig. 5) (84,89,91,151,152). Nonetheless, acyclovir prophylaxis effectively prevents herpes zoster during the early post-transplant period, when patients are most severely immunosuppressed and are at highest risk for VZV-related complications (153). Studies of prophylactic acyclovir administered for 12 months following transplantation showed the regimen to be highly effective and suggested that the risk of postprophylaxis zoster recurrence may be lower following 12 months of prophylaxis compared with 6 months of prophylaxis (88). Although short-term (≤3 months) acyclovir prophylaxis is almost universally recommended by transplant specialists, there is currently no consensus regarding the relative merits of long-term acyclovir prophylaxis (154).

Prevention of VZV Infections

Serological screening of transplant candidates to determine susceptibility to VZV is essential to guide decision-making regarding immunoprophylaxis. Seronegative transplant patients with a defined exposure to VZV (either to chickenpox or to herpes zoster) should receive varicella-zoster immune globulin (VZIG) to provide passive immunity (155,156). In most cases, VZIG adminis-

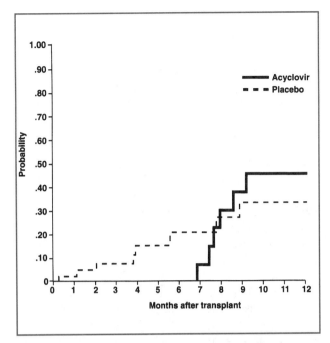

Figure 5. Time-to-event curves showing cumulative risk of herpes zoster in BMT patients receiving prophylaxis with acyclovir (*solid line*) or placebo (*dashed line*) for 6 months (*p* = 0.006 at 6 months; *p* = 0.34 overall). Modified from Selby et al. (153), with permission.

tration will not prevent infection in the susceptible host but will significantly reduce the severity of the resulting illness. Placebo-controlled trials in immunocompromised children have clearly demonstrated that VZIG ameliorates the severity of chickenpox and significantly reduces the risk of disseminated infection (155,156). A single treatment will reduce the risk of disseminated infection by about 75% and will provide 4 weeks of passive immunity. For maximal efficacy, VZIG must be administered as soon as possible after exposure (within at most 96 hours). VZIG is administered by deep intramuscular injection at a dose of 125 units/10 kg, to a maximum of 625 units. Intravenous immunoglobulin (IVIG) also contains substantial amounts of VZV-specific IgG and can be used if VZIG is not immediately available. VZIG is not useful for treatment of established varicella or herpes zoster. Unfortunately, if the VZV exposure is unrecognized, which is often the case, the opportunity for VZIG administration will be missed. The advisability of using acyclovir for postexposure prophylaxis (or preemptive therapy) in seronegative transplant patients who have been exposed to VZV has not determined (157).

A more attractive option for VZV prevention is to use a vaccine to provide active immunity. The VZV$_{Oka}$ live-attenuated virus vaccine has been in use around the world for more than 20 years and was approved in 1995 for administration to immunocompetent children in the United States (158). Concerns about use of the live-attenuated virus vaccine in immunocompromised patients have focused on the potential for the vaccine virus to cause disease and on the possibility that immunocompromised patients will fail to mount a protective immune response (159). Careful trials of VZV_Oka vaccine in leukemic children demonstrated that the vaccine was safe and immunogenic if the patients were at least 1 year away from induction chemotherapy, if they had lymphocyte counts of more than 700/mm³, and if chemotherapy was temporarily suspended around the time of vaccination (160,161). Because of the diminished immune response, administration of two doses of vaccine 3 months apart is recommended.

Preliminary data suggest that VZV_Oka vaccine is safe and effective in SOT patients (162–164). In a study conducted in France, all seronegative renal transplant candidates were given a single dose of the VZV_Oka vaccine; patients who failed to seroconvert received a second dose of the vaccine (162). After vaccination, seropositivity rates at 1 year and 10 years were 62% and 42%, respectively. Following renal transplantation, the incidence of varicella was 12% among vaccinees and 45% among unvaccinated patients with no history of chickenpox (162). Varicella was clinically less severe in the vaccinated population (no deaths) than in the seronegative unvaccinated population (three deaths). Herpes zoster subsequently developed in 13% of the patients with a history of varicella, in 7% of the vaccine recipients, and in 38% of the seronegative unvaccinated patients who developed primary varicella after grafting (162). Another study conducted in Spain showed that VZV_Oka could be safely administered to renal transplant recipients after grafting with good antibody response and with minimal risk (164). In this study, the live-attenuated vaccine was administered without modifying immunosuppressive therapy. Although further studies are necessary, vaccination may play an important role in protecting seronegative transplant patients from VZV infections (165). The safety of live virus vaccines in highly immunosuppressed patients (e.g., allogeneic BMT recipients) has not yet been assessed. Compared with the expense of VZIG or treatment of varicella, immunization would be highly cost-effective (166).

Adult transplant patients are latently infected with VZV and at risk for herpes zoster. Due to concerns regarding use of live virus vaccine after BMT a novel approach to preventing herpes zoster is the use of a heat-inactivated VZV vaccine to boost cellular immune response and, thus, prevent virus reactivation (167). Seventy-five BMT patients were randomized to receive heat-inactivated VZV vaccine or placebo at 1, 2, and 3 months after transplantation. Compared with the placebo group, the vaccine recipients had an identical incidence of herpes zoster (22%), but disease severity was dramatically decreased (167). T-cell recognition of VZV proteins in BMT patients does not usually recover until there has been a reexposure to VZV antigens via reactivation (111). Use of the heat-inactivated vaccine could provide an alternative method of antigen exposure, leading to early restoration of immunity and modification of the severity of subsequent herpes zoster.

HUMAN HERPESVIRUS-6

A previously unknown virus was isolated from peripheral blood lymphocytes from six patients with lymphoproliferative disorders in 1986 (168). The presence of an icosahedral nucleocapsid containing 162 capsomeres plus a genome of double-stranded DNA marked the isolate as a herpesvirus, now known as human herpesvirus-6. HHV-6 is classified as a beta herpesvirus and is most closely related to CMV and HHV-7 (169). Two antigenically distinct variants of HHV-6 have been identified, designated as HHV-6A and HHV-6B (170). HHV-6B was proven to be the etiologic agent of exanthem subitum (roseola), a common and benign childhood disease (171). Although information remains incomplete, a growing body of data has linked HHV-6 to disease in the immunocompromised host, including patients with AIDS and organ transplant recipients (172).

Epidemiology

HHV-6 infection is endemic in humans, with high seroprevalence rates in all populations studied to date. The vast majority of primary HHV-6 infections occur during the first year of life (173). Seroprevalence rates are 90% by age 12 months and virtually 100% by age 3 years (174,175). Infection is likely transmitted by virus shed in the oral secretions of adults or other children (176).

Pathogenesis

The cell types that support initial viral replication and subsequent latency have not been fully identified. Potential sites of latency include epithelial cells of the oropharynx or the upper respiratory tract, salivary glands, or mononuclear cells (lymphocytes, monocytes, or macrophages) in blood or lymphoidal tissue (177). The primary target cells for HHV-6 replication is CD4⁺ T-lymphocytes, although the virus can replicate in human CD8⁺ lymphocytes, NK cells, and macrophages (178). HHV-6 is a potent inducer of cytokine production, and infection can result in profound suppression of the cellular immune system (179,180). A potential role for HHV-6 as a cofactor in the pathogenesis of AIDS is undergoing active investigation (181–184). By virtue of its immunosuppressive activity, HHV-6 may predispose the host to enhanced pathogenic effects of other viruses such as CMV or EBV (185–187).

Clinical Course and Natural History of HHV-6 Disease

Primary HHV-6 infections are usually asymptomatic. The most common clinical manifestation of infection is exanthem subitum, a self-limited illness of small children characterized by fever and a macular rash (188). HHV-6 is also the probable cause of a syndrome of childhood encephalitis with febrile convulsions (189,190) and of a mononucleosis-like syndrome in older children and adults (191). An etiologic role for HHV-6 in neurological disorders, including multiple sclerosis, has been postulated (192).

HHV-6 has been linked to a variety of clinical manifestations in organ transplant recipients, although a causal role for HHV-6 was not always proven. HHV-6 typically becomes detectable in blood about 2–4 weeks following transplantation. Infection has been documented in 38% to 60% of BMT recipients, 38% to 55% of renal transplant recipients, and 28% to 31% of liver transplant recipients (186,193–200). HHV-6 infection in adult organ transplant recipients likely results from reactivation of latent infection (194,197,201). However, at least two instances of probable HHV-6 transmission via the donor organ have been reported (198,202,203).

HHV-6 disease in transplant patients may present with high fever, often with temperatures in excess of 40–41°C (204,205). In BMT patients, a diffuse, erythematous, macular rash has been reported in many patients with documented HHV-6 viremia, although the virus has not been isolated from skin biopsies (194,195). In studies reported from Japan, HHV-6 was isolated from peripheral blood or bone marrow of 18 of 44 (41%) and 10 of 25 (40%) BMT patients. Fever with rash was reported from 33% of the viremic patients (194,195). Initiation or exacerbation of GVHD by HHV-6 has been suggested (206).

In BMT patients, HHV-6 infection has been associated with bone marrow suppression (193,207), although other investigators have failed to confirm the observation (200). HHV-6 was isolated from blood of six of 16 (38%) adult BMT patients; four of the six viremic patients (67%) experienced idiopathic marrow suppression, compared with one of 10 nonviremic patients (193). HHV-6-associated marrow suppression is characterized by leukopenia (83% of cases), thrombocytopenia (67%), and anemia (50%), and ranges from mild and transient to severe and protracted suppression (172,208). Febrile illness with cytopenias has also been associated with HHV-6 disease in liver and renal transplant patients (205,209–211). The clinical course of HHV-6-induced marrow suppression may differ according to the HHV-6 variant involved. HHV-6B is most commonly associated with mild to moderate chronic marrow suppression, whereas HHV-6A may cause acute, severe aplastic anemia (207,208,212,213).

Interstitial pneumonia occurring within the first month after bone marrow transplantation has been attributed to HHV-6 infection (214–216). Investigators have identified HHV-6 in lung tissue by immunohistochemical staining, PCR, and viral cultures of bronchoalveolar lavage fluid. However, HHV-6 infection is universal, and asympto-

matic reactivation is common in immunocompromised patients, so viral isolation in the setting of pneumonitis does not necessarily prove an etiologic association. The importance of HHV-6 as a pulmonary pathogen in transplant patients has not yet been fully delineated (217).

Accumulating evidence suggests that HHV-6 may also be an important cause of encephalitis in transplant patients. In a retrospective study, investigators used PCR to assay cerebrospinal fluid (CSF) from BMT patients with CNS symptoms of unknown etiology and found six of 12 positive for HHV-6 DNA (218). The six PCR-positive patients had clinical evidence of encephalitis, including altered mental status, focal neurological abnormalities, seizures, abnormal EEGs, and elevated CSF protein. One case report described an allogeneic BMT patient with HHV-6 viremia who was admitted with progressive deterioration in mental status and subsequently died. Histopathological studies showed necrosis in the gray matter of the left hippocampal gyrus and of the white matter of the frontal lobe with associated loss of neurons and demyelination; HHV-6B-infected cells were detected throughout the necrotic tissue by immunohistochemical staining (219). Anecdotal reports have suggested clinical benefit from ganciclovir or foscarnet therapy in transplant patients with HHV-6 encephalitis (218,220). Further studies are required to define the incidence and spectrum of HHV-6 infection of the central nervous system in transplant patients.

Diagnosis of HHV-6 Infection

Susceptibility to HHV-6 infection can be determined serologically by ELISA (221,222). However, virtually all transplant patients have been seropositive since early childhood, so serological testing is not helpful in the diagnosis of active HHV-6 disease. HHV-6 can be cultured *in vitro* in a variety of cell lines of lymphocyte origin (207,223). Unfortunately, HHV-6 culture is slow (median time to appearance of CPE is 11 days), technically demanding, and not widely available (172). A rapid shell-vial culture using monoclonal antibodies against HHV-6 immediate-early proteins to detect virus has been described (224). PCR can be used to detect HHV-6 DNA in tissues or body fluids (196,225). Unfortunately, neither culture nor PCR can reliably distinguish between subclinical viral shedding and active disease. PCR detection of free virus in plasma may provide a more specific method for diagnosing active disease (196).

Therapy of HHV-6 Infection

No prospective controlled trials of antiviral therapy for HHV-6 infections in transplant patients have been published. *In vitro*, antiviral susceptibility patterns of HHV-6 closely resemble those of CMV. Both ganciclovir and foscarnet have good activity against HHV-6 at concentrations readily achievable in human plasma by standard dosing (226–228). There are anecdotal reports of successful ganciclovir therapy of HHV-6 disease in transplant patients (204,205). Concentrations of acyclovir required to inhibit HHV-6 are beyond the achievable therapeutic range, although one study has reported efficacy of acyclovir for prophylaxis of HHV-6 infections in allogeneic BMT patients (229). Prophylactic approaches to HHV-6 disease using ganciclovir (intravenous or oral) have not been tested.

HUMAN HERPESVIRUS-7

HHV-7 was first isolated in 1990 from cultures of CD4$^+$ T-lymphocytes (230). As seen with HHV-6, HHV-7 primarily infects CD4$^+$ T-cells and the CD4 molecule appears to be a component of the HHV-7 receptor (231,232). Potential interactions among HHV-6, HHV-7, and HIV (all of which infect CD4$^+$ lymphocytes) are under investigation (232,233).

HHV-7 is probably transmitted by oral secretions. Using PCR techniques, HHV-7 DNA can be detected in saliva specimens from 55% to 95% of healthy adults (234). Primary HHV-7 infection usually occurs in early childhood, although the median age at seroconversion for HHV-7 (17 months) is slightly older than that reported for HHV-6 (11 months) (235). More than 90% of adults are seropositive for HHV-7 (236).

Clinical manifestations of HHV-7 infection are poorly defined (237). A few cases of a roseola-like syndrome occurring in conjunction with primary HHV-7 have been described (235). HHV-7 may also account for some cases of febrile convulsions in children (238). What diseases, if any, HHV-7 may cause in organ transplant recipients remain to be elucidated. There are currently no recommendations for therapy or prophylaxis of HHV-7 infections.

HUMAN HERPESVIRUS-8

Prior to the onset of the AIDS pandemic, Kaposi's sarcoma (KS) was a well-described but rare skin tumor occurring in a classic form in elderly men of Mediterranean extraction and an endemic form in subpopulations of African men (239). In the early 1980s, large numbers of cases of KS were noted in patients subsequently shown to be infected with HIV (240). Kaposi's sarcoma rapidly emerged as the most common opportunistic malignancy among HIV-infected patients, although the incidence of KS now appears to be declining with the advent of more effective antiretroviral therapy. In 1994 researchers using the technique of representational difference analysis isolated two novel DNA fragments from KS lesions of AIDS patients (241). Sequence analysis of these fragments demonstrated a high degree of homology with known sequences from gamma herpesviruses such as EBV. The

new virus was labeled Kaposi's sarcoma–associated herpesvirus (KSHV), or human herpesvirus-8 (HHV-8). A growing body of evidence implicates HHV-8 as the probable etiologic pathogen for KS and body cavity lymphomas in patients with AIDS (242–244), endemic and classical KS (245–247), and multicentric Castleman's disease (248).

Epidemiology

Serological studies of the prevalence and incidence of HHV-8 infection have been hampered by the lack of a sensitive and specific assay. There are some discrepancies among the available seroepidemiological reports, but a pattern appears to be emerging (249–251). HHV-8-specific antibody is detectable in 83% to 100% of patients with KS, including AIDS patients and HIV-negative African patients with endemic KS. Among homosexual American men with AIDS but without KS, the HHV-8 seroprevalence rates have ranged from 30% to 90% (249–251). However, much lower rates are reported for women with AIDS and for patients who acquired HIV infection by parenteral blood exposure such as hemophiliacs (0 to 3% HHV-8 positive) and recipients of HIV-positive blood (5%) (249,250). Similarly, the incidence of KS in homosexual men with AIDS is higher than that in HIV-positive hemophiliacs (242,252). Seroprevalence rates in the general population (e.g., blood donors) have ranged from 0 to 25%, likely representing differences in antibody assay methodology (249–251). In one study, HHV-8 seroprevalence in healthy children was 2% to 8%, but increased to 25% by adulthood (251).

Pathogenesis of HHV-8 Infections

The route of transmission of HHV-8 is not known with certainty, although the seroepidemiology studies cited earlier strongly suggest sexual transmission and the virus has been identified in human semen and prostatic tissue (253). The tissues that support primary viral replication and latency have not yet been identified. HHV-8 sequences can be detected in peripheral blood mononuclear cells of patients with KS, and the virus appear to preferentially infect CD19$^+$ B-lymphocyte subsets (243). In cells of KS lesions, HHV-8 gene expression is highly limited, suggesting a latent rather than a lytic infection (254). Studies of the biology of HHV-8 will be greatly assisted by newly described methods for *in vitro* culture of the virus (255).

In vitro studies have revealed a tight association between HHV-8 and KS. Using PCR, HHV-8 DNA was identified in 97% of 224 KS lesions, but in only 2% of 449 control tissues (242). An etiologic role for HHV-8 is also suggested by the presence of the virus in peripheral blood mononuclear cells, which precedes and predicts the risks of subsequent development of KS (242). HHV-8 is present in virtually all body cavity lymphomas from AIDS patients but not in lymphomas of other histologic types (256). Among organ transplant recipients, HHV-8 sequences can be identified from KS lesions but not from other opportunistic malignancies (257,258). KS biopsies from SOT recipients were analyzed by PCR and HHV-8 sequences were identified in 27 of 28 specimens (259).

KS in Organ Transplant Patients

A study from the Toronto Hospital of 2,099 SOT recipients transplanted between 1981 and 1985 found 12 cases of KS, for an incidence of 0.5% (260). In that series of 12 KS patients, eight were male, nine were of Italian origin, six had cutaneous KS only (all renal transplant patients), and three had visceral KS (260). Transplant-associated KS has been most frequently reported among renal transplant patients (261–263), but smaller numbers of cases have also been reported following liver (264–267), heart (261), lung (268), and both autologous and allogeneic bone marrow transplants (269–272). The usual presentation of KS in transplant patients is the appearance of painless purplish cutaneous macules or plaques, usually occurring months to years after transplantation (273,274). In most cases, the initial lesion is solitary or limited to a few lesions in a localized area. These may remain localized or progress to further cutaneous or visceral dissemination. Occasionally, patients will present with a more aggressive form of KS characterized by large numbers of lesions and rapid progression (273,274). Cases of visceral KS without cutaneous involvement also occasionally occur and may be very difficult to diagnose (266,268).

Patients who have had previous episodes of KS are at high risk for recurrence if resubjected to intensive immunosuppressive therapy. In a series reported from Belgium, four patients with prior histories of KS underwent a second renal transplant (263). KS had been in remission for periods ranging from 5 months to 19 years, yet all four patients developed recurrent KS within months of retransplantation. All required reduced immunosuppression for control of the KS, and three of the patients lost the grafts (263). Careful consideration of the risks of KS recurrence must be given when considering retransplanting a patient with a history of KS.

Diagnosis of HHV-8 Infections

HHV-8-induced malignancies such as KS are routinely diagnosed by lesion biopsy and histopathological examination. Serological assays to assess prior HHV-8 infection have been described (251) but are not widely available and require further validation to fully document their sensitivity and specificity. Quantitative competitive PCR methodologies for detection of HHV-8 have been developed and represent a promising diagnostic approach (275). In one case report, HHV-8 viral load in blood correlated with the clinical course of KS in a renal transplant patient (275). Culture of HHV-8 is currently a research tool only (255).

Treatment and Prevention of HHV-8 Infection

From the limited information available regarding the pathogenesis of HHV-8 disease, there is little to suggest that lytic viral replication plays an active role in the process of malignant transformation. Mechanisms by which HHV-8 might contribute to KS tumorigenesis are not known but are the subject of active investigation. Since available antiviral drugs are only active against replicating virus, it seems unlikely that antiviral therapy will play a major role in treatment of HHV-8-induced malignancies. A more likely role for antiviral drugs would be as prophylaxis to suppress HHV-8 and prevent KS development. Some retrospective observational studies in AIDS patients showed a trend toward reduction of KS risks in patients receiving ganciclovir or foscarnet, although the differences were not statistically significant (276). *In vitro*, HHV-8 is susceptible to ganciclovir, foscarnet, and cidofovir but is resistant to acyclovir (277). At this time, there is no indication for antiviral treatment or prophylaxis for HHV-8 infection.

The primary therapeutic approach for KS lesions in organ transplant recipients is reduction in immunosuppressive therapy (260). Although approximately 50% of KS lesions will regress or disappear with reduction of immunosuppression, this places the patient at significant risk for organ rejection (260). Patients who fail to improve with reduced immunosuppression can be treated with conventional chemotherapy (e.g., doxyrubicin plus bleomycin plus vincristine), local radiation therapy, or interferon (260,265,278,279).

REFERENCES

1. Armstrong JA, Evans AS, Raon HM. Viral infections in renal transplant recipients. *Infect Immun* 1976;14:970–975.
2. Zaia JA. Infections in organ transplant recipients. In: Richman DD, Whitley RJ, Hayden FG, eds. *Clinical virology.* New York: Churchill-Livingston; 1997:87–112.
3. Roizman B. The family Herpesviridae. In: Roizman B, Whitley RJ, Lopez C, eds. *The human herpesvirus.* New York: Raven Press; 1993: 1–9.
4. Roizman B, Sears AE. Herpes simplex viruses and their replication. In: Fields BN, Knipe DM, Howley PM, eds. *Field's virology,* 3rd ed. Philadelphia: Lippincott-Raven; 1995:2231–2295.
5. Corey L, Spear PG. Infections with herpes simplex viruses (Part 1). *N Engl J Med* 1986;314:686–691.
6. Bader C, Crumpacker CS, Schnipper LE, et al. The natural history of recurrent facial-oral infection with herpes simplex virus. *J Infect Dis* 1978;879–905.
7. Spruance SL, Overall JC, Kern ER, Krueger GG, Pliam V, Miller W. The natural history of recurrent herpes simplex labialis. *N Engl J Med* 1977;297:69–75.
8. Corey L, Adams HG, Brown ZA, Holmes KK. Genital herpes simplex virus infections: clinical manifestations, course, and complications. *Ann Intern Med* 1983;98:958–972.

9. Mertz GJ, Benedetti J, Ashley R, Selke SA, Corey L. Risk factors for the sexual transmission of genital herpes. *Ann Intern Med* 1992;116: 197–202.

10. Fleming DT, McQuillan GM, Johnson RE, et al. Herpes simplex virus type 2 in the United States, 1976 to 1994. *N Engl J Med* 1997;337: 1105–1111.

11. Rosenthal SL, Stanberry LR, Biro FM, et al. Seroprevalence of herpes simplex virus types 1 and 2 and cytomegalovirus in adolescents. *Clin Infect Dis* 1997;24:135–139.

12. Meyers JD. Treatment of herpesvirus infections in the immunocompromised host. *Scand J Infect Dis* 1985;47:128–136.

13. Saral R, Burns WH, Laskin OL, Santos GW, Lietman PS. Acyclovir prophylaxis of herpes simplex virus infections: a randomized, double-blind controlled trial in bone marrow transplant recipients. *N Engl J Med* 1981;305:63–67.

14. Korsager B, Spencer ES, Mordhorst CH. Herpesvirus hominis infection in renal transplant recipients. *Scand J Infect Dis* 1975;7:11–19.

15. Naraqi S, Jackson GG, Jonasson OM. Viremia with herpes simplex type 1 in adults. *Ann Intern Med* 1976;85:165–169.

16. Koneru B, Tzakis AG, Depuydt LE, et al. Transmission of fatal herpes simplex infection through renal transplantation. *Transplantation* 1988;45:653–666.

17. Kusne S, Schwartz M, Breinig MK, et al. Herpes simplex hepatitis after solid organ transplantation in adults. *J Infect Dis* 1991;163: 1001–1007.

18. Pass RF, Long WK, Whitley RJ, et al. Productive infection with cytomegalovirus and herpes simplex in renal transplant recipients: role of source of kidney. *J Infect Dis* 1978;137:556–563.

19. Dummer JS, Armstrong J, Somers J, et al. Transmission of infection with herpes simplex virus by renal transplantation. *J Infect Dis* 1987; 155:202–206.

20. Holland HK, Wingard JR, Saral R. Herpesvirus and enteric viral infections in bone marrow transplantation; clinical presentations, pathogenesis, and therapeutic strategies. *Cancer Invest* 1990;8: 509–521.

21. Wade JC, Day LM, Crowley JJ, Meyers JD. Recurrent infections with herpes simplex virus after marrow transplantation: role of the specific immune response and acyclovir treatment. *J Infect Dis* 1984;149: 750–756.

22. Englehard D, Marks MI, Good RA. Infections in bone marrow transplant recipients. *J Pediatr* 1986;108:335–346.

23. Rand KH, Rasmussen LE, Pollard RB, Arvin AM, Merigan TC. Cellular immunity and herpes virus infections in cardiac transplant patients. *N Engl J Med* 1977;296:1372–1377.

24. Meyers JD, Flournoy N, Thomas ED. Infection with herpes simplex virus and cell-mediated immunity after marrow transplantation. *J Infect Dis* 1980;142:338–346.

25. Prentice HG, Hann IM. Antiviral therapy in the immunocompromised patient. *Br Med J* 1985;41:367–373.

26. Breinig MK, Zitelli B, Starzl TE, Ho M. Epstein-Barr virus, cytomegalovirus, and other viral infections in children after liver transplantation. *J Infect Dis* 1987;156:273–279.

27. Winston DJ, Emmanouiliades C, Busuttil RW. Infections in liver transplant recipients. *Clin Infect Dis* 1995;21:1077–1091.

28. Kusne S, Dummer JS, Singh N, et al. Infections after liver transplantation: an analysis of 101 consecutive cases. *Medicine* 1988;67: 132–143.

29. Winston DJ, Ho WG, Champlin RE, Gale RD. Infectious complications of bone marrow transplantation. *Exp Hematol* 1984;12:205–215.

30. Chou S, Gallagher JG, Merigan TC. Controlled trial of intravenous acyclovir in heart transplant patients with mucocutaneous herpes simplex infections. *Lancet* 1981;1:1392–1394.

31. Singh N, Dummer JS, Kusne S, et al. Infections with cytomegalovirus and other herpesviruses in 121 liver transplant recipients: transmission by donated organ and effect of OKT3 antibodies. *J Infect Dis* 1988;158:124–131.

32. Whitley RJ, Levin M, Barton N, et al. Infections caused by herpes simplex virus in the immunocompromised host: natural history and topical acyclovir therapy. *J Infect Dis* 1984;150:323–329.

33. Crosby DL, Jones JH, Sussman M. Herpetic naso-oral ulcers after renal transplantation. *Lancet* 1969;2:1191–1191.

34. Stone WJ, Scowden EB, Spannuth CL, Lowry SP, Alford RH. Atypical herpesvirus hominis type 2 infection in uremic patients receiving immunosuppressive therapy. *Am J Med* 1977;63:511–516.

35. Winston DJ, Gale RP, Meyer DV, Young LS. Infectious complications of human bone marrow transplantation. *Medicine* 1979;58:1–31.

36. Sable CA, Donowitz GR. Infections in bone marrow transplant recipients. *Clin Infect Dis* 1994;18:273–284.

37. Bhart CG. Persistent cutaneous herpes simplex infection. *Int J Dermatol* 1981;20:552–554.

38. Linneman CC, First MR, Alvira MM, Alexander JW, Schiff GM. Herpesvirus hominis type 2 meningoencephalitis following renal transplantation. *Am J Med* 1976;61:703–708.

39. Rubin RH, Tolkoff-Rubin NE. Viral infection in the renal transplant patient. *Proc Eur Dial Transplant Assoc* 1982;19:513–528.

40. Gomez E, Melon S, Aguado S, et al. Herpes simplex virus encephalitis in a renal transplant patient: diagnosis by polymerase chain reaction detection of HSV DNA. *Am J Kidney Dis* 1997;30:423–427.

41. McDonald GB, Sharma P, Hackman RC, Meyers JD, Thomas ED. Esophageal infections in immunosuppressed patients after marrow transplantation. *Gastroenterology* 1985;88:1111–1117.

42. Warren KG, Brown SM, Wroblewska Z, Gilden D, Koprowski H, Subak-Sharpe J. Isolation of latent herpes simplex virus from the superior cervical and vagus ganglion of human beings. *New Engl J Med* 1978;298:1068–1070.

43. Nash G, Ross JS. Herpetic esophagitis—a common cause of esophageal ulceration. *Hum Pathol* 1974;5:339–345.

44. Naik HR, Siddique N, Chandrasekar PH. Foscarnet therapy for acyclovir-resistant herpes simplex virus 1 infection in allogeneic bone marrow transplant recipients. *Clin Infect Dis* 1995;21:1514–1515.

45. Ramsey PG, Fife KH, Hackman RC, Meyers JD, Corey L. Herpes simplex virus pneumonia: clinical, virological, and pathological features in 20 patients. *Ann Intern Med* 1982;97:813–820.

46. Smyth RL, Higenbottam TW, Scott JP, et al. Herpes simplex virus infection in heart-lung transplant recipients. *Transplantation* 1990; 49:735–739.

47. Ramsey PG, Rubin RH, Tolkoff-Rubin NE, Cosimi AB, Russell PS, Greene R. The renal transplant patient with fever and pulmonary infiltrations: etiology, clinical manifestations, and management. *Medicine* 1980;59:206–222.

48. Scott JP, Fradet G, Smyth RL, Solis E, Higenbottam TW, Wallwork J. Management following heart and lung transplantation: five years experience. *Eur J Cardiothorac Surg* 1990;4:197–200.

49. Douglas RG, Anderson MS, Weg JG, et al. Herpes simplex virus pneumonia-occurrence in an allotransplanted lung. *JAMA* 1969;210: 902–904.

50. Dummer JS, Montero CG, Griffith BP, Hardesty RL, Paradis IL, Ho M. Infections in heart-lung transplant recipients. *Transplantation* 1986;41:725–729.

51. Johnson JR, Egaas S, Gleaves CA, Hackman R, Bowden RA. Hepatitis due to herpes simplex virus in marrow transplant recipients. *Clin Infect Dis* 1992;14:38–45.

52. Montgomerie JZ, Becroft DMO, Croxson MC, Doak PB, North JDK. Herpes simplex virus infection after renal transplantation. *Lancet* 1969;2:867–871.

53. Sopko J, Anuras S. Liver disease in renal transplant recipients. *Am J Med* 1978;64:139–146.

54. Elliott WC, Houghton DC, Bryant RE, Wicklund R, Barry JM, Bennett WM. Herpes simplex type 1 hepatitis in renal transplantation. *Arch Intern Med* 1980;140:1656–1660.

55. Taylor RJ, Saul SH, Dowling JN, Hakala TR, Peel RL, Ho M. Primary disseminated herpes simplex infection with fulminant hepatitis following renal transplantation. *Arch Intern Med* 1981;141:1519–1521.

56. Anuras S, Summers R. Fulminant herpes simplex hepatitis in an adult: report of a case in renal transplant recipient. *Gastroenterology* 1976; 70:425–428.

57. Holdsworth SR, Atkins RC, Scott DF, Hayes K. Systemic herpes simplex infection with fulminant hepatitis post-transplantation. *Aust NZ J Med* 1976;6:588–590.

58. Chase RA, Pottage JC, Haber MH, Kistler G, Jensen D, Levin S. Herpes simplex viral hepatitis in adults: two case reports and review of the literature. *Rev Infect Dis* 1987;9:328–333.

59. Arvin AM, prober CC. Herpes Simplex Viruses. In: Murray PR, Baron EJ, Pfaller MA, Tenover FC, Yolken RH, eds. *Manual of clinical m microbiology,* 6th ed. Washington, D.C.: ASM Press; 1995: 876–883.

60. Lafferty WE, Krofft S, Remington M, et al. Diagnosis of herpes simplex virus by direct immunofluorescence and viral isolation from

samples of external genital lesions in a high prevalence population. *J Clin Microbiol* 1987;25:323–326.

61. Lakeman FD, Whitley RJ, the NIAID Collaborative Antiviral Study Group. Diagnosis of herpes simplex encephalitis: application of polymerase chain reaction to cerebrospinal fluid from brain biopsied patients and correlation with disease. *J Infect Dis* 1995;171:857–863.

62. Cone RW, Hobson AC, Palmer J, Remington M, Corey L. Extended duration of herpes simplex virus DNA in genital lesions detected by the polymerase chain reaction. *J Infect Dis* 1991;164:757–760.

63. Cheeseman SH, Rubin RH, Stewart JA, et al. Controlled clinical trial of human leucocyte interferon in renal transplantation. Effect on cytomegalovirus and herpes simplex virus infection. *N Engl J Med* 1979;300:1345–1349.

64. Whitley RJ, Spruance S, Hayden FG. Vidarabine therapy for mucocutaneous herpes simplex virus infections in the immunocompromised host. *J Infect Dis* 1984;149:1–8.

65. Selby PJ, Powles RL, Jameson B, et al. Parenteral acyclovir therapy for herpesvirus infections in man. *Lancet* 1979;12:1267–1270.

66. Straus SE, Smith HA, Brickman C, Miranda DP, McLaren C, Keeney RE. Acyclovir for chronic mucocutaneous herpes simplex virus infection in immunosuppressed patients. *Ann Intern Med* 1982;96:270–277.

67. Meyers JD, Wade K, Mitchell CD, et al. Multicenter collaborative trial of intravenous acyclovir for treatment of mucocutaneous herpes simplex virus infection in the immunocompromised host. *Am J Med* 1982;73[Suppl 1A]:229–235.

68. Shepp DH, Newton BA, Dardliker PS, Flournoy N, Meyers JD. Oral acyclovir therapy for mucocutaneous herpes simplex virus infections in immunocompromised marrow transplant recipients. *Ann Intern Med* 1985;102:783–785.

69. Beutner KR, Friedman DJ, Forszpaniak C, Anderson PL, Wood MJ. Valaciclovir compared with acyclovir for improved therapy for herpes zoster in immunocompetent adults. *Antimicrob Agents Chemother* 1995;39:1546–1553.

70. Cirelli R, Herne K, McCrary M, Lee P, Tyring SK. Famciclovir: a review of clinical efficacy and safety. *Antiviral Res* 1996;29:141–151.

71. Gäbel H, Flamholc L, Ahlfors K. Herpes simplex virus hepatitis in a renal transplant recipient: successful treatment with acyclovir. *Scand J Infect Dis* 1988;20:435–438.

72. Wade JC, McLaren C, Meyers JD. Frequency and significance of acyclovir-resistant herpes simplex virus isolated from marrow transplant patients receiving multiple course of treatment with acyclovir. *J Infect Dis* 1983;148:1077–1082.

73. Ljungman P, Ellis MN, Hackman RC, Shepp DH, Meyers JD. Acyclovir-resistant herpes simplex virus causing pneumonia after marrow transplantation. *J Infect Dis* 1990;162:244–248.

74. Englund JA, Zimmerman ME, Swierkosze U, Goodman JL, Scholl DR, Balfour HH. Herpes simplex virus resistant to acyclovir: a study in a tertiary care center. *Ann Intern Med* 1990;112:416–422.

75. Reusser P, Cordonnier C, Einsele H, et al. European survey of herpesvirus resistance to antiviral drugs in bone marrow transplant recipients. *Bone Marrow Transplant* 1996;17:813–817.

76. Sacks SL, Wanklin RJ, Reece DE, Hicks KA, Tyler KL, Coen DM. Progressive esophagitis from acyclovir-resistant herpes simplex: clinical roles for DNA polymerase mutants and viral heterogeneity? *Ann Intern Med* 1989;111:893–899.

77. Ambinder RF, Burns WH, Lietman PS, Saral R. Prophylaxis: a strategy to minimise antiviral resistance. *Lancet* 1984;1:1154–1155.

78. Burns WH, Saral R, Santos GW, et al. Isolation and characterisation of resistant herpes simplex virus after acyclovir therapy. *Lancet* 1982;1:421–423.

79. Crumpacker CS, Schnipper PN, Hershey BJ, Levin MJ. Resistance to antiviral drugs of herpes simplex virus isolated from a patient treated with acyclovir. *N Engl J Med* 1982;306:343–346.

80. Chatis PA, Miller CH, Schrager LE, Crumpacker CS. Successful treatment with foscarnet of an acyclovir-resistant mucocutaneous infection with herpes simplex virus in a patient with acquired immunodeficiency syndrome. *N Engl J Med* 1989;320:297–300.

81. Safrin S, Crumpacker C, Chatis P, et al. A controlled trial comparing foscarnet with vidarabine for acyclovir resistant mucocutaneous herpes simplex in the acquired immunodeficiency syndrome. *N Engl J Med* 1991;325:551–555.

82. Taylor CE, Sviland L, Pearson ADJ, et al. Virus infections in bone marrow transplant recipients: a three years prospective study. *J Clin Pathol* 1990;43:633–637.

83. Engelhard D, Morag A, Naparsteck E, et al. Prevention of herpes simplex virus (HSV) infection in recipients of HLA-matched T-lymphocyte-depleted bone marrow allografts. *Isr J Med Sci* 1988;24:145–150.

84. Lundgren G, Wilczek H, Lönnqvist B, Lindholm A, Wahren B, Ringden O. Acyclovir prophylaxis in bone marrow transplant recipients. *Scand J Infect Dis* 1985;47:137–144.

85. Hann IM, Prentice HG, Blacklock HA, et al. Acyclovir prophylaxis against herpes virus infections in severely immunocompromised patients: randomised double blind trial. *Br Med J* 1983;287:384–388.

86. Wade JC, Newton B, Flournoy N, Meyers JD. Oral acyclovir for prevention of herpes simplex virus reactivation after marrow transplantation. *Ann Intern Med* 1984;100:823–828.

87. Shepp DH, Dardliker PS, Flournoy N, Meyers JD. Sequential intravenous and twice-daily oral acyclovir for extended prophylaxis of herpes simplex virus infection in marrow transplant patients. *Transplantation* 1987;43:654–658.

88. Meyers JD. Chemoprophylaxis of viral infection in immunocompromised patients. *Eur J Can Clin Oncol* 1989;25:1369–1374.

89. Perren TJ, Powles RL, Easton D, Stolle K, Selby PS. Prevention of herpes zoster in patients by long-term oral acyclovir after allogenic bone marrow transplantation. *Am J Med* 1988;85 [Suppl. 2A]:99–101.

90. Gold D, Corey L. Acyclovir prophylaxis for herpes simplex virus infections. *Antimicrob Agents Chemother* 1987;31:361–367.

91. Pettersson E, Hovi T, Ahonen J, et al. Prophylactic oral acyclovir after renal transplantation. *Transplantation* 1985;39:279–281.

92. Paya CV, Hermans PE, Washington JA, et al. Incidence, distribution, and outcome of episodes of infection in 100 orthotopic liver transplantations. *Mayo Clin Proc* 1989;64:555–564.

93. Burke RL. Current status of HSV vaccine development. In: Roizman B, Whitley RJ, Lopez C, eds. *The human herpesviruses.* Philadelphia: Lippincott-Raven; 1993:367–379.

94. Yorke JA, London WP. Recurrent outbreaks of measles, chickenpox and mumps II. Systematic differences in contact rates and stochastic effects. *Am J Epdemiol* 1973;469–482.

95. Weller TH. Varicella and herpes zoster: a perspective and overview. *J Infect Dis* 1992;140:S1–S6.

96. Preblud SR, Orensetin WA, Bart KJ. Varicella: clinical manifestations, epidemiology and health impact in children. *Pediatr Infect Dis J* 1984;3:505–509.

97. Donahue JG, Choo PW, Manson JE, Plat R. The incidence of herpes zoster. *Arch Intern Med* 1995;155:1605–1609.

98. Straus SE, Ostrove JM, Inchauspe G, et al. Varicella-zoster virus infections. *Ann Intern Med* 1988;108:221–237.

99. Sawyer MH, Wu YN, Chamberlin CJ, et al. Detection of varicella-zoster virus DNA in the oropharynx and blood of patients with varicella. *J Infect Dis* 1992;166:885–888.

100. Gordon JE. Chickenpox: an epidemiologic review. *Am J Med Sci* 1962;244:362–389.

101. Grose C. Variation on a theme by Fenner: the pathogenesis of chickenpox. *Pediatrics* 1981;68:735–737.

102. Gilden DH, Dueland AN, Devlin ME, Mahalingam R, Cohrs R. Varicella-zoster virus reactivation without rash. *J Infect Dis* 1992;166:S30–S34.

103. Schuchter LM, Wingard JR, Piantadosi S, Burns WH, Santos GW, Saral R. Herpes zoster infection after autologous bone marrow transplantation. *Blood* 1989;74:1424–1427.

104. Christiansen N, Haake R, Hurd D. Early herpes zoster in adult patients with Hodgkin's disease undergoing autologous bone marrow transplantation. *Bone Marrow Transplant* 1991;7:435–437.

105. Locksley RM, Flournoy N, Sullivan KM, Meyers JD. Infection with varicella-zoster virus after marrow transplantation. *J Infect Dis* 1985;152:1172–1181.

106. Atkinson K, Meyers JD, Storb RL, Prentice RL, Thomas ED. Varicella-zoster virus infection after marrow transplantation for aplastic anemia or leukemia. *Transplantation* 1980;29:47–50.

107. Webster A, Grint P, Brenner MK, Prentice HG, Griffiths PD. Titration of IgG antibodies against varicella zoster virus before bone marrow transplantation is not predictive of future zoster. *J Med Virol* 1989;27:117–119.

108. Luby JP, Ramirez-Ronda C, Rinner S, Hull A, Verge-Marini P. A longitudinal study of varicella-zoster virus infections in renal transplant recipients. *J Infect Dis* 1977;135:659–663.

109. Wahren B, Gahrton G, Linde A, et al. Transfer and persistence of viral

antibody-producing cells in bone marrow transplantation. *J Infect Dis* 1984;150:358–365.

110. Meyers JD, Flournoy N, Thomas ED. Cell-mediated immunity to varicella-zoster after allogeneic marrow transplant. *J Infect Dis* 1980; 141(4):479–487.

111. Wilson A, Sharp M, Koronpchak CM, Ting SF, Arvin AM. Subclinical varicella-zoster virus viremia, herpes zoster, and T lymphocyte immunity to varicella-zoster viral antigens after bone marrow transplantation. *J Infect Dis* 1992;165:119–126.

112. Ljungman P, Lönnqvist B, Gahrton G, Ringden O, Sundquist VA, Wahren B. Clinical and subclinical reactivations of varicella-zoster virus in immunocompromised patients. *J Infect Dis* 1986;153(5): 840–847.

113. Rifkind D. The activation of varicella-zoster virus infections by immunosuppressive therapy. *J Lab Clin Med* 1966;68:463–474.

114. Spenser ES, Anderson HK. Clinically evident, non-terminal infection with herpesvirus and wart virus in immunosuppressed renal transplant recipients. *Br Med J* 1970;3:251–254.

115. Tzeng CH, Liu JH, Fan S, et al. Varicella zoster virus infection after allogeneic or autologous hemopoietic stem cell transplantation. *J Formosan Med Assoc* 1995;94:313–317.

116. Schimpff S, Serpick A, Stolar B. Varicella-zoster infection in patients with cancer. *Ann Intern Med* 1972;76:241–254.

117. Atkinson K, Strob R, Prentice RL, et al. Analysis of late infections in 89 long-term survivors of bone marrow transplantation. *Blood* 1979; 53:720–731.

118. Morgan ER, Smalley LA. Varicella in immunocompromised children. *Am J Dis Child* 1983;137:883–885.

119. Parnham AP, Flexman JP, Saker BM, Thatcher GN. Primary varicella in adult renal transplant recipients: a report of three cases plus a review of the literature. *Clin Transplant* 1995;9:115–118.

120. Feldman S, Hughes WT, Daniel CB. Varicella in children with cancer: seventy-seven cases. *Pediatrics* 1975;56:388–397.

121. McGregor RS, Zitelli BJ, Urbach AH, Malatack JJ, Gartner JC. Varicella in pediatric orthotopic liver transplant recipients. *Pediatrics* 1989;83:256–261.

122. Naraqi S, Jackson GG, Jonasson O, Yamashiroya HM. Prospective study of prevalence, incidence, and source of herpesvirus infections in patients with renal allografts. *J Infect Dis* 1977;136:531–540.

123. Clift RA, Buckner CD, Fefer A, et al. Infectious complications of marrow transplantation. *Transplant Proc* 1974;6:389–393.

124. Saral R. Viral infections in bone marrow transplantation recipients. *Plasma Ther Transfus Technol* 1985;6:275–284.

125. Schiller GJ, Nimer SD, Gajewski JL, Golde DW. Abdominal presentation of varicella-zoster infection in recipients of allogenic bone marrow transplantation. *Bone Marrow Transplant* 1991;7:489–491.

126. Gallagher JG, Merigan TC. Prolonged herpes-zoster infection associated with immunosuppressive therapy. *Ann Intern Med* 1979;91: 842–846.

127. Garweg J, Böhnke M. Varicella-zoster virus is strongly associated with atypical necrotizing herpetic retinopathies. *Clin Infect Dis* 1997; 24:603–608.

128. Stemmer SM, Kinsman K, Tellschow S, Jones RB. Fatal noncutaneous visceral infection with varicella-zoster virus in a patient with lymphoma after autologous bone marrow transplant. *Clin Infect Dis* 1993; 16:497–499.

129. Rogers SY, Irving W, Harris A, Russell NH. Visceral varicella zoster infection after bone marrow transplantation without skin involvement and the use of PCR for diagnosis. *Bone Marrow Transplant* 1995;15: 805–807.

130. Gershon AA, Larussa P, Steinberg SP. Varicella-zoster virus. In: Murray PR, Baron EJ, Pfaller MA, Tenover FC, Yolken RH, eds. *Manual of clinical microbiology*, 6th ed. Washington, D.C.: ASM Press; 1995.

131. Weigle KA, Grose C. Common expression of varicella-zoster viral glycoprotein antigens *in vitro* and in chickenpox and zoster vesicles. *J Infect Dis* 1983;148:630–638.

132. Drew WL, Mintz L. Rapid diagnosis of varicella-zoster virus infection by direct immunofluorescence. *Am J Clin Pathol* 1980;73:699–701.

133. Rawlinson WD, Dwyer DE, Gibbons VL, Cunningham AL. Rapid diagnosis of varicella-zoster virus infection with a monoclonal antibody based direct immunofluorescence technique. *J Virol Methods* 1989;23:13–18.

134. Nahass GT, Goldstein BA, Zhu WY, Serfling U, Penneys NS, Leonardi CL. Comparision of Tzanck smear, viral culture, and DNA

135. Shoji J, Honda Y, Murai I, Sata Y, Oizumi K, Hondo R. Detection of varicella-zoster virus DNA by polymerase chain reaction in cerebrospinal fluid of patients with herpes zoster meningitis. *J Neurol* 1992;239:69–70.

136. Schlupen EM, Korting HC, Nachbar F, Volkenandt M. Molecular evidence for the existence of disseminated zoster as a distinct entity in an immunosuppressed renal transplant patient. *J Mol Med* 1995;73: 525–528.

137. Dlugosch D, Eis-Hubinger AM, Kleim JP, Kaiser R, Bierhoff E, Schneweis KE. Diagnosis of acute and latent varicella-zoster virus infections using the polymerase chain reaction. *J Med Virol* 1992;35: 136–141.

138. Wasmuth EW, Miller WJ. Sensitive enzyme-linked immunosorbent assay for antibody to varicella-zoster virus using purified VZV glycoprotein antigen. *J Med Virol* 1990;32:189–193.

139. Shepp DH, Dandliker PS, Meyers JD. Treatment of varicella-zoster infection in severely immunocompromised patients: a randomized comparison of acyclovir and vidarabine. *N Engl J Med* 1986;314: 208–212.

140. Whitley RJ, Gnann JW, Hinthorn D, et al. Disseminated herpes zoster in the immunocompromised host: a comparative trial of acyclovir and vidarabine. *J Infect Dis* 1992;165:450–455.

141. Prober CG, Kirk LE, Keeney RE. Acyclovir therapy of chickenpox in immunosuppressed children—a collaborative study. *J Pediatr* 1982; 101:622–625.

142. Feldman S, Lott L. Varicella in children with cancer: impact of antiviral therapy and prophylaxis. *Pediatrics* 1987;80:465–472.

143. Balfour HH, Bean B, Laskin OL, et al. Acyclovir halts progression of herpes zoster in immunocompromised patients. *N Engl J Med* 1983; 308:1448–1453.

144. Serota FT, Starr SE, Bryan CK, Koch PA, Plotkin SA, August CS. Acyclovir treatment of herpes zoster infections: use in children undergoing bone marrow transplantation. *JAMA* 1982;247:2132–2135.

145. Meyers JD, Wade JC, Shepp DH, Newton B. Acyclovir treatment of varicella-zoster virus infection in the compromised host. *Transplantation* 1984;37:571–574.

146. Ljungman P, Lonnqvist B, Ringden O, Skinhoj P, Gahrton G, and the Nordic Bone Marrow Transplant Group. A randomized trial of oral versus intravenous acyclovir for treatment of herpes zoster in bone marrow transplant recipients. *Bone Marrow Transplant* 1989;4: 613–615.

147. Tyring S, Boon R, Saltzman R. The efficacy and safety of famciclovir for the treatment of herpes zoster in immunocompromised patients. 20th International Congress of Chemotherapy. Sydney, Australia; 1997.[Abstract]

148. Gnann J, Tyring S, Burdge D, et al. Oral antiviral therapy for herpes zoster in immunocompromised patients: soriviudine vs. acyclovir. 35th IDSA. San Francisco; 1997. [Abstract 511]

149. Jacobson MA, Berger TG, Fikrig S, et al. Acyclovir-resistant varicella zoster virus infection after chronic oral acyclovir therapy in patients with the acquired immunodeficiency syndrome (AIDS). *Ann Intern Med* 1990;112:187–191.

150. Smith KJ, Kahlter DC, Davis C, James WD, Skelton HG, Angritt P. Acyclovir-resistant varicella zoster responsive to foscarnet. *Arch Dermatol* 1991;127:1069–1071.

151. Ljungman P, Wilczek H, Gahrton G, et al. Long-term acyclovir prophylaxis in bone marrow transplant recipients and lymphocyte proliferation responses to herpes virus antigens in vitro. *Bone Marrow Transplant* 1986;1:185–192.

152. Sempere A, Sanz GF, Senent L, et al. Long-term acyclovir prophylaxis for prevention of varicella zoster virus infection after autologous blood stem cell transplantation in patients with acute leukemia. *Bone Marrow Transplant* 1992;10:495–498.

153. Selby PJ, Powles RL, Easton D, et al. The prophylactic role of intravenous and long-term oral acyclovir after allogenic bone marrow transplantation. *Br J Cancer* 1989;59:434–438.

154. Momin F, Chandrasekar PH. Antimicrobial prophylaxis in bone marrow transplantation. *Ann Intern Med* 1995;123:205–215.

155. Orenstein WA, Heymann DL, Ellis RJ, et al. Prophylaxis of varicella in high-risk children: dose response effect of zoster immunoglobulin. *J Pediatr* 1981;98:368–373.

156. Zaia JA, Levin MJ, Preblud SR, et al. Evaluation of varicella-zoster

immune globulin: protection of immunosuppressed children after household exposure to varicella. *J Infect Dis* 1983;147:737–743.

157. Asano Y, Yoshikawa T, Suga S, et al. Postexposure prophylaxis of varicella in family contact by oral acyclovir. *Pediatrics* 1993;92:219–222.

158. Committee on Infectious Diseases. Recommendations for the use of live attenuated varicella vaccine. *Pediatrics* 1995;95:791–796.

159. White CJ. Varicella-zoster virus vaccine. *Clin Infect Dis* 1997;24: 753–763.

160. Gershon AA, Steinberg SP, Gelb L, et al. Live attenuated varicella vaccine: efficacy for children with leukemia in remission. *JAMA* 1984;252:355–362.

161. Arbeter AM, Granowetter L, Starr SE, Lange B, Wimmer R, Plotkin SA. Immunization of children with acute lymphoblastic leukemia with live attenuated varicella vaccine without complete suspension of chemotherapy. *Pediatrics* 1990;85:338–344.

162. Broyer M, Tete MJ, Guest G, Gagnadoux MF, Rouzioux C. Varicella and zoster in children after kidney transplantation: long-term results of vaccination. *Pediatrics* 1997;99:35–39.

163. Giacchino R, Marcellini M, Timitilli A, et al. Varicella vaccine in children requiring renal or hepatic transplantation. *Transplantation* 1995;60:1055–1056.

164. Zamora I, Simon JM, DaSilva ME, Piqueras AI. Attenuated varicella virus vaccine in children in renal transplants. *Pediatr Nephrol* 1994;8: 190–192.

165. Gershon AA. Immunizations for pediatric transplant patients. *Kidney Int* 1993;43[Suppl]:S87–S90.

166. Kitai IC, King S, Gafni A. An economic evaluation of varicella vaccine for pediatric liver and kidney transplant recipients. *Clin Infect Dis* 1993;17:441–447.

167. Redman RL, Nader S, Zerboni L. Early reconstitution of immunity and decreased severity of herpes zoster in bone marrow transplant recipients immunized with inactivated varicella vaccine. *J Infect Dis* 1997;176:578–585.

168. Salahuddin SZ, Ablashi DV, Markham PD, et al. Isolation of a new virus, HBLV, in patients with lymphoproliferative disorders. *Science* 1986;234:596–601.

169. Lawrence GL, Chee M, Craxton MA, Gompels UA, Honess RW, Barrell BG. Human herpesvirus 6 is closely related to human cytomegalovirus. *J Virol* 1990;64:287–299.

170. Aubin J-T, Agut H, Collandre H, Chandran B, Montagnier L, Huraux J-M. Antigenic and genetic differentiation of two putative types of human herpesvirus-6. *J Virol Methods* 1993;41:223–234.

171. Yamanishi K, Okuno T, Shiraki K, et al. Identification of human herpesvirus-6 as a causal agent for exanthem subitum. *Lancet* 1988;1: 1065–1067.

172. Singh N, Carrigan DR. Human herpesvirus-6 in transplantation: an emerging pathogen. *Ann Intern Med* 1996;124:1065–1071.

173. Yoshikawa T, Suga S, Asano Y, Yazaki T, Kodama H, Ozaki T. Distribution of antibodies to a causative agent of exanthem subitum (human herpesvirus-6) in healthy individuals. *Pediatrics* 1989;84:675–677.

174. Leach CT, Sumaya CV, Brown NA. Human herpesvirus-6: clinical implications of a recently discovered, ubiquitous agent. *J Pediatr* 1992;121:173–181.

175. Yanagi K, Harada S, Ban F, Oya A, Okaba N, Tobinai K. High prevalence of antibody to human herpesvirus-6 and decrease in titers with increase in age in Japan. *J Infect Dis* 1990;161:153–154.

176. Levy JA, Greenspan D, Ferro F, Lennette ET. Frequent isolation of HHV-6 from saliva and high seroprevalence of the virus in the population. *Lancet* 1990;335:1047–1050.

177. Jarrett RF, Clark DA, Josephs SF, Onions DE. Detection of human herpesvirus-6 DNA in peripheral blood and saliva. *J Med Virol* 1990;32:73–76.

178. Lusso P, Malnati M, De Maria A, et al. Productive infection of CD4$^+$ and CD8$^+$ mature human T cell populations and clones by human herpesvirus 6. Transcriptional down-regulation of CD3. *J Immunol* 1991;147:685–691.

179. Flamand L, Gosselin J, Stefanescu I, Ablashi D, Menezes J. Immunosuppressive effect of human herpesvirus 6 on T-cell functions: suppression of interleukin-2 synthesis and cell proliferation. *Blood* 1995;85:1263–1271.

180. Knox KK, Pietryga D, Harrington DJ, Franciosi R, Carrigan DR. Progressive immunodeficiency and fatal pneumonitis associated with human herpesvirus-6 infection in an infant. *Clin Infect Dis* 1995; 20:406–413.

181. Lusso P, De Maria A, Malnati M, et al. Induction of CD4 and susceptibility to HIV-1 infection in human CD8$^+$ T lymphocytes by human herpesvirus 6. *Nature* 1991;349:533–535.

182. Horvat RT, Wood C, Josephs SF, Balachandran N. Transactivation of the human immunodeficiency virus promoter by human herpesvirus 6 (HHV-6) strains GS and Z-29 in primary human T lymphocytes and identification of transactivating HHV-6 (GS) gene fragments. *J Virol* 1991;65:2895–2902.

183. Wang J, Jones C, Norcross M, Bohnlein E, Razzaque A. Identification and characterization of a human herpesvirus 6 gene segment capable of transactivating the human immunodeficiency virus type 1 long terminal repeat in an Sp1 binding site-dependent manner. *J Virol* 1994;68:1706–1713.

184. Fairfax MR, Schacker T, Cone RW, Collier AC, Corey L. Human herpesvirus 6 DNA in blood cells of human immunodeficiency virus-infected men: correlation of high levels with high CD4 cell counts. *J Infect Dis* 1994;169:1342–1345.

185. Dockrell DH, Prada J, Jones MF, et al. Seroconversion to human herpesvirus 6 following liver transplantation is a marker of cytomegalovirus disease. *J Infect Dis* 1997;176:1135–1140.

186. Herbein G, Strasswimmer J, Altieri M, Woehl-Jaegle ML, Wolf P, Obert G. Longitudinal study of human herpesvirus-6 infection in organ transplant recipients. *Clin Infect Dis* 1996;22:171–173.

187. Desjardin JA, Falagas ME, Gibbons L, et al. Human herpes virus 6 (HHV-6) infection is associated with development of primary cytomegalovirus (CMV) infection and CMV disease in kidney transplantation. 37th ICAAC. Toronto; 1997. [Abstract #H-116]

188. Ueda K, Kushuraha K, Hirose M, et al. Exanthem subitum and antibody to human herpesvirus-6. *J Infect Dis* 1989;159:750–752.

189. Hall CB, Long CE, Schnabel KC, et al. Human herpesvirus-6 infection in children: a prospective study of complications and reactivation. *N Engl J Med* 1994;331:432–438.

190. McCullers JA, Lakeman FD, Whitley RJ. Human herpesvirus 6 is associated with focal encephalitis. *Clin Infect Dis* 1996;21:571–576.

191. Irvin WL, Cunningham AL. Serologic diagnosis of infection with human herpesvirus type 6. *Br Med J* 1990;300:156–159.

192. Soldan SS, Berti R, Salem N, et al. Association of human herpesvirus 6 (HHV-6) with multiple sclerosis: increased IgM response to HHV-6 early antigen and detection of serum HHV-6 DNA. *Nature Med* 1997;3:1394–1397.

193. Drobyski WR, Dunne WM, Burd EM, et al. Human herpesvirus-6 (HHV-6) infection in allogeneic bone marrow transplant recipients: evidence of a marrow-suppressive role for HHV-6 in vivo. *J Infect Dis* 1993;167:735–739.

194. Yoshikawa T, Suga S, Asano Y, et al. Human herpesvirus-6 infection in bone marrow transplantation. *Blood* 1991;78:1381–1384.

195. Frenkel N, Katsafanas GC, Wyatt LS, Yoshikawa T, Asano Y. Bone marrow transplant recipients harbor the B variant of human herpesvirus 6. *Bone Marrow Transplant* 1994;14:839–843.

196. Wilborn F, Brinkmann V, Schmidt CA, Neipel F, Gedlerblom H, Siegert W. Herpesvirus type 6 in patients undergoing bone marrow transplantation: serologic features and detection by polymerase chain reaction. *Blood* 1994;83:3052–3058.

197. Okuno T, Higashi K, Shiraki K, et al. Human herpesvirus 6 infection in renal transplantation. *Transplantation* 1990;49:519–522.

198. Yoshikawa T, Suga S, Asano Y, et al. A prospective study of human herpesvirus-6 infection in renal transplantation. *Transplantation* 1992;54:879–883.

199. Schmidt C, Wilborn F, Oettle H, et al. A prospective study of human herpesvirus type-6 detected by polymerase chain reaction after liver transplantation. *Transplantation* 1996;61:662–664.

200. Kadakia MP, Rybka WB, Stewart JA, et al. Human herpesvirus 6: infection and disease following autologous and allogeneic bone marrow transplantation. *Blood* 1996;87:5341–5354.

201. Robert C, Agut H, Lunell-Fabiani F, P. L. Human herpesvirus-6 and hepatitis in heart transplant recipients. *Presse Med* 1994;23: 1209–1210.

202. Ward KN, Gray JJ, Efstathiou S. Primary human herpesvirus 6 infection in a patient following liver transplantation from a seropositive donor. *J Med Virol* 1989;28:67–72.

203. Hoshino K, Nishi T, Adachi H, et al. Human herpesvirus-6 infection in renal allografts: retrospective immunohistochemical study in Japanese recipients. *Transplant Int* 1995;8:169–173.

204. Jacobs U, Ferber J, Klehr HU. Severe allograft dysfunction after

OKT3-induced human herpes virus-6 reactivation. *Transplant Proc* 1994;26:3121–3121.

205. Singh N, Carrigan DR, Gayowski T, Singh J, Marino IR. Variant B human herpesvirus-6 associated febrile dermatosis with thrombocytopenia and encephalopathy in a liver transplant recipient. *Transplantation* 1995;60:1355–1357.

206. Appleton AL, Sviland L, Peiris JS, et al. Human herpesvirus-6 infection in marrow graft recipients: role in pathogenesis of graft-versus-host disease. *Bone Marrow Transplant* 1995;16:777–782.

207. Carrigan DR, Knox KK. Human herpesvirus-6 (HHV-6) isolation from bone marrow: HHV-6-associated bone marrow suppression in bone marrow transplant patients. *Blood* 1994;84:3307–3310.

208. Knox KK, Carrigan DR. Chronic myelosuppression associated with persistent bone marrow infection due to human herpesvirus-6 in a bone marrow transplant recipient. *Clin Infect Dis* 1996;22:174–175.

209. Morris DJ, Littler E, Arrand J, Jordan D, Mallick NP, Johnson RW. Human herpesvirus 6 infection in renal-transplant recipients (letter). *N Engl J Med* 1989;320:1560–1561.

210. Singh N, Carrigan DR, Gayowski T, Marino IR. Human herpesvirus-6 infection in liver transplant recipients: documentation of pathogenicity. *Transplantation* 1997;64:674–678.

211. Chang FY, Singh N, Gayowski T, Wagener MM, Marino IR. Fever in liver transplant recipients: changing spectrum of etiologic agents. *Clin Infect Dis* 1998;26:59–65.

212. Rosenfeld CS, Rybka WB, Weinbaum D, et al. Late graft failure due to dual bone marrow infection with variant A and B of human herpesvirus-6. *Exp Hematol* 1995;23:626–269.

213. Carrigan DR. Human herpesvirus-6 and bone marrow transplantation (letter). *Blood* 1995;85:294–295.

214. Carrigan DR, Drobyski WR, Russler SK, Tapper MA, Knox KK, Ash RC. Interstitial pneumonitis associated with human herpesvirus-6 infection after marrow transplantation. *Lancet* 1991;338:147–149.

215. Cone RW, Huang ML, Hackman RC. Human herpesvirus 6 and pneumonia. *Leuk Lymphoma* 1994;15:235–241.

216. Cone RW, Hackman RC, Huang ML, et al. Human herpesvirus 6 in lung tissue from patients with pneumonitis after bone marrow transplantation. *N Engl J Med* 1993;329:156–161.

217. Cone RW. Human herpesvirus 6 as a possible cause of pneumonia. *Semin Respir Infect* 1995;10:254–258.

218. Ljungman P, Wang F-Z, Linde A, et al. Human herpesvirus 6 (HHV-6) encephalitis in allogeneic BMT recipients [Abstract]. *Blood* 1997;90 [Suppl 1]:543a.

219. Drobyski WR, Knox KK, Majewski D, Carrigan DR. Brief report: fatal encephalitis due to variant B human herpesvirus-6 infection in a bone marrow-transplant recipient. *N Engl J Med* 1994;330:1356–1360.

220. Rieux C, Gautheret-Dejean A, Challine-Lehman D, et al. Human herpes virus 6 (HHV6) disseminated infection with meningoencephalitis in an allogeneic bone marrow transplant patient. 37th ICAAC. Toronto; 1997. [Abstract # H-117]

221. Chou SW, Scott KM. Rises in antibody to human herpesvirus 6 detected by enzyme immunoassay in transplant patients with primary cytomegalovirus infection. *J Clin Microbiol* 1990;28:851–854.

222. Sloots TP, Kapeleris JP. Evaluation of a commercial enzyme-linked immunosorbent assay for detection of serum immunoglobulin-G response to human herpesvirus-6. *J Clin Microbiol* 1996;34:675–679.

223. Drobyski WR, Eberle M, Jajewski D, Baxter-Lowe LA. Prevalence of human herpesvirus 6 variant A and B infections in bone marrow transplant recipients as determined by polymerase chain reaction and sequence-specific oligonucleotide probe hybridization. *J Clin Microbiol* 1993;31:1515–1520.

224. Carrigan DR, Milburn G, Dienglewicz R, Kemen N, Papdopoulas E, Singh N. Diagnosis of active human herpesvirus six (HHV-6) infections in immunosuppression and patients with a rapid shell-vial assay.96th General Meeting of the American Society for Microbiology. New Orleans: American Society of Microbiology; 1996. [Abstract]

225. Secchiero P, Carrigan DR, Asano Y, et al. Detection of human herpesvirus 6 in plasma of children with primary infection and immunosuppressed patients by polymerase chain reaction. *J Infect Dis* 1995;171:273–280.

226. Agut H, Collandre H, Aubin J-T, et al. *in vitro* sensitivity of human herpesvirus-6 to antiviral drugs. *Res Virol* 1989;140:219–228.

227. Russler SK, Tapper MA, Garrigan DR. Susceptibility of human herpesvirus 6 to acyclovir and ganciclovir (letter). *Lancet* 1989;2:382.

228. Burns WH, Sandford GR. Susceptibility of human herpesvirus 6 to antivirals *in vitro*. *J Infect Dis* 1990;162:634–637.

229. Wang F-Z, Dahl H, Linde A, Brytting M, Ehrnst A, Ljungman P. Lymphotropic herpesviruses in allogeneic bone marrow transplantation. *Blood* 1996;88:3615–3620.

230. Frenkel N, Schirmer EC, Wyatt LS, et al. Isolation of a new herpesvirus from human CD4+ T cells. *Proc Natl Acad Sci U S A* 1990;87:748–752.

231. Berneman ZN, Blashi DV, Li G, Eger-Fletcher M, Reitz MS, Jr. Human herpesvirus 7 is a T-lymphotropic virus and is related to, but significantly different from, human herpesvirus 6 and human cytomegalovirus. *Proc Natl Acad Sci U S A* 1992;89:10552–10556.

232. Lusso P, Secchiero P, Drowley RW, Garzino-Demo A, Berneman ZN, Gallo RC. CD4 is a critical component of the receptor for human herpesvirus 7: interference with human immunodeficiency virus. *Proc Natl Acad Sci U S A* 1994;91:3872–3876.

233. Osman HK, Peiris JS, Taylor CE, Warwicker P, Jarrett RF, Madeley CR. "Cytomegalovirus disease" in renal allograft recipients: is human herpesvirus 7 a co-factor for disease progression? *J Med Virol* 1996; 48:295–301.

234. Wilborn F, Schmidt CA, Lorenz F, et al. Human herpesvirus type 7 in blood donors: detection by the polymerase chain reaction. *J Med Virol* 1995;47:65–69.

235. Torigoe S, Kumamoto T, Koide W, Taya K, Yamanishi K. Clinical manifestations associated with human herpesvirus 7 infection. *Arch Dis Child* 1995;72:518–519.

236. Wyatt LS, Rodriguez WJ, Balachandran N, Frenkel N. Human herpesvirus 7: antigenic properties and prevalence in children and adults. *J Virol* 1991;65:6260–6265.

237. Grose C. Childhood infections with human herpesviruses types 6, 7, and 8. *Adv Pediatr Infect Dis* 1996;12:181–208.

238. Caserta M, Hall C, Schnabel K, D'Heron N. Human herpesvirus-7 (HHV-7) infection in U.S. children. *Pediatr Res* 1996;39:168A.

239. Safai B, Good RA. Kaposi's sarcoma: a review and recent developments. *Clin Bull* 1980;10:62–68. [Abstract]

240. Friedman-Kien A, Laubenstin LJ, Rubenstein P, et al. Disseminated Kaposi's sarcoma in homosexual men. *Ann Intern Med* 1982;96: 693–700.

241. Chang Y, Cesarman F, Pessin MS, et al. Identification of herpesvirus-like DNA sequences in AIDS-associated Kaposi's sarcoma. *Science* 1994;266:1865–1869.

242. Moore PS, Chang Y. Detection of herpesvirus-like DNA sequences in Kaposi's sarcoma in patients with and without HIV infection. *N Engl J Med* 1995;332:1181–1185.

243. Ambroziak JA, Blackbourn DJ, Herndier BG, et al. Herpesvirus-like sequences in HIV-infected and uninfected Kaposi's sarcoma patients. *Science* 1995;268:582–583.

244. Cesarman E, Chang Y, Moore PS, Said JW, Knowles DM. Kaposi's sarcoma-associated herpesvirus-like DNA sequences in AIDS-related body cavity-based lymphomas. *N Engl J Med* 1995;332:1186–1191.

245. Boshoff C, Whitby D, Hatziioannou T, et al. Kaposi's sarcoma-associated herpesvirus in HIV-negative Kaposi's sarcoma. *Lancet* 1995;345:1043–1044.

246. DeLellis L, Fabris M, Cassai E, et al. Herpesvirus-like DNA sequences in non-AIDS Kaposi's sarcoma. *J Infect Dis* 1995;172: 1605–1607.

247. Huang YQ, Li JJ, Kaplan MH. Human herpesvirus-like nucleic acid in various forms of Kaposi's sarcoma. *Lancet* 1995;345:759–761.

248. Soulier J, Grollet L, Oksenhendler E, Cacoub P, Casals-Haten D, Babinet P. Kaposi's sarcoma-associated herpesvirus-like DNA sequences in multicentric Castleman's disease. *Blood* 1995;86:1995.

249. Kedes DH, Opetskalski E, Busch M, R. K, Flood J, Ganem D. The seroepidemiology of human herpesvirus 8 (Kaposi's sarcoma-associated herpesvirus): distribution of infection in KS risk groups and evidence for sexual transmission. *Nature Med* 1996;2:918–924.

250. Gao SJ, Kingsley L, Li M, et al. KSHV antibodies among Americans, Italians, and Ugandans with and without Kaposi's sarcoma. *Nature Med* 1996;2:925–928.

251. Lennette ET, Blackbourn DJ, Levy JA. Antibodies to human herpesvirus type 8 in the general population and in Kaposi's sarcoma patients. *Lancet* 1996;348:858–856.

252. Bigoni B, Dolcetti R, de Lellis L. Human herpesvirus 8 is present in the lymphoid system of healthy persons and can reactivate in the course of AIDS. *J Infect Dis* 1996;173:542–549.

253. Monini P, DeLellis L, Fabris M, Rigolin F, Cassai E. Kaposi's sarcoma-associated herpesvirus DNA sequences in prostate tissue and human semen. *N Engl J Med* 1996;334:1168–1172.

254. Moore PS, Gao SJ, Dominguez G, et al. Primary characterization of a herpesvirus agent associated with Kaposi's sarcoma. *J Virol* 1996;70:549–558.

255. Foreman KE, Friborg J, Wing-Pui K, Nickoloff BJ, Nabel GJ. Propagation of a human herpesvirus from AIDS-associated Kaposi's sarcoma. *N Engl J Med* 1997;336:163–171.

256. Corbellino M, Poirel L, Bestetti G, et al. Human herpesvirus-8 in AIDS-related and unrelated lymphomas. *AIDS* 1996;10:545–546.

257. Cathomas G, Tamm M, McGandy CE, et al. Transplantation-associated malignancies: restriction of human herpesvirus 8 to Kaposi's sarcoma. *Transplantation* 1997;64:175–178.

258. Kedda MA, Margolius L, Kew MC, Swanepoel C, Pearson D. Kaposi's sarcoma-associated herpesvirus in Kaposi's sarcoma occurring in immunosuppressed renal transplant recipients. *Clin Transplant* 1996;10:429–431.

259. Alkan S, Karcher DS, Ortiz A, Khalil S, Akhtar M, Ali MA. Human herpesvirus-8/Kaposi's sarcoma-associated herpesvirus in organ transplant patients with immunosuppression. *Br J Haematol* 1997;96:412–414.

260. Shepherd FA, Maher E, Cardella C, et al. Treatment of Kaposi's sarcoma after solid organ transplantation. *J Clin Oncol* 1997;15:2371–2377.

261. Aebischer MC, Zala LB, Braathen LR. Kaposi's sarcoma as manifestation of immunosuppression in organ transplant recipients. *Dermatology* 1997;195:91–92.

262. Vella JP, Mosher R, Sayegh MH. Kaposi's sarcoma after renal transplantation (letter). *N Engl J Med* 1997;336:1761.

263. Doutrelepont JM, De Pauw L, Gruber SA, et al. Renal transplantation exposes patients with previous Kaposi's sarcoma to a high risk of recurrence. *Transplantation* 1996;62:463–466.

264. Rezeig MA, Fashir BM. Kaposi's sarcoma in liver transplant recipients on FK506: two case reports. *Transplantation* 1997;63:1520–1521.

265. Besnard V, Euvard S, Kanitakis J, et al. Kaposi's sarcoma after liver transplantation. *Dermatology* 1996;193:100–104.

266. Colina F, Lopez-Rios F, Lumbreras C, Martinez-Laso J, Garcia IG, Moreno-Gonzalez E. Kaposi's sarcoma developing in a liver graft. *Transplantation* 1996;61:1779–1781.

267. Hertzler G, Gordon SM, Piratzky J, Henderson JM, Gal AA. Case report: fulminant Kaposi's sarcoma after orthotopic liver transplantation. *Am J Med Sci* 1995;309:278–281.

268. Sleiman C, Mal H, Roue C, et al. Bronchial Kaposi's sarcoma after single lung transplantation. *Eur Respir J* 1997;10:1181–1183.

269. Erer B, Angelucci E, Muretto P, et al. Kaposi's sarcoma after allogeneic bone marrow transplantation. *Bone Marrow Transplant* 1997;19:629–631.

270. Vivancos P, Sarra J, Palou J, Valls A, Garcia J, Granena A. Kaposi's sarcoma after autologous bone marrow transplantation for multiple myeloma. *Bone Marrow Transplant* 1996;17:669–671.

271. Gluckman E, Parquet N, Scieux C, et al. KS-associated herpesvirus-like DNA sequences after allogeneic bone marrow transplantation (letter). *Lancet* 1995;346:1558–1559.

272. Helg C, Adatto M, Salomon D, et al. Kaposi's sarcoma following allogeneic bone marrow transplantation. *Bone Marrow Transplant* 1994;14:999–1101.

273. Penn I. Kaposi's sarcoma in transplant recipients. *Transplantation* 1997;64:669–673.

274. Gotti E, Remuzzi G. Post-transplant Kaposi's sarcoma. *J Am Soc Nephrol* 1997;8:130–137.

275. Lock MJ, Griffiths PD, Emery VC. Development of a quantitative competitive polymerase chain reaction for human herpesvirus 8. *J Virol Methods* 1997;64:19–26.

276. Glesby MJ, Hoover DR, Weng S, et al. Use of antiherpes drugs and the risk of Kaposi's sarcoma: data from the multi-center AIDS cohort study. *J Infect Dis* 1996;173:1477–1480.

277. Kedes DH, Ganem D. Sensitivity of Kaposi's sarcoma-associated herpesvirus replication to antiviral drugs. *J Clin Invest* 1997;99.

278. Halmos O, Inturri P, Galligioni A, et al. Two cases of Kaposi's sarcoma in renal and liver transplant recipients treated with interferon. *Clin Transplant* 1996;10:374–378.

279. Brambilla L, Boneschi V, Fossati S, Ferrucci S, Finzi AF. Vinorelbine therapy for Kaposi's sarcoma in a kidney transplant patient. *Dermatology* 1997;194:281–283.

Transplant Infections edited by
Raleigh A. Bowden, Per Ljungman, and Carlos V. Paya.
Lippincott–Raven Publishers, Philadelphia © 1998

CHAPTER 20

Adenovirus, Parvovirus B19, and Papillomavirus

Michael Green and Marian G. Michaels

ADENOVIRUS

Adenoviruses are common pediatric pathogens responsible for a wide variety of infectious syndromes. Although adenoviral infection results in self-limited disease in the majority of immunocompetent children, it can result in life-threatening illness in immunocompromised hosts (1).

Age and Immunity

The highest incidence of adenoviral infection occurs in children between the ages of 6 months and 5 years (2,3), although outbreaks have been noted among military recruits and adolescents at summer camp (4,5). Explanations for the infrequent incidence of disease in the very young or in older individuals include the presence of transplancentally acquired maternal antibody in the young infant and the development of neutralizing antibody to the most common adenoviral strains (serotypes 1, 2, and 5) in the majority of children older than 5 years. A risk factor for infection in the preschool age group is the increased likelihood of person-to-person spread resulting from intimate contact between children in the absence of well-developed sanitary habits, especially those in day care or other closed environments (2). Similarly, it is thought that the relative lack of hygiene and crowding in military barracks explains the increased risk of adenoviral spread among recruits.

Adenovirus has been found to cause disease in 10% of children undergoing liver transplantation (LT) under cyclosporine-based immunosuppression (6) compared with the infrequent recognition of adenovirus among adult LT recipients. Presumably, this difference is due to

adults having protective type-specific antibody against adenovirus. However, serological evidence of previous infection does not confer complete protection against invasive adenovirus disease (e.g., adenovirus hepatitis has occurred in pediatric LT recipients with type-specific antibody) (7). Sporadic cases of adenovirus infection have also been reported in adult renal transplant (RT) recipients (8–16). Prior antibody status studies were not available for these patients and disease has typically been caused by serotype 11, an infrequent isolate in children.

In contrast to solid-organ transplant recipients, the dramatic alterations in immunologic status that occur in the early period after bone marrow transplantation (BMT) render patients susceptible to a variety of infectious pathogens to which they may have previously developed immunity. Accordingly, it is not surprising that significant adenoviral disease has been reported in both adults and children who have undergone BMT, although reported rates are still higher in pediatric BMT recipients (17,18).

Mode of Transmission

Among normal hosts, adenovirus is typically transmitted from person to person. Among transplant recipients, infection tends to occur within the first few months after transplantation, while the patient is often still hospitalized and, in the case of BMT recipients, often still in isolation. Although outbreaks of adenovirus infections among transplant recipients have been reported (19), attempts to document nosocomial person-to-person spread in two large series were unsuccessful (6,17). Adenovirus has not been reported to spread through the use of blood products, thereby eliminating another potential source of viral transmission. These facts, as well as the stereotypical timing of adenoviral infection within the first several months after transplantation (6,14,17,18), have led to the suggestion that reactivation of latent virus and/or donor organ–associated

From the Division of Allergy, Immunology, and Infectious Diseases, Children's Hospital of Pittsburgh, University of Pittsburgh School of Medicine, Pittsburgh, PA 15213.

transmission are the major sources of infection in transplant recipients. In support of this hypothesis is the capacity of adenovirus to remain latent and the striking similarities, in terms of both timing of infection and relationships between serostatus and severity of disease (7), that exist between adenovirus and cytomegalovirus. Of greatest similarity is the significant increase in organ-specific adenoviral disease in the transplanted organ.

Clinical Disease

Only a limited number of clinical series describing adenovirus infection after transplantation have been published. The largest of these series detail infections in pediatric LT (6) and BMT recipients of all ages (17,20). Additionally, a large number of single-case reports have described adenoviral infection after RT (8–16), and one recent report describes four cases of fatal adenovirus infection after lung transplantation (21). An overview of the frequency and sites of adenovirus infection after liver, lung, and bone marrow transplantation is shown in Table 1.

Liver Transplantation

Adenovirus is the third most important virus after CMV and Epstein-Barr virus following pediatric LT. Although no cases of adenoviral infection have been reported in adult recipients, we found a 10% incidence of adenovirus infection in our review of 484 pediatric LT recipients under cyclosporine A (6). Of interest, we have observed a dramatic decrease in the incidence and severity of adenovirus infection under tacrolimus. Median age at the time of diagnosis of adenoviral disease was 3.0 years (range 0.8–17.2 years). The median time of adenoviral isolation was 25.5 days after LT, with severe infections typically presenting in the first 50 days. The occurrence of infection within the first 3 months of transplantation is similar to published reports from other centers (22–24). Nonetheless, it is important to note that one of our recent LT recipients presented with rapidly

TABLE 1. *Overview of frequency and sites of adenovirus infection after liver, lung, and bone marrow transplantation*

Organ (references)	Liver (6)	Lung (21)	Bone marrow (17,18,20)
Patients reviewed	484	308	1248
Total infections	53	NR[a]	110
Tissue—invasive episodes	20	NR	19
Pneumonia	7	4	14
Renal	2	NR	8
Gut	NR	NR	2
Liver	16	NR	7
Adenovirus-associated mortality	10	4	7

[a]Not reported.

fatal adenoviral hepatitis 6 months after transplantation. A prolonged history of very intense immunosuppression may explain both the severity and the unusual timing of this infectious episode.

Serotypes 1, 2, and 5 were the most common isolates from these children, with serotype 5 causing most cases of hepatitis and serotype 2 causing most cases of pneumonia. It is interesting to note that adenovirus type 5 (which is associated with hepatitis in both immunocompetent and immunocompromised hosts) accounted for 30% of adenoviral infections in this series compared with only 5% of isolates obtained from nontransplant patients at our institution during the same time period.

Analysis for potential risk factors identified the use of OKT3 as showing a trend toward more severe infection (6). A second potential risk factor for severe disease appears to be the presence of seropositivity against adenovirus in donors whose grafts were given to seronegative recipients (7). Similar to CMV infection, this serological mismatching resulted in the most severe disease in a series of 10 pediatric LT recipients who developed adenoviral infection (7).

Symptomatic disease, ranging from self-limited fever, gastroenteritis, or cystitis to devastating illness with hepatitis or pneumonia, occurred in 60% of infected patients in our series. Hepatitis, the most common form of invasive infection, was identified in 14 of our 34 children with symptomatic adenoviral infection. All of these children experienced prolonged high-grade fevers (mean = 16 days). Eight of these 14 children recovered, four without the loss of their graft. Four of the survivors underwent successful retransplantation and had immediate resolution of their fever. One of the four had a mild episode of recurrent disease. Three additional patients died during the attempted retransplantation operation; the remaining three patients died without an effort at retransplantation. Although replacement of the liver appears to be a promising treatment in children with severe adenoviral hepatitis, it should be noted that Varki and colleagues reported a child who developed recurrent adenovirus hepatitis and died 5 days after retransplantation (23). Because of the possibility of infection of the new graft, retransplantation should be delayed as long as possible after adenoviral hepatitis. Serial liver biopsies can be used to document the absence of adenovirus prior to retransplantation.

Adenovirus pneumonia is a serious infection for pediatric LT recipients. A probable diagnosis of adenoviral pneumonia was made in eight children in our series, resulting in six deaths. Two of six fatalities occurred in children with concurrent hepatitis. None of these patients were retransplanted.

Renal Transplantation

The reported experience of adenovirus infections after RT is limited to case reports that have accumulated over the last 20 years. The most frequently recorded infection has been hemorrhagic cystitis due to adenovirus type 11 (12–16). Each episode was self-limited despite the fact that many of these patients were initially treated as having rejection with augmented immunosuppression. More serious illness, consisting of interstitial pneumonia due to adenovirus types 34 and 35, has been less frequently reported and was associated with fatal, disseminated disease in at least one patient (9–11). Additionally, a single case of fatal hepatitis due to adenovirus type 5 has been reported following RT (8).

Similar to adenoviral infections after pediatric LT, the vast majority of adenovirus infections after RT have developed within the first 6 months after transplantation (range, 17 days to 9 months; median, 2.5 months) (8–16). However, all the reported cases of adenoviral infection in RT recipients have occurred in adults (range 17–61 years; median, 30.5 years) (8–16). The early timing after transplantation and the predilection for infection of the transplanted organ has again led to the hypothesis that these cases may be due to donor-associated transmission.

Cardiac Transplantation

There is little information about adenoviral infection following cardiac transplantation. However, adenovirus genome has been identified by polymerase chain reaction in endomyocardial biopsy specimens of eight of 40 pediatric cardiac transplant recipients who had histologic evidence of inflammation indistinguishable from rejection (25). Of interest, several of the children with this finding had recent or concurrent histories of upper respiratory tract infections. Two of the eight patients presented with cardiogenic shock and were felt to have histologic evidence of high-grade rejection. They were treated for rejection with improved clinical status and adenovirus could not be identified on subsequent biopsies. Whether adenovirus was the sole cause of the inflammation, a promoter of rejection, or an innocent bystander in these patients was not established in this report.

Lung Transplantation

Limited data describing the frequency and outcome of adenovirus infections among lung transplant recipients are available. Ohori and colleagues reported the outcome of four cases of adenovirus pneumonia among 308 lung transplant recipients at the University of Pittsburgh (21). As with other organ transplant recipients, the incidence was much higher among children (three of 40) than among adults (one of 268) (21). Disease occurred in the first 6 weeks following transplantation and was uniformly fatal. Dissemination beyond the respiratory tree was not demonstrated despite the performance of an autopsy in each of the patients. The authors speculated that the presence of ischemic harvest injury predisposed

their patients to the development of adenovirus pneumonitis.

Bone Marrow Transplantation

The overall reported incidence of adenovirus infection following BMT has ranged from 5% to 21% (17–20). Shields and colleagues documented a frequency of adenoviral infection in 5% of BMT recipients of all age groups (17). More recently, Flomenberg and colleagues found an overall incidence rate of 20.9%, with a significantly higher rate of recovery for children (31%) than for adults (13.6%) followed in their series ($p < 0.01$) (20). Similarly, Wasserman and colleagues identified a high incidence (18%) of adenovirus infection in pediatric BMT recipients (18).

Adenovirus was most commonly isolated from cultures of urine, stool, and throat swabs and was frequently recovered from more than one site in these series (17,18). Although earlier studies suggest that the most frequent time of isolation of adenovirus is within the first 3–4 months after transplantation (17,18), Flomenberg and colleagues found a significant difference in the timing of adenovirus infection according to the age of the patients (20). Similar to the previous studies, the vast majority of adenoviral infection in pediatric BMT recipients developed in the first 3 months (including a large number in the first month following transplantation). However, adult cases of adenovirus infection were much more likely to present at least 3 months following transplantation (20). The most frequent serotypes isolated were 1, 2, 5, and members of subgenus B (types 11, 34, and 35) (17,18,20). The distribution of adenovirus serotypes was similar in adults and children (20).

Clinical manifestations of adenoviral infection after BMT range from fever associated with gastroenteritis or cystitis to fatal, disseminated disease. Of interest is the finding in one study that eight of 16 patients with culture-proven adenoviral infection and cystitis (gross hematuria or at least 10 red cells per high power field on urinalysis) did not have adenovirus isolated from their urine (17). This finding suggests the need to culture for the presence of adenovirus from multiple sites in patients with cystitis. However, it is important to note that cystitis was documented in only eight of 22 patients with a positive urine culture for adenovirus, suggesting that at least some patients demonstrate asymptomatic shedding of adenovirus in their urine. It is also important to note that there are other causes of hemorrhagic cystitis following BMT. Therefore potential etiologies other than adenovirus should be considered in patients with negative cultures.

Invasive adenovirus infection has been reported in about 20% of infected patients (17–20). Adenovirus was identified as a major contributor to death in more than half of the patients with invasive disease (17–20). Interstitial pneumonia, associated with positive cultures for adenovirus, was observed in most patients with invasive infection. Other frequent sites of invasive disease included the kidney, colon, and liver. Of interest, despite the relative frequency of hepatic involvement, only four cases of adenovirus hepatitis with subsequent liver failure have been reported among BMT recipients (26).

Diagnosis and Management

It is very difficult to presumptively diagnose infection due to adenovirus in transplant recipients, as fever and hepatitis or pneumonitis may represent infection (with adenovirus or other pathogens), rejection, or graft-versus-host disease. The presence of high-grade fevers and symptoms suggestive of infection should prompt serial culturing for viruses (including adenovirus) from the buffy coat, stool, throat, and urine. Unexplained elevations of hepatocellular enzymes suggestive of hepatitis warrant consideration of performance of a liver biopsy in any patient who has undergone solid-organ transplantation and after BMT in patients without graft-versus-host disease. Histologic examination for the presence of adenoviral inclusions, as well as the use of immunohistochemical stains, will help confirm this diagnosis in most cases. Viral cultures should also be obtained from respiratory secretions (including bronchoalveolar lavage fluid) in patients with clinical and radiographic evidence of pneumonia. The presence of unexplained hemorrhagic cystitis (even in the absence of fever) should lead to collection of urine specimens for viral cultures.

Unfortunately, there is no definitive or specific treatment for adenoviral infection at this time. The most important component of therapy is supportive care along with a decrease in immunosuppression. Although no clear response to withdrawal of immunosuppression in transplant recipients with adenoviral infection has been demonstrated, the logic of this approach prompts our strong recommendation to decrease or stop immunosuppressive therapy in all patients with invasive adenoviral infection. Management of patients with hemorrhagic cystitis after RT is less clear because of the apparent self-limited nature of these infections; many reported episodes resolved despite initial augmentation of immunosuppression.

The role of antiviral agents in adenoviral infection is unproven at this time. A small number of case reports describe the use of ribavirin (27–29) and ganciclovir (23) in the treatment of single patients with adenoviral infection after transplantation. *In vitro* evidence supports the theoretical role of ribavirin but not that of ganciclovir in the treatment of these infections. In addition to these published reports, an adult patient with disseminated adenovirus type 7 improved after treatment with cidofovir (HPMPC) and pooled, high-titered immunoglobulin against respiratory syncytial virus (Respigam) along with decreased immunosuppression (personal communication,

P.A. Williams, M.D., University of Pittsburgh). Unfortunately, no conclusive evidence of the efficacy of any of these antiviral agents can be drawn from these reports.

A possible role for intravenous immunoglobulin has been suggested by a single case of apparent improvement after treatment of pneumonia in a child with severe combined immunodeficiency (24). The immunoglobulin preparation had a high titer of antibody to the adenovirus serotype causing pneumonia. Once again we are unable to generalize the potential efficacy of this treatment to adenoviral infections occurring in the post-transplant patient.

Another single report describes the use of donor leukocyte infusions as therapy for life-threatening adenoviral infections after T-cell-depleted BMT (30). This strategy, which has been applied to the treatment of EBV infections in BMT recipients, was used in a single patient with persistent hemorrhagic cystitis after T-cell-depleted BMT. In contrast to the uniformly fatal outcome the authors had seen in T-cell-depleted BMT patients with a similar clinical course, the patient survived.

PARVOVIRUS B19 INFECTION

Parvovirus B19, a small, single-stranded DNA virus, is a common cause of infection typically acquired during childhood. The virus was first recognized as causing pure red cell aplasia in people with underlying sickle cell anemia in 1981 (31). Shortly thereafter, it was associated with the common childhood disease, erythema infectiosum, and the rare occurrence of stillbirths due to hydrops fetalis. It has increasingly been recognized as a cause of red cell aplasia (and possibly pancytopenia) in immunosuppressed patients.

Epidemiological studies show that parvovirus B19 is usually acquired during the school-age period. Serological evidence of past infection increases substantially between the ages of 5 and 15 years; by adulthood, 30% to 60% of people are seropositive (31). Infection appears to confer lifelong immunity in immunocompetent hosts.

Clinical Manifestations

Most infections of immunocompetent children are asymptomatic or result in a mild illness characterized by a "slapped cheek" rash with or without a lacy erythematous exanthem of the extremities (31,32). Occasionally, arthritis is noted, although this is more common in adults (31,32). Individuals with shortened red blood cell life spans, such as sickle cell disease or thalassemia, are at risk for severe anemia during acute infection. Further studies demonstrated that even those with normal hematopoietic systems suffer a transient period of red blood cell aplasia during acute parvovirus B19 infection. However, the usual longevity of circulating red blood cells prevents this abnormality from becoming clinically apparent or even demonstrable by analysis of peripheral blood counts (33).

Diagnosis of parvovirus B19 infection in immunocompetent children is typically made clinically, based upon the presence of a classic rash. Demonstration of IgM directed against parvovirus in a single specimen is evidence of recent infection. Shortly after the onset of illness, IgG and IgM antibodies can be present; both peak by 30 days. IgM antibody generally becomes undetectable by 2–3 months after onset of disease (34), but IgG persists lifelong. The finding of inclusions in giant pronormoblasts in bone marrow biopsies of patients with red cell aplasia is strongly suggestive of the diagnosis (35). Nucleic acid hybridization and polymerase chain reaction have been used for more sensitive detection of virus, particularly in immunosuppressed hosts (32–34, 36,37).

Parvovirus in Transplant Recipients

Chronic parvovirus B19 infections, characterized by symptomatic red blood cell aplasia, were initially described in immunodeficient patients, including children with acute leukemia or congenital deficiencies, recipients of bone marrow transplantation, and individuals with AIDS (38–40). It was not until 1993 that Nour and colleagues reported red cell aplasia in children who had received organ transplantation (41). Subsequent to this, increasing numbers of organ transplant recipients have been diagnosed with persistent parvovirus B19 infection. During this same time period, only a low number of BMT recipients have been found to have symptomatic B19 infection (42,43). The reason for this finding lies with understanding the natural history of disease and immunity to virus. Infection in healthy human volunteers revealed viremia beginning 5–7 days after intranasal challenge that persisted for 10–15 days. IgM antibodies were detectable on days 10–13, and IgG antibody by day 13 (32). Viremia decreases coincident with the rise in IgG antibody. Immunosuppressed individuals, despite an increase in IgM antibody, are at risk for persistence of virus and chronic anemia because of the lack of an effective IgG response. Many investigators have reported the disease to be aborted by administration of exogenous antibody, such as intravenous immunoglobulin (31,32, 35–37,38–44). Currently, many BMT protocols routinely include prophylaxis with intravenous immunoglobulin around the time of maximum immunosuppression as a method of preventing cytomegalovirus disease. This strategy has been hypothesized to give passive added protection against parvovirus B19 infection or reactivation. A prospective study of 51 BMT recipients who received IVIG by protocol around the time of transplantation failed to find any disease caused by parvovirus B19, supports the hypothetical benefit of IVIG use (43). Case reports of recipients of bone marrow or autologous peripheral stem cell who develop red cell aplasia associated with parvovirus infection have been limited to those who did not receive IVIG (36,45). In this group of patients, parvovirus disease has usually been early, when the patient is most immunosuppressed, prior to establishment of the transplanted hematopoietic system. However, later disease has been reported in individuals who continue to receive immunosuppressive drugs to combat graft-versus-host disease (36,39). Although the preceding reports make the use of IVIG prophylaxis theoretically attractive, its efficacy is not established. At least one series of 66 BMT recipients who did not receive IVIG prophylaxis did not document any episodes of symptomatic parvovirus disease, though eight of these patients had asymptomatic infection (46). Thus other protective factors (including differences in immunosuppressive regimens) may explain the perceived protection associated with the use of IVIG.

Organ transplant patients who do not routinely receive immunoglobulin after transplantation or who remain chronically immunosuppressed continue to have a lifelong risk for parvovirus infection. This is particularly true for pediatric transplant recipients, who are more likely to be seronegative to parvovirus prior to transplantation. Accordingly, they are at increased risk to experience a primary infection after transplantation without the benefit of previous immunity. Nour and colleagues reported on four pediatric recipients of liver transplantation and one child who had undergone a heart transplant who developed parvovirus B19 infection 2–34 months after transplantation (41). One child had spontaneous recovery of bone marrow within 4 weeks of hemoglobin nadir, whereas the other four were treated with IVIG and had improved reticulocyte counts and hemoglobin levels within 2–4 weeks. Subsequent reports of severe anemia have been found for liver, renal, and cardiac transplantation (35,37,41). Patients have ranged in age between 1.4 and 62 years. However, as expected, a preponderance of disease was found in the younger patients.

Disease was manifested by chronic anemia, with or without accompanying decrease in platelets and white blood count. Systemic signs of illness were found in approximately half of the reported patients, including fever and malaise. Rash and arthritis were uncommon. Several adult patients have also presented with pancytopenia. Parvovirus B19 infection should be included in the differential diagnosis in any transplant recipient who has pancytopenia regardless of the absence of other signs or symptoms.

Treatment

Outcome of infection has been reported for a limited number of transplant recipients. Several patients cleared the B19 infection with spontaneous resolution of anemia (37,41,45). However, most patients reported in the literature who were treated with IVIG had temporal clinical responses. Varying doses and intervals of IVIG were employed, making it difficult to offer recommendations on the amount and timing of IVIG therapy. Doses varied between 0.4 and 1 g/kg/day given for 3–10 days (35, 37,40,41,44). Continued IVIG use was reported in some patients over the course of months (37). The lack of sufficient cases of parvovirus B19-associated anemia in any one center hampers the ability to perform clinical controlled trials to identify the optimal prescription regimen. Cooperation between centers coupled with improved detection methods of circulating parvovirus DNA in the peripheral blood should lead to better understanding of the pathogenesis and treatment of this virus in transplant recipients.

PAPILLOMAVIRUS

Human papillomavirus (HPV) is a double-stranded DNA virus with more than 60 different subtypes. HPV has been associated with a variety of clinical syndromes, including cutaneous warts, anogenital warts, and epidermodysplasia verruciformis. HPV has also been implicated in the development of cervical cancer and squamous cell carcinoma. Patients with deficiencies of cell-mediated immunity have been shown to be at an increased risk of developing HPV-associated warts and cancers (47).

Cutaneous Warts in Transplant Recipients

Several reports have documented an increased rate of HPV-associated cutaneous warts among adult renal transplant recipients (48,49). The overall incidence of HPV-associated warts in these patients has been reported to range from 25% to 50%. However, the incidence increases with increasing duration of immunosuppression. Gassenmaier and colleagues found that the incidence of warts rose from 3.3% prior to transplant to 25% in the first 2 years after transplant (48). Subsequent incidence of HPV-associated warts rose to greater than 70% among renal transplant recipients at least 8 years from the time of transplantation (48). Similarly, Rudlinger and colleagues found that nearly 90% of adult renal transplant recipients in their series who had survived for at least 5 years after transplant suffered from HPV-associated warts (50). Most patients developed multiple warts that tended to disseminate over the entire body and to recur after excision (48). Although similar experiences have not been reported from adult recipients of other organ transplant procedures, it is logical to assume that these patients will also be predisposed to developing HPV-associated warts following transplantation.

Published experience from pediatric transplant recipients is much more limited. Ingelfinger and colleagues reported that 18 of 49 children undergoing renal transplantation developed warts (51). Thirteen of the 18 children had numerous warts involving multiple body parts. Successful eradication after treatment was accomplished in only five of the affected children. In contrast to the descriptions of HPV-associated warts in adult transplant recipients, an increase in the prevalence of warts with increasing time of immunosuppression in these children was not demonstrated. However, only a small number of the children were followed for more than 3 years after transplantation in this study.

Several risk factors for the development of cutaneous warts have been identified among transplant recipients. Warts are more likely to be found in sun-exposed areas. Patients with skin prone to the development of sunburn are more likely to develop warts than those with a tendency to tan (52). Additional risk factors for the development of warts include prolonged sun exposure and increasing duration of immunosuppression. The role of different immunosuppressive regimens on the risk of developing warts has also been studied. McLelland and colleagues found that patients on azathioprine and prednisone alone were at increased risk of developing warts compared with those on cyclosporine-based immunosuppression (49). However, this difference may be an artifact of the shorter period of follow-up observation for the cyclosporine patients at the time of that report. Experience describing warts in patients treated with tacrolimus has not been published.

It is interesting to note that there is no literature reporting the incidence of papillomavirus following BMT. Anecdotally, the incidence appears to be quite low (personal communication: R. Bowden, M.D.). Although specific explanations are not clear, it may be that the relatively limited period of immunosuppression associated with BMT is not long enough to predispose to this problem. Alternatively, similar to solid-organ transplantation, warts may develop late after transplant at a time when specialists at BMT centers may be unaware of the frequency or importance of this problem.

A wide variety of HPV serotypes have been associated with cutaneous wart lesions on transplant recipients (48,53). HPV serotypes 1, 2, 3, 4, 5, 6, 10, 16, 27, and 49 have been identified in wart lesions from renal transplant recipients (48,53). Although only one type of HPV DNA has been simultaneously recovered from a given wart, individuals may have different HPV types recovered from separate warts suggesting infection with different HPV types (54).

Management of cutaneous warts in transplant recipients typically parallels the treatment in immunocompetent individuals. Unfortunately, lesions tend to be either refractory to treatment or to recur. Where possible, reduction of immunosuppression at the time of treatment may enhance the likelihood of success.

Urogenital and Anal Warts

Infection with papillomaviruses has also been associated with the development of urogenital and anal warts. These lesions appear as classical condylomata acuminata. HPV types 6, 11, and 42 have been identified in these lesions. Rudlinger and colleagues found that 10% of female renal transplant recipients had genital warts (47,50). Similar to HPV-associated cutaneous warts, management of these lesions has been very difficult in immunosuppressed transplant recipients.

Oncogenicity

HPV are one of several classes of double-stranded DNA viruses that are thought to be oncogenic in organ transplant recipients. HPV DNA has been detected in premalignant lesions, as well as squamous cell carcinoma, transitional cell carcinoma, and cervical cancers in recipients of organ and bone marrow transplantation.

Investigators have found that squamous cell carcinomas are about 36 times more frequent in renal transplant recipients than in normal individuals (55). Similar to the prevalence of HPV-associated warts, the rate of squamous cell carcinomas increases with increasing duration of immunosuppression following transplantation (56,57). Rates as high as 45% have been reported 15 years after transplant (57). Squamous cell carcinoma of the skin tends to arise in beds of flat warts.

Specific types of HPV are more associated with malignant transformation than others, including HPV 16, 18, 31, 33, and 35 (58). In addition to the role of immunosuppression, chronic sun exposure is thought to be a cofactor in the development of skin cancers in these patients. Accordingly, transplant recipients, particularly those experiencing problems with warts, should avoid excess sun and ultraviolet light exposure (48). HPV 16 and 18 have also been identified in transitional cell carcinoma in renal transplant recipients (57).

There is also an increased rate of urogenital cancers, including cervical carcinoma and carcinoma of the bladder, in association with HPV infections in recipients of organ transplantation.

Management of HPV-associated carcinomas of the skin, cervix, and urinary tract consists of combinations of resection, reduction, or withdrawal of immunosuppression, radiation, and chemotherapy. Overall outcome from these cancers is difficult to estimate because of the limited number of reported cases in the literature.

REFERENCES

1. Zahradnik JM, Spencer MJ, Porter DD. Adenovirus infection in the immunocompromised patient. *Am J Med* 1980;68:725–732.
2. Bell JA, Huebner RJ, Rosen L, et al. Illness and microbial experiences of nursery children at junior village. *Am J Hyg* 1961;74:267–292.
3. Bell TM, Turner G, MacDonald A, et al. Type-3 adenovirus infection. *Lancet* 1960;2:1327–1329.
4. Forsyth BR, Bloom HH, Johnson KM, et al. Patterns of adenovirus infection in Marine Corps personnel. II. Longitudinal study of successive advanced recruit training. *Am J Hyg* 1964;80:343–355.
5. McNamara MJ, Pierce WE, Crawford YE, et al. Patterns of adenovirus infection in respiratory diseases of naval recruits. A longitudinal study of two companies of naval recruits. *Am Rev Respir Dis* 1962;86:485–494.
6. Michaels MG, Green M, Wald ER, Starzl TE. Adenovirus infection in pediatric liver transplant recipients. *J Infect Dis* 1992;165:170–174.
7. Koneru B, Atchison R, Cassavilla A, Van Thiel DH, Starzl TE. Serologic studies of adenoviral hepatitis following pediatric liver transplantation. *Transplant Proc* 1990;22:1547–1548.
8. Norris SH, Butler TC, Glass N, Tran R. Fatal hepatic necrosis caused by disseminated type 5 adenovirus infection in a renal transplant recipient. *Am J Nephrol* 1989;9:101–105.
9. Hierholzer JC, Atuk NO, Gwaltney JM Jr. New human adenovirus isolated from renal transplant recipient: description and characterization of candidate adenovirus type 34. *J Clin Microb* 19756;1:366–376.
10. Keller EW, Rubin RH, Black PH, Hirsch MS, Hierholzer JC. Isolation of adenovirus type 34 from a renal transplant recipient with interstitial pneumonia. *Transplantation* 1977;23:188–191.
11. Stalder H, Hierholzer JC, Oxman MN. New human adenovirus (candidate adenovirus type 35) causing fatal disseminated infection in a renal transplant recipient. *J Clin Microb* 1977;6:257–265.
12. Shindo K, Kitayama T, Ura T, et al. Acute hemorrhagic cystitis caused by adenovirus type 11 after renal transplantation. *Urol Int* 1986;41:152–155.
13. Shiramizu T, Satoh T, Jinushi K, Oka N, Inokuchi K. Renal allograft dysfunction with acute hemorrhagic cystitis caused by adenovirus in a recipient of a transplanted kidney. *Tokai J Exp Clin Med* 1986;11:371–375.
14. Yagisawa T, Takahashi K, Yamaguchi Y, et al. Adenovirus induced nephropathy in kidney transplant recipients. *Transplant Proc* 1989;21:2097–2099.
15. Harnett GB, Bucens MR, Clay SJ, Saker BM. Acute hemorrhagic cystitis caused by adenovirus 11. *Med J Aust* 1982;1:565–567.
16. Buchanan W, Bowman JS, Jaffers G. Adenoviral acute hemorrhagic cystitis following renal transplantation. *Am J Nephrol* 1990;10:350–351.
17. Shields AF, Hackman RC, Fife KH, Corey L, Meyer JD. Adenovirus infections in patients undergoing bone-marrow transplantation. *N Engl J Med* 1985;312:529–533.
18. Wasserman R, August CS, Plotkin SA. Viral infections in pediatric bone marrow transplant patients. *Pediatr Dis J* 1988;7:109–115.
19. Yolken RH, Bishop CA, Townsend TR, et al. Infectious gastroenteritis in bone-marrow transplant recipients. *N Engl J Med* 1982;306:1009–1012.
20. Flomenberg P, Babbitt J, Brobyski WR, et al. Increasing incidence of adenovirus disease in bone marrow transplant recipients. *J Infect Dis* 1994;169:775–781.
21. Ohori NP, Michaels MG, Jaffe R, Williams P, Yousem SA. Adenovirus pneumonia in lung transplant recipients. *Hum Pathol* 1995;26:1073–1079.
22. Cassano WF. Intravenous ribavirin therapy for adenovirus cystitis after allogenic bone marrow transplantation. *Bone Marrow Transplant* 1991;7:247–248.
23. Wreghitt TG, Gray JJ, Ward KN, et al. Disseminated adenovirus infection after liver transplantation and its possible treatment with ganciclovir. *J Infect* 1989;19:88–89.
24. Dagan R, Schwartz RH, Insel RA, Menegua MA. Severe diffuse adenovirus 7a pneumonia in a child with combined immunodeficiency: possible therapeutic effect of human immune serum globulin containing specific neutralizing antibodies. *Pediatr Infect Dis J* 1984;3:246–251.
25. Schowengerdt KO, Ni J, Denfield SW, et al. Diagnosis, surveillance and epidemiologic evaluation of viral infections in pediatric cardiac transplant recipients with use of polymerase chain reaction. *J Heart Lung Transplant* 1995;15:111–123.
26. Bertheau P, Parquet N, Ferchal F, Gluckman E, Brocheriou C. Fulminant adenovirus hepatitis after allogeneic bone marrow transplantation. *Bone Marrow Transplant* 1996;17:295–298.

27. Kapelushnik J, Or R, Delukina A, et al. Intravenous ribavirin therapy for adenovirus gastroenteritis after bone marrow transplantation. *J Pediatr Gastroenterol Nutr* 1995;21:110–112.

28. Murphy GF, Wood DP Jr, McRoberts JW, Henslee-Downey PJ. Adenovirus-associated hemorrhagic cystitis treated with intravenous ribavirin. *J Urol* 1993;149:565–566.

29. Liles WC, Cushing H, Holt S, Bryan C, Hackman RC. Severe adenoviral nephritis following bone marrow transplantation: successful treatment with intravenous ribavirin. *Bone Marrow Transplant* 1993;14:663–664.

30. Hromas R, Cornetta K, Srour E, Blanke C, Broun ER. Donor leukocyte infusion as therapy for life-threatening adenoviral infection after T-cell-depleted bone marrow transplantation. *Blood* 1994;84:1689–1690.

31. Anderson LJ. Role of parvovirus B19 in human disease. *Pediatr Infect Dis J* 1987;6:711–718.

32. Anderson LJ. Human parvoviruses. *J Infect Dis* 1990;61:603–608.

33. Anderson LJ, Higgins PG, Davis LR, et al. Experimental parvoviral infection in humans. *J Infect Dis* 1985;152:257–265.

34. Anderson LJ, Tsou C, Parker RA, et al. Detection of antibodies and antigens of human parvovirus B19 by enzyme-linked immunosorbent assay. *J Clin Microbiol* 1986;24: 522–526.

35. Bergen GA, Sakalosky PE, Sinnot JT. Transient aplastic anemia caused by parvovirus B19 infection in a heart transplant recipient. *J Heart Lung Transplant* 1996;15:843–845.

36. Weiland HT Salimans MMM, Fibbe WE, Kluin PM, Cohen BJ. Prolonged parvovirus B19 infection with severe anemia in a bone marrow transplant recipient [letter]. *Br J Haematol* 1989;71:300.

37. Chang FY, Singh N, Gayowski T, Mariono IR. Parvovirus B19 infection a liver transplant recipient: case report and review in organ transplant recipients. *Clin Transplant* 1996;10:243–247.

38. Kurtzman GJ Ozawa K, Cohen B, Hanson G, Oseas R, Young NS. Chronic bone marrow failure due to persistent B19 parvovirus infection. *N Engl J Med* 1987;317:287–294.

39. Kurtzman GJ, Cohen B, Meyers P, Ammunullah, Young NS. Persistent B19 parvovirus infection as a cause of severe chronic anaemia in children with acute lymphocytic leukemia. *Lancet* 1988;2:1159–62.

40. Kurtzman GJ, Frickhofen N, Kimball J, Jenkins DW, Nienhuis AW, Young NS. Pure red-cell aplasia of 10 years' duration due to persistent Parvovirus B19 infection and its cure with immunoglobulin therapy. *N Engl J Med* 1989;321:519–523.

41. Nour B, Green M, Michaels M, et al. Parvovirus B19 infection in pediatric transplant patients. *Transplantation* 1993;56:835–838.

42. Frickhofen N, Arnold R, Hertenstein B, Wiesneth M, Young NS. Parvovirus B19 infection and bone marrow transplantation. *Ann Hematol* 1992;64:A121–A124.

43. Azzi A, Fanci R, Ciappi S, Zakrzewska K, Bosi A. Human parvovirus B19 infection in bone marrow transplantation patients. *Am J Hematol* 1993;44:207–209.

44. Janner D, Bork J, Baum M, Chinnock R. Severe pneumonia after heart transplantation as a result of human parvovirus B19. *J Heart Lung Transplant* 1994;13:336–338.

46. Ang HA, Apperley JF, Ward KN. Persistence of antibody to human parvovirus B19 after allogenic bone marrow transplantation: role of prior recipient immunity. *Blood* 1997;89:4646–4651.

45. Itala M, Kotilainen P, Nikkari S, Remes K, Nikoskelainen J. Pure red cell aplasia caused by B19 parvovirus infection after autologous blood stem cell transplantation in a patient with chronic lymphocytic leukemia [Letter]. *Leukemia* 1997;11:171.

47. Barnett N, Mak H, Winkelstein JA. Extensive verrucosis in primary immunodeficiency diseases. *Arch Dermatol* 1983;119(1):5–7.

48. Gassenmaier A, Fuch P, Schell H, Pfister H. Papillomavirus DNA in warts of immunosuppressed renal allograft recipients. *Arch Dermatol Res* 1986;278:219–223.

49. McLelland J, Rees A, Williams G, Chu T. The incidence of immunosuppression-related skin disease in long-term transplant patients. *Transplantation* 1988;46:871–874.

50. Rudlinger R, Smith IW, Bunney MH, Hunter JAA. Human papillomavirus infections in a group of renal transplant recipients. *Br J Dermatol* 1986;115:681–692.

51. Ingelfinger JR, Grupe WE, Topor M, Levey RH. Warts in pediatric renal transplant population. *Dermatologica* 1977;155:7–12.

52. Boyle J, Briggs JD, Mackie RM, Junor BJR, Aitchison TC. Cancer, warts, and sunshine in renal transplant patients. *Lancet* 1984;1(8379):702–704.

53. Van der Leest RJ, Zachow KR, Ostrow RS, Bender M, Pass F, Faras AJ. Human papillomavirus heterogeneity in 36 renal transplant recipients. *Arch Dermatol* 1987;123:354–357.

54. Wilson CAB, Holmes SC, Campo MS, White SI, Tillman D, Mackie RM, Thomson J. Novel variants of human papillomavirus type 2 in warts from immunocompromised individuals. *Br J Dermatol* 1989;121, 571–576.

55. Hoxtell EO, Mandel JS, Murray SS, Schuman LM, Goltz RW. Incidence of skin carcinoma after renal transplantation. *Arch Dermatol* 1977;113(4):436–438.

56. Shuttleworth D, Roberts E, Griffin PJA. Renal transplantation and the skin. *Lancet* 1988;1(8580):293–294.

57. Leigh IM, Glover MT. Skin cancer and warts in immunosuppressed renal transplant recipients. *Recent Results Cancer Res* 1995;139:69–86.

58. Noel JC, Thiry L, Verhest A, et al. Transitional cell carcinoma of the bladder: evaluation of the role of human papillomaviruses. *Urology* 1994;44:671–675.

Transplant Infections edited by
Raleigh A. Bowden, Per Ljungman, and Carlos V. Paya.
Lippincott–Raven Publishers, Philadelphia © 1998

CHAPTER 21

Community Respiratory Virus Infections in Transplant Recipients

Estella E. Whimbey and Janet A. Englund

Respiratory disease in the transplant recipient has traditionally been attributed to bacteria, fungii, *Pneumocystis carinii*, mycobacteria, and a variety of other exotic, opportunistic pathogens. In terms of viruses, the focus has been almost exclusively on the herpesviruses (particularly cytomegalovirus [CMV]) and an occasional adenovirus. However, more than 30% of pneumonias in the transplant recipient have not had a defined etiology and have been relegated to a poorly understood category variously called the "idiopathic" pneumonia or pneumonia of unknown etiology, or have been attributed to regimen-related toxicity or to the acute respiratory distress syndrome (ARDS). In a classic study of 215 nonbacterial, nonfungal pneumonias in 525 allogeneic hematopoetic cell transplant (HCT) recipients transplanted between 1969 and 1979, 47% of the pneumonias were attributed to CMV, HSV, or VZV; 0.5% were attributed to adenovirus; and 44% of the pneumonias remained undiagnosed. The overall mortality with idiopathic pneumonia was high (60%) (1).

Over the last decade, there has been a growing recognition that the viruses that commonly cause acute respiratory illness in the global community are also a common cause of respiratory disease in transplant recipients (2–11). These community respiratory viruses (CRV) include respiratory syncytial virus (RSV), influenza viruses, parainfluenza viruses (PIV), adenoviruses, rhinoviruses, coronaviruses, echoviruses, and coxsackie viruses. In the general community, these viruses produce a wide range of clinical syndromes, including the common cold, pharyngitis, tracheobronchitis, laryngotracheo-

bronchitis (croup), bronchiolitis, and pneumonia. Each of these viruses can produce several different syndromes, and otherwise healthy persons typically experience two to six illnesses each year. "All ages, all seasons, all populations, and all geographic locations experience illnesses caused by respiratory viruses; an extraordinary amount of time is lost from school and work because of the acute respiratory illnesses. The impact of these illnesses on human health is difficult to overestimate" (12).

CRV also have an enormous impact on the health of the transplant recipient, causing numerous illnesses, ranging from self-limited upper respiratory tract illnesses (URIs) to life-threatening pneumonias (and occasionally other organ disease or disseminated disease), depending largely on the virus, the type of transplant, and the type, degree, and duration of immunodeficiency. The pneumonias may be primarily viral, bacterial/fungal, or mixed in origin.

The emergence of these viruses in the transplant setting largely reflects our developing knowledge of the frequency and significance of infections that have existed. Their emergence also reflects the increasing population of severely immunodeficient patients; the more aggressive attempts to identify high-risk patients with URIs and to obtain samples of their respiratory secretions for viral studies; the more widespread implementation of a different type of sampling of respiratory secretions (the nasopharyngeal wash or aspirate); and a growing effort on the part of clinical virology and pathology laboratories to identify these viruses as well as the traditional herpesviruses in clinical specimens. Of note, the potential seriousness of CRV infections in immunocompromised children has been recognized since the 1970s, more than a decade earlier than in immunocompromised adults (13–20). This earlier recognition probably reflects the dominating role played by such viruses, particularly by RSV and PIV, in serious respiratory disease in children.

EEW: From the M.D. Anderson Cancer Center, University of Texas, Houston, TX 77030. JAE: From the Departments of Microbiology and Immunology and Pediatrics, Baylor College of Medicine, Houston, TX 77030.

VIRION CHARACTERISTICS AND EPIDEMIOLOGY

The CRV comprise a diverse group of viruses belonging to several distinct families, including the orthomyxoviridae (influenza viruses), the paramyxoviridae (RSV and PIV), the picornaviridae (rhinoviruses and enteroviruses), the coronaviridiae (coronaviruses), and the adenoviridae (adenoviruses) (12). They are all single-stranded RNA viruses, except for adenovirus, which is a double-stranded DNA virus. Adenovirus is assembled in the nucleus, and, similar to CMV, morphological abnormalities can frequently be visualized in clinical material with light microscopy as the presence of intranuclear inclusions in infected cells. By contrast, the RNA viruses are assembled in the cytoplasm. In some cases, morphological abnormalities can be visualized with light microscopy as the presence of intracytoplasmic inclusions. This occurs frequently with RSV, less frequently with PIV, and occasionally with influenza viruses. The histologic diagnosis of RSV or PIV infection may be further suggested by the presence of multinucleated syncytia (the fusion of adjacent infected cells). In many cases of pneumonia due to CRV, however, there are no distinguishing cytological abnormalities visualizable with light microscopy. In these cases, the histopathological abnormalities in the lung might be categorized by the pathologist as idiopathic or ARDS unless the clinical scenario and viral cultures point to a more specific etiology, or more sophisticated diagnostic tools such as electron microscopy or PCR are used to examine the lung tissue.

The CRV are acquired exogenously, except for adenovirus, which is thought to be acquired by endogenous reactivation as well. The infections are transmitted from person to person or through fomites by the transfer of virus-containing respiratory secretions. Transmission may occur through aerosols, large droplets, or direct or indirect contact with infected secretions. Contamination of hands followed by autoinoculation of the mucosal surfaces of the eye, mouth, or nose is a common mode of transmission. Although a virus may have a predominating mode of transmission (e.g., influenza is primarily transmitted through small-particle aerosols; RSV is primarily transmitted through contact), each of these viruses can be transmitted by more than one route. Nosocomial transmission is common, and devastating hospital outbreaks have occurred (21). Because these viruses are transmitted from person to person, infection control measures are critical in controlling the spread of these infections.

The temporal occurrence of these infections in immunocompromised patients tends to mirror their occurrence in the community. Community outbreaks of RSV infections typically occur during the late fall, winter, and early spring, and influenza outbreaks typically occur during the winter in temperate climates. PIV infections occur throughout the year, with outbreaks occurring primarily in the spring, summer, and fall. The other viruses typically occur year round, although sporadic outbreaks of all CRV may occur.

OVERVIEW OF THE FREQUENCY AND IMPACT OF CRV INFECTIONS IN TRANSPLANT RECIPIENTS

Hematopoetic Stem Cell Transplantation

Over the last decade, the cumulative experience reaped from surveillance studies for CRV from several transplant centers has established the high frequency and the significant clinical impact of CRV infections in HCT recipients (2–11).

At The Children's Hospital of Philadelphia, a retrospective review from 1979 to 1986 revealed a CRV infection in 11 (12%) of 96 pediatric HCT patients, including PIV ($n = 5$); adenoviruses ($n = 3$); RSV ($n = 1$)); influenza virus ($n = 1$); and rhinovirus ($n = 1$) (2). Interstitial pneumonia developed in two children with adenovirus infection (both of whom also had CMV and both of whom died), and one patient with PIV infection. This study confirmed earlier studies demonstrating the importance of CRV in immunocompromised children.

At the Fred Hutchinson Cancer Research Center (FHCRC), a prospective surveillance study conducted between January and April, 1987 documented a CRV infections in 15 (19%) of 78 mostly adult immunocompromised patients who were followed from before transplant until 60 days after transplant or until hospital discharge (3). The viruses included PIV ($n = 8$); adenovirus ($n = 5$); RSV ($n = 1$); and influenza virus ($n = 1$). This study demonstrated the high frequency and the considerable morbidity and mortality associated with CRV infections in immunocompromised adults. Five (33%) patients developed pneumonia: PIV ($n = 2$); adenovirus ($n = 2$); and RSV ($n = 1$). Two (13%) patients died: one with RSV, the other with adenovirus. Because this study included pretransplant recipients, these findings probably represented a minimal estimate of the risk for pneumonia and death.

A subsequent prospective surveillance study conducted at FHCRC among HCT recipients from 1990 to 1996 revealed 127 CRV infections, including RSV (35%), PIV (30%), rhinoviruses (25%), and influenza viruses (11%) (10). The overall frequency of CRV infections was approximately 4%. It was observed that the frequency of isolation from BAL specimens varied considerably among the different viruses and that this probably reflected different frequencies of progression to lower respiratory tract disease. For example, 49% of RSV isolates were from BAL, compared with 22% of PIV isolates, 10% of influenza virus isolates, and 3% of rhinovirus isolates.

At the Huddinge University Hospital, Sweden, a prospective surveillance study conducted among HCT recipients between 1989 and 1996 detected 39 (7.1%) CRV infections in 545 patients, including influenza viruses (38%), RSV (21%), PIV (21%), and adenoviruses (21%) (11). The frequency was 9.3% in allogeneic and 1.8% in autologous HCT recipients.

At M.D. Anderson Cancer Center (MDACC) a prospective surveillance study conducted among hospitalized adult HCT recipients during two 6-month periods in the late fall, winter, and early spring of 1992–1993 and 1993–1994 detected 67 (31%) CRV infections in 217 patients hospitalized with an acute respiratory illness (7). These 67 cases constituted approximately 21% of the patients undergoing transplant during that time period. This was a minimum estimate of the frequency because all cases were confirmed by culture rather than by serology or rapid detection assays, and only hospitalized patients were cultured. Approximately half (49%) of these infections were due to RSV; the remainder were due to influenza viruses (18%), picornaviruses (18%), PIV (9%), or adenoviruses (6%). Half of these infections were acquired nosocomially. The various infections were interspersed throughout this time period so that a precise prediction of a particular pathogen based on the epidemiology was not possible. The impact of these illnesses was considerable: 58% of the infections were complicated by pneumonia, and 51% of the pneumonias were fatal. The overall pneumonia-associated mortality was similarly high among autologous (12/20, 60%) and allogeneic HCT recipients (8/19, 42%). In an era of reasonably effective prophylactic and/or preemptive strategies for CMV disease, CRV were observed to have assumed a dominating role in the etiology of viral pneumonia (Table 1). During this 12-month period, the frequency of CRV-associated pneumonias was more than four times as high as CMV-associated pneumonias (18% vs 4%, respectively), and the overall mortality associated with these pneumonias was more than four times as high (9% vs 2%, respectively). Of interest, it was not uncommon for patients to have dual CRV infections or dual CMV-CRV infection. It was also not uncommon for patients to have perplexingly prolonged respiratory illnesses that upon virologic analysis revealed sequential infections with different viruses.

TABLE 1. *Pneumonias associated with community respiratory viruses and cytomegalovirus in 217 adult bone marrow transplant recipients hospitalized[a] with an acute respiratory illness*

	Community respiratory viruses	Cytomegalovirus
Pneumonia	39 (18%)	9 (4%)
Deaths	20 (9%)[b]	5 (2%)[c]

[a]Nov. 1 to May 1, 1992–93, 1993–94.

[b]12/20 autologous and 8/19 allogeneic bone marrow transplant (BMT) recipients died.

[c]0/3 autologous and 5/6 allogeneic BMT recipients died.

Reprinted, with permission, from ref. 9.

The wide divergence reported in the overall frequency of CRV infections, the frequency of individual viral infections, and the associated morbidity and mortality largely reflects differences in the intensity of the surveillances; the time of year when the surveillance was performed and the viruses prevalent in the community; the type and degree of immunosuppression of the patients being evaluated; the type of infection control and influenza vaccination policies; the inclusion of potential as well as actual transplant recipients; the inclusion of outpatients as well as inpatients; the types of viruses routinely assayed for in the laboratory (e.g., some laboratories have not specifically assayed for rhinoviruses); the multiplicity of laboratory methods used to identity different viruses (e.g., culture and/or rapid antigen assays and/or PCR and/or histopathology); and the definition of a case (i.e., confirmed by culture and/or rapid detection assays).

Solid Organ Transplant Recipients

Comprehensive surveillances of solid organ transplant (SOT) recipients for CRV infections have not been reported. A few studies have focused on specific viruses (22–24).

At the Children's Hospital of Pittsburgh, a retrospective review revealed 45 infections due to PIV ($n = 32$) or influenza virus ($n = 13$) in pediatric SOT recipients between 1985 and 1992 (22). The frequency of infections varied with the type of transplant, ranging from 3% with renal transplants to 8% with liver transplants and 29% with small bowel transplants. The infections were associated with considerable morbidity and mortality. Eight (18%) children died (five with PIV, three with influenza virus), half of whom had serious concurrent infections. Differences in clinical presentations and outcomes could not be discerned between the two viruses or between the different types of organ transplanted. Risk factors for poor outcome included young age, onset of infection within 1 month after transplant, and augmented immunosuppression.

At the University of Minnesota, a retrospective review revealed 19 infections due to RSV ($n = 9$) or PIV ($n = 10$) infection in 18 (21%) of 84 lung transplant recipients between 1986 and 1993 (23,24). Most patients were adults. Most infections occurred many months post-transplant (range, 24–2,056 days; median, 260 days). The illnesses were associated with considerably morbidity. All patients developed lower respiratory tract disease and six (33%) patients developed a decline in spirometry, which was irreversible in two patients. The high frequency of lower respiratory tract infections in the late post-transplant period was thought to reflect the persistence of abnormal lung defenses. In contrast to HCT recipients, the mortality was relatively low. Only one patient (with RSV infection) died. In addition to lower respiratory tract disease, a possible association with allograft rejection was suggested.

Studies such as these have made it apparent that CRV are an underappreciated cause of morbidity and mortality in SOT recipients. A full understanding of the impact of these infections will need to take into consideration the age of the patient, the specific virus causing the infection, the type of organ transplanted, the type and degree of immunosuppression, and the time following transplant.

RESPIRATORY SYNCYTIAL VIRUS

RSV is a major cause of lower respiratory tract disease in infants and young children, causing tracheobronchitis, bronchiolitis, and pneumonia. Most persons are infected during the first years of life (25,26). Natural immunity is incomplete, and repeated infections are common. In older children and adults, RSV infections are seldom severe and are usually manifested as URIs or tracheobronchitis. In the elderly, RSV infections may be complicated by lower respiratory tract illnesses similar to influenza. In immunocompromised adults as well as children, RSV infections are associated with substantial morbidity and mortality, the frequency of which varies considerably, depending on the type and degree of underlying immunodeficiency.

Hematopoetic Stem Cell Transplant Recipients

The significant morbidity and mortality of RSV infections in HCT recipients was brought to focus in 1988 in a study describing six HCT recipients with serious RSV disease (27). Subsequent studies from several transplant centers in the United States and Europe have established a fairly consistent picture of the epidemiology, frequency, and clinical course of RSV infections in HCT recipients (28–34). These studies have established that RSV is a frequent cause of acute respiratory illness in autologous as well as allogeneic pediatric and adult HCT recipients during community outbreaks. These outbreaks typically occur during the late fall, winter, and early spring, but occasionally occur at other times of the year. Devastating nosocomial outbreaks of fatal pneumonia have occurred, highlighting the need for aggressive hospital infection control strategies. At the University of Minnesota, eight (11%) of 74 HCT recipients were diagnosed to have acute RSV-induced lung injury between March, 1987 and April, 1988 (29). Four (50%) pneumonias were fatal. At FHCRC, 31 (16%) of 199 HCT recipients were diagnosed with RSV infections during a 13-week winter outbreak in 1989–1990 (31). Three-quarters of the infections were acquired nosocomially. Fourteen (78%) of 18 pneumonias were fatal. At MDACC, 19 (17%) of 111 hospitalized adult HCT recipients were diagnosed with RSV infections during a 9-week winter outbreak in 1992–1993 (33). These 19 patients constituted 45% of the adult HCT recipients hospitalized with an acute respiratory illness. Two-thirds of the infections were acquired nosocomially and nine (56%) of 16 pneumonias were fatal.

RSV infections in adult HCT recipients follow the same clinical sequence as in children: signs and symptoms of a URI (rhinorrhea, sinus congestion, sore throat, otitis media) almost always precede pneumonia, and provide the clue that the pneumonia may be due to a CRV such as RSV. The frequency of progression of URI to pneumonia is highest in patients who are early (<1 month) post-transplant or preengrafted (70% to 80%). In patients who are late (>2 months) post-transplant or postengrafted, the frequency is reported to be 25% to 40% (31,33). The latter figures are probably an overestimate because patients are followed less closely in the late post-transplant period, and there is a tendency for more severe cases to come to medical attention. Once RSV disease has progressed to pneumonia, however, the mortality is similarly high (over 80%) in pre- and post-engrafted HCT recipients.

Controlled trials of therapy for RSV disease in immunocompromised patients have not been conducted. In an open trial in adult HCT recipients with "RSV-induced acute lung injury," monotherapy with aerosolized ribavirin has been reported to be of benefit if initiated prior to the development of radiographic infiltrates (29). In another open trial in adult HCT recipients with radiographically visible RSV pneumonia, combination therapy with aerosolized ribavirin and high RSV-titered IVIG has been reported to be of benefit if initiated prior to the onset of respiratory failure (9,33). Regardless of the type of therapeutic intervention, the mortality of RSV pneumonia has approached 100% when therapy has been initiated after the onset of respiratory failure. Exceptions have raised the possibility of superimposed pulmonary hemorrhage, pulmonary edema, or bacterial superinfection precipitating the intubation, rather than progressive viral pneumonia.

Because the frequency of progression of RSV URIs to pneumonia has been observed to be exceptionally high in some subsets of patients and because the overall pneumonia-associated mortality has been high regardless of the therapeutic intervention, "preemptive" strategies are being investigated (9,10), similar to the preemptive approach to CMV pneumonia. In the case of RSV, this has meant treating the infections at the URI stage. Preliminary results of two open preemptive therapeutic trials have suggested that although this approach may be more effective than waiting for the onset of frank pneumonia, the morbidity and mortality remain high. The need to investigate prophylactic strategies has become apparent.

Of note, some types of rapid RSV antigen detection assays performed on nasopharyngeal secretions may be relatively insensitive in immunocompromised adults compared with young children due to the relatively low quantity of virus shed in the nasal secretions (35). Since a favorable outcome hinges on the prompt initiation of therapy, it is crucial to be cognizant of the possibility of falsely negative antigen detection assays and to pursue the diagnosis by other means, such as BAL.

Solid Organ Transplant Recipients

RSV disease has been less well studied in SOT recipients. Aside from scattered case reports, case series have been reported primarily in lung transplant, renal transplant and pediatric liver transplant recipients (23,27,36–38). In these patients, the illnesses have ranged from URIs characterized by rhinorrhea, sinus congestion, and mild cough to bronchiolitis and life-threatening pneumonias.

Lung transplant recipients have been reported to have a high frequency of RSV lower respiratory tract disease but a relatively low mortality. As described earlier, at the University of Minnesota, nine (11%) of 84 lung transplant recipients were documented to have RSV infections, and all infections were complicated by lower respiratory tract disease (23). Most patients were treated with aerosolized ribavirin, and all these patients survived. The one death occurred in an untreated patient with bronchiolitis obliterans. RSV infections in lung transplant recipients have also been associated with organ rejection and bronchiolitis obliterans, both of which have been observed to be seasonally related (24).

Adult renal transplant recipients have also been reported to develop RSV-associated lower respiratory tract disease. The mortality has been low, and most patients have recovered without specific antiviral therapy (27,37).

In pediatric liver transplant recipients, RSV infections have been associated with significant morbidity but a relatively low mortality (38). Among 483 pediatric liver transplant recipients cared for at the University of Pittsburgh between 1985 and 1991, 17 (3.4%) children developed RSV infections, three-quarters of which were nosocomially acquired. The majority (71%) of the children had lower respiratory tract involvement, and two (12%) children died. None of the children received specific antiviral therapy. The risk factors for more severe disease included onset of infection early after transplant, preexisting lung pathology, augmented immunosuppression prompted by rejection, and younger age. Infections occurring late after transplantation in the absence of rejection were usually not severe.

In summary, these limited data suggest that RSV is an important cause of morbidity in SOT recipients, causing lower respiratory tract disease as well as possibly other types of morbidity, such as organ rejection and bronchiolitis obliterans. The mortality was relatively low compared with HCT recipients. It is unclear whether the favorable outcome in lung transplant recipients was related to therapy with ribavirin or whether it simply reflected the natural course of the disease as with renal transplant and pediatric liver transplant recipients.

Prophylaxis and Therapy of RSV

Options for the Prophylaxis of RSV Infections

An aggressive infection control strategy can be highly effective in reducing the nosocomial acquisition of RSV by transplant recipients (21). Active immunoprophylaxis is not an option because an effective vaccine is not currently available. Passive immunoprophylaxis has been studied in placebo-controlled trials in high-risk infants and children. In these children, the monthly administration of RSV-IVIG, a human polyclonal IgG immune globulin with high RSV microneutralization titers (Respigram, Medimmune), has been effective in decreasing the risk of serious RSV disease (39). A similar trial in children of the monthly administration of monoclonal RSV antibody, a humanized monoclonal antibody (investigational, MEDI-493, Medimmune) is currently being conducted and appears promising (40). Passive immunoprophylaxis in immunocompromised patients has not been studied.

Options for Preventing the Progression of RSV Upper Respiratory Tract Illnesses to Pneumonia or "Preemptive Therapy"

In patients who have not yet received conditioning therapy, consideration should be given to postponing the transplant until the illness resolves. In patients who have received conditioning therapy and who are at risk for fatal viral pneumonia, it is generally agreed that it may be beneficial to begin therapy at the URI stage. As controlled trials have not been conducted, however, there is considerable divergence of opinion on the optimal preemptive regimen. The available options showing promise are aerosolized ribavirin with or without immunotherapy (high-titered or standard IVIG).

At FHCRC, 25 HCT recipients with RSV-URIs were treated with aerosolized ribavirin at a high concentration (60 mg/ml) for 2 hours each day (total: 2 g/day) (10). The advantage of this regimen was that it could be administered as an outpatient. Eight (32%) patients developed pneumonia, and seven (29%) patients died. At MDACC, 12 HCT recipients with RSV-URIs were treated with a combination of aerosolized ribavirin and IVIG (500 mg/kg qod) (9). The daily dose of ribavirin was higher (6 g/day), and the duration of therapy each day was considerably longer. Ribavirin was administered at 20 mg/ml for 18 hours/day to five patients, and at 60 mg/ml for 2 hours three times per day to seven patients (41,42). Two (17%) patients developed pneumonia (one in each dosage regimen) and both died. Although both studies were limited by the lack of controls, the overall findings suggest that the frequency of pneumonia and death may be decreased by promptly treating URIs. Whether higher daily doses and longer daily durations of therapy are more effective needs to be further evaluated.

The decision to initiate therapy with aerosolized ribavirin and/or IVIG for a simple RSV-URI is complex and needs to take into consideration many factors, including the patient's risk of developing serious lower respiratory tract disease, the unproven efficacy of these drugs in transplant recipients, the potential for environmental contamination and exposure of health care workers, the psychological and physical discomfort to the patients of prolonged aerosol therapy and confinement within a scavenging tent, the adverse effects of aerosolized ribavirin, such as bronchospasm, the high cost of these drugs as well as the intensive respiratory therapy needed to safely administer aerosolized ribavirin, and the need for hospitalization with more frequent or prolonged ribavirin dosing regimens. Studies are under way to define more closely the patients at risk and to identify the simplest to administer and least costly yet effective regimen.

Options for the Therapy of RSV Pneumonia

Aerosolized ribavirin is approved by the FDA for the therapy of RSV bronchiolitis and pneumonia in infants and young children. In HCT recipients with RSV disease, the reported benefit of monotherapy with aerosolized ribavirin has been conflicting. Favorable responses have been reported primarily when therapy was initiated at an early stage of the respiratory illness (either at the URI, tracheobronchitis, or early pneumonia stage). In an open trial at the University of Minnesota, none of four adult HCT recipients with "RSV-induced acute lung injury" died when monotherapy was initiated prior to the onset of radiographic infiltrates, compared with all four HCT recipients in whom monotherapy was initiated afterwards (29). At FHCRC, monotherapy with aerosolized ribavirin was associated with a high mortality (69%) in 13 HCT recipients with radiographically visible RSV pneumonia, but it was felt that the early initiation of therapy may have been beneficial (31). In SOT recipients, favorable responses have been reported in an open trial of lung transplant recipients with lower respiratory tract disease who received monotherapy with aerosolized ribavirin (23).

Whether passive immunotherapy is of benefit alone or in combination with antiviral therapy is being investigated (43–48). In one placebo-controlled trial in 35 hospitalized RSV-infected infants and children (not transplant recipients), monotherapy with IVIG containing substantial RSV neutralizing antibody titers resulted in significant reductions in nasal RSV shedding and improvement in oxygenation (46). In a larger placebo-controlled trial in 105 hospitalized high-risk children with RSV lower respiratory illness, however, monotherapy with RSV-IVIG was not found to be efficacious (48).

In an open trial at MDACC, combination therapy with aerosolized ribavirin (18 hours/day) and high RSV-titered IVIG (0.5 g/kg every other day) has been associated with a favorable response in adult HCT recipients with RSV pneumonia in whom therapy was initiated prior to respiratory failure (Table 2) (9). Thus the mortality was 31% in 13 patients in whom combination therapy was initiated prior to respiratory failure and 100% in nine patients who did not receive specific antiviral therapy or who were started on therapy after respiratory failure. Similarly, none of eight adults with leukemia with RSV pneumonia died in whom combination therapy with aerosolized ribavirin and IVIG was initiated prior to respiratory failure, compared with eight (89%) of nine patients who did not receive specific antiviral therapy or who could not tolerate the therapy or were started on therapy after respiratory failure (9,49). In subsequent years, MDACC has continued to use a combined regimen with similar response, although standard IVIG in frequent and large doses (500 mg/kg QOD) has been substituted for high-titered IVIG. At the Dana Farber Cancer Institute, combination therapy with aerosolized ribavirin (18 hours/day) and RSV-IVIG (1.5 g/kg for one dose) was similarly associated with a favorable response in 2 HCT recipients with clinically severe RSV pneumonia occurring early following transplant (47).

Other options being investigated either alone or in combination with aerosolized ribavirin include IV ribavirin (an investigational drug, ICN) and topical immunoglobulins (50–52). The relative ease of administration of IV ribavirin is attractive. However, in a recent study at FHCRC, the mortality was 80% in 10 HCT recipients with RSV pneumonia treated with IV ribavirin alone, and 20% of the patients developed significant hemolytic anemia. This suggests that monotherapy with IV ribavirin was not adequate and that IV ribavirin may

TABLE 2. *Mortality associated with respiratory syncytial virus pneumonia in adult bone marrow transplant recipients and adults with leukemia*

Therapy[a]	Mortality (%) BMT (n=23)	Mortality (%) Leukemia (n=17)
Early[b]	4/13 (31)	0/8 (0)
Early (noncompliant)	—	2/2 (100)
Early (6 h/day)	1/1 (100)	—
Late[b]	5/5 (100)	4/4 (100)
None	4/4 (100)	2/3 (66)

BMT, bone marrow transplant.
[a]Therapy consisted of aerosolized ribavirin (20 mg/ml for 18 h/day) and intravenous immunoglobulin (IV Ig; 500 mg/kg every other day). One patient received aerosolized ribavirin (60 mg/ml for 2 h every 8 h) and IV Ig.
[b]Therapy was classified as "early" or "late" depending on whether it was initiated >24 h or <24 h prior to respiratory failure requiring mechanical ventilation, respectively.
Reprinted, with permission, from ref. 9.

be more toxic in these patients than has been previously reported in patients with hemorrhagic fevers (53,54). In contrast, the European experience with combination aerosolized/intravenous ribavirin has been favorable (55).

The optimal duration of therapy has not been defined. Among the factors to be considered are the immunologic status of the patient (HCT recipients who are preengrafted, and leukemia patients who are myelosuppressed are at higher risk and may need more prolonged therapy) and the response to therapy of the respiratory illness. Of note has been the observation that some patients may recover in spite of persistence of viral shedding.

INFLUENZA VIRUSES

Influenza is considered to be one of the most important respiratory diseases of mankind, having a significant impact on persons of all ages in all parts of the global community (56). Because of the frequent antigenic variation of its surface glycoproteins (hemagglutinin and neuraminidase), influenza continues to challenge clinicians with the problem of an "emerging virus." Outbreaks of influenza of variable extent and severity occur nearly annually during the winter in temperate climates and are associated with considerable morbidity and mortality.

Although the Centers for Disease Control and Prevention (CDC) has long recommended that immunocompromised patients receive annual influenza vaccination and be considered for chemoprophylaxis during influenza outbreaks, this has been an unpopular practice in many cancer and transplant centers (57). Perhaps the most compelling reason has been the lack of data documenting significant influenza-associated morbidity and mortality in these patients. Over the last decade, the impact of influenza in transplant patients and patients with hematologic malignancies has become increasingly appreciated, though the reported frequency and severity of illness has varied considerably among different types of transplant and different transplant centers (58–64).

Hematopoetic Stem Cell Transplantation

The highest frequency of symptomatic illness and serious disease has been reported among HCT recipients cared for at MDACC, where influenza infections have been aggressively searched for prospectively (9,62). Over the course of six winter seasons (1991–1992 to 1996–1997), influenza type A and B viruses were isolated from approximately 60 hospitalized adult HCT recipients. These infections occurred during 7–18-week periods. Similar to RSV, the temporal occurrence of these infections mirrored their occurrence in the community. During these outbreaks, influenza was isolated from approximately 10% to 30% of the transplant recipients hospitalized with an acute respiratory illness. This was a minimal estimate of the frequency of influenza because these infections were diagnosed by

culture only. During the first few winters, many infections were acquired nosocomially. Subsequent to the institution of rigorous infection control measures, most infections were acquired in the community. This highlights the need to develop prophylactic strategies beyond those in the hospital.

The impact of influenza in this patient population was evident in its morbidity as well as its mortality, as reflected in the secondary bacterial and fungal sinusitis and pneumonias, and the prolonged hospitalizations and extensive evaluations for generalized debility and fevers. Approximately 60% of the patients with influenza developed pneumonia, and approximately 25% of the patients with influenza died of progressive respiratory failure.

The frequency of progression of uncomplicated influenza to pneumonia during the preengraftment period was considerably lower than that with RSV. However, the spectrum of patients at risk for fatal influenza-associated pneumonia was broad, and included autologous transplant recipients in remission who were more than 1 year after transplant without other known risk factors for serious influenza. Appreciation of the risk for serious influenza in late transplant recipients is important so that the appropriate prophylactic and therapeutic measures can be instituted in these patients as well as more immunodeficient transplant recipients.

The mortality of HCT recipients with influenza-associated pneumonia was considerably lower than that with RSV- or CMV-associated pneumonias (40% versus 80%, respectively). This was primarily because many of the influenza-associated pneumonias appeared to be secondary bacterial or fungal superinfections rather than primary viral pneumonias, and resolved with antibacterial/antifungal therapy. A similar situation exists in the global community. However, among patients who actually had influenza viral pneumonia, the clinical course was as fulminant and lethal as with these other viral pneumonias.

At MDACC the frequency of pneumonia and death was similar among patients who were and who were not treated with amantadine or rimantadine (A/R), the only FDA-approved drugs for the therapy of influenza A. One reason monotherapy with A/R was not effective in preventing the progression of uncomplicated influenza type A to pneumonia, or halting the progression of pneumonia in these immunocompromised patients appeared to be due to the rapid development of viral resistance to the drug (65). This has already been well demonstrated in otherwise healthy people with influenza, one-third of whom develop resistant strains of virus within a few days of starting A/R (66–68). As in immunocompetent patients, the development of resistance has been through single amino acid changes on the transmembrane of the M2 protein (65).

The high frequency of influenza and the severity of the illness in HCT recipients cared for at MDACC has not been uniformly observed in other HCT centers. Among 18 HCT recipients with influenza A and B infections cared for in European centers from 1989 to 1996, approximately one-third of the patients developed pneumonia, and three (17%) patients died (11). Among 10 HCT recipients with influenza A or B infections cared for in Stockholm during the 1988–1989 and/or 1989–1990 influenza seasons, two (20%) patients developed pneumonia (both during the aplastic phase) and both died (58,61). In contrast, among HCT recipients cared for at FHCRC from 1990 to 1996, influenza pneumonia was reported to occur infrequently compared with RSV, based on the finding that influenza virus was isolated from the BAL of two (10%) of 21 patients with influenza while RSV was isolated from the BAL of 23 (49%) of 47 patients with RSV infections (10).

Solid Organ Transplant Recipients

Scant data exist on the frequency and clinical course of influenza in SOT recipients. Aside from scattered case reports of serious influenza in various organ transplant recipients, most case series have been in pediatric SOT recipients and renal transplant recipients (22,58,61,69,70). Among pediatric SOT recipients, influenza has been reported to cause fairly severe disease. Among 12 pediatric SOT recipients with influenza B cared for at the University of Minnesota from 1989 to 1992, 10 children required hospitalization, and two children required mechanical ventilation. Five (42%) children developed neurological complications, and one (8%) died (70). Similarly, as described earlier, among 13 pediatric SOT recipients with influenza cared for at the University of Pittsburgh from 1985 to 1992, three (23%) children died (22).

In contrast, among renal transplant recipients, influenza has generally been reported to cause only mild self-limited illness (58,61). Among 15 renal transplant recipients (mostly adults) with influenza A or B infections cared for in Stockholm during the 1988–1989 and/or 1989–1990 influenza seasons, only one patient developed pneumonia and none died. Another type of morbidity observed has been an association with acute graft rejection (71,72).

Surprisingly, case series of serious influenza in lung transplant recipients have not been reported thus far, although their susceptibility to serious RSV and PIV infections has been demonstrated. It has been suggested that this may reflect the aggressiveness with which these patients are targeted for annual influenza vaccination, rather than underrecognition of the problem (24). A seasonal increased frequency of bronchiolitis obliterans, however, has been observed, suggesting that influenza may be a contributing factor to this serious complication of lung transplantation (73).

In summary, in view of the high annual attack rate of influenza in the global community during outbreaks, ranging from 10% to 50% or higher in semiclosed settings with a large number of susceptible people, it is not surprising that transplant recipients also become infected with influenza frequently. HCT recipients and pediatric SOT recipients have been reported to be at high risk for life-threatening complications; however, other types of SOT recipients need be studied, particularly those with known risk factors for serious influenza such as cardiac and lung transplant recipients. The validity of negative studies needs to be questioned, unless there is a rational explanation, such as confinement in protected environments or effective immunization or chemoprophylaxis. Documentation of a high frequency of infection requires an appreciation of the strong likelihood of the occurrence of influenza during outbreaks; obtaining optimal samples of respiratory secretions; and processing the samples in a laboratory capable of isolating these viruses. The wide spectrum of observations on the severity of influenza illnesses in transplant recipients largely reflects the wide spectrum of ages and immunodeficiencies in the patients being studied. In addition, some studies have focused on hospitalized patients, thereby selecting for more severe cases. In less immunocompromised patients, the clinical course of influenza may be more comparable to that in immunocompetent people. It is also noteworthy that influenza viruses undergo frequent antigenic variation and prevalent types and stereotypes vary, so the morbidity and mortality may be expected to vary from year to year.

Prophylaxis and Therapy for Influenza

Options for the Prophylaxis of Influenza

Prophylaxis and therapy for influenza (74) include aggressive infection control measures and active immunoprophylaxis through annual vaccination of patients and their families, close contacts, and health care workers and chemoprophylaxis. Although some subsets of transplant recipients (such as HCT recipients in the early post-transplant period or those with chronic GVHD) are unlikely to respond to vaccination (75–77), other subsets of patients may benefit from vaccination. Because these patients continue to be at risk for serious influenza disease, immunization would seem prudent. The benefit of immunomodulation with GM-CSF administered concomitantly with influenza vaccination has recently been evaluated in HCT recipients (78). Although there was a trend toward higher-antibody titers, the frequency of seroconversion was not increased. Immunization of the donor is another theoretically promising intervention currently being investigated. Because of the potential for suboptimal responses to vaccination, chemoprophylaxis with A/R may be considered for transplant recipient for the duration of influenza A activity in the community. Though its efficacy has not been established in immunocompromised patients, this has been an effective strategy in the general community. Unimmunized close contacts in the home or the hospital may also be considered for chemoprophylaxis during the duration of influenza A activity in the community or until 2 weeks after vaccination. New classes of antiviral agents (neuraminidase inhibitors) may offer other options in the future as prophylactic agents (79,80).

Options for Preventing the Progression of Uncomplicated Influenza to Serious Disease, or "Preemptive Therapy"

The available options for preventing the progression of uncomplicated influenza to serious disease, or "preemptive therapy," include postponing the transplant until the illness has resolved, aggressively treating bacterial/fungal superinfections, and promptly beginning antiviral therapy. Amantadine and rimantadine have been shown to be of benefit in the therapy of uncomplicated influenza A in healthy young adults if therapy is initiated promptly; however, their benefit in preventing the progression of uncomplicated infection to pneumonia or in treating serious influenza has not been established. Monotherapy with A/R is inherently limited by the rapid development of resistant virus, the lack of efficacy against type B virus, and the lack of a parenteral formulation. The MDACC experience suggests that monotherapy with A/R is not sufficient to prevent the progression of uncomplicated influenza to pneumonia in HCT recipients. Other options will need to be investigated, such as neuraminidase inhibitors and/or ribavirin and/or immunotherapy.

Options for Treating Serious Influenza Disease

Though influenza has been studied for decades, there are no quidelines for the treatment of influenza pneumonia in either immunocompetent or immunocompromised patients. In the MDACC experience, monotherapy with A/R was not effective in preventing the progression of early pneumonia to fatal pneumonia. Monotherapy with A/R is inherently limited by the factors outlined above. There are other potentially promising drugs to investigate, including ribavirin and the neuraminidase inhibitors (79–89). Both drugs have the advantage that they are active against type B as well as type A virus and that the emergence of resistant virus in people treated with these drugs has not been reported. Aerosolized ribavirin is active against influenza *in vitro* and in animal studies. Several controlled studies of uncomplicated influenza in healthy young adults and one in children have demonstrated a beneficial effect of aerosolized ribavirin therapy, which is commercially available but not FDA approved for this indication. Aerosolized ribavirin therapy has also been associated with a favorable response in several

anecdotal case reports of severe influenza virus pneumonia, including a case series of six immunocompetent adults (85). Intravenous ribavirin (investigational, ICN) has also been associated with a favorable response in several cases of serious influenza, as has the combination of aerosolized and intravenous ribavirin (55). Recent controlled studies in healthy young adults with experimental and naturally occurring uncomplicated influenza have also demonstrated a beneficial effect with the inhalational/intranasal neuraminidase inhibitor, Zanamivir or GG167 (investigational, Glaxo Wellcome). An oral neuraminidase inhibitor, GS 4104 (investigational, Gilead Sciences), looks promising *in vitro* and in animals models and is currently being studied in humans (79,80).

In vitro and animal studies suggest that combinations of anti-viral drugs (such as A/R and/or ribavirin (iv and/or aerosolized) and/or neuraminidase inhibitors) may have enhanced antiviral efficacy (90). Combination therapy may have the added advantage of deterring the emergence of resistant virus. This will need to be investigated, as well as the potential additive benefit of immunotherapy.

PARAINFLUENZA VIRUSES

PIV types 1, 2, and 3 were first recovered in 1956 and recognized as the major causes of croup, or laryngotracheobronchitis, in young children (91,92). PIV types 1 and 3 have been the most frequent types identified in immunocompromised patients. PIV type 4 has been recovered from both adults and children with URIs but is generally more difficult to isolate, and relatively little is known about its epidemiology, particularly in immunocompromised patients.

The duration of viral shedding following PIV infection in healthy people is approximately 1 week, although this is dependent on many variables, including age and severity of infection. In children, PIV type 3 may be excreted for as long as 4 weeks, and in 17% of infected children, virus is excreted during the third week after the onset of symptoms (92). Prolonged PIV shedding (>4 weeks) has been documented in children with compromised immune status, organ transplant recipients, and individuals receiving prolonged steroid therapy.

Hematopoetic Cell Transplant Recipients

The importance of PIV infections in adult as well as pediatric HCT recipients was initially highlighted in a 16-year retrospective review conducted at the University of Minnesota from 1974 to 1990 (93). In that study, 12 of 580 adults and 15 of 673 children (2.2% overall) who underwent HCT were documented to be infected with PIV. Six of 19 (32%) patients with lower respiratory tract involvement died. Similar findings have been reported at other centers (9,10,11,94,95). A 3-year prospective study at MDACC from 1991 to 1994 involving 61 adult HCT recipients with PIV infections demonstrated an overall frequency of 5% and highlighted the highly epidemic nature of PIV infections (95). More than half of the cases occurred in the late spring and early summer of 1 year. During that time, PIV were isolated from one-third (32/96) of the adult HCT recipients hospitalized with acute respiratory illnesses.

The clinical course and outcome of PIV infection among hospitalized adults with leukemia have mirrored the experience with hospitalized adult HCT recipients (9). Among 45 consecutive HCT recipients and nine adults with leukemia hospitalized at MDACC with PIV infections, the respiratory illnesses were complicated by pneumonia in 26 (58%) and six (60%) patients, respectively. Nearly all patients initially presented with signs or symptoms of URIs. Relatively high mortality rates were noted in patients with pneumonia (39% and 66%, respectively). Autopsies revealed findings consistent with viral pneumonia. However, more than half of the patients had serious concurrent opportunistic infections, stressing their profound underlying immunodeficiency.

Solid Organ Transplant Recipients

Relatively limited data are available on the incidence and significance of PIV infections in SOT recipients (22,23,96,97). The largest case series have been described in pediatric SOT recipients and lung transplant recipients (described earlier). In addition, an epidemic of PIV type 3 infections has been documented among 16 recent renal transplant recipients (97). Although these illnesses were not complicated by lower respiratory tract disease, they were associated with an increased frequency of acute rejection.

Prophylaxis and Therapy of PIV

The use of passive immunoprophylaxis has not been studied in humans, despite its benefit in an animal model. Although there are high rates of PIV infection, hospitalization and accompanying morbidity in young children, vaccine development has been relatively slow. Evaluation of live attenuated PIV vaccines in adults and children is ongoing, but this approach is likely to be limited in immunocompromised patients (52,92).

There is no licensed or proven therapy for PIV infections. The treatment of PIV pneumonia in a cotton rat model using topical antibody and corticosteroids has been reported indicating that specific immunotherapy may ultimately be possible (98). Questions relating to mechanisms of action and timing and dosing of these agents require further study. Ribavirin has antiviral effects against PIV in cell culture and has been used for the treatment of lower respiratory tract disease in immunocompromised hosts. Case reports documenting

decreased viral load and clinical improvement in several children with severe combined immunodeficiency following multiple treatments with aerosolized ribavirin have been described (52). Ribavirin has also been used in lung transplant recipients with PIV-associated pneumonias with a favorable response (23).

The risk factors for the progression of PIV-URI to pneumonia in HCT recipients remains to be elucidated, as does the efficacy of therapy with ribavirin. Among the 27 HCT recipients with PIV-associated upper and lower respiratory tract disease at the University of Minnesota, the mortality was the same (22%) among nine patients treated and 18 patients not treated with aerosolized ribavirin (93). Among the 26 adult HCT recipients with PIV-associated pneumonias at MDACC, three patients treated with combination aerosolized ribavirin and IVIG before the onset of respiratory failure survived, while two patients treated after the onset of respiratory failure died (9). However, more than 60% of the patients who did not receive specific antiviral therapy also survived, suggesting that many of these pneumonias were either self-limited viral pneumonias or bacterial or fungal superinfections, similar to the situation with influenza. The high frequency of PIV-associated pneumonias that resolve without antiviral therapy and the high frequency of concurrent opportunistic infections will render it difficult to judge the benefit of any therapeutic intervention except in a controlled trial.

RHINOVIRUSES AND CORONAVIRUSES

Rhinoviruses are the most commonly isolated viruses in people with the common cold. They typically cause an afebrile, self-limited coryzal syndrome characterized by rhinorrhea and nasal congestion and less frequently sore throat, mild cough and hoarseness (99–102). Evidence is accumulating that rhinoviruses may also be associated with exacerbations of sinusitis, chronic bronchitis and asthma, and with lower respiratory tract syndromes and atypical pneumonias in otherwise healthy people and the elderly. The specific mechanisms by which rhinoviruses produce disease are not well understood. It is hypothesized that rhinoviruses may give rise to clinical illness through inflammatory mediators and neurogenic reflexes.

Limited data exist on the role of rhinoviruses in immunocompromised patients. A recent 5-year study at MDACC has suggested that rhinovirus infections may be associated with considerable more morbidity and mortality in these patients. In approximately one-third of the adult HCT recipients who developed symptomatic rhinovirus infections prior to engraftment, the respiratory illness progressed to unexplained pneumonias, and all the pneumonias were fatal. In almost all cases, lung biopsies and autopsies only revealed findings consistent with interstitial pneumonitis and/or ARDS. Whether these pneumonias were induced by direct viral invasion of the lung tissue or by an immunologic response in the lung remains to be elucidated.

Coronaviruses are one of the most frequent causes of the common cold (103,104). Little is known about the role of coronaviruses in immunocompromised patients. This is in part due to the difficulty of isolating these viruses in culture as well as the lack of a characteristic histopathology. The availability of more sophisticated diagnostic tools, such as PCR, should facilitate the elucidation of their clinical significance.

PREVENTION OF CRV INFECTIONS THROUGH INFECTION CONTROL

Infection control strategies play a crucial role in the prevention of CRV infection (21). At the core of an effective strategy is an appreciation of the potential seriousness of CRV infections in transplant recipients; the knowledge of the CRV currently prevalent in the community; and ongoing surveillance for CRV infections in high-risk patients. This entails continuing education of patients, family members, visitors and staff regarding the potential seriousness of these infections, their epidemiology, their modes of transmission, and means of control. Also, frequent clinical screening of high-risk patients for an acute upper and/or lower respiratory tract illness or flulike illness must be ongoing and sampling of respiratory secretions of symptomatic patients for viral cultures and rapid diagnostic testing undertaken. Samples with high yield include the nasopharyngeal wash and aspirate and the BAL.

In general, infection control strategies need to be designed to prevent spread by several different modes of transmission, because several different CRV may circulate in the community concurrently and because CRV can be spread by several modes of transmission. Infection control measures may need to be intensified during community or hospital outbreaks of CRV infections. The intensity and duration of the infection control measures should be tailored to the risk of serious CRV in different subsets of transplant recipients, and to what works in the "real world." For instance, although handwashing may be as effective as gloving in a controlled setting, handwashing is notoriously difficult to enforce in clinical practice, and gloves may help ensure "clean hands." Among patients at high risk for life-threatening CRV infections, such as HCT recipients early after transplant, it would seem prudent to err on the side of overcautiousness.

That it is possible to prevent the nosocomial acquisition of CRV infections in HCT recipients has been demonstrated in a prospective study at MDACC by their rare occurrence among patients cared for in a "protected environment" compared with patients cared for on a transplant unit where infection control measures were strongly encouraged, but not rigidly enforced (7). The effectiveness of infection control interventions has also

been demonstrated by the dramatic decline in the frequency of nosocomial CRV infections among HCT recipients cared for in this transplant unit after the implementation of an aggressive, multifaceted infection control strategy (21). The measures included were that

1. All people entering a patient's room wore masks and gloves. Gloves were changed between patients and hands were washed thoroughly before entering the room and after removing the gloves.
2. The number of visitors was restricted, as was visitation by people with respiratory or flulike illnesses, and visitation by children.
3. Hospital personnel with respiratory or flulike illnesses were restricted from directly caring for HCT recipients.
4. Health care workers and close contacts were encouraged to receive annual influenza vaccination.
5. HCT recipients wore masks and gloves when exiting their room.
6. The time spent by HCT recipients in crowded areas, such as waiting rooms and elevators was minimized.
7. HCT recipients with CRV illnesses were isolated and cohorted on other wards.

Although this aggressive multifaceted approach has been effective in our experience, a less rigorous strategy may have sufficed. Moreover, it is often not feasible or desirable to protect so intensively patients for the duration of increased susceptibility to serious CRV disease, because immunosuppression may continue for months to years, and such strategies are costly and cumbersome, and pose unpleasant restrictions on the freedom and quality of life of the patient and their families. This problem is further compounded by the growing trend to discharge patients from the hospital sooner, and to perform transplants in the outpatient setting.

Among high-risk transplant recipients living in the community, the prevention of exposure to CRV is particularly challenging because these infections are so prevalent in the community and so contagious. Because many situations of exposure to infected people are beyond the control of the patient, the aim can only be to minimize these exposures. Examples of protective measures for outpatients include washing hands frequently and thoroughly and avoiding close contact with individuals suffering from respiratory illnesses. In many cases, however, such as mothers caring for small children, this is not possible. The rigorousness and duration of prophylactic measures need to be individualized in accordance with the immunologic status of the patient and the risk for serious CRV disease, the needs of the patient, and quality-of-life issues.

SUMMARY AND CONCLUSION

Growing appreciation of the profound impact that CRV have on the health and well-being of transplant recipients has stimulated widespread efforts to elucidate the pathogenesis and natural history of these infections, to identify the specific immunodeficiencies predisposing to serious disease, and to develop effective diagnostic, prophylactic, and therapeutic strategies. Effectively caring for transplant recipients with CRV infections poses an exceptional challenge because "CRV" are comprised of a wide diversity of viruses each one of which needs to be approached individually, and "transplant recipients" are comprised of a wide spectrum of patients with a broad range of immunologic and anatomic immunodeficiencies associated with different susceptibilities to serious CRV disease. Even within a particular type of transplant, such as HCT recipients, there is a wide range of vulnerability to serious CRV disease, and this vulnerability is often in a state of flux. Because the vast majority of transplant recipients with a "common cold" or a "flulike illness" will recover without antiviral therapy, it is essential to identify the risk groups within each type of transplant so that prophylaxis and therapy can be targeted judiciously.

Because these infections are so common and contagious, optimal prevention of CRV infections through infection control measures is only feasible in short-term situations. Active immunoprophylaxis through vaccination is only available for influenza, and the capacity to respond to immunization is often quite limited. Passive immunoprophylaxis is awaiting further evaluation. The chemoprophylactic and therapeutic options currently available are limited in number and often have unproven efficacy. Use of these agents is complicated, in some instances, by the rapid development of resistance (with A/R), cost, and cumbersomeness. Uncontrolled studies are difficult to interpret because many CRV infections are self-limited or resolve with antibacterial and antifungal therapy, and because the potential beneficial effects of antiviral therapy may be masked by the presence of multiple other serious concurrent infections and medical problems. Placebo-controlled studies raise ethical dilemmas in subsets of patients in whom the infections are known to be highly lethal and other potentially beneficial drugs are available, as is the case of aerosolized ribavirin for RSV pneumonia. Prompt intervention is often limited by the lack of routine rapid diagnostic assays. Awaiting the results of culture often culminates in interventions that are little more than well-meaning, futile gestures. Broad-scale use of empiric therapy, a common approach in immunocompromised patents, is difficult to endorse with costly and cumbersome-to-administer drugs whose efficacy is still undergoing investigation.

The challenges ahead are immense, yet fascinating. The major breakthrough in the last decade has been the widespread appreciation of the existence, the frequency, and the potential seriousness of CRV infections in immunocompromised patients, and the burgeoning of a concerted effort by the medical community to understand and master all aspects of these infections.

REFERENCES

1. Meyers JD, Flournoy N, Thomas ED. Nonbacterial pneumonia after allogeneic marrow transplantation: a review of ten years experience. *Rev Infect Dis* 1982;4:1119–1132.
2. Wasserman R, August CS, Plotkin SA. Viral infections in pediatric bone marrow transplant patients. *Pediatr Infect Dis* 1988;7:109–115.
3. Ljungman P, Gleaves CA, Meyers JD. Respiratory virus infections in immunocompromised patients. *Bone Marrow Transplant* 1989;4:35–40.
4. Whimbey E, Bodey GP. Viral pneumonia in the immunocompromised adult with neoplastic disease: the role of common community respiratory viruses. *Semin Respir Infect* 1992;7:122–131.
5. Bowden RA. Other viruses after marrow transplantation. In: Forman SJ, Blume KG, Thomas ED, eds. *Bone marrow transplantation.* Cambridge, MA: Blackwell Scientific Publication; 1994:443–453.
6. Sable CA, Haydn FG. Orthomyxoviral and paramyxoviral infections in transplant patients. *Dis Clin North Am* 1995;9:987–1003.
7. Whimbey E, Champlin R, Couch R, et al. Community respiratory virus infections among hospitalized adult bone marrow transplant recipients. *Clin Infect Dis* 1996;22:778–782.
8. Couch RB, Englund JA, Whimbey E. Respiratory viral infections in immunocompetent and immunocompromised persons. *Am J Med* 1997;102(3A):2–8.
9. Whimbey E, Englund JA, Couch RB. Community respiratory virus infections in immunocompromised patients with cancer. *Am J Med* 1997;102(3A):10–18.
10. Bowden RA. Respiratory virus infections after marrow transplant: the Fred Hutchinson Cancer Research Center experience. *Am J Med* 1997;102(3A):27–30.
11. Ljungman P. Respiratory virus infections in bone marrow transplant recipients: the European perspective. *Am J Med* 1997;102(3A):44–47.
12. Couch RB. Respiratory diseases. In: Galasso GJ, Whitley RJ, Merigan TC, eds. *Antiviral agents and viral diseases of man,* 3rd ed. New York: Raven Press; 1990:327–372.
13. Karp D, Willis J, Wilfert CM. Parainfluenza virus II and the immunocompromised host. *Am J Dis Child* 1974;127:592–593.
14. Feldman S, Webster RG, Sugg M. Influenza in children and young adults with cancer. *Cancer* 1977;39:350–353.
15. Craft AW, Reid MM, Gardner PS, et al. Virus infections in children with acute lymphoblastic leukaemia. *Arch Dis Child* 1979;54:755–759.
16. Bruce E, Reid MM, Craft AW, Kernahan J, Gardner PS. Multiple virus isolations in children with acute lymphoblastic leukaemia. *J Infect Dis* 1979;1:243–248.
17. Jarvis WR, Middleton PJ, Gelfand EW. Parainfluenza pneumonia in severe combined immunodeficiency disease. *J Pediatr* 1979;94(3):423–425.
18. Delage G, Brochu P, Pelletier M, Jasmin G, Lapointe N. Giant-cell pneumonia caused by parainfluenza virus. Brief clinical and laboratory observations. *J Pediatr* 1979;94(3):426–429.
19. Fishaut M, Tubergen D, McIntosh K. Cellular response to respiratory viruses with particular reference to children with disorders of cell-mediated immunity. *J Pediatr* 1980;96(2):179–186.
20. Frank JA, Warren RW, Tucker JA, Zeller J, Wilfert CM. Disseminated parainfluenza infection in a child with severe combined immunodeficiency. *Am J Dis Child* 1983;137:1172–1174.
21. Raad I, Abbas J, Whimbey E. Infection control of nosocomial respiratory viral disease in the immunocompromised host. *Am J Med* 1997; 102(3A):48–52.
22. Apalsch AM, Green M, Ledesma-Medina J, Nour B, Wald ER. Parainfluenza and influenza virus infections in pediatric organ transplant recipients. *CID* 1995;20:394–399.
23. Wendt CH, Fox JMK, Hertz MI. Paramyxovirus infection in lung transplant recipients. *J Heart Lung Transplant* 1995;14(3):479–485.
24. Wendt CH. Community respiratory viruses: organ transplant recipients. *Am J Med* 1997;102(3A):31–36.
25. Hall CB, Powell KR, MacDonald NE, et al. Respiratory syncytial viral infection in children with compromised immune function. *N Engl J Med* 1986;315:77–81.
26. Hall CB, McCarthy AJ. Respiratory syncytial virus. In: Mandell GL, Bennett JE, Dolin R, eds. *Principles and practice of infectious diseases.* New York: Churchill-Livingstone; 1997:1501–1518.
27. Englund JA, Sullivan CJ, Jordan C, Dehner LP, Vercellotti GM, Bal-

four HH. Respiratory syncytial virus infections in immunocompromised adults. *Ann Intern Med* 1988;109:203–208.

28. Martin MA, Bock MJ, Pfaller MA, Wenzel RP. Respiratory syncytial virus infections in adult bone marrow transplant recipients. *Lancet* 1988;1396–1397.

29. Hertz MI, Englund JA, Snover D, Bitterman PB, McGlave PB. Respiratory syncytial virus-induced acute lung injury in adult patients with bone marrow transplants: a clinical approach and review of the literature. *Medicine* 1989;68:269–281.

30. Fouillard L, Mouthon L, Laporte JP, et al. Severe respiratory syncytial virus pneumonia after autologous bone marrow transplantation: a report of three cases and review. *Bone Marrow Transplant* 1992;9:97–100.

31. Harrington RD, Hooton RD, Hackman RC, et al. An outbreak of respiratory syncytial virus in a bone marrow transplant center. *J Infect Dis* 1992;165:987–993.

32. Winn N, Mitchell D, Pugh S, Russell NH. Successful therapy with ribavirin of late onset respiratory syncytial virus pneumonitis complicating allogeneic bone marrow transplantation. *Clin Lab Haematol* 1992;14:29–32.

33. Whimbey E, Champlin R, Englund JA, et al. Combination therapy with aerosolized ribavirin and intravenous immunoglobulin for respiratory syncytial virus disease in adult bone marrow transplant recipients. *Bone Marrow Transplant* 1995;16:393–399.

34. Wendt CH, Hertz MI. Respiratory syncytial virus and parainfluenza virus infections in the immunocompromised host. *Semin Respir Infect* 1995;10:224–231.

35. Englund JA, Piedra PA, Jewell A, et al. Rapid diagnosis of respiratory syncytial virus infection in immunocompromised adults. *J Clin Microbiol* 1996;34:1649.

36. Sinnott JT, Cullison JP, Sweeney MS, Hammond M, Holt DA. Respiratory syncytial virus pneumonia in a cardiac transplant recipient. *J Dis* 1988;158(3):650–651.

37. Peigue-Lafeuille H, Gazuy N, Mignot P, Deteix P, Beytout D, Baguet JC. Severe respiratory syncytial virus pneumonia in an adult renal transplant recipient: successful treatment with ribavirin. *Scand J Infect Dis* 1990;22:87–89.

38. Pohl C, Green M, Wald ER, Ledesma-Medina J. Respiratory syncytial virus infections in pediatric liver transplant recipients. *J Dis* 1992; 165:166–169.

39. Groothuis JR, Simoes EAF, Levin MJ, et al. Prophylactic administration of respiratory syncytial virus immune globulin to high-risk infants and young children. *N Engl J Med* 1993;329:1524–1530.

40. Johnson S, Oliver C, Prince GA, et al. Development of a humanized monoclonal antibody (MEDI-493) with potent *in vitro* and *in vivo* activity against respiratory syncytial virus. *J Dis* 1997;176:1215–1224.

41. Englund JA, Piedra PA, Ahn Y, et al. High-dose, short-duration ribavirin aerosol therapy compared with standard ribavirin therapy in children with suspected respiratory syncytial virus infection. *J Pediatr* 1994;125:636–641.

42. Whimbey E, Champlin R, Englund J, et al. High-dose, short-duration aerosolized ribavirin for respiratory syncytial virus disease in adult BMT recipients. *Abstracts of the 34th Interscience Conference on Antimicrobials Agents and Chemotherapy*, Orlando, Florida 1994. [Abstract #H88]

43. Hemming VS, Prince GA, Horswood RL, et al. Studies of passive immunotherapy for infections of respiratory syncytial virus in the respiratory tract of a primate model. *J Infect Dis* 1985;152:1083–1087.

44. Prince GA, Hemming GV, Horswood RL, Chanock RM. Immunoprophylaxis and immunotherapy of respiratory syncytial virus infection in the cotton rat. *Virus Res* 1985;3:193–206.

45. Gruber WC, Wilson SZ, Throop BJ, Wyde PR. Immunoglobulin administration and ribavirin therapy: efficacy in respiratory syncytial virus infection of the cotton rat. *Pediatr Res* 1987;21:270–275.

46. Hemming VG, Rodriguez W, Kim HW, et al. Intravenous immunoglobulin treatment of respiratory syncytial virus infections in infants and young children. *Antimicrob Agents Chemother* 1987;31: 1882–1886.

47. DeVincenzo JP, Leombuno D, Soiffer RJ, Siber GR. Immunotherapy of respiratory syncytial virus infection following bone marrow transplantation. *Bone Marrow Transplant* 1996 17:1051–1056.

48. Rodriquez WJ, Gruber WC, Welliver RC, et al. Respiratory syncytial virus (RSV) immune globulin intravenous therapy for RSV lower respiratory tract infection in infants and young children at high risk for severe RSV infections. *Pediatrics* 1997;99: 454–461.

49. Whimbey E, Couch R, Englund J, et al. Respiratory syncytial virus pneumonia among hospitalized adult patients with leukemia. *Clin Infect Dis* 1995;21:376–379.

50. DeVincenzo JP, Musrsthy K, Skornick WA. Aerosolized respiratory syncytial virus antibody treatment of RSV infected cotton rats. Abstracts of the 34th Annual Meeting of the Infectious Disease Society of America, New Orleans, Louisiana, 1996 (#101).

51. Lewinsohn DM, Bowden RA, Mattson D, Crawford SW. Phase I study of intravenous ribavirin treatment of respiratory syncytial virus pneumonia after marrow transplantation. *Antimicrob Agents Chemother* 1996;40: 2555–2557.

52. Englund JA, Piedra A, Whimbey E. Prevention and treatment of respiratory syncytial virus and parainfluenza viruses in immuncompromised patients. *Am J Med* 1997;102(3A):61–70.

53. McCormick JB, King LJ, Webb PA, et al. Lassa fever: effective therapy with ribavirin. *N Engl J Med* 1986;314:20–26.

54. Huggins JW, Hsiang CM, Cosgriff TM, et al. Prospective double-blind concurrent placebo-controlled clinical trial of intravenous ribavirin therapy of hemorrhagic fever with renal syndrome. *J Infect Dis* 1991; 164:1119–1127.

55. Sparrelid E, Ljungman P, Ekelof-Andstrom E, et al. Ribavirin therapy in bone marrow transplant recipients with viral respiratory tract infections. *Bone Marrow Transplant* 1997;19:905–908.

56. Glezen WP, Couch RB. Influenza virus. In: Evans AS, Kaslow RA, eds. *Viral infections in humans*. New York: Plenum; 1997:473–505.

57. Center for Disease Control. Prevention and control of influenza: Recommendations of the Advisory Committee on Immunization Practices (ACIP). *Morbid Mortal Weekly Rep* 1997;46(RR-9):1–25.

58. Aschan J, Ringden O, Ljungman P, Andersson J, Lewensohn-Fuchs I, Forsgren M. Influenza B in transplant patients. *Scand J Infect Dis* 1989;21:349–350.

59. Kempe A, Hall CB, MacDonald NE, et al. Influenza in children with cancer. *J Pediatr* 1989;115:33–39.

60. Hirschhorn LR, McIntosh K, Anderson KG, Dermody TS. Influenza pneumonia as a complication of autologous bone marrow transplantation. *Clin Infect Dis* 1992;14:786–787.

61. Ljungman J, Andersson J, Aschan J, et al. Influenza A in immunocompromised patients. *Clin Infect Dis* 1993;17:244–247.

62. Whimbey E, Elting LS, Couch RB, et al. Influenza A virus infection among hospitalized adult bone marrow transplant recipients. *Bone Marrow Transplant* 1994;13:437–440.

63. Elting LS, Whimbey E, Lo W, Andreff M, Bodey GP. Epidemiology of influenza A virus infection in patients with acute or chronic leukemia. *Support Care Cancer* 1995;3:198–202.

64. Yousuf HM, Englund J, Couch R, et al. Influenza among hospitalized adults with leukemia. *Clin Infect Dis* 1997;24:1095–1099.

65. Englund J, Champlin RE, Wyde PR, et al. Common emergence of amantadine- and rimantadine-resistant influenza A viruses in symptomatic immunocompromised adults. *CID (in press)*.

66. Hayden FG, Belshe RB, Clover RD, Hay AJ, Oakes MG, Soo W. Emergence and apparent transmission of rimantadine-resistant influenza A virus in families. *N Engl J Med* 1989;321:1696–1702.

67. Mast EEL, Harmon MW, Gravenstein S, et al. Emergence and possible transmission of amantadine-resistant viruses during nursing home outbreaks of Influenza A (H3N2). *Am J Epidemiol* 1991;134:988–997.

68. Klimov AI, Rocha E, Hayden FG, Shult PA, Roumillat LF, Cox NJ. Prolonged shedding of amantadine-resistant influenza A viruses by immunodeficient patients: detection by polymerase chain reaction-restriction analysis. *J Infect Dis* 1995;172:1352–1355.

69. Embrey RP, Geist LJ. Influenza A pneumonitis following treatment of acute cardiac allograft rejection with murine monoclonal anti-CD3 antibody (OKT3). *Chest* 1995;108(5):1456–1459.

70. Mauch TJ, Bratton S, Myers T, Krane E, Gentry SR, Kashtan CE. Influenza B virus infection in pediatric solid organ transplant recipients. *Pediatrics* 1994;94(2):225–229.

71. Briggs JD, Timbury MC, Paton AM, Bell PRF. Viral infection and renal transplant rejection. *Br Med J* 1972;4:520–522.

72. Gabriel R, Selwyn S, Brown D, et al. Virus infections and acute renal transplant rejection. *Nephron* 1976;16:282–286.

73. Hohlfeld J, Niedermeyer J, Hamm M, Schafers HJ, Wagner TOF, Fabel H. Seasonal onset of bronchiolitis obliterans syndrome in lung transplant recipients. *J Heart Lung Transplant* 1996;15(9):888–894.

74. Hayden FG. Prevention and treatment of influenza in immunocompromised patients. *Am J Med* 1997;102(3A):55–60.

75. Engelhard D, Nagler A, Hardan I, et al. Antibody response to a two-dose regimen of influenza vaccine in allogeneic T cell depleted and autologous BMT recipients. *Bone Marrow Transplant* 1993;11:1–5.

76. Somani J, Larson RA. Reimmunization after allogeneic bone marrow transplantation. *Am J Med* 1995;98:389–398.

77. Ljungman P, Cordonnier C, de Bock R, et al. Immunisations after bone marrow transplantation: results of a European survey and recommendations from the infectious diseases working party of the European Group for Blood and Marrow Transplantation. *Bone Marrow Transplant* 1995;15(3):455–460.

78. Pauksen K, Hammarstrom V, Linde A, et al. Immunomodulation with GM-CSFat Influenza Vaccination of Bone Marrow Transplant Recipients. *Abstracts of the 37th Interscience Conference on Antimicrobials Agents and Chemotherapy,* Toronto, Ontario, Canada 1997. [Abstract #H-138]

79. Hayden FG, Treanor JJ, Betts RF, Lobo M, Esinhart JD, Hussey EK. Safety and efficacy of the neuraminidase inhibitor GG167 in experimental human influenza *JAMA* 1996;275:295–299.

80. Hayden FG, Osterhaus ADME, Treanor JJ, et al. Efficacy and safety of the neuraminidase inhibitor Zanamivir in the treatment of influenza virus infections. *N Engl J Med* 1997;337(13):874–880.

81. Knight V, McClung HW, Wilson SZ, et al. Ribavirin small-particle aerosol treatment of influenza. *Lancet* 1981;2:945–949.

82. McClung HW, Knight V, Gilbert BE, et al. Ribavirin aerosol treatment of influenza B virus infection. *JAMA* 1983;249:2671–1674.

83. Wilson SZ, Gilbert BE, Quarles JM, et al. Treatment of influenza A (H1N1) virus infection with ribavirin aerosol. *Antimicrob Agents Chemother* 1984: 26: 200–203.

84. Gilbert BE, Wilson SZ, Knight V, et al. Ribavirin small-particle aerosol treatment of infections caused by influenza virus strains A/Victoria/7/83 (H1N1) and B/Texas/1/84. *Antimicrob Agents Chemother* 1985;27:309–313.

85. Knight V, Gilbert BE. Ribavirin aerosol treatment of influenza. *Antiviral Chemother* 1987;1:441–457.

86. Bell M, Hunter JM, and Mostaf SM. Nebulised ribavirin for influenza B viral pneumonia in a ventilated immunocompromised adult. *Lancet* 1988;2: 1084–1085.

87. Rodriguez WJ, Hall CB, Welliver R et al. Efficacy and safety of aerosolized ribavirin in young children hospitalized with influenza: a double-blind, multicenter, placebo-controlled trial. *J Pediatr* 1994; 125:129–135.

88. Ray CG, Icenogle TB, Minnich LL, Copeland JH, Grogan TM. The use of intravenous ribavirin to treat influenza virus-associated acute myocarditis. *J Infect Dis* 1989;159:829–836.

89. Hayden FG, Sabie CA, Connor JD, Lane J. Intravenous ribavirin by constant infusion for serious influenza and parainfluenza virus infection. *Antiviral Ther* 1996;1:51–56.

90. Hayden FG. Combination antiviral therapy for respiratory virus infections. *Antiviral Res* 1996;96:45–48.

91. Chanock RM, Parrott RH, Johnson KM, Kapikian.Z, Bell JA. Myxoviruses: Parainfluenza. *Am Rev Respir Dis* 1963;88:152–166.

92. Piedra PA, Englund JA, Glezen WP. Respiratory syncytial virus and parainfluenza viruses. In: Richman DD, Whitley RJ, Hayden FG, eds. *Clinical virology.* New York: Churchill-Livingstone; 1997: 787–819,

93. Wendt CH, Weisdorf DJ, Jordan MC, Balfour HH Jr,Hertz MI. Parainfluenza virus respiratory infection after bone marrow transplantation. *N Engl J Med* 1992;326:921–926.

94. Whimbey E, Vartivarian SE, Champlin R, Elting LS, Luna M, Bodey GP. Parainfluenza virus infection in adult bone marrow transplant patients. *Eur J Clin Microbiol Infect Dis* 1993;12:699–701.

95. Lewis V, Champlin R, Englund J., et al. Respiratory disease due to parainfluenza virus in adult bone marrow transplant recipients. *Clin Dis* 1996;23:1033–1037.

96. Cobian L, Houston S, Greene J, Sinnott JT. Parainfluenza virus respiratory infection after heart transplantation: successful treatment with ribavirin. *CID* 1995;21:1040–1041.

97. DeFabritus AM, Tittio RR, David DS, Senterfit LB, Cheigh JS, Stenzel KH. Parainfluenza type 3 in a transplant unit. *JAMA* 1979; 241(4):384–386.

98. Ottolini MG, Hemming VG, Piazza FM, Johnson SA, Darnell MER, Prince GA. Topical immunoglobulin is an effective therapy for parainfluenza type 3 in a cotton rat model. *J Infect Dis* 1995;172:243–245.

99. Couch RB. Rhinoviruses. *Fields virology,* 3rd ed. 1996;23:713–733.

100. Gwaltney JM, Rueckert RR. Rhinovirus. In: Richman DD, Whitley RJ, Hayden FG, eds. *Clinical virology.* New York: Churchill-Livingstone; 1997:1025–1047.

101. Johnston SL. Natural and experimental rhinovirus infections of the lower respiratory tract. *Am J Respir Crit Care Med* 1995;152:S46–S52.

102. Gern JE, Galagan DM, Jarjour NN, Dick EC, Busse WW. Detection of rhinovirus RNA in lower airway cells during experimentally induced infection. *Am J Respir Crit Care Med* 1997;155:1159–1161.

103. McIntosh K. Coronaviruses. In: Richman DD, Whitley RJ, Hayden FG, eds. *Clinical virology.* New York: Churchill-Livingstone; 1997: 1123–1132.

104. Monto AS. Coronavirus. In: Evans AS, Kaslow RA, eds. *Viral infections of humans: epidemiology and control.* New York: Plenum Publishing; 1997:211–228.

Transplant Infections edited by
Raleigh A. Bowden, Per Ljungman, and Carlos V. Paya.
Lippincott–Raven Publishers, Philadelphia © 1998

CHAPTER 22

Viral Hepatitis in the Transplant Patient

Natalie H. Bzowej and Teresa L. Wright

Chronic viral hepatitis secondary to hepatitis B (HBV), hepatitis D (HDV), and HCV (HCV) is a very common cause of varying degrees of liver disease in the transplant setting. In recent years there has been much interest in establishing the epidemiology, diagnosis, natural history, and treatment of these different viral infections. Great strides have been made, but our understanding of the mechanisms of viral replication, liver injury, and oncogenesis lags behind. The patient who undergoes transplantation offers a unique opportunity to study the natural history of disease in an immunocompromised population and provides a framework to examine host/viral interactions that can provide clues to the pathogenesis of viral-related liver damage.

This chapter highlights the importance of hepatotropic viruses as pathogens in patients undergoing transplantation, their contribution to morbidity and mortality after transplantation, and the approach to treatment of these pathogens when they cause disease. Although many advances have been made in the management of viral hepatitis in the transplant setting, there remain unanswered questions about the long-term natural history of disease. Understanding of the pathogenesis of infection in the setting of transplantation is emerging slowly, but complete understanding requires further investigation. New approaches to treating disease in patients with either HBV or HCV infection are under development and will likely focus on the use of combinations of antiviral and immunomodulatory agents.

We review the spectrum of viral infections in organ transplantation, with particular emphasis on HBV and HCV, because HDV is much less common and hepatitis G virus (HGV) has been shown not to be hepatotropic. Because much more is known about HBV and HCV in liver and kidney than in bone marrow and heart transplantation, this chapter focuses on these two transplant settings. Because minimal information exists about viral hepatitis in other solid organ transplant settings (e.g., pancreas, lung), these will not be discussed. Prevalence of infection, the natural history of disease, and current options for management are outlined. This information is vital if we are to make rational decisions about transplantation of patients infected with viral infections and the use of organs infected with hepatotropic viruses.

HBV INFECTION

HBV Infection and Liver Transplantation

Natural History

Prior to the availability of treatment, a high rate of recurrence of HBV infection after liver transplantation with severe graft infection and decreased survival of patients and grafts was observed (1,2). The advent of long-term immunoprophylaxis with hepatitis B immune globulin (HBIG) has greatly improved this outcome (see later). The natural history of recurrent HBV infection is variable and dependent upon a number of pretransplantation factors. A large study (2) that evaluated patients from 17 European centers showed that replicative state of HBV prior to transplantation has prognostic importance. In this study, the risk of recurrence was greatest in patients with chronic infection and active viral replication (detectable HBV DNA and/or HBeAg) at the time of transplantation. The recurrence rate was lower in patients with fulminant HBV and in those co-infected with HDV. Patients with fulminant HBV present during a phase of active elimination of the virus, often with no detectable HBV DNA in their serum at the time of transplantation. Patients who are co-infected with HDV fare better than those with HBV alone because HDV suppresses HBV replication.

Further support of the prognostic importance of the HBV replicative state prior to transplantation in predict-

NHB: From the Department of Gastroenterology, University of California, San Francisco, San Francisco, California 94121.

TLW: From the Gastroenterology Section, Veterans Affairs Medical Center, San Francisco, California 94121.

ing the severity of HBV recurrence comes from observations of patients with "occult" pretransplantation HBV infection (3). Of 207 patients who were HBsAg negative prior to transplant, 20 (10%) became HBsAg positive after transplantation. Using molecular techniques, low-level pretransplantation infection was detected in five patients with end-stage liver disease who were HBsAg negative and two donors who lacked all serological markers for HBV. Post-transplantation survival of those patients who had apparently acquired HBV in the peri-transplantation period was significantly greater than that of patients with overt pretransplantation HBV infection. The level of virus in patients with "occult" pretransplantation infection was uniformly low, detectable only by sensitive molecular assays, such as amplification by polymerase chain reaction (PCR).

The presence of pretransplantation replication is not the only factor that determines the severity of post-transplantation disease. One group (4) has reported that post-transplantation infection with pre-Core mutant strains of HBV carry a greater risk of developing graft loss from recurrent HBV disease than does infection with wild-type virus. This finding has recently been challenged (5).

Prevention and Treatment

Generally, there are two main approaches to the patient with HBV infection undergoing liver transplantation: (a) prevention of recurrent infection and (b) treatment of disease when and if it occurs. These strategies can be implemented prior to transplantation, as the patient is awaiting a donor organ (e.g., with the use of nucleoside analogs), at the time of transplantation (e.g., with the use of HBIG), and following transplantation (e.g., with the use of HBIG and/or nucleoside analogs).

Immunoprophylaxis Following Transplantation

Early studies of the natural history of post-transplantation HBV infection in patients who did not receive immunoprophylaxis revealed that delayed mortality is increased in patients with disease recurrence (1).

Most of the experience in preventing recurrent HBV infection in patients who were infected with HBV pre-transplant has been with hepatitis B immune globulin (anti-HBsIg/HBIG) (2,6–8). The presumed mode of action of this polyclonal antibody is to neutralize circulating virus and prevent infection of the transplanted liver. The usual protocol entails using 10,000 IU of HBIG at the time of transplantation, daily for the first 6 postoperative days and then approximately monthly thereafter. With this regimen most patients will achieve trough anti-HBs titers in serum of at least 500 IU/ml, with median titers of 1,250 IU/ml (9). Some investigators have used data from early pharmacokinetic measurements to determine the dose necessary to achieve adequate protective titers of anti-HBs (10). It

should be noted that with other therapeutic agents on the horizon (see later), the use of long-term, post-transplant HBIG treatment will likely diminish.

Passive immunization with HBIG has been a significant first step in the development of treatment strategies for lowering this recurrence (2). The strongest support for the use of prophylactic HBIG comes from a large European study involving 17 countries that involved treating patients with short-term HBIG (<2 months), long-term HBIG (at least 6 months), or not at all (2). Three-year actuarial risk of recurrence was significantly lower and survival was significantly higher in patients receiving long-term HBIG than in those receiving either short-term or no HBIG therapy. It should be noted, however, that although HBIG is effective in preventing recurrent HBV infection, failures or "breakthroughs" (defined as HBsAg positivity) occur in 20% to 50% of patients, and in the European study HBIG was not effective at preventing recurrence in patients with active pretransplantation replication (2). Experience with HBIG from U.S. centers supports the efficacy of this approach in reducing post-transplantation infection, even in those with active pre-transplantation viral replication (see Fig. 1) (9).

Causes of breakthrough are likely multifactorial, and include (a) inadequate post-transplantation anti-HBs titers (9), (b) mutations in the region of the surface gene that encodes the "a" determinant (11,12), and (c) high levels of viral replication, although the third explanation is controversial (2,9,10). The "a" determinant is the region of the surface protein where anti-HBs binds. Mutations in the surface gene encoding this region have been reported in association with monoclonal and polyclonal HBIG therapy, and are thought to reduce the binding of the antibody to the virus (11,12). Recently, Terrault and colleagues (9) reported a G-to-A mutation encoding for amino acid 145 in association with late failures (at approximately 1 year after transplantation), but not early failures. No mutations were observed in control patients with HBV recurrence who never received HBIG. The absence of these mutations in virus amplified from serum obtained prior to exposure to HBIG suggests that mutations result from immune pressure exerted by the antibody, rather than from selection by the antibody of preexisting variants (9). To resolve whether HBV variants are selected for or merely emerge under treatment, sensitive molecular techniques that can detect minor populations of virus (representing less than 5% of the total population) will need to be applied broadly. Few studies have used techniques with adequate sensitivity to establish incontrovertibly that HBV variants emerge. Nevertheless, the weight of data, whether in the setting of liver transplantation or in the setting of HBV escape mutants in association with vaccination of infants, suggests that variants emerge as a result of therapy, rather than that they are selected for by therapy from minor populations that preexist.

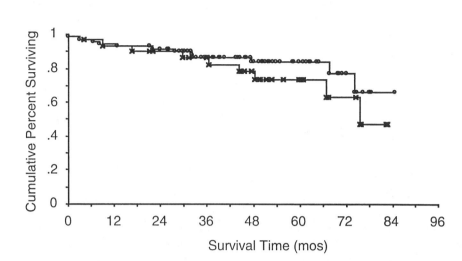

Figure 1. Recurrence of HBV infection (defined as detection of HBsAg) in patients undergoing liver transplantation with and without hepatitis B immune prophylaxis. Fifty-two patients underwent liver transplantation with hepatitis B immune prophylaxis (⊖⊖⊖) (*n* = 24) and without hepatitis B immune prophylaxis (✕✕✕) (*n* = 28). The *x* axis shows the duration of follow-up and the *y* axis shows the probability of recurrence. The rate of reinfection was significantly less in the immune prophylaxis group than in the no treatment group (*p* = 0.0002), despite the presence of pretransplantation replication in a large percentage of the former group (46% versus 22%, respectively, were HBeAg positive). Reproduced from Terrault et al. Prophylaxis in liver transplant recipients using schedule of hepatitis B immunoglobulin. *Hepatology* 1996; 24:1327–1333. With permission.

Treatment of HBV-Infected Patients Before Transplantation

The goal with treatment of HBV-infected patients before transplantation is to treat patients with an antiviral agent so as to suppress viral replication (i.e., cause a patient who is positive for HBeAg and HBV-DNA to become negative for both markers), and in so doing to reduce the risk of post-transplantation disease. Interferon alpha, famciclovir, and lamivudine have been used in patients awaiting liver transplantation, although the information on the use of all three of these drugs in this setting is limited. Interferon must be used cautiously in patients with decompensated HBV-induced liver disease, because treatment may precipitate further progression (13,14). If interferon is used in such patients, liver transplantation must be available in case of deterioration, and low doses should be administered (2–3 million units subcutaneously three times per week). In one study of pretransplantation interferon used in combination with perioperative HBIG, interferon appeared to have little influence on rates of post-transplantation recurrence, although any beneficial effects may have been overridden by the effect of HBIG (13). Famciclovir is a guanosine analog that has significant HBV-inhibitory effects in preclinical studies. Uncontrolled data from patients treated with this drug (500 mg orally three times daily) before and after transplantation suggest that HBV replication is suppressed, but not permanently eradicated. Lamivudine is a negative enantiomer of 3-thiacytadine that blocks replication of HBV. Pilot and ongoing open label studies using 100 mg daily for at least 1 month before transplantation suggest that lamivudine suppresses viral replication in virtually all patients (15). When patients receive lamivudine in transplantation, although the post-trans-

plantation follow-up is still limited, resistance to lamivudine would be predicted to emerge (see later) (16,17).

Treatment of HBV-Infected Patients After Transplantation

There are limited data regarding the safety and efficacy of interferon therapy for post-transplantation HBV recurrence. In an uncontrolled series of 14 patients, all of whom had evidence of active viral replication before treatment, elimination of HBV DNA was seen in four, elimination of HBeAg in two, and elimination of HBsAg in one patient after treatment (18). A theoretical risk associated with use of interferon in patients with transplants is that enhanced HLA expression on epithelial cells of the bile duct by interferon could lead to allograft rejection. The magnitude of this risk (if any) is controversial (18).

Nucleoside analogs, described earlier for prevention, have also been used for the treatment of recurrence. Ganciclovir suppresses HBV DNA to 90% of pretreatment levels associated with reduction in serum alanine aminotransferase levels (to 83% of pretreatment levels), and stabilization and/or improvement in liver histology (19). However, this drug has already been replaced by newer agents that have greater oral bioavailability. Famciclovir, initially promising, suppresses HBV DNA levels to only 50% of pretreatment levels, although results are still preliminary (20). The suppressive effect of lamivudine may be greater. Preliminary data recently reported suggest that lamivudine at a dose of 100 mg daily results in an elimination of HBV DNA in all patients after 2 months of therapy (21). More recently, therapy with lamivudine has been extended (22,23). In one report (22), patients were treated with 100 mg of lamivudine per day orally before transplantation, and this was continued for 12 months after transplantation. In another report (23), patients with recurrent HBV infection after transplantation were treated with lamivudine 100 mg daily for 12 months. In those patients who were treated with lamivudine before and after transplantation, there were significant decreases in HBsAg and HBeAg. In both, there were also significant decreases in HBV DNA. However, prolonged therapy was also associated with development of resistance. Breakthrough of serum HBV DNA occurred in 14 of 67 patients after a mean of 8 months of therapy. Seven of the 14 had increasing ALT levels at the time of breakthrough, but all have remained clinically stable to date. Breakthrough was associated with mutations at the YMDD locus, the same position in the viral polymerase that is associated with lamivudine resistance in HIV infection (16,17). To overcome this, future treatment strategies will be aimed not only at designing new antiviral therapies, but also at designing combination therapy with other agents.

HBV Infection and End-Stage Renal Disease

HBV Infection in Dialysis Patients

In the 1970s, HBV accounted for a large number of cases of hepatitis among hemodialysis patients. The incidence and prevalence of HBsAg in 1976 were 3.0% and 7.8%, respectively. In contrast, in 1989 the numbers had fallen to 0.1% and 1.4%. This has likely occurred as a result of patient monitoring for HBV infection, provision of separate rooms and dialysis machines for HBV-infected people, use of universal precautions, screening of blood products for anti-HBc, and widespread use of HBV vaccination (24,25).

When staff get infected in the dialysis unit with hepatitis B, they generally become symptomatic and then eventually clear the virus. This is in contrast to the effect on dialysis patients, who generally are asymptomatic but often become chronic carriers (26). Although data are limited, HBV-infected dialysis patients do not seem to have increased mortality as compared with noninfected dialysis patients (26).

HBV Infection and Renal Transplantation

The safety and efficacy of renal transplantation in HBsAg-positive patients have been debated for almost two decades. Thus, the criteria for acceptance of HBV-infected candidates for renal transplantation vary throughout the United States. In one study published recently (27), U.S. transplant centers were evaluated and found to exclude 22% of patients from transplantation if they are HBsAg-positive. Twenty-nine percent perform liver biopsy in HBsAg-positive patients if liver tests are abnormal for more than 6 months, whereas 16% per-

form a liver biopsy regardless of liver test abnormalities. Furthermore, in 31% there is no specific policy about HBsAg-positive patients. Although 53% encourage all hepatitis B surface antigen- and antibody-negative potential transplant recipients to receive HBV vaccination, 10% do not advocate such intervention. As many as 37% have no specific policy regarding hepatitis B vaccination.

In one natural history study, 151 HBsAg-positive kidney transplant recipients, who were followed for a median follow-up of 125 months, were found to have a high rate of persistent viral replication (50%) and reactivation (30%) (28). Noteworthy, was the high frequency of histologic deterioration (85.3%), accompanied by cirrhosis in 28% and by hepatocellular carcinoma in 23% of the patients with cirrhosis. Co-infection of hepatitis B with hepatitis C was associated with histologic worsening. Liver disease was the leading cause of death in this series (36.6%). Paradoxically, in the same study, there was no significant difference in the survival of these 151 HBsAg-positive recipients, as compared with 1247 HBsAg-negative kidney recipients.

With the shortage of organs, the use of HBV-positive donors has been reconsidered. One small study examined 12 patients who had been immunized to HBV (by natural infection or vaccine) before transplantation (29). After transplantation of these patients with HBsAg-positive organs, none developed clinical hepatitis or became HBsAg-positive. However, ALT levels did rise in two and anti-HBc appeared transiently in patients whose immunity was elicited by vaccination. Post-transplant appearance of HBV DNA was not evaluated. Policies regarding renal transplantation in HBV-infected individuals and the use of HBV-infected organs must be reevaluated in the light of therapeutic advances.

Treatment of HBV Infections in Renal Failure Patients

The most effective means of managing HBV infection in patients with renal failure is prevention with vaccination. Among dialysis patients immunized with twice the usual dose of recombinant HBV (40 μg), 60% develop adequate anti-HBs titers, compared with only 40% in renal transplant patients (30). Among patients responding to vaccination before transplantation, more than 85% develop increased anti-HBs levels in response to booster doses of vaccine following surgery (31).

Antiviral therapy of HBV infection following renal transplantation is of unproven efficacy and safety, and thus cannot be advocated at this time. One recent small, uncontrolled study tested ganciclovir in the treatment of HBV-induced liver disease (32). Six patients with severe liver disease were treated with 10 mg/kg/day for 15 days, followed by a half dose daily for 15 days and then a half dose two or three times per week for 5 months. With treatment serum aminotransferase activity was improved at the end of therapy. HBV DNA was negative in three patients followed for at least 3 months and significantly lower in the rest. Liver histology at the end of treatment showed some improvement in activity score, but not of fibrosis. Given these promising results, the role of orally available nucleoside analogs, such as lamivudine, is under evaluation.

HBV Infection and Bone Marrow Transplantation

The occurrence of hepatic complications in bone marrow transplantation (BMT) recipients is a well-known cause of transplant-related morbidity and mortality (33). HBV infection can be a serious problem in the BMT setting, either because of infection as a result of the transplant process or because of the use of chemotherapy and immunosuppression that can reactivate latent hepatitis B. Early studies reported high mortality associated with reactivation (34), and increased prevalence of veno-occlusive disease (VOD), graft-versus-host disease (GVHD), and graft failure in HBsAg-positive BMT patients (33).

Although HBV infection in the BMT setting is a frequent cause of liver dysfunction, subsequent studies have shown that the course of the disease is not fatal. In one report, 145 BMT patients were evaluated and 30 (21%) were found to be HBsAg positive either before or after BMT (35). Twenty-one (14.4%) patients became HBsAg positive after transplant, but subsequently cleared the antigen. Nine of the 21 patients had mild or asymptomatic hepatitis. Twelve of the 21 had clinically overt hepatitis, but none had life-threatening liver disease. Of interest, none of the 30 patients developed VOD. Another study that examined the clinical course of 20 HBsAg-positive patients who underwent BMT also showed no increased incidence of VOD (36). These data suggest that HBsAg positivity should not be considered an absolute contraindication to BMT.

Little information exists regarding the risk of infusion of HBsAg-positive marrow. Thus there is wide variability in BMT policy about the use of HBsAg-positive donors (37). In a recent study, a total of 24 of 2,586 patients (0.9%) received HBsAg-positive marrow (38). HBsAg became detectable in 22% of patients who were HBsAg-negative before BMT, but only 5.5% became chronic carriers. Severe liver failure with death occurred in a large number of patients (21%). Antigenemia developed more frequently in anti-HBs-negative patients than in those who were anti-HBs positive, independently of passive prophylaxis with hyperimmune anti-HBs Ig, although the difference was not significant. Further prospective study is required to confirm these results.

To prevent HBV acquisition or reactivation following BMT, various approaches have been attempted. Attempts to immunize the BMT patient have been unsuccessful, likely secondary to deficient T-cell-dependent B-cell responses that generally persist for 1 year after transplant.

In contrast, adoptive transfer of immunity to HBV has recently been accomplished by BMT from donors who are immune to HBV because of past infection or active immunization (39). In this study, bone marrow donor BALB/c mice were immunized with recombinant HBV vaccine and demonstrated seroconversion to HBs antibody within 4 weeks of primary immunization. Bone marrow recipient mice, conditioned by sublethal irradiation, were injected intravenously with bone marrow cells from the HBs-antibody-positive donors. Antibody was detected in 10% of the recipients within 30 days and in 56% within 1 month after a booster injection that led to a secondary rise in HBs antibody. Subsequently, the same investigators studied adoptive immunity in BMT (40). Two groups were examined. Group A consisted of 12 pairs of BMT donors and recipients, in which all bone marrow donors were positive for antibodies to HBc and HBs, as a result of previously acquired HBV infection and resolution. Group B consisted of eight pairs of donors and recipients in which all the donors were actively immunized against HBV between 30 and 11 days before BMT. Of note is that all recipients were negative for HBV markers before transplant. In group A, after BMT all recipients developed protective anti-HBs levels that were detected 30–120 days after transplant. In group B, all eight recipients seroconverted to anti-HBs 9–42 days after transplantation.

Furthermore, in a very recent study, BMT from immune donors was shown to result not only in transfer immunity, but in actual clearance of hepatitis B virus in patients with chronic HBV infection (41). To determine the serological and clinical outcome of HBsAg-positive BMT recipients in relation to the HBV status (carrier/immune/seronegative) of the donors, their group examined 226 patients who received allogeneic BMT. Twenty-one of the 226 were HBsAg positive before BMT. Of these 21 patients, five patients received anti-HBs-positive marrow and 16 received anti-HBs-negative marrow. Two of the five patients who received anti-HBs-positive marrow had persistent clearance of HBsAg, in contrast to none of the 16 patients who received anti-HBs-negative marrow ($p < 0.05$). One additional patient who received anti-HBs-positive marrow had transient HBsAg seroconversion. Taken together, these data have led to the suggestion that adoptive immunity transfer may be employed to treat chronic HBV infection.

HBV Infection and Heart Transplantation

Studies examining HBV infection in heart transplantation are extremely limited. In one study of 80 transplanted patients followed for 60 months, sustained liver dysfunction was seen in 50 patients (62.5%), HBV infection was found in 13 of the 50, or 26%, and HBV-related deaths occurred in two patients (42). This prevalence of post-transplantation HBV infection is unusually high but may be related to transfusion of blood products contaminated with hepatitis B. At the time of this study blood banks were not yet using anti-HBc or ALT testing in France. Clearly, studies with larger numbers and longer follow-up are necessary to document the actual severity of HBV infection in this setting. From our knowledge of the severity of recurrent HBV liver disease in the liver transplant setting, one might anticipate similar outcomes in the heart transplant setting. If true, studies testing various treatment regimens, such as nucleoside analogs, will be warranted. To date, treatment with these agents is anecdotal (43).

HCV INFECTION

Diagnosis of HCV Infection and Disease Prior To and Following Transplantation

Currently, there is no gold standard for diagnosis of HCV infection in immunosuppressed patients. Infection can be diagnosed by tests that detect the presence of antibodies to HCV (serological assays) and by tests that detect presence of HCV RNA (virologic assays). It is important when interpreting results from a study to establish which method for detection was used, because these methods vary greatly in sensitivity and specificity. Serological tests (anti-HCV) are based on the detection of antibodies to antigens encoded by specific sequences of the genome. Typically, antigens from highly conserved regions are used in serological assays to ensure broad reactivity. Two serological tests, the second-generation enzyme-linked immunoassay (EIA2) and the recombinant immunoblot assay (RIBA2), are both sensitive and specific in the immunocompetent patient. EIA2 detects antibodies to antigens C-22 (core region) and C-200—a composite antigen of C-33 (NS3) and C-100-3—and has replaced the earlier EIA1, which only detected antibodies to the C-100-3 antigen of the NS4 region. RIBA2 detects antibodies to C-100-3, C-33, C-22, and 5-1-1 antigens (NS4/NS5 region) and is considered a supplemental test. Because of the fall of antibody titer to certain HCV antigens with immunosuppression, these tests become less reliable in the setting of transplantation, resulting in frequent false-negative results. Thus, for accurate detection of HCV infection, virologic techniques must be used (44). Two such assays that have been widely employed are (a) PCR amplification using primers to the conserved 5' untranslated region and (b) branched-chain DNA assay (b-DNA), in which the signal used to detect viral RNA, rather than the target RNA itself, is amplified. PCR amplification offers the advantage over bDNA of being more sensitive for detection of low levels of virus and is less expensive to perform. However, bDNA not only detects virus, but can quantitate the amount of viral RNA, is standardized and reproducible, and is less labor intensive to perform than PCR-based methodologies. One study in liver transplant recipients compared the sensitivity and specificity of serological and virologic techniques (45). Serological assays (EIA2 and RIBA2) failed to detect infection in 12% and 17%, respectively, of patients with HCV infection detected by both PCR and bDNA (45).

Diagnosis of HCV disease is dependent on detection of infection as well as on demonstration of end-organ damage. This may be difficult because there is overlap in the histologic features of recurrent hepatitis from HCV and allograft rejection. Bile duct injury and portal lymphocytic infiltration are common to both conditions. In addition, susceptibility to disease or disease severity is likely dependent on a number of factors. Viral RNA levels rise with immunosuppression (46), and patients with high pretransplantation levels of virus tend to have high posttransplantation levels. However, the relationship between levels of post-transplantation viremia and degree of histologic liver injury is complex and controversial. In one series, increased levels were associated with acute hepatitis invoking direct cytotoxicity of the virus as the mechanism of liver damage (47). Other series have failed to show a strong association between viral levels and disease (46,48,49). It is likely that patients with severe recurrence have high titers of virus but that not all patients with high titers of virus have severe recurrence.

Organ Transplantation: Prevalence and Transmission of HCV

The prevalence of HCV infection following solid organ transplantation in large part depends upon the method used for diagnosis. This has been clearly demonstrated in a large national collaborative study, in which 3,078 cadaveric organs from eight U.S. organ procurement centers were tested for prevalence of HCV RNA and anti-HCV by ELISA1 and ELISA2 (50). Anti-HCV was detected by ELISA1 in 5.1% of the 3,078 donors, whereas the prevalence of ELISA2 and HCV RNA was lower, with values of 4.2% and 2.4%, respectively (Table 1).

The transmission of HCV by transfusion of blood products from anti-HCV-positive donors has been demonstrated unequivocally (51). After parenteral exposure to HCV, seroconversion usually occurs within 3 months, but may take as long as 1 year. Transmission by organ transplantation has been observed to be significant (52–54). In the New England Organ Bank study (52), of 716 organ donors, 13 were positive for anti-HCV, for a prevalence of almost 2%. These HCV-infected organs were then transplanted into 29 recipients. HCV (as detected by ELISA, enzyme immunoassay, and HCV RNA) was the cause of hepatitis in 12 of these patients. In a subsequent study from the New England Organ Bank, using PCR to detect HCV RNA, HCV was detected in 9 of 11 organs (82%) with positive first-generation ELISA for anti-HCV (53). Among the HCV RNA-negative recipients of organs from HCV RNA-pos-

TABLE 1. *Prevalence of HCV infection in cadaveric organ donors*

	#Pts	E1A1%	E1A2%	PCR%
New England Organ Bank, MA	1,012	2.9	2.4	1.7
Regional Organ Bank, IL	596	6.0	3.2	2.7
Lifelink, Inc, FL	521	7.7	7.3	4.0
Center for Organ Recovery and Ed, PA	516	5.8	5.4	2.1
Midwest Organ Bank, KS	172	4.7	4.1	2.0
Louisiana Organ Procurement Agency, LA	129	2.3	2.3	0.8
Oregon Health Services University, OR	67	1.5	NA	NA
Washington Hospital Center, DC	66	16.7	8.3	4.2
TOTAL	**3,078**	**5.1**	**4.2**	**2.4**

From Pereira BJG, Wright TL, Schmid CH, et al. Screening and confirmatory testing of cadaver organ donors for hepatitis C virus infection. A US National Collaborative Study. Used with permission from *Kidney Int* 1994;46:887.

1A1, first-generation enzyme-linked immunoassay; E1A2, second-generation enzyme-linked immunoassay; PCR, polymerase chain reaction.

itive donors, there was an observed 100% incidence of post-transplantation HCV infection. Furthermore, none of the HCV RNA-negative recipients of organs from HCV-negative donors had HCV RNA or liver disease after transplantation.

Based on this high documented prevalence of HCV infection among recipients of organs from anti-HCV and HCV RNA-positive donors, it has been suggested that these organs only be transplanted for life-saving transplant, such as heart and lung (52). Alternatively, others have suggested only transplanting HCV-positive donors into HCV-positive recipients (55). However, anti-HCV is not a neutralizing antibody, and thus exposures to different strains of hepatitis C could lead to multiple HCV infections in a single recipient. These recommendations continue to evolve as more outcome studies emerge that examine long-term consequences of hepatitis C and severity of liver disease in the transplant setting (54).

HCV Infection and Liver Transplantation

Natural History

Annually, approximately 1,000 patients undergo liver transplantation for HCV disease, and post-transplantation infection is almost universal. One of the first reports of recurrence documented progressive graft dysfunction in one of six patients with pretransplantation disease (56). A larger study that used both serological and virologic assays for diagnosis, demonstrated that HCV viremia persists in more than 95% of patients, with liver disease in approximately half at 1 year (57). Conclusive evidence of HCV recurrence came from a study that, via sequencing of the hypervariable region (E2/NS1) of the HCV genome in patients who were HCV-PCR positive, demonstrated a high degree of homology (>95%) and between pairs of pre- and post-transplantation samples, with much lower sequence homology between viruses infecting different patients (48).

Many studies suggest that the natural history of HCV infection in liver transplant recipients may be accelerated when compared with that in immunocompetent patients, although a side-by-side comparison of these two groups has never been performed. Although the disease course in many liver transplant patients is benign, progressive liver injury has been documented (56). However, the extent of the influence of HCV infection itself on patient and graft survival is difficult to ascertain, because many pre- and post-transplant factors that may alter outcome (such as age of the patient, severity of liver disease at the time of transplantation, type and amount of administered immunosuppression) have not been analyzed in most series. One study showed that moderate chronic hepatitis developed in 27% of patients with HCV infection after transplant after a median of 35 months and that the disease progressed to cirrhosis in 8% after a median of 51 months (47). Although the rates of both graft survival and patient survival at 5 years were similar in patients with and without HCV infection, published series to date have not included sufficient patients to detect minor differences in outcome (differences, for example, of 5% or less). Moreover, the duration of follow-up in most series has been short (less than 5 years). A large experience in the United States comes from the data from the United Network for Organ Sharing (UNOS), in which 5-year graft but not patient survival was significantly lower in patients transplanted for HCV infection than in those transplanted for alcoholic liver disease (58). These results suggest that with long-term follow-up, HCV-infected patients may experience more problems than those without infection. However, in a recently published study with the longest duration of follow-up published to date (12 years), most HCV-infected liver transplantation recipients developed chronic hepatitis of the graft, but the disease was mild in most cases (59). Furthermore, no excess mortality from hepatitis C infection in the first decade after transplantation was observed. Cumulative survival at 2, 5, and 10 years after transplantation was 67%, 62%, and

62%, respectively, and not significantly different from that in patients transplanted for other nonmalignant liver diseases without HCV infection (Fig. 2). The main factor determining long-term survival was the presence or absence of hepatocellular carcinoma (HCC) at transplantation. The 5-year survival rate for HCV patients was 35% with HCC and 73% without HCC ($p < 0.05$) (Fig. 3). No deaths because of viral hepatitis of the graft were observed. This study, unlike previous studies, did analyze the possible confounding effects of a number of variables on the severity of HCV hepatitis and found no association with age, sex, severity of liver disease before liver transplantation, cold ischemic time of graft, duration of operation, transfusions, number of rejection episodes, or long-term immunosuppressive regime. Only initial short-term therapy with interleukin 2 receptor antibodies adversely influenced inflammatory activity. These data suggest that with medium-term follow-up, the disease course closely resembles that seen in nontransplanted hepatitis C patients. Assessment of the full impact of HCV infection on post-transplantation outcome will require prolonged follow-up (10–20 years) of large numbers of patients.

Recent data suggest that different genotypes (HCV isolates from genetically distinct groups that have arisen during the evolution of this virus) may influence disease severity, but this remains controversial. Some studies have implicated genotype 1, and in particular subtype 1b, in causing progressive liver injury when compared with non-1 genotype (48). However, a recent study that followed 110 patients for 25 months could demonstrate no such association (49). Actuarial graft survival and the histologic severity of liver disease did not differ between

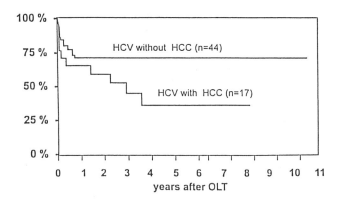

Figure 3. Cumulative survival of HCV-infected patients with and without HCC at transplantation. *Straight line,* patients without HCC ($n = 44$); *dotted line,* patients with HCC ($n = 17$). The difference between the groups is statistically significant; $p = 0.049$ (log rank test). (From Boker et al. Long-term outcome of hepatitis C virus in infection after liver transplantation. *Hepatology* 1997;25:203–210. With permission.)

those with and those without infection with genotype 1 (Fig. 4) (49).

The explanation for these different findings is not immediately apparent, although these studies differed in distribution of genotype in the study population, in the type and amount of administered immunosuppression, and in the method used to quantify the degree of liver damage. Probably more important, in the negative study

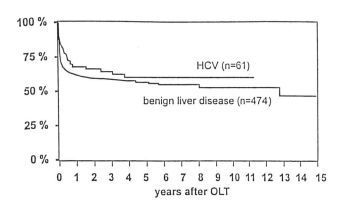

Figure 2. Cumulative survival of patients transplanted for hepatitis C-related disease versus patients transplanted for other nonmalignant indications. Patients with concomitant HCC are not excluded from the hepatitis C group. Patients with hepatitis B-related diseases are included in the nonmalignant indication group. *Dotted line,* HCV ($n = 61$); *straight line,* nonmalignant indications except HCV ($n = 474$). The difference between the groups is not statistically significant; $p = 0.25$ (log rank test). (From Boker et al. Long-term outcome of hepatitis C virus in infection after liver transplantation. *Hepatology* 1997;25:203. With permission.)

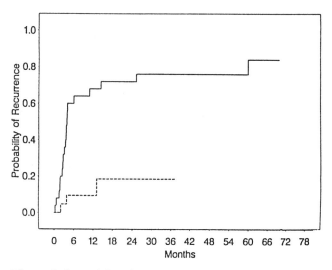

Figure 4. Actuarial graft survival in patients undergoing liver transplantation for HCV disease according to genotype responsible for infection. The actuarial survival following transplantation (in months) was compared in patients infected with HCV genotype 1a and 1b (–x–) ($n = 72$) and patients infected with other genotypes (–o–) ($n = 40$). There were no significant differences in survival ($p = 0.48$, Gehan's Wilcoxon test). (From Zhou et al. Severity of liver disease in liver transplantation with hepatitis C virus infection: relationship to genotype and level of viremia. *Hepatology* 1996; 24:1041–1046. With permission.)

from the United States, severe liver disease was infrequent, even though the duration of follow-up was comparable to that of the European study, marking that demonstration of a minor effect is difficult. In the more recent study with a 12-year post-transplantation follow-up, genotype was also not correlated with survival. In this case, the distribution of genotypes revealed 1b to be present in 73.6%, 1a to be present in 7.5%, and 3a to be present in 3.8%. The small number of patients with the latter genotypes may explain the lack of association. Thus, if this is an effect of genotype on the severity of post-transplantation liver injury, it is likely to be a minor one, and other factors clearly play a role in the pathogenesis of post-transplantation disease.

With an individual infected with a certain genotype, further heterogeneity exists. The closely related yet significantly different viral genomes produced over time in response to host pressures in an individual known as quasispecies are characterized by extensive genetic mutation with the second envelope gene (E2) hypervariable region (HVR) (60). Data suggest that HCV quasispecies mutation may play a role in pathogenesis of progressive HCV infection. Gretch and colleagues (1996) recently tracked HCV quasispecies major and minor variants before and after liver transplantation in five individuals, three of whom developed severe recurrent hepatitis C and two of whom developed mild post-transplantation infections. In the three with severe recurrent disease, quasispecies major variants present in the pretransplant serum were efficiently propagated immediately after liver transplantation and were propagated throughout the course of acute and chronic hepatitis. In contrast, in the two mild cases, there was rapid depletion of pretransplant quasispecies major variants from post-transplant serum, and minor species present pretransplantation became dominant after transplantation. These results are intriguing but do not clearly show a relationship between dominance of certain viral species and disease severity, thus highlighting the need for further examination of this question in large populations of immunocompetent, as well as immunocompromised patient groups.

Treatment of Post-Transplant HCV Infection and Disease

The standard by which to judge or measure response to treatment to antivirals is evolving. Ideally, one would like to utilize measures such as morbidity and mortality when determining beneficial effects of therapy. However, the lack of specific complaints and the indolent natural history of chronic HCV make these end points of therapy both difficult and impractical to measure. Therefore, traditionally intermediate assessments of disease such as normalization of transaminases, histologic improvement, and loss of detectable virus have been used. These end points are less satisfactory because there

is no proof that achieving these end points changes the long-term natural history of disease. Moreover, there are often discrepancies between biochemical, histologic, and virologic markers within a study. The method used for viral detection will influence whether virologic clearance is achieved, because assays differ in their sensitivity and reproducibility, particularly at the lower end of their range (see earlier). Moreover, the time at which treatment end points are assessed will influence the rate of response because many patients who appear to respond initially will relapse when therapy is discontinued. Although logically elimination of virus would seem to be better than mere normalization of serum transaminases, with current therapies, elimination of virus is uncommon in immunosuppressed transplant recipients. Thus, it is difficult to compare treatment response when no consistent criteria exist.

There are three possible strategies for prevention and/or treatment of HCV infection in the setting of liver transplantation. The first involves the use of prophylactic therapy at the time of transplantation in an attempt to prevent recurrence. The second is to treat patients early in the post-transplant period before histologic liver injury has occurred. The third is to wait until post-transplantation hepatitis has been demonstrated histologically before instituting treatment. Unlike HBV-infected patients undergoing liver transplantation who can be treated successfully with prophylactic therapy, HCV-infected patients lack this option. There is only a weak neutralizing humoral immune response to HCV (in contrast to the very effective neutralizing response to HBV infection), so that administration of a hepatitis C immune globulin (if one were available) would be predicted to be less effective than for HBV. Moreover, HCV is a highly mutable virus, so that immune escape to prophylaxis would be predicted to occur very rapidly.

Treatment options for HCV infection are still severely limited. Interferon is the only approved drug for this disease, and its use in immunocompromised patients has not been approved by the U.S. Food and Drug Administration. Moreover, interferon is less effective in patients with advanced liver disease (such as those undergoing liver transplantation) than in those with early disease. Thus, pretransplantation treatment with interferon would be predicted to eradicate viremia rarely and treatment could precipitate further decompensation. For these reasons, treatment with interferon cannot be recommended in patients with clinically decompensated HCV disease.

Therapy following transplantation has been studied in a few uncontrolled case series with two agents, interferon and ribavirin. Interferon alpha therapy in nonimmunocompromised patients results in transient normalization of serum aminotransferase levels in only half the patients treated, and sustained clearance of virus in only about 10%. Treatment results in liver transplant recipients would be predicted to be worse than this, because factors associated with treatment nonresponse (high levels of virus and infection with genotype 1) are common in this patient group. In one prospective trial, interferon alpha-2b (3 million units three times per week for at least 4 months) was administered to 18 patients (61). At the end of therapy, although there was no significant histologic response, five patients (28%) had complete normalization of transaminases (defined as responders), and both responders and nonresponders had reduced HCV RNA levels. With the cessation of treatment, both biochemical and virologic relapses were noted. Responders were more likely than nonresponders to have low pretreatment levels of HCV RNA and to have low serum bilirubin (i.e., they tended to have mild disease). Side effects resulted in treatment cessation in two patients and dosage reduction in six. Of note, no clear-cut episodes of allograft rejection were seen. In a second open trial of interferon (62), the course with treatment of 14 patients with recurrent HCV was compared with that of 32 patients who were not treated. In contrast to the previous study, five of the 14 treated patients developed chronic rejection, leading to retransplantation in three. Rejection occurred less frequently in the untreated group ($p < 0.005$). Among the nine treated patients who did not experience rejection, a decrease of transaminases or of HCV RNA levels to more than 50% of pretreatment levels was observed in eight and four patients, respectively. Two patients had a complete response and one did not relapse after discontinuation of interferon.

A preliminary report has suggested that treatment with interferon alpha-2b begun early after transplantation is effective at decreasing viral burden without increasing the rate of allograft rejection (63). Sixty-five patients received 1.5 million units of interferon three times per week for 3 weeks beginning at 1 week after transplantation. The dosage was then escalated to 3 million units of interferon three times per week for 52 weeks. Patients were followed for up to 1 year. At 6 months, 16 of 48 patients (33%) were negative for HCV RNA, and at 1 year, 25% remained negative. However, the long-term efficacy of early treatment with interferon requires further investigation. Taken together these results indicate that interferon therapy for patients with post-transplantation HCV recurrence has a transient antiviral effect, which is somewhat less than that seen in the immunocompetent patient. Moreover, treatment carries some risk, albeit probably a low risk, of precipitating allograft rejection. A second recombinant interferon, interferon alpha-2a, has recently been approved by the FDA for treatment of HCV. Preliminary data from a randomized controlled trial of this agent support the prior findings from uncontrolled studies (64).

Alternatives to interferon are few and are considered experimental at the present time. Ribavirin, a guanosine analog, is a broad-spectrum antiviral agent with activity against DNA and RNA viruses and has the advantage

over interferon of oral administration. Recently, ribavirin as monotherapy was shown in the immunocompetent patient to have beneficial effects on serum aminotransferase levels and histologic findings, but no effect on HCV RNA levels (65). These data suggest that ribavirin alone is not an effective antiviral agent against hepatitis C. In the immunocompromised host, ribavirin has recently been found in a pilot study to normalize transaminases but to have no antiviral effect (66). Although the data are limited, ribavirin monotherapy does not appear to have a major beneficial effect in the treatment of post-transplantation disease.

Because of the limited efficacy of ribavirin alone in the treatment of HCV disease, combination therapy with interferon has recently been tested in immunocompetent patients, and several studies have consistently shown that ribavirin reduces the relapse rate after interferon therapy (67–70). In the immunocompromised setting, a pilot study was reported on the use of interferon in combination with ribavirin after liver transplantation (71). Twenty-one patients were treated after transplantation with interferon (3 million units weekly for 6 months) in combination with 1,200 mg of ribavirin daily, followed by ribavirin alone for an additional 6 months. After combination therapy, all patients had normalization of ALT levels and improved histology. Ten patients (48%) had undetectable serum levels of HCV RNA, as assessed by PCR, and HCV RNA levels decreased significantly (more than 50%) in the others ($p = 0.0013$). During the period of ribavirin monotherapy, ALT remained normal in all but one of the 18 patients who tolerated therapy ($p = 0.004$). HCV RNA reappeared in five of the 10 patient responders, but HCV RNA levels did not return to pretreatment levels ($p = 0.0004$). Most important, there was complete absence of graft rejection. Although uncontrolled, these data suggest that combination therapy with interferon alpha and ribavirin following liver transplantation is an effective and safe treatment modality for recurrent HCV infection. Moreover, these positive results are prolonged by ribavirin maintenance. Unfortunately, no follow-up data on these 21 patients after cessation of ribavirin were included. Thus, the question of continued response versus relapse was not addressed. Nevertheless, these preliminary results do offer a novel potential treatment option to prevent progression of HCV-related graft disease and warrant future study.

The inability of currently available antiviral therapy to eliminate HCV in liver transplantation recipients suggests that more effective therapies, administered either alone or in combination with current therapies, will be necessary. The feasibility of such an approach will depend not only on a clear demonstration that therapy results in improvement in biochemical, virologic, and/or histologic markers of disease activity, but more important, on the fact that therapy results in improved graft and patient survival. Successful treatment will also depend on the availability of an antiviral agent, or combination of agents, that have low toxicity, few side effects, and a high rate of patient compliance. Since at present it is not clear which patients are at risk of developing serious sequelae from recurrent HCV, future studies should attempt to select those patients in greatest need for therapeutic intervention.

HCV Infection and End-Stage Renal Disease

HCV Infection and Dialysis Patients

The incidence and prevalence of hepatitis C infection among patients is steadily declining (72). Nonetheless, the 0.4% to 15% incidence of anti-HCV hemodialysis (HD) units continues to be a cause for concern. Although nosocomial transmission of HCV infection in HD has been demonstrated, the Centers for Disease Control and Prevention (CDC) does not recommend dedicated machines, patient isolation, or a ban on reuse in HD patients with HCV infection (72). Conventional cleansing and sterilization procedures for reprocessing the dialyzers appear to be adequate to inactivate the virus (72). The duration of time on HD is correlated with presence of HCV infection (73,74). Lower anti-HCV seroprevalence rates are seen in patients on peritoneal dialysis (73), suggesting that transmission in this setting is less efficient than that for hemodialysis.

Several reports have shown that abnormal liver enzymes are more common in anti-HCV-positive dialysis patients than in anti-HCV-negative patients (75–77). Furthermore, HCV RNA-positive dialysis patients have been shown to display higher hepatic enzyme levels than dialysis patients with no detectable HCV RNA (78). In one of the few series of HCV-infected patients on hemodialysis in which liver histology was determined, most patients had histologic evidence of liver injury even though most also had normal serum ALT (79). Larger studies are needed to corroborate this finding. If ALT is confirmed to be a poor marker of the stage of liver disease, it will be necessary to perform biopsies in dialysis patients to determine severity of disease.

HCV Infection and Renal Transplantation

As mentioned earlier, there exists a high prevalence of HCV infection in dialysis patients, and thus many referred for transplant will be infected with HCV. The optimal approach to the HCV-infected end-stage renal disease patient remains unknown (80). A recent survey showed that 89% of transplant centers in the United States are currently transplanting kidneys into HCV-positive recipients (81), although in the same survey 37% of these centers did require that the patient have no histologic evidence of chronic liver disease. Other studies have suggested expansion of the pretransplant work-up to

include biopsy for histologic staging, interferon therapy if there is histologic evidence of significant hepatitis, and HCV RNA testing by PCR (82–84). Most studies comparing HCV-positive with HCV-negative renal transplant recipients have failed to show any difference in graft or patient survival (83,85). One study (54) has shown an increased risk of death from sepsis for HCV-positive patients after renal transplantation. The extent of liver disease was not assessed at the time of transplantation, but it is likely that active liver disease contributed to the poor outcome observed. In contrast, a recent study that examined HCV-positive patients with at least 2 years follow-up showed better survival for those who underwent renal transplant (33 patients) than similar patients who remained on dialysis awaiting transplantation (25 patients) (74). These two small groups of patients were similar with respect to age, race, duration of dialysis, cause of renal failure, prevalence of heart disease, and results of liver function tests. The true impact of HCV infection in end-stage renal failure and further recommendations regarding transplantation of HCV-infected patients and organs will be determined only by further large, prospective outcome studies comparing dialysis and transplantation patients.

Treatment of HCV Infection in Renal Failure Patients

The use of interferon alpha in HCV-positive transplantation candidates is controversial, because of its questionable efficacy and its potential to impair renal function. To date no large series or controlled studies have been performed. In two small studies, a biochemical response was observed in some patients, but relapses were common, and renal impairment was reported (84,86). Acute and subacute renal failure have been reported in many studies, often secondary to rejection (86–88). Given this significant side effect profile and the lack of convincing data that show improved outcome with interferon therapy for chronic hepatitis C in renal transplant patients, the use of interferon in this setting cannot be firmly recommended.

In a search for an alternative treatment, ribavirin therapy has been tested in one uncontrolled trial, which showed a biochemical response in approximately 57% of those treated (89). In this preliminary study, no detrimental side effects of graft function were observed. These data suggest that future studies with ribavirin in this setting can be proposed.

HCV Infection and Bone Marrow Transplantation

In recent years, significant liver disease in the bone marrow patient has been shown to be common and is most often secondary to veno-occlusive disease (VOD), graft-versus-host disease (GVHD), drug toxicity, recurrent hematologic malignancy, and infectious hepatitis (90). The overall mortality from liver failure in 63 European BMT centers has been shown to be 4.5% (258 of 5,788) (37). VOD of the liver occurs after about 20% of allogeneic BMT and about 10% of autologous BMT. As many as 50% of patients who develop VOD die of fulminant hepatic failure. HCV infection may be a risk factor for development of VOD, but this relationship remains controversial.

Although HCV has emerged as a common cause of mild liver disease in this setting in the short term (91–93), the long-term risk of chronic hepatitis C virus infection remains to be determined. One report examined 181 patients undergoing BMT and assessed HCV status by using both a second-generation ELISA and a confirmatory RIBA2 (94). In this study, biochemical evidence of chronic hepatitis was more frequent in the patients who were HCV-positive before BMT (86% versus 32%, respectively). However, the proportion of those who developed VOD, or in whom liver failure contributed to death, was similar regardless of the presence of anti-HCV before BMT or documented seroconversion with BMT. In a second study (95), of 128 patients who were tested for HCV positivity following transplant, only two (one anti-HCV-positive and one anti-HCV-negative) experienced VOD. A later report by the same group compared 31 patients who died of severe liver failure after BMT with 26 matched BMT controls who did not develop liver failure (96). Causes of liver failure included VOD ($n = 7$), liver GVHD ($n = 5$), or hepatitis ($n = 19$). Despite a high prevalence of HCV positivity (47% as determined by PCR), HCV-RNA was equally prevalent in patients with or without liver failure (48% versus 46%, respectively), and positive HCV status was shown once again not to be a predictor of VOD. Furthermore, a recent study found no correlation between HCV genotype and type or severity of post-transplant liver disease (97).

In contrast, another study evaluated 61 patients who underwent BMT (98). Six of these patients had been infected with HCV before and three acquired HCV during or shortly after BMT. All six infected with HCV before BMT died within 10 weeks of transplantation. Five of these six (83%) died of VOD, compared with nine of 52 (17%) not infected with HCV ($p < 0.005$). Parallel to the development of VOD, replication of HCV increased, as demonstrated by rising concentrations of viral RNA. These data suggested that patients with liver disease caused by HCV infection are at high risk of developing lethal VOD after BMT. Thus, further studies are needed to prospectively evaluate the contribution of HCV to the development of VOD and other liver complications after BMT. Although the rate of HCV infection has decreased with the screening of blood products for HCV antibodies, multiply transfused patients will continue to acquire HCV infection. HCV RNA positivity in blood components has been shown to be a more effective test of HCV transmissibility than the tests that check for HCV antibodies (second-generation ELISA or the sec-ond-generation RIBA). It is important not only to develop criteria for estimating the risk of post-transplant liver disease in HCV-infected patients, but to develop new treatment strategies of HCV infection and prophylaxis of associated complications.

There are anecdotal reports of acute liver failure related to exacerbation of preexisting HCV infection in association with withdrawal of immunosuppressive therapy after BMT (92,99–101). This is analogous to the relationship between HBV and immunosuppressive therapy and suggests that the liver injury occurring with HCV infection is at least in part immune-mediated. Such adverse effects of withdrawal of immunosuppression may be avoided with ribavirin (102). Three allogeneic BMT patients were treated with ribavirin. Therapy was started between 10 days and 3 weeks before transplant, continued through the transplant period, and further continued for 4–18 months after transplant. The duration of ribavirin therapy was determined in such a way that immunosuppression was stopped before ribavirin was discontinued. Patients who were HCV RNA positive became HCV RNA negative with treatment, and remained negative between 6 and 12 months off therapy during follow-up. The exact role for ribavirin in this setting requires further study.

HCV Infection and Heart Transplantation

Very little is known about the clinical course of HCV in heart transplant recipients. In a recently reported retrospective survey (103), 96 patients who underwent heart transplant between 1983 and 1995 were confirmed to be HCV positive by a second-generation antibody test and/or PCR for HCV RNA viremia following transplantation. Actuarial survival of these 96 transplanted patients was compared with 7,302 UNOS Public Use Data patients transplanted between 1987 and 1991. There was no statistical difference in the Kaplan Meier actuarial survival for the HCV-positive group as compared with the UNOS control group ($p = 0.40$). In another study (104), a high prevalence (63%) of liver dysfunction was reported in 80 heart transplant recipients who were followed for 60 months (median; range, 1.5–98 months). Causes included NANBH (32%), hepatitis B (26%), hepatitis D (2%), drugs (12%), and cardiac failure (14%). Anti-HCV antibodies were found in more than half of the patients with NANBH and in 20% of the patients with HBV infection. In contrast, a more recent study (105) showed only a 7% (four of 59) prevalence rate of HCV infection according to a serum HCV RNA detection in their heart transplant recipients. The long-term outcome of patients with biochemical or histologic evidence of hepatitis in this setting is not known. Reports of cholestatic liver disease leading to liver failure are anecdotal (105,106). Whether interferon alpha plays a role in the setting of HCV-induced liver failure post-transplantation setting remains to be established.

OTHER VIRAL INFECTIONS

HDV Infection

Natural History

Liver transplant patients with chronic HDV infection are at lower risk for post-transplantation HBV recurrence than those with HBV infection alone, and if reinfection does occur, the disease is less devastating. The inhibitory effect of HDV infection on HBV replication (107) results in low pretransplantation levels of HBV DNA, which likely decreases the risk of post-transplantation recurrence, and low levels of HBV DNA following transplantation, which likely results in mild liver disease (2,108–110). An early study (110) described the natural history of seven patients with HDV who underwent liver transplantation. Although two patients cleared infection, post-transplantation recurrence was observed in five, hepatitis in three, death from recurrent hepatitis in one, and retransplantation for reasons unrelated to viral hepatitis in the fifth. Subsequently, the same investigators reported recurrence of HDV in 22 of 27 transplant recipients (108). Two patients died of coexisting HDV and HBV infection, and five (18%) cleared both viruses. Overall survival was good at 78%, despite the inconsistent use of HBIG prophylaxis. Disease recurrence (defined as evidence of histologic hepatitis) was only seen in those patients with HBV as well as HDV infection, not in those with HDV infection alone (108). Interestingly, in many patients HDV infection was detected before any evidence of HBV infection, but HDV disease only occurred when HBV infection reactivation occurred. These clinical observations support the experimental findings that HDV is dependent on HBV for viral packaging (and presumably for disease pathogenesis).

In a small study from the United States, HBV recurrence was high, regardless of the presence of HDV coinfection, but death from liver failure was more frequent in those with HBV infection alone than in those with concomitant HDV infection (111). In a larger study from Europe, three 3-year actuarial risk of HBV recurrence after transplantation was lower in those with HDV-related cirrhosis (32%, $n = 110$) and those with fulminant HDV (40%, $n = 14$), compared with those with HBV-related cirrhosis with detectable HBV DNA (83%, $n = 58$) (2). Coexistent infection with HDV was shown to be associated with improved survival (relative risk 3.92; 95% confidence interval 2.48–6.21; $p < 0.001$). As in the U.S. study, the use of HBIG prophylaxis was inconsistent.

Treatment

Currently, there are no effective therapies specific for HDV infection, and treatment strategies have largely paralleled those developed for HBV infection. As for patients with HBV-infection alone, long-term immuno-prophylaxis with HBIG is associated with decreased recurrence rates and improved survival (2). The 3-year risk of recurrence is reduced significantly in patients receiving long-term immunoprophylaxis compared with those receiving short-term immunoprophylaxis or no therapy (17% versus 56% and 70%, respectively, $p < 0.001$). In multivariate analysis, long-term administration of HBIG (relative risk 2.22; 95% confidence interval (CI), 1.13–4.33, $p < 0.001$) and HDV superinfection (relative risk 6.25; 95 per CI, 3.13–12.42, $p < 0.001$) was independently predictive of a better survival in all patients with HBV infection (2).

Little is known regarding the use of interferon for the treatment of HDV in either immunocompetent or immunocompromised patients. In a randomized controlled trial of chronic HDV, 42 patients were assigned to receive 9 million or 3 million units of interferon alpha-2a (three times a week for 48 weeks), or no treatment (107). Normalization of transaminases and a loss of HDV RNA occurred in 50% treated with 9 million units, as compared with 21% treated with 3 million units ($p = 0.118$), and none in untreated controls ($p = 0.004$). In addition, treatment with the higher dose resulted in histologic improvement, whereas there was histologic deterioration in the control patients. Although biochemical responses persisted for up to 4 years, early virologic relapses (within 12 months of completion of therapy) were common. In a pilot study, 11 patients undergoing liver transplantation with HBV/HDV infection were treated with interferon for 2–3 months, between the first and the thirteenth months after transplantation (112). Reinfection of the graft was observed in seven patients, with histologic signs of acute hepatitis in five and transition to chronic hepatitis in one. Although treatment with interferon did not appear to prevent or reduce of HBV replication, it may have had a beneficial effect on HDV replication in liver allografts.

SUMMARY

This chapter highlights the importance of hepatotropic viruses as pathogens in patients undergoing transplantation, their contribution to morbidity and mortality after transplantation, and the approach to treatment of these pathogens when they cause disease. Although many advances have been made in the management of viral hepatitis in the transplant setting, unanswered questions remain about the long-term natural history of the disease. Understanding of the pathogenesis of infection in the setting of transplantation is emerging slowly, but complete understanding requires further investigation. New approaches to treating disease in patients with either HBV or HCV infection are under development and will likely focus on the use of combinations of antiviral and immunomodulatory agents.

REFERENCES

1. Todo S, Demetris A, Van Thiel D, Teperman L, Fung J, Starzl T. Orthotopic liver transplantation for patients with hepatitis B virus-related liver disease. *Hepatology* 1991;13:619–626.

2. Samuel D, Muller R, Alexander G, et al. Liver transplantation in European patients with the hepatitis B surface antigen. *N Engl J Med* 1993; 329:1842–1847.

3. Chazouilleres O, Mamish D, Kim M, et al. Occult hepatitis B virus as source of infection in liver transplant recipients. *Lancet* 1994;43: 142–146.

4. Angus P, Locarnini S, McCaughan G, Jones R, McMillan J, Bowden D. Hepatitis B virus precore mutant infection is associated with severe recurrent disease after liver transplantation. *Hepatology* 1995;21: 14–18.

5. Naumann U, Protzer-Knolle U, Berg T, et al. A pretransplant infection with precore mutants of hepatitis B virus does not influence the outcome of orthotopic liver transplantation in patients on high dose anti-hepatitis B virus surface antigen immunoprophylaxis. *Hepatology* 1997;26:478–484.

6. Lauchart W, Muller R, Pichlmayr R. Long-term immunoprophylaxis of hepatitis B virus reinfection in recipients of human liver allografts. *Transplant Proc* 1987;19:4051–4053.

7. Mora N, Klintmalm G, Poplawski S, et al. Recurrence of hepatitis B after liver transplantation. Does hepatitis-B-immunoglobulin modify the recurrent disease? *Transplant Proc* 1990;22:1549–1550.

8. Samuel D, Bismuth A, Mathieu D, et al. Passive immunoprophylaxis after liver transplantation in HBsAg-positive patients. *Lancet* 1991; 337:813–815.

9. Terrault N, Zhou S, Combs C, et al. Prophylaxis in liver transplant recipients using schedule of hepatitis B immunoglobulin. *Hepatology* 1996;24:1327–1333.

10. McGory R, Ishitani M, Oliveira W, et al. Improved outcome of orthotopic liver transplantation for chronic hepatitis B cirrhosis with aggressive passive immunization. *Transplantation* 1996;61:1358–1364.

11. Terrault N, Zhou S, Singleton S, et al. Mutational analysis of surface (S) and polymerase (P) genes in liver transplant (OLT) recipients failing HBIG immunoprophylaxis. *Hepatology* 1996;24:181A.

12. Carman W, Trautwein C, Van Deursen F, et al. Hepatitis B virus envelope variation after transplantation with and without hepatitis B immune globulin prophylaxis. *Hepatology* 1996;24:489–493.

13. Marcellin P, Samuel D, Areias J, et al. Pretransplantation interferon treatment and recurrence of hepatitis B virus infection after liver transplantation for hepatitis B-related end-stage liver disease. *Hepatology* 1994;19:6–12.

14. Rakela J, Wooten R, Batts K, Perkins J, Taswell H, Krom R. Failure of interferon to prevent recurrent hepatitis B infection in hepatic allograft. *Mayo Clin Proc* 1989;64:429–432.

15. Grellier L, Brown D, McPhilips P, Burroughs A, Rolles K, Dusheiko G. Lamivudine prophylaxis new strategy for prevention of reinfection in liver transplantation for hepatitis B DNA positive cirrhosis. *Hepatology* 1995;22:224A.

16. Ling R, Mutimer D, Ahmed M, et al. Selection of mutations in the hepatitis B virus polymerase during therapy of transplant recipients with lamivudine. *Hepatology* 1996;24:711–713.

17. Tipples G, Ma M, Fischer K, Bain VG, Kneteman NM, Tyrrell DL. Mutation in HBV RNA-dependent DNA polymerase confers resistance to lamivudine *in vivo*. *Hepatology* 1996;24:714–717.

18. Terrault N, Holland C, Ferrell L, et al. Interferon alpha for recurrent hepatitis B infection following liver transplantation. *Liver Transplant Surg* 1996;2:132.

19. Gish R, Lau JYN, Brooks L, et al. Ganciclovir treatment of hepatitis B virus infection in liver transplant recipients. *Hepatology* 1996;23:1–7.

20. Rabinovitz M, Dodson F, Rakela J. Famciclovir for recurrent hepatitis B (HBV) infection after liver transplantation (OLTX). *Hepatology* 1996;24:282A.

21. Perrillo R, Rakela J, Martin P, et al. Lamivudine for hepatitis B following liver transplantation. *Hepatology* 1996;24:182A.

22. Perrillo R, Rakela J, Martin P, et al. Lamivudine for suppression and/or prevention of hepatitis B when given pre/post transplantation (OLT). *Hepatology* 1997;26:261A.

23. Perrillo R, Rakela J, Martin P, et al. Long term lamivudine therapy of patients with recurrent hepatitis B post liver transplantation. *Hepatology* 1997;26:177A.

24. Alter M, Favero M, Moyer L, et al. National surveillance of dialysis-associated diseases in the United States. *ASAIO J* 1991;37:97.

25. Mioli V, Balestra E, Bibiano L, et al. Epidemiology of viral hepatitis in dialysis centers: a national survey. *Nephron* 1992;61:278.

26. London W, Drew J, Lustbader E, Werner BG, Blumberg BS. Host response to hepatitis B infection in patients in a chronic hemodialysis unit. *Kidney Int* 1977;12:51–58.

27. Ramos E, Kasiske B, Alexander S, et al. The evaluation of candidates for renal transplantation. *Transplantation* 1994;57:490–497.

28. Fornairon S, Pol S, Legendre C, et al. The long-term virologic and pathologic impact of renal transplantation on chronic hepatitis B virus infection. *Transplantation* 1996;62:297–299.

29. Bedrossian J, Akposso K, Metvier F, Moal M, Pruna A, Idatte J. Kidney transplantations with HBsAg+ donors. *Transplant Proc* 1993;25: 1481–1482.

30. Grob P. Hepatitis B vaccination of renal transplant and hemodialysis patients. *Scand J Infect Dis* 1983;38[Suppl]:28–32.

31. Lefebure A, Verpooten G, Couttenye M, De Broe M. Immunogenicity of a recombinant DNA hepatitis B vaccine in renal transplant patients. *Vaccine* 1993;11:397–399.

32. Garnier J, Chossegros P, Daoud S, et al. Treatment of hepatitis B virus replication by Ganciclovir in kidney transplant patients. *Transplant Proc* 1997;29:817.

33. McDonald G, Shulman H, Wolford J, Spencer G. Liver disease after human marrow transplantation. *Semin Liv Dis* 1987;7:210–229.

34. Chen P, Fan S, Hsieh R, et al. Liver disease in patients with liver dysfunction prior to bone marrow transplantation. *Bone Marrow Transplant* 1992;9:415–419.

35. Locasciulli A, Bacigalupo A, Van Lint MT, et al. Hepatitis B virus (HBV) infection and liver disease after allogeneic bone marrow transplantation: a report of 30 cases. *Bone Marrow Transplant* 1990;6: 25–29.

36. Reed EC, Myerson D, Corey L, Meyers JD. Allogeneic marrow transplantation in patients positive for hepatitis B surface antigen. *Blood* 1991;77:195–200.

37. Locasciulli A, Alberti A, de Bock R, et al. Impact of liver disease and hepatitis infections on allogeneic bone marrow transplantation in Europe: a survey from the European Bone Marrow Transplantation (EBMT) Group-Infectious Diseases Working Party. *Bone Marrow Transplant* 1994;14:833–837.

38. Locasciulli A, Alberti A, Bandini G, et al. Allogeneic bone marrow transplantation from HBsAg+ donors: a multicenter study from the Gruppo Italiano Trapianto di Midollo Osseo (GITMO). *Blood* 1995;86:3236–3240.

39. Shouval D, Adler R, Ilan Y. Adoptive transfer immunity to hepatitis B virus in mice by bone marrow transplantation from immune donors. *Hepatology* 1993;17:955–959.

40. Ilan Y. Nagler A, Adler R, et al. Adoptive transfer immunity to hepatitis B virus after T cell-depleted allogeneic bone marrow transplantation. *Hepatology* 1993;18:246–252.

41. Lau G, Lok A, Liang R, et al. Clearance of hepatitis B surface antigen after bone marrow transplantation: role of adoptive immunity transfer. *Hepatology* 1997;25:1497–1501.

42. Cadranel J, Grippon O, Lunel F, et al. Chronic liver dysfunction in heart transplant patients, with special reference to viral B, C, and non-A, non-B, non-C hepatitis. A retrospective study in 80 patients with follow-up of 60 months. *Transplantation* 1991;52:645–650.

43. Anand B, Yoffe B, Young J. Ganciclovir treatment of active hepatitis B virus infection in a heart transplant patient. *J Clin Gastroenterol* 1996;22:144–146.

44. Lok A, Chien D, Choo Q, et al. Antibody response to core, envelope and nonstructural hepatitis C virus antigens: comparison of immunocompetent and immunosuppressed patients. *Hepatology* 1993;18: 497–502.

45. Donegan E, Wright TL, Roberts J, et al. Detection of hepatitis C after liver transplantation. Four serologic tests compared. *Am J Clin Pathol* 1995;104:673–679.

46. Chazouilleres O, Kim M, Combs C, et al. Quantitation of hepatitis C virus RNA in liver transplant recipients. *Gastroenterology* 1994;106: 994–999.

47. Gane EJ, Portmann BC, Naoumov N, et al. Long-term outcome of hepatitis C infection after liver transplantation. *N Engl J Med* 1996;334:815–820.

48. Feray C, Gigou M, Samuel D, et al. Influence of the genotypes of

hepatitis C virus on the severity of recurrent liver disease after liver transplantation. *Gastroenterology* 1995;108:1088–1096.

49. Zhou S, Terrault NA, Ferrell L, et al. Severity of liver disease in liver transplantation recipients with hepatitis C virus infection: relationship to genotype and level of viremia. *Hepatology* 1996;24:1041–1046.

50. Pereira B, Wright T, Schmid C, et al. Screening and confirmatory testing of cadaver organ donors for hepatitis C virus infection: a US national collaborative study. *Kidney Int* 1994;46:886–892.

51. Alter H, Purcell R, Shih J, et al. Detection of antibody to hepatitis C virus in prospectively followed transfusion recipients with acute and chronic non-A, non-B, hepatitis. *N Engl J Med* 1989;321:1494–1500.

52. Pereira B, Milford E, Kirkman R, Levey A. Transmission of hepatitis C virus by organ transplantation. *N Engl J Med* 1991;325:454–460.

53. Pereira B, Milford E, Kirkman R, et al. Prevalence of hepatitis C virus RNA in organ donors positive for hepatitis C antibody and in the recipients of their organs. *N Engl J Med* 1992;327:910–915.

54. Pereira B, Wright TL, Schmid C. A controlled study of hepatitis C transmission by organ transplantation. The New England Organ Bank Hepatitis C Study Group. *Lancet* 1995;345:484–487.

55. Pirsch J, Belzer F. Transmission of HCV by organ transplantation. *N Engl J Med* 1992;326:412.

56. Martin P, Munoz S, Di Bisceglie A, et al. Recurrence of hepatitis C virus infection following orthotopic liver transplantation. *Hepatology* 1991;13:719–721.

57. Wright TL, Donegan E, Hsu H, et al. Recurrent and acquired hepatitis C viral infection in liver transplant recipients. *Gastroenterology* 1992;103:317–322.

58. Detre K. Liver transplantation for chronic viral hepatitis. A.A.S.L.D. Single Topic Conference, Reston, VA 1995.

59. Boker K, Dalley G, Bahr M, et al. Long-term outcome of hepatitis C virus infection after liver transplantation. *Hepatology* 1997;25:203–210.

60. Bukh J, Miller R, Purcell R. Genetic heterogeneity of hepatitis C virus: quasispecies and genotypes. *Semin Liver Dis* 1995;15:41–63.

61. Wright TL, Combs C, Kim M, et al. Interferon-alpha therapy for hepatitis C virus infection after liver transplantation. *Hepatology* 1994;20:773–779.

62. Feray C, Samuel DMG, et al. An open trial of interferon alpha recombinant for hepatitis C after liver transplantation. *Hepatology* 1995;22:1084–1089.

63. Reddy K, Weppler D, Zervos X, et al. Recurrent HCV infection following OLTX: the role of early post OLTX interferon treatment. *Hepatology* 1996;24:295A.

64. Crippin J, Huang K, Wright TL, et al. Efficacy of interferon alpha 2A (Roferon A) in the treatment of hepatitis C and G following liver transplantation; A prospective, randomized study. *Hepatology* 1996; 24:294A.

65. DiBisceglie A, Conjeevaram H, Fried M, et al. Ribavirin as therapy for chronic hepatitis C. *Ann Intern Med* 1995;123:897–903.

66. Rezieg M, Altraif I, Roach C, et al. Treatment of hepatitis C viral infection (HCV) in the transplanted patient with ribavirin. *Hepatology* 1993;18:342A.

67. Chemello L, Bernardineelo E, Guido M, Pontisso P, Alberti A. The effect of interferon alpha and ribavirin combination therapy in naive patients with chronic hepatitis C. *J Hepatology* 1995;23[Suppl 2]:8–12.

68. Brillanti S, Miglioli M, Barbara L. Combination antiviral therapy with ribavirin and interferon alpha in interferon alpha relapsers and non-responders: Italian experience. *J Hepatol* 1995;23[Suppl 2]:13–16.

69. Schvarcz R, Ando Y, Sonnerborg A, Weiland O. Combination treatment with interferon alpha-2b and ribavirin for chronic hepatitis C in patients who have failed to achieve sustained response to interferon alone: Swedish experience. *J Hepatol* 1995;23[Suppl 2]:17–21.

70. Lai M, Yang P, Wang JT, et al. Long-term efficacy of ribavirin plus interferon alpha in the treatment of chronic hepatitis C. *Gastroenterology* 1996;111:1307–1312.

71. Bizollon T, Palazzo U, Chevallier M, Ducerf C, Trepo C. HCV recurrence after OLTX: a pilot study of ribavirin therapy following initial combination with INF. *Hepatology* 1996;24:293A.

72. Murthy B, Pereira B. A 1990's perspective of hepatitis C, human immunodeficiency virus, and tuberculosis infections in dialysis patients. *Semin Nephrol* 1997;17:346–363.

73. Cantu P, Mangano S, Masini M, Limido A, Crovetti G, DeFilippo C. Prevalence of antibodies against hepatitis C virus in a dialysis unit. *Nephron* 1992;61:337–338.

74. Knoll G, Tankersley M, Lee J, Julian B, Curtis J. The impact of renal transplantation on survival in hepatitis C-positive end-stage renal disease patients. *Am J Kid Dis* 1997;29:608–614.

75. Zeldis J, Depner T, Kuramoto I, Gish R, Holland P. The prevalence of hepatitis C antibodies among hemodialysis patients. *Ann Intern Med* 1990;112:958–960.

76. Alivanis P, Derveniotis V, Dioudis C, et al. Hepatitis C virus antibodies in hemodialysed and in renal transplant patients: correlation with chronic liver disease. *Transplant Proc* 1991;23:2662–2663.

77. Chan T, Lok A, Cheng I, Chan R. Prevalence of hepatitis C virus infection in hemodialysis patients: a longitudinal study comparing the results of RNA and antibody assays. *Hepatology* 1993;17:5–8.

78. Fabrizi F, Lunghi G, Andrulli S, et al. Influence of hepatitis C virus (HCV) viremia upon aminotransferase activity in chronic dialysis patients. *Nephrol Dial Transplant* 1997;12:1394–1398.

79. al-Wakeel J, al-Mohaya S, Mitwalli A, Baroudi F, Gamal H, Kechrid M. Liver disease in dialysis patients with antibodies to hepatitis C virus. *Nephrol Dial Transplant* 1996;11:2265–2268.

80. Kasiske B, Ramos E, Gaston R, et al. The evaluation of renal transplant candidates: clinical practice guidelines. *J Am Soc Nephrol* 1995;6:1–34.

81. Schweitzer E, Bartlett ST, Keay S, Hadley GA, Cregar J, Stockdreher DD. Impact of hepatitis B or C infection on the practice of kidney transplantation in the United States. *Transplant Proc* 1993;25:1456–1457.

82. Glicklich D, Kapoian T. Should the hepatitis C positive end stage renal disease patient be transplanted? *Semin Dial* 1996;9:5–8.

83. Roth D, Zucker K, Cirocco R. The impact of hepatitis C virus infection on renal allograft recipients. *Kidney Int* 1994;45:238–244.

84. Rosen H, Friedman L, Martin P. Hepatitis C and the renal transplant patient. *Semin Dial* 1996;9:39–46.

85. Ynares C, Johnson H, Kerlin T, Crowe D, MacDonell R, Richie R. Impact of pretransplant hepatitis C antibody status upon long-term patients and renal allograft survival. A 5- and 10-year follow-up. *Transplant Proc* 1993;25:1466–1468.

86. Yasamura T, Nakajima H, Hamashima T, et al. Long-term outcome of recombinant INF-alpha treatment of chronic hepatitis C in kidney transplant recipients, *Transplant Proc* 1997;29:784–786.

87. Magnone M, Holley J, Shapiro R, et al. Interferon-a-induced acute renal allograft rejection. *Transplantation* 1995;59:1068–1070.

88. Rostaing L, Modesto A, Baron E, Cisterne J, Chabannier M, Durand D. Acute renal failure in kidney transplant patients treated with interferon alpha 2b for chronic hepatitis C. *Nephron* 1996;74:512–516.

89. Garnier J, Chevallier P, Dubernard J, Trepo C, Touraine J, Chossegros P. Treatment of hepatitis C virus infection with ribavirin in kidney transplant patients. *Transplant Proc* 1997;29:783.

90. Terrault NA, Wright TL, Pereira BJ. Hepatitis C infection in the transplant recipient. *Infect Dis Clin North Am* 1995;9:943–964.

91. Shuhart M, Myerson D, Childs B, et al. Marrow transplantation from hepatitis C virus seropositive donors: Transmission rate and clinical course. *Blood* 1994;84:3229–3235.

92. Ljungman P, Johansson N, Aschan J, et al. Long-term effects of hepatitis C virus infection in allogeneic bone marrow transplant recipients. *Blood* 1995;86:1614–1618.

93. Shuhart M, Myerson D, Spurgeon C, Bevan C, Sayers M, McDonald GB. Hepatitis C virus (HCV) infection in bone marrow transplant patients after transfusions from anti-HCV positive blood donors. *Bone Marrow Transplant* 1996;17:601–606.

94. Norol F, Roche B, Saint Marc Girardin M, et al. Hepatitis C virus infection and allogeneic bone marrow transplantation. *Transplant* 1994;57:393–397.

95. Locasciulli A, Bacigalupo A, Van Lint MT, et al. Hepatitis C virus infection in patients undergoing allogeneic bone marrow transplantation. *Transplant* 1991;52:315–318.

96. Locasciulli A, Bacigalupo A, Van Lint MT, et al. Hepatitis C virus infection and liver failure in patients undergoing allogeneic bone marrow transplantation. *Bone Marrow Transplant* 1995:16:407–411.

97. Locasciulli A, Testa M, Pontisso P, et al. Hepatitis C virus genotypes and liver disease in patients undergoing allogeneic bone marrow transplantation. *Bone Marrow Transplant* 1997;19:237–240.

98. Frickhofen N, Wiesneth M, Jainta C, et al. Hepatitis C infection is a risk factor for liver failure from veno-occlusive disease after bone marrow transplantation. *Blood* 1994;83:1998–2004.

99. Kanamori H, Fukawa H, Maruta A, et al. Case report: fulminant hepatitis C viral infection after allogeneic bone marrow transplantation. *Am J Med Sci* 1992;303:109–111.

100. Fan FS, Tzeng CH, Hsiao KI, Hu ST, Liu WT, Chen PM. Withdrawal of immunosuppressive therapy in allogeneic bone marrow transplantation reactivates chronic viral hepatitis C. *Bone Marrow Transplant* 1991;8:417–420.

101. Shuhart M, Myerson D, Childs B, et al. Marrow transplantation from hepatitis C virus seropositive donors. *Blood* 1994;84:3229–3235.

102. Ljungman P, Anderson J, Aschan J, et al. Oral ribavirin for prevention of severe liver disease caused by hepatitis C virus during allogeneic bone marrow transplantation. *Clin Infect Dis* 1996;23:167–169.

103. Lake K, Smith C, Milfred-La Forest S, Pritzker MR, Emery RW. Outcomes of hepatitis C positive (HCV+) heart transplant recipients. *Transplant Proc* 1997;29:581–582.

104. Cadranel J, Grippon P, Lunel F, et al. Chronic liver dysfunction in heart transplant recipients, with special reference to viral B, C and non-A, non-B, non-C hepatitis. *Transplantation* 1991;52:645–650.

105. Zein N, McGregor C, Wendt N, et al. Prevalence and outcome of hepatitis C infection among heart transplant recipients. *Transplantation* 1995;14:865–869.

106. Lim H, Lau G, Davis G, Dolson D, Lau J. Cholestatic hepatitis leading to hepatic failure in a patient with organ-transmitted hepatitis C virus infection. *Gastroenterology* 1994;106:248–251.

107. Farci P, Mandas A, Coiana A, et al, Treatment of hepatitis D with interferon alpha-2a. *N Engl J Med* 1994;330:88–94.

108. Ottobrelli A, Marzano A, Smedile A, et al. Patterns of hepatitis delta virus reinfection and disease in liver transplantation. *Gastroenterology* 1991;101:1649–1655.

109. Samuel D, Zignego A, Arulnaden J, et al. Liver transplantation for post hepatitis delta cirrhosis. *Hepatology* 1992;16:45A.

110. Rizzetto M, Chiaberge E, Negro F, et al. Liver transplantation in hepatitis delta virus disease. *Lancet* 1987;2:469–471.

111. Lucey M, Graham D, Martin P, et al. Recurrence of hepatitis B and delta hepatitis after orthotopic liver transplantation. *Gut* 1992;33:1390–1396.

112. Hopf U, Neuhaus P, Lobeck H, et al. Follow-up of recurrent hepatitis B and delta infection in liver allograft recipients after treatment with recombinant interferon-alpha. *J Hepatol* 1991;13:339–346.

Transplant Infections edited by
Raleigh A. Bowden, Per Ljungman, and Carlos V. Paya.
Lippincott–Raven Publishers, Philadelphia © 1998

CHAPTER 23

Fungal Infections After Marrow Transplantation

Raleigh A. Bowden

Over the past decade, invasive fungal infections have become an increasingly important problem in patients following bone marrow transplantation (BMT). Although candidiasis has been the most common cause of invasive fungal infections (1,2), data from single institutions have shown significant increases in aspergillosis in recent years (1,3). Further, with the progress made in prevention of cytomegalovirus (CMV) infection and CMV pneumonia, aspergillosis has now become, and will likely continue to be, the leading infectious cause of death after allogeneic transplant in the near future (3,4). The development of invasive aspergillosis has been reported to be the strongest risk factor for death by multivariate analysis of risk factors predicting death after BMT (2), again highlighting the importance of this pathogen.

The types of fungal organisms that cause disease following BMT can be divided into three general categories. The first includes infections caused by yeasts that are distinguished from other fungi by the absence of true hyphae and their propensity to colonize mucous membranes. The most common yeast infections in the BMT setting are the *Candida* spp. The second group of fungi are the molds, distinguished by their ability to form true hyphae. Molds are generally acquired through the inhalation of aerosolized spores. *Aspergillus* spp. are by far the most common cause of mold infections; less common molds include the Mucorales order (e.g., *Rhizopus*, *Rhizomucor*, and *Absidia*) as well as a variety of rarer molds including *Fusarium*, *Bipolaris*, and *Pseudoallescheria*, just to name a few examples. The timing of candidal and mold infections after allogeneic transplantation is shown in Figure 1. Patients undergoing autologous transplantation have a similar risk period for candidiasis, but their risk for

aspergillosis is confined to the neutropenic period. The final group of fungi are the dimorphic fungi, which have both a yeast and a hyphael stage (e.g., *Histoplasma*, *Coccidiodomycetes*, and *Blastomycetes*) and which are quite rare after BMT.

This chapter will address the epidemiology, pathogenesis, risk factors, and prevention and treatment of invasive fungal disease associated with BMT. Data on how the spectrum of fungal infections has changed over the past decade will be highlighted, and areas for which future investigative efforts are needed will be discussed. Although brief mention of diagnosis specific to BMT will be included in this chapter, the reader is referred to Chapter 7 for a more extensive review of diagnostic techniques for fungal infection pertinent to both the BMT setting as well as the solid organ transplant population.

PATHOGENESIS

The pathogenesis varies for the different types of fungal organisms seen in the BMT setting. Unfortunately, apart from an understanding of how these infections are acquired and what spectrum of disease they cause, little is known about the specific host defense defects in the clinical setting other than neutropenia or which fungal virulence factors are important in the BMT setting.

Candida spp. are normal commensal organisms residing on mucous membrane surfaces. Local or systemic disease occurs when the normal host-commensal relationships, particularly at the gastrointestinal (GI) epithelial lining, are disrupted. The use of broad-spectrum antibiotics, usually given for fever during neutropenia, results in an overgrowth of yeast that increases the likelihood of infection and disease. Mucositis due to the conditioning regimen or GVHD disrupts the integument of the GI (or other mucous membranes such as the genital tract), leading to portals of entry for these organisms into the bloodstream. Further, infection with herpes simplex

From the Clinical Research Division, Fred Hutchinson Cancer Research Center, Seattle, WA 98109–1024.

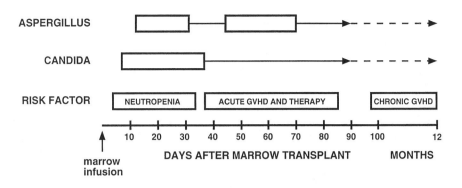

Figure 1. Risk periods for invasive fungal infection after allogeneic HCT.

virus or CMV can also facilitate access to otherwise sterile sites in the body. It is not unusual to see overgrowth of yeast on the base of the viral ulcers upon direct inspection of the upper GI tract using endoscopy. Finally, because neutrophils are required to maintain the normal integument of the GI epithelium and are the first line of defense against *Candida* spp., it is not surprising that neutropenia is an important risk factor for the development of systemic candidiasis (5).

The fact that the abdominal visceral organs are such a common location for disseminated candidiasis (6,7) suggests that much of the access of *Candida* spp. is through the portal circulation, with the liver and spleen serving as a filter for the organisms. This may explain why many cases of hepatosplenic candidiasis occur in the absence of positive blood cultures (1). The kidney is a less frequent site of visceral disease. Invasive candidal disease above the diaphragm is unusual. *Candida* spp. are the second most common cause of central nervous system (CNS) infection in the BMT setting (8) and infection of the CNS results from dissemination via the bloodstream, often presenting in a miliary pattern. Infection in the skin is also observed, although infrequently in the BMT patient, and is usually seen in the setting of candidemia.

In contrast to candidal infection, molds most commonly result from inhalation of spores. Therefore the pattern of distribution of mold infections is quite different from that observed for the *Candida* spp. The route of access also explains why most of the infection one sees with *Aspergillus* spp. and other molds occurs in the sinuses and lungs (9,10). As infection progresses, invasion of the blood vessels in the pulmonary vasculature may occur, resulting in infection in the heart or CNS. *Aspergillus* spp. are the most common cause of CNS infection in the BMT setting (8). CNS infection can also develop from direct extension from the sinuses and may extend to the periorbital area as well. Late in the course of infection, *Aspergillus* spp. spread to the abdominal visceral organs.

The less common mold infections—including *Rhizopus* and other species in the Mucorales order, *Bipolaris* and other dermatiaceous fungi, and *Fusarium*—also presumably result from inhalation of spores. An unusual case

of orally acquired *Mucor* hepatic abscesses was reported in a patient with GVHD who had ingested naturopathic medication containing *Mucor* spores identical to the species found in the abscesses by DNA analysis (11). This case highlights the principle that, given the appropriately immunosuppressed host and a high inoculum size, portals of entry for molds other than the respiratory tract are possible.

Each of the molds appears to have a different tissue tropism, which might explain why *Fusarium* is more commonly found in the blood with associated skin lesions than other molds. In contrast, *Mucor* spp. and other fungi from the Mucorales group are often found in the oral cavity, particularly the hard palate and the sinuses. Reasons for different tissue tropism of the different molds is poorly understood.

DIAGNOSIS

For the purposes of discussing the topic of fungal infections after BMT, the definitions of fungal infection and disease must be clarified. *Fungal infection* is a broad term used to describe the presence of any fungus by culture, or histologic laboratory techniques, including potassium hydroxide preparations, from secretions, dermal surfaces, bloodstream, visceral organs, or sterile body fluids in the presence of clinical symptoms.

Superficial fungal infection is distinguished from invasive fungal disease. *Superficial fungal infection* is a term that is usually limited to infections of the skin or mucous membranes caused by yeast or dermatophytes. Invasive fungal disease describes culture and/or histologic evidence of fungi in a normally sterile body site (or sites), including blood. The diagnosis of invasive aspergillosis is often referred to in the literature as "proven invasive" and "probable invasive" disease (12). Proven invasive fungal disease is supported by biopsy (culture or histology) or blood culture, whereas probable invasive disease refers to fungi in the respiratory tract diagnosed by bronchoalveolar lavage (BAL) or sputum with compatible clinical and radiographic evidence for invasive *Aspergillus* spp. or other mold infection. In many reports of clinical trial results, proven and probable fungal disease are grouped together. Fungal colonization is defined by the presence of fungal growth or infection from a nonsterile site, including genitourinary or gastrointestinal (GI) tract cultures in the absence of clinical, radiographic, or histologic evidence for superficial or invasive disease, defined later.

Although Chapter 7 provides a more extensive review of diagnostic techniques for invasive fungal infection, several points regarding diagnosis will be emphasized here. Early diagnosis of invasive fungal infection remains the single most important limitation to successful treatment of infections. In general, and as noted earlier, diagnosis relies on culture of the organism from a sterile site or identification by histologic methods in cases where the organism does not grow. There is no role at present for antibody-based serological assays in the diagnosis of invasive fungal infection (13). Diagnosis by antigen detection or polymerase chain reaction technology (14–17) from blood, urine, or other specimens remains experimental. Although antigen detection for *Aspergillus* spp. showed promise in initial clinical studies (18) and despite the availability of commercial kits for *Aspergillus* antigen detection in Europe (19), this technique has not been routinely applied in most clinical laboratories in the United States.

Diagnosis of tissue or bloodstream infection can be difficult because the culture of biopsy material may be negative. Histologic diagnosis also can be difficult, especially from tissue. Because up to 10% of all biopsies of tissue containing fungal disease will result in positive histology without a positive culture in the BMT setting (2), as many as 10% of cases of *Aspergillus* spp. may actually be caused by other molds. Further, it is likely that many of the reports that have described the incidence figures of aspergillosis underestimate the true incidence after BMT, not only because of the uncertainty of negative cultures but also because of the fact that the autopsy rate in most studies is well below 100%. In fact, in the recent retrospective study by Wald and colleagues, 23% of invasive aspergillosis in the BMT setting was diagnosed only at autopsy (2).

Cultures, and particularly blood cultures, have remained the gold standard for the diagnosis of invasive candidal infection, but they remain relatively insensitive for the diagnosis of hepatosplenic candidiasis. In this setting, approximately 50% of cultures will be negative. Lysis centrifugation cultures have increased the yield of candidemias in recent years and are now being largely replaced by the automated blood culture systems (see Chapter 7 for more details).

BAL is a relatively insensitive method for diagnosing pulmonary aspergillosis and may be negative in up to 50% of cases. However, any positive isolate from the respiratory tract has a strong association with proven invasive infection (20). In the study by Wald and colleagues, there were no significant differences in the course of infection or outcome between patients whose pulmonary aspergillosis was diagnosed by lung biopsy compared with BAL, supporting the practice of combining proven and probable cases in defining invasive disease of the lung (2). Yeast species identified from BAL rarely predict invasive candidal pneumonia, a relatively rare entity in the BMT setting. Better rapid diagnostic tests applicable to the clinical laboratory are clearly needed.

Radiographic techniques can be quite helpful in identifying the patient at high risk for invasive aspergillosis in the sinuses, lungs, and central nervous system (CNS) as well as for the identification of patients with probable visceral involvement with *Candida* spp. However, it cannot be overemphasized that no radiographic finding is pathopneumonic for invasive fungal infection, and a confirming diagnostic procedure should be performed whenever possible. Computerized tomography (CT) scans are more sensitive for aspergillosis in the lungs than are standard radiographs and in some centers the use of high-resolution CT is increasing to detect early stages of infection.

EPIDEMIOLOGY AND RISK FACTORS

The frequency and types of fungi that cause infection and disease in the BMT setting and their timing following BMT have been well described. Because infections with *Candida* and *Aspergillus* spp. are most common, much has been described regarding their epidemiology. The incidence of invasive candidal infection varies from 10% to 20% prior to the use of fluconazole prophylaxis (1). With the introduction of fluconazole in the early 1990s, the incidence of *C. albicans* and *C. tropicalis* has dropped substantially, whereas the incidence of other non-*albicans Candida* spp. is increasing (21). The incidence of invasive aspergillosis varies from 10% to 20%, depending on the center reporting the data and the year of BMT. It may be as high as 22% in patients receiving unrelated donor grafts (Bowden, unpublished data). Several investigators have reported a consistent increase in recent years (3,4).

In contrast to the relatively common occurrence of *Candida* and *Aspergillus* spp., fungal disease caused by *Cryptococcus* is as unusual as infection caused by the dimorphic fungi in the BMT setting. Although infections with these organisms do occur, the frequency is lower than one might expect when comparing the frequency in other immunocompromised patients such as those undergoing solid organ transplant (22) or those infected with human immunodeficiency virus (HIV).

Candida albicans has accounted for more than half of all candidal species identified after BMT (23), with *C. tropicalis* being the second most common species identified (21,23,24). Infections due to *C. glabrata*, *C. krusei*, *C. parapsilosis*, *C. lusitaniae*, and *C. guillermondi* are seen less commonly. The latter two species are quite rare in most reported series.

With fluconazole prophylaxis, *C. albicans* and *C. tropicalis* have become much less common, whereas infections with *C. glabrata* and *C. parapsilosis* have increased in some centers (21,24,25). In addition, while initial reports suggested that *C. krusei*, which is inherently resistant to fluconazole, was increasing in centers where fluconazole was used (26), this has been more of a problem in some centers than others. Table 1 shows the impact of fluconazole prophylaxis (beginning routinely in 1992) at Fred Hutchinson Cancer Research Center (FHCRC) over a 5-year period. Although the frequency of the different candidal species may have been changing recently because of the availability of fluconazole, it is not entirely clear that this change is due solely to the introduction of fluconazole, because it is being seen in centers where fluconazole is not being used (21,25,27). Further, the increase of non-*albicans Candida* spp. was noted more than 10 years before fluconazole was available (28).

Timing of Fungal Infections

Figure 1 shows the timing and associated risk periods for *Candida* spp. and *Aspergillus* spp. after allogeneic marrow transplantation. Historically, *Candida albicans* has been the most common cause of invasive fungal disease in the immunocompromised host in general, including in the BMT setting (23,29). The most significant risk period for candidal infection is from the time the neutrophil count drops below 500/mm^3 until the point it which the count recovers with engraftment. Prior to the availability of fluconazole, the median time of onset of all candidal infection was 15 days (range day −13 to day +89) after BMT and the median time to deep tissue disease was 20 days (range day −10 to day +97) (23).

Patients undergoing autologous BMT have a relatively short risk for invasive candidal infection, which is confined almost exclusively to the neutropenic period. For autologous BMT recipients, once the neutrophil count has recovered, immunity quickly returns to near normal function because these patients are not at risk for graft-versus-host disease (GVHD) or the risks associated with it, including fever and repeated antibiotic courses or

steroid therapy. In contrast, allogeneic BMT patients with GVHD are at risk not only during the neutropenic period but after engraftment, especially when corticosteroids are used for GVHD prophylaxis or treatment.

With the availability of fluconazole prophylaxis, *Aspergillus* spp. have become the most common cause of invasive fungal infections in many BMT centers (3,4,30). A recent large review of more than 250 cases of *Aspergillus* spp. infection and disease from FHCRC showed a bimodal incidence distribution after BMT (2). As one can see from Figure 2, the earlier peak occurs coincident with neutropenia (median, day 16 after BMT; quartile range, day 10–25). Both autologous and allogeneic BMT patients are at risk during this earlier peak. The earlier peak may represent infection acquired (but not recognized) prior to transplant or acquired early in the post-transplant course. The later peak was comprised of allogeneic BMT patients with a median time of onset of day 96 after BMT (quartile range, day 26–95), coinciding with the timing of GVHD and its treatment.

Risk Factors for Invasive Fungal Infection

The knowledge of risk factors is important for defining the patient populations and timing infection following BMT so that preventative measures can be appropriately and cost-effectively introduced to cover these high-risk periods. The risk for both invasive candidal and fungal disease caused by *Aspergillus* spp. is 10 times higher in allogeneic BMT patients than for patients undergoing autologous BMT (1,2,23). As mentioned earlier, the most obvious explanation for this difference is the immunosuppression experienced in the allogeneic setting due to GVHD and its therapy.

Neutropenia, including both the depth of the nadir and its duration, is an important risk factor for both *Candida* and *Aspergillus* spp. (2,5,23,31–33). However, the association of neutropenia with invasive aspergillosis is much higher in the autologous than in the allogeneic BMT setting. Twelve out of 14 (86%) of all autologous BMT patients developed aspergillosis during neutropenia, compared with only 38 of 144 (28%) of allogeneic BMT patients with aspergillosis diagnosed during the neutropenic period in one study (2). In contrast, in the allo-

TABLE 1. *Number of BMT patients with positive blood/tissue cultures (first isolate only) Fred Hutchinson Cancer Research Center, 1991–1995*

Candida species	1991	1992	1993	1994	1995	Total
C. albicans	19	16	2	4	4	45
C. glabrata	2	3	5	3	8	21
C. parapsilosis	4	3	6	17	3	33
C. krusei	1	1	2	4	5	13
Other or NOS[a]	11	7	11	12	6	47
Total	37	30	26	40	26	159
Total # BMT	**412**	**462**	**443**	**441**	**451**	**2128**

[a]NOS, not otherwise specified.

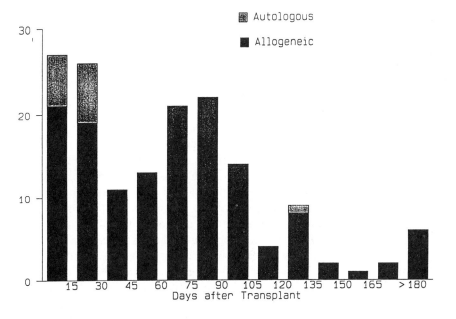

Figure 2. Timing of first positive *Aspergillus* spp. culture after BMT in 2,496 patients.

geneic setting, the risk of neutropenia appears to be more important for candidiasis than for aspergillosis in one study (34).

In addition to neutropenia, other risk factors for invasive candidal infection include increasing age, HLA mismatch between the donor and recipient, and time to engraftment (23). Interestingly, the use of laminar air flow (LAF) was not protective against invasive candidal infection in that study. Additional risk factors significant in multivariate analysis included the use of fractionated total body irradiation and cyclophosphamide, the underlying diagnosis of aplastic anemia or acute myeloid leukemia, the occurrence of acute GVHD, and the initial treatment of GVHD with cyclosporine. Other studies have also found acute GVHD and corticosteroid therapy (5,23) to be significant risk factors for invasive candidiasis. Corticosteroids can affect both neutrophil and macrophage function (35). Finally, factors that increase mucosal overgrowth with *Candida* spp. (e.g., broad-spectrum antibiotics and poor nutrition) or breakdown in the normal mucosal barrier (chemotherapy used for conditioning, GVHD) are also risk factors specific to the *Candida* spp.

Risk factors for progression from candidal fungemia to visceral candidiasis have also been examined (23). Total days of fungemia were strong predictors for invasive visceral disease, with 80% of patients with more than 7 days of fungemia developing organ involvement compared with 50%, 33%, and 57% with either 1, 2, or 3–7 days of fungemia, respectively (*p* = .03). The absence of engraftment was also strongly associated with visceral fungal disease in patients with fungemia.

Some risk factors are common for both candidal infection and aspergillosis in the BMT setting; others are more specific to one or the other group of infections (Table 2). In addition, as shown in Table 1, the risks for invasive aspergillosis may vary according to when the infection develops after BMT (2). For example, increasing donor age and donor HLA-matching were risk factors for aspergillosis regardless of when the infection occurred

TABLE 2. *Risk factors[a] for candidiasis and aspergillosis after BMT*

	Candidiasis (1)	Aspergillosis (2)	
		Early peak	Late peak
Increasing age	Yes	Yes	Yes
HLA mismatch donor	Yes	Yes	Yes
Acute GVHD	Yes	No	Yes
Laminar air flow	No	Yes	No
Underlying disease	Yes	Yes	Yes
Corticosteroid use	Yes	No	Yes
Building construction	No	No	Yes
Season	No	Yes	No
Neutropenia	Yes	No	Yes

[a]Multivariate analysis.
[b]Nd, not done.

following BMT. Factors such as the season and LAF had more of an effect on the incidence during the early peak, whereas corticosteroid use and GVHD were risks for the late but not the early peak. The role of construction in increasing the risk for aspergillosis remains somewhat controversial, because at least one study has shown that outbreaks during construction are not associated with a predominant species (36). Finally, in contrast to the associated risk of invasive fungal infection and CMV in the solid organ transplant setting (22), CMV was not found to be a significant risk for invasive aspergillosis after BMT in the Wald study (2).

CLINICAL SPECTRUM OF FUNGAL INFECTIONS AFTER BMT

Clinical Presentation of Candidal Infection and Aspergillosis

Candidiasis

The clinical significance of the differing species of *Candida* is related to their apparent difference in risk for dissemination and visceral involvement (31). *C. albicans* and *C. tropicalis* are well-known causes of disseminated candidiasis associated with high mortality, especially prior to the use of fluconazole prophylaxis (21,23). On the other hand, *C. parapsilosis* is a catheter-associated infection and has been linked to contaminated hyperalimentation fluid. For unclear reasons, this candidal species is rarely associated with disseminated visceral infection. In a recent unpublished experience at FHCRC, an outbreak of *C. parapsilosis* fungemia in 32 patients over a 15-month period was associated with a contaminated hyperalimentation set-up procedure. Despite multiple positive blood cultures in these patients and in some up to 14 days of persistent fungemia, only one patient

showed evidence of visceral involvement, which was limited to microscopic evidence at autopsy. *C. albicans*, *C. tropicalis*, and *C. krusei* were more likely to occur with neutropenia than *C. glabrata* and *C. parapsilosis* (24).

Before the days of effective candidal prophylaxis, the spectrum of candidal infection included thrush, esophagitis, and fungemia. Disseminated infection with visceral organ involvement was less common but occurred in up to half of patients with fungemia (see Table 2) (23). Infection of the mucous membranes occurred primarily during the first several weeks after BMT, when patients experienced both neutropenia and mucositis related to the conditioning therapy used to prepare patients for BMT. A significant number of patients also developed direct extension of the infection to the esophagus, although the exact incidence of candidal esophagitis has not been well described.

Mucosal candidiasis has become a rare problem in centers that use fluconazole prophylaxis, presumably because *Candida albicans*, the candidal species most commonly associated with this infection, is sensitive to fluconazole. For some patients (e.g., patients undergoing autologous transplantation where fluconazole may not be used routinely), topical antifungal agents such as nystatin or clotrimazole can be effective in preventing local mucous membrane infection, although there is no evidence that these topical agents reduce the incidence of systemic candidiasis.

The frequency of bloodstream infection with or without visceral involvement has been well described and is also shown in Table 3. These data are derived from a review of 171 cases of candidal disease in more than 1,500 BMT patients performed at FHCRC (23). During this time, topical nystatin swish and swallow was used during the period of neutropenia, empirical amphotericin B was added for persistent febrile neutropenia, and neither fluconazole, itraconazole, nor lipid-based ampho-

TABLE 3. *Organ Involvement and Mortality of Invasive Candidal Infection After BMT (1)*

Syndrome	Number of patients	(% all patients)	% mortality
Fungemia	102	(6.8)	66
Alone	46		39
With tissue involvement	56		88
Tissue-invasive disease[a]	125	(8.3)	90
Pneumonia only	18		78
Liver, spleen, kidney only	4		75
Brain only	4		100
Other syndrome[b]	8		25
Multiple organ	59		98
Mixed infection			
Candida + CMV pneumonia	21		100
Candida + *Aspergillus*	7		100
Candida + *Aspergillus* + CMV pneumonia	4		100
All candidal disease	171	(11.4)	73

CMV cytomegalovirus.
[a]Includes the 56 patients with fungemia.
[b]Includes patients with positive peritoneal cultures (3) and sinus, knee, mesenteric nodes, multiple nodular skin lesions, and myocardial abscess (1 each).

tericin B formulations were available. In this review, more than 90% of BMT patients had allogeneic donors. One hundred seventy-one patients (11.4%) had documented invasive fungal infection demonstrated by blood or tissue specimen. As shown in Table 3, approximately 45% of fungemias occurred without documented tissue involvement, and the mortality rate for patients with candidemia alone was 39%. For patients with fungemia-associated visceral organ involvement, the mortality rate was 88%. Patients with multiple organ or brain involvement had 100% mortality (1).

Fungemia usually involves a single candidal organism, but in rare cases, more than one species may be identified (23,24). Although most patients have only 1–2 days of positive blood cultures per episode, the duration of fungemia may be affected by whether or not the central indwelling intravenous catheter is removed. Unfortunately, no well-controlled prospective studies have been performed addressing the need to remove the indwelling catheter in patients with candidemia in the BMT setting. Most clinicians routinely remove the catheter when blood cultures remain positive for more than 48 hours on amphotericin B therapy.

The exact incidence of deep-tissue involvement with *Candida* spp. has been difficult to characterize for the various candidal species because of the difficulty of diagnosis. The blood cultures are negative in approximately half of patients with tissue infection documented later by biopsy or at autopsy. The best estimate is that deep-tissue involvement represents slightly more than half of all cases of invasive candidal infection (23). The spectrum of tissue involvement in patients with documented disseminated infection from the FHCRC study (23) is also shown in Table 3. Involvement of multiple organs was most common, with liver and spleen with or without renal involvement being the typical finding (37). The mortality rate was uniformly poor, varying from 80% to 100% (1). CNS infection with *Candida* spp. is usually diagnosed at autopsy only, because the infection often results in small, multifocal areas of infection not visible on CT scan and often not associated with typical clinical CNS symptoms (8).

Since the advent of fluconazole prophylaxis, both fungemia and visceral infection with *C. albicans* have become quite uncommon. Although fungemia continues to occur with other candidal species such as *C. glabrata*, *C. krusei*, and *C. parapsilosis*, the dramatic reduction in visceral disease suggests that these species do not have a high predilection for establishing infection in visceral organs. Most of the hepatosplenic candidiasis observed prior to fluconazole prophylaxis was due to *C. albicans* (1,23).

Aspergillosis

Aspergillosis most commonly involves the respiratory track (10). Invasive aspergillosis in the lungs appears to

be more common than sinus involvement, but the true incidence of *Aspergillus* spp. as a cause of sinusitis has not been well described and is likely underrepresented in the BMT literature. *Aspergillus* infection of the lung may be confined to a single lesion (i.e., aspergilloma) or may involve multiple lesions in a single or multiple lobes. As with candidiasis, the spectrum of infection with *Aspergillus* spp. ranges from local colonization to multi-organ-system involvement. However, 80% of disease is confined to the respiratory tract (Table 4). CNS infection is most commonly observed in patients with established lung or sinus infection. CNS lesions most commonly present as solitary abscesses on CT scan; occasionally, multiple abscesses are observed (8). The literature reports that blood cultures are rarely positive for *Aspergillus* spp. (9), and any positive blood culture report from the laboratory must be considered contamination in the absence of supportive clinical data.

Aspergillus fumagatus continues to account for most cases of invasive aspergillosis after BMT (Table 5) despite the development of newer antifungal agents with activity against *Aspergillus* spp. (e.g., itraconazole). Although most morbidity and mortality appear to be associated with *A. fumagatus*, other species can be associated with fatal infections (38). *Aspergillus flavus* was the second most common species identified in patients with invasive disease in the FHCRC series (16 of 133 isolates [12%]) (2). Isolates of *A. flavus* were significantly associated with skin involvement. Of interest in this study, only 10 patients had *Aspergillus* spp. isolated from blood. All were single blood cultures and no patient had evidence for invasive aspergillosis at any time during his or her post-transplant course.

Colonization

Colonization with *Candida* spp. is very common in patients coming to BMT. Among 300 patients cultured prior to BMT and weekly thereafter until day 100 as part of a randomized trial of fluconazole prophylaxis, 80%

TABLE 4. *Aspergillosis and other molds after BMT transplantation: clinical syndromes and mortality*

Syndrome	Number of patients	% mortality
Aspergillus only		
Pneumonia	21	62
Brain	1	100
Oral invasive	2	0
Multiple organ	17	100
Other syndrome	2	50
Total	43	74
Other molds		
Mucomycosis	1	100
Rhizopus	2	50
Fusarium	2	100
Petriellidium	1	100
Total	6	83
TOTAL	**49**	**84**

TABLE 5. *Anatomic site and* Aspergillus *species in BMT patients with invasive disease (2)*

Site	A. fumagatus n = 107 (80%)	A. flavus n = 16 (12%)	A. terreus n = 9 (7%)	A. niger n = 1 (1%)	Total n = 134
Pulmonary[a]	88	6	6	1	101
Rectum	2	0	0	0	2
Sinus and nose	0	2	0	0	2
Skin	5	6	2	0	13
Internal organs[b]	11	2	1	0	15

[a]Includes sputum (48), BAL (9), and lung (44).
[b]Includes brain (6), heart (1), kidney (5), intestine (1), and spleen (1).

were colonized at the time of transplant and 80% of those not given prophylactic fluconazole remained colonized during the post-BMT period (39). For this reason, the value of colonization with *Candida* spp. as a predictor for subsequent invasive candidal disease is of limited value. The value of surveillance cultures for identifying patients at high risk for invasive candidal disease is still questionable and thus they are not routinely recommended (40).

The true incidence of colonization with *Aspergillus* spp. or the predictive value of a positive surveillance culture for aspergillosis has not been well described because routine surveillance for this organism is not performed in most centers. In the study by Wald and colleagues, data describing the incidence of colonization as a component of all *Aspergillus* spp. in 2,496 consecutive BMT patients showed that 44 (2%) were colonized only (2). Of all patients where *Aspergillus* spp. were recovered, 21% were colonized only. Because routine surveillance for *Aspergillus* spp. was not performed as part of this study, these numbers likely underestimate the true incidence of colonization. As with surveillance for *Candida* spp., there are no studies to date providing data to support the use of routine surveillance for *Aspergillus* spp. However, when a colonizing species is present, the risk of invasive disease appears to be at least 50%; the data from the study by Wald and colleagues suggest this risk is 79% (2).

A. niger was the second most common isolate from colonizing sites (11 of 44 isolates [25%]) in the Wald study (2) (Table 6). Here isolates from the lung were significantly more likely to be associated with invasive disease, whereas isolates from the rectum were significantly more likely to be associated with colonization only. None of seven rectal *A. flavus* isolates were from patients with demonstrated invasive disease. Therefore many centers treat colonization, when identified, as presumptive evi-

dence of invasive disease, despite the fact that the positive predictive value is low. Clearly, better tests to predict invasive infection are needed.

PREVENTION OF INVASIVE FUNGAL INFECTION

As with many infections after BMT, treatment of established infection is clearly more difficult and is associated with poorer outcomes than prevention of the disease. This is particularly true for invasive fungal infections where the diagnosis is often delayed until disseminated disease is well established.

Prevention of Invasive Fungal Infection

The challenge in the prevention of invasive fungal infection after BMT is that the relative frequency of infection is low (10% to 20%) compared with some other infections after transplant (such as CMV). Further, the paucity of strong predictive risk factors and/or diagnostics tests, which would focus our attention on those patients at highest risk, means preventive strategies must currently be provided to most BMT patients (41). For example, to prevent invasive candidiasis with fluconazole, one currently must give all allogeneic patients prophylaxis during the early post-BMT period even though the risk for invasive disease may be only 10% to 20%. Universal prophylaxis becomes particularly challenging when the cost, inconvenience, or toxicity of the therapy is high.

Successful control of invasive fungal infection will likely come from the prevention, rather than treatment, of invasive fungal disease. Preventing exposure would be ideal, particularly when the organism comes from the

TABLE 6. *Anatomic site and* Aspergillus *species in colonized patients (2)*

Site	A. fumagatus n = 26 (63%)	A. flavus n = 2 (5%)	A. terreus n = 2 (5%)	A. niger n = 11 (27%)	Total n = 41
Pulmonary	18	1	1	2	22
Rectum	5	0	0	7	12
Nose and pharynx	2	1	0	2	5
Ear	1	0	1	0	2

environment (e.g., *Aspergillus* spp.), in contrast to when the organism comes from endogenous flora of the patient, as is the case with candidal infection. Further, the prevention of invasive fungal disease may more importantly involve measures that improve host defense, such as the reduction of immunosuppressive or neutropenia-inducing therapy, which is not always possible in the BMT setting. Because the pathogenesis and periods of risk differ between candidiasis and aspergillosis, prevention of each will be discussed separately. Empirical therapy for persistent fever during neutropenia will be discussed in the section on treatment.

Prevention of Acquisition of Candida Spp. and Invasive Candidal Disease

Prevention of exposure to *Candida* spp. is generally not effective. As discussed, infection with *Candida* spp. is usually caused by acquisition of the organism from the patient's own endogenous flora. There is no evidence to date that reducing colonization will result in prevention of invasive candidal disease, as with such topical agents as clotrimazole or nystatin. One exception is *C. parapsilosis*, which can be introduced via contaminated hyperalimentation fluid and is therefore amenable to prevention by careful infection control procedures regarding the preparation of hyperalimentation fluids. Finally, because there is growing evidence that *Candida* spp. can be transmitted by the hands of health care workers (42), a strong emphasis should be placed on careful handwashing. The most effective means of preventing fungal infection after BMT has been the prevention of candidiasis with fluconazole. Fluconazole has now been shown in several controlled studies to be highly effective for the prevention of disease due to *C. albicans* and *C. tropicalis* (39,43). A dose of 400 mg given once daily from the time of conditioning until either engraftment (43) or day 75 (43) significantly reduced superficial infection, invasive disease, and the use of empirical amphotericin B. In the latter study, where fluconazole was continued until day 75, it significantly improved survival, although this improvement was not clearly related to a reduction in fungal-related deaths. The optimal dose of fluconazole for prophylaxis has not been defined. However, data have shown that 100 mg/day is not effective (44). Until further data are available, 400 mg/day should be used. The ideal duration of prophylaxis has not been established. It may be that selected patients with GHVD who continue on high doses of immunosuppressive drugs, especially corticosteroids, should be considered for an extended duration of therapy. Although fluconazole resistance has now been reported after BMT (45,46), its occurrence appears to be infrequent. There is debate as to whether patients undergoing autologous transplantation should receive fluconazole prophylaxis, because they are at substantially lower risk for invasive infection. In general, fluconazole pro-

phylaxis is probably not needed in the autologous setting. Consideration might be given to providing prophylaxis to those patients whose conditioning regimens are associated with a high degree of mucositis, and prophylaxis should only be given for the early post-transplant period until both neutropenia and mucositis have been resolved. There are currently no effective ways to ensure the prevention of *Candida* spp. other than *C. albicans* and *C. tropicalis* with fluconazole. However, because they have been the two most common species of candidal infection after BMT, fluconazole prophylaxis continues to have a significant impact.

Prevention of Acquisition of *Aspergillus* spp. and Invasive Aspergillosis

Aspergillus spp. lend themselves much better to prevention of acquisition strategies than do the candidal species because *Aspergillus* spp. come directly from the environment through the inhalation of spores. However, except for the use of LAF, which effectively reduces the risk of aspergillosis for the period patients are confined to LAF rooms (2,47), preventing exposure has been difficult to achieve or at least difficult to demonstrate conclusively that such means are effective. Despite the attractiveness of such a preventive approach, including the use of masks or instillation of amphotericin B directly into the airways, there remain little controlled human data to support the use of any such strategies to date. Despite this, because such means may be commonly used in some parts of the BMT community, the data regarding such strategies will be reviewed briefly.

Regular masks provide no protection against the acquisition of *Aspergillus* spp. spores, presumably because of the fact that the masks are not fitted tightly enough to provide effective barriers against the spores. Also, patients cannot wear them absolutely continually. The same holds true of the use of masks for many respiratory pathogens, including community-acquired respiratory viruses, and many centers have abandoned the use of masks for their patients and health care workers altogether.

The use of LAF remains controversial because of increasing pressure to manage patients outside of the hospital environment for cost reasons. Some centers choose to use LAF rooms for patients at highest risk for invasive aspergillosis, such as patients with aplastic anemia or those with graft failure awaiting a second transplant where the duration of neutropenia is anticipated to be longer than normal.

There has also been interest in the use of aerosolized amphotericin B instilled into the airways based on encouraging studies in animal models. In humans there are no controlled studies to date that evaluate its use in the clinical setting. Conneally and colleagues published a study using the aerosolized route in 34 leukemic patients during 144 episodes of neutropenia and showed no cases of aspergillosis (48). Meunier and colleagues reported that 10 mg/ml daily of amphotericin B instilled by aerosolization into the nose resulted in only two cases of aspergillosis in 34 consecutive patients, which is an incidence of 6% without a comparison group (49). A third study, by Jorgensen and colleagues, where 10 mg/ml was given daily intranasally resulted in five cases of aspergillosis in 15 patients (50). Another study of 56 patients over 3 years who received 7 mg/ml of nasal drops four times daily showed no aspergillosis, although again without a comparison group. Although some of these reports may be encouraging, results are not consistent and therefore difficult to interpret without a concurrent control group.

An alternative method for prevention of both aspergillosis and candidiasis after BMT that might be associated with reduced toxicity is the use of low-dose prophylactic amphotericin B. Most published studies have evaluated this strategy using data derived from historical comparisons. An example is the study by O'Donnell and colleagues in which low-dose amphotericin B, 5–10 mg/day, was initiated after a sudden increase in fungal infections (30% of patients) occurred in their BMT unit (51). Institution of low-dose amphotericin B resulted in an apparent decrease in fungal infections in the following years (9%; $p = .01$). However, many centers normally observe an incidence of 5% to 10% without such therapy. Data showing the effect of low-dose amphotericin B on reducing the incidence of candidiasis or renal toxicity associated with that therapy were not reported. Rousey and colleagues reported no change in the incidence of both aspergillosis and invasive candidal infection compared with data from historical records using 0.1–0.25 mg/kg/day of amphotericin B, except in a subset of patients with GHVD (52). Finally, Perfect and colleagues performed a concurrently controlled randomized study in patients undergoing autologous transplantation and showed no significant difference in invasive fungal infections in patients receiving 0.1 mg/kg/day (8.8%) compared with controls (14.3%) (53). Additional work is needed to clarify the efficacy and safety of low-dose amphotericin B, including specifically whether this approach truly results in a decrease in aspergillosis and a decrease in renal toxicity when a low dose of amphotericin B is used, especially in the highest-risk allogeneic BMT patients.

Itraconazole is potentially useful for prevention of a variety of fungal infections, including aspergillosis (12). Its difficulties include poor absorption, especially in the BMT setting, and numerous drug/drug interactions, including with cyclosporin, dilantin, rifampin, astemizole, oral hypoglycemics, and warfarin-like anticoagulants, some of which are commonly used in the early post-BMT period. In addition, it is not available intravenously to date, which may limit its use for prophylaxis in the early post-BMT setting. Although initial studies using the capsule formulation for prophylaxis were discouraging (54), the newer formulation of oral itraconazole solution, which uses a cyclodextran vehicle, has a higher absorption rate and may prove to be more useful for prophylaxis or treatment (55). The major side effect of itraconazole solution is GI upset and a bad taste. Absorption is dependent on acidic gastric pH. Studies are under way to evaluate this preparation for prophylaxis after BMT.

Newer antifungal drugs are under development. One of these is voriconazole, which has excellent activity against *Aspergillus* spp. as well as non-*albicans Candida* spp. (56). The role of this azole and that of drugs with other mechanisms of action in both prevention and treatment are currently under evaluation.

Growth Factors

Despite data that growth factors (granulocyte colony-stimulated factor and granulocyte/macrophage colony-stimulating factor) have shortened the time of neutropenia, no data show that prophylactic use of growth factors after BMT has significantly affected the incidence of invasive fungal disease (57). Theoretically, growth factors may be of benefit (e.g., stimulation of the numbers or function of monocytes, macrophages, and neutrophils), and further studies are warranted. The use of macrophage stimulating factor showed some benefit in the treatment of invasive fungal infections after BMT in a phase I/II trial, but unfortunately it is no longer under development (58). (See Chapter 27 for a more in-depth review of growth factors.)

BMT Patients with a History of Proven Fungal Infections

Patients with a history of documented fungal infections prior to transplantation appear to be at higher risk for invasive fungal infection in the early post-BMT period. With the use of increasingly intense regimens for induction of various leukemias, more patients are coming to BMT with a history of prolonged neutropenia. Associated with this has been the observation that more patients are being evaluated for BMT with a history of invasive disease with either *Candida* or *Aspergillus* spp. before transplantation. Several attempts have been made to determine whether these patients can be safely transplanted under any condition (59,60). In one such study, Bjerke and colleagues demonstrated that patients with documented candidiasis who were treated with at least a gram of amphotericin B prior to transplantation and who subsequently had stabilization or improvement of CT evidence of disease, had no appreciably increased risk for post-transplant recurrence of candidiasis as long as they were treated with 0.5 mg/kg/day of amphotericin B during the preengraftment phase (60).

Similar attempts to safely transplant patients with documented invasive aspergillosis have met with mixed results. Offner and colleagues reported that patients with documented aspergillosis prior to transplant did not have a worse outcome as long as treatment was continued (61). In contrast to the experience with candidiasis, the unpublished experience at FHCRC has not been as favorable. In the past 2 years, more than 20 patients undergoing unrelated or mismatched BMT with proven aspergillosis prior to BMT have resulted in close to 100% mortality. In the early post-transplant period, only two of these patients died as a direct result of aspergillosis progressive fungal infection; the remainder died from multiple causes. These experiences suggest that less immunocompromised patients with a history of aspergillosis may do better during the transplant than the more severely immunocompromised patients undergoing BMT already infected with aspergillosis, or simply that invasive aspergillosis prior to BMT is a poor prognostic factor for survival in general.

TREATMENT OF INVASIVE FUNGAL INFECTION

Treatment of established fungal infections after BMT remains difficult and largely depends on recovery of granulocyte count and other host immunity. The major challenge in the treatment of invasive fungal infections in this setting is the lack of available diagnostic tests that allow identification of patients at the earliest stages of infection. The choice of antifungal agent and the dose and duration of therapy remain empirical in most cases without available controlled studies to assist in defining the treatment strategy. Thus patients are often treated based on clinical signs and symptoms of fungal infection (e.g., persistent fever, characteristic chest CT scan) without confirmation by culture or histologic examination.

Empirical Therapy for Persistent Febrile Neutropenia Unresponsive to Broad-Spectrum Antibiotics

Empirical antifungal therapy is most often given during persistent fever in the setting of neutropenia that has not responded to a broad-spectrum antibiotics (62,63). The standard practice is to initiate therapy with amphotericin B, either at a dose of 0.5 mg/kg daily if one suspects candidal infection or at a higher dose of 1.0–1.5 mg/kg/day if one suspects aspergillosis or other disseminated mold infection (62,64). Clearly, not every persistent fever after transplant is due to invasive fungal infection. Other common causes of fever include an occult viral infection (e.g., respiratory viruses during the winter months, CMV in patients not on ganciclovir prophylaxis), fever associated with tissue damage from the conditioning therapy, drug fever, or GVHD. Further, the widespread use of corticosteroids for the management of GVHD or regimen-related toxicity often ablates the febrile response such that routine blood cultures or radiographs can be the only way an occult invasive fungal infection may be identified. The use of prophylactic fluconazole has made the management of persistent fever during neutropenia even more challenging because it has excellent coverage against *Candida albicans* but unreliable coverage against a number of the other candidal species and offers no protection against the *C. krusei* or the molds. Thus when persistent fever develops in patients on fluconazole prophylaxis, amphotericin is often added as secondary empirical therapy. In this situation, one should consider adding the higher dose of amphotericin B (1.0 mg/kg), especially when the likelihood is higher that the infection is caused by a mold.

There are few prospective randomized controlled studies demonstrating the optimal antifungal agent, dose, or duration of therapy for any invasive fungal infection following BMT. Therefore the drug, dose, and duration selected and recommended are often based on observational data or clinical experience. A recent preliminary report comparing liposomal amphotericin B with conventional amphotericin B for the management of fever during neutropenia in cancer patients showed no advantage in terms of resolution of fever or survival, although it did demonstrate significant reduction in nephrotoxicity in patients receiving liposomal amphotericin B (65).

Treatment of Invasive *Candida* Spp.

The recommended treatment of neutropenic patients with systemic candidiasis remains amphotericin B at a dose of 0.5 mg/kg, for a total dose of approximately 1.5 g in the normal-sized adult (66). In the engrafted, stable patient, alternatives include lipid-complexed amphotericin B or fluconazole. Several lipid-complexed drugs have become available worldwide in the past several years (67). Although the initial hope was that the lipid vehicle would allow the delivery of higher doses with better therapeutic outcome and less toxicity, this hope has been only partially realized. As an example, Anaissie and colleagues have presented preliminary data showing that the amphotericin lipid complex had equivalent efficacy but improved renal safety in cancer patients with invasive candidiasis (68). Renal safety continues to be the major advantage of all the lipid/amphotericin products, but variable infusion-related toxicity continues to be observed with several of the preparations (67,69,70). Given the high cost of the lipid products, one should consider using the standard preparation of amphotericin B as first-line therapy because renal toxicity can often be avoided with careful hydration. In many cases, renal toxicity due to amphotericin B can be handled successfully by giving careful attention to fluid management (71). Alternatively, fluconazole at a dose of 400 mg/kg was studied in a noncontrolled study in cancer patients with systemic candidiasis and appeared to have good efficacy when used for treatment of established infection (7).

Adjunctive therapy, either surgical or chemotherapeutic, plays little role in the treatment of invasive candidiasis, and most reports of combined therapeutic agents or modalities remain descriptive. Surgical excision, because the infection is generally disseminated at presentation, plays no role in candidiasis, except possibly in the case of isolated splenic candidal infection. Combination therapy has also not been studied in controlled trials in the BMT setting. Amphotericin B plus 5-fluorocytosine (5-FC) is perhaps the most widely used combination for visceral *Candida* spp. (66), usually used only in the setting of the engrafted patient, but data are lacking to support the added benefit of 5-FC. The potential benefit of 5-FC must be balanced with its risk for marrow toxicity.

Treatment of Aspergillus and Other Molds

Despite the recent availability of itraconazole and lipid complex amphotericin B preparations, the mortality of patients with established invasive aspergillosis remains high. The standard therapy for this infection remains amphotericin B, given at a dose of 1.0–1.5 mg/kg for a total dose of 3–4 g in the normal-sized adult. Several studies using historical data comparing amphotericin B with amphotericin B lipid complex (67) or amphotericin B colloidal dispersion (70) have now been published showing a significant renal sparing effect of the lipid preparation and suggesting improved outcome. However, such studies include patients identified at autopsy and often lack the rigorous controls of prospectively controlled studies so that no firm conclusions about efficacy are possible. Preliminary analysis of a blinded, randomized controlled study of Amphotericin B versus Amphotericin B colloidal dispersion for first line treatment of established invasive aspergillosis showed no difference in outcome, although renal impairment was, again, reduced in the colloidal dispersion arm (72). Further, the optimal dose of these preparations for treatment of established infection has not been determined. The recommended dose is approximately 5 mg/kg for most preparation; however, small numbers of patients have been cured using lower doses (69). Duration of therapy is usually empirical. Some argue that patients with visceral disease should be treated until CT lesions have disappeared or have been shown to be stable for some period of time.

Itraconazole also has potentially attractive features for use in treating aspergillosis after transplantation, because it has good activities against *Aspergillus* spp. and is available orally. Efficacy has been demonstrated in a noncontrolled trial in a variety of immunocompromised patient settings (12). However, its unreliable absorption and drug/drug interactions make it a challenging drug to administer and achieve adequate drug levels, especially early after BMT. One way the drug is currently being used,

again without controlled data, is for therapy following initial induction and control of infection with amphotericin B. However, following blood levels will likely be critical based on our unpublished experience at FHCRC, where approximately 50% of BMT patients who take the standard dose of 400 mg/day do not have measurable blood levels of drug after treatment for 2 weeks. Again, newer antifungal drugs under development may provide safer and more effective therapeutic alternatives in the future.

Treatment of other types of mold infections remains largely anecdotal as a result of the small number of cases. Successful outcome of treatment of *Fusarium* spp. appears particularly sensitive to the recovery of adequate numbers of neutrophils, and limited experience in combining amphotericin B with granulocyte transfusions for infection occurring during neutropenia appears promising (73).

Surgery may have an adjunctive role in the treatment of aspergillosis and disease with other molds. However, studies defining the optimal settings are lacking. The most common way surgery is used for therapy of mold infections is for drainage of sinus infections and removal of isolated lung nodules in combination with antifungal therapy.

Granulocyte Transfusions

The use of granulocyte transfusions for treating invasive fungal infections during neutropenia after BMT is considered an adjunctive treatment to standard antifungal therapy despite the availability of controlled data. The use of G-CSF to stimulate granulocyte donors has resulted in granulocyte transfusions with appreciable numbers of neutrophils compared with nonstimulated collections (74,75). Preliminary phase I/II data evaluating community donors as a source of granulocytes for patients with proven invasive fungal infection in the first few weeks after transplant showed poor survival, particularly in patients treated for aspergillosis (76). Controlled trials are needed to determine the role of granulocyte transfusions in the management of invasive fungal infection during the preengraftment period after BMT.

CONCLUSION

Invasive fungal infections have become an increasingly important cause of morbidity and mortality after BMT. Progress has been made in understanding the importance of these infections in the BMT setting and in considering these pathogens in the differential diagnosis of fever. Furthermore, fluconazole prophylaxis is associated with successful control of *C. albicans* and *C. tropicalis*. Newer antifungal agents for treatment and prevention are becoming available. Much work is needed in the development of early diagnostic tests so that therapy can not only be initiated in earlier stages of infection, but be targeted to patients who need it most. Invasive aspergillosis remains the leading infectious cause of death after allogeneic transplantation, and there are currently no reliable ways to prevent it. The development of more effective and safer drugs for *Aspergillus* spp., particularly those that are well absorbed orally, will have a major impact on the successful outcome of BMT in the years to come.

REFERENCES

1. Meyers JD. Fungal infections in bone marrow transplant patients. *Semin Oncol* 1990;17(3):10–13.
2. Wald A, Leisenring W, van Burik J-A, Bowden RA. Epidemiology of *Aspergillus* infections in a large cohort of patients undergoing bone marrow transplantation. *J Infect Dis* 1997;175:1459–1466.
3. Pannuti C, Gingrich R, Pfaller MA, Kao C, Wenzel RP. Nosocomial pneumonia in patients having bone marrow transplant: attributable mortality and risk factors. *Cancer* 1992;69(11):2653–2662.
4. Peterson PK, McGlave P, Ramsay NKC, et al. A prospective study of infectious diseases following bone marrow transplantation: emergence of *Aspergillus* and cytomegalovirus as the major causes of mortality. *Infect Control* 1983;4(2):81–89.
5. Gerson SL, Talbot GH, Hurwitz S, Strom BL, Lusk EJ, Cassileth PA. Prolonged granulocytopenia: the major risk factor for invasive pulmonary aspergillosis in patients with acute leukemia. *Ann Intern Med* 1984;100:345–351.
6. Thaler M, Pastakia B, Shawker TH, O'Leary T, Pizzo PA. Hepatic candidiasis in cancer patients: the evolving picture of the syndrome. *Ann Intern Med* 1988;108:88–100.
7. Torres-Valdivieso MJ, Lopez J, Melero C, et al. Hepatosplenic candidosis in an immunosuppressed patient responding to fluconazole. *Mycoses* 1994;37:443–446.
8. Hagensee ME, Bauwens JE, Kjos B, Bowden RA. Brain abscess following marrow transplantation: the Fred Hutchinson Cancer Research Center experience 1984–1992. *Clin Infect Dis* 1994;19:402–408.
9. Denning DW, Stevens DA. Antifungal and surgical treatment of invasive aspergillosis: review of 2,121 published cases. *Rev Infect Dis* 1990;12(6):1147–1201.
10. Morrison VA, Haake RJ, Weisdorf DJ. Non-candidal fungal infections after bone marrow transplantation: risk factors and outcome. *Am J Med* 1994;96(6):497–503.
11. Oliver MR, Van Voorhis WD, Boeckh M, Mattson D, Bowden R. Hepatic Mucormycosis in a bone marrow transplant recipient who ingest naturopathic medicine. *Clin Infect Dis* 1996;22:521–524.
12. Denning DW, Lee JY, Hostetler JS, et al. NIAID mycoses study group multicenter trial of oral itraconazole therapy for invasive aspergillosis. *Am J Med* 1994;97:135–144.
13. Young RC, Bennett JE. Invasive aspergillosis: absence of detectable antibody response. *Am Rev Respir Dis* 1971;104:710–716.
14. Van Deventer AJM, Goessens WHF, van Belkum HJA, van Vliet EWM, Verbrugh HA. Improved detection of *Candida albicans* by PCR in blood of neutropenic mice with systemic candidiasis. *J Clin Microbiol* 1995;32:2962–2967.
15. Einsele H, Hebart H, Roller G, et al. Detection and identification of fungal pathogens in blood by using molecular probes. *J Clin Microbiol* 1997;35(6):1353–1360.
16. Hopfer RL, Walden P, Setterquist S, Highsmith WE. Detection and differentiation of fungi in clinical specimens using PCR amplification and restriction enzyme analysis. *J Med Vet Mycol* 1993;31:65–75.
17. Hebart H, Loffler J, Hartmann M, et al. Polymerase chain reaction for early diagnosis of fungal infections following allogeneic bone marrow and peripheral blood stem cell transplantation. 39th Annual Meeting of the American Society of Hematology. San Diego, CA 1997.
18. Patterson TF, Miniter P, Patterson JE, Rappeport JM, Andriole VT. Aspergillus antigen detection in the diagnosis of invasive aspergillosis. *J Infect Dis* 1995;171:1553–1558.
19. Hurst SF, McLaughlin DW, Reyes G, Reiss E, Morrison CJ. Development of an inhibition EIA to detect galactomannanemia/uria: Comparison to Pastorex Aspergillus Latex Agglutination Test (PALA) for the diagnosis of invasive aspergillosis. 34th Interscience Conference on Antimicrobial Agents Chemotherapy. Orlando, FL 1994.
20. Yu VL, Muder RR, Poorsattar A. Significance of isolation of *Aspergillus* from the respiratory tract in diagnosis of invasive pulmonary aspergillosis: results from a three-year prospective study. *Am J Med* 1986;81:249–254.
21. Wingard JR. Importance of *Candida* species other than *C. albicans* as pathogens in oncology patients. *Clin Infect Dis* 1995;20:115–125.
22. Paya CV. Fungal infections in solid-organ transplantation. *Clin Infect Dis* 1993;16:677–88.
23. Goodrich JM, Reed EC, Mori M, et al. Clinical features and analysis of risk factors for invasive candidal infection after marrow transplantation. *J Infect Dis* 1991;164:731–740.
24. Abi-Said D, Anaissie E, Uzun O, Raad I, Pinzcowski H, Vartivarian S. The epidemiology of hematogenous candidiasis caused by different Candida species. *Clin Infect Dis* 1997;24:1122–1128.
25. Kunova A, Trupl J, Dluholucky S, Galova G, Krcmery VJ. Use of fluconazole is not associated with a higher incidence of *Candida krusei* and other non-*albicans Candida* species. *Clin Infect Dis* 1995;21(1):226–227.
26. Wingard JR, Merz WG, Rinaldi MG, Johnson TR, Karp JE, Saral R. Increase in *Candida krusei* infection among patients with bone marrow transplantation and neutropenia treated prophylactically with fluconazole. *N Engl J Med* 1991;325:1274–1277.
27. White MH. Editorial response: the contribution of fluconazole to the changing epidemiology of invasive candidal infections. *Clin Infect Dis* 1997;24:1129–1130.
28. Meunier-Carpentier F, Kiehn TE, Armstrong D. Fungemia in the immunocompromised host: changing patterns, antigenemia, high mortality. *Am J Med* 1981;71(3):363–370.
29. Verfaillie C, Weisdorf D, Haake R, Hostetter M, Ramsay NK, McGlave P. *Candida* infections in bone marrow transplant recipients. *Bone Marrow Transplant* 1991;8(3):177–184.
30. Walsh TJ, Dixon DM. Nosocomial aspergillosis: environmental microbiology, hospital epidemiology, diagnosis and treatment. *Eur J Epidemiol* 1989;5(2):131–142.
31. Komshian SV, Uwaydah AK, Sobel JD, Crane LR. Fungemia caused by *Candida* species and *Torulopsis glabrata* in the hospitalized patient: frequency, characteristics, and evaluation of factors influencing outcome. *Rev Infect Dis* 1989;11(3):379–390.
32. Paulin T, Ringden O, Nilsson B, Lonnqvist B, Gahrton G. Variables predicting bacterial and fungal infections after allogeneic marrow engraftment. *Transplantation* 1987;43(3):393–398.
33. Bodey GP, Buckley M, Sathe YS, Freireich EJ. Quantitative relationships between circulating leukocytes and infection in patients with acute leukemia. *Ann Intern Med* 1966;64:328.
34. De Bock R. Epidemiology of invasive fungal infections in bone marrow transplantation. EORTC Invasive Fungal Infections Cooperative Group. *Bone Marrow Transplant* 1994;14[Suppl. 5]:S1–S2.
35. Rinehart JJ, Balcerzak SP, Sagone AL, LoBuglio AF. Effects of corticosteroids on human monocyte function. *J Clin Invest* 1974;54:1337–1343.
36. Ribaud P, Chastang C, Latge JP, et al. Invasive aspergillosis (IA) after allogeneic marrow transplantation: survival, prognostic factors and molecular epidemiology in 27 cases observed in a single center. 37th Annual Meeting of the American Society of Hematologists. Seattle, WA 1995.
37. Rossetti F, Brawner DL, Bowden R, et al. Fungal liver infection in marrow transplant patients: prevalence at autopsy, predisposing factors, and clinical features. *Clin Infect Dis* 1995;20:801–811.
38. Tritz DM, Woods GL. Fatal disseminated infection with *Aspergillus terreus* in immunocompromised hosts. *Clin Infect Dis* 1993;16:118–122.
39. Slavin MA, Osborne B, Adams R, et al. Efficacy and safety of fluconazole for fungal infections after marrow transplant—a prospective, randomized, double-blind study. *J Infect Dis* 1995;171:1545–1552.
40. Walsh TJ. Role of surveillance cultures in prevention and treatment of fungal infections. *NCI Monogr* 1990;9:43–45.
41. Uzun O, Anaissie EJ. Antifungal prophylaxis in patients with hematologic malignancies: a reappraisal. *Blood* 1995;86(6):2063–2072.
42. Doi M, Homma M, Iwaguchi S-I, Horibe K, Tanaka K. Strain relatedness of *Candida albicans* strains isolated from children with leukemia and their bedside parents. *J Clin Microbiol* 1994;32:2253–2259.
43. Goodman JL, Winston DJ, Greenfield RA, et al. A controlled trial of fluconazole to prevent fungal infections in patients undergoing bone marrow transplantation. *N Engl J Med* 1992;326:845–851.
44. Donowitz G, Harman C. Low dose fluconazole prophylaxis in neutropenia. The Ninth International Symposium on Infections in the Immunocompromised Host. Assisi, Italy 1996.

45. Marr KA, White TC, van Burik J-AH, Bowden RA. Development of fluconazole resistance in *Candida albicans* causing disseminated infection in a patient undergoing marrow transplantation. *Clin Infect Dis* 1997;25:908–910.

46. Nolte FS, Parkinson T, Falconer DJ, et al. Isolation and characterization of fluconazole- and amphotericin B-resistant *Candida albicans* from blood of two patients with leukemia. *Antimicrob Agents Chemother* 1997;41:196–199.

47. Petersen FB, Buckner CD, Clift RA, et al. Laminar air flow isolation and decontamination: a prospective randomized study of the effects of prophylactic systemic antibiotics in bone marrow transplant patients. *Infection* 1986;14:115–121.

48. Conneally E, Cafferkey MT, Daly PA, Keane CT, McCann SR. Nebulized amphotericin B as prophylaxis against invasive aspergillosis in granulocytopenic patients. *Bone Marrow Transplant* 1990;5:403–406.

49. Meunier-Carpentier F, Snoeck R, Gerain J, Muller C, Klastersky J. Amphotericin B nasal spray as prophylaxis against aspergillosis in patients with neutropenia. *N Engl J Med* 1984;311(16):1056.

50. Jorgensen CJ, Dreyfus F, Vaixeler J, et al. Failure of amphotericin B spray to prevent aspergillosis in granulocytopenic patients. *Nouv Rev Fr Hematol* 1989;31(5):327–328.

51. O'Donnell MR, Schmidt GM, Tegtmeier BR, et al. Prediction of systemic fungal infection in allogeneic marrow recipients: impact of amphotericin prophylaxis in high-risk patients. *J Clin Oncolol* 1994;12:827–834.

52. Rousey SR, Russler S, Gottlieb M, Ash RC. Low-dose amphotericin B prophylaxis against invasive Aspergillus infections in allogeneic marrow transplantation. *Am J Med* 1991;91:484–492.

53. Perfect JR, Klotman ME, Gilbert CC, et al. Prophylactic intravenous amphotericin B in neutropenic autologous bone marrow transplant recipients. *J Infect Dis* 1992;165:891–897.

54. Tam JY, Hamed KA, Blume K, Prober CG. Use of itraconazole in treatment or prevention of invasive aspergillosis in bone marrow transplant recipients. ICAAC Session 75 1993:268.

55. Prentice AG, Morgenstern GR, Prentice HG, Ropner JE, Schey SA, Warnock DW. Fluconazole v itraconazole prophylaxis in neutropenia following therapy for hematological malignancy. 39th Annual Meeting of the American Society of Hematology. San Diego, CA 1997.

56. Murphy M, Bernard EM, Ishimaru T, Armstrong D. Activity of voriconazole (UK-109,496) against clinical isolates of *Aspergillus* species and its effectiveness in an experimental model of invasive pulmonary aspergillosis. *Antimicrob Agents Chemother* 1997;41(3):696–698.

57. Nemunaitis J, Rosenfeld CS, Ash R, et al. Phase III randomized, double-blind placebo-controlled trial of rhGM-CSF following allogeneic bone marrow transplantation. *Bone Marrow Transplant* 1995;15(6):949–954.

58. Nemunaitis J, Anasetti C, Storb R, et al. Phase II trial of recombinant human granulocyte macrophage colony stimulating factor in patients undergoing allogeneic bone marrow transplantation from unrelated donors. *Blood* 1992;79:2572–2577.

59. Katamaya Y, Koizumi S, Yamagami M, et al. Successful peritransplant therapy in children with active hepatosplenic candidiasis. *Int J Hematol* 1994;59(2):125–130.

60. Bjerke J, Meyers JD, Bowden RA. Hepatosplenic candidiasis—a contraindication to marrow transplantation? *Blood* 1994;84:2811–2814.

61. Offner F, Cordonnier C, Ljungman P, et al. Impact of previous aspergillosis on the outcome of bone marrow transplantation. *Clin Infect Dis* 1998 (*in press*).

62. Pizzo PA, Robichaud KJ, Gill FA, Witebsky FG. Empiric antibiotic and antifungal therapy for cancer patients with prolonged fever and granulocytopenia. *Am J Med* 1982;72:101–111.

63. Schimpff SC. Empiric antibiotic therapy for granulocytopenic cancer patients. *Am J Med* 1986;80:13.

64. Hughes WT, Armstrong D, Bodey GP, et al. Guidelines for the use of antimicrobial agents in neutropenic patients with unexplained fever. *J Infect Dis* 1990;161:381–396.

65. Walsh T, Bodensteiner D, Hiemenz J, et al. A randomized, double-blind trial of AmBisome (liposomal amphotericin B) versus Amphotericin B in the empirical treatment of persistently febrile neutropenic patients. 37th Interscience Conference on Antimicrobial Agents Chemotherapy. Toronto, Canada 1997.

66. Edwards JE Jr, Bodey GP, Bowden RA, et al. International conference for the development of a consensus on the management and prevention of severe candidal infections. *Clin Infect Dis* 1997;25(1):43–59.

67. Hiemenz JW, Walsh TJ. Lipid formulations of amphotericin B: recent progress and future directions. *Clin Infect Dis* 1996;22(Suppl 2):S133–44.

68. Anaissie EJ, White M, Uzun O, et al. Amphotericin B lipid complex vs. amphotericin B for treatment of invasive candidiasis: a prospective, randomized, multicenter trial. 35th Interscience Conference on Antimicrobial Agents Chemotherapy. San Francisco, CA 1995:330.

69. Bowden R, Cays M, Gooley TA, Mamelok RD, van Burik J-A. Phase I study of Amphotericin B colloidal dispersion for the treatment of invasive fungal infections after marrow transplant. *J Infect Dis* 1996;173:1208–1215.

70. White MH, Anaissie EJ, Kusne S, et al. Amphotericin B colloidal dispersion vs. Amphotericin B as therapy for invasive aspergillosis. *Clin Infect Dis* 1997;24:635–642.

71. van Burik JH, Bowden RA. Standard antifungal treatment including role of alternative modalities to administer amphotericin B. In: Meunier F, ed. *Current issues and recent developments on invasive fungal infections in cancer patients*, vol 2. London: Bailliere Tindall; 1995:89–109.

72. Bowden R, Chandrasekar P, White M, van Burik J-A, Wingard J, and the Multicenter Aspergillus Study Group. A double-blind, randomized controlled trial of amphocil (ABCD) vs. Amphotericin B (AmB) for treatment of invasive aspergillosis in immunocompromised patients. *10th International Symposium in Infections in the Immunocompromised Host.* Davos, Switzerland, June 21–24, 1998.

73. Anaissie E, Kantarjian H, Ro J, et al. The emerging role of *Fusarium* infections in patients with cancer. *Medicine* 1988;67:77–83.

74. Chatta GS, Price TH, Allen RC, Dale DC. Effects of *in vivo* recombinant methionyl human granulocyte colony-stimulating factor on the neutrophil response and peripheral blood colony-forming cells in healthy young and elderly adult volunteers. *Blood* 1994;84:2923–2929.

75. Dale DC, Liles WC, Summer WR, Nelson S. Review: granulocyte colony-stimulating factor-role and relationships in infectious diseases. *J Infect Dis* 1995;172:1061–1075.

76. Bowden R, Price T, Boeckh M, Liles C, Cays M, Dale D. Phase I/II study of granulocyte transfusions from G-CSF-stimulated unrelated donors for treatment infections in neutropenic blood and marrow transplant (BMT) patients. 39th Annual Meeting of the American Society of Hematology. San Diego, CA 1997.

Transplant Infections edited by
Raleigh A. Bowden, Per Ljungman, and Carlos V. Paya.
Lippincott–Raven Publishers, Philadelphia © 1998

CHAPTER 24

Fungal Infections in Solid Organ Transplant Recipients

Jan G. Tollemar

Invasive fungal infections remain a substantial cause of morbidity and mortality in solid organ transplant (SOT) recipients and occur in all types of transplant recipients. The fungal species and type of infection differ, depending on the organ transplanted and geographic residence (1–3). Fungal infection is common in transplant recipients, and as many as 20% of kidney recipients, 35% of heart/lung recipients, 38% of pancreas recipients, and 42% of liver recipients have in previous studies been reported to develop significant fungal infections after the transplant (4–7). However, advances in immunosuppression and in patient care with improved surgical technique have reduced the incidence of fungal infections to, for example, 5% for renal allograft recipients, but still a high 53% among small bowel transplant recipients (8–9). The pace of an infection in immunosuppressed patients is accelerated and mortality is higher than that for most other infections, with a maximum mortality rate that ranges between 70% for candidiasis and 100% in aspergillosis (2). The occurrence of invasive fungal infections in these patients depends on several factors, such as the underlying disease, surgical procedures, immunosuppressive regimen, other types of infection, epidemiological exposure and efficacy, and whether antifungal prophylaxis has been given. Besides the host's predisposition, management of fungal infections involves other challenges, including the lack of reliable diagnostic methods and a limited therapeutic arsenal associated with drug/drug interactions and side effects. Fungal infections are therefore a challenge for the clinician.

INCIDENCE, EPIDEMIOLOGY, AND OUTCOME OF FUNGAL INFECTIONS IN SOLID ORGAN TRANSPLANTATION

The principal fungal pathogens causing fungal infections in transplant recipients can be divided into two categories. First there are opportunistic infections due to *Candida* spp., *Aspergillus* spp., *Cryptococcus neoformans*, Mucoraceae, and occasionally other rare fungi such as the dermatophytes and *Penicillum*. Then there are geographically restricted systemic mycoses causing infections in any patient living in endemic areas. They may particularly have an intense impact on transplant recipients with *de novo* infections or reactivation of residual infections, such as blastomycosis, coccidioidomycosis, and histoplasmosis (6).

The true incidence of and mortality rate associated with invasive fungal infections have not been clearly defined because of difficulties in establishing the exact diagnosis. Table 1 shows the widely varying incidences of fungal infections, pathogen proportion, and mortality reported in SOT recipients. The wide range depends on which organ was transplanted, but it is also affected by the clinical progress made over the years, with reduced immunosuppression, better supportive care, and improved surgical techniques. This progress is obvious in kidney transplant recipients, in whom studies during the 1960s reported incidences as high as 45% caused by *Candida* spp. in 52%, *Aspergillus* spp. in 22% and other fungi or a mixture in 26% (4). However, in more recent years, incidence figures below 10% have been reported. *Candida, Cryptococci,* and *Aspergillus* spp. are still the commonest pathogens, with proportions ranging up to 76%, 39%, and 30%, respectively (8,10). The mortality rate ranges between 23% and 71% for candidiasis, 0 and 60% for cryptococcosis, and 20% to 100% in cases of aspergillosis (10–17).

From the Department of Transplantation Surgery, Huddinge Hospital, Karolinska Institute, S-141 86 Huddinge, Sweden.

TABLE 1. *Incidence, relative proportion of pathogens, and mortality in invasive fungal infections in solid-organ transplant recipients*

Transplantation, ref.	Incidence of fungal infection (%)	Relative proportion of pathogen (%)		Mortality (%)
Kidney, 4,10–17	0–20	15–76	*Candida* spp.	23–71
		0–39	*Cryptococcus neoformans*	0–60
		5–30	*Aspergillus* spp.	20–100
		0–39	Other fungi	55
Liver, 7,8,18–27	4–42	47–100	*Candida* spp.	6–77
		0–53	*Aspergillus* spp.	50–100
		3–7	*Cryptococcus neoformans*	0–22
		3–15	Other fungi	100
Pancreas with or without kidney, 6,28–30	6–38	100*	*Candida* spp.	20–27
Heart/lung, 5,8,31–37	10–35	36–53	*Aspergillus* spp.	21–100
		18–26	*Cryptococcus neoformans*	
		4–5	*Candida* spp.	27
		11–16	Other fungi	
Small bowel, 9,38	33–53	66–78	*Candida* spp.	0–5
		11–33	*Aspergillus* spp.	0–100
		0–11	Other fungi	33

[a]Intra-abdominal infections.

In liver transplant recipients, the incidence ranges between 4% and 42%, *Candida* and *Aspergillus* spp. being the commonest pathogens with a low proportion of *Cryptococci*, up to 100%, 53%, and 7%, respectively (7,8,18–27). The mortality rate among liver transplant recipients ranges between 6% and 77%, 50% and 100%, and 0 and 22% for candidiasis, aspergillosis, and cryptococcosis, respectively (6,18,19,25).

In pancreas transplant recipients, the incidence of fungal infections ranges between 6% and 38%, with *Candida* as the only pathogen group found in intra-abdominal infections, with a mortality ranging between 22% and 27%. However, most patients lost their graft (6,28–30).

Unlike all other types of transplants, heart and lung recipients suffer mainly from invasive fungal infection caused by *Aspergillus* spp. The incidence ranged between 10% and 35% (5,8,31–33). *Aspergillus* spp. followed by *Cryptococcus neoformans* were the commonest pathogens, followed by *Candida*, with proportions of up to 53%, 26%, and 5%, respectively. Mortality rates for aspergillosis and candidiasis were reported to be 21% to 100% and 27%, respectively, among lung and heart/lung recipients, compared with a lower mortality of 32% to 64% for aspergillosis in heart transplant recipients (8,34–37).

At present transplantation of the small bowel is still a rather uncommon procedure, but two papers have reported incidence of fungal infections of 33% and 53% with *Candida* as the most common pathogen occurring in 66% and 78%, followed by *Aspergillus*, in 11% and 33%. Mortality for *Candida* and *Aspergillus* infections ranged between 0 to 5% and 0 to 100%, respectively (9,38).

As new antifungal drugs become available, these figures will improve. At our center, liposomal amphotericin B has been used since 1989 in 121 adult and 25 pediatric

SOT recipients. Cure rates in SOT recipients with verified invasive fungal infections were, for adults, 25 out of 27 (93%) and, for children, eight of nine (89%), respectively (39,40).

FUNGAL DEFENSE AND RISK FACTORS

Defenses against fungi are both fungal specific and nonspecific. Nonspecific defenses include phagocytic cells such as neutrophils, monocytes, and macrophages, which provide the major host defenses against *Candida* spp., *Aspergillus* spp., and Mucoraceae (41). Granulocytopenia and its duration are well-known risk factors for fungal infections in bone marrow transplant recipients (42). Also in organ transplant recipients, myelosuppression due to azathioprin treatment or as a result of a cytomegalovirus infection may be present. Cell function may be poor, and phagocytic cells have been shown to have both defective chemotactic and phagocytic capacity after corticosteroid treatment (41,43). In renal transplant recipients a relationship between the total dose of corticosteroids and rejections and infectious (aspergillosis) complications and patient survival has been shown (10,44).

Integument barriers—such as the skin and mucosal membranes of the respiratory, gastrointestinal, and urinary tracts—are also part of the nonspecific host defense and are important for protection from colonization to gain systemic access. These anatomic barriers are disrupted in organ transplant recipients by extensive surgery; bladder, biliary, and drainage catheters; intravenous lines; and herpesvirus lesions. Colonization resistance is reduced because the intense treatment with broad-spectrum antibiotics lessens the number of normal microbiological flora, thus increasing endogenous fungal colonization.

Fungal-specific defense includes humoral and cellular immunity that provides important safeguards against infections like cryptococcosis and histoplasmosis (45). Late after organ transplantation, these defenses are impaired by the chronic immunosuppressive therapy. At present, more modern selective immunosuppressive agents have reduced overall immunosuppression but still improved long-term patient and graft survival rates, thus widening the indications for transplantation regarding both recipient and immunologic barriers. As more difficult cases are transplanted, treatment with T-cell antibody will be given increasingly for acute rejection or as induction therapy. The risk for infection will probably increase. Another factor leading to chronic immunosuppression is the presence or absence of infections by immunomodulating viruses like cytomegaloviruses and the Epstein-Barr virus (41,46,47). Prophylactic gancilovir treatment in heart transplant recipients significantly reduces the incidence of fungal infections as well as the incidence of cytomegalovirus infections (48).

In patients, all host defense systems are activated simultaneously and function synergistically to prevent and cure an infection; thus any transplant recipient may present with several defects. The disease that results in transplantation, the degree of immunosuppression, metabolic changes, and invasive surgical procedures influence the risk of fungal infection. It would be of value to distinguish patients at risk and thus identify those who would benefit from early intervention or even from prophylaxis. Several analyses have been performed, especially of liver transplant recipients, to identify specific risk factors. Table 2 shows factors from four separate studies found with multivariate analysis that can be regarded as true risk factors. Most of them are common to the different transplant centers and concern the patient's condition before transplantation and the course of pre-, intra-, and postoperative events (7,18,19,22).

TABLE 2. *Significant risk factors for invasive fungal infections in liver transplant recipients, based on multivariate analysis of findings in four studies (7,18,19,22)*

Time	Risk factor
Preoperative	Low hemoglobin level pretransplant High bilirubin level pretransplant Preoperative steroid treatment Preoperative antibiotic treatment Male donor sex
Intraoperative	Duration of first transplant operation Choledochojejunostomy anastomosis Blood transfusions during operation
Postoperative	Duration of ICU stay Reoperation and duration of operation Bacterial infections CMV infection Postoperative steroid treatment Rejection treatment Prolonged ciprofloxacin treatment

FUNGAL PATHOGENS

Candida Spp.

Candida spp. accounts for most fungal infections in organ transplant recipients. Resolution of an infection does not confer protection, and reinfection or reactivation may occur if host resistance is lowered. Healthy individuals are often colonized in the gastrointestinal (GI) tract; colonization has been reported in up to 70%. Colonization increases during hospitalization (49). In most transplant patients, infection with *Candida* spp. originates from the individual's endogenous reservoir (49). Treatment or prophylaxis of mucosal colonization might reduce the risk of a more serious infection, but no solid data have yet been presented supporting this (50). Nosocomial sources such as another person, food, intravenous catheters, and parenteral fluids have, however, also been reported to cause infections (51).

More than 200 *Candida* spp. are pathogenic to man. The two most common that cause serious infection in transplanted patients are *C. albicans* and *C. tropicalis*. *C. parapsilosis* occasionally develops in patients requiring prolonged total parenteral nutrition (49,52). We might in the future see a shift in pathogens because the increased use of prophylactic fluconazole and the incidence of non-*Candida albicans* strains like *C. krusei* and *C. glabrata*, which are less susceptible or even resistant to therapy, has increased (53,54).

The clinical syndromes range from minimal mucosal colonization/infection to more serious invasive infections, like candidemia, including life-threatening disseminated infection. Candidemia is defined as *Candida* in blood with or without visceral involvement. A disseminated infection means that several deep-seated organs or one organ together with blood are infected. The term *systemic candidiasis* has been used in a more general setting, also when only one organ or a site of nonhematogenous spread like the peritoneum is affected (55).

Oral colonization is the most frequent superficial candidiasis of the mouth, and *Candida* is then a harmless commensal in healthy individuals (49,55). But in transplant recipients with predisposing factors the most common form is oral candidiasis with white lesions of the buccal mucosa, gums, or tongue that if untreated can develop into confluent plaques. Symptoms may be absent or the patient may complain of burning or dryness of the mouth, loss of taste, and sometimes even dysphagia. *C. esophagitis* occurs often in conjunction with oral candidiasis and presents with dysphagia, retrosternal chest pain, burning, nausea, and vomiting that may be hemorrhagic. It can lead to mediastinitis after a perforation with stenosis as a late complication but also to candidemia or disseminated infection. GI tract disorders due to candidiasis have been difficult to prove and the possibility of *Candida* inducing diarrhea is controversial. *Candida* pseudomembrane of the mucosa or ulcerations with perforation and deep infections have been seen (56). However, *Candida* can interact in the GI tract by colonization, invasion, and persorption (49,51). Invasion has been reported after chemotherapy/irradiation in neutropenic patients. Extensive abdominal surgery, as in liver transplantation, is also a significant risk factor in this setting. Persorption, on the other hand, means that fungi obtain access to the bloodstream via a normal, intact intestinal wall, which has been shown in healthy individuals ingesting large amounts of fungi and might occur during periods of increased colonization (57).

Candida peritonitis occurs as a complication to peritoneal dialysis, as a result of GI perforation, or after contamination during surgery. Symptoms include fever, abdominal pain, and tenderness. Dissemination from peritonitis is rare but can occur in patients treated with corticosteroids (55).

The organs most often affected during hematogenous dissemination of *Candida* spp. are the kidneys, brain, heart, lungs, eyes, skin, skeletal muscle, liver, spleen, bone, and joints. The clinical manifestations are usually nonspecific. Patients mostly present with fever, but it can be low grade or even absent during corticosteroid therapy. Other signs and symptoms rarely occur, apart from abdominal tenderness, when intra-abdominal organs are affected. Eye involvement must be suspected in case of a sudden impairment of vision. Macronodular cutaneous lesions may develop as a manifestation of disseminated candidiasis. They vary from a single nodule to a widespread rash that can be mistaken for an allergic reaction (49,55).

Renal candidiasis is more often a result of hematogenous spread than a result of an ascending infection. Symptoms include fever, rigor, and lumbar and abdominal pain. Candiduria may cause asymptomatic bladder colonization or a low-urinary-tract infection that may be complicated by an ascending urethral infection and/or obstruction by a fungus ball (58). Renal parenchymal infections can cause candiduria and are thought to have their origin in hematogenous dissemination (58,59). In one report, 80% of patients with disseminated candidiasis had a renal infection and almost all had candiduria (60). Candidal cystitis runs with symptoms similar to those of bacterial cystitis.

Cerebral candidiasis is seldom diagnosed during life and includes meningeal candidiasis, diffuse metastatic candidiasis, or brain abscesses. In addition to fever, symptoms may include meningeal irritation, confusion in patients with a disseminated infection, or, those with abscess, focal neurological signs (55).

Candidal endocarditis is the most common form of cardiac complication after a dissemination, occurring in patients with predisposition, as is found in those with native valve diseases or prosthetic heart valves (55).

Pulmonary candidiasis can arise following hematogenous dissemination, with a diffuse pneumonia affecting both lungs. Infection can also arise as a result of endotracheal inoculation from oropharyngeal candidiasis, in which case the appearance is that of a bronchopneumonia (55).

Hepatic candidiasis can be seen after hematogenous spread and is characterized by small abscesses randomly spread throughout the organ. Candidal cholecystitis has also been described, and in liver transplant recipients candidal cholangitis is not uncommon (39,55,61).

Aspergillus Spp.

Aspergillus spp. are ubiquitous, soil-dwelling molds that, in contrast to *Candida* spp., can often be isolated from air samples, dust, food, and potted plants in hospitals. The infection is nosocomial and usually hospital acquired by airborne transmission to the respiratory tract (62). Outbreaks of *Aspergillus* infections have been reported when construction work has been done in or near hospital premises (50,62,63). Only a few species are associated with disease in man. Twenty-one have been listed, but the most pathogenic species of *Aspergillus* are *fumigatus*, *flavus*, *niger*, and *terreus* (63,64).

Clinical syndromes include hypersensitivity syndromes, local infections like aspergilloma, and invasive aspergillosis. Invasive infection is the most common type of aspergillosis in immunosuppressed patients and causes hemorrhagic bronchopneumonia, pulmonary infection with solitary or multiple abscesses, invasion of the pulmonary arteries with distal infarction and/or hemorrhages. Symptoms are few and nondescript, including fever with cough and sometimes pleural pain in case of infarction (65). Another form of invasive aspergillosis in immunosuppressed patients is paranasal sinusitis. Initially, there is headache or facial pain; later, visual disturbance may arise. Both pulmonary and paranasal sinus infections may be the portal of entry for dissemination to other major organs. The isolation of *Aspergillus* spp. from biological specimens in such patients indicates presence of an invasive infection or a high risk for developing it (65).

In the case of a dissemination, clinical presentation is characterized by fever that does not respond to broad-spectrum antibacterial antibiotics and usually pulmonary infiltrates, nodules, or cavitation—sometimes having a triangular wedge shape resulting from blood vessel occlusion with thrombosis and necrosis. The classical second site for lesions is the central nervous system (CNS); other metastatic sites include the heart, kidney, liver, and spleen (64). When cerebral aspergillosis occurs in an immunocompromised host, the outlook is very poor. Cortical disease is most common, with solitary or multiple abscesses and subcortical hemorrhagic infarct reminiscent of the lesions found in the lung (66). Cardiac aspergillosis goes with infarction and necrosis after thrombosis of vessels. Also in the kidney, liver, and spleen complications of dissemination include areas with infarction, necrosis, and abscess formation (64).

Cryptococcus neoformans

Cryptococcosis caused by *Cryptococcus neoformans* is an exogenous infection, acquired by inhalation of fungal spores. *Cryptococcus neoformans*, distributed worldwide, is found in soil, vegetable matter, and bird excrement (67). It is a common cause of fungal infection in immune-compromised patients, especially in those with impaired cellular defense. Cryptococcosis in the organ transplant recipient typically occurs more than 6 months after transplant (68). CNS infection is the predominant finding in most patients and most likely represents extrapulmonary spread of the primary infection. Signs and symptoms of CNS infection include headache, fever, neurological, or psychiatric disturbances. The onset of the infection may, however, be insidious and without dramatic neurological findings other than headache (67). Pulmonary infection may present with a pulmonary infiltrate with flulike symptoms; chest pain and dyspnea have been described in 33% of patients, and cough has been seen in 20%. Extrapulmonary sites besides CNS include mucous membranes, bone marrow, and skin. Skin lesions may be present in up to 30% of the cases (68–70).

Rare Fungal Infections

Zygomycosis

Zygomycosis is caused by fungi of the Mucorales order, which belongs to the Zygomycetes class. The three commonest genera of Mucoraceae are *Absidia*, *Rhizomucor*, and *Rhizopus* (71). These fungi, common in soil, can be found in decomposing plant and animal matter. The usual route of infection is inhalation of spores. An infection is primarily seen in patients with poorly controlled diabetes mellitus or immunosuppression, with acidosis and uremia as risk factors. The most common clinical manifestation is rhinocerebral infection, which has been reported in 11 renal and one heart transplant recipient (72–74). Signs and symptoms correspond to the anatomic site and consist of fever, headache, facial and sinus swelling with pain, nasal discharge, stupor, or coma. Other forms include primary pulmonary, gastrointestinal, and cutaneous infections, all of which may disseminate in debilitated patients (71).

Coccidioidomycosis

Coccidioidomycosis is caused by *Coccidioides immitis*, a soil-dwelling fungus with endemic areas in the southwestern United States (75). The infection is acquired by airborne transmission, causing primarily a pulmonary infection with fever, cough, chest pain, and malaise. In transplanted patients the infection is more common to disseminate to the CNS, the genitourinary tract, liver, spleen, soft tissues, and skeletal system. Common clinical symptoms include meningitis, pyelonephritis, hepatitis, and arteritis. Incidences of 6.9% and 9%, respectively, have been reported in renal and heart transplant recipients resident in Arizona. The mortality was 72% for a disseminated infection and 25% in case of pulmonary infection (76,77). In renal transplant recipients, dissemination has been seen up to 4 years after the transplant, but it is most common during the first post-transplant year (77).

Histoplasmosis

Histoplasmosis is the mycosis caused by *Histoplasma capsulatum* most commonly affecting transplant recipients resident in endemic areas (6). Histoplasmosis is commonest in river valleys throughout the United States and in Central and South America. It is rare in Europe and nonexistent in Australia. The fungus is soil-dwelling and the primary infection is located in the lung and may be followed by a flulike illness characterized by fever, myalgia, and cough. The infection may disseminate to major organs. Symptoms may then include skin and mucosal lesions, as well as a febrile headache caused by CNS infection (6). Histoplasmosis has so far been described only in renal transplant recipients at an incidence of between 0.5% and 2.1%, of which 77% of the infections disseminated (78).

Miscellaneous Infections

Other rare fungi that have been reported to affect organ transplant recipients include *Blastomyces dermatitidis*, that causes blastomycosis; *Fusarium oxysporum*; *Acremonium falciforme*, causing hyalohyphomycosis; *Alternaria* or *Bipolaris* spp., causing phaeohyphomycosis; *Pseudallescheria boydii*, causing pseudallescheriosis; *Sporothrix schenckii*, causing sporotrichosis; and *Kluyveromyces fragilis* (1–3,21,75,76,79).

TIMING AND TYPE OF FUNGAL INFECTIONS IN SOT

Timing

The post-transplant course can be divided into three periods in terms of risk for infection: the first month, the 1–6-month period, and the period of more than 6 months after transplantation (1–3). During the first month after transplant, *Candida* infections—mainly wound infections and, in case of contamination of vulnerable sites during surgery, invasive infections—may develop. Other fungal infections are rare, but especially aspergillosis may occur in patients colonized before transplantation, a particular concern in patients with underlying diseases like cystic fibrosis. In the period 1–6 months after transplant, patients are susceptible to aspergillosis or geographically restricted mycoses, even in those with limited exposure. *Candida* infections are uncommon unless technical problems requiring drains or indwelling catheters are still present. Finally, more than 6 months following transplant, patients with chronic poor graft function due, for example, to chronic rejection requiring high immunosuppression are at risk for both opportunistic and endemic mycoses.

Kidney Recipients

In kidney transplant recipients the most important factor is the degree of immunosuppression, which influences if and which fungal disease will develop (10,41–44). The commonest clinical syndrome with *Candida* spp. is mucocutaneous colonization/infection that involves the oral cavity, esophagus, intertriginous skin folds, and vagina (59). Candiduria is not uncommon in kidney recipients. A less common finding is *Candida* fungemia, which carries a substantial risk of dissemination, leading to metastatic infections like renal infection, endocarditis, and candidal pneumonia (80). In general, all candidemias should be treated in organ transplant recipients (6). Also patients with repeated candiduria must be treated because of a significant risk for obstructive uropathy and pyelonephritis.

Aspergillus spp., the most common presentation includes pulmonary infections that can disseminate throughout the body. The clinical findings include low-grade fever, unproductive cough, dyspnea, pleural chest pain, and pulmonary infiltrates, nodules, or cavitation (14,15,80).

Cryptococcal infections usually develop late in this patient population, causing subacute chronic meningitis, with headache and fever as the commonest symptoms (3). Cutaneous cryptococcosis, a manifestation of disseminated cryptococcal disease, has also been described (81).

Pancreas and Pancreas–Kidney Recipients

There are only a few reports regarding fungal infections in pancreas recipients. The highest risk patient for fungal infections following pancreas transplant recipients is the diabetic patient with *Candida* colonization, poor GI tract function, and extensive abdominal surgery. *Candida* spp. have been the commonest fungal pathogens, mainly causing superficial and/or deep-wound or intra-abdominal infections around the organ, peritonitis, urinary tract infections, and fungemias, regardless of the surgical technique used for pancreas exocrine drainage. Infections usually occur in the early post-transplant period and require graft removal for cure (28–30). *Aspergillus* infections presumably do not differ from those in kidney recipients.

Liver Recipients

In liver transplant recipients many factors govern which fungal infection will arise; however, the often protracted extensive abdominal surgery is an important factor (7,18,19,22). Most infections occur early, within the first month, with *Candida* spp. as the major pathogen. The commonest infections are intra-abdominal candidiasis, resulting in abscess formation; candidemia, with possible dissemination; candidal pneumonia; and urinary tract infection. In patients with indwelling biliary drains or stents and poor graft function, infections in the biliary tract with cholangitis and liver parenchymal manifestations may develop (7,18–22,82). *Aspergillus* infections develop late, up to 6.5 years after the transplant, and are in most cases fatal, with the same infectious panorama as for kidney transplant recipients (83).

Heart and Lung Recipients

Unlike all other organ transplant recipients, in heart/lung transplant recipients most infections are caused by *Aspergillus* spp., followed by *Candida* spp., which reflects the colonization pattern during the preceding chronic illness (2). Fungal infections are reported to be commoner in heart/lung transplant than in heart transplant recipients. The common *Aspergillus* infection is a local airway or invasive pulmonary infection, with abscess formation and dissemination to the CNS. Mediastinitis and necrotizing bronchopneumonia have also been described with ulceration, necrosis, cartilage invasion, and pseudomembrane formation at the site of the bronchial anastomosis (84).

With candidal infections the primary concern is colonization, which may affect healing of the bronchial anastomosis, causing tracheobronchitis and leakage with mediastinitis, which in many cases are fatal. Other manifestations of candidal infections include *Candida* endocarditis, aortic mycotic aneurysm with rupture, pneumonia, and dissemination (31,32,85).

Small Bowel Recipients

Recipients of small bowel have poor GI tract function before transplantation, with increased risk of fungal colonization in combination with bowel surgery and ischemic injuries. Bowel transplantation is still rare, and only a few reports on fungal infections in bowel recipients have been presented, with *Candida* spp. followed by *Aspergillus* spp. as the commonest pathogens. The candidal infections described were candidal esophagitis followed by intra-abdominal infections and candidemia with dissemination (9,38). *Aspergillus* infections presumably do not differ from those in kidney recipients, but there is only one patient reported with *Aspergillus* isolated in bronchoalveolar lavage (BAL) fluid (38).

ANTIFUNGAL TREATMENT AND PREVENTION

Antifungal Agents

The choice of antifungal treatment for patients with organ transplants must be guided by the toxicity of the drugs and their interactions with the immunosuppressives used. Three types of antifungal treatment are given: prophylaxis, preemptive therapy guided by laboratory tests or clinical characteristics in high-risk patients, and treatment of an established or suspected fungal infection (86). We are currently witnessing an intense development of new antifungal drugs, but some drugs cannot be used in transplant recipients because of drug/drug interactions. Some of the antifungal drugs that can be used in transplant recipients are presented in Table 3.

After more than 30 years of intravenous administration of amphotericin B, it remains the gold standard for most invasive fungal infections (87). Amphotericin B is a polyene antibiotic, active against most commonly encountered fungi, and entails a low risk for the development of resistance (88). The usual dose of amphotericin B for systemic infections ranges between 0.7 and 1 mg/kg daily, or every other day, depending on renal function for a period of 2–4 weeks, and a total dose of 1–1.5 g, depending on the signs and symptoms (1,2,89). Amphotericin B and nystatin can be given orally to treat local infections and colonization without toxicity, because they are not absorbed. However, when given intravenously, a number of adverse events, especially renal impairment that becomes worse when amphotericin B is combined with cyclosporine, may contraindicate the use of therapeutic doses (90). Approaches to handling toxicity include low-dose therapy in combination with 5-flucytosine (5-FC), which is synergistic with amphotericin B; administration of calcium channel blockers; pentoxiphylline; or sodium loading of the patient prior to therapy (91,92). However, 5-FC should be used with caution because of its suppressive effect on the bone marrow. Development of resistance to 5-FC is also common, especially when used as a single agent.

TABLE 3. *Antifungal drugs available for prophylaxis and treatment of fungal infections in solid organ transplant recipients*

Not absorbed orally	Amphotericin B
	Nystatin
Absorbed orally	Itraconazole
	Fluconazole
Intravenous	Amphotericin B
	Liposomal amphotericin B (L-AMB)
	Amphotericin B lipid complex (ABLC)
	Amphotericin B colloidal dispersion (ABCD)
	Fluconazole

Another approach was the development of various lipid formulations of the drug that provided new methods of delivery with less toxicity and enhanced efficacy in immunosuppressed patients (39,40,93–100). At present, three preparations are commercially available: the true liposome AmBisome (L-amB) (NeXstar, Inc., Boulder, Colorado), the colloidal dispersion Amphocil/tec (ABCD) (Sequus, Inc., Menlo Park, CA), and the lipid complex Abelcet (ABLC) (Liposome Company, Inc., Princeton, NJ). All these preparations differ in size, structure, pharmacokinetics, antifungal activity, and probably clinical efficacy. Nephrotoxicity in general, but also in conjunction with cyclosporine, was reportedly reduced with all three preparations (97,98). However, acute toxicity, with fever and chills, was common with both ABLC and ABCD, but not with L-amB (97,98). Very little data from randomized trials regarding efficacy have been reported in organ transplant recipients. But all three lipid formulations have shown what may be interpreted as an improved therapeutic index, especially in bone marrow but also in SOT recipients (39,40,99,100). Approvals for the use of lipid formulations have generally been given for rescue treatment when conventional treatment has failed.

In our department we have used L-amB treatment for more than 7 years in 121 SOT recipients—83 liver, 21 kidney, 16 kidney and pancreas, and one pancreas recipient. AmBisome was given to 27 patients for a documented invasive infection, to 42 patients for a suspected infection, and to 58 patients as prophylaxis for a fungal infection. The median maximum dose given for proven infections was 1.8 mg/kg/day (range 0.8–4.3), median total dose was 0.9 g (range 0.5–8.1), and treatment was given for a median of 17 days (range 4–63). Treatment was safe, and efficacy in patients with proven infections was mycological cure in 93% (39). For the other two lipid preparations, so far no data on treatment in SOT recipients have been published.

The azole drugs represent an important part of antifungal therapy. They act by inhibiting the fungal cytochrome P-450 enzyme, which causes poor ergosterol synthesis and a defective cell membrane (101). As a result of their varying interaction with human cytochrome P-450 enzyme, the azoles also interact to a greater or lesser extent with immunosuppressive drugs by down-regulation of both cyclosporine and FK 506 metabolism (102–104). The azoles available for treatment of transplant recipients include the triazoles, itraconazole, and fluconazole. However, careful monitoring of cyclosporine and FK 506 levels is warranted in the case of azole therapy to prevent toxicity. The triazoles have a very wide spectrum of activity, including many of the dimorphic fungi; however, they also have some important differences and limitations (105). Itraconazole is active against *Aspergillus* spp. Because no parenteral preparation is widely available and absorption is unpredictable, itraconazole is mainly used as maintenance therapy in patients with aspergillosis or histoplasmosis, in whom disease control has been achieved with amphotericin B or its lipid preparations (2). Fluconazole is fungistatic and has activity against most species of *Candida* and *Cryptococcus* but not against those of *Aspergillus*. Fluconazole has proved to be useful in transplant recipients as primary treatment of candidiasis and cryptococcosis (3). Of 74 consecutive organ transplant patients treated with fluconazole, 71% were cured, 15% improved, and 14% showed no improvement. This study, however, has not been published but referred to; therefore the conclusion must be that fluconazole treatment seems promising and might be suitable therapy in stable patients with candidiasis that is not life-threatening (89). However, in the event of widespread use of fluconazole, resistant species may develop (53,54). Randomized trials are needed to evaluate all the new fungal agents and their place in the antifungal arsenal. Failures were caused by infections with unsusceptible strains like *Candida glabrata* and/or the presence of anatomic/technical problems requiring long-term percutaneous drainage (3).

Antifungal Treatment

Suggestions for antifungal treatment of invasive fungal infections are presented in Table 4. The duration of treatment and the doses used have not been defined and must be based on type of fungi, patient's immune status, toxicity, interactions, clinical findings, and, most important, improvement in the signs and symptoms. Few recommendations for treatment have been established in randomized trials; instead, most are based on clinical findings in a few patients in an uncontrolled fashion. However, sufficient data from SOT recipients have been accumulated on the use of fluconazole and L-amB and for ABLC and ABCD from bone marrow transplant recipients to prove their value, but well-planned and performed trials are needed to establish optimal treatment regimes.

Candidosis

Mucocutaneous candidiasis may be treated topically with amphotericin B or nystatin solutions, systemically with fluconazole 200–400 mg/day, or in special cases with low-dose amphoptericin B, 5–10 mg/day iv. (89). Lower doses of fluconazole between 50 and 100 mg for 7–14 days has proven clinical efficacy in organ transplant recipients but has been documented only in AIDS patients (2). Lower dosing may lead to the development of resistance.

Candiduria may be treated with bladder irrigation or low doses of intravenous amphotericin B ± 5-FC and, in case of susceptible *Candida* strains, with oral fluconazole (3,89,104).

In candidemia and invasive infections treatment with amphotericin B in a dose of 0.5–1.0 mg/kg/day is recommended as first-line therapy with or without 5-FC (2,90). In case of toxicity, L-amB in a dose of 1–3 mg/kg/day, ABLC in a dose of 5 mg/kg ABCD in a dose of 4 mg/kg may be tried (39,40,99,100). A disseminated infection may benefit from escalation of both the dose

TABLE 4. *Treatment of systemic fungal infections in solid organ transplant recipients (2,3,25,39,89,94,97,104–111)*

Infection	Drug	Dose/day	Duration of treatment
Candida			
Candiduria	Amph.B	0.3–0.5 mg/kg	Clinical picture
	Fluconazole	100–200 mg	2–4 weeks[a]
Candidemia	Amph.B	0.5–1 mg/kg	2–4 weeks[a]
Invasive candidos	Lipid-Amph[b]	1–5 mg/kg	For at least 2 weeks
	Fluconazole	200–400 mg	For at least 11 weeks
Disseminated	Amph.B	1 mg/kg	Not known, clinical picture must guide
	Lipid-Amph B	2–5 mg/kg	
Aspergillus			
Invasive	Amph.B + 5-flucytosin	1–1.5 mg/kg	
	Lipid-Amph B	3–5 mg/kg	Not known, clinical picture must guide
	Itraconazole[c]	400 mg/day	
Cryptococcosis			
	Amph.B + 5-flucytosin	≥0.7 mg/kg	For 2 weeks and then
	+Fluconazole	200–400 mg	for 2 more weeks
	Lipid-Amph B	3–5 mg/kg	For around 4 weeks
Other fungi			
	Amph.B or Lipid-Amph B, depending on type of infection		

[a]At least 2 weeks after negative culture.
[b]Lipid-Amph B, Lipid formulations of Ampho.B: L-amB, 1–5 mg/kg/day, ABLC, 5 mg/kg/day & ABCD, 4 mg/kg/day.
[c]itraconazole, not first-line therapy, check serum concentration.

and the duration of therapy. The duration has not been specifically studied; it probably differs between drugs and must be guided by the clinical findings. Fluconazole has so far been used with caution in immunosuppressed patients having invasive candidal infections. In nonneutropenic patients, however, fluconazole was shown to be effective in treating candidemia (105). Fluconazole has also proved to be useful in organ transplant recipients with invasive candidal infections, in doses between 200 and 400 mg/day for 11 weeks of treatment (2,106,107). In case of severe infections in patients in poor condition, fluconazole must be used with caution.

Aspergillosis

Treatment of invasive aspergillosis requires higher doses of amphotericin B, between 1 and 1.5 mg/kg/day (2,25,89,108). Itraconazole has not yet been considered as first-line therapy. The duration of treatment is not known and patients often receive long-term maintenance treatment with itraconazole afterward. There is one report of successful treatment of an intra-abdominal *Aspergillus* abscess in a liver transplant recipient with itraconazole, 400 mg/day for 3 months (109).

Cryptococcosis

Primary therapy does not differ from that recommended for other immunocompromised patients and includes amphotericin B, combined with 5-FC for about 2 weeks, followed by 4 weeks of fluconazole treatment (110,111). Alternatively, L-amB has proved effective in AIDS patients in a dose of 3 mg/kg for a mean of 27 days (112). Fluconazole has also proved to be effective in a renal transplant recipient in a dose of 200 mg on the first day and then 100 mg daily for 68 days (106).

Miscellaneous Infections

In most other fungal infections amphotericin B is the drug of choice, but more data are accumulating regarding patients treated with lipid formulations or azoles, which in future will probably become the established treatment of choice (2,3,89). In patients with zygomycosis, surgical removal of infected tissue must be combined with amphotericin B (2), when possible.

Prophylaxis

Reducing the risk of fungal infection in organ transplant recipients is the same as in other types of patients at risk. It consists mainly of elimination and reduction of risk factors and exposure and the optimization of hospital care. A more controversial issue is primary antifungal chemoprophylaxis, because few well-designed trials have

been done. Many centers use selective bowel decontamination, including antifungal agents, but hitherto unabsorbed antifungal drugs have shown no prophylactic effect against invasive fungal disease using this method (113). Controlled trials of systemically given or orally absorbed drugs have proved effective in liver transplant recipients (114–116). In one study liver transplant recipients who required treatment in an intensive care unit or had had encephalopathy before transplantation or had been found to have a positive fungal surveillance culture before transplantation received 10 mg/day i.v. of amphotericin B during the first 10–14 postoperative days (25). Using this regimen, the incidence of invasive fungal infections was 7.5%. This study was performed in a nonrandomized way, without controls. The incidence given was low, compared with historical data, but not compared with our most recent incidence of 9% without any consistent systemic fungal prophylaxis being given.

However, two controlled trials have proved that the prophylactic approach is effective in liver transplant recipients. The first was a randomized, blinded trial of L-amB prophylaxis, 1 mg/kg/day or placebo for 5 days starting during the transplantation in 77 patients (114–116). During the first month no invasive fungal infections developed in liposomal-treated patients compared with six infections (five candidiasis and one aspergillosis) among the control patients ($p < 0.01$). At 1 year, the probability of fungal infection was significantly lower: 11% in the L-amB group (three aspergillosis and one candidiasis), compared with 29% in the placebo group (nine candidiasis and two aspergillosis) ($p < 0.05$).

In another study of liver transplant patients fluconazole 100 mg/day was compared with nystatin (4×10^6 U) from day 3 to day 28 after transplantation (116). Fungal colonization was significantly lower in fluconazole-treated patients, 25% versus 53% in nystatin-treated patients. The incidence of fungal infections was significantly lower in the fluconazole group, 13% versus 34% in the nystatin group; of these, 2.6% and 9%, respectively, were invasive. There was no emergence of resistant fungal pathogens in the fluconazole group, but one must beware of the risk for development of resistance (53,54,116).

Preemptive Therapy

Preemptive therapy might be a more efficient approach to antifungal therapy, and such an approach has been suggested in 4 situations (1,6). Treatment would then be reserved for a subgroup of patients at particularly high risk of an invasive infection, based on clinical epidemiological data or a laboratory test. The three proposals are the following (to date these have not been tested):

1. Fluconazole or amphotericin B + 5-FC would be given to eliminate candiduria to prevent obstruction by fungus balls in renal transplants.

2. Fluconazole or itraconazole would be given to prevent disseminated cryptococcosis or *H. capsulatum* infection triggered by surgical excision of a pulmonary nodule.

3. Long-term fluconazole therapy would be given to patients with a complicated post-transplant course requiring high levels of immunosuppression over a long time period. In all these cases, lipid compounds could be considered instead of the preceding drugs.

Environmental Control

The route of acquisition of the common fungal pathogens must be taken into consideration if environmental control is to be effective. *Candida* is present in the subject's endogenous reservoir (49,50). However, exogenous sources—such as another person, food, intravenous catheters, and parenteral fluids—have also been reported (50). Aspergillosis is an airborne infection, and spores can be isolated from air samples, dust, food, and potted plants at hospitals, with outbreaks of infections after construction work in hospitals (62). Cryptococcosis is an exogenous infection, usually acquired prior to hospitalization by inhalation of fungal spores found in soil, vegetable matter, and bird excrement.

Therefore separate environmental control must be considered for prevention. Such measures consist mainly of a reduction in risk factors, such as reducing *Candida* colonization of a patient, eliminating plants and construction sites in the close vicinity, or improving hospital care by isolation and careful nursing, with strict hygiene. Proper cooking of food and avoidance of raw vegetables, pepper, and flowers in the patient's environment may also be important. No potted plants should be allowed on the ward, and construction work in the near vicinity is a warning. Patients should be followed and checked for colonization, and in general, no fungal pathogens found in patient populations at risk should be regarded as contaminants or as nonpathogenic fungi. Furthermore, the patient must be told about risks and risk behavior on discharge from the hospital (113). (See Chapter 3 for more specific details.)

SUMMARY AND CONCLUSION

Invasive fungal infections in SOT recipients are still an important cause of morbidity and mortality. Each type of SOT must be considered separately because of the different risk factors, fungal pathogens, and infectious panoramas in each case. Knowledge of epidemiological risk factors is of the utmost importance. The ways to improve the outcome of invasive fungal infections in organ transplant recipients include a high degree of observation, aggressive use of diagnostic methods available, and early institution of antifungal therapy, preemptively, or the use of systemic antifungal prophylaxis in high-risk patients.

REFERENCES

1. Rubin HR. Infection in the organ transplant recipient. In: Rubin RH, Young LS, eds. *Clinical approach to infection in the compromised host,* 3rd ed. New York: Plenum; 1994:629–705.
2. Hadley S, Karchmer AW. Fungal infections in solid organ transplant recipients. *Infect Dis Clin North Am* 1995;4:1045–1074.
3. Hibberd PL, Rubin RH. Clinical aspects of fungal infections in organ transplant recipients. *Clin Infect Dis* 19[Suppl 1]:S33–S40.
4. Rifkind D, Marchcioro TL, Schneck SA, et al. Systemic fungal infections complicating renal transplantation and immunosuppressive therapy. *Am J Med* 1967;43:28.
5. Baumgartner WA, Peitz BA, Oyer PE, et al. Cardiac homotransplantation. *Curr Probl Surg* 1979;16:1–61.
6. Fishman JA, Rubin RG. Fungal infections in the organ transplant recipient: challenges and opportunities. In: Vincent JL, ed. *Yearbook of intensive care and emergency medicine.* Berlin: Springer-Verlag; 1996:555–566.
7. Wajszczuk CP, Dummer JS, Ho M, et al. Fungal infections in liver transplant recipients. *Transplantation* 1985;40:347–353.
8. Dummer JS, Hardy A, Poorsatter A, et al. Early infections in kidney, heart, and liver transplant recipients on cyclosporine. *Transplantation* 1983;36:259–267.
9. Kusne S, Abu-Elmagd K, Hutson W, et al. Invasive fungal infections after adult small bowel transplantation (SBTX). Fifth International Symposium on Small Intestinal Transplantation, Cambridge, UK, July 31–August 2, 1997. [Abstract no. O34]
10. Masur H, Cheigh JS, Stubenbord WT. Infection following renal transplantation: a changing pattern. *Rev Infect Dis* 1982;4:1208–1219.
11. Gustafson TL, Schaffner W, Lavely GB, et al. Invasive aspergillosis in renal transplant recipients: correlation with corticosteroid therapy. *J Infect Dis* 1983;148:220–238.
12. Chugh KS, Sakhuja V, Jain S, et al. High mortality in systemic fungal infections following renal transplantation in third-world countries. *Nephrol Dial Transplant* 1993;8:168–172.
13. Petterson PK, Ferguson R, Fryd DS, et al. Infectious diseases in hospitalized renal transplant recipients: a prospective study of a complex and evolving problem. *Medicine* 1982;61:360–372.
14. Gallis HA, Berman RA, Cate TR, et al. Fungal infections following renal transplantation. *Arch Intern Med* 1975;135:1163–1172.
15. Weiland D, Ferguson RM, Peterson PK, et al. Aspergillosis in 25 renal transplant patients: epidemiology, clinical presentation, diagnosis and management. *Ann Surg* 1983;198:622–629.
16. Gallis HA, Berman RA, Cate TR, et al. Fungal infection following renal transplantation. *Arch Intern Med* 1975;135:1163–1172.
17. Murphy JF, McDonald FD, Dawson M, Reite A, Turcotte J, Fekey FR Jr. Factors affecting the frequency of infection in renal transplant recipients. *Arch Intern Med* 1976;136:670–677.
18. Tollemar J, Ericzon B-G. Invasive *Candida albicans* infections in orthotopic liver graft recipients. Incidence and risk-factors. *Clin Transplant* 1991;5:306–312.
19. Collins LA, Samore MH, Roberts MS, et al. Risk factors for invasive fungal infections complicating orthotopic liver transplantation. *J Infect Dis* 1994;170:644–651.
20. Kusne S, Dummer JS, Singh N, et al. Infections after liver transplantation: an analysis of 101 consecutive cases. *Medicine* 1988;67: 132–143.
21. Wade JJ, Rolando N, Hayllar K, Philpott-Howard J, Casawell MW, Williams R. Bacterial and fungal infections after liver transplantation: an analysis of 284 patients. *Hepatology* 1995;5:1328–1336.
22. Patel R, Portela D, Badley AD, et al. Risk factors of invasive *Candida* and non-*Candida* fungal infections after liver transplantation. *Transplantation* 1996;62:926–934.
23. Castaldo P, Stratta RJ, Wood RP, et al. Clinical spectrum of fungal infections after orthotopic liver transplantation. *Arch Surg* 1991;126: 149–156.
24. Hadley S, Samore MH, Lewis DW, et al. Major infectious complications after orthotopic liver transplantation and comparison of outcomes in patients receiving cyclosporine or FK506 as primary immunosuppression. *Transplantation* 1995;59:851–859.
25. Mora NP, Klintmalm G, Solomon RM, et al. Selective amphotericin B prophylaxis in the reduction of fungal infections after liver transplant. *Transplant Proc* 1993;24(1):154–155.
26. Schröter GPJ, Hoelscher M, Putnam CW, et al. Fungus infections after liver transplantation. *Ann Surg* 1976:156:115–122.

27. Rossi G, Tortorano AM, Viviani MA, et al. *Aspergillus fumigatus* infections in liver transplant patients. *Transplant Proc* 1989;21:2268–2270.
28. Hesse UJ, Sutherland DER, Najarian JS, et al. Intra-abdominal infections in pancreas transplant recipients. *Ann Surg* 1986;203:153–162.
29. Benedetti E, Gruessner AC, Troppmann C, et al. Intra-abdominal fungal infections after pancreatic transplantation: incidence, treatment and outcome. *J Am Coll Surg* 1996;183:307–316.
30. Perkins JD, Frohnert PP, Servise FJ, et al. Pancreas transplantation at Mayo: III. Multidisciplinary management. *Mayo Clin Proc* 1990;65:496–508.
31. Dummer JS, Montero CG, Griffith BP, Hardesly RL, Paradis IL, Ho M. Infections in heart-lung transplant recipients. *Transplantation* 1986;41:725–729.
32. Brooks RG, Hofflin JM, Jamiesson SW, et al. Infectious complications in heart-lung transplant recipients. *Am J Med* 1985;79:412–422.
33. Britt RH, Enzmann DR, Remmington JS. Intracranial infection in cadaveric transplant recipients. *Ann Neurol* 1981;9:107–119.
34. Kramer MR, Marshall SE, Starnes VA, et al. Infectious complications in heart-lung transplantation. *Arch Intern Med* 1993;153:2010–2016.
35. Dowling RD, Baladi N, Zenati M, et al. Disruption of the aortic anastomosis after heart-lung transplantation. *Ann Thorac Surg* 1990;49:118–122.
36. Grossi P, De Maria R, Caroli A, et al. Infections in heart transplant recipients: the experience of the Italian heart transplantation program. *J Heart Lung Transplant* 1992;11:847–866.
37. Hofflin JM, Potasman I, Baldwin JC, et al. Infectious complications in heart transplant recipients receiving cyclosporine and corticosteroids. *Ann Intern Med* 1987;106:209–216.
38. Reyes J, Abu-Elmagd K, Tzakis A, et al. Infectious complication after human small bowel transplantation. *Transplant Proc* 1992;24:1249–1250.
39. Tollemar J, Svahn BM, Remberger M, Ringdén O. Invasive fungal infections in solid organ transplant recipients, incidence and treatment efficacy of liposomal amphotericin B treatment (AmBisome). Eighth Congress of the European Society for Organ Transplantation, Budapest, Hungary, September 2–6, 1997. [Abstract no. 392]
40. Ringdén O, Ekelöf Andström E, et al. Prophylaxis and therapy using liposomal amphotericin B (AmBisome) for invasive fungal infections in children undergoing organ or allogeneic bone-marrow transplantation. *Pediatr Transplant* 1997;1;124–129.
41. Richardson MD, Shankland GS. Pathogenesis of fungal infection in the non-compromised host. In: Warnock DW, Richardson MD, eds. *Fungal infection in the compromised patient,* 2nd ed. New York: John Wiley; 1991:1–23.
42. Martin DH, Counts GW & Thomas ED. Fungal infections in human bone marrow transplant recipients. Seventeenth Interscience Conference on Antimicrobial Agents and Chemotherapy, American Society for Microbiology, New York, 1977. [Abstract 406]
43. Cupps TR, Fauci AS. Corticosteroid-mediated immunoregulation in man. *Immunol Rev* 1982;56:134–155.
44. Vincenti F, Amend W, Feduska NJ, Duca RM, Salvatierra O Jr. Improved outcome following renal transplantation with reduction in the immunosuppression therapy for rejection episodes. *Am J Med* 1980;69:107–112.
45. Khardori N. Host-parasite interaction in fungal infections. *Eur J Clin Microbiol Infect Dis* 1989;8:331–351.
46. Oh CS, Stratta RJ, Fox BC, et al. Increased infections associated with the use of OKT3 for treatment of steroid-resistant rejection in renal transplantation. *Transplantation* 1988;45:68–73.
47. Stratta RJ, Shaefer MS, Markin RS, et al. Clinical pattern of cytomegalovirus disease after liver transplantation. *Arch Surg* 1989;124:1443–1450.
48. Wagner JA, Ross H, Hunt S, et al. Prophylactic ganciclovir treatment reduces fungal as well as cytomegalovirus infections after heart transplantation. *Transplantation* 1995;60:1473–1477.
49. Odds FC. *Candida and candidiasis: a review and bibliography,* 2nd ed. London: Bailliere Tindall; 1988.
50. Meunier F. Prevention of *Mycoses* in immunocompromised patients. *Rev Infect Dis* 1987;2:408–416.
51. Hay RJ. Dimorphism and candidiasis: clinical and therapeutic implications. diagnosis and treatment of *Mycoses.* In: Vanden Bossche H, Odds FC, Kerridge D, eds. *Dimorphic fungi in biology and medicine.* New York: Plenum Press; 1993:373–379.
52. Piper JP, Rinaldi MG, Winn RI. *Candida parapsilosis:* an emerging problem. *Infect Dis Newslett* 1988;7:49–52.
53. Wingard JR, Merz WG, Rinaldi MG, et al. Increase in *Candida krusei* infection among patients with bone marrow transplantation and neutropenia treated prophylactically with fluconazole. *N Engl J Med* 1991;325:1274–1277.
54. Wingard JR, Merz WG, Rinaldi MG, et al. Association of *Torulopsis glabrata* infections with fluconazole prophylaxis in neutropenic bone marrow transplant patients. *Antimicrob Agents Chemother* 1993;37:1847–1849.
55. Dupont B. Clinical manifestations and management of candidiasis in the compromised patient. In: Warnock DW, Richardson MD, eds. *Fungal infection in the compromised patient,* 2nd ed. New York: John Wiley; 1991:56–83.
56. Eras P, Golstein MJ, Sherlock P. *Candida* infection of the gastrointestinal tract. *Medicine* 1972;51:367–379.
57. Krause W, Mathies H, Wulf K. Fungaemia and fungiuria after oral administration of Candida albicans. *Lancet* 1969;1:598–599.
58. Fisher JF, Chew WH, Shadomy S, et al. Urinary tract infections due to Candida albicans. *Rev Infect Dis* 1982;4:1107–1118.
59. Rubin RH. Infectious disease complications of renal transplantation. *Kidney Int* 1993;44:221–236.
60. Kozinn PJ, Taschdjian CL, Goldberg PK, Wise GJ, Toni EF, Seelig MS. Advances in the diagnosis of renal candidiasis. *J Urol* 1978;119:184–187.
61. Gomez-Mateos JM, Porto AS, Parra DM, Balbutin AR, Serrano AL, Lugne JA. Disseminated candidiasis and gangrenous cholecystitis due to *Candida* spp. *J Infect Dis* 1988;158:653–655.
62. Bodey GP, Vartivarian S. Aspergillosis. *Eur J Clin Microbiol Infect Dis* 1989;8:413–437.
63. Rinaldi MG. Invasive aspergillosis. *Rev Infect Dis* 1983;5:1061–1077.
64. Cohen J. Clinical manifestation and management of aspergillosis in the compromised patient. In: Warnock DW, Richardson MD, eds. *Fungal infection in the compromised patient,* 2nd ed. New York: John Wiley; 1991:118–152.
65. Young RC, Bennet JE, Vogel CL, Carbone PP, DeVita VT. Aspergillosis: the spectrum of the disease in 98 patients. *Medicine* 1970;49:147–173.
66. Walsh TJ, Hier DB, Caplan LR. Aspergillosis of the central nervous system: clinicopathological analysis of 17 patients. *Ann Neurol* 1985;18:574–582.
67. Hay RJ. Clinical manifestations and management of cryptococcosis in the compromised patient. In: Warnock DW, Richardson MD, eds. *Fungal infection in the compromised patient,* 2nd ed. New York: John Wiley; 1991:85–116.
68. Wheat LJ, Fungal infection in the immunocompromised host. In: Rubin RH, Young LS, eds. *Clinical approach to infection in the compromised host,* 3rd ed. New York: Plenum; 1994:211–237.
69. Wolfson JS, Sober AJ, Rubin RH. Dermatologic manifestations of infections in immunocompromised patients. *Medicine* 1985;64:115–133.
70. Schröter GPJ, Temple DR, Husberg BS, et al. Cryptococcosis after renal transplantation: report of ten cases. *Surgery* 1976;79:268–277.
71. Skahan KJ, Wong B, Armstrong D. Clinical manifestation and management of mucormycosis in the compromised patient. In: Warnock DW, Richardson MD, eds. *Fungal infection in the compromised patient,* 2nd ed. New York: John Wiley; 1991:154–190.
72. Hammer GS, Bottone EJ, Hirschman SZ. Mucormycosis in a transplant recipient. *Am J Clin Pathol* 1975;64:389–398.
73. Fisher J, Tuazon CU, Geelhoed GW. Mucormycosis in transplant patients. *Am Surg* 1980;46:315–322.
74. Morduchowicz G, Pitlik SD, Shapira Z, Shmueli AY, Djalovski S, Rosenfeld JB. Infection in renal transplant recipients in Israel. *Isr J Med Sci* 1985;21:791–797.
75. Cohen IM, Galgiani JN, Potter D, Ogden DA. Coccidioidomycosis in renal replacement therapy. *Arch Intern Med* 1982;489–494.
76. Cohen IM, Galgiani JN, Potter D, Ogden DA. Coccidioidomycosis in renal replacement therapy. *Arch Intern Med* 1982;142:489–494.
77. Calhoun DL, Galgiani JN, Zvkoski C, et al. Coccidioidomycosis in recent renal or cardiac transplant recipients, In Einstein HE, Catanzaro A, eds. *Proceedings of the 4th International Conference on coccidioidomycosis.* Washington, DC, National Foundation for Infectious Diseases; 1985:312–318.
78. Wheat LJ, Smith EJ, Sathapatyavongs B, et al. Histoplasmosis in renal allograft recipients: two large urban outbreaks. *Arch Intern Med* 1983;143:703–707.
79. Warnock DW, Johnson EM. Clinical manifestation and management

of hyalohyphomycosis, phaeohyphomycosis and other uncommon forms of fungal infection in the compromised patient. In: Warnock DW, Richardson MD, eds. *Fungal infection in the compromised patient,* 2nd ed. New York: John Wiley; 1991:247–310.

80. Zeluff JZ. Fungal pneumonia in transplant recipients. *Semin Respir Infect* 1990;1:80–89.

81. Rubin RH, Wolfson JS, Cosimi AB, Tolkoff-Rubin ME. Infection in the renal transplant recipient. *Am J Med* 1981;70:405–411.

82. Paya CV, Hermans PE, Washington JA, et al. Incidence, distribution, and outcome of episodes of infection in 100 orthotopic liver transplantations. *Mayo Clin Proc* 1989;64:555–564.

83. Singh N, Arnow PM, Bonham A, et al. Invasive aspergillosis in liver transplant recipients in the 1990s. *Transplantation* 1997;64:716–720.

84. Kramer MR, Denning DW, Marshall SE, et al. Ulcerative tracheobronchitis after lung transplantation: a new form of invasive aspergillosis. *Am Rev Respir Dis* 1991;144:552–556.

85. Masur H, Rosen PP, Armstrong D. Pulmonary disease caused by candida species. *Am J Med* 1977;63:914–925.

86. Rubin RH, Tolkoff-Rubin NE. Antimicrobial strategies in the care of organ transplant recipients. *Antimicrob Agents Chemother* 1993;37:619–624.

87. Gallis HA, Drew RH, Pickard WW. Amphotericin B: 30 years of clinical experience. *Rev Infect Dis* 1990;12:308–329.

88. Warnock DW. Amphotericin B: an introduction. *J Antimicrob Chemother* 1991;28[Suppl. B]:27–38.

89. Edwards JE Jr, Bodey GP, Bowden RA, et al. International conference for the development of a consensus on the management and prevention of severe candidal infections. *Clin Infect Dis* 1997;25:43–59.

90. Shulman H, Striker G, Deeg HJ, et al. Nephrotoxicity of cyclosporine A after allogeneic marrow transplantation. *N Engl J Med* 1981;305:1392–1395.

91. Francis P, Walsh TJ. Evolving role of flucytocin in immunocompromised patients: new insights into safety, pharmacokinetics, anti antifungal therapy. *Clin Infect Dis* 1992;15:1003–1018.

92. Bianco JA, Appelbaum FR, Nemunaitis J, et al. Phase I-II trial of pentoxifylline for the prevention of transplant-related toxicity following bone marrow transplantation. *Blood* 1991;78:1205–1211.

93. Meunier F, Prentice HG, Ringdén O. Liposomal amphotericin B (AmBisome): safety data from a phase II/III clinical trial. *J Antimicrob Chemother* 1991;28[Suppl. B]:83–91.

94. Tollemar J. Diagnosis and treatment of invasive fungal infections in transplant recipients. In: *Workshop, prophylaxis and treatment of invasive fungal infections,* by the Medical Products Agency of Sweden 1995;2:89–102.

95. Wingard JR. Efficacy of amphotericin B lipid complex injection (ABLC) in bone marrow transplant recipients with life-threatening systemic mycoses. *Bone Marrow Transplant* 1997;19:343–347.

96. Lister J. Amphotericin B lipid complex (Abelcet) in the treatment of invasive mycoses: the North American experience. *Eur J Haematol* 1996;56[Suppl 57]:18–23.

97. Tollemar J, Ringdén O. Lipid formulations of amphotericin B: less toxicity but at what economic cost? *Drug Safety* 1995;13(4):207–218.

98. Janknegt R, de Marie S, Bakker-Woudenberg IAJM, et al. Liposomal and lipid formulations of amphotericin B clinical pharmacokinetics. *Clin Pharmacokinet* 1992;23(4):279–291.

99. White MH, Anaissie EJ, Kusne S, et al. Amphotericin B colloidal dispersion vs. amphotericin B as therapy for invasive aspergillosis. *Clin Infect Dis* 1997;24:635–642.

100. Wingard JR. Efficacy of amphotericin B lipid complex injection (ABLC) in bone marrow transplant recipients with life-threatening systemic mycoses. *Bone Marrow Transplant* 1997;19:343–347.

101. Bodey GP. Azole antifungal agents. *Clin Infect Dis* 1992;14[Suppl 1]:S161–S169.

102. Sugar AM, Saunders C, Idelson BA, et al. Interaction of fluconazole and cyclosporine. *Ann Intern Med* 1989;110:844.

103. Kwan JTC, Foxall PJD, Davidson DCG, et al. Interaction of cyclosporine and itraconazole. *Lancet* 1987;2:282.

104. Manez R, Martin M, Raman V, et al. Fluconazole therapy in transplant recipients receiving FK506. *Transplantation* 1994;57:1521–1535.

105. Rex JH, Bennett JE, Sugar AM, et al. A randomized trial comparing fluconazole with amphotericin B for the treatment of candidemia in patients without neutropenia. *N Engl J Med* 1994;331:1325–1330.

106. Conti DJ, Tolkoff-Rubin NE, Baker GP, et al. Successful treatment of invasive fungal infection with fluconazole in organ transplant recipients. *Transplantation* 1989;48:692–694.

107. Bren A, Kandus A, Lindic J, Vari J. Fluconazole in the treatment of fungal infections in kidney-transplanted patients. *Transplant Proc* 1992;24:2765–2766.

108. Armstrong D. Treatment of opportunistic fungal infections. *Clin Infect Dis* 1993;16:1–7.

109. Durand F, Bernau J, Dupont B, et al. *Aspergillus* intraabdominal abscess after liver transplantation successfully treated with itraconazole. *Transplantation* 1992;54:734–735.

110. Dismukes WE, Cloud G, Gallis HA, et al. Treatment of cryptococcal meningitis with combination amphotericin B and flucytocin for four as compared with six weeks. *N Engl J Med* 1987;317:334–341.

111. Saag MS, Powderly WG, Cloud GA, et al. Comparison of amphotericin B with fluconazole in the treatment of acute AIDS-associated cryptococcal meningitis. *N Engl J Med* 1992;326:83–89.

112. Coker RJ, Viviani M, Gazzard BG, et al. Treatment of cryptococcosis with liposomal amphotericin B (AmBisome) in 23 patients with AIDS. *AIDS* 1993;7:829–835.

113. Tollemar J, Prophylaxis against fungal infections in transplant recipients. *Clin Immunotherapeut* 1997 (in press).

114. Tollemar J, Höckerstedt K, Ericzon BG, Jalanko H, Ringdén O. Liposomal amphotericin B prevents invasive fungal infections in liver transplant recipients: a randomized, placebo controlled study. *Transplantation* 1995;59:1:45–50.

115. Tollemar J, Höckerstedt K, Ericzon B-G, Jalanko H, Ringdén O. Prophylaxis with liposomal amphotericin B (AmBisome) prevents fungal infections in liver transplant recipients: long-term results of a randomized, placebo controlled trial. *Transplant Proc* 1995;27:1195–1198.

116. Lumbreras C, Cuervas-Mons V, Jara P, et al. Randomized trial of fluconazole versus nystatin for the prophylaxis of *Candida* infection following liver transplantation. *J Infect Dis* 1996;174:583–588.

Transplant Infections edited by
Raleigh A. Bowden, Per Ljungman, and Carlos V. Paya.
Lippincott–Raven Publishers, Philadelphia © 1998

CHAPTER 25

Immunization of Transplant Recipients

Per Ljungman

During the last 25 years the numbers of solid organ and blood and bone marrow transplant (BMT) patients have increased rapidly. Infections have been major obstacles for successful transplantations. Thus infection prevention is very important in transplant recipients. Until recently, most attention has been focused on preventing infections that occur during the early phase after transplantation with conventional chemoprophylaxis. As the results of transplantation have improved, the number of long-term survivors have increased. Many patients remain immunosuppressed for a long time either because of the interaction between the graft and the host (i.e., graft-versus-host disease [GVHD]) in BMT recipients or because of the immunosuppressive therapy given to prevent graft rejection in solid organ transplant recipients. Immunizations, which have for various reasons not been used consistently at many transplant centers, are important for two main reasons. Obviously, the most important is the need to protect the transplant recipient against serious infections that may occur during the early or late post-transplant period. However, another reason is the public health point of view—namely, that it is important not to have an increasing number of individuals vulnerable to important infectious agents (e.g., poliovirus). Both reasons require analysis of risks and benefits for the transplant recipient.

IMMUNIZATIONS AFTER BLOOD AND MARROW TRANSPLANTATION

Allogeneic BMT

Transfer and Persistence of Immunity in Allogeneic BMT Recipients

After an allogeneic BMT, the immune system of the recipient is replaced by the immune system of the host.

The immune deficiency after BMT is caused by the preparative regimen before BMT, GVHD, and immunosuppressive therapy given after transplantation. Many studies have shown that immunity to some infectious agents is transferred by the graft and can be detected in the patient early after the BMT (1–8). Thus it would make sense to immunize the donor before donation to improve the transfer of immunity. Studies of pretransplant donor immunization have shown that pretransplant immunization of the marrow donor to some antigens such as tetanus toxoid, diphtheria toxoid, and hepatitis B virus increases the probability of transfer of B-cell immunity by the marrow graft (5,9). Two recent case reports suggest that transfer of immunity from a hepatitis B virus (HBV)–immune donor can clear virus from an HBV-antigen and DNA-positive recipient (10,11). Whether this immunity from recently immunized donors will protect against infection in the recipient or clear infection already present in the recipient needs further study.

However, no effective and safe vaccines are available for most infections that are common and serious early after BMT. The infections for which pretransplant immunizations could be considered are cytomegalovirus (CMV), influenza, and varicella-zoster virus (VZV). CMV has caused major morbidity and mortality after BMT. Currently, no vaccines against CMV are available, although vaccines based on new vaccine technology such as subunit vaccines and vaccines using other viruses as vectors are currently in early clinical development. No studies have been performed with donor immunization against influenza or varicella-zoster virus.

However, despite the transfer of specific immunity after allogeneic BMT, the long-term presence of specific antibodies after BMT is dependent not only on the donor's immune status but also on the recipient's immune status before BMT (6,12,13). In most patients, immunity is usually progressively weakened over time, and an increasing number of patients become susceptible to

From the Department of Hematology, Huddinge University Hospital, Karolinska Institute, S-14186 Huddinge, Sweden.

infections such as tetanus (3,13), poliovirus (14,15), and measles (12) during extended follow-up. The loss of protective immunity is more rapid in patients who obtained immunity by immunization against measles than in those who became immune after natural measles disease (12). Thus the immune status of the donor is important for transfer of B-cell immunity, but the transfer usually has a finite duration. It should also be remembered that many patients are transplanted because of hematologic malignancies, and these patients have received intensive immunosuppressive therapy before they come to transplantation. Hammarström and colleagues have shown that 41% of nontransplanted acute leukemia patients were nonprotected against tetanus (16). Risk factors for loss of immunity were acute lymphoblastic leukemia (ALL) when compared with acute myelogenous leukemia (AML), more advanced disease, and increasing age.

Studies of Immunizations After Allogeneic BMT

Recommendations for vaccination of BMT recipients are shown in Table 1. These are based on a consensus of US and European experts on infectious diseases and updated with reference to more recently published information. The aim of the recommendations is to achieve the same level of protection for BMT recipients as for the general population. The recommendations are divided into three grades:

++ = *Strongly recommended for all patients.* (The recommendation is based on studies showing efficacy safety of vaccination. Immunizations are recommended for the general population in most countries.)

+ = *Recommended for all patients.* (The recommendations are based on the fact that an increased risk of severe infection is documented in BMT recipients and the risk of immunization is regarded to be low.)

± = *Recommended on an individual basis.* (The decision regarding vaccination must be based on individual assessment of benefit—for example, depending on the epidemiological situation in the country, presence of GVHD, or ongoing immunosuppression.)

Influenza Vaccine

Influenza A and B infections can be severe and life-threatening in BMT recipients (17–19). Whether pretransplant immunization of the recipient would be protective has not been studied. Immunization with two doses of influenza vaccine can elicit an immune response, but in a study by Engelhard and colleagues, the time after BMT was shown to be important for the efficacy of the immunization (20). No patient could respond when immunizations were given less than 6 months after BMT; approximately 25% of the patients responded when immunizations were given between 6 months and 2 years after BMT; and more than 60% of patients responded when immunizations were given more than 2 years after BMT. We have recently performed a randomized study investigating the addition of GM-CSF to influenza vaccine given between 4 and 12 months after BMT (Pauksen and Ljungman, unpublished data). Unfortunately, there was no difference between the two groups, and only approximately 30% of the patients in both groups responded to immunization. Another option for protecting patients against influenza would be to immunize family members and hospital staff, thereby reducing the risk for transmission of the infection to the patient.

Varicella-zoster Virus Vaccine

Primary VZV infections can be very severe early after allogeneic transplantation. The existing vaccine is live, attenuated, and therefore impossible to use early in the post-transplant period. It would be logical to immunize a seronegative patient before transplantation, because the vaccine has been proven safe and effective in children with leukemia in remission, providing that enough time has elapsed from the vaccination to the transplant procedure. No data are available allowing assessment of the

TABLE 1. *Recommendations for immunizations of allogeneic and autologous BMT recipients*

Vaccine	Allogeneic BMT recipients	Autologous BMT recipients	Recommended time for immunization
Tetanus toxoid	++	++	6–12 months after BMT
Diphtheria toxoid	++	++	6–12 months after BMT
Inactivated poliovirus	++	++	6–12 months after BMT
Measles (attenuated)	±	±	Individual not <24 months after BMT
Rubella (attenuated)	±	±	Individual not <24 months after BMT
Influenza	+	+	6 months (during season)
Haemophilus Influenzae	++	+	4–6 months after BMT
Hepatitis B	+	+	pre-BMT, 6–12 months after BMT
Pneumococci	+	±	8–12 months after BMT
VZV (attenuated)	+	+	pre-BMT (seronegative patients)

++, Strongly recommended for all patients. Benefit >> Risk.
+, Recommended. Benefit > Risk.
±, Individual recommendation. Benefit and risk must be assessed in individual cases.

minimum interval needed between immunization and transplantation. However, this strategy has not been tested in a clinical study, although it is likely that children with acute leukemia who have been immunized with the varicella vaccine have subsequently undergone allogeneic BMT. However, no data are available regarding the protective efficacy of pretransplant immunization against VZV. One small study with immunization of eight children who had undergone allogeneic BMT has been published (21). Four patients were seronegative and four had low antibody titers against VZV before vaccination. The vaccine was well tolerated, but only three of eight children developed an antibody response against VZV. Furthermore, the data are too limited to allow any conclusions regarding protection against primary VZV in allogeneic BMT recipients. A high proportion of BMT patients develop herpes zoster that occasionally becomes severe. The risk for herpes zoster is strongly influenced by the presence of GVHD. Redman and colleagues used heat-inactivated varicella vaccine and showed no reduction in the risk for developing herpes zoster but a reduced severity of the herpes zoster in the immunized group (22).

Hepatitis B Virus Vaccine

HBV infection is a major cause of morbidity in many parts of the world. One specific problem occurs when a seronegative BMT patient is scheduled to receive a HBsAg-positive marrow graft. Immunization against HBV in normal individuals usually requires three injections spread over a couple of months to ensure protective immunity. This might cause a problem when scheduling a BMT. Furthermore, a subset of 5% to 15% of normal individuals will not respond to HBV immunization. No data exist about eventual protective efficacy of pretransplant immunization of the marrow recipient.

Pneumococcal and Haemophilus influenzae Vaccines

Protective immunity against Streptococcus pneumoniae and Haemophilus influenzae type B (HIB) is mediated through antibodies directed against polysaccharides from the bacterial capsule. The risk for severe pneumococcal infections is increased in patients with chronic GVHD (23–25). Immunization with the currently available pneumococcal vaccines can elicit good antibody responses 6–12 months after BMT in patients without GVHD but has been ineffective in eliciting adequate immune responses in patients with chronic GVHD (26–30). In particular, the specific IgG2 responses have been poor (29,31). The immune response was not significantly improved by two doses of pneumococcal vaccine as compared with one dose (28). In contrast, immunization with HIB vaccines conjugated with tetanus toxoid or diphtheria toxoid were able to elicit protective immune responses (28,30). In a study where the donor was immu-

nized with vaccines against H. influenzae and pneumococci and the recipient was immunized with the same vaccines after the transplantation, the recipients's immune response was improved against H. influenzae when vaccinated at 3 months after transplant but not against pneumococci given at 12 and 24 months after BMT (32). There are also new conjugate vaccines against pneumococci in early testing, and these may be more effective in mediating protection against pneumococcal disease in BMT recipients with chronic GVHD.

Tetanus Toxoid, Diphtheria Toxoid, and Poliovirus Vaccine

Several studies have shown loss of immunity to tetanus, poliovirus, and diphtheria during extended follow-up after BMT (13–15,33). Large epidemics with diphtheria have occurred in Russia. Small outbreaks of poliomyelitis still occur in nonimmune populations. Tetanus is a rare but life-threatening disease preventable by immunization. Thus there are good medical reasons for having an immunization strategy against these infections in BMT recipients.

A few studies on effectiveness of reimmunization programs have been published (13–15,34). Repeated doses of tetanus toxoid, diphtheria toxoid, and inactivated poliovirus vaccine were needed to obtain stable protective immunity (13,34). In most of these studies reimmunization was initiated approximately 1 year after BMT. However, Parkkali and colleagues have recently shown that good immune responses against both tetanus toxoid and poliovirus can be obtained when the first dose is given at 6 months after BMT (35,36). The inactivated poliovirus vaccine should be used to prevent vaccine-induced paralytic disease. It is also recommended that the oral live poliovirus vaccine not be used in family members of BMT patients.

Measles, Mumps, and Rubella Vaccine

Most patients become seronegative to measles during extended follow-up (12). Measles can cause severe disease in immunocompromised patients. Recently, a large measles epidemic occurred in Sao Paolo, Brazil (37). The available measles vaccines are live, attenuated, and not recommended for immunocompromised patients. Thus immunization can only be considered in allogeneic BMT patients without chronic GVHD or ongoing immunosuppression. Data in such patients indicate that measles vaccine can be given without severe side effects at 2 years after BMT (38). No data exist on the safety of immunization earlier after transplantation, although earlier immunizations were given during the epidemic in Brazil (37). However, no data about efficacy or side effects are yet available. Measles immunization could be considered prior to 2 years on an individual basis, depending on the epidemiological situation in the community. Data indicate that rubella vaccine can be given without severe side effects at 2 years after BMT in patients without chronic GVHD or ongoing immunosuppression (38). Rubella vaccine could be indicated in female patients who have retained the potential for becoming pregnant.

Other Vaccines

Other immunizations that can be discussed in allogeneic stem cell transplantation are those for meningococci and yellow fever. The vaccine against meningococci is prepared in a way similar to the pneumococcal vaccine and can therefore be used without any risk for significant side effects in epidemic situations. Yellow fever is a life-threatening infection primarily occurring in South America and southern and central Africa. The vaccine is live and attenuated. Rio and colleagues have presented three cases that were immunized at 5 years after BMT without severe side effects (39). Immunization can be considered in patients who must travel to endemic regions for yellow fever.

BCG vaccine can cause severe infections in patients with depressed T-cell function and is not recommended in BMT recipients.

Autologous Bone Marrow Transplantation

Persistence of Immunity in Autologous BMT Recipients

In autologous BMT recipients the immune system is depressed by high doses of chemo- and radiotherapy but there is no immunologic disparity between the graft and the host. The immune regeneration is, in most patients, quicker than that after allogeneic BMT and even more so after peripheral blood stem cell transplantation. Less is known about late immune deficiency after autologous BMT than after allogeneic BMT.

Several studies have shown that autologous BMT recipients also lose protective immunity to tetanus, poliovirus, and measles during extended follow-up (15,40,41). There are no published data on retainment of long-term immunity in peripheral stem cell transplant recipients. Similar to allogeneic BMT recipients, poor responses to immunization are elicited if immunizations are given early after transplantation (20). One option to obtain better immune responses in ABMT recipients is to immunize the patient either before marrow harvest or just before the transplantation. Immunization against HBV could elicit protective immune response when one dose was given before and one dose early after autologous BMT (42). However, in one-third of the responding patients the seroconversion was only transient. Immunization with conjugated *H. influenzae* type B vaccine and tetanus toxoid before marrow harvest followed by immunization at 3, 6, 12, and 24 months after ABMT improved the antibody titers to both

H. influenzae and tetanus toxoid already at 3 months after the transplantation (43). However, when immunizations were given with pneumococcal vaccines given in the same schedule, there was no difference in antibody titer at any time after the ABMT.

Immunization of Autologous BMT Recipients

Fewer studies of immunization have been performed in autologous than in allogeneic BMT recipients. Recommendations for vaccination of ABMT recipients are shown in Table 1 and are based on a consensus of European experts on infectious diseases and updated with reference to more recently published information. If no specific knowledge exists regarding autologous BMT recipients, the recommendations are based on those given for allogeneic BMT recipients.

Influenza

Immunization against influenza A and B could be considered in autologous BMT recipients. However, no patient responded if immunizations were performed earlier than 6 months after autologous BMT (20). In a recent study, we have shown that GM-CSF does not improve the response to immunization against influenza given between 4 and 12 months after autologous BMT (Pauksen and Ljungman, unpublished data). Moreover, for ABMT patients immunization of family members and hospital staff could be considered, thereby reducing the risk for transmission of influenza to the patient.

Pneumococcal and HIB Vaccines

Limited data exist regarding the need for and efficacy of immunization with pneumococcal and HIB vaccines in autologous BMT recipients. Hammarström and colleagues showed that most autologous BMT patients retained normal antibody levels to Pneumococcus (29).

Tetanus Toxoid, Diphtheria Toxoid, and Poliovirus Vaccine

Autologous BMT recipients have a greater risk than the normal population for losing protective immunity to poliovirus and tetanus (15,41,44). Reimmunizations with repeated dose schedules of inactivated poliovirus vaccine and tetanus toxoid effectively restore protective immunity in autologous BMT recipients (15,41,44).

Measles, Mumps, and Rubella Vaccine

Children who have been immunized to measles before autologous BMT frequently become seronegative during follow-up, but adults who before the autologous BMT had experienced natural measles disease usually remain immune to measles during a follow-up of 3 years after transplant (40). Immunization results show that immunization with measles vaccine is effective in seronegative children who have undergone autologous BMT (40,45). Immunization can be initiated at 12 months after autologous BMT. Rubella vaccine could be indicated in female patients who have retained the potential for becoming pregnant.

SOLID ORGAN TRANSPLANT RECIPIENTS

The need for immunization in solid organ transplant recipients can arise from three components, each of which causes a suppression of the immune system: the immunosuppressive activity of the underlying disease (e.g., chronic renal failure), the immunologic reactivity between graft and host (i.e., rejection), and the immunosuppressive therapy given after the transplantation. The first two mechanisms are similar to the situation in allogeneic BMT. However, there is an important difference concerning the immunosuppressive therapy, namely, that it must be given life-long in solid organ transplant recipients but is usually given only for a limited time after allogeneic BMT. This life-long immunosuppression is of importance when reimmunization programs for solid organ transplant recipients are designed. The different transplant types will be discussed together in this chapter because there are no data on possible different immunization efficacy in the separate solid organ transplant groups. Suggested recommendations for vaccination are shown in Table 2.

Immunizations can be given either before solid organ transplantation, with the aim to prevent infections occurring during the early post-transplant phase, or after transplantation, with the aim of preventing late infections. Infections that might be prevented by pretransplant immunization include CMV and hepatitis B, whereas infections that might prevent post-transplant immunizations include influenza and pneumococci.

Immunizations Given Before Transplantation

HBV can be transmitted either by a hepatitis B-antigen-positive organ graft or through blood transfusions. HBV vaccination is recommended in HBV-negative patients before organ transplantation because there is an increased risk of severe HBV infections in transplant patients. The efficacy of HBV vaccine is lower in patients on hemodialysis than in healthy individuals (46,47). However, in children with biliary atresia awaiting liver transplantation, HBV vaccine elicited an immune response in 73% of the patients (48). Whether HBV vaccination also protects against challenge with HBV is unknown. On the other hand, three doses of HBV vaccine gave an antibody response in only 44% to 54% of patients with other forms of end-stage liver disease (49).

Data are lacking about the vaccine's protective efficacy against HBV acquisition if an antigen-positive organ donor is used. There is one published case report of combined HBV vaccination and HBV immune globulin where the patient did not develop HBV infection despite an HBV-positive organ donor (50). Another possible indication for HBV vaccination would be to prevent reinfection of a liver allograft in HBV-positive patients. However, this strategy has been ineffective (51).

CMV is an important pathogen after solid organ transplantation. Randomized studies with the currently unavailable vaccine based on the Towne strain have showed a reduction in the severity of CMV disease and a reduction in graft rejection. The effect was strongest in the patient group with highest risk for CMV disease, namely, the seronegative recpients getting organs from seropositive donors (52,53). Today, however, antiviral chemoprophylaxis is more effective for preventing CMV disease and the vaccine is unavailable for use. There is ongoing work with new CMV vaccines that may change this situation in the future.

VZV can cause severe and fatal disease in organ transplant patients. Varicella vaccine given to uremic children awaiting renal transplantation was safe and able to reduce the post-transplant risk for both varicella in prevaccination seronegative patients and herpes zoster in prevaccination seropositive patients (54). Recently, a follow-up study was published showing that the protection was long-lasting, with 42% of patients still having antibodies at more than 10 years after immunization. Furthermore, the risk for varicella was lower in immunized patients and the disease was significantly less severe than in nonimmunized patients (55).

TABLE 2. Recommendations for immunizations in solid organ transplant recipients

Vaccine	Before transplantation	After transplantation	Comments
Hepatitis B virus	++		Seronegative patients
VZV vaccine (attenuated)	++		Seronegative patients
Influenza	+	++	Seasonal
Haemophilus influenzae	+	±	Children
Pneumococci	++	±	Children
Hepatitis A vaccine	++	±	Liver transplant patients

++, Strongly recommended for all patients. Benefit >> risk.
+, Recommended. Benefit > risk.
±, Individual recommendation. Benefit and risk must be weighed in individual cases.

Immunizations against *S. pneumoniae* and *H. influenzae* can be considered in children waiting for a solid organ transplantation (56,57).

Hepatitis A virus has increasingly been recognized as a potential cause of severe and even fulminant hepatitis, in particular in patients waiting for liver transplantation (1). An effective, inactivated vaccine exists although there is no published data. The knowledge regarding other vaccines suggests that this new vaccine should be given as early as possible in patients who might become candidates for liver transplantation.

In addition to the above mentioned vaccines it is important to update the vaccinations in a patient, in particular children, waiting for organ transplantation with additional doses of diphtheria toxoid, tetanus toxoid, and poliovirus vaccine (58).

Immunization Given After Transplantation

The efficacy of HBV vaccination is low after solid organ transplantation, with response rates between 5% and 15% (59,60). Thus pretransplant immunization is recommended (see earlier).

Influenza can cause severe infections in renal transplant patients (17,18). Immunization is recommended by the U.S. Public Health Service Advisory Committee on Immunization Practices (61). The reported results of immunization vary. Versluis and colleagues reported that renal transplant patients treated with cyclosporine had a significantly lower antibody response than patients treated with azathioprine, who had responses comparable to those of healthy individuals (62). In a study of young adults after solid organ transplantation, the transplant patients had lower antibody titers and lower response rates than immunocompetent patients. No improvement was seen with a second dose of vaccine (63). In contrast, two studies have shown normal responses to influenza immunization in children after organ transplantation (64,65).

Immunizations against *S. pneumoniae* and HIB could also be considered (56). The efficacy of the 23-valent pneumococcal polysaccharide vaccine was similar to normal immunocompetent controls (66). However, the benefit of immunizations with these vaccines is uncertain in solid organ transplant recipients, although it is logical to assume that reducing the risk for infection with *S. pneumoniae* and HIB could be beneficial in, for example, lung transplant recipients. There are no data concerning the need or efficacy of immunization against tetanus or poliovirus in solid organ transplant recipients.

Immunization with live vaccines is not recommended without further study in solid organ transplant patients because of the risk for vaccine-associated complications. A small study of varicella vaccination in kidney-transplanted children has shown good serological responses and no severe side effects (67). Vaccination is an attractive alternative for prevention because varicella can be severe in renal transplant recipients and vaccine strain

dissemination can be treated with antiviral drugs. However, further studies are needed. A small series of liver transplant patients immunized with measles vaccine showed a rather poor response (seven of 18 immunized seroconverted), but no vaccine associated side effects were found (68).

REFERENCES

1. Lum L, Seigneuret M, Storb R. The transfer of antigen-specific humoral immunity from marrow donors to marrow recipients. *J Clin Immunol* 1986;6:389–396.
2. Lum L. The kinetics of immune reconstitution after human marrow transplantation. *Blood* 1987;69:369–380.
3. Lum L, Noges J, Beatty P, et al. Transfer of specific immunity in marrow recipients given HLA-mismatched, T cell-depleted, or HLA-identical marrow grafts. *Bone Marrow Transplant* 1988;3:399–406.
4. Lum L. Effects of acute and chronic GVHD on immune recovery after BMT. In: Burakoff SJ, et al., eds. *Graft-vs-host disease.* New York: Marcel Dekker; 1990:369–380.
5. Saxon A, Mitsuyaso R, Stevens R, et al. Transfer of specific immune responses after bone marrow transplantation. *J Clin Invest* 1986;78:959–967.
6. Wahren B, Gahrton G, Linde A, et al. Transfer and persistence of viral antibody-producing cells in bone marrow transplantation. *J Infect Dis* 1984;150:358–365.
7. Witherspoon R, Storb R, Ochs H, et al. Recovery of antibody production in human allogeneic marrow graft recipients: influence of time posttransplantation, the presence or absence of chronic graft-versus-host disease, and antithymocyte globulin treatment. *Blood* 1981;58:360–368.
8. Witherspoon R, Matthews D, Storb R, et al. Recovery of *in vivo* cellular immunity after human marrow grafting. Influence of time postgrafting and acute graft-versus-host disease. *Transplantation* 1984;37:145–150.
9. Wimperis J, Brenner M, Prentice H, et al. Transfer of a functioning humoral immune system in transplantation of T-lymphocyte-depleted bone marrow. *Lancet* 1986;1:339–343.
10. Ilan Y, Nagler A, Adler R, et al. Ablation of persistent hepatitis B by bone marrow transplantation from a hepatitis B-immune donor. *Gastroenterology* 1993;104:1818–1821.
11. Brugger S, Oesterreicher C, Hofmann H, et al. Hepatitis B virus clearance by transplantation of bone marrow from hepatitis B immunized donor. *Lancet* 1997;349:996–997.
12. Ljungman P, Levensohn-Fuchs I, Hammarström V, et al. Long-term immunity to measles, mumps and rubella after allogeneic bone marrow transplantation. *Blood* 1994;84:657–664.
13. Ljungman P, Wiklund HM, Duraj V, et al. Response to tetanus toxoid immunization after allogeneic bone marrow transplantation. *J Infect Dis* 1990;162:496–500.
14. Ljungman P, Duraj V, Magnius L. Response to immunization against polio after allogeneic marrow transplantation. *Bone Marrow Transplant* 1991;7:89–93.
15. Engelhard D, Handsher R, Naparstek E, et al. Immune responses to polio vaccination in bone marrow transplant recipients. *Bone Marrow Transplant* 1991;8:295–300.
16. Hammarström V, Pauksen K, Svensson H et al. Tetanus immunity in patients with haematological malignancies. *Support Care Cancer* 1998 (*in press*).
17. Aschan J, Ringdén O, Ljungman P, et al. Influenza B in transplant patients. *Scand J Infect Dis* 1989;21:349–50.
18. Ljungman P, Andersson J, Aschan J, et al. Influenza A in immunocompromised patients. *Clin Infect Dis* 1993;17:244–247.
19. Whimbey E, Elting L, Couch R, et al. Influenza A virus infections among hospitalized adult bone marrow transplant recipients. *Bone Marrow Transplant* 1994;13:437–440.
20. Engelhard D, Nagler A, Hardan I. Antibody response to a two-dose regimen of influenza vaccine in allogeneic T cell-depleted and autologous BMT recipients. *Bone Marrow Transplant* 1993;11:1–5.
21. Sauerbrei A, Prager J, Hengst U, et al. Varicella vaccination in children after bone marrow transplantation. *Bone Marrow Transplant* 1997;20:381–383.

22. Redman R, Nader S, Zerboni L, et al. Early reconstitution of immunity and decreased severity of herpes zoster in bone marrow transplant recipients immunized with inactivated varicella vaccine. *J Infect Dis* 1997;176:578–585.

23. Cordonnier C, Bernaudin J, Bierling P, et al. Pulmonary complications occurring after allogeneic bone marrow transplantation. A study of 130 consecutive transplanted patients. *Cancer* 1986;58:1047–1054.

24. Aucotourier P, Barra A, Intrator I, et al. Long-lasting IgG subclass and antibacterial polysaccharide antibody deficiency after allogeneic bone marrow transplantation. *Blood* 1987;70:779–785.

25. Winston D, Schiffman L, Wang D, et al. Pneumococcal infection after human bone marrow transplantation. *Ann Intern Med* 1979;91: 835–841.

26. Parkkali T, Kayhty H, Ruutu T, et al. A comparison of early and late vaccination with *Haemophilus influenzae* type B conjugate and pneumococcal polysaccharide vaccines after allogeneic BMT. *Bone Marrow Transplant* 1996;18:961–967.

27. Avanzini M, Carra A, Macccario R, et al. Antibody response to pneumococcal vaccine in children receiving bone marrow transplantation. *J Clin Immunol* 1995;15:137–144.

28. Guinan E, Molrine D, Antin J, et al. Polysaccharide conjugate vaccine response in bone marrow transplant recipients. *Transplantation* 1994;57:677–684.

29. Hammarström V, Pauksen K, Azinge J, et al. The influence of graft versus host reaction on the response to pneumococcal vaccination in bone marrow transplant patients. *J Support Care Cancer* 1993;1:195–199.

30. Barra A, Cordonnier C, Preziosi M, et al. Immunogenicity of *Haemophilus influenzae* type B conjugate vaccine in allogeneic bone marrow recipients. *J Infect Dis* 1992;166:1021–1028.

31. Lortan J, Vellodi A, Jurges E, et al. Class- and subclass-specific pneumococcal antibody levels and response to immunization after bone marrow transplantation. *Clin Exp Immunol* 1992;88:512–519.

32. Molrine D, Guinan E, Antin J, et al. Donor immunization with *Haemophilus influenzae* type B (HIB)-conjugate vaccine in allogeneic bone marrow transplantation. *Blood* 1996;87:3012–3018.

33. Lum L, Munn N, Schanfield M, et al. The detection of specific antibody formation to recall antigens after human bone marrow transplantation. *Blood* 1986;67:582–587.

34. Prager J, Baumert A, Thilo W, et al. Untersuchungen zur Kinetik der Impfantikörper gegen Tetanustoxoid, Diphterietoxoid, Masern-virus, Poliomyelitis-virus und Pneumokokken nach allogener und autologer Knochenmarktransplantation und Wiederholungsimpfung. Teil 3: Kinetik der Impfantikörper gegen Tetanustoxoid nach allogener und autologer Knochenmarktransplantation und kombinierter Wiederholungsimpfung gegen Diphterie and Tetanus. *Kinderarztl Prax* 1992;60: 230–238.

35. Parkkali T, Ölander R-M, Ruutu T, et al. A randomized comparison between early and late vaccination with tetanus toxoid vaccine after allogeneic BMT. *Bone Marrow Transplant* 1997;19:933–938.

36. Parkkali T, Stenvik M, Ruutu T, et al. Randomized comparison of early and late vaccination with inactivated poliovirus vaccine after allogeneic BMT. *Bone Marrow Transplant* 1997;20:663–668.

37. Machado C, Goncalves F, Pannuti C, et al. Measles in BMT recipients during an outbreak in Saol Paulo, Brazil. ICAAC abstract LB-24, Toronto, Canada, 1997.

38. Ljungman P, Fridell E, Lönnqvist B, et al. Efficacy and safety of vaccination of marrow transplant recipients with a live attenuated measles, mumps, and rubella vaccine. *J Infect Dis* 1989;159:610–615.

39. Rio B, Marjanovic Z, Lévy V, et al. Vaccination for yellow fever after bone marrow transplantation. *Bone Marrow Transplant* 1996;17[Suppl. 1]:S95– .

40. Pauksen K, Duraj V, Ljungman P, et al. Immunity to and immunization against measles, rubella and mumps in patients after autologous bone marrow transplantation. *Bone Marrow Transplant* 1992;9:427–432.

41. Pauksen K, Hammarström V, Ljungman P, et al. Immunity to poliovirus and immunization with inactivated poliovaccine after autologous bone marrow transplantation. *Clin Infect Dis* 1994;18:547–552.

42. Nagler A, Ilan Y, Adler R, et al. Successful immunization of autologous bone marrow transplantation recipients against hepatitis B virus by active vaccination. *Bone Marrow Transplant* 1995;15:475–478.

43. Molrine D, Guinan E, Antin J, et al. *Haemophilus influenzae* type B (HIB)-conjugate immunization before bone marrow harvest in autologous bone marrow transplantation. *Bone Marrow Transplant* 1996;17: 1149–1155.

44. Hammarström V, Pauksen K, Björkstrand B, Simonsson B, Öberg G,

Ljungman P. Tetanus immunity in autologous bone marrow and blood stem cell transplant recipients. *Bone Marrow Transplant* 1998;22:67–72.

45. Pauksen K, Linde A, Lönnerholm G, et al. Influence of the specific T-cell response on seroconversion after measles vaccination in autologous bone marrow transplant patients. *Bone Marrow Transplant* 1996;18: 969–973.

46. Crosnier J, Junges P, Courouce A-M, et al. Randomized placebo-controlled trial of hepatitis B surface antigen vaccine in French haemodialysis units. II. Haemodialysis patients. *Lancet* 1981;2:797–800.

47. Stevens C, Alter H, Taylor P, et al. Hepatitis B virus vaccine in patients receiving hemodialysis: immunogenecity and efficacy. *N Engl J Med* 1984;311:496–501.

48. Sokal E, Ulla L, Otte J. Hepatitis B vaccine response before and after transplantation in 55 extrahepatic biliary atresia children. *Dig Dis Sci* 1992;37:1250–1252.

49. Van Thiel D, el-Ashmawy L, Love K, et al. Response to hepatitis B vaccination by liver transplant candidates. *Dig Dis Sci* 1992;37: 1245–1249.

50. Turik M, Markowitz S. A successful regimen for the prevention of seroconversion after transplantation of a heart positive for hepatitis B surface antigen. *J Heart Lung Transplant* 1992;11:781–783.

51. Carey W, Pimentel R, Westweer M, et al. Failure of hepatitis B immunization in liver transplant patients: results of a prospective trial. *Am J Gastroenterol* 1990;85:1590–1592.

52. Plotkin S, Higgins R, Kurtz J, et al. Multicenter trial of Towne Strain attenuated virus vaccine in seronegative renal transplant recipients. *Transplantation* 1994;58:1176–1178.

53. Plotkin SA, Starr S, Friedman H, et al. Effect of Towne live virus vaccine on cytomegalovirus disease after renal transplant. A controlled trial. *Ann Intern Med* 1991;114:525–531.

54. Broyer M, Boudailliez B. Varicella vaccine in children with chronic renal insufficiency. *Postgrad Med J* 1985;61[Suppl 4]:103–106.

55. Broyer M, Tete M, Guest G, et al. Varicella and zoster in children after kidney transplantation: long-term results of vaccination. *Pediatrics* 1997;99:35–39.

56. Linnemann CJ, First M, Schiffman G. Response to pneumococcal vaccine in renal transplant and hemodialysis patients. *Arch Intern Med* 1981;141:pp# TK

57. Furth S, Neu A, Case B, et al. Pneumococcal polysaccharide vaccine in children with chronic renal disease: a prospective study of antibody response and duration. *J Pediatr* 1996;128:99–101.

58. Vento S, Garofano T, Renzini C, et al. Fulminant hepatitis associated with hepatitis A virus superinfection in patients with chronic hepatitis C. *N Engl J Med* 1998;338:286–290.

59. Wagner D, Wagenbreth I, Stachan-Kunstyr R, et al. Failure of vaccination against hepatitis B with Gen H-B-Vax-D in immunosuppressed heart transplant patients. *J Infect Dis* 1992;166:1021–1028.

60. Wagner D, Wagenbreth I, Stachan-Kunstyr R, et al. Hepatitis B vaccination of immunosuppressed heart transplant recipients with the vaccine Hepa gene 3 containing pre-S1, pre-S2, and S gene products. *Clin Invest* 1994;72:240–252.

61. CDC. Prevention and control of influenza. Recommendations of the Immunization Practices Advisory Committee (ACIP). *Morb Mortal Wkly Rep* 1992;41:1–17.

62. Versluis D, Beyer W, Masurel N, et al. Impairment of the immune response to influenza vaccination in renal transplant recipients by cyclosporine, but not azathioprine. *Transplantation* 1986;42:376–379.

63. Blumberg E, Albano C, Pruett T, et al. The immunogenecity of influenza virus in solid organ transplant recipients. *Clin Infect Dis* 1996;23:295–302.

64. Mauch T, Crouch N, Freese D, et al. Antibody response of pediatric solid organ transplant recipients to immunization against influenza virus. *J Pediatr* 1995;127:957–960.

65. Furth S, Neu A, McColley S, et al. Immune response to influenza vaccination in children with renal disease. *Pediatr Nephrol* 1995;9: 566–568.

66. Dengler T, Strnad N, Zimmermann R, et al. Pneumococcal vaccination after heart and liver transplantation. Immune responses in immunosuppressed patients and in healthy controls. *Deutsche Medizinische Wochenschrift* 1996;121:1519–1525.

67. Zamora I, Simon J, Da Silva M, et al. Attenuated varicella virus vaccine in children with renal transplants. *Pediatr Nephrol* 1994;8: 190–192.

68. Rand E, McCarthy C, Whitington P. Measles vaccination after orthoptic liver transplantation. *J Pediatr* 1993;123:87–89.

Transplant Infections edited by
Raleigh A. Bowden, Per Ljungman, and Carlos V. Paya.
Lippincott–Raven Publishers, Philadelphia © 1998

CHAPTER 26

Granulocyte Transfusions

David C. Dale

Granulocyte transfusions—or, more precisely, neutrophil transfusions—have been considered for many years as a direct approach to correcting the problem of neutropenia. Ideally, it should be possible to replace these cells in the blood and their function in preventing and containing infection by collecting cells from a normal donor and transfusing them to a deficient host. For a number of reasons, however, supportive care for neutrophil transfusions has not developed to parallel erythrocyte and platelet transfusions. Recently, the discovery and development of the colony-stimulating factors, particularly granulocyte colony-stimulating factor (G-CSF), has revived interest in this area. This chapter reviews the physiological principles underlying the collection and transfusion of neutrophils, the results of clinical trials, and the current status of this therapy.

NEUTROPHIL PHYSIOLOGY

All blood cells are derived from common hematopoietic stem cells. At an early stage in differentiation some of these cells become committed to the granulocyte-monocyte lineage from which neutrophils develop. It is estimated that normally 10–14 days are required for a neutrophil to form from the earliest identifiable cell of the neutrophilic lineage (1,2). For the first 4–8 days of this period, cells are dividing and recognizable as myeloblasts, promyelocytes, and myelocytes (the mitotic pool), after which cell division stops and the cells mature sequentially to metamyelocytes, bands, and mature neutrophils (the postmitotic pool). For many years it has been recognized that the time periods for the steps in cell development are variable. With stress or infection, cell formation can accelerate considerably (3). In the basal state the bone marrow of the normal adult produces about 1.0×10^{11}

neutrophils per day (4). When the cells are fully mature as recognized by the segmentation of the nuclear chromatin, they leave the extravascular space of the marrow and enter the blood, where they circulate with a blood halflife, usually estimated to be around 6–10 hours (4). Etiocholanolone, endotoxin, and corticosteroids are well-studied agents that raise neutrophil levels principally by accelerating the movement of neutrophils and "bands" from the marrow to the blood (5). In the blood only about half of the total population of neutrophils is freely circulating; the other half is in the microcirculation or loosely adherent to vascular walls from which it can be mobilized by stimuli that increase cardiac output, such as exercise or epinephrine infusion. The freely circulating cells are usually regarded as being in the circulating pool, and those in the microcirculation and adherent to vascular walls are considered to belong to the marginal pool. In man the spleen sequesters neutrophils in some pathological states, but ordinarily does not contain a disproportionate number of marginated cells (Table 1).

Neutrophils serve predominantly as tissue phagocytic cells, accumulating in the first phase of the normal tissue response to infection or injury and many types of inflammatory stimuli. At the tissue site, bacteria and foreign debris are phagocytized, and the neutrophil's cytoplasmic granules fuse with the phagosome, which contains the ingested material. Microbes are killed by the combined actions of reactive oxygen species, halide ions, and microbicidal proteins contained in the neutrophil granules (6).

COLONY-STIMULATING FACTORS

Over recent decades many details have been added to our understanding of neutrophil physiology and function. The discovery of the hematopoietic growth factors was one of the most important developments (7). It is now recognized that several factors regulate neutrophil development (Fig. 1). Granulocytic colony-stimulating factor

From the Department of Medicine, University of Washington, Seattle, WA 98117-6422.

TABLE 1. *Key blood cell kinetic measurements related to neutrophil transfusion therapy*

Neutrophil Kinetics		
	Average life span: 10 hours	
	T_{fi}: 6.6 hours	
	Turnover rate (daily production): 180×10^7/kg body weight/day	
	Released into circulation daily: 1.0×10^{11}/l	
Comparison	Average Life Span	% of Circulating Cells Consumed Daily
Red Blood Cell:	90 days	0.8%
Platelet:	10 days	10%
Neutrophils:	0.4 days	200% to 300%
Approximate Quantities of Neutrophils in Various Pools		
Marrow storage pool (mobilizable)	1.3×10^{11}/l	
Circulating pool (available for collection)	2.0×10^{10}/l	
Marginating pool (unavailable for collection)	2.0×10^{10}/l	

From Maakestad et al. (Ref. 31).
Adapted from Athens, J.W. (1961) Leukokinetic studies. IV. The total blood, circulating, and marginal granulocyte pools and the granulocyte turnover rate in normal subjects. *J Clin Invest* 40:989–95; and Wright, D. G. (1984) Symposium on infectious complications of neoplastic disease (part II). Leukocyte transfusions: thinking twice. *Am J Med* 76:637–44.

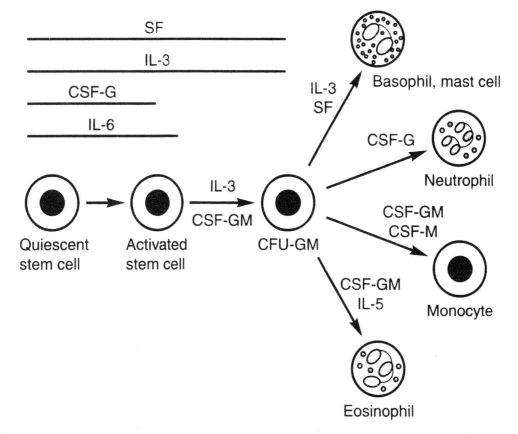

Figure 1. Schema for formation of basophils, neutrophils, monocytes, and eosinophils from hematopoietic stem cells. Figure illustrates probable sites for major effects of stem cell factor (SCF) interleukin-3 (IL-3), granulocyte colony-stimulating factor (G-CSF), interleukin-6 (IL-6), granulocyte-macrophage colony-stimulating factor (GM-CSF), macrophage colony-stimulating factor (M-CSF), and interleukin-5 (IL-5). G-CSF is the critical factor for maintaining the neutrophil supply (see text).

(G-CSF) regulates all phases of neutrophil development, including the time spent in the postmitotic pool in the marrow and the number of neutrophils in the blood (8–11). Granulocyte-macrophage colony-stimulating factor (GM-CSF) shares many *in vitro* properties with G-CSF (12), but data from gene "knock-out" experiments and other studies indicate that it is not necessary for maintenance of normal neutrophil production or blood levels (13). The finding that both neutrophil precursors and the mature cells have receptors for both G-CSF and GM-CSF suggests that these factors may act in concert in regulating the early stages of neutrophil production as well as the function of mature cells at inflammatory foci. *In vivo* studies have shown that both G-CSF and GM-CSF accelerate neutrophil development through the differentiation and maturation process in the marrow (11,14). *In vitro* exposure of mature neutrophils to either cytokine primes the cells for an accentuated response when exposed *in vitro* to particles or bacteria. In addition, both G-CSF and GM-CSF prolong neutrophil survival through an antiapoptotic effects (15).

When normal subjects are administered G-CSF or GM-CSF, there is a dose-dependent and time-dependent increase in the blood neutrophil levels. Initially, a modest decrease in neutrophil levels may occur, followed by a rapid increase in blood neutrophil counts, attributable to influx of cells from the postmitotic marrow pool or marrow neutrophil "reserves." These effects are quite similar to those observed after endotoxin administration. Of importance for collecting cells for transfusion, the physiologic limits of this acute response are not fully known. When G-CSF administration is continued on a daily basis, there is a further dose-dependent increase in the counts because of the stimulation of cell production (16). The levels measured in the blood are thus dependent both on the duration of treatment and on the time after the dose when the blood cell count is measured. With daily dosing, large-scale oscillations recur with peak levels occurring 6–12 hours after the dose; counts then decline toward the previous day's level and return to normal in 2–3 days (16).

GM-CSF administration causes an increase in blood neutrophils that is substantially less than G-CSF (1,17). It also increases blood monocytes and eosinophils. Because the marrow does not normally have a storage pool of monocytes and eosinophils, these increases generally take several days to develop. Because of its lesser potency in acutely raising blood neutrophil levels, plus greater frequency and severity of side effects in normal subjects, GM-CSF generally has not been used as a stimulus of donors for neutrophil transfusion therapy.

STUDIES OF NEUTROPHIL TRANSFUSIONS

The historical development of neutrophil transfusion therapy can be divided into four eras. In the first era (the 1930s and 1940s), a few reports indicate that "buffy coats" were collected from peripheral blood and injected intramuscularly or intravenously. In 1934, Strumia reported that these "leukocyte cream" injections increase the blood neutrophil levels in nine of 10 patients with neutropenia (18). The benefits of this treatment are unknown. In 1953, Brecher and colleagues demonstrated in experimental animals that transfused neutrophils could circulate and migrate to a site of inflammation (19). These were the first studies providing a clear physiological basis for neutrophil transfusion therapy.

No clinically important developments occurred until Freireich and colleagues began using cells from patients with chronic myelogenous leukemia in support of febrile neutropenic cancer patients around 1960 (20). These investigators then reported that approximately 54% of transfused patients receiving approximately 3×10^{11} cells became afebrile with 36 hours of transfusion. The lack of donors, the risk of transferring infectious diseases, and concern about transplantation of the malignancy, however, limited the use of this therapy (21).

The third era began with the development of methods for neutrophil collection from normal donors by centrifuge leukapheresis. In the mid-1960s investigators at the National Institute of Health, with support from the International Business Machines Corporation, developed the continuous-flow centrifuge for separating blood cells on the basis of their density (22). They found that they could achieve a blood flow rate of approximately 40 ml/min through the centrifuge and that they could collect an average of 5×10^9 granulocytes from a normal donor in a 3–4-hour period. This represented a 14% efficiency of collection (cells collected divided by cells passing through the centrifuge) (21) (Fig. 2). The efficiency of lymphocyte collection was actually better than the collection of neutrophils because these cells are denser and separate faster from the erythrocytes than the neutrophils. Soon thereafter corticosteroids (usually prednisone or dexamethasone) or the androgen metabolite etiocholanolone was introduced to raise the count of the donor and increase the harvest of cells (23). To improve collections further, hydroxyethyl starch was added to the blood before it entered the centrifuge (24). It accelerated red blood cell sedimentation, causing rouleaux formation. By the early 1970s routine use of hydroxyethyl starch and pretreatment of donors with corticosteroids allowed collection of up to $1-3 \times 10^{10}$ neutrophils in a 3-hour leukapheresis (21).

In retrospect, it is unfortunate that a competing technology for neutrophil collection, filtration leukapheresis, developed in this same era. Filtration of leukapheresis involved passing heparinized blood through a nylon-fiber filter, collecting neutrophils selectively because of their adherence to the fibers (25). This allowed the collection of larger numbers of cells with higher efficiency than continuous blood centrifugation, but the cells were damaged in

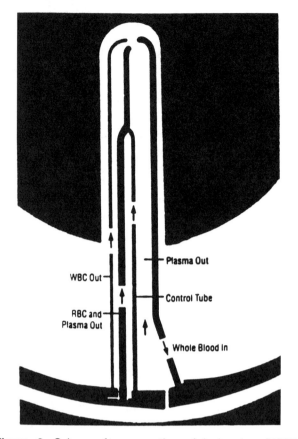

Figure 2. Schema for separation of leukocytes (WBC), plasma, and erythrocytes from peripheral blood by continuous-flow centrifugation. As blood enters the centrifuge bowl, hydroxyethyl starch is added and erythrocytes move quickly to the periphery. Leukocytes are somewhat lighter and move more slowly, forming a band at the interfaces of the RBCs and plasma. WBC are removed with some RBCs and a substantial number of platelets by the port set at this interface.

the collection procedure (26,27). Without full appreciation of the damage done to the cells, a number of clinical trials were done with cells collected by this method or with some donors collected by centrifugation and others by filtration leukapheresis. This contributed to confusion in interpreting the results of these studies and probably caused some of the negative results that were observed.

Over the next few years, several clinical trials of granulocyte transfusions were conducted and have been summarized in several reports (28–31). The results of controlled trials of neutrophil transfusions in adults between 1972 were summarized by Strauss (Table 2) (30). The first major trial reported 100% survival of cancer patients receiving four transfusions, versus 30% survival in a control group, a contemporary group without a suitable donor (32). A second study largely confirmed these findings (76% survival in the transfused group versus 26% for the controls), but subsequent studies showed lesser benefits (33). As shown in Table 1, survival for the control groups in all subsequent studies varied substantially, although overall survival for all studies after the initial trial by Graw was much higher. Vogler and Winton (34) reported that patients with prolonged neutropenia seemed to benefit most and that patients receiving less than 0.3×10^{10} neutrophils showed no response to this therapy. In the trial by Alavi and colleagues, patients with a relatively good prognosis were included, and no differences were observed (35). In the study by Winston and colleagues, survival in the control group was also high (36), and it is not surprising that there was no higher survival with the transfusion therapy. In this study a mean of only 0.5×10^{10} cells were transfused.

By the late 1970s the results of these trials had dampened enthusiasm for neutrophil transfusions in adults. There was a brief period of enthusiasm for prophylactic neutrophil transfusions (37,38), but this passed because the cost of this treatment was so high and the benefits uncertain. For children, however, including those with chronic granulomatous disease and neonates with presumed sepsis, results were considerably more promising (39,40). This is because large numbers of cells could be collected from healthy adults and transfused into the small recipients.

The fourth era began in the early 1990s with studies of administration of G-CSF to normal subjects, studies that showed in greater detail than those earlier how G-CSF can induce neutrophilia with minimal adverse effects (11). In 1993, Bensinger and colleagues reported on the effects of daily administration of G-CSF to eight normal volunteers who then became donors of neutrophils for

TABLE 2. *Controlled trials of neutrophil transfusions in adults*

| First author | Year | No. of patients transfused | % Survival | | Efficacy |
			Transfused	Control	
Graw	1972	76	46%	30%	Partial
Higby	1975	36	76%	26%	Yes
Fortuny	1975	39	78%	80%	No
Vogler	1977	30	59%	15%	Yes
Alavi	1977	31	80%	62%	Partial
Herzig	1977	27	75%	36%	Yes
Winston	1982	95	63%	72%	No

From Maakestad et al. (Ref. 31).
Adapted from Strauss RG (30).

their relatives undergoing bone marrow transplantation (41). The neutrophil donors were syngeneic (5), HLA-identical (2), or haplo-identical (1) twins. The donors were given G-CSF (3.5–6 μg/kg/day) for 9–14 days, so that a series of collections was done from each donor (mean 7.6 donations, range 4–12). The treatment of the donors was well tolerated except that they became mildly anemic from having donated both bone marrow and substantial numbers of red cells through the neutrophil collection procedures. Although the precollection neutrophil levels varied considerably (11.8–79.8 × 10^9/L, mean 29.6 × 10^9/L), the blood neutrophil counts were considerably higher than previously achieved with steroid treated donors. Similarly, the number of neutrophils collected was substantially larger (mean 41.6 × 10^9, range 1.3–144 × 10^9). Most remarkably, by comparison with earlier studies, the mean neutrophil level was 0.95 × 10^9/L at 24 hours after a transfusion of these cells into the severely neutropenic recipients. The greater number of cells collected could easily be attributed to the higher circulating counts of the donors. The higher levels in the recipients were attributed to the large number of cells that were transfused and the anti-apoptotic effects of G-CSF. The unique aspect of this study was the use of syngeneic twins and HLA-identical donors, thus avoiding concern about alloimmunization. Good transfusion increments were seen throughout the period in which the neutrophil transfusions were administered. This study thus showed that it is feasible to collect neutrophils repeatedly from the same donor without depleting the donor's neutrophil supply.

Casper and colleagues performed a similar study using normal community volunteers as donors (42). They collected a mean of 44 ± 16 × 10^9 cells per leukapheresis performed 12–16 hours after 300 μg of G-CSF. As in almost all recent studies, including the studies of Bensinger, they utilized hydroxyethyl starch in the collection procedure, but in contrast to this study they irradiated the cells to prevent graft-versus-host disease. With serial counts, they estimated a blood halflife of the transfused cells of about 9–12 hours. They also evaluated neutrophil function and found that cells from the G-CSF treated donors functioned normally (42).

Subsequently, several studies have now confirmed that 40–50 × 10^9 neutrophils can be collected from donors treated with daily doses of 300–600 μg of G-CSF with essentially normal functional properties of the cells. To try to collect even larger numbers of neutrophils, investigators have reexamined the use of starch (43,44) and studied the combination of G-CSF plus dexamethasone for the mobilization of neutrophils in normal subjects. In one study, five normal subjects were randomly assigned to receive (a) G-CSF 300 μg subcutaneously, (b) G-CSF 600 μg subcutaneously, (c) dexamethasone 800 mg orally, (d) G-GSF 300 μg subcutaneously plus dexamethasone 8 mg orally, and (e) G-CSF 600 μg subcuta-

neously plus dexamethasone 8 mg orally. Blood counts were performed at 0, 6, 12, and 24 hours. The results showed that the greatest increases in blood neutrophils occurred with the higher dose of G-CSF plus dexamethasone. The mean baseline counts were 3.5 × 10^9/L and increased to 43 × 10^9/L at 12 hours with this treatment. These results suggested that this combination of agents with the accompanying greater degree of neutrophilia would permit collection of twice as many neutrophils as with G-CSF alone.

Using a pretreatment protocol of G-CSF 600 μg subcutaneously and dexamethasone 8 mg orally 12 hours before leukapheresis, recent studies have shown that 75–100 × 10^9 neutrophils can be routinely collected from community donors without significant adverse effects (46). Studies of the morphological and functional properties of these cells—including their *in vitro* surface properties, metabolic burst responses to several stimuli, and bactericidal functions—showed that the neutrophils had a normal morphology, maintained a normal inducible respiratory burst, and had a normal bactericidal activity against *Staphylococcus aureus*. There was some decrease in cell surface expression of the leukocyte adhesion protein CD11b/CD18 and reduced expression of L-selectin and CD16 on the cell surface, as has been noted previously for neutrophils from G-CSF-treated subjects. When the neutrophils were labeled radioisotopically and reinfused, they had prolonged blood halflife. Preliminary data on transfusion of cells from donors stimulated with G-CSF plus dexamethasone indicate that recipients have very substantial increments in their counts, and these increases last for 24 hours or more.

Using this protocol, which raises the neutrophil count so quickly, makes it feasible to locate and treat donors and to collect and transfuse enough cells to potentially give clinical benefit within less than 24 hours. As yet, however, there are no controlled trials critical for defining the benefits of transfusing the large number of neutrophils that can be collected from G-CSF/dexamethasone-stimulated donors. A few preliminary reports, however, suggest that this may be an efficacious approach to the problem of severe bacterial and fungal infections after bone marrow transplantation (47–49). They have not been studied for treatment of infections after solid organ transplantation, when the risk of neutropenia is low.

UNRESOLVED ISSUES

Many old and new questions are raised by these recent findings, and a sense of urgency to answer them is engendered by the severity of the susceptibility to infection that accompanies severe neutropenia and immunosuppression after bone marrow transplantation. Some important issues are the following:

1. What is the optimal treatment for the donors? Is one or are several doses of G-CSF better to optimize the

number and function of the cells that can be collected? Some data suggest that neutrophils may acquire enhanced functional properties if the donor is treated for several days with G-CSF. The magnitude and significance of this effect need to be evaluated.

2. How important is the dose of G-CSF? Higher doses give higher cell numbers but add to the cost of cell collection. With higher G-CSF doses, the fully mature neutrophils with the greatest functional properties may be diluted by the influx to the blood of less mature cells recruited from the marrow.

3. Is the combination of G-CSF with a corticosteroid truly beneficial? It is clear that the combination of agents improves cell collection, but does it have a deleterious effect on cell function? Further studies are needed.

4. Are there adverse effects or significant risks to treating normal donors with these agents? G-CSF is produced endogenously and is the natural regulator of the blood neutrophil count. It has very few acute side effects. It will be extremely difficult to evaluate long-term risk of treating donors with this cytokine. Several experts have, however, recommended that long-term data should be collected to evaluate the safety (50).

5. Which patients could benefit from high-dose neutrophil transfusions? Intuitively, patients with severe bacterial and fungal infections after bone marrow transplantation are at extremely high risk, but they often have a poor prognosis because of graft failure, recurrence of their underlying disease and other factors. Defining the proper patient population for transfusion should be investigated through controlled trials.

6. Is it necessary to match donors and recipients for neutrophil transfusions? A number of reports indicate that, as for platelet and red blood cell transfusions, histocompatibility is important for neutrophil transfusions. For short-term support, however, unmatched donors may prove satisfactory, as with random donor platelet support. Studies are under way to address this question.

7. What is the optimal frequency of transfusion? Can the blood neutrophil level be used as a surrogate similar to the platelet count for platelet support? Heretofore, neutrophils were transfused as frequently as possible because of the low numbers that could be collected and their short survival as reflected by serial counts after transfusions. With cells from G-CSF-treated donors considerable data will be needed to establish transfusion frequency. Conceivably, transfusion at more than 24-hour intervals will prove efficacious and may be more cost-effective.

8. How much will neutrophil transfusion therapy add to the cost of bone marrow transplantation? This will undoubtedly be an expensive modality of supportive care because of the specialized equipment required for cell collection, the cost of the drugs, and the expertise required. If transfusions prove efficacious, however, prevention or accelerated recovery from serious infection in the bone marrow transplant unit could prove to be both a life-saving and a cost-saving therapy.

9. Would patients without neutropenia (i.e., patients after marrow or solid organ transplant with abnormal neutrophil function secondary to immunosuppressive therapy) benefit from transfusion of neutrophils from normal donors?

SUMMARY

Neutrophil transfusion therapy is a logical approach to preventing or treating infection in the neutropenic host. Despite many innovations, it has proven very difficult to collect and transfuse enough cells from normal subjects to prove that this is an efficacious therapy. Recently, however, several groups have shown that mobilization of neutrophils from the bone marrow to the blood with G-CSF raises the blood neutrophil count several-fold and allows the collection of large numbers of normally functioning neutrophils. Even greater numbers can be collected from normal donors treated with a combination of G-CSF plus a corticosteroid (e.g., dexamethasone). Forty to 80×10^9 neutrophils can be collected after administration of these agents. This is a sufficient quantity to raise the blood neutrophil count to a normal level in a severely neutropenic patient. In addition, these cells have a long blood halflife, allowing for the maintenance of a near normal neutrophil level in the blood for many hours after the transfusions are administered. Preliminary data suggest that this approach may be an important advance in supportive care of neutropenic bone marrow transplant patients, but carefully controlled clinical trials are needed to prove the efficacy of this approach to therapy.

REFERENCES

1. Babior BM, Golde DW. Production, distribution, and fate of neutrophils. In: Beutler E, Lichtman MA, Coller BS, Kipps TJ, eds. *Williams hematology.* New York: McGraw-Hill; 1995:773–779.
2. Athens JW, Raab SO, Haab OP, et al. The distribution of granulocytes in the blood of normal subjects. *J Clin Invest* 1961;40:159–164.
3. Marsh JC, Boggs DR, Cartwright GE, Wintrobe MM. Neutrophil kinetics in acute infection. *J Clin Invest* 1967;46:1943–1953.
4. Dancey JT, Deubelbeiss KA, Harker LA, Finch CA. Neutrophil kinetics in man. *J Clin Invest* 1976;58:705–715.
5. Dale DC, Fauci AS, Guerry D, Wolff SM. Comparison of agents producing a neutrophilic leukocytosis in man: hydrocortisone, prednisone, endotoxin and etiocholanolone. *J Clin Invest* 1975;58:808–813.
6. Smolen JE, Boxer LA. Functions of neutrophils. In: Beutler E, Lichtman MA, Coller BS, Kipps TJ, eds. *Williams hematology.* New York: McGraw-Hill; 1995:779–798.
7. Lieschke GJ, Burgess AW. Granulocyte colony-stimulating factor and granulocyte-macrophage colony-stimulating factor. *N Engl J Med* 1992;327:28–35, 99–106.
8. Demetri GD, Griffin JD. Granulocyte colony-stimulating factor and its receptor. *Blood* 1991;78:2791–2808.
9. Hammond WP, Sciba E, Canin A, Sousa LM, Dale DC. Chronic neu-

tropenia: a new canine model induced by G-CSF. *J Clin Invest* 1991;87: 704–710.

10. Lieschke GJ, Grail D, Hodgson G, et al. Mice lacking granulocyte colony-stimulating factor have chronic neutropenia, granulocyte and macrophage progenitor cell deficiency, and impaired neutrophil mobilization. *Blood* 1994;84:1737–1746.

11. Price TH, Chatta GS, Dale DC. The effect of recombinant granulocyte colony-stimulating factor on neutrophil kinetics in normal young and elderly humans. *Blood* 1996;88:335–340.

12. Gasson JC. Molecular physiology of granulocyte-macrophage colony-stimulating factor. *Blood* 1991;77:1131–1145.

13. Stanley E, Lieschke GJ, Grail D, et al. Granulocyte/macrophage colony-stimulating factor-deficient mice show no major perturbation of hematopoiesis but develop a characteristic pulmonary pathology. *Proc Natl Acad Sci U S A* 1994;91:5592–5596.

14. Aglietta M, Piacibello W, Sanavio F, et al. Kinetics of human haematopoietic cells after *in vivo* administration of granulocyte-macrophage colony-stimulating factor. *J Clin Invest* 1989;83:551.

15. Dale DC, Liles WC, Summer W, Nelson S. Granulocyte-colony-stimulating factor: role and relationships in infectious diseases. *J Dis* 1995; 172:1061–1075.

16. Chatta GS, Price TH, Allen RC, Dale DC. The effects of *in vivo* recombinant methionyl human granulocyte colony stimulating factor (rhG-CSF) on the neutrophil response and peripheral blood colony forming cells in healthy young and elderly volunteers. *Blood* 1994;84: 2923–2929.

17. Hill ADK, Naama HA, Calvano SE, Daly JM. The effect of granulocyte-macrophage colony-stimulating factor on myeloid cells and its clinical applications. *J Leukoc Biol* 1995;58:634.

18. Strumia MM. The effect of leukocytic cream injections in the treatment of the neutropenias. *Am J Med Sci* 1934;187:527–544.

19. Brecher G, Wilbur KM, Cronkite EP. Transfusion of separated leukocytes into irradiated dogs with aplastic marrows. *PSEBM* 1953;84:54–56.

20. Freireich EJ, Levin RH, Whang J, et al. The function and fate of transfused leukocytes from donors with chronic myelocytic leukemia in leukopenic recipients. *Ann NY Acad Sci* 1964;113:1081–1089.

21. Boggs DR. Transfusion of neutrophils as prevention or treatment of infection in patients with neutropenia. *N Engl J Med* 1974;290: 1055–1062.

22. Graw RG Jr, Herzig GP, Eisel RJ, et al. Leukocyte and platelet collection from normal donors with the continuous flow blood cell separator. *Transfusion* 1971;11:94–101.

23. Mishler JM, Moser AM, Carter JB. The safety of dexamethasone and hydroxyethyl starch in the multiply leukapheresed donor. *Transfusion* 1976;16:170–173.

24. Mishler JM, Hadlock DC, Fortuny IE, Nicora RW, McCullough JJ. Increased efficiency of leukocyte collection by the addition of hydroxyethyl starch to the continuous flow centrifuge. *Blood* 1974;44: 571–581.

25. Buchholz DH, Schiffer CA, Wiernik PH, Betts SW, Reilly JA. Granulocyte harvest for transfusion: donor response to repeated leukapheresis. *Transfusion* 1975;15:96–106.

26. Klock JC, Stossel TP. Detection, pathogenesis, and prevention of damage to human granulocytes caused by interaction with nylon wool fiber. *J Clin Invest* 1977;60:1183–1190.

27. Price TH, Dale DC. Neutrophil transfusion: the effect of storage and collection method on neutrophil blood kinetics. *Blood* 1978;51: 789–798.

28. Schiffer CA. Granulocyte transfusions: an overlooked therapeutic modality. *Trans Med Rev* 1990;5:2–7.

29. Quie PG. The white cells: use of granulocyte transfusions. *Rev Infect Dis* 1987;9:189–193.

30. Strauss RG. Therapeutic granulocyte transfusions in 1993. *Blood* 1993;7:1675–1678.

31. Makestad K, Mazanet R, Liles WC, Dale DC. Neutrophil transfusions for treatment of infections. In: Morstyn G, Sheridan WP, eds. *Cell therapy.* Cambridge: Cambridge University Press; 1996:510–526.

32. Graw RG, Herzig G, Perry S, et al. Normal granulocytes transfusion therapy: treatment of septicemia due to gram-negative bacteria. *N Engl J Med* 1972;287:367–371.

33. Higby DJ, Yates DW, Henderson ES, et al. Filtration leukapheresis for granulocyte transfusion therapy. *N Engl J Med* 1975;292:761–766.

34. Vogler WR, Winton EF. A controlled study of the efficacy of granulocyte transfusions in patients with neutropenia. *Am J Med* 1977;63: 548–555.

35. Alavi JB, Root RK, Djerassi I, et al. A randomized clinical trial of granulocyte transfusions for infection in acute leukemia. *N Engl J Med* 1977;296:706–711.

36. Winston DJ, Ho WG, Gale RP, et al. Therapeutic granulocyte transfusions for documented infections. *Ann Intern Med* 1982;97:509–515.

37. Winston DJ, Ho WG, Gale RP, et al. Prophylactic granulocyte transfusion therapy during chemotherapy of acute nonlymphocytic leukemia. *Ann Intern Med* 1981;96:616–622.

38. Clift RA, Sanders JE, Thomas ED, et al. Granulocyte transfusions for the prevention of infection in patients receiving bone-marrow transplants. *N Engl J Med* 1978;298:1052–1057.

39. Strauss, RG. Current status of granulocyte transfusions to treat neonatal sepsis. *J Clin Apheresis* 1989;5:25–29.

40. Cairo MS. The role of granulocyte transfusions as adjuvant therapy in the treatment of neonatal sepsis. *Transfus Sci* 1991;12:247–256.

41. Bensinger WI, Price TH, Dale DC, et al. The effects of daily recombinant human granulocyte colony-stimulating factor administration on normal granulocyte donors undergoing leukapheresis. *Blood* 1993;81: 1883–1888.

42. Casper CB, Seger RA, Burger J, et al. Effective stimulation of donors for granulocyte transfusions with recombinant methionyl granulocyte colony-stimulating factor. *Blood* 1993;81:2866–2871.

43. Lee JH, Leitman SF, Klein HG. A controlled comparison of the efficacy of hetastarch and pentastarch in granulocyte collections by centrifugal leukapheresis. *Blood* 1995;86:4662–4666.

44. Lee JH, Cullis H, Leitman SF, Klein HG. Efficacy of pentastarch in granulocyte collection by centrifugal leukapheresis. *J Clin Apheresis* 1995;10:198–202.

45. Liles WC, Huang JE, Llewellyn C, SenGupta D, Price TH, Dale DC. A comparative trial of granulocyte-colony-stimulating factor and dexamethasone, separately and in combination, for the mobilization of neutrophils in the peripheral blood of normal volunteers. *Transfusion* 1997;37:182–187.

46. Dale DC, Liles WC, Llewellyn C, Rodger E, Bowden R, Price TH. Neutrophil transfusion therapy: characteristics and kinetics of cells from donors treated with a combination of G-CSF and dexamethasone. *Blood* 1996;88[Suppl 1]:627a.

47. Fleming R, Anaissie E, O'Brien S, et al. Treatment of neutropenia related fungal infections with G-CSF mobilized granulocytes transfusions in patients with severe neutropenia and life threatening infections. *Blood* 1996;88[Suppl 1]:331a.

48. Leitman SF, Obiltas JM, Emmons R, Dunn DE, Young NS. Clinical efficacy of daily G-CSF-recruited granulocyte transfusions in patients with severe neutropenia and life threatening infections. *Blood* 1996: 88[Suppl 1]:331a.

49. Taylor K, Moore D, Kelly C, et al. Safety and logistical use of filgrastim (FG) mobilised granulocytes (FMG) in early management of severe neutropenic sepsis (SNS) in acute leukemia (AL)/autograft. *Blood* 1996;88[Suppl 1]:349a.

50. Anderlini P, Korbling M, Stoncek D, et al. Consensus conference on the safety of recombinant human granulocyte colony-stimulating factor (rhG-CSF) treatment in normal stem cell donors. *Blood* 1997;90: 903–908.

Transplant Infections edited by
Raleigh A. Bowden, Per Ljungman, and Carlos V. Paya.
Lippincott–Raven Publishers, Philadelphia © 1998

CHAPTER 27

Growth Factors and Other Immunomodulators

John R. Wingard

The risk for infection in the transplant recipient is a function of the interplay between host susceptibility, exposure to an opportunistic microorganism, and inherent virulence of a given microorganism. A variety of pharmacologic agents have been developed to combat pathogenic microorganisms, primarily interfering with their growth and replication. Infection control measures are designed to reduce exposure of a susceptible host to opportunistic pathogens and to prevent nosocomial transmission. Even with these measures, constant threats to the transplant recipient remain: the ever-present problem of antibiotic resistance, the increasing reliance on invasive technology to support patients through medical crises, and the improved capacity to support patients through critical illnesses that once were fatal, leaving survivors even more vulnerable for novel pathogens. For these reasons, enhancement of the host immunity is an important facet of minimizing the risk for developing infection, reducing its severity, and optimizing its resolution. Improvements in our understanding of specific deficits of host defenses and their contribution to various infections coupled with the introduction into clinical practice of several modulators of host immunity have led to important therapeutic advances.

BASIS FOR CONSIDERATION OF IMMUNE ENHANCEMENT

Following solid organ and bone marrow transplant (BMT), immune responses of the transplant recipient are profoundly altered. Several factors influence this (Table 1 and Chapter 1).

Immunosuppressive therapy is given to facilitate graft acceptance. In BMT recipients, the prevention of graft-versus-host disease (GVHD) is also necessary because the donor graft contains lymphoid progenitors that may be stimulated by histoincompatibility differences between donor and recipient and react against recipient antigens expressed on a variety of host tissues. As a consequence of the immunosuppressive agents employed, marked suppression of cell-mediated immune responses is universal. The depth of the deficiency of cell-mediated responses is influenced by several factors: the number and type of immunosuppressive agents employed, the dose of corticosteroids and other immunosuppressive agents, whether or not antithymocyte globulin is used, and the degree of mismatch between donor and recipient. Moreover, the occurrence of a rejection episode and the need to intensify immune suppression augment the immunodeficiency. The occurrence of GVHD in the BMT recipient similarly profoundly increases the degree of immunodeficiency. Certain viral infections, especially members of the herpesvirus family, also add to the degree of immunodeficiency.

Humoral immunity is frequently impaired in the post-transplant setting because of the use of corticosteroids and as a consequence of deficient cell-mediated responses that are necessary for T-dependent humoral responses. Impaired opsonization has been noted in patients with chronic GVHD following BMT. Hypogammaglobulinemia has similarly been noted in some BMT recipients, and IgG subclass deficiencies, even in the face of normal IgG levels, have been observed.

Neutropenia occurs as a matter of course after BMT where the pretransplant conditioning regimen includes cytoreductive agents that not only are immunosuppressive but also are myeloablative, destroying the host hematopoietic system in preparation for the donor hematopoietic progenitors. Following this conditioning regimen there is a period of 2–4 weeks during which there is profound deficiency of neutrophils, monocytes, macrophages, lymphocytes, and plasma cells. As the donor hematopoietic stem

From the Department of Medicine, University of Florida College of Medicine, Gainesville, FL 32610-0277.

TABLE 1. *Factors that influence immunodeficiency following organ or hematopoietic transplantation*

Factor	Immune Defense Suppressed[a]						Infectious Sequelae
	Integument	Mucosal Barrier	Phagocytes	Humoral Immunity	Cell-Mediated Immunity	Reiculoendothelial Cells	
Immuosuppressive agents							Viruses (especially herpesvirus), fungi
Corticosteroids			++	+	++++	++	
Alkylating agents, antimetabolites	+	++	+	+	+++		Fungi, viruses, bacteria
Donor recipient mismatch					++++		Viruses, fungi
Graft rejection							
Solid organ				++	++++		Bacterial, fungi, virus
Bone marrow			++++		++++		Bacteria, fungi
Graft-vs-host disease	++	+++	+	+	++++	+++	Viruses, fungi, bacteria
Viruses	+	++	+		++++		Bacteria, fungi
Transplant surgical trauma	+++	+					Bacteria
Myeloablative conditioning regimen	++	++++	++++	+	+	+	Bacteria, fungi

[a]The number of +'s denotes the relative degree of suppression.

cells engraft, the numbers of phagocytes are gradually restored. During the neutropenic interval, the patient is vulnerable for pathogens that can exploit weakened phagocytosis. Even after engraftment, with restoration of normal numbers of phagocytes in the circulation, reserves may be reduced; stressful events, such as infection, may be accompanied by a fall in the number of phagocytes, as the nascent hematopoietic system is not capable of increasing production of phagocytic precursors to replace those that are consumed. Moreover, even in the face of normal numbers of phagocytes, their function may be impaired. This is especially problematic in patients receiving corticosteroids where neutrophil and monocyte functions of ingesting and destroying microorganisms are compromised.

In solid organ transplant recipients, neutropenia is occasionally noted but not routinely encountered. Its occurrence results from the use of certain cytoreductive immunosuppressive medications, hypersplenism, the occurrence of cytomegalovirus (CMV) or other viral infections, or the use of ganciclovir as treatment of CMV infection. The duration and depth of neutropenia are highly variable.

Pulmonary alveolar macrophages, Kupfer cells, and the remainder of the reticuloendothelial system play important roles in clearing pathogens that have entered the circulation. The function of these cells is impaired following transplantation, and the use of corticosteroids or the occurrence of chronic GVHD exacerbate this deficit.

The mucosal barrier is an important defense against microorganisms that normally reside on their surface. Severe mucosal damage is frequently noted in the BMT patient in which cytoreductive agents such as total body irradiation, alkylating chemotherapeutic agents, or antimetabolites are employed that damage mucosal stem cells, which are especially vulnerable to the effects of cell cycle active agents because of their rapid turnover. The mucosal barrier also may be compromised by a reduction in the numbers of phagocytes and impaired cellular and humoral immunity because these are second-line defenses at the mucosa. The mucosal damage may render the patient vulnerable to commensal microorganisms residing on the mucosal surface.

Changes in host defenses take place over time. Following solid organ transplantation, in the perisurgical period, the changes that are most prominent are those related to the surgery. The surgical incision disrupts the integumentary barrier, rendering the patient susceptible to wound infections. Localized collections of blood and/or serum from vascular or lymphatic disruption can lead to enclosed environments where seeded microorganisms can flourish. Ischemia or an inadequate vascular supply may render tissue vulnerable to pathogens. Clots at the graft anastomotic site may also become infected. Intravenous, urinary, or other types of catheters or surgical drains offer conduits by which microorganisms may cause local or invasive bacterial infections. Intubation and ventilator support during and after surgery render the patient susceptible to respiratory pathogens. With the use of multiple antibiotics, fungal superinfections can also occur.

Following this acute postoperative period, integumentary and mucosal barrier deficits become less problematic, as the need for nosocomial invasive procedures is reduced and the use of perioperative antibiotics decreases. Increasingly prominent is the suppression of humoral and cell-mediated immunity from the immunosuppressive regimen. Thus viral and fungal infections are increasingly problematic. Acute rejection episodes are most common during the first 3 months following transplantation. Increased intensity of immunosuppression is given during a rejection episode and renders the patient more vulnerable to an infectious episode. Invasive fungal infections, CMV, and other viral infections are prominent infectious complications during this interval.

The type of transplanted organ is an important factor that determines the site and type of infection. Thus, for example, the urinary tract in renal transplant patients, the biliary tree in liver transplants, and the lung and thoracic cavity in heart and lung transplant are frequent sites of infection. Moreover, CMV tends to cause its most striking damage in the transplanted organ. Thus, for example, CMV hepatitis is particularly problematic in liver transplant recipients, and CMV pneumonitis is problematic in heart and lung transplant recipients.

Following BMT, the use of intensive cytoreductive chemotherapy or radiotherapeutic conditioning regimens designed to immunosuppress the recipient, ablate the host hematopoietic system, and treat the neoplastic disease (if that is the reason for which the transplant is being performed) characteristically incapacitate phagocytic host defenses and damage the gastrointestinal mucosal barrier during the first several weeks after transplant. Infections due to Gram-negative bacteria, *Candida* species, and *Aspergillus* species are common sequelae. Because of the widespread use of indwelling central venous catheters, Gram-positive bacterial infections due to staphylococcal species and *Corynebacteria* are frequent. Infections due to *Streptococcus viridans,* especially *S. mitis,* are also frequent due to mucosal damage. As the donor hematopoietic graft restores hematopoiesis, susceptibility to bacterial and fungal pathogens decreases. During the second and third months following BMT, invasive fungal infections and CMV infections are frequent complications due to the routine use of immunosuppressive agents to suppress GVHD. After the first 3 months, there is gradual recovery of humoral and cell-mediated immunity. Generally, immunosuppressive therapy is discontinued 6 months after an allogeneic BMT, in contrast to solid organ transplantation, where immunosuppressive therapy usually is continued indefinitely. If chronic GVHD occurs, however, prolonged immunosuppressive therapy for an additional 6–12 months or even longer may be required. In such individuals, a chronic immunodeficiency state occurs with poor immune responses to infectious pathogens, including impaired humoral and cell-mediated immunity and deficient reticuloendothelial function. Susceptibility to repeated infections from varicella-zoster virus, CMV, respiratory viral pathogens, and encapsulated bacterial organisms may occur. Even in the absence of chronic GVHD, recipients of unrelated donor marrow grafts or mismatched family donor grafts may have delayed reconstitution of immune responses and continued susceptibility to infectious pathogens that may persist up to 1 or more years.

IMMUNOMODULATORY MOLECULES

During the last decade several molecules with the potential of bolstering host defenses have become available. Because of their susceptibility for infections, organ transplant recipients have been groups in which a number of these agents have been evaluated and for whom clinical applications appear appropriate and beneficial. For reasons noted earlier, the utility may vary widely from one type of transplant recipient to another and may also vary within a given patient group over time. Table 2 lists such immunomodulatory agents.

TABLE 2. *Immunomodulatory molecules capable of enhancing host defenses with proven or potential roles in transplant recipients*

Agent	Host defense enhanced
G-CSF	Phagocytosis
GM-CSF	Phagocytosis
IVIG	Humoral immunity
Hyperimmune globulins	Humoral immunity (to specific pathogens)
Interferon α,β,γ	Phagocytosis, cell-mediated immunity
Interleukin 2	Cell-mediated immunity
Interleukin 7[a]	Cell-mediated immunity
Interleukin 12[a]	Cell-mediated immunity
Transforming growth factor (TGF)β[a]	Mucosal barrier
Keratinocyte-stimulating factor (KGF)[a]	Mucosal barrier

[a]Investigational.

HEMATOPOIETIC GROWTH FACTORS

A number of low-molecular-weight glycoprotein molecules, collectively referred to as hematopoietic growth factors, or cytokines, are now known to regulate blood cell production. Proliferation and differentiation of hematopoietic progenitors along different differentiation pathways are both positively and negatively modulated by multiple cytokines in accordance with constantly changing day-to-day needs and consumption.

Granulocyte colony-stimulating factor (G-CSF) and granulocyte-macrophage colony-stimulating factor (GM-CSF) are currently available for clinical use to enhance the production of myeloid precursors and to bolster host phagocytic defenses. In our current understanding, pluripotent hematopoietic stem cells have the capacity for multilineage differentiation, proliferation, and self-renewal. The earliest steps of division of the pluripotent stem cell and the factors that regulate this are poorly understood. G-CSF and GM-CSF appear to not influence these early events. However, the progeny of the stem cell are dependent on G-CSF and GM-CSF for survival, proliferation, and further differentiation. These hematopoietic progenitors have cell membrane receptors for multiple hematopoietic growth factors.

G-CSF is an O-glycosylated polypeptide produced by monocytes, fibroblasts, and endothelial cells. Its major target cells appear to be primarily late myeloid progenitors enhancing production and function (1–6). It has only modest effects on monocyte or macrophages.

GM-CSF is an N-glycosylated glycoprotein produced by T-lymphocytes, fibroblasts, and endothelial cells. GM-CSF has a broader array of effects than G-CSF (2,7,8). The development of both granulocytes and macrophages is influenced by GM-CSF. Moreover, GM-CSF enhances the function of macrophages (9–11).

In early clinical trials, a dose-dependent effect on the number of circulating neutrophils was noted with both G-

CSF and GM-CSF. These effects were observed both in patients with baseline normal numbers of neutrophils (so that elevated neutrophil numbers would result) and in patients with decreased numbers of neutrophils (with resulting recovery of normal numbers of neutrophils).

Several strategies for the use of G-CSF and GM-CSF have been evaluated in clinical trials (Table 3). In general, they are given for infection prophylaxis or treatment. Neutropenia has long been recognized to be associated with bacterial and fungal infections. The incorporation of cytoreductive chemotherapeutic regimens into cancer treatments reinforced this association. This understanding has led to the operational presumption that fever during chemotherapy-induced neutropenia should be treated as bacterial infection until proven otherwise. Both the depth and duration of neutropenia are important influences on the risk for infection. With the recognition that G-CSF and GM-CSF could increase bone marrow production of neutrophils, the utility of these agents for reducing the severity and duration of neutropenia was evaluated extensively. It was presumed that shortening or decreasing the depth of neutropenia would result in reduction in infectious morbidity. Thus, studies were designed to test whether these molecules could reduce the duration of chemotherapy-induced neutropenia and thereby decrease the risk for infection or infectious morbidity. As corollaries, the duration of antibiotic utilization, length of hospital stay, and cost were also evaluated.

In transplant patients, the use of growth factors has been most extensively evaluated in the BMT setting, where severe neutropenia is a universal occurrence following the conditioning regimen during the interval that host hematopoiesis has been abrogated but before engraftment of donor hematopoiesis. The duration of severe neutropenia ranges from 10 to 30 days in general.

A number of studies have evaluated the effects of G-CSF and GM-CSF to speed engraftment of the donor hematopoiesis (12–30). Three categories of outcome variables have been examined: the effect on blood counts, the impact on resource utilization, and the influence on infectious events. As shown in Table 4, a consistent finding in these studies was a reduction in the duration of neutropenia. In allogeneic BMT recipients, the number of days of neutropenia reduced ranged from 2 to 6. In autologous BMT recipients, the shortening of neutropenia was greater, ranging from 3 to 13 days. In most trials, these differences were statistically significant. Similarly, in general, reductions in the duration of antibiotic use and a decrease in duration of hospital stay were observed in a number of these studies. There was a concomitant decrease in hospital charges in several studies. The reduction in resource utilization and cost is not surprising when one considers that the guidelines for antibiotic utilization and duration are that they be administered (even though an infection might never be documented) until recovery from neutropenia. Because infection is documented in only a small minority of patients, continuation of antibiotics beyond recovery of neutropenia occurs only infrequently.

G-CSF and GM-CSF are widely used in the field of BMT based on their effects on recovery of neutropenia and a reduction in resource utilization. The use of G-CSF or GM-CSF is almost universal in the autologous transplant setting. There is debate as to whether the magnitude of shortening of the duration of neutropenia in the allogeneic transplant setting is sufficient to warrant its expense, and many centers do not routinely use growth factors for this group of patients. Indeed, in a subset of allogeneic transplant recipients where the donor is an unrelated volunteer (as opposed to the more common use of a sibling donor), two trials (29,31) observed trends toward reduced survival rates in patients receiving hematopoietic growth factors. Reassuringly, in no study has there been a suggestion of higher rates of GVHD or graft rejection in BMT recipients.

The effect of G-CSF and GM-CSF on reducing infectious events in the BMT setting is poorly documented. Indeed, no decreases in bacterial or fungal infection rates have been demonstrated in most studies (see Table 4). No reduction in infectious mortality has been demonstrated. Unfortunately, many of the clinical trials were insufficiently powered to appropriately document such a bene-

TABLE 3. *Strategies for the use of G-CSF and GM-CSF in transplant recipients*

Strategy	Goal
Prophylaxis of infection	
Hasten hematopoietic engraftment[a]	Decrease resource utilization and infectious morbidity
Treat delayed hematopoietic engraftment[a]	Decrease resource utilization and infectious morbidity
Enrich hematopoietic stem cell product[a]	Decrease resource utilization
Facilitate use of myelosuppressive, immunosuppressive, antifungal, antiviral agents	Optimize effectiveness of those strategies as an adjunctive measure
Counter myelosuppressive effects of viral infections	Decrease risk for superinfections
Counter consumption by hypersplenism	Decrease risk for infection
Treatment of infection	
Treat presumed infection (i.e., neutropenic fever)	Decrease resource utilization and infectious morbidity
Treat documented infection	Decrease resource utilization and infectious morbidity

[a]Primarily used for bone marrow transplant recipients.

TABLE 4. *Randomized clinical trials of G-CSF or GM-CSF to reduce duration of neutropenia and their effects on resource utilization and infectious complications in bone marrow transplant recipients*

Author	Ref. no.	BMT type	Stem cell source	Growth factor	Number of Days Neutrophil <500		Effect on severe neutropenia (neutrophils <100)	Effect on Resource Utilization			Effect on Clinical Events			
					Growth factor	Control		Antibiotic duration	Amphotericin duration	Hosp. stay**	Fever duration	Infection	Bacteremia	Fungal infection
Linch	12	Allo & Auto	Marrow	G-CSF[a]	13–17++[b]	19	NA	+[b]	–	+	–	–	–	NA
Khwaja	13	Auto	Marrow	GM-CSF	14++	20	–	–	NA	+	–	–	–	–
Gorin	14	Auto	Marrow	GM-CSF	14++	21	NA	–	NA	++	NA	–	–	–
Gulati	15	Auto	Marrow	GM-CSF	12	16	NA	NA	NA	++	NA	–	–	–
Link	16	Auto	Marrow	GM-CSF	15++	28	NA	–	NA	+	–	+	–	–
Nemunaitis	17	Auto	Marrow	GM-CSF	19++	26	–	++	–	+	–	–	–	–
Schmitz	18	Auto	Marrow	G-CSF[a]	12–14++	20	NA	–	NA	–	–	–	–	–
Stahel	19	Auto	Marrow	G-CSF	10++	18	NA	–	NA	–	+	–	–	–
Advani	20	Auto	Blood/Marrow	GM-CSF	12+	16	NA	NA	NA	–	NA	+	–	–
Legros	21	Auto	Marrow	GM-CSF	13.7	18.5	NA	–	NA	–	+	–	NA	NA
Spitzer	22	Auto	Marrow	G-& GM-CSF	10++	16	++	NA	NA	+	–	NA	–	NA
Klumpp	23	Auto	Marrow	G-CSF	10.5++	16	NA	+	NA	++	–	NA	NA	NA
Linch	24	Auto	Marrow	G-CSF	9++	12	NA	NA	NA	++	NA	NA	NA	NA
Gisselbrecht	25	Allo & Auto	Blood/Marrow	G-CSF	14++ / 14++	20 (AU) / 20 (AL)	NA	++	NA	+	+	+	–	NA
de Witte	26	Allo	Marrow	GM-CSF	15.8	19.9	++	–	NA	–	–	–	–	–
Nemunaitis	27	Allo	Marrow	GM-CSF	13++	17	++	–	–	+	–	++	+	–
Powles	28	Allo	Marrow	GM-CSF	13	16	NA	<	NA	–	<	–	–	NA
Blaise	30	Allo & Auto	Marrow	G-CSF	10.5	13.5 (AU)	NA	–	NA	+	+	NA	NA	NA
					15	17 (AL)	NA	+	NA	–	+	NA	NA	NA
Anasetti	29	Allo	Marrow	GM-CSF	20++	22	–	NA	NA	NA	NA	NA	–	NA

[a]Several different dosages were used; [b]+ = favorable at a significant level of p<0.05; ++ = favorable at a significant level of p<0.01; – = not significantly different; NA = not assessed; < = growth factor inferior to control.

fit, if it exists. Thus today we are uncertain of the true benefit of these agents. Indeed, one could argue that if there is a benefit, it must be small. The basis for this reasoning is that 90% of neutropenic infections occur when the number of circulating neutrophils is less than 100 cells/μl (13,32,33). Only 10% of infections occur when the circulating neutrophil count ranges between 100 and 500 cells/μl. Yet G-CSF and GM-CSF have minimal effect on the duration of severe neutropenia prior to engraftment (the interval that the neutrophil count is below 100). Most of the shortening of neutropenia is in the speed of recovery of neutrophils between 100 and 1000 cells/μl. Thus most clinical trials in BMT recipients have shown a dramatic reduction in the time to achieving a count of 500 or 1,500 cells/μl, but little or no reduction in the time to achieving a neutrophil count of 100/μl. Because few infections occur during this time of neutrophil recovery, one could reasonably question whether speeding a recovery already under way is really all that clinically useful. A number of studies in recent years have shortened the duration of empiric antibiotic administration by discontinuing antibiotics at neutrophil levels lower than 500/μl (34–42). Several studies have discontinued antibiotics at 250 neutrophils/μl with no ill effect. Moreover, with the increasing practice of managing uncomplicated neutropenic fevers in the outpatient setting, including BMT recipients (41,42), and with the introduction of broad-spectrum agents that can be effectively and safely used for management of neutropenic fever, the assumptions about resource utilization, hospitalization duration, and costs all should be reexamined.

Both the dose schedule and the route of administration have varied between different studies and for the two different molecules. The FDA-approved dose schedule for GM-CSF (sargramostim) is 250 μg m²/day for 21 days given as a 2-hour intravenous infusion starting 2–4 hours after the marrow stem cell infusion, but not less than 24 hours after the last dose of chemotherapy or 12 hours after the dose of radiotherapy. GM-CSF is continued until the circulating neutrophil count exceeds 1,500/μl for three consecutive days, at which time it is stopped or the dose is adjusted. For G-CSF (filgrastim), the FDA-approved dose schedule is 10 μg/kg/day given intravenously over a 4–24-hour interval or as a continuous 24-hour subcutaneous infusion starting at least 24 hours after the last dose of chemotherapy or marrow infusion. Once the circulating neutrophil count exceeds 1,000/μl for 3 consecutive days, the dose is reduced to 5 μg/kg/day and then discontinued if it persists above 1,000/μl. If there is a decline in the neutrophil count below 1,000/μl, then G-CSF is resumed at 5 μg/kg/day at the clinician's discretion.

In clinical practice, the dose schedules and routes of administration vary considerably from center to center and from one group of patients to another. Most clinicians use similar doses of G-CSF or GM-CSF inter-

changeably. Subcutaneous injection is usually the preferred route of administration because of convenience. Some clinicians prefer the intravenous route in patients with severe thrombocytopenia because of the concern for hemorrhage or bruising at the injection site. Others continue to use subcutaneous administration even in severely thrombocytopenic patients and report few problems. Although higher rates of toxicity for *Escherichia coli*–derived GM-CSF have been been reported than with either G-CSF or yeast-derived GM-CSF, there is a widespread perception that yeast-derived GM-CSF is more toxic than G-CSF. This has not been evaluated in any published controlled clinical trial, but one abstracted report of a randomized trial in nontransplant patients suggests that the toxicities are comparable (43).

Multiple clinical trials have employed different start-and-stop criteria. Delaying the initiation of the growth factor for 5–7 days has been evaluated in several trials (44–49). The rationale is that a benefit of a growth factor might not be evident until sufficient numbers of progenitors are present. Such studies suggest that this appears to be the case: delayed initiation of growth factor affects the engraftment similarly as early initiation. An additional consideration is whether growth factors need to be given to the transplant recipient after stem cell infusion if they are used prior to the collection of the stem cells (to enhance the numbers of committed myeloid progenitors, as noted in Table 3). Several studies have evaluated this question (21–23,50–53). These data suggest that if the number of stem cells used is optimal, the benefit of giving the patient growth factors following the stem cell infusion is negligible. However, if the content of the stem cell graft is suboptimal, growth factors may enhance the rapidity of engraftment.

Other benefits have been proposed for the routine use of G-CSF and GM-CSF in the BMT setting. Because neutrophils are an important component of the mucosal barrier, an effect on mucositis, related to cytoreductive chemotherapy or total body irradiation, methotrexate in the immunosuppressive regimen, or reactivation of herpes simplex virus, is possible. Although several uncontrolled studies have suggested a reduced severity of mucositis in chemotherapy-treated patients receiving G-CSF or GM-CSF (54–58), no such benefit has been demonstrated in controlled trials in BMT, although only a few of the clinical trials have examined this question (12,17,21,25,27) and the adequacy of evaluation is questionable. Although an influence of G-CSF and GM-CSF on other proinflammatory cytokines such as IL-1, Il-6, IL-2, TNF, and interferon is possible, to date no study has investigated these interactions or their clinical significance.

Patients with poor hematopoietic graft function are ideal candidates for an empiric trial of hematopoietic growth factors. Certainly, poor hematopoietic graft function after the first 2 weeks has been shown to be associated with an adverse relationship with survival (59). Although there are no randomized control trials to demonstrate their effectiveness, several anecdotal reports have shown improved hematopoietic graft function in patients with sluggish engraftment following autologous or allogeneic BMT (60–65).

The potential for G-CSF or GM-CSF to be used as adjuncts to antibiotics in patients with suspected or proven infection is an attractive consideration. Certainly, neutropenic patients with bacteremia in whom the neutrophil count rises have better success rates than those with persistent neutropenia (32,66,67). Similar observations for candidal infections (68) and aspergillosis (69) have also been observed. G-CSF, GM-CSF, and monocyte colony-stimulating factor (M-CSF) have all been evaluated as adjuncts to antibiotic treatment during infection (70–72). Although M-CSF was shown to enhance a variety of monocyte and macrophage function—including migration, expression of Fc receptors, cytotoxicity, respiratory burst activity, and bacterial and fungal killing—it is no longer under clinical development. As noted earlier, GM-CSF and G-CSF potentiate function and survival of neutrophils and enhance killing of microorganisms by increased phagocytosis and superoxide production. Preclinical animal models similarly demonstrate such benefits *in vivo*. Unfortunately, no clinical trials have evaluated these molecules as treatment of established infection in transplant recipients. In one randomized trial in children undergoing BMT with presumed infection, no shortening of fever duration was noted, but a reduction in duration of antibiotic use and hospital stay was noted (73). Several randomized controlled trials in nontransplant chemotherapy-treated cancer patients have failed to demonstrate a reduction in infectious mortality (reviewed in ref. 74). However, as in the BMT trial, shortening of neutrophil recovery and duration of antibiotic use have been seen (75–80).

Several uncontrolled trials have evaluated G-CSF and GM-CSF in solid organ as well as BMT patients as therapy for neutropenic episodes that occur as a result of viral infection, the use of myelosuppressive drugs such as ganciclovir, the use of myelosuppressive and immunosuppressive drugs, or hypersplenism (81–87). Because of their uncontrolled nature, the precise benefit is not certain, but certainly several patients appear to have benefited.

Two other potential applications of G-CSF and GM-CSF enhancing transplant recipient immunity bear mentioning. The first is that growth factor mobilization of hematopoietic stem cells from the bone marrow into the peripheral blood is feasible, is widely practiced in the autologous BMT setting, and is being evaluated in the allogeneic BMT setting. Large numbers of hematopoietic progenitor cells can be obtained, rapid hematopoietic engraftment is routinely seen, and long-term follow-up shows that engraftment is durable. In animal models, pretreatment of donors with G-CSF prior to collection of hematopoietic stem cells has resulted in lower rates of GVHD-associated mortality than expected, given that much higher numbers of T-lymphocytes are used (88). Further testing has indicated a polarization from a Th1 immunophenotype to a Th2 immunophenotype with increased IL4 production and decreased IL2 and interferon-γ production (89). Since interferon-γ appears to play a role in the development of acute GVHD (90–92), the lower level of interferon production may in part explain less severe GVHD. A second potential use is the coadministration of GM-CSF as an adjuvant for vaccines to enhance immune responses. The administration of GM-CSF along with peptide-based vaccines in a rat model has been demonstrated to enhance such immune responses (93). The clinical significance of these two potential applications remains to be seen.

INTERFERONS

The interferons are families of small-molecular-weight proteins first identified as substances produced by cells in response to viral infection. In addition to being a first-line defense against infectious pathogens, they enhance monocyte and natural killer (NK)–cell function and have antiproliferative effects on experimental and human tumors. Interferons also stimulate the production of interleukin-2 (IL-2), which in turn has additional immunomodulatory properties. There are at least three families of interferons (α, β, γ), and each family has a number of subtypes. Interferon's antiviral activities are complex, are multifactorial, and vary with host cell type, virus type and innoculum, and the type of interferon. Production of interferon after stimulation is impaired in BMT recipients up to 1 year after transplant (94), and this deficient response has been suggested as a contributor to deficient cellular immune responses.

In immunocompetent patients, randomized controlled trials evaluating the therapeutic use of exogenous interferon-α have demonstrated a reduction in the replication of hepatitis B virus (95–102). An improvement in histologic findings has been noted in some instances (103), but sustained clinical benefit has been less well assessed. In one study (103), a long-term benefit was noted in those individuals who cleared the hepatitis B e-antigen after treatment with interferon-α. Similarly, benefits with interferon-α have been noted with chronic hepatitis C infections in randomized controlled trials conducted in immunocompetent patients (104,105). In those individuals in which a loss of hepatitis C RNA was noted, and this antiviral effect persisted, sustained clinical improvements were also noted. However, whether this has an impact on overall survival or prevention of hepatic cirrhosis remains to be demonstrated (106). In one study, proliferative responses to hepatitis C in immunocompetent patients with chronic hepatitis C infection were enhanced by interferon-α (107). It has been speculated that the ultimate clinical benefit of interferon may depend on not only the effects on viral replication but the generation of protective immune responses. Once interferon therapy ceases, the durability of the clinical benefit may be determined by whether or not an effective T-cell response has been generated and persists (107).

Because interferon is believed to have a role in the pathogenesis of GVHD (90–92), as noted earlier, caution should be exercised in the use of interferon in allogeneic BMT recipients.

In organ transplant recipients, in contrast to immunocompetent patients, there are few studies of interferon and no randomized trials. Efficacy has been noted in some liver transplant patients treated for hepatitis B (108,109). In renal transplant recipients, interferon-α has been noted to have only a limited benefit in a series of patients treated for hepatitis B and hepatitis C infections (110). Graft rejection may occur with interferon treatment (111), perhaps as a result of up-regulation of class II histocompatibility antigens; thus caution should be exercised.

In one randomized controlled trial in BMT recipients treated for acute lymphoblastic leukemia, interferon-α was given in an attempt to reduce CMV infection rates and mortality from CMV disease (112). No antiviral benefits were noted; however, a reduction in the recurrence rate of leukemia was incidentally noted.

Another biological activity of interferon that may reduce the risk for transplant infection is its capacity to enhance cytotoxicity of neutrophils and macrophages and to induce or enhance natural killer (NK) activity. Interferon-γ has been demonstrated to be useful in the treatment of chronic granulomatous disease, a disorder of bactericidal activity by neutrophils and monocytes (113). Infections caused by intracellular pathogens such as mycobacteria, Leishmania, and Toxoplasma have also been responsive to interferon-γ (114,115). Beneficial effects on oxidative responses and damage to Aspergillus hyphae by neutrophils treated by G-CSF and interferon-γ (4) have been noted. In in vitro assays of monocytes, interferon-γ, M-CSF and GM-CSF can restore impaired phagocytosis and killing of Aspergillus organisms caused by corticosteroids (116–121). Thus there is interest in evaluating the adjunctive use of interferon along with antifungal agents. However, to date, no clinical trial has been performed to evaluate these interesting preclinical observations.

INTERLEUKINS 2, 7, AND 12

In vitro studies suggest that IL-2, IL-7, and IL-12, either alone or in combination, generate substantial cytotoxicity that is particularly active against malignancies. Much of the interest in these three cytokines relates to efforts to enhance host antitumor immune responses and reduce the risk for relapse in BMT patients treated for

neoplasia. However, their immunomodulatory activity also has potentially important roles in augmenting the transplant recipient's defenses against infection.

Interleukin-2 (IL-2) is a glycoprotein produced by activated T cells that promote proliferative and cytotoxic responses of both T and NK cells, and the generation of nonspecific lymphokine-activated killer (LAK) cells from heterogeneous mononuclear blood cells. Cytotoxic effects against selected tumor cell lines and in animal models of certain epithelial tumors have been demonstrated by administration of LAK cells plus IL-2 or IL-2 alone. Clinical trials have shown evidence of antitumor activity in several trials. IL-2 administration has been shown to produce sustained increases in CD4 lymphocyte counts in HIV-infected patients (122). Targets of IL-2 stimulation include activated T and B cells, NK cells, and monocytes. Defective IL-2 production and correction of functional T-cell deficits in vitro by IL-2 have been demonstrated in patients after BMT (123). Thus it has been speculated that the abnormal immune function in patients after BMT may be, at least in part, attributable to this. In other studies, IL-2 responses did not appear impaired, suggesting that other pathogenic mechanisms for the immunodeficiency (124). One cautionary note is that patients receiving exogenous IL-2 have been noted to have higher-than-expected rates of bacteremia (125). Certainly, the need for an indwelling venous catheter is contributory, but a profound, reversible effect in neutrophil chemotaxis has also been noted with IL-2 therapy and may be contributory also (126).

IL-7 promotes the generation of B- and T-cell precursors and to a lesser extent plays a role in activating mature T cells. IL-7 stimulates natural killer (NK) activity. In one study, in an animal model of BMT, IL-7-treated animals demonstrated enhanced cytotoxic T-cell activity against influenza and improved survival (127).

IL-12 is produced by phagocytic cells, B cells, and other antigen-presenting cells. Monocytes and macrophages are the major producers of IL-12. IL-12 plays a role in activating phagocytes in response to infection and contributes to the generation of T helper type 1 (Th1) cells, which in turn produce IL-2 and interferon-γ and for the maturation of cytotoxic T cells. Natural killer activity is also enhanced by IL-12. In addition to its role in inducing interferon-γ production, it has synergistic activity with IL-2 in this regard. IL-12 is emerging as an important mediator of host defenses against infections (128–131). In experimental animal models, IL-12 has an important role in inducing the acute production of interferon-γ and facilitating phagocytes to produce GM-CSF and TNF-α as protective host responses. Endogenous production of IL-12 has been noted in animal models to be crucial for the survival of mice infected by Listeria monocytogenes and Toxoplasma gondii. Animals treated with IL-12 had a dramatic response to experimental infection by Leishmania. Although IL-12 messenger

RNA transcripts are readily detected in macrophages from mice with healing *Candida albicans* infections (and not in mice with progressive disease) and antibodies to IL-12 abrogate the development of anticandidal resistance, administration of IL-12 does not appear to favorably affect the course of infection in mice with progressive infection (132,133). Although IL-12 would be expected to have an important role in antiviral cytotoxic T-cell responses, little information is currently available.

MUCOSAL GROWTH FACTORS

Several molecules have been noted to play roles in the wound-healing process by stimulation of epithelial cell division. Such growth factors as epidermal growth factor, basic fibroblast growth factor, and transforming growth factor β (TGF β) stimulate the growth of human keratinocytes. The growth of mucosal epithelial cells are also regulated by TGF β and a member of the fibroblast growth factor family, keratinocyte growth factor (KGF).

TGF β is a cytokine found principally in platelets and in bone. It has been shown to reversibly inhibit the cycling of human buccal mucosal epithelial cells and pretreatment of such cells with TGF β protects them from toxicity mediated by a variety of chemotherapy agents. In an animal trial, it was reasoned that a transient inhibition of the basal epithelial cell proliferation during chemotherapy administration would reduce mucosal toxicity. TGF β was found to reduce the incidence, severity, and duration of chemotherapy-induced ulcerative mucositis (134). KGF has also been noted to affect proliferative activity of mucosal epithelial cells in animal models and cell lines (135–137). In an animal model of radiation and chemotherapy-induced gastrointestinal mucositis and mortality, KGF was found to have protective effects with reduced weight loss, mortality, and a marked increase in the intestinal proliferative crypt activity during the healing phase. Both molecules are currently undergoing clinical trials to ascertain whether host mucosal barrier function can be bolstered in chemotherapy-treated patients.

REFERENCES

1. Begley CG, Lopez AF, Nicola NA, et al. Purified colony-stimulating factors enhance the survival of human neutrophils and eosinophils *in vitro*. *Blood* 1986;68:162.
2. Metcalf D. Control of granulocytes and macrophages: molecular, cellular, and clinical aspects. *Science* 1991;254:529.
3. Anderlini P, Przepiorka D, Champlin R, Korbling M. Biologic and clinical effects of granulocyte colony-stimulating factor in normal individuals. *Blood* 1996;88:2819–2825.
4. Roilides E, Uhlig K, Venzon D, et al. Enhancement of oxidative response and damage caused by human neutrophils to *Aspergillus fumigatus* hyphae by granulocyte colony-stimulating factor and gamma interferon. *Infect Immunol* 1993;61:1185–1193.
5. Roilides E, Holmes A, Blake C, Pizzo PA, Walsh TJ. Effects of granulocyte colony-stimulating factor and interferon-γ on antifungal activity of human polymorphonuclear neutrophils against pseudohyphae of different medically important *Candida* species. *J Leukocyte Biol* 1995;57:651–656.
6. Vecchiarelli A, Monari C, Baldelli F, et al. Beneficial effect of recombinant human granulocyte colony-stimulating factor on fungicidal activity of polymorphonuclear leukocytes from patients with AIDS. *J Infect Dis* 1995;171:1448–1454.
7. Gough NM, Nicola NA. *Colony-stimulating factors*. New York: Dekker 1990;111.
8. Mayer P, Schutze E, Lam C, Kricek F, Liehl E. Recombinant murine granulocyte-macrophage colony-stimulating factor augments neutrophil recovery and enhances resistance to infections in myelosuppressed mice. *J Infect Dis* 1991;163:584–590.
9. Smith PD, Lamerson CL, Banks SM, et al. Granulocyte-macrophage colony-stimulating factor augments human monocyte fungicidal activity for *Candida albicans*. *J Infect Dis* 1990;161:999–1005.
10. Weiser WY, VanNiel A, Clark SC, David JR, Remold HG. Recombinant human granulocyte/macrophage colony-stimulating factor activates intracellular killing of *Leishmania donovani* by human monocyte-derived macrophages. *J Exp Med* 1987;166:1436–1446.
11. Reed SG, Nathan CF, Pihl DL, et al. Recombinant granulocyte/macrophage colony-stimulating factor activates macrophages to inhibit *Trypanosoma cruzii* and release hydrogen peroxide. *J Exp Med* 1987;166:1734–1746.
12. Linch DC, Scarffe H, Proctor S, et al. Randomized vehicle-controlled dose-finding study of glycosylated rhG-CSF after bone marrow transplantation. *Bone Marrow Transplant* 1993;11:307.
13. Khaja A, Linch DC, Goldstone AH, et al. rhG-CSF after bone marrow transplantation for malignant lymphoma: a BNLI double-blind placebo-controlled trial. *Br J Haematol* 1992;82:317.
14. Gorin NC, Coiffier B, Hayat M, et al. rhGM-CSF after high dose chemotherapy and ABMT with unpurged and purged marrow in non-Hodgkin's lymphoma: a double-blind placebo-controlled trial. *Blood* 1992;80:1149.
15. Gulati SC, Bennett CL. GM-CSF as adjunct therapy in relapsed Hodgkin disease. *Ann Intern Med* 1992;116:177.
16. Link H, Boogaerts MA, Carella AM. A controlled trial of rhGM-CSF after TBI, high-dose chemotherapy, and ABMT for ALL or malignant lymphoma. *Blood* 1992;80:2188.
17. Nemunaitis J, Rabinowe SN, Singer JW, et al. rhGM-CSF after ABMT for lymphoid cancer. *N Engl J Med* 1991;324:1773.
18. Schmitz N, Dreger P, Zander AR. Results of a randomized controlled multicenter study of rhG-CSF in patients with Hodgkin's disease and non-Hodgkin's lymphoma undergoing ABMT. *Bone Marrow Transplant* 1995;15:261.
19. Stahel RA, Jost LM, Cerny T, et al. Randomized study of rhG-CSF after high-dose chemotherapy and ABMT for high-risk lymphoid malignancies. *J Clin Oncol* 1994;12:1931.
20. Advani R, Chao NJ, Horning SJ, et al. GM-CSF as an adjunct to autologous hematopoietic stem cell transplantation for lymphoma. *Ann Intern Med* 1992;116:183.
21. Legros M, Fleury J, Cure H, et al. rhGM-CSF after high dose chemotherapy and PBPC: a unicenter randomized study of 50 patients. *Blood* 1994;84:62a.
22. Spitzer G, Adkins DR, Spencer V, et al. Randomized study of growth factors post PBPC transplant. Neutrophil recovery is improved with modest clinical benefit. *J Clin Oncol* 1995;13:1323.
23. Klumpp TR, Mangan KF, Goldberg SL, et al. G-CSF accelerates neutrophil engraftment following PBSC transplantation: a prospective, randomized trial. *J Clin Oncol* 1995;13:1323.
24. Linch DC, Milliagan DW, Winfield DA, et al. G-CSF significantly accelerates neutrophil recovery after PBSC transplantation in lymphoma patients and shortens the time in hospital: Preliminary results of a randomized BNLI trial. *Blood* 1995;86:102a.
25. Gisselbrecht C, Prentice HG, Bacigalupo A, et al. Placebo-controlled phase III trial of lenograstim in bone marrow transplantation. *Lancet* 1994;343:696.
26. DeWitte T, Gratwohl A, Van Der Lely N, et al. rhGM-CSF accelerates neutrophil and monocyte recovery after allogeneic T-cell-depleted bone marrow transplantation. *Blood* 1992;79:1359.
27. Nemunaitis J, Rosenfeld CS, Ash R, et al. Phase III randomized, double-blind placebo-controlled trial of rhGM-CSF following allogeneic bone marrow transplantation. *Bone Marrow Transplant* 1995;15:949.
28. Powles R, Smith C, Milan S, et al. rhGM-CSF in allogeneic bone marrow transplantation for leukaemia: double-blind, placebo-controlled trial. *Lancet* 1990;336:1417.
29. Anasetti C, Anderson G, Appelbaum FR, et al. Phase III study of rh-

GM-CSF in allogeneic bone marrow transplantation from unrelated donors. *Blood* 1993;82:454a.

30. Blaise D, Vernant JP, Fiere D, et al. A randomized, controlled, multicenter trial of recombinant human granulocyte colony stimulating factor (filgrastim) in patients treated by bone marrow transplantation (BMT) with total body irradiation (TBI) for acute lymphoblastic leukemia (ALL) or lymphoblastic leukemia (LL). *Blood* 1992;80: 248a. [Abstract 982]

31. Schriber JR, Chao NJ, Long GD. Granulocyte colony-stimulating factor after allogeneic bone marrow transplantation. *Blood* 1989;84: 1047–1050.

32. Bodey GP, Buckley M, Sathe YS, et al. Quantitative relationship between circulating leukocytes and infection in patients with acute leukemia. *Ann Intern Med* 1966;64:328–340.

33. Tsakona CP, Khwaja A, Goldstone AH. Does treatment with haematopoietic growth factors affect the incidence of bacteraemia in adult lymphoma transplant recipients? *Bone Marrow Transplant* 1993;11: 433–436.

34. Talcott JA, Finberg R, Mayer RJ, Goldman L. The medical course of cancer patients with fever and neutropenia: clinical identification of a low-risk subgroup at presentation. *Arch Intern Med* 1988;148: 2561–2568.

35. Mullen CA, Buchanan GR. Early hospital discharge of children with cancer treated for fever and neutropenia: identification and management of the low-risk patient. *J Clin Oncol* 1990;8:1998–2004.

36. Talcott JA, Siegel RD, Finberg R, Goldman L. Risk assessment in cancer patients with fever and neutropenia: a prospective, two-center validation of a prediction rule. *J Clin Oncol* 1992;10:316–322.

37. Rubenstein EB, Rolston K, Benjamin RS, et al. Outpatient treatment of febrile episodes in low-risk neutropenic patients with cancer. *Cancer* 1993;71:3640–3646.

38. Buchanan GR. Approach to treatment of the febrile cancer patient with low-risk neutropenia. *Hematol Oncol Clin North Am* 1993;7: 919–935.

39. Weiser MA, Frisbee-Hume S, Manzullo E, Escalante C, Rubenstein EB. Identification and outpatient management for the low-risk febrile neutropenic patient with cancer. *Home HealthCare Consultant* 1996;3:35–49.

40. Rolston K, Rubenstein E, Frisbee-Hume S, et al. Outpatient treatment of febrile episodes in low-risk neutropenic cancer patients. *Proc Am Soc Clin Oncol* 1993;12:436.

41. Gilbert C, Meisenberg B, Vrendenburgh J, et al. Sequential prophylactic oral and empiric once-daily parenteral antibiotics for neutropenia and fever after high-dose chemotherapy and autologous bone marrow support. *J Clin Oncol* 1994;12:1005–1011.

42. Meisenberg B, Gollard R, Brehm T, McMillan R, Miller W. Prophylactic antibiotics eliminate bacteremia and allow safe outpatient management following high-dose chemotherapy and autologous stem cell rescue. *Support Care Cancer* 1996;4:364–369.

43. Miller JA, Beveridge RA. A comparison of efficacy of GM-CSF versus G-CSF in the therapeutic setting of chemotherapy induced neutropenia. *Blood* 1994;84:22a. [Abstract #78]

44. Faucher C, le Carroller AG, Chabannon C, et al. Administration of G-CSF can be delayed after transplantation of autologous G-CSF-primed blood stem cells: a randomized study. *Bone Marrow Transplant* 1996;17:533–536.

45. Sobrevilla-Calvo P, Cortes P, Solano P, et al. Starting G-CSF on day -7 or on day 0 is equally effective in accelerating neutrophil recovery after autologous peripheral blood stem cell transplantation. *J Clin Oncol* 1996;15:272.

46. Vey N, Molnar, Faucher C, et al. Delayed administration of granulocyte colony-stimulating factor after autologous bone marrow transplantation: effect of granulocyte recovery. *Bone Marrow Transplant* 1994;14:779.

47. Khwaja A, Mills W, Leveridge K, Goldstone AH, Linch DC. Efficacy for a delayed granulocyte colony-stimulating factor after autologous bone marrow transplantation. *Bone Marrow Transplant* 1993;11: 479–482.

48. Viret F, Molina L, Plantaz D, Chabannon C, Hollard D. Impact of delayed start (day -5) G-CSF after allogeneic bone marrow transplantation: a pilot study. *Blood* 1994;84:63. [Abstract 369]

49. Masaoka T, Takaku F, Kato S, et al. rhG-CSF in allogeneic bone marrow transplantation. *Exp Hematol* 1989;17:1047.

50. Cortelazzo C, Viero P, Bellavita P, et al. G-CSF following PBPC transplant in non-Hodgkin's lymphoma. *J Clin Oncol* 1995;13:935.

51. Szilvassy SF, Hoffman R. Hematopoietic growth factors do not accelerate neutrophil recovery after transplantation of optimally mobilized peripheral blood stem cells. *Biol Blood Marrow Transplant* 1996;2:2.

52. Brandwein JM, Callum J, Sutcliffe SB, et al. Analysis of factors affecting hematopoietic recovery after ABMT. *Bone Marrow Transplant* 1995;16:139–140.

53. Klumpp TR, Goldberg SL, Magdalinski AT, Mangan KF. Effect of hematopoietic growth factors on the rate of neutrophil recovery following peripheral blood stem cell transplantation. *Biol Blood Marrow Transplant* 1996;2:1.

54. Lieschke GJ, Ramenghi U, O'Connor MP, Sheridan W, Szer J, Morstyn G. Studies of oral neutrophil levels in patients receiving G-CSF after autologous marrow transplantation. *Br J Haematol* 1992; 82:589–595.

55. Gordon B, Spadinger A, Hodges E, Ruby E, Stanley R, Coccia P. Effect of granulocyte-macrophage colony-stimulating factor on oral mucositis after hematopoietic stem cell transplantation. *J Clin Oncol* 1994;12:1917–1922.

56. Chi K, Chen C, Chan W, et al. Effect of granulocyte-macrophage colony stimulating factor on oral mucositis in head and neck cancer patients after cisplatin, fluorouracil, and leucovorin chemotherapy. *J Clin Oncol* 1995;13:2620–2628.

57. Throuvalas N, Antonadou D, Pulizzi M, et al. Evaluation of the efficacy and safety of GM-CSF in the prophylaxis of mucositis in patients with had and neck cancer treated with RT. European Cancer Conference, Paris, France 1995;Oct. 29–Nov. 2:S93. [Abstract 431]

58. Wardley AM, Scarffe JH. Role of granulocyte-macrophage colony-stimulating factor in chemoradiotherapy-induced oral mucositis. *J Clin Oncol* 1996;14:1741–1744.

59. Offner F, Schoch G, Fisher LD, Torok-Storb B, Martin PJ. Mortality hazard functions as related to neutropenia at different times after marrow transplantation. *Blood* 1996;88:4058–4062.

60. Weisdorf D, Verfaillie CM, Davies SM. Hematopoietic growth factors for graft failure after bone marrow graft failure: a randomized trial of granulocyte macrophage colony-stimulating factor (GM-CSF) plus granulocyte CSF. *Blood* 1995;85:3452–3456.

61. Nemunaitis J, Singer JW, Buckner CD, et al. Use of rhGM-CSF in graft failure after BMT. *Blood* 1990;76:245.

62. Vose JM, Bierman PJ, Kessinger A, et al. The use of rhGM-CSF for the treatment of delayed engraftment following high dose therapy and autologous hematopoietic stem cell transplantation for lymphoid malignancies. *Bone Marrow Transplant* 1991;7:139.

63. Brandwein JM, Nayar R, Baker MA, et al. GM-CSF therapy for delayed engraftment after ABMT. *Exp Hematol* 1991;19:191.

64. Ippoliti C, Przepiorka D, Giralt S, et al. Low-dose non-glycosylated rhGM-CSF is effective for the treatment of delayed hematopoietic recovery after ABMT or PBSC transplantation. *Bone Marrow Transplant* 1993;11:55.

65. Klingemann HG, Eaves AC, Barnett MJ, et al. rGM-CSF in patients with poor graft function after bone marrow transplantation. *Clin Invest Med* 1990;13:77.

66. Gurney H. The problem of neutropenia resulting from cancer therapy. *Clinician* 1989;7:2–10.

67. Dejongh CA, Joshi JH, Newman KI, et al. Antibiotic synergism and response in gram-negative bacteraemia in granulocytopenic cancer patients. *Am J Med* 1986;80:96–100.

68. Maksymiuk AW, Thongprasert S, Hopfer R, Luna M, Fainstein V, Bodey GP. Systemic candidiasis in cancer patients. *Am J Med* 1984;77:20–27.

69. Bodey GP, Vartivarian S. Aspergillosis. *Eur J Clin Microbiol Infect Dis* 1989;8:413–437.

70. Bodey GP, Anaissie EJ, Gutterman J, et al. Role of GM-CSF as adjuvant therapy for fungal infection in patients with cancer. *Clin Dis* 1993;17:705.

71. Nemunaitis J, Meyers JD, Buckner CD, et al. Phase I trial of recombinant human macrophage colony-stimulating factor in patients with invasive fungal infections. *Blood* 1991;78:907–913.

72. Nemunaitis J, Shannon-Dorcy K, Appelbaum FR, et al. Long-term follow-up of patients with invasive fungal disease who received adjunctive therapy with recombinant human macrophage colony-stimulating factor. *Blood* 1993;82:1422–1427.

73. Mitchell PLR, Morland B, Stevens MCG, et al. Granulocyte colony-stimulating factor in established febrile neutropenia: a randomized study of pediatric patients. *J Clin Oncol* 1997;15:1163–1170.

74. ASCO Ad Hoc Colony-Stimulating Factor Guideline Expert Panel. American Society of Clinical Oncology Recommendations for the Use of hematopoietic colony-stimulating factors: Evidence-based, clinical practice guidelines. *J Clin Oncol* 1994;12:2471–2508.

75. Maher D, Green M, Bishop J, et al. Randomized, placebo-controlled trial of filgrastim (rmetHuG-CSF) in patients with febrile neutropenia (FN) following chemotherapy (CT). *Proc Am Soc Clin Oncol* 1993; 12:434.

76. Mayordomo JI, Rivera F, Diaz-Puente MT, et al. Decreasing morbidity and cost of treating febrile neutropenia by adding G-CSF and GM-CSF to standard antibiotic therapy: results of a randomized trial. *Proc Am Soc Clin Oncol* 1993;12:437.

77. Anaissie EJ, Vartivarian S, Bodey GP, et al. Randomized comparison between antibiotics alone and antibiotics plus granulocyte-macrophage colony stimulating factor (*E. coli*-derived) in cancer patients with neutropenia and fever. *Am J Med* 1997 (in press).

78. Biesma B, de Vries ER, Willemse PH, et al. Efficacy and tolerability of recombinant human granulocyte-macrophage colony-stimulating factor in patients with chemotherapy-related leukopenia and fever. *Eur J Cancer* 1990;26:932–936.

79. Riikonen P, Saarinen UM, Makipernaa A, et al. rhGM-CSF in the treatment of fever and neutropenia: a double-blind, placebo-controlled study in children with malignancy. *Proc Am Soc Clin Oncol* 1993; 12:442.

80. Valenga E, Uyl-de Groat CA, de Wit R, et al. Randomized placebo controlled trial of granulocyte-macrophage colony-stimulating factor in patients with chemotherapy-related febrile neutropenia. *J Clin Oncol* 1996;14:619–627.

81. Ishizone S, Makuuchi M, Kawasaki S, et al. Effect of granulocyte colony-stimulating factor on neutropenia in liver transplant recipients with hypersplenism. *J Pediatr Surg* 1994;29:510–513.

82. Wasler A, Iberer F, Auer T, et al. Treatment of leukopenia with granulocyte-macrophage colony-stimulating factor after heart transplantation. *Transplant Proc* 1995;27:2633–2634.

83. Diflo T, Kuo P, Lewis WD, Jenkins R. Simultaneous use of ganciclovir and granulocyte colony stimulating factor in liver transplant recipients. *Blood* 1997 (in press).

84. Peddi VR, Hariharan S, Schroeder TJ, First MR. Role of granulocyte colony stimulating (G-CSF) in reversing neutropenia in renal allograft recipients. *Clin Transplant* 1996;10:20–23.

85. Wang JC, Gordon B, Cheigh JS, Riggio RR, Stenzel KH, Suthanthiran M. Use of granulocyte colony-stimulating factor (G-CSF) in leukopenic renal transplant recipients. *J Am Soc Nephrol* 1992;3:887. [Abstract 106P]

86. Page B, Morin MP, Mamzer MF, et al. Use of granulocyte-macrophage colony-stimulating factor in leukopenic renal transplant recipients. *Transplant Proc* 1994;16:283.

87. Jin DC, Yoon YS, Kim SY, et al. Use of granulocyte-macrophage colony stimulating factor (GM-CSF) in azathioprine-induced leukopenic renal transplant recipients. *Kidney Int* 1993;44:1191. [Abstract.]

88. Pan L, Bressler S, Cooke KR, Krenger W, Karandikar M, Ferrara JLM. Long-term engraftment, graft-vs-host disease, and immunologic reconstitution after experimental transplantation of allogeneic peripheral blood cells from G-CSF-treated donors. *Biol Blood Marrow Transplant* 1996;2:126–133.

89. Pan L, Delmonte J, Jalonen CK, Ferrara JLM. Pretreatment of donors with granulocyte colony-stimulating factor polarized donor T lymphocytes toward type 2 cytokine production and reduces severity of experimental graft versus host disease. *Blood* 1995;86:4422.

90. Mowat A. Antibodies to IFN-gamma prevent immunological mediated intestinal damage in murine graft-versus-host reactions. *Immunology* 1989;68:18.

91. Nestel FP, Price KS, Seemayer TA, Lapp WS. Macrophage priming and lipopolysaccharide-triggered release of tumor necrosis factor alpha during graft-versus-host disease. *J Exp Med* 1992;175:405.

92. Rus V, Svetic A, Nguyen P, Gause WC, Via CS. Kinetics of Th1 and Th2 cytokine production during the early course of acute and chronic murine graft-versus-host disease. *J Immunol* 1995;155:2396.

93. Disis ML, Bernhard H, Shiota FM, et al. Granulocyte-macrophage colony-stimulating factor: an effective adjuvant for protein and peptide-based vaccines. *Blood* 1996;88:202–210.

94. Koscielniak E, Bruchelt G, Treuner J, et al. Kinetics of restoration of interferon production after bone marrow transplantation in man. *Bone Marrow Transplant* 1987;1:379–387.

95. Hoofnagle JH, Peters M, Mullen KD, et al. Randomized, controlled trial of recombinant human alpha-interferon in patients with chronic hepatitis B. *Gastroenterology* 1988;95:1318–1325.

96. Alexander GJM, Brahm J, Fagan EA, et al. Loss of HBsAg with interferon therapy in chronic hepatitis B virus infection. *Lancet* 1987;2: 66–69.

97. Brook MG, McDonald JA, Karayiannis P, et al. Randomized controlled trial of interferon alfa 2A (rbe) (Roferon A) for the treatment of chronic hepatitis B virus (HBV) infection: factors that influence response. *Gut* 1989;130:1116–1122.

98. Saracco G, Mazzella G, Rosina F, et al. A controlled trial of human lymphoblastoid interferon in chronic hepatitis B in Italy. *Hepatology* 1989;10:336–341.

99. Perillo RP, Schiff ER, Davis GL, et al. A randomized, controlled trial of interferon alfa-2b alone and after prednisone withdrawal for the treatment of chronic hepatitis B. *N Engl J Med* 1990;323:295–301.

100. Perillo RP. Antiviral therapy of chronic hepatitis B: past, present, and future. *J Hepatol* 1993;17: S56–S63.

101. Tine F, Liberati A, Craxi A, Almasio P, Pagliaro L. Interferon treatment in patients with chronic hepatitis B: a meta-analysis of the published literature. *J Hepatol* 1993;18:154–162.

102. Perillo RP, Brunt EM. Hepatic histologic and immunohistochemical changes in chronic hepatitis B after prolonged clearance of hepatitis B e antigen and hepatitis B surface antigen. *Ann Intern Med* 1991;115: 113–115.

103. Niederau C, Heintges T, Lange S, et al. Long-term follow-up of HBeAg-positive patients treated with interferon alfa for chronic hepatitis B. *N Engl J Med* 1996;334:1422–1427.

104. Davis GL, Balart LA, Schiff ER, et al. Treatment of chronic hepatitis C with recombinant interferon alpha: a multicenter randomized, controlled trial. *N Engl J Med* 1989;321:1501–1506.

105. Di Bisceglie AM, Martin P, Kassianides C, et al. Recombinant interferon alfa therapy for chronic hepatitis C: a randomized, double-blind, placebo-controlled trial. *N Engl J Med* 1989;321:1506–1510.

106. Hoofnagle JH, Lau D. Chronic viral hepatitis: benefits of current therapies. *N Engl J Med* 1996;334:1470–1471.

107. Zhang Z, Milich DR, Peterson DL, et al. Interferon alfa treatment induces delayed CD4 proliferative responses to the hepatitis C virus nonstructural protein 3 regardless of the outcome of therapy. *J Infect Dis* 1997;175:1294–1301.

108. Terrault NA, Holland CC, Ferrell L, et al. Interferon alfa for recurrent hepatitis B infection after liver transplantation. *Liver Transplant Surg* 1996;2:132–138.

109. Poterucha JJ, Weisner RH. Liver transplantation and hepatitis B. *Ann Intern Med* 1997;126:805–806.

110. Rodrigues A, Morgado T, Areias J, et al. Limited benefits of INF-alfa therapy in renal graft candidates with chronic viral hepatitis B or C. *Transplant Proc* 1997;29:777–780.

111. Dousset B, Conti F, Houssin D, Calmus Y. Acute vanishing bile duct syndrome after interferon therapy for recurrent HCV infection in liver transplant recipients [letter]. *N Engl J Med* 1994;330:1160–1161.

112. Meyers JD, Fournoy N, Sanders JE, et al. Prophylactic use of human leukocyte interferon after allogeneic marrow transplantation. *Ann Intern Med* 1987;107:809–816.

113. The International Chronic Granulomatous Disease Cooperative Study Group. A controlled trial of interferon-gamma to prevent infection in chronic granulomatous disease. *N Engl J Med* 1991;324:509–516.

114. Murray HW. Interferon-gamma and host antimicrobial defense: current and future clinical applications. *Am J Med* 1994;97:459–467.

115. NIH Conference. Interferon-gamma in the management of infectious diseases. *Ann Intern Med* 1995;123:216–224.

116. Schaffner A. Therapeutic concentrations of glucocorticoids suppress the antimicrobial activity of human macrophages without impairing their responsiveness to gamma interferon. *J Clin Invest* 1985;76: 1755–1764.

117. LoVelle B. Fungicidal activation of murine macrophages by recombinant gamma interferon. *Infect Immunol* 1987;55:2951–2955.

118. Szefler SJ, Norton CE, Ball B, Gross JM, Aida Y, Pabst MJ. IFN-γ and

LPS overcome glucocorticoid inhibition of priming for superoxide release in human monocytes. *J Immunol* 1989;142:3985–3992.

119. Roilides E, Holmes A, Blake C, Venzon D, Pizzo PA, Walsh TJ. Antifungal activity of elutriated human monocytes against *Aspergillus fumigatus hyphae*: enhancement by granulocyte-macrophage colony-stimulating factor and interferon-γ. *J Infect Dis* 1994;170:894–899.

120. Roilides E, Sein T, Holmes A, et al. Effects of macrophage colony-stimulating factor on antifungal activity on mononuclear phagocytes against *Aspergillus fumigatus*. *J Infect Dis* 1995;172:1028–1034.

121. Roilides E, Blake C, Holmes A, Pizzo PA, Walsh TJ. Granulocyte-macrophage colony-stimulating factor and interferon-γ prevent dexamethasone-induced immunosuppression of antifungal monocyte activity against *Aspergillus fumigatus hyphae*. *J Med Vet Mycol* 1996;34:63–69.

122. Kovacs JA, Vogel S, Albert JM, et al. Controlled trial of interleukin-2 infusions in patient infected with the human immunodeficiency virus. *N Engl J Med* 1996;335:1350–1356.

123. Welte K, Ciobanu N, Moore MAS, Gulati S, O'Reilly RJ, Mertelsmann R. Defective interleukin 2 production in patient after bone marrow transplantation and *in vitro* restoration of defective T lymphocyte proliferation by highly purified interleukin 2. *Blood* 1984;64:380–385.

124. Abdul-Hai A, Lorberboum-Gliski H, Mechushtan A, et al. Involvement of interleukin-2 in immunologic reconstitution following bone marrow transplantation. *J Interferon Cytokine Res* 1995;15:95–101.

125. Snydman DR, Sullivan B, Gill M, Gould JA, Parkinson DR, Atkins MD. Nosocomial sepsis associated with interleukin-2. *Ann Intern Med* 1990;112:102–107.

126. Klempner MS, Noring R, Mier JW, Atkins MB. An acquired chemotactic defect in neutrophils from patients receiving interleukin-2 immunotherapy. *N Engl J Med* 1990;322:959–965.

127. Abdul-Hai A, Ben-Yehuda A, Weiss L, et al. Interleukin-7-enhanced cytotoxic T lymphocyte activity after viral infection in marrow transplanted mice. *Bone Marrow Transplant* 1997;19:539–543.

128. Trinchieri G. Interleukin-12: a proinflammatory cytokine with immunoregulatory functions that bridge innate resistance and antigen-specific adaptive immunity. *Ann Rev Immunol* 1995;13:251–276.

129. Locksley RM. Interleukin 12 in host defense against microbial pathogens. *Proc Natl Acad Sci U S A* 1993;90:5879–5880.

130. Scott P. IL-12: initiation cytokine for cell-mediated immunity. *Science* 1993;260:496–497.

131. Trinchieri G. Interleukin-12: a cytokine produced by antigen-presenting cells with immunoregulatory functions in the generation of T-helper cells type 1 and cytotoxic lymphocytes. *Blood* 1994;84:4008–4027.

132. Romani L, Mencacci A, Tonnetti, et al. Interleukin-12 but not interferon-γ production correlated with induction of T helper type-1 phenotype in murine candidiasis. *Eur J Immunol* 1994;24:909.

133. Romani L, Mencacci A, Tonnetti L, et al. Interleukin-12 is both required and prognostic *in vivo* for T helper type 1 differentiation in murine candidiasis. *J Immunol* 1994;153:5167–5175.

134. Sonis ST, Lindquist L, Van Vugt A, et al. Prevention of chemotherapy-induced ulcerative mucositis by transforming growth factor 3. *Cancer Res* 1994;54:1135–1138.

135. Housley RM, Morris CF, Boyle W, et al. Keratinocyte growth factor induced proliferation of hepatocytes and epithelial cells throughout the rat gastrointestinal tract. *J Clin Invest* 1994;94:1764–1777.

136. Yi ES, Shabaik AS, Lacey DL, et al. Keratinocyte growth factor causes proliferation of urothelium *in vivo*. *J Urol* 1995;154:1566–1570.

137. Yi ES, Yin S, Harclerode DL, et al. Keratinocyte growth factor induces pancreatic ductal epithelial proliferation. *Am J Pathol* 1994;145:80–85.

Transplant Infections edited by
Raleigh A. Bowden, Per Ljungman, and Carlos V. Paya.
Lippincott–Raven Publishers, Philadelphia © 1998

CHAPTER 28

Cellular Adoptive Immunotherapy for Viral Infection with Unmodified or Genetically Modified T Cells

Stanley R. Riddell and Philip D. Greenberg

Cellular immunotherapy can be broadly defined as the administration of effector cells of the immune system for the treatment of disease. This approach has been investigated in humans predominantly as a therapy for malignant diseases. However, a primary function of the cellular immune system is to afford protection against pathogens, including acute and persistent viral infections. Thus allogeneic hematopoietic cell transplant (HCT) and solid organ transplant recipients who receive immunosuppressive therapy to interfere with cellular immune functions are prone to severe and potentially fatal viral infection, and efforts to restore protective immune responses by cellular immunotherapy could be beneficial. Despite the conceptual attraction of immunotherapeutic approaches to viral infections in transplant recipients and the success of immunotherapy in experimental animal models, efforts to translate the basic principles established in animal model studies to clinical infections remain in the very early stages. The objective of this chapter is to review the principles underlying cellular immunotherapy for viral infections and the results of the initial clinical efforts with this approach in transplant recipients.

Transplant recipients are vulnerable to progressive infection following the acquisition of a primary viral infection and after the reactivation of viruses that have previously established a latent or persistent infection in the host. Primary infection with acute seasonal respiratory viruses such as influenza, respiratory syncytial virus, and parainfluenza is a relatively unusual cause of serious infection in immunocompromised hosts except during periods when infections with these viruses are prevalent in the community (1–4). Acute infection of transplant recipients with such respiratory viruses can be self-limiting, as in immunocompetent hosts, but often progresses to severe pneumonitis and death (1–4). Studies in murine models suggest that both B-cell and T-cell immunity are important in preventing and resolving these infections, but the unpredictable occurrence of outbreaks and the antigenic diversity of the causative viruses make them less attractive candidates for initial studies of cellular immunotherapy to restore potentially protective immune responses (5,6).

Historically, a more prevalent problem for transplant recipients was the acquisition of primary infection with cytomegalovirus (CMV) and Epstein-Barr virus (EBV), both of which could be transmitted to previously unexposed recipients by blood products and/or the hematopoietic stem cells or solid organ. If the transplant donor and recipient are both seronegative for CMV, primary infection of the recipient can be prevented by the use of blood products from CMV seronegative donors for transfusion (7). However, CMV- or EBV-seronegative HCT or solid organ transplant recipients receiving HCT or an organ from a CMV- or EBV-seropositive donor are at risk for the development of progressive disease caused by these viruses.

Reactivation of endogenous latent viruses of the herpes group—including herpes simplex virus (HSV), varicella-zoster virus (VZV), CMV, and EBV—also results in significant morbidity and mortality in immunocompromised transplant recipients. The use of acyclovir was highly effective for preventing or treating reactivations of HSV and VZV and caused minimal toxicity but was only partially effective for preventing CMV disease and was inef-

SRR: From the Immunology Program, Fred Hutchinson Cancer Research Center, Seattle, WA 98104. PDG: From the departments of Medicine and Immunology, the University of Washington, Seattle, WA 98104.

fective for EBV (8–10). The administration of ganciclovir for CMV infection—either prophylactically to prevent reactivation or after reactivation was detected by periodic screening of the recipient by culture, antigenemia, or PCR methodology—was highly effective for preventing disease in both allogeneic HCT and solid organ transplant recipients but frequently caused neutropenia, especially after HCT (11–16). Studies in HCT recipients also demonstrated that the use of ganciclovir early after transplant to prevent CMV disease was associated with a delay in reconstitution of CMV-specific T-cell immunity and with an increased incidence of late-onset (occurring >100 days after transplant) CMV disease (17). Late CMV disease was also observed in solid organ transplant recipients after ganciclovir was discontinued (18). Unlike infection with HSV, VZV, and CMV, effective antiviral drugs for prophylaxis or preemptive therapy of EBV infection have not been identified.

Although antiviral drugs have constituted an important advance for prevention or resolution of herpes viral infections, especially those occurring in the early post-transplant period, long-term control of persistent herpes viruses will probably depend on the ability of the host to mount an adequate immune response to the respective pathogen. The discussion here will focus on the role of cellular effectors in controlling viral infections and their potential use in immunotherapy.

EFFECTOR CELL POPULATIONS AND CONTROL OF VIRAL INFECTION

The development of cellular immunotherapy for individual viral infections should be predicated on an understanding of the nature of the host response(s) responsible for protective immunity in immunocompetent hosts. After acute infection with a pathogen the normal host mounts a multifaceted and coordinated immune response. The cellular components of this response can be broadly divided into two categories—effector cells that are not antigen-specific, such as natural killer (NK) cells and macrophages, which may be important in the initial containment of infection, and effector cells that express surface receptors that convey a high degree of specificity for antigens expressed by the virus, such as $\gamma\delta^+$ T cells, $\alpha\beta^+$ T cells, and antibody-producing B cells.

NK cells recognize and lyse target cells expressing low levels of class I major histocompatibility complex (MHC) molecules and might be expected to participate in the host response against viruses such as CMV, HSV, and adenovirus, which down-regulate the expression of class I MHC in the infected cell (19–22). NK cells exhibit antiviral activity *in vivo*, as demonstrated by studies in mice and in humans with selective NK deficiency, and may be important during the early phase of infection prior to the development of virus-specific T cells (23,24). However, viruses such as CMV express genes that inhibit

NK activation and lysis of the infected cell, potentially limiting the efficacy of NK cells in established infection (25). The administration of activated NK cells to patients with malignant disease has also been associated with significant toxicity (26). Thus to justify the use of this effector population for adoptive immunotherapy of infections in transplant recipients, additional studies are necessary to define the degree to which deficiencies of NK cells contribute to the progression of individual viral infections and to identify measures that may reduce the toxicity of therapy.

$\gamma\delta^+$ T cells that recognize virus-infected cells have been identified and could be of benefit in adoptive immunotherapy (27,28). However, strategies to isolate and expand virus-specific $\gamma\delta^+$ T cells are not well defined, and their role in controlling viral infection is uncertain. Thus as with NK cells it is premature at the present time to consider utilizing $\gamma\delta^+$ T cells for adoptive immunotherapy.

The consensus from studies in animal models of experimental infection is that the induction and maintenance of virus-specific CD4$^+$ and CD8$^+$ $\alpha\beta^+$ T-cell responses is sufficient and often essential for the resolution of infection (28,29). Furthermore, $\alpha\beta^+$ T cells provide immunologic memory that may be of major significance in settings where the patient will experience repeated exposure to the virus or where the virus has established a latent infection in the host (30,31). The methodology to isolate and expand clonal populations of $\alpha\beta^+$ T cells with defined specificity for viral antigens is well established for several viruses that cause disease in transplant recipients (29). Thus strategies to develop adoptive cellular immunotherapy for transplant recipients have primarily focused on the use of virus-specific $\alpha\beta^+$ T cells.

Experiments performed in animal models to examine the cellular requirements for an effective host response to viral infection have included a detailed analysis of the contributions of the two broad subsets of $\alpha\beta^+$ T cells—class II MHC-restricted CD4$^+$ helper T cells (Th) and class I MHC-restricted CD8$^+$ T cytotoxic T cells (CTL). Initially, the adoptive transfer of purified T-cell subsets or T-cell clones to augment individual responses or the administration of monoclonal antibodies to deplete the activity of a single T-cell subset was used as a strategy to examine the role of CD4$^+$ and CD8$^+$ T cells (32–35). Later studies utilized mice rendered deficient in expression of class I or class II MHC molecules by gene knock-out technology and thus unable to generate CD8$^+$ or CD4$^+$ T cells, respectively, to examine the contribution of these T-cell subsets in viral infections (36–39). The results of these experiments demonstrated that, depending on the dose, route, timing, pathogenesis, virulence, and type of challenge virus, either CD8$^+$ or CD4$^+$ virus-specific T cells could provide protective immunity to virus challenge and resolve acute infection (32–39). This analysis in animal models demonstrated the crucial role of CD8$^+$ and CD4$^+$ antiviral T cells and not only provided important insights into the cooperativity between these subsets but also indicated that the development of adoptive immunotherapy in humans should be guided by an understanding of the pathogenesis of infection and examination of the antiviral activity of CD4+ and CD8+ T-cell subsets for individual viruses.

EFFECTOR MECHANISMS OF αβ+ T CELLS

Basic studies of T-cell biology have provided an understanding of the effector mechanisms that can be mediated by CD4+ and CD8+ T cells and insights into how these cells contribute to the resolution of viral infections.

CD4+ αβ+ Th Effector Functions

Antigen recognition by virus-specific CD4+ T cells involves an interaction between the αβ+ T-cell receptor and the class II MHC heterodimer containing a peptide fragment derived from a viral protein in its binding groove (40,41). The expression of class II MHC is primarily restricted to professional antigen-presenting cell (APC) such as dendritic cells, macrophages, and B cells but can be induced on other cell types, including endothelial cells. The antigens presented to CD4+ T cells are usually endocytosed by the APC and degraded by proteolysis in endosomal compartments where the resulting peptides encounter and bind to class II MHC molecules that traffic to the cell surface (Fig. 1A). Because the viral antigens can be obtained by endocytosis at the site of infection or in the draining lymph nodes, the APC does not actually need to be infected with the virus to activate CD4+ Th. Several viruses, including HIV, CMV, EBV, and measles, do productively infect cells bearing class II MHC molecules, and in this circumstance, endogenously synthesized viral proteins may also enter the class II processing pathway and directly activate CD4+ Th (40,42).

The primary function of activated CD4+ Th is to produce cytokines that by autocrine and paracrine effects orchestrate a local and systemic host response to the pathogen. Mature differentiated CD4+ Th are categorized into two major subsets—Th1 and Th2—with distinct profiles of cytokine production and functional roles in the immune response (43,44). A third subset of CD4+ Th cells termed *Th0* appears to represent an intermediate stage of CD4+ T-cell differentiation between naive T cells and either Th1 or Th2 cells and exhibits a mixed pattern of cytokine production. The precise signals involved in determining the commitment of CD4+ T cells to the Th1 or Th2 phenotypes are not fully delineated, but it is well established that the differentiation pathway can be influenced by other cytokines. Interferon-γ (IFN-γ) and IL-12 in the milieu will favor the development of the Th1 phenotype, and IL-4 and IL-10 favor the development of the Th2 phenotype (45–47).

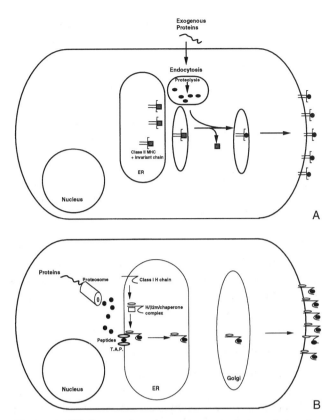

Figure 1. (A) Processing of exogenous protein antigens for presentation to CD4+ class II MHC–restricted T-helper cells. Viral proteins are endocytosed by professional antigen-presenting cells and are degraded to peptides in acidic endosomal compartments. Class II MHC molecules are bound to an invariant chain in the endoplasmic reticulum to prevent their association with peptides in the ER. The class II MHC/invariant chain complex encounters antigenic peptides in the endosomal compartment during transit to the cell surface, and the invariant chain is cleaved from the class II molecule, allowing the binding of antigenic peptides that are then displayed at the cell surface. **(B)** Processing of endogenous protein antigens for presentation to CD8+ class I MHC–restricted cytotoxic T cells. Viral proteins in the cytosol are degraded by the proteosome complex to peptide fragments, which are transported into the ER by the heterodimeric TAP complex. In the ER the peptides associate with class I MHC and the complex is transported to the cell surface.

The CD4+ Th1 subset produces IL-2, IFN-γ, and TNF, and preferentially promotes cell-mediated immune responses (43). IL-2 activates and induces the proliferation of NK cells and is the major growth factor for CD8+ CTL (48,49). Indeed, in an animal model of persistent viral infection, the ability to mount a virus-specific CD4+ Th response was essential to sustain virus-specific CD8+ CTL responses (50). IFN-γ and TNF activate nonspecific effector cells such as macrophages and NK cells, exert direct inhibitory effects on virus replication, and promote resistance of uninfected cells to viral infection (51,52). The Th2 subset of CD4+ Th produces IL-4, IL-5, and IL-10, and promotes the development of humoral immunity and the activation and differentiation of eosinophils and mast cells (53,54).

Although there is little information concerning the role of distinct CD4+ Th subsets in the immune response to individual viral infections in humans, insights derived from murine models suggest that the subtype of CD4+ T cells used in adoptive therapy may affect both efficacy and safety. For example, in a murine model of influenza infection, the transfer of an influenza-specific CD4+ Th1 clone was protective, whereas the transfer of an influenza-specific Th2 clone failed to confer protective immunity (55). In the RSV model both RSV-specific Th1 and Th2 cells exhibited antiviral activity and promoted clearance of virus, but the Th2 cells induced an eosinophil-rich infiltrate in the lungs and worsened morbidity (56). These results indicate that, depending on the viral infection being treated, the selection of CD4+ T cells for use in therapy may be a decisive factor in success or failure.

CD8+ αβ+ CTL Effector Functions

CD8+ cytotoxic T cells recognize peptides complexed to class I MHC molecules on the surface of cells (57). In distinction to recognition by CD4+ Th, where the peptides presented by class II MHC molecules are derived from proteins entering the endocytic pathway in the APC, the antigenic peptides displayed with class I MHC are primarily derived by the proteolytic cleavage of intracellular proteins by the proteosome complex (58). These peptides are then transported from the cytosol into the endoplasmic reticulum (ER) by a heterodimeric protein complex termed the *transporter associated with antigen presentation* (TAP) (59). In the ER, the peptides bind to the class I MHC heavy chain, leading to the formation of a stable trimolecular peptide/class I H chain/β2 microglobulin complex that is transported via the Golgi to the cell surface (Fig. 1B). Because class I MHC molecules are constitutively expressed or are inducible in most cell types, CD8+ CTL serve as a surveillance mechanism for detecting and eliminating virus-infected cells and appear to be required for clearance and resolution of most viral infections (28).

The interaction between the T-cell receptor and the relevant class I/peptide complex usually results in direct lysis of the target cell and the production of Th1-type cytokines, including IFN-γ and TNF. However, in contrast to CD4+ Th1 cells, differentiated effector CD8+ CTL do not produce IL-2 following antigen stimulation but are dependent on IL-2 producing CD4+ Th for proliferation. The lytic signal delivered by CD8+ CTL involves the directed exocytosis of cytolytic granules containing perforin and serine esterases (granzymes) or Fas/Fas ligand (Fas L) interactions (60). Perforin disrupts the target cell cytoplasmic and nuclear membranes, facilitating the entry of the granzymes that induce DNA fragmentation

and ensuring destruction of the target cell and cessation of virus replication. Activated CD8+ CTL also express Fas L and may induce programmed cell death in virus-infected target cells expressing Fas.

The contribution of cytolytic granules to the antiviral activities of CD8+ CTL has most clearly been demonstrated in the murine LCMV model. Mice generated with a disruption in the perforin gene cannot induce the membrane injury and lyse the target cell (61). CD8+ T cells from perforin-deficient mice inoculated with LCMV will proliferate in response to virus challenge but exhibit only weak LCMV-specific cytolytic activity *in vitro,* possibly mediated by Fas/FasL interactions (61). Perforin-deficient mice fail to clear LCMV infection *in vivo*, illustrating the requirement for perforin-mediated lytic events for resolution of this infection (61).

T-CELL IMMUNOTHERAPY OF POST-TRANSPLANT CMV INFECTIONS

CMV is a ubiquitous herpesvirus that infects 50% to 70% of the population. Primary infection in immunocompetent hosts is largely unrecognized except as an occasional cause of mononucleosis, and viral persistence is not associated with any clinical sequelae. However, in patients with iatrogenic or acquired immunodeficiency, reactivation of CMV in CMV-seropositive hosts or the acquisition of primary CMV infection from blood products or the donated organ often leads to progressive infection and visceral disease and represents a major obstacle to a successful outcome for transplant recipients.

The clinical manifestations of CMV infection may differ, depending on the type of transplant and associated clinical factors. Solid organ transplant recipients who are CMV seronegative and receive an organ from a CMV-seropositive donor often develop a CMV syndrome consisting of fever, leukopenia, hepatosplenomegaly, myalgias, and occasionally pneumonitis (62,63). Reactivation of CMV in seropositive solid organ transplant recipients may also progress to visceral infection, especially in those patients who require intense therapy with immunosuppressive drugs to treat episodes of rejection. Allogeneic HCT recipients who develop a primary or reactivation infection with CMV may also develop fever and leukopenia, but interstitial pneumonitis or enteritis are the most common manifestations of CMV disease in these patients (8).

CMV-Specific T-Cell Immunity and CMV Disease in Immunosuppressed Transplant Recipients

A critical role for αβ+ T cells in human CMV infection was first suggested by studies in the murine cytomegalovirus (MCMV) model. MCMV is genetically distinct from human CMV, but the pathogenesis of infection in immunosuppressed mice is similar to that for human CMV. In the MCMV model, the transfer of CD8⁺ MCMV-specific CTL alone was sufficient to protect mice from fatal CMV infection, although the administration of CD4⁺ Th was essential for eliminating salivary gland infection (35,64–66). CD8⁺ CTL specific for the MCMV major IE protein alone were sufficient to provide protective immunity from lethal virus challenge, suggesting that restoring even a limited repertoire of the host CTL response can be therapeutically beneficial (64).

The hypothesis that progressive human CMV infection in HCT and organ transplant recipients is related to a quantitative deficiency of virus-specific $\alpha\beta^+$ T-cell responses has been examined in several studies. Quinnan and colleagues showed that the recovery of cytolytic activity for CMV-infected fibroblasts in samples of peripheral blood lymphocytes obtained from allogeneic HCT and renal transplant recipients was associated with resolution of CMV infection (67). Recent studies have cultured the peripheral blood lymphocytes from allogeneic HCT recipients *in vitro* to more clearly distinguish the recovery of CD4⁺ and CD8⁺ CMV-specific T-cell responses and to improve the sensitivity for detecting these responses (17,68,69). In all published reports a correlation was observed between the presence of MHC-restricted $\alpha\beta^+$ T-cell responses to CMV and protection from the subsequent occurrence of CMV disease, supporting the concept that $\alpha\beta^+$ T-cell responses are an essential component of protective immunity to CMV.

Specificity of $\alpha\beta^+$ CD8⁺ CMV-Specific T Cells

The CMV genome may encode more than 200 proteins. Thus in permissively infected cells there are a large number of antigens that could be presented for recognition by CD8⁺ cytotoxic T cells. Definition of the specificity of CTL responses in individuals with protective immunity to CMV is a critical prelude to the development of effective adoptive immunotherapy to ensure that the T cells to be transferred are selected to represent the protective responses in immunocompetent hosts. CMV expresses its genes in a temporal sequence with discrete phases of gene expression termed the *immediate early* (IE), *early* (E), and *late* (L) phases (70). Infected cells expressing a limited array of viral proteins can be prepared by the timed addition of inhibitors to block viral protein or RNA synthesis, and this methodology was employed to determine if CTL preferentially recognized proteins produced at IE, E, or L stages of the replicative cycle. Surprisingly, the introduction of an RNA synthesis inhibitor to target cells just prior to virus exposure to prevent the production of newly synthesized viral proteins after viral entry did not prevent recognition by CD8⁺ CMV-specific CTL lines and the majority of CTL clones isolated from normal CMV-seropositive individuals (71). This demonstrated that viral gene expression in the target cell was not required at all to sensitize the cell for lysis

and that virion proteins introduced into the target cell cytosol following viral entry rather than newly synthesized IE, E, or L proteins were the immunodominant target antigens of the host CTL response. The specificity of the CD8⁺ CMV-specific CTL that recovered after allogeneic BMT and were associated with protection from subsequent CMV disease was similarly analyzed, and these CTL were also specific for epitopes derived from structural virion proteins (17).

The contribution of individual virion proteins as antigens for CTL was assessed by pulsing peptide fragments of purified proteins onto target cells or infecting target cells using recombinant vaccinia viruses encoding a single CMV gene. The matrix protein pp65 has been identified as the target of the immunodominant host response most frequently, although major responses to a second matrix protein pp150 are observed in some individuals (72–74; S. Riddell, unpublished data). Insight into the biological importance of CTL for structural virion proteins was suggested by studies evaluating the ability of these CTL to kill CMV-infected cells at different stages of the replication cycle. CMV-infected target cells are rapidly (<1 hour following virus inoculation) sensitized for lysis by CD8⁺ CTL specific for either pp65 or pp150, and the infected cell remains a target throughout the entire replicative cycle (Fig. 2). Thus such CTL should be effective in limiting virus dissemination after reactivation by promptly eliminating newly infected cells. However, the rapid recognition of structural proteins such as pp65

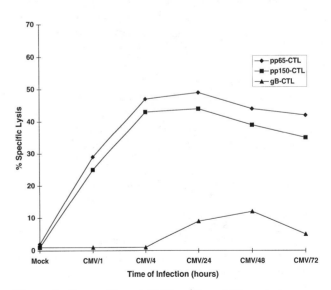

Figure 2. Recognition of CMV pp65, pp150, and glycoprotein B (gB) at different stages of the virus replication cycle. Autologous fibroblasts were either uninfected (mock) or infected with CMV for 1, 4, 24, 48, and 72 hours, and assessed as targets for lysis by CD8⁺ CTL clones specific for pp65, pp150, or gB. To enhance the sensitivity for detecting killing by gB-specific CTL, the infected fibroblasts were preincubated with interferon γ for 24 hours. The effector to target ratio is 10:1.

and pp150 is not observed with CTL specific for virus envelope gB protein (see Fig. 2). CTLs specific for gB lyse CMV-infected cells poorly at all stages of the replicative cycle and are present in CMV-seropositive individuals at substantially lower frequency than CTL for pp65 or pp150 (74–76). The fact that CTL specific for pp65 and/or pp150 are maintained at very high frequency for life in normal CMV-seropositive individuals suggests that even in these immunocompetent hosts virus reactivation occurs intermittently but remains subclinical because of rapid control by the host immune response.

Specificity of αβ⁺ CD4⁺ CMV-Specific T-Cell Responses

CD4⁺ Th responses to antigen preparations extracted from CMV-infected cells are readily demonstrable in healthy CMV-seropositive individuals. Recombinant gB, pp65, IE-2, p52 and IE-1 CMV proteins have been generated and used to determine the specificity of CD4⁺ Th responses. Detectable responses have been observed to all the antigens studied, with approximately 70% of individuals responding to gB, pp65, and IE-2 and a smaller proportion responding to IE-1 and the DNA-binding protein p52 (77–80). Although additional studies are needed, the available data suggest that considerable diversity exists in the CD4⁺ Th response to CMV.

Animal model studies have illustrated the potential importance of characterizing the cytokine profile of CD4⁺ Th to be used in adoptive immunotherapy for the safety and efficacy of therapy. The cytokine profile of CD4⁺ CMV-specific Th clones isolated from CMV-seropositive individuals has been analyzed, and all clones tested produced IL-2 and IFN-γ characteristic of Th1 cells but many also produced IL-4 consistent with an overlapping or Th0 phenotype (S. Riddell, unpublished data). It remains to be determined if the phenotype of these cells can be fixed to a Th1 or Th2 pattern *in vitro* and if this will be necessary for the safety and/or efficacy of immunotherapy with CD4⁺ CMV-specific T cells.

Immune Evasion Strategies Employed by Cytomegalovirus

Several viruses have evolved strategies for evading recognition by the host immune response, and identification of the mechanisms utilized by CMV should assist in selecting the appropriate effector cells to use in adoptive immunotherapy to restore protective immunity. It is generally accepted that CMV can enter a latent state that allows the virus to persist even during the height of the immune response, although the cellular sites of latency and the status of viral gene expression in such cells are not completely defined (70,81).

Once the virus reactivates from latency and initiates replication, infection is likely to progress in the absence

of a host response to limit dissemination. One strategy CMV uses to elude destruction of permissively infected cells by CD8⁺ CTL is to inhibit the cellular processes involved in delivering class I MHC molecules bearing antigenic peptides to the cell surface. Studies of cells replicating CMV demonstrated a reduced surface expression of class I MHC at the E and L stages of the replicative cycle (19,22). The mechanisms involved in the downregulation of class I MHC were elucidated with the identification of four viral genes—US2, US3, US6, and US1—which interfere in a coordinated fashion at discrete steps in the antigen presentation pathway (82–86). US3 is an ER-resident glycoprotein encoded by an IE gene and hinders antigen presentation by binding to class I MHC and retaining these molecules in the ER (84). US2 and US11 are encoded by E genes and direct the reverse translocation of class I MHC molecules from the ER into the cytosol, where they are rapidly degraded (83,85). US6 is encoded by an E/L gene and inhibits, via effects on the luminal side of the ER, the transport of antigenic peptides into the ER, where they are normally loaded onto class I molecules (86). These diverse maneuvers directed by virus-encoded proteins collectively impede the efficient presentation of viral proteins expressed after the IE stage of replication and provide a biological basis for the immunodominance of CD8⁺ CTL directed against structural virion proteins that are presented before this global blockade in class I antigen presentation (Fig. 3). Moreover, these findings suggest that CD8⁺ CTL against structural proteins may be essential for eliminating newly

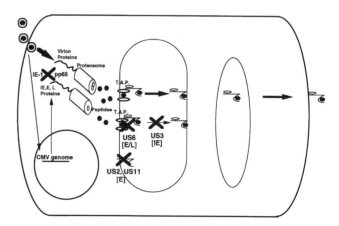

Figure 3. Sites of CMV interference in class I antigen processing and presentation of newly synthesized viral proteins. The virion protein pp65 selectively interferes with the presentation of the major immediate early protein presumably at a step prior to proteolytic degradation. The viral proteins US3, US6, US2, and US11 act to retain class I in the ER, block peptide transport, and expel class I from the ER into the cytosol, thereby inducing a global blockade in the presentation of newly synthesized viral antigens. The major source of peptides that bind class I and transit to the cell surface is from proteolysis of the structural virion proteins that enter the cytosol following virus penetration.

infected cells because viral proteins synthesized at E or L times are unlikely to be efficiently presented.

The IE protein is made in abundance immediately after infection and prior to the decline in cell surface class I MHC expression. Conceptually, it would be a good antigen to target in adoptive immunotherapy. Studies using vaccinia recombinant viruses encoding the 72-kD major immediate early (IE) protein have identified IE-specific CTL in normal CMV-seropositive individuals (75,76). Surprisingly, these CTL fail to lyse permissively infected target cells even if virus replication is arrested at the IE stage of replication (Fig. 4) (75). This suggested an additional mechanism by which CMV interfered with the presentation of IE. Recent studies have demonstrated that the pp65 protein that is introduced into the cytosol after virion entry and prior to IE synthesis selectively interferes with the presentation of IE peptides (see Fig. 4) (87). The elucidation of these virus evasion strategies provides important insights into the role CTL of different specificities might have in the host response and suggests that the use of CD8+ CTL specific for structural virion proteins that recognize newly infected cells rapidly after viral entry represents the most logical choice for initial studies to reconstitute protective immunity to CMV.

The early and sustained decrease in surface class I MHC expression in CMV-infected cell should enhance the susceptibility of these cells to recognition by NK cells and suggests a potential role for this effector population in eliminating permissively infected target cells. However, the arsenal of stealth tactics employed by CMV also extends to evasion of NK recognition. CMV encodes a molecule, UL18, which is homologous to class I MHC and when expressed on the cell surface delivers an inhibitory signal to the NK cell and prevents NK-mediated lysis (25).

Clinical Studies of Adoptive Immunotherapy with CMV-Specific T Cells

At the present time, the investigation of adoptive immunotherapy with CMV-specific T cells is impractical for some subgroups of transplant recipients. In solid organ transplantation, T cells isolated for use in therapy should be derived from the recipient because donor T cells could elicit recipient immune responses to donor major or minor histocompatibility antigens. For CMV-seronegative solid organ transplant recipients it is technically difficult to isolate and expand autologous virus-specific T cells before transplant for use in immunotherapy after transplant because of the extremely low precursor frequency of such cells in the peripheral blood in the absence of prior natural infection. One potential strategy would be to induce virus-specific T-cell responses in the CMV-seronegative recipient by vaccination prior to transplant and then isolate such cells for use in therapy to augment the endogenous response during the period of post-transplant immunosuppression. Examination of such an approach will have to await the design of safe and effective vaccines to elicit CMV-specific T-cell responses. In the setting of HLA-identical allogeneic HCT, the CMV-specific T cells for post-transplant immunotherapy should be derived from the donor because the immune system that develops in the host after transplant is derived from donor hematopoietic cells. Thus for CMV-seropositive transplant recipients receiving HCT from a CMV-seronegative donor it would again be necessary to first vaccinate the donor to elicit virus-specific T-cell responses that could then be isolated for use in therapy (88).

Recipients receiving HCT from a CMV-seropositive donor provide the most favorable setting to investigate CMV-specific T-cell therapy because T cells with reactivity for CMV antigens can be readily isolated from the donor by *in vitro* stimulation with autologous APC expressing CMV antigens. The generation of polyclonal populations of CMV-reactive T cells from the donor is technically feasible, but these polyclonal populations may also contain T cells that are not reactive with CMV, including T cells that could recognize recipient minor histocompatibility antigens. Thus one concern with the use of polyclonal donor T cells for adoptive transfer is the potential for inducing graft-versus-host disease (GVHD). Indeed, GVHD was frequently observed when polyclonal

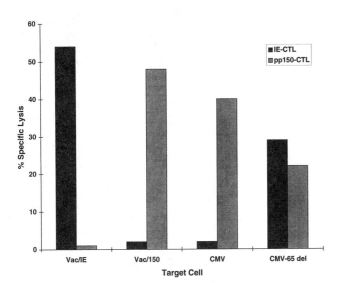

Figure 4. The major immediate early protein is not recognized in CMV-infected cells because of a selective inhibition by pp65. Autologous target cells were infected with a vaccinia recombinant virus encoding IE, a vaccinia recombinant virus encoding pp150, CMV, or a mutant CMV that is deleted in pp65 and contains no pp65 in its matrix. CD8+ CTL clones specific for IE or pp150 were used as effector cells. The IE CTL lyses the vac/IE-infected and the CMV-del65-infected target cells efficiently but does not lyse the wild-type CMV-infected target. The control CTL specific for pp150 lyses vac/pp150, CMV, and CMV-del65.

T cells were administered to HCT recipients to treat EBV-induced lymphomas (89). This potential problem could be avoided if individual T-cell clones were isolated and selected for recognition of recipient APC presenting CMV antigens but not recipient APC alone.

The first evaluation of adoptive immunotherapy in humans with virus-specific T cells was performed in allogeneic HCT recipients and examined the safety and immunomodulatory properties of administering CD8+ class I MHC-restricted CMV-specific cytotoxic T-cell clones (90). CD8+ CTL were selected for initial investigation because data from animal models of CMV infection and reconstitution studies in humans suggested CD8+ CTL were both necessary and sufficient for protective immunity (17,35,68). CD8+ CMV-specific T-cell clones were isolated by limiting dilution cloning from polyclonal T-cell lines established from the bone marrow donor. The T-cell clones were cultured *in vitro* by intermittent stimulation of the T-cell receptor in the presence of donor-derived γ irradiated feeder cells followed by the addition of low doses of IL-2 to promote numerical expansion. Clones were tested for cell surface expression of the αβ T-cell receptor, CD3, CD8, and CD4 and for class I MHC-restricted lysis of CMV-infected target cells. Clones that were αβTcR+, CD3+, CD8+, and CD4−, and recognized epitopes derived from structural virion proteins in the context of class I MHC were selected for intravenous administration to the recipient.

Each patient received a weekly infusion of CD8+ CTL for 4 weeks beginning 28–42 days after transplant at cell doses of $3.3 \times 10^7/m^2$ body surface area, $1 \times 10^8/m^2$, $3.3 \times 10^8/m^2$, $1 \times 10^9/m^2$, respectively. No serious acute toxicities were observed even at the highest cell dose in any of the 14 patients treated, and the patients did not require

hospitalization for the infusions. Minor side effects that included transient fever and chills were observed in two patients (91).

The ability of adoptively transferred CD8+ CTL clones to restore CMV-specific immune responses in the recipient was examined by evaluating the generation of class I MHC-restricted CMV-specific cytolytic activity in cultures of lymphocytes obtained from the peripheral blood before and at intervals after each infusion. Eleven of the 14 patients did not have detectable CMV-specific CTL responses in the blood immediately prior to the first infusion; however, CTL responses were evident 2 days after the first infusion and increased with each subsequent infusion such that the responses measured 2 days after the fourth infusion were equivalent to those present in PBL obtained from the healthy donor (Fig. 5). The T-cell receptor Vβ gene rearrangement was used as a molecular marker to identify infused CTL clones in samples of blood obtained up to 12 weeks after therapy was completed. This analysis determined that the infused CTL were capable of persisting *in vivo* for at least 12 weeks and were responsible for the CMV-specific lytic activity observed in the cultures (91).

CMV-specific CTL responses equivalent in magnitude to those of the donor were achieved in all patients following the fourth infusion, but longitudinal analysis revealed a decline in these responses during the next 12 weeks in the subset of patients who developed grade 2 GVHD as a consequence of the HCT and required combination immunosuppressive therapy with cyclosporine and prednisone (Fig. 6A). This subset of patients also failed to recover endogenous CD4+ CMV-specific Th (see Fig. 6A). In contrast, patients who recovered CD4+ CMV-specific Th responses maintained strong CD8+ CTL

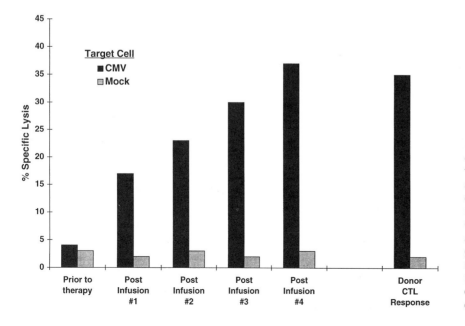

Figure 5. Reconstitution of CMV-specific CD8+ T-cell immunity by adoptive transfer of CTL clones. CTL generation assays were performed on lymphocytes obtained from the blood of HCT recipients prior to therapy with CD8+ CMV-specific T-cell clones and 2 days after each of the four infusions. The target cells included autologous CMV and mock-infected fibroblasts. The CTL response in normal immunocompetent donors is shown for comparison. The effector to target ratio is 10:1.

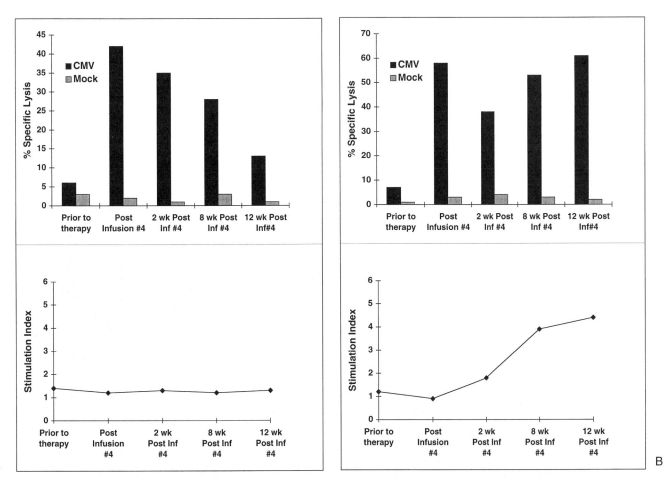

Figure 6. Requirement for CD4+ CMV-specific Th responses to sustain adoptively transferred CTL. The upper panel shows the results of the CD8+ CTL assays at intervals up to 12 weeks after completing the four T-cell infusions, and the lower panel shows the response of CD4+ Th cells expressed as a stimulation index for cells exposed to CMV antigen versus media control. A stimulation index of less than 2 is indicative of a deficiency of CMV-specific Th cells. The patient depicted in **A** fails to recover CD4+ CMV-specific Th and exhibits a gradual decline in the magnitude of the CD8+ CTL response. In contrast, the patient depicted in **B** recovers CD4+ CMV-specific Th and sustains a strong CD8+ CTL response.

responses (Fig. 6B). The loss of transferred CTL in the patients with severe GVHD may have been due to either direct inhibitory effects of combined therapy with the immunosuppressive drugs cyclosporine and prednisone on CD8+ CTL or the absence of Th function, which may be essential for persistence of CD8+ CTL (50,91).

Reactivation of CMV, as assessed by culture of CMV from throat, urine, or blood samples, occurs in up to 90% of CMV-seropositive allogeneic HCT recipients (92). One patient receiving therapy with CD8+ CTL had a positive throat culture for CMV before the T-cell infusions were initiated but was culture negative after the first infusion. Two other patients excreted CMV from the urine after the initiation of T-cell infusions but none of the 14 patients on the phase 1 study developed CMV viremia or disease (91).

This initial study of adoptive immunotherapy with CD8+ CMV-specific T-cell clones in allogeneic HCT recipients

demonstrated that the approach was safe and effective for the rapid restoration of CD8+ CMV-specific CTL immunity and provided sufficiently encouraging evidence of antiviral activity to proceed with additional investigation. Several issues were also identified for investigation in future studies, including the apparent requirement for CD4+ Th to sustain adoptively transferred CD8+ CTL and the potential adverse effects of immunosuppressive therapy with high-dose prednisone on the survival and/or function of transferred T cells. A phase 2 study of adoptive immunotherapy in which both CMV-specific CD8+ CTL and CD4+ Th are administered prophylactically to allogeneic HCT recipients is now in progress and should provide insights into these issues. The primary end point selected for the phase 2 study is CMV viremia, and it is anticipated that the results of this and future studies should assist in defining the efficacy of cellular immunotherapy for CMV in the HCT setting.

T-CELL IMMUNOTHERAPY OF POST-TRANSPLANT EBV INFECTIONS

EBV infects approximately 90% of the adult population and establishes a persistent latent infection in oropharyngeal epithelium and in B-lymphocytes (93). In immunocompetent hosts EBV infection can be associated with the later development of malignancies, including Burkitt's lymphoma, a proportion of cases of Hodgkin's disease, and nasopharyngeal carcinoma (94). These EBV-associated malignancies in immunocompetent hosts typically express very few EBV proteins and in addition exhibit decreased expression of class I MHC molecules, and absence of adhesion molecules to evade immune recognition (94).

In immunodeficient hosts such as allogeneic solid organ and HCT recipients, and patients with AIDS, EBV infection of B-lymphocytes induces their proliferation and can progress to a monoclonal immunoblastic lymphoma (95–99). These EBV-associated lymphoproliferations in immunodeficient hosts typically occur in B cells of the recipient in solid organ transplants and B cells of the donor in HCT. Several EBV proteins that are targets of the CD8$^+$ CTL response in normal immunocompetent hosts are expressed in the EBV-infected proliferating B cells, and these cells are not deficient in expression of class I MHC or adhesion molecules. Indeed, the phenotype is strikingly similar to that of EBV-transformed B cells (EBV-LCL) that will spontaneously grow out of the blood of EBV-seropositive individuals if T cells are depleted from the culture or if cyclosporine A is added (100). Thus the pathogenesis of EBV lymphomas in immunodeficient hosts appears to reflect the absence of sufficient T-cell immunity to control reactivation of EBV, and adoptive immunotherapy with EBV-specific T cells has the potential to restore the host with the requisite effector cells to promote tumor regression.

EBV-Specific T-Cell Immunity and the Pathogenesis of EBV-Induced Lymphoproliferation (EBV-LPD)

The major recognized clinical syndrome of EBV reactivation in immunodeficient hosts is EBV-LPD, and this usually occurs in the most severely immunosuppressed of these individuals. Thus patients receiving T-cell-depleted bone marrow to prevent GVHD or T-cell-specific antibodies to treat organ rejection or GVHD are at high risk for EBV-LPD (98,101–105). In recipients of allogeneic T-cell-depleted bone marrow, the risk of EBV-LPD varies from 11% to 26%, depending on the method of T-cell depletion and the type of post-transplant immunosuppression (98,102). Recipients of unmodified bone marrow rarely (<1%) develop EBV-LPD unless they require intense post-transplant immunosuppression with anti-T-cell monoclonal antibodies or antithymocyte globulin (ATG) to treat GVHD. The type of solid organ transplant and the intensity of immunosuppression influence the risk of EBV-LPD. Solid organ transplant recipients who

are EBV seronegative and acquire EBV as a primary infection from the donor organ or blood products are at particularly high risk of developing EBV LPD following transplant, presumably because these individuals have no preexisting T-cell immunity to EBV (99,106). For all solid organ transplant patients, the incidence of EBV-LPD is increased if OKT3 is used as prophylaxis or therapy for rejection episodes (105). Methods for monitoring reactivation of EBV after solid organ or HCT have not been evaluated as rigorously as those for CMV, although a recent study suggested that assessing EBV load by PCR may be useful in predicting the subsequent occurrence of EBV lymphoproliferative disease (107).

A strong EBV-specific CD8$^+$ cytotoxic T-cell response is elicited in immunocompetent hosts following primary infection with EBV and correlates with the resolution of the clinical manifestation of EBV. Lucas and colleagues have analyzed the temporal recovery of EBV-specific cytotoxic T-cell responses following unmodified or T-cell-depleted HCT using EBV-transformed B-lymphocytes as stimulator cells (108). Profound deficiencies of EBV-specific cytotoxic T cells were observed at 3 months after transplant in the majority of individuals but recovered in most patients by 6 months after transplant (108). Most cases of post-transplant EBV-LPD develop in the first 4 months after transplant coincident with the most severe deficiency of EBV-specific CTL. Moreover, those patients who developed EBV-LPD have weak or undetectable EBV-specific cytolytic activity (108). These observations combined with the occasional spontaneous regression of established EBV-LPD after reduction in the intensity of immunosuppressive drug therapy suggest a critical role for T cells in preventing the outgrowth of EBV-infected B cells.

Insights into the role of different effector populations in controlling EBV-LPD have also been derived from studies in SCID mice inoculated intravenously or subcutaneously with EBV-transformed LCL. Depending of the route of inoculation, these mice develop disseminated or localized EBV lymphomas and have been used as models to assess the role of αβ$^+$ T-cell subsets and NK cells for promoting tumor regression. The infusion of CD8$^+$ EBV-specific T-cell lines or clones delayed or completely prevented the outgrowth of EBV lymphoma. CD4$^+$ EBV-specific Th also mediated protection in some instances; however, NK or LAK cells were ineffective (109–111). Studies in mice with established subcutaneous EBV lymphomas have demonstrated that infusion of EBV-specific CTL lines results in preferential migration of the infused T cells to sites of tumor and tumor regression (112).

Specificity of αβ$^+$ CD8$^+$ and CD4$^+$ EBV-Specific CTL

EBV-specific CD8$^+$ CTL responses can readily be elicited *in vitro* from EBV-seropositive donors using autologous EBV-LCL as stimulator cells. Only a minority of these EBV-transformed B cells are undergoing full EBV replication and lytic infection. The majority express only six EBV nuclear antigens (EBNA-1, EBNA-2, EBNA-3A, EBNA-3B, EBNA-3C, and EBNA-LP) and two membrane antigens (LMP-1 and LMP-2) (113,114). These eight EBV antigens are also those expressed in the B cells of EBV-LPD in immunosuppressed hosts. Vaccinia recombinant viruses encoding these individual EBV proteins have been constructed and used to assess the specificity of EBV-reactive CTL elicited after stimulation of peripheral blood lymphocytes with EBV-LCL. In most individuals studied, one or more of EBNA-3A, -3B, and -3C antigens were immunodominant, with lesser responses against EBNA-2, LP, LMP-1 and LMP-2 (113,114). Of interest, EBNA-1 was not recognized as a target antigen by any EBV-specific CD8$^+$ CTL.

Detailed studies of the role of individual EBV proteins expressed in EBV-LCL as target antigens for CD4$^+$ EBV-specific Th have not been reported. CD4$^+$ T cells reactive with EBNA-1 have been isolated, but the epitopes recognized are not presented by EBV-LCL, suggesting that uptake and processing by professional APC is required for activation of these T cells (115).

EBV Evasion of T-Cell Recognition

The establishment of latency appears to be an important mechanism of immune evasion for EBV. The viral genome persists in latently infected cells as an episome, and three distinct forms of EBV latency have been distinguished based on the expression of different viral proteins (115). The EBNA-1 protein is expressed in all EBV-associated malignancies and thus would be an attractive target antigen for a host T-cell response. However, the expression of EBNA-1 protein is also essential in all three forms of EBV latency, suggesting there must be a mechanism for preventing presentation of this protein to CD8$^+$ CTL. Recent studies have shown that the presence of a region containing repetitive sequences of glycine and alanine in the EBNA-1 protein prevent the processing and presentation of EBNA-1, and render this protein invisible to host CD8$^+$ CTL (116).

Clinical Studies of Adoptive Immunotherapy of Post-transplant EBV-LPD

EBV-LPD occurs more frequently in solid organ transplant recipients than in HCT recipients, but the use of adoptive immunotherapy with EBV-reactive T cells has not been reported, partly because of the absence of a source of T cells for use in therapy. However, in allogeneic HCT recipients the marrow donor can be used as a source of T cells for immune reconstitution. This strategy was first evaluated in a study by Papadopoulos and colleagues in which five recipients of T-cell-depleted bone marrow transplants who had developed EBV-LPD received infusions of peripheral blood mononuclear cells from their EBV-seropositive donors. The dose of T cells administered was 1×10^6 CD3$^+$ cells/kg, and this therapy resulted in the complete regression of EBV-LPD in all five patients within 30 days, and three of the five patients became long-term survivors (89). Acute and chronic GVHD were observed consistent with the presence of alloreactive T cells as well as EBV-reactive T cells in the infused population. The patients receiving this therapy experienced dramatic increases in circulating EBV-specific CTL consistent with rapid expansion of this subset after antigen stimulation *in vivo*. Fourteen additional patients have been treated utilizing cell doses as low as 1×10^5/kg, and 89% of the patients have had complete eradication of the EBV-LPD (111). The incidence of acute and chronic GVHD was 16% and 42%, respectively (111).

Recently, the administration of EBV-specific T-cell lines that exhibit cytolytic activity for EBV-LCL has been used for the treatment and prevention of EBV-LPD after T-cell-depleted HCT (117). The enrichment of polyclonal T cells for EBV reactivity by *in vitro* culture has been effective in eliminating GVHD as a toxicity of therapy (118). In these studies, the T-cell lines were transduced with a retroviral vector encoding neomycin phosphotransferase to permit analysis of the persistence and migration of T cells after adoptive transfer. These studies have demonstrated that infused gene marked CTL at cell doses of 1×10^8/m^2 induce regressions of established EBV-LPD and prevent the development of EBV-LPD in susceptible individuals. Moreover, the marked CTL persisted for more than 18 months after infusion, suggesting that the therapy conferred immunologic memory (118).

GENETIC MODIFICATION OF T CELLS TO IMPROVE SAFETY AND EFFICACY OF CELLULAR ADOPTIVE IMMUNOTHERAPY

The early investigations of cellular immunotherapy for viral infections in transplant recipients have affirmed the therapeutic potential of this approach. The introduction of a marker gene into infused T cells has assisted in the rapid analysis of *in vivo* persistence of transferred effector cells and suggested that gene transfer may be useful to alter the functional properties of T cells to improve either the safety or efficacy of therapy. A study of adoptive immunotherapy for HIV infection with CD8$^+$ HIV-specific T-cell clones utilized retrovirus-mediated gene transfer to introduce the HSV-thymidine kinase gene into the T-cell clones (119). HSV-TK-modified T cells are exquisitely sensitive to ganciclovir *in vitro* and could be eliminated *in vivo* if the therapy caused toxicity by administering ganciclovir to the patient. No serious toxicity occurred in the HIV study, and ganciclovir was not required. However, this study did reveal a potential limitation for gene therapy. The transfer of T cells containing the TK gene and the hygromycin phosphotransferase gene resulted in the induction of CD8[+] CTL responses to epitopes derived from the TK and Hy proteins (Hy) in five of six patients. The immune response to TK and Hy limited the *in vivo* survival of modified cells and prevented successful transfer of immunity with reinfusions (120). The immunogenicity of transgene products may be less problematic in the hosts with more severe immunodeficiency. In a subsequent study, polyclonal donor T-lymphocytes transduced with HSV-TK were used to treat relapsed leukemia or EBV-LPD occurring in eight T-cell-depleted HCT recipients, and immune responses to TK were observed in only one patient. Of interest, GVHD developed in three of these eight patients and was reversed in two by treatment with ganciclovir (121).

An obstacle to effective immunotherapy with CD8[+] CTL alone identified in the CMV study is the requirement for CD4[+] Th cells to support the survival and proliferation of CD8[+] CTL. CD8[+] CTL could be modified to function independent of CD4[+] T cells by the introduction of genes to provide an autocrine growth signal. One strategy being evaluated is to modify the IL-2 receptor to make the cell responsive to cytokines such as GM-CSF that are produced by the CD8[+] T cell after antigen stimulation. Signaling via the IL-2 receptor (IL-2R) after IL-2 binding requires dimerization of the cytoplasmic regions of the IL-2R β and γ chains (122). Thus chimeric IL-2R chains containing the signaling cytoplasmic portions of the IL-2 β and γ chains but the extracellular domains of the GMCSF receptor α and β chains fused to the transmembrane domains of IL-2R β and γ have been shown to deliver an IL-2-like proliferative signal following binding of IL-2 (122). The introduction of such novel receptor constructs into CD8[+] CTL could provide an antigen-regulated autocrine growth loop.

T-cell therapy for CMV and EBV in solid organ transplant recipients who are seronegative for these viruses and receive an organ from a seropositive donor could be of significant therapeutic benefit but is currently difficult because of the inability to obtain T cells from the recipient for therapy. T-cell recognition involves an interaction of the αβ[+] T-cell receptor with the MHC peptide complex on the target cell. Thus it should be possible to engineer T cells to express a desired specificity by introducing the T-cell receptor α and β genes. This strategy would require cloning of T-cell receptor genes from EBV- or CMV-specific T cells with defined MHC restriction to generate a bank of receptor genes. The appropriate T-cell receptor genes could then be introduced into recipient T cells, and the cells could be tested for virus specificity and expanded for use in therapy.

CONCLUSIONS

Considerable progress has been made in our understanding of the immunobiology of viral infections in immunocompromised hosts. Insights derived from animal model and human studies have provided the rationale to investigate immunotherapy with αβ[+] T cells to restore responses considered essential for protective immunity to CMV and EBV. The use of genetically modified T cells has already been evaluated clinically and offers the potential for improving safety and efficacy and removing obstacles to successful immunotherapy. Although these studies are in the early stages and present considerable technical challenges, the results suggest that cellular immunotherapy will be a fruitful area for investigation in future years.

REFERENCES

1. Whimbey E, Elting LS, Couch RB, et al. Influenza A virus infections among hospitalized adult bone marrow transplant recipients. *Bone Marrow Transplant* 1994;13:437–440.
2. Lewis VA, Champlin R, Englund J, et al. Respiratory disease due to parainfluenza virus in adult bone marrow transplant recipients. *Clin Infect Dis* 1996;23:1033–1037.
3. Whimbey E, Champlin RE, Couch RB, et al. Community respiratory virus infections among hospitalized adult bone marrow transplant recipients. *Clin Infect Dis* 1996;22:778–782.
4. Ljungman P, Gleaves CA, Meyers JD. Respiratory virus infection in immunocompromised patients. *Bone Marrow Transplant* 1989;4: 35–40.
5. Ada GL, Jones PD. The immune response to influenza infection. *Curr Top Microbiol Immunol* 1986;128:1–54.
6. Cannon MJ, Openshaw PJ, Askonas BA. Cytotoxic T cells clear virus but augment lung pathology in mice infected with respiratory syncytial virus. *J Exp Med* 1988;168:1163–1168.
7. Bowden RA, Sayers M, Flournoy N, et al. Cytomegalovirus immune globulin and seronegative blood products to prevent primary cytomegalovirus infection after marrow transplantation. *N Engl J Med* 1986;314:1006–1010.
8. Meyers JD. Infections in marrow transplant recipients. Mandell GL, Douglas RG Jr, Bennett JE, eds. *Principles and practices of infectious diseases,* New York: Churchill Livingstone; 1990:2291–2294.
9. Winston DJ. Prophylaxis and treatment of infection in the bone marrow transplant recipient. *Curr Clin Top Infect Dis* 1993;13:293–321.
10. Meyers JD, Reed EC, Shepp DH, et al. Acyclovir for prevention of cytomegalovirus infection and disease after allogeneic marrow transplantation. *N Engl J Med* 1988;318:70–75.
11. Goodrich JM, Mori M, Gleaves CA, et al. Early treatment with ganciclovir to prevent cytomegalovirus disease after allogeneic bone marrow transplantation. *N Engl J Med* 1991;325:1601–1607.
12. Schmidt GM, Horak DA, Niland JC, Duncan SR, Forman SJ, Zaia JA. A randomized, controlled trial of prophylactic ganciclovir for cytomegalovirus pulmonary infection in recipients of allogeneic bone marrow transplants: the City of Hope–Stanford–Syntex CMV Study Group. *N Engl J Med* 1991;324:1005–1011.
13. Goodrich JM, Bowden RA, Fisher L, Keller C, Schoch G, Meyers JD. Ganciclovir prophylaxis to prevent cytomegalovirus disease after allogeneic marrow transplant. *Ann Intern Med* 1993;118:173–178.
14. Winston DJ, Ho WG, Bartoni K, et al. Ganciclovir prophylaxis of cytomegalovirus infection and disease in allogeneic bone marrow transplant recipients. Results of a placebo-controlled, double-blind trial. *Ann Intern Med* 1993;118:179–184.
15. Merigan TC, Renlund DG, Keay S, et al. A controlled trial of ganciclovir to prevent cytomegalovirus disease after heart transplantation. *N Engl J Med* 1992;326:1182–1186.
16. Crumpacker CS. Ganciclovir. *N Engl J Med* 1996;335:721–729.
17. Li CR, Greenberg PD, Gilbert MJ, Goodrich JM, Riddell SR. Recov-

ery of HLA-restricted cytomegalovirus (CMV)-specific T-cell responses after allogeneic bone marrow transplant: correlation with CMV disease and effect of ganciclovir prophylaxis. *Blood* 1994;83: 1971–1979.

18. Van den Berg AP, van Son WJ, Haagsma EB, et al. Prediction of recurrent cytomegalovirus disease after treatment with ganciclovir in solid-organ transplant recipients. *Transplantation* 1993;55:847–851.

19. Beersma MF, Bijlmakers MJ, Ploegh HL. Human cytomegalovirus down-regulates HLA class I expression by reducing the stability of class I H chains. *J Immunol* 1993;151:4455–4464.

20. Rawle FC, Tollefson AE, Wold WS, Gooding LR. Mouse anti-adenovirus cytotoxic T lymphocytes. Inhibition of lysis by E3 gp19K but not E3 14.7K. *J Immunol* 1989;143:2031–2037.

21. York IA, Roop C, Andrews DW, Riddell SR, Graham FL, Johnson DC. A cytosolic herpes simplex virus protein inhibits antigen presentation to CD8+ T lymphocytes. *Cell* 1994;77:525–535.

22. Warren AP, Ducroq DH, Lehner PJ, Borysiewicz LK. Human cytomegalovirus-infected cells have unstable assembly of major histocompatibility complex class I complexes and are resistant to lysis by cytotoxic T lymphocytes. *J Virol* 1994;68:2822–2829.

23. Biron CA, Byron KS, Sullivan JL. Severe herpesvirus infections in an adolescent without natural killer cells. *N Engl J Med* 1989;320: 1731–1735.

24. Welsh RM, Brubaker JO, Vargas-Cortes M, O'Donnell CL. Natural killer (NK) cell response to virus infections in mice with severe combined immunodeficiency. The stimulation of NK cells and the NK cell-dependent control of virus infections occur independently of T and B cell function. *J Exp Med* 1991;173:1053–1063.

25. Reybum HT, Mandelboim O, Vales-Gomez M, Davis DM, Pazmany L, Strominger JL. The class I MHC homologue of human cytomegalovirus inhibits attack by natural killer cells. *Nature* 1997;386:514–517.

26. Rosenberg SA, Lotze MT, Muul LM, et al. Observations on the systemic administration of autologous lymphokine-activated killer cells and recombinant interleukin-2 to patients with metastatic cancer. *N Engl J Med* 1985;313:1485–1492.

27. Sciammas R, Johnson RM, Sperling AI, et al. Unique antigen recognition by a herpesvirus-specific TCR-gamma delta cell. *J Immunol* 1994;152:5392–5397.

28. Doherty PC, Allan W, Eichelberger M, Carding SR. Roles of alpha beta and gamma delta T cell subsets in viral immunity. *Annu Rev Immunol* 1992;10:123–151.

29. Riddell SR, Greenberg PD. Principles for adoptive T cell therapy of human viral diseases. *Annu Rev Immunol* 1995;13:545–586.

30. Ahmed R. Immunological memory against viruses. *Semin Immunol* 1992;4:105–109.

31. Hou S, Hyland L, Ryan KW, Portner A, Doherty PC. Virus-specific CD8+ T-cell memory determined by clonal burst size. *Nature* 1994;369:652–654.

32. Mackenzie CD, Taylor PM, Askonas BA. Rapid recovery of lung histology correlates with clearance of influenza virus by specific CD8+ cytotoxic T cells. *Immunology* 1989;67:375–381.

33. Nash AA, Jayasuriya A, Phelan J, Cobbold SP, Waldmann H, Prospero T. Different roles for L3T4+ and Lyt 2+ T cell subsets in the control of an acute herpes simplex virus infection of the skin and nervous system. *J Gen Virol* 1987;68:825–833.

34. Moskophidis D, Cobbold SP, Waldmann H, Lehmann-Grube F. Mechanism of recovery from acute virus infection: treatment of lymphocytic choriomeningitis virus-infected mice with monoclonal antibodies reveals that Lyt-2+ T lymphocytes mediate clearance of virus and regulate the antiviral antibody response. *J Virol* 1987;61:1867–1874.

35. Reddehase MJ, Weiland F, Munch K, Jonjic S, Luske A, Koszinowski UH. Interstitial murine cytomegalovirus pneumonia after irradiation: characterization of cells that limit viral replication during established infection of the lungs. *J Virol* 1985;55:264–273.

36. Raulet DH. MHC class I-deficient mice. Adv Immunol 1994;55: 381–421.

37. Eichelberger M, Allan W, Zijlstra M, Jaenisch R, Doherty PC. Clearance of influenza virus respiratory infection in mice lacking class I major histocompatibility complex-restricted CD8+ T cells. *J Exp Med* 1991;174:875–880.

38. Bender BS, Croghan T, Zhang L, Small PA, Jr. Transgenic mice lacking class I major histocompatibility complex-restricted T cells have delayed viral clearance and increased mortality after influenza virus challenge. *J Exp Med* 1992;175:1143–1145.

39. Cardell S, Merkenschlager M, Bodmer H, et al. The immune system of mice lacking conventional MHC class II molecules. *Adv Immunol* 1994;55:423–440.

40. Long EO. Antigen processing for presentation to CD4+ T cells. *New Biol* 1992;4:274–282.

41. Yewdell JW, Bennink JR. The binary logic of antigen processing and presentation to T cells. *Cell* 1990;62:203–206.

42. Malnati MS, Marti M, LaVaute T, et al. Processing pathways for presentation of cytosolic antigen to MHC class II-restricted T cells. *Nature* 1992;357:702–704.

43. Mosmann TR, Cherwinski H, Bond MW, Giedlin MA, Coffman RL. Two types of murine helper T cell clone. I. Definition according to profiles of lymphokine activities and secreted proteins. *J Immunol* 1986;136:2348–2357.

44. Maggi E, Del-Prete G, Macchia D, et al. Profiles of lymphokine activities and helper function for IgE in human T cell clones. *Eur J Immunol* 1988;18:1045–1050.

45. Maggi E, Parronchi P, Manetti R, et al. Reciprocal regulatory effects of IFN-gamma and IL-4 on the *in vitro* development of human Th1 and Th2 clones. *J Immunol* 1992;148:2142–2147.

46. Mosmann TR, Moore KW. The role of IL-10 in cross-regulation of TH1 and TH2 responses. *Immunol Today* 1991;12:A49–A53.

47. Seder RA, Gazzinelli R, Sher A, Paul WE. Interleukin 12 acts directly on CD4+ T cells to enhance priming for interferon gamma production and diminishes interleukin 4 inhibition of such priming. *Proc Natl Acad Sci U S A* 1993;90:10188–10192.

48. Farrar JJ, Benjamin WR, Hilfiker ML, Howard M, Farrar WL, Fuller-Farrar J. The biochemistry, biology, and role of interleukin 2 in the induction of cytotoxic T cell and antibody-forming B cell responses. *Immunol Rev* 1982;63:129–166.

49. Biron CA, Young HA, Kasaian MT. Interleukin 2-induced proliferation of murine natural killer cells *in vivo*. *J Exp Med* 1990;171:173–188.

50. Matloubian M, Concepcion RJ, Ahmed R. CD4+ T cells are required to sustain CD8+ cytotoxic T-cell responses during chronic viral infection. *J Virol* 1994;68:8056–8063.

51. Staeheli P. Interferon-induced proteins and the antiviral state. *Adv Virus Res* 1990;38:147–200.

52. Wong GH, Goeddel DV. Tumour necrosis factors alpha and beta inhibit virus replication and synergize with interferons. *Nature* 1986;323:819–822.

53. Paul WE. Interleukin-4: a prototypic immunoregulatory lymphokine. *Blood* 1991;77:1859–1870.

54. Lopez AF, Sanderson CJ, Gamble JR, Campbell HD, Young IG, Vadas MA. Recombinant human interleukin 5 is a selective activator of human eosinophil function. *J Exp Med* 1988;167:219–224.

55. Graham MB, Braciale VL, Braciale TJ. Influenza virus-specific CD4+ T helper type 2 lymphocytes do not promote recovery from experimental virus infection. *J Exp Med* 1994;180:1273–1282.

56. Alwan WH, Kozlowska WJ, Openshaw PJ. Distinct types of lung disease caused by functional subsets of antiviral T cells. *J Exp Med* 1994; 179:81–89.

57. Yewdell JW, Bennink JR. Cell biology of antigen processing and presentation to major histocompatibility complex class I molecule-restricted T lymphocytes. *Adv Immunol* 1992;52:1–123.

58. Driscoll J, Brown MG, Finley D, Monaco JJ. MHC-linked LMP gene products specifically alter peptidase activities of the proteasome. *Nature* 1993;365:262–264.

59. Spies T, DeMars R. Restored expression of major histocompatibility class I molecules by gene transfer of a putative peptide transporter. *Nature* 1991;351:323–324.

60. Doherty PC. Cell-mediated cytotoxicity. *Cell* 1993;75:607–612.

61. Kagi D, Ledermann B, Burki K, et al. Cytotoxicity mediated by T cells and natural killer cells is greatly impaired in perforin-deficient mice. *Nature* 1994;369:31–37.

62. Suwansirikul S, Rao N, Dowling JN, Ho M. Primary and secondary cytomegalovirus infection. *Arch Intern Med* 1977;137:1026–1029.

63. Betts RF, Freeman RB, Douglas RG Jr, Talley TE. Clinical manifestations of renal allograft derived primary cytomegalovirus infection. *Am J Dis Child* 1977;131:759–763.

64. Reddehase MJ, Mutter W, Munch K, Buhring HJ, Koszinowski UH. CD8-positive T lymphocytes specific for murine cytomegalovirus immediate-early antigens mediate protective immunity. *J Virol* 1987; 61:3102–3108.

65. Reddehase MJ, Mutter W, Koszinowski UH. *In vivo* application of

recombinant interleukin 2 in the immunotherapy of established cytomegalovirus infection. *J Exp Med* 1987;165:650–656.

66. Lucin P, Pavi'c I, Poli'c B, Jonji'c S, Koszinowski UH. Gamma interferon-dependent clearance of cytomegalovirus infection in salivary glands. *J Virol* 1992;66:1977–1984.

67. Quinnan GV Jr, Kirmani N, Rook AH, et al. Cytotoxic T cells in cytomegalovirus infection: HLA-restricted T-lymphocyte and non-T-lymphocyte cytotoxic responses correlate with recovery from cytomegalovirus infection in bone-marrow-transplant recipients. *N Engl J Med* 1982;307:7–13.

68. Reusser P, Riddell SR, Meyers JD, Greenberg PD. Cytotoxic T-lymphocyte response to cytomegalovirus after human allogeneic bone marrow transplantation: pattern of recovery and correlation with cytomegalovirus infection and disease. *Blood* 1991;78:1373–1380.

69. Krause H, Hebart H, Jahn G, Muller CA, Einsele H. Screening for CMV-specific T cell proliferation to identify patients at risk of developing late onset CMV disease. *Bone Marrow Transplant* 1997;19: 1111–1116.

70. Mocarski ES Jr. Cytomegalovirus biology and replication. In: Roizman B, Whitley RJ, Lopez C, eds. *The human herpes viruses.* New York: Raven Press; 1993:173–193.

71. Riddell SR, Rabin M, Geballe AP, Britt WJ, Greenberg PD. Class I MHC-restricted cytotoxic T lymphocyte recognition of cells infected with human cytomegalovirus does not require endogenous viral gene expression. *J Immunol* 1991;146:2795–2804.

72. McLaughlin-Taylor E, Pande H, Forman S, et al. Identification of the major late human cytomegalovirus matrix protein pp65 as a target antigen for CD8+ virus-specific cytotoxic T lymphocytes. *J Med Virol* 1994;43:103–110.

73. Wills MR, Carmichael AJ, Mynard K, et al. The human cytotoxic T-lymphocyte (CTL) response to cytomegalovirus is dominated by structural protein pp65: frequency, specificity, and T-cell receptor usage of pp65-specific CTL. *J Virol* 1996;70:7569–7579.

74. Boppana SB, Britt WJ. Recognition of human cytomegalovirus gene products by HCMV-specific cytotoxic T cells. *Virology* 1996;222: 293–296.

75. Gilbert MJ, Riddell SP, Li CR, Greenberg PD. Selective interference with class I major histocompatibility complex presentation of the major immediate-early protein following infection with human cytomegalovirus. *J Virol* 1993;67:3461–3469.

76. Borysiewicz LK, Hickling JK, Graham S, et al. Human cytomegalovirus-specific cytotoxic T cells. Relative frequency of stage-specific CTL recognizing the 72-kD immediate early protein and glycoprotein B expressed by recombinant vaccinia viruses. *J Exp Med* 1988;168:919–931.

77. He H, Rinaldo CR, Jr., Morel PA. T cell proliferative responses to five human cytomegalovirus proteins in healthy seropositive individuals: implications for vaccine development. *J Gen Virol* 1995;76: 1603–1610.

78. Van Zanten J, Harmsen MC, van der Meer P, et al. Proliferative T cell responses to four human cytomegalovirus-specific proteins in healthy subjects and solid organ transplant recipients. *J Infect Dis* 1995;172: 879–882.

79. Davignon JL, Clement D, Alriquet J, Michelson S, Davrinche C. Analysis of the proliferative T cell response to human cytomegalovirus major immediate-early protein (IE1): phenotype, frequency and variability. *Scand J Immunol* 1995;41:247–255.

80. Liu YN, Klaus A, Kari B, Stinski MF, Eckhardt J, Gehrz RC. The N-terminal 513 amino acids of the envelope glycoprotein gB of human cytomegalovirus stimulates both B-and T-cell immune responses in humans. *J Virol* 1991;65:1644–1648.

81. Kondo K, Xu J, Mocarski ES. Human cytomegalovirus latent gene expression in granulocyte-macrophage progenitors in culture and in seropositive individuals. *Proc Natl Acad Sci U S A* 1996;93: 11137–11142.

82. Jones TR, Hanson LK, Sun L, Slater JS, Stenberg RM, Campbell AE. Multiple independent loci within the human cytomegalovirus unique short region down-regulate expression of major histocompatibility complex class I heavy chains. *J Virol* 1995;69:4830–4841.

83. Wiertz EJ, Jones TR, Sun L, Bogyo M, Geuze HJ, Ploegh HL. The human cytomegalovirus US11 gene product dislocates MHC class I heavy chains from the endoplasmic reticulum to the cytosol. *Cell* 1996;84:769–779.

84. Jones TR, Wiertz EJ, Sun L, Fish KN, Nelson JA, Ploegh HL. Human

cytomegalovirus US3 impairs transport and maturation of major histocompatibility complex class I heavy chains. *Proc Natl Acad Sci U S A* 1996;93:11327–11333.

85. Wiertz EJ, Tortorella D, Bogyo M, et al. Sec61-mediated transfer of a membrane protein from the endoplasmic reticulum to the proteasome for destruction. *Nature* 1996;384:432–438.

86. Hengel H, Koopmann JO, Flohr T, et al. A viral ER-resident glycoprotein inactivates the MHC-encoded peptide transporter. *Immunity* 1997;6:623–632.

87. Gilbert MJ, Riddell SR, Plachter B, Greenberg PD. Cytomegalovirus selectively blocks antigen processing and presentation of its immediate-early gene product. *Nature* 1996;383:720–722.

88. Diamond DJ, York J, Sun JY, Wright CL, Forman SJ. Development of a candidate HLA A*0201 restricted peptide-based vaccine against human cytomegalovirus infection. *Blood* 1997;90:1751–1767.

89. Papadopoulos EB, Ladanyi M, Emanuel D, et al. Infusions of donor leukocytes to treat Epstein-Barr virus-associated lymphoproliferative disorders after allogeneic bone marrow transplantation [see comments]. *N Engl J Med* 1994;330:1185–1191.

90. Riddell SR, Watanabe KS, Goodrich JM, Li CR, Agha ME, Greenberg PD. Restoration of viral immunity in immunodeficient humans by the adoptive transfer of T cell clones [see comments]. *Science* 1992;257: 238–241.

91. Walter EA, Greenberg PD, Gilbert MJ, et al. Reconstitution of cellular immunity against cytomegalovirus in recipients of allogeneic bone marrow by transfer of T-cell clones from the donor. *N Engl J Med* 1995;333:1038–1044.

92. Meyers JD, Ljungman P, Fisher LD. Cytomegalovirus excretion as a predictor of cytomegalovirus disease after marrow transplantation: importance of cytomegalovirus viremia. *J Infect Dis* 1990;162:373–380.

93. Straus SE, Cohen JI, Tosato G, Meier J. NIH conference. Epstein-Barr virus infections: biology, pathogenesis, and management. *Ann Intern Med* 1993;118:45–58.

94. Rickinson AB, Kieff E. Epstein-Barr virus. In: Fields BN, Knipe DM, Howley PM, eds. *Field's virology.* Philadelphia: Lippincott-Raven; 1996:2397–2446.

95. Cohen JI. Epstein-Barr virus lymphoproliferative disease associated with acquired immunodeficiency. *Medicine* 1991;70:137–160.

96. Zutter MM, Martin PJ, Sale GE, et al. Epstein-Barr virus lymphoproliferation after bone marrow transplantation. *Blood* 1988;72:520–529.

97. Shapiro RS, McClain K, Frizzera G, et al. Epstein-Barr virus associated B cell lymphoproliferative disorders following bone marrow transplantation. *Blood* 1988;71:1234–1243.

98. Caldas C, Ambinder R. Epstein-Barr virus and bone marrow transplantation. *Curr Opin Oncol* 1995;7:102–106.

99. Basgoz N, Preiksaitis JK. Post-transplant lymphoproliferative disorder. *Infect Dis Clin North Am* 1995;9:901–923.

100. Young L, Alfieri C, Hennessy K, et al. Expression of Epstein-Barr virus transformation-associated genes in tissues of patients with EBV lymphoproliferative disease. *N Engl J Med* 1989;321:1080–1085.

101. Martin PJ, Shulman HM, Schubach WH, et al. Fatal Epstein-Barr-virus-associated proliferation of donor B cells after treatment of acute graft-versus-host disease with a murine anti-T-cell antibody. *Ann Intern Med* 1984;101:310–315.

102. Antin JH, Bierer BE, Smith BR, et al. Selective depletion of bone marrow T lymphocytes with anti-CD5 monoclonal antibodies: effective prophylaxis for graft-versus-host disease in patients with hematologic malignancies. *Blood* 1991;78:2139–2149.

103. Opelz G, Henderson R. Incidence of non-Hodgki's lymphoma in kidney and heart transplant recipients. *Lancet* 1993;342:1514–1516.

104. Renard TH, Andrews WS, Foster ME. Relationship between OKT3 administration, EBV seroconversion, and the lymphoproliferative syndrome in pediatric liver transplant recipients. *Transplant Proc* 1991;23:1473–1476.

105. Swinnen LJ, Costanzo-Nordin MR, Fisher SG, et al. Increased incidence of lymphoproliferative disorder after immunosuppression with the monoclonal antibody OKT3 in cardiac-transplant recipients. *N Engl J Med* 1990;323:1723–1728.

106. Walker RC, Paya CV, Marshall WF, et al. Pretransplantation seronegative Epstein-Barr virus status is the primary risk factor for posttransplantation lymphoproliferative disorder in adult heart, lung, and other solid organ transplantations. *J Heart Lung Transplant* 1995;14: 214–221.

107. Savoie A, Perpete C, Carpentier L, Joncas J, Alfieri C. Direct correla-

tion between the load of Epstein-Barr virus-infected lymphocytes in the peripheral blood of pediatric transplant patients and risk of lymphoproliferative disease. *Blood* 1994;83:2715–2722.

108. Lucas KG, Small TN, Heller G, Dupont B, O'Reilly RJ. The development of cellular immunity to Epstein-Barr virus after allogeneic bone marrow transplantation. *Blood* 1996;87:2594–2603.

109. Rencher SD, Slobod KS, Smith FS, Hurwitz JL. Activity of transplanted CD8+ versus CD4+ cytotoxic T cells against Epstein-Barr virus-immortalized B cell tumors in SCID mice. *Transplantation* 1994;58:629–633.

110. Buchsbaum RJ, Fabry JA, Lieberman J. EBV-specific cytotoxic T lymphocytes protect against human EBV-associated lymphoma in scid mice. *Immunol Lett* 1996;52:145–152.

111. O'Reilly RJ, Small TN, Papadopoulos E, Lucas K, Lacerda J, Koulova L. Biology and adoptive cell therapy of Epstein-Barr virus-associated lymphoproliferative disorders in recipients of marrow allografts. *Immunol Rev* 1997;157:195–216.

112. Lacerda JF, Ladanyi M, Louie DC, Fernandez JM, Papadopoulos EB, O'Reilly RJ. Human Epstein-Barr virus (EBV)–specific cytotoxic T lymphocytes home preferentially to and induce selective regressions of autologous EBV-induced B cell lymphoproliferations in xenografted C.B-17 scid/scid mice. *J Exp Med* 1996;183:1215–1228.

113. Murray RJ, Kurilla MG, Brooks JM, et al. Identification of target antigens for the human cytotoxic T cell response to Epstein-Barr virus (EBV): implications for the immune control of EBV-positive malignancies. *J Exp Med* 1992;176:157–168.

114. Khanna R, Burrows SR, Kurilla MG, et al. Localization of Epstein-Barr virus cytotoxic T cell epitopes using recombinant vaccinia: implications for vaccine development. *J Exp Med* 1992;176:169–176.

115. Moss DJ, Schmidt C, Elliott S, Suhrbier A, Burrows S, Khanna R. Strategies involved in developing an effective vaccine for EBV-associated diseases. *Adv Cancer Res* 1996;69:213–245.

116. Levitskaya J, Coram M, Levitsky V, et al. Inhibition of antigen processing by the internal repeat region of the Epstein-Barr virus nuclear antigen-1. *Nature* 1995;375:685–688.

117. Rooney CM, Smith CA, Ng CY, et al. Use of gene-modified virus-specific T lymphocytes to control Epstein-Barr-virus-related lymphoproliferation. *Lancet* 1995;345:9–13.

118. Heslop HE, Ng CY, Li C, et al. Long-term restoration of immunity against Epstein-Barr virus infection by adoptive transfer of gene-modified virus-specific T lymphocytes. *Nature Med* 1996;2:551–555.

119. Riddell SR, Greenberg PD, Overell RW, et al. Phase I study of cellular adoptive immunotherapy using genetically modified CD8+ HIV-specific T cells for HIV seropositive patients undergoing allogeneic bone marrow transplant. The Fred Hutchinson Cancer Research Center and the University of Washington School of Medicine, Department of Medicine, Division of Oncology. *Hum Gene Ther* 1992; 3:319–338.

120. Riddell SR, Elliott M, Lewinsohn DA, et al. T-cell mediated rejection of gene-modified HIV-specific cytotoxic T lymphocytes in HIV-infected patients. *Nature Med* 1996;2:216–223.

121. Bonini C, Ferrari G, Verzeletti S, et al. HSV-TK gene transfer into donor lymphocytes for control of allogeneic graft-versus-leukemia. *Science* 1997;276:1719–1724.

122. Nelson BH, Lord JD, Greenberg PD. Cytoplasmic domains of the interleukin-2 receptor beta and gamma chains mediate the signal for T-cell proliferation. *Nature* 1994;369:333–336.

Transplant Infections edited by
Raleigh A. Bowden, Per Ljungman, and Carlos V. Paya.
Lippincott–Raven Publishers, Philadelphia © 1998

CHAPTER 29

Clinical Applications of Immune Globulin in Stem Cell and Solid Organ Transplant Recipients

David Emanuel

Over the past 25 years stem cell and organ transplantation has been successfully applied as therapy for a wide variety of malignancies, bone marrow and organ failure syndromes, immune deficiency syndromes, and genetic diseases. Despite remarkable progress in our overall clinical management of this patient population, infections and their complications are still the primary causes of non-relapse-related morbidity and mortality following transplantation. Profound and prolonged immune system dysfunction remains an inherent and integral part of the post-transplant period for almost all patients. Clinically relevant immune recovery usually occurs within 12–18 months in most patients. However, quantifiable deficiencies within the immune system repertoire may be detectable for years. These include the ability to mount a vigorous antigen-specific response, resulting in the production of functional antibodies to a variety of bacterial and viral pathogens. This chapter will review the use of passive immunotherapy with immune globulin to prevent and treat infectious complications in the post-transplant period. The rationale for the use of passive antibody immunotherapy in this patient population is self-evident. However, despite the continued widespread use of these products in most transplant units worldwide, the overall clinical and cost efficacy of passive immunotherapy with immune globulin for the prevention and treatment of infections during the post-transplant period remains a subject of intense debate and investigation.

ONTOGENY OF B-LYMPHOCYTE DEVELOPMENT AND THE RECONSTITUTION OF HUMORAL IMMUNITY FOLLOWING STEM CELL TRANSPLANTATION

The sole effector function of a B-lymphocyte is the production of antibody. The primary function of the humoral immune response is to destroy extra-cellular microorganisms and to prevent the spread of intra-cellular infections. Antibodies utilize basically three functional mechanisms to destroy microorganisms and toxins: neutralization, opsonization, and complement activation. The effector mechanism utilized by an antibody depends on its isotype (IgG, IgM, IgA, etc.).

B cells are selected during the immune response to a foreign antigen instead of during ontogeny (viz. T cells), and the selecting antigen is the foreign antigen itself. B-cell development essentially occurs in three phases: antigen independence, antigen dependence, and terminal differentiation (1). B cells develop within the marrow, and production continues throughout life. The stages of development are characterized by progressive immunoglobulin gene rearrangements that are responsible for the almost infinite diversity of antibody specificities. The end result of this process is the production of a B cell that is monoclonal and monospecific in its antibody production. Each B cell produced possesses a unique surface receptor that is generated through somatic mutations of the heavy and light immunoglobulin genes. Separate rearrangement sequences result in the production of the two chains of the immunoglobulin molecule. The process is strictly regulated, resulting in the production of one heavy chain and one light chain that combine to produce an antibody surface receptor of single specificity.

From the Stem Cell Transplantation Program, Indiana University School of Medicine, Indianapolis, IN 46202.

Immunoglobulin gene rearrangement begins with the heavy-chain genes, resulting in the production of heavy chain on the cell surface (pre–B-cell stage). Rearrangement of the light-chain genes then begins, resulting in the expression of a complete IgM on the cell surface (immature B-cell stage). Once surface immunoglobulin is expressed, these molecules begin to function as antigen receptors. Immature B cells that bind self-antigen either become anergic or undergo apoptosis, thereby ensuring tolerance to self. Self-tolerance is augmented by the dependence of most B cells on T-cell help. Mature naive B cells that now coexpress IgM and IgD leave the marrow to enter the periphery to circulate through lymphnodes and Peyer's patches in the gut until they encounter antigen. Following antigen binding and subsequent stimulation, B cells accumulate within germinal centers in lymphnodes, coming into contact with follicular dendritic cells. These cells are responsible for amplification of the antibody response by (a) the binding of high concentrations of antigen on their cell surface with multiple B-cell receptor molecules, and (b) binding of CD23 with the CD19/Tapa-1/CR2 complex on the B-cell surface. This co-stimulation mechanism induces a much lower stimulus threshold to accomplish subsequent B-cell activation. B cells will now differentiate either into terminal plasma cells that secrete antibody or into memory B cells. This is determined by signaling via the CD23 and CD40 molecules. B cells signaled through CD23 alone induce differentiation into plasma cells, whereas co-stimulation via CD23 and CD40 ligand induces the production of memory B cells expressing high-affinity surface immunoglobulin. Plasma cells, which can no longer respond to antigen, will migrate back to the bone marrow or remain in the medulla of the lymphoid organ, where T-cell-dependent isotype switching occurs, resulting in the production of IgG, IgE, or IgA of identical specificity.

The primary properties of immune reconstitution following stem cell transplantation are the following:

1. Absence of sustained transfer of T- and B-cell immune function from the donor to the recipient;
2. Recapitulation of ontogeny of both B cells and T cells;
3. Effect of immunosuppressive drugs and graft-versus-host disease on the process of immune reconstitution;
4. Influence of donor-recipient HLA compatibility (2–4).

B-cell Reconstitution Following Stem Cell Transplantation

The capacity of B-lymphocytes to respond to mitogen stimulation (e.g., using protein A or anti-IgM antibodies) parallels the emergence of B-lymphocytes into the peripheral circulation and may be normal as soon as 2–3 months after transplant (5-6). Antigen-specific antibody responses are markedly reduced for at least 3 months after transplant and are dependent on the type of transplant (autologous versus allogeneic), HLA compatibility between donor and recipient and graft manipulation procedures (T-cell depletion). Recipients of marrow from an HLA-compatible sibling may exhibit normal IgM production by 4–6 months after transplant and normal IgG production by 9 months. In contrast, recipients of T-cell-depleted marrow grafts do not exhibit normal immunoglobulin production for at least 12 months after transplantation. Antibody production arising from mature B cells contained within the marrow graft is not sustained for longer than 3 months after transplant. The in vivo production of specific antibodies is dependent on (a) the generation of antigen-specific T cells arising from donor stem cells and (b) appropriate interactions between professional antigen-presenting cells with both B and T cells. The interaction of T and B cells with each other and with other antigen-presenting cells is progressively attenuated in the context of increasing HLA donor/host disparities. A primary antigen-specific immune response (e.g., to a neoantigen such as phage ϕX174) is not demonstrable within the first 3 months after transplant. A normal response to a neoantigen is dependent on the absence of graft-versus-host disease (GVHD) (i.e., patients with chronic GVHD have an impaired capacity to generate an antigen-specific response and to switch antibody isotype following secondary immunization). The ability of stem cell transplant recipients to respond to polysaccharide antigens is impaired. Failure to demonstrate an antibody response to a polysaccharide antigen challenge indicates a need for antibiotic prophylaxis or the prophylactic use of intravenous immunoglobulin (IVIG) containing functional antibodies to encapsulated respiratory bacteria.

Immunodeficiencies Secondary to Graft-Versus-Host Disease

Acute Graft-Versus-Host Disease

Acute GVHD has no overt effect on the number or phenotype of circulating B or T cells and does not impact on CD3$^+$ T-cell recovery. In addition, acute GVHD in the absence of chronic GVHD may cause sustained immunodeficiency secondary to prolonged thymus dysfunction (2–4).

Chronic Graft-Versus-Host Disease

Chronic GVHD is associated with (a) a decrease in antigen-specific T-cell responses and (b) a markedly depressed response to immunization with neo-antigens. In addition, there is a marked decrease in production of specific antibodies, especially to polysaccharide antigens, with a subsequent high incidence of infection with encapsulated respiratory bacteria (e.g., sepsis, pneumonia, and sinusitis). Patients with chronic GVHD also demonstrate an increased production of autoantibodies.

INTRAVENOUS IMMUNOGLOBULIN PRODUCTS

Intravenous immunoglobulin products are concentrated human immunoglobulin preparations, predominantly containing IgG, that are purified from pooled plasma collected from screened donors. IVIG was originally developed in the early 1980s as passive replacement therapy for children and adults with primary humoral immune deficiencies. Prior to this time IgG was administered intramuscularly. The development of IVIG facilitated the administration of high doses of human IgG over a short period of time with significantly fewer side effects compared with the intramuscular preparations. IVIG products are expensive, with an average wholesale drug cost of $42 to $104 per gram (7). Nine manufacturers

produce and market standard or hyperimmune IVIG products in the United States (Table 1). All IVIG products are prepared from pooled human sera collected from both paid and unpaid donors. The number of donors in a plasma pool varies from manufacturer to manufacturer and ranges from 1,000 to 50,000. Hyperimmune IVIG products licensed for sale in the United States include Cytogam (CMV immune globulin) and Respigam (RSV immune globulin). These products are produced from pools of plasma collected from prescreened donors with high antibody titers to the pathogen of interest. Donor serum samples are screened for antibodies to HIV, hepatitis B and C, hepatitis B surface antigen, and elevated levels of alanine aminotransferase. Samples that test positive are discarded. All U.S. manufacturers use Cohn-Oncley cold ethanol fractionation (fraction 2), which produces a very pure immunoglobulin preparation. Subsequent preparation methodologies are manufacturer-specific and include ion exchange chromatography, ultrafiltration, pH manipulation, enzyme treatment, and adjustment of salt

TABLE 1. *Standard and hyperimmune IVIG preparations available in the United States*

Trade name (manufacturer)	Formulation	FDA labeled indications	Virus inactivation procedures
Gamimune N 5%	Liquid	1. Primary humoral immune deficiencies	Purification Procedure
Gamimune N 10%	Liquid	2. ITP	*Plus*
(Bayer Biological)		3. BMT	Solvent/Detergent Treatment
		Infections	
		Interstitial pneumonia	
		Acute GvHD+	
		4. Pediatric HIV infection	
Gammagard S/D 5%	Freeze-dried powder	1. Primary humoral immune deficiencies	Purification Procedure
Gammagard S/D 10%	Freeze-dried powder	2. ITP	*Plus*
(Baxter Healthcare)		3. CLL	Solvent/Detergent Treatment
		Bacterial infections	
Gammar-P 5%	Lyophilized powder	1. Primary humoral immune deficiencies	Purification Procedure
Gammar-P 10%	Lyophilized powder		*Plus*
(Centeon)			Heat treatment
Sandoglobulin 3%	Lyophilized powder	1. Primary humoral immune deficiencies	Purification Procedure
Sandoglobulin 6%	Lyophilized powder	2. ITP	
Sandoglobulin 12%	Lyophilized powder		
(Sandoz)			
Iveegam 5%	Freeze-dried powder	1. Primary humoral immune deficiencies	Purification Procedure
(Immuno-US)		2. Kawasaki syndrome	
Polygam S/D 5%	Freeze-dried powder	1. Primary humoral immune deficiencies	Purification Procedure
Polygam S/D 10%	Freeze-dried powder	2. ITP	*Plus*
(American Red Cross)		3. CLL	Solvent/Detergent Treatment
		Bacterial infection	Treatment
Venoglobulin-S 5%	Liquid	1. Primary humoral immune deficiencies	Purification Procedure
Venoglobulin-S 10%	Liquid	2. ITP	*Plus*
(Alpha Therapeutics)			Solvent/Detergent Treatment
Respigam (RSV Immune Globulin) 5%	Liquid	1. RSV prophylaxis <2 years of age with BPD or prematurity	Purification Procedure *Plus* Solvent/Detergent Treatment
(Medimmune)			
Cytogam (CMV Immune Globulin) 5%	Liquid	1. CMV prophylaxis Renal transplantation only	Purification Procedure *Plus* Solvent/Detergent Treatment
(Medimmune)			

ITP, idiopathic thrombocytopenic purpura; BMT, bone marrow transplantation; CLL, chronic lymphocytic leukemia; RSV, respiratory syncytial virus; CMV, cytomegalovirus.

concentrations. Some manufacturers recently have introduced an additional viral inactivation step for safety purposes, following hepatitis C contamination of a commercially available IVIG product in 1994 and transmission of the virus to recipients of infected product lots. Viral inactivation procedures currently in use include heat treatment and treatment with solvent/detergent. All IVIG products produced in the United States consist predominantly of intact monomeric IgG with an IgG subclass distribution reflecting that in normal human serum. Trace amounts of IgM and IgA are present at differing concentrations, dependent on the product. IVIG is produced from pooled plasma collected from multiple donors. The IVIG product will thus contain antibody specificities representative of the pool of donors. Recently, the University Hospital Consortium, an alliance of 66 leading academic centers in the United States, published a technology assessment of IVIG products available in the United States. It recommended that in the absence of adequate data demonstrating the existence of clinically significant differences, it is reasonable to assume that IVIG preparations commercially available in the United States are therapeutically interchangeable (8).

INTRAMUSCULAR IMMUNOGLOBULIN PRODUCTS

Product characteristics for the three most commonly prescribed intramuscular immunoglobulin (IMIG) products for prophylaxis following infectious exposure are outlined in Table 2. These include hepatitis B immune globulin, tetanus immune globulin, and varicella-zoster immune globulin. The clinical uses of these products are discussed later in this chapter.

CLINICAL USES OF INTRAVENOUS IMMUNOGLOBULIN AND INTRAMUSCULAR IMMUNOGLOBULIN IN STEM TRANSPLANT RECIPIENTS

IVIG and IMIG are utilized in stem cell transplant recipients in the context of two general indications:

1. Deficiencies of humoral immune function in the post-transplant period; antibody replacement therapy for prophylactic or therapeutic purposes;

2. Immune modulation; use of IVIG to modulate immune-mediated tissue injury or immune-mediated cell destruction.

The therapeutic use of IVIG for the treatment of CMV pneumonia will not be addressed in this chapter. This application is discussed in detail in those chapters specifically addressing CMV infections in solid organ and marrow transplant recipients.

Deficiencies of Humoral Immune Function in the Post-transplant Period

Hypogammaglobulinemia

Deficiencies in humoral immune function (hypogammaglobulinemia) in the post-transplant period can either be primary following failure of B-cell engraftment or secondary to a wide variety of causes, including GVHD and its therapy, viral infections, use of immunosuppressive medications, and immunologically relevant HLA disparities between donor and recipient.

Primary Hypogammaglobulinemia: Failure of Donor B-cell Engraftment

The consistent development of humoral immunity in the post-transplant period is dependent either on the presence of full donor chimerism with donor B- and T-lymphocytes or on a successful immunologic interaction between host B cells and donor T cells. This phenomenon has been most closely studied in children with severe combined immunodeficiency disease (SCID) receiving T-cell-depleted marrow transplants from haplotype-disparate parental donors (9–11). Full reconstitution of T-cell immunity is regularly observed in children with SCID receiving T-cell-depleted HLA-mismatched marrow grafts. In contrast, humoral immunity develops in only half of these patients. This may be due to failure of engraftment of donor B-lymphocytes or subsequent to HLA disparities between donor T cells and host antigen-presenting cells, including B-lymphocytes (11). Consistent engraftment of B-lymphocytes is only seen in patients receiving myeloablative preparative regimens (e.g., busulfan and cyclophosphamide) (11).

IVIG therapy is indicated for all patients following a stem cell transplant who have demonstrable failure of B-

TABLE 2. *Immunoglobulin Products (intramuscular) for Infection Prophylaxis in Transplant Recipients*

Trade name (manufacturer)	Formulation	FDA labeled indications	Virus inactivation procedures
Hepatitis B immune globulin (Abbott, MSD, Cutter)	Liquid For intramuscular use only	Post-hepatitis B exposure prophylaxis	Purification procedure
Tetanus immune globulin (Cutter Biological)	Liquid For intramuscular use only	Post-tetanus exposure prophylaxis	Purification procedure
Varicella-zoster immune globulin (American Red Cross)	Liquid For intramuscular use only	Post-varicella-zoster exposure prophylaxis	Purification procedure

cell engraftment with hypogammaglobulinemia (IgG < 200 mg/dl). The therapeutic goal is to bring the serum IgG level into the normal range for age (generally >500 mg/dl). Because of the difference in half-life of IgG in individual patients, serum IgG levels should be measured before each infusion and the dose of IVIG should be adjusted accordingly. Trough levels 2–4 weeks following an infusion should be maintained at 400–600 mg/dl, which is a value close to the lower limit of normal. Following infusion of IVIG, the serum IgG level increases initially by 250 mg/dl for each 100 mg/kg of IVIG infused (12). Recommended dose schedules range widely, from 100–200 mg/kg/month through 400–600 mg/kg per dose every 1–2 weeks (12–14).

Secondary Hypogammaglobulinemia

Following stem cell transplantation, B-cell dysfunction and consequent secondary hypogammaglobulinemia can persist from months to years, especially in patients with chronic GVHD (4–6,15). B-cell recovery in the post-transplant period tends to recapitulate normal B-cell ontogeny except in patients with chronic GVHD, where their severe humoral immunodeficiency might be explained by a failure to follow normal ontogenetic B-cell development and differentiation (6,15,16). Based on the successful use of IVIG for the prophylaxis of infectious complications in patients with primary hypogammaglobulinemia, initial studies in stem cell transplant recipients with secondary hypogammaglobulinemia were directed primarily at the prevention of major infectious complications affecting these patients, especially CMV infection and associated diseases.

Prophylaxis of Cytomegalovirus Infection and Disease in Stem Cell Transplant Recipients Using CMV Immune Plasma and Intravenous Immunoglobulin (Tables 3 and 4)

CMV Immune Plasma

In 1982 Winston reported data from the first CMV immunoprophylaxis trial, which utilized CMV immune plasma. This randomized controlled study enrolled both CMV-seronegative and CMV-seropositive recipients to receive CMV immune plasma prepared from plasma donors with CMV complement fixation antibody (CFA) titers of ≥1:64. The plasma utilized in the study had a CMV CFA titer of 1:128 and a CMV neutralizing antibody titer of 1:256. Plasma was administered at a dose of 10 ml/kg prior to the start of the conditioning regimen and at days 3, 30, 45, 60, 75, 90, and 120 following transplant. Patients were further randomized to either receive post-transplant leukocyte infusions or not receive them. Leukocyte infusions have been implicated as a major cause for post-transplant CMV infections, particularly in

CMV-seronegative recipients (17). Most patients (87.5%) were CMV-seronegative and received CMV-seronegative marrow. Primary end points for this study were the incidence of CMV infection, the incidence of interstitial pneumonitis, and mortality. The use of CMV immune plasma did not significantly impact on the overall incidence of CMV infection or survival. However, in patients receiving CMV immune plasma who developed viremia, the incidence of CMV interstitial pneumonia was significantly reduced. CMV-seropositive plasma recipients had a lower incidence of symptomatic CMV infections. CMV-seronegative recipients did not have a significant reduction in either CMV interstitial pneumonia or symptomatic CMV infection with plasma use. The greatest benefit of CMV immune plasma infusions was noted in those patients who did not receive leukocyte infusions. The incidence of both symptomatic CMV disease and CMV interstitial pneumonia was significantly reduced in this subgroup. The authors concluded that CMV immune plasma appeared to impact on the incidence of both symptomatic CMV infection and interstitial pneumonitis, although neither reached statistical significance, except in patients receiving leukocyte infusions (18).

In 1987, Ringdén and colleagues reported the results of a study conducted by the Nordic Bone Marrow Transplant Group in which CMV-immune plasma was given to predominantly CMV-seropositive patients receiving seropositive marrow (19). Fifty-four patients were randomized to receive CMV plasma or to receive no therapy. In contrast to the Winston study, these authors noted no decrease in either the incidence or severity of CMV infection or associated disease in CMV plasma recipients. In addition, overall survival was not affected by plasma infusions (19). Thus CMV immune plasma does not impact on either the incidence of CMV infection or that of CMV disease in CMV-seropositive recipients, but it may reduce the incidence of CMV infection and disease in CMV-seronegative marrow recipients not receiving leukocyte transfusions.

CMV Immune Globulin

The potential use of CMV immune globulin to prevent CMV infection and disease following stem cell transplantation has been intensively studied over the past 10 years (17,20–25). Meyers and colleagues at the Fred Hutchinson Cancer Research Center in Seattle were the first to report the use of an intramuscular preparation of CMV immune globulin for the prevention of CMV infection and disease in CMV-seronegative marrow transplant recipients (17). Sixty-two CMV-seronegative recipients were randomized to receive CMV immune globulin or receive no treatment. Of these recipients, 63% also received marrow from a CMV-seronegative donor. Patients received two doses (6 ml/m^2) before transplant, followed by weekly intramus-

TABLE 3. *Immune plasma and globulin studies in allogeneic and autologous stem cell transplant recipients: patient populations and products used*

Study	No. of Patients	Transplant type	CMV serology	Risk factors for CMV	Product	Dosage
Winston 1982 (18)	48 24 treatment 24 no Rx	Allogeneic	81% R– 87% D–	Leukocyte transfusions	CMV immune plasma	10 ml/kg days 3, 30, 45, 60, 75, 90, 120
Meyers 1983 (17)	62 30 treatment 32 no Rx	Allogeneic	100% R– 63% D–	Leukocyte transfusions	CMV immune globulin (i.m.)	6 ml/m^2 days -4, -2, weekly through day 77
Condie 1984 (23)	55 20 no Rx, 18 IVIG, 17 CMV-IgG	Allogeneic	33% R+	Leukocyte transfusions	IVIG and CMV-IVIG	200 mg/kg days 25, 50, 75
Kubanek 1985 (24)	49 23 IVIG 26 CMV-IgG	Allogeneic	59% R+	Unscreened blood donors	IVIG and CMV-IVIG	2 ml/kg days 13, 33, 73, 93
Bowden 1986 (21)	97 24 no Rx, 28 (screened blood), 22 (CMV-IgG), 23 (CMV-IgG +screened blood)	Allogeneic	100% R– 68% D–	None	CMV-IVIG (Mass. Public Health Labs)	150 mg/kg, days 6, 130, 34; 00 mg/kg, days 48, 62
Ringdén 1987 (19)	54 27 No Rx 27 Treatment	Allogeneic	83% D+ 83% R+	None	CMV immune plasma	30 ml/kg, days 3, 35, 50, 75
Winston 1987 (25)	75 37 No Rx 38 treatment	Allogeneic	83% D–84% R–	None	IVIG (Gamimune N)	1,000 mg/kg, weekly to day +120
Sullivan 1990 (22)	382 191 No Rx 191 Treatment	Allogeneic 90% Autologous 10%	81% R+ 68% D+	None	IVIG (Gamimune N)	500 mg/kg, weekly to day 90; monthly to day 360
Bowden 1991 (26)	120 60 No Rx 60 treatment	Allogeneic	100% R– 100% D–	Unscreened blood products	IVIG (Gamimune N)	200 mg/kg, days -8, -6, 7, 14, 28, 42, 56, 70
Emanuel 1992 (30)	92 46 No Rx 46 Treatment	Allogeneic	D/R Neg/Neg 43.4% Pos/Neg 14.2% Neg/Pos 19.6% Pos/Pos 22.8%	None	IVIG (Gammagard)	500 mg/kg every 2 weeks to day 100; 250 mg/kg every 2 weeks to day 180
Winston 1993 (27)	48 23 CMV blood; 25 CMV blood plus IVIG	Allogeneic	100% R– 56.9% D– 43.1% D+	None	IVIG (Sandoglobulin)	1,000 mg/kg, weekly to day +120
Wolff 1996 (33)	170 82 IVIG 88 No Rx	Autologous	Unknown	None	IVIG (Sandoglobulin)	500 mg/kg, weekly from start of chemotherapy to ANC > 500
Wolff 1996 (32) Winston 1996 (31)	627 1/3 low-dose IVIG 1/3 mid-dose IVIG 1/3 high-dose IVIG	Allogeneic	Unknown	None	IVIG (Venoglobulin-S)	100 mg/kg, 250 mg/kg, 500 mg/kg, weekly to day 100; monthly to day 360

cular injections through day +77. Thirty-nine percent of patients overall developed CMV infection. Similar to the finding of Winston and colleagues in their CMV immune plasma study, the use of CMV immune globulin did not prevent CMV infection in patients receiving granulocyte transfusions. However, in patients not receiving granulocytes, a significant reduction in CMV infections was noted in the immune globulin recipients (12% versus 42% in the control group). There was a particularly striking decrease in the incidence of CMV infection in those globulin recipients who had a CMV-seronegative marrow donor, where no CMV infections were observed. Thus, similar to the Winston study,

patients at lowest risk for the development of CMV infection and disease (CMV-seronegative donor and recipient, without granulocyte exposure), appeared to benefit most from the use of CMV immune globulin. This same group reported data in 1986 from a three-arm study in which CMV-seronegative marrow transplant recipients were randomized to receive either no treatment (no globulin or screened blood products), CMV-seronegative blood products alone, or CMV-seronegative blood products and intravenous CMV immune globulin (21). The product used for this study was a CMV immune globulin prepared by Massachusetts Public Health Biologic Laboratories. Two doses (150

TABLE 4. *Immune plasma and globulin studies in allogeneic and autologous stem cell transplant recipients: summary of clinical results*

Study	Products dosage	Treatment group	CMV infection (%)	CMV interstitial pneumonia (%)	Bacterial infection (%)	Acute GvHD (%)	Survival (%)
Winston 1982 (18)	CMV immune plasma 10 ml/kg, days 3, 30, 45, 60, 75, 90, 120	Control arm Treatment arm	50 21 (NS)	33 13 (NS)	NA NA	NA NA	38 50 (NS)
Meyers 1983 (17)	CMV-IVIG 6 ml/M^2, Days -4, -2; weekly through day 77	Control arm Treatment arm	44 33 (NS)	6 7 (NS)	NA NA	NA NA	NA NA
Condie 1984 (23)	CMV-IVIG IVIG 200 mg/kg, days 25, 50, 75	Control arm CMV-IVIG	50 0*	30 0*	NA NA	60 41	NA NA
Kubanek 1985 (24)	CMV-IVIG IVIG 2 ml/kg, days 13, 33, 73, 93	IVIG CMV-IVIG	NA NA	26 4*	NA NA	NA NA	
Bowden 1986 (21)	CMV-IVIG 150 mg/kg, days 6, 30, 34; 100 mg/kg, days 48, 62	Control arm CMV-IVIG	40 24 (NS)	15 9 (NS)	NA NA	NA NA	NA NA
Ringden 1987 (19)	CMV immune plasma 30 ml/kg, Days 3, 25, 50, 75	Control arm Treatment arm	22 41	11 11	NA NA	NA NA	56 70
Winston 1987 (25)	IVIG 1,000 mg/kg, weekly to day +120	Control arm Treatment arm	46 21*	32 16 (NS)	NA NA	65 34*	NA NA
Sullivan 1990 (22)	IVIG 500 mg/kg, weekly to day 90; monthly to day 360	Control arm Treatment arm	NS NS	NS NS	33 11*	52 42 (NS)	35 (2 years) 33 (2 years)
Bowden 1991 (26)	IVIG 200 mg/kg, days -8, -6, 7, 14, 28, 42, 56, 70	Control arm Treatment arm	15 15	15 13	NA NA	NA NA	68 67
Emanuel 1992 (30)	IVIG 500 mg/kg every 2 weeks to day 100; 250 mg/kg, every 2 weeks to day 180	Control arm Treatment arm	10.7 8.7	NS NS	13 26 (Gram Negative sepsis)	64.7 31.3*	NS NS
Winston 1993 (27)	IVIG 1,000 mg/kg, weekly to day +120	CMV-negative blood products CMV-negative blood plus IVIG	9 7	0 0	8 13	48 20*	46 41
Wolff 1996 (33)	IVIG 500 mg/kg weekly from start of chemotherapy to ANC > 500	Control Arm Treatment Arm	NA NA	NA NA	34 35	NA NA	96.6 86.6*
Wolff 1996 (32)	IVIG	100 mg/kg	NS	NS	NS	39	NS
Winston 1996 (31)	100 mg/kg, 250 mg/kg, 500 mg/kg weekly to day 100; monthly to day 360	250 mg/kg 500 mg/kg	NS NS	NS NS	NS NS	43 35	NS NS

NS, not statistically significant; *, statistically significant ($p=0.05$); NA, not applicable or no data available.

mg/kg) were given before transplant and every 14 days thereafter through day +62. CMV-seronegative blood products were given through day +100. Sixty-two percent of patients developed CMV infection. As in their previous study, a seronegative donor significantly reduced the incidence of both CMV infection and disease (3% versus 32%; 0 versus 16%, respectively), but only if CMV-seronegative blood products were used as well. Of note was the observation that CMV globulin therapy did not provide prophylaxis against CMV infection, independent of the effect of donor marrow serology. In addition, the use of CMV globulin did not protect against CMV pneumonia following development of a CMV infection. The authors concluded that CMV globulin added little to CMV prophylaxis over and above the use of CMV-seronegative blood products, which alone were extremely effective in preventing CMV infection and disease in CMV-seronegative marrow transplant recipients (21). In 1991 this same group reported a study that addressed the question of whether intravenous CMV immunoglobulin could reduce the incidence of CMV infection and disease in CMV-seronegative marrow recipients receiving CMV-seropositive marrow and CMV unscreened blood products (26). Patients were randomized to receive CMV immunoglobulin (Gamimune N) at a dose of 200 mg/kg (infused on days 8 and 6 prior to transplantation, followed by infusions on days 7, 14, 28, 42, 56, and 70 following transplant) or no treatment. The primary end points were the incidence of both CMV infection and disease within the first 100 days following transplant. CMV immunoglobulin did not affect the incidence of CMV pneumonitis, CMV infection, or survival. Administration of immunoglobulin significantly reduced the incidence of CMV viremia. The conclusion of this study was that the use of CMV immune globulin does not appear to significantly modify the incidence of CMV infection or disease during the first 100 days following transplant (26).

Prophylaxis of Infectious Complications and GVHD with Intravenous Immunoglobulin Following Stem Cell Transplantation

Two large controlled CMV and infection prophylaxis studies in allogeneic marrow transplant recipients, utilizing the same off-the-shelf intravenous immunoglobulin product (Gamimune N), were reported from UCLA and Seattle in 1987 and 1990 by Winston and Sullivan, respectively (22,25). The UCLA study enrolled CMV-seronegative marrow transplant recipients who were randomized to receive either Gamimune N or no treatment. The dose used in this study was much higher than that used in previous trials. IVIG was given at a dose of 1,000 mg/kg, starting prior to the conditioning regimen and continued on a weekly basis through day 120 following transplant. The primary end points for this study were the incidence of CMV infection and interstitial pneumonia. GVHD prophylaxis regimens were balanced in the two treatment arms. The overall incidence of CMV infection was similar in the two study arms (47% versus 62%). However, the incidence of symptomatic CMV infection (fever, symptomatic viruria, or pneumonia) was significantly reduced in recipients of IVIG (21% versus 46%). The overall incidence of interstitial pneumonia (18% versus 46%) was statistically significantly reduced in the

IVIG arm of the study. However, the observed reduction in the incidence of CMV pneumonia in IVIG recipients was not statistically significant. The maximum benefit for IVIG therapy was again observed in CMV-seronegative recipients receiving CMV-seronegative marrow. Of greater potential significance was the observation that recipients of high-dose IVIG appeared to have a lower incidence of acute GVHD (34% in IVIG recipients, 65% in controls). The overall severity or grade of GVHD was not reported. The reduction in the overall incidence of interstitial pneumonia in the IVIG group was independent of the presence or absence of GVHD. The important by-product of this study was the first-time observation that high-dose IVIG may have immune-modulating properties, manifest by the reduction in the overall incidence of GVHD in IVIG recipients (25). This same group in 1993 reported results from a prospective randomized trial comparing high-dose IVIG (Sandoglobulin, 1,000 mg/kg weekly through day +120) plus CMV-seronegative blood products with CMV-seronegative blood products alone, to prevent CMV infection and disease in CMV-seronegative allogeneic BMT recipients (27). This trial was conducted to evaluate the benefits of IVIG for CMV prophylaxis in the context of CMV-seronegative recipients receiving screened blood products. The efficacy of CMV-seronegative blood products to prevent CMV infection and disease in CMV-seronegative recipients receiving CMV-seronegative marrow is well established (21,28). Twenty-three patients received CMV-negative blood products alone, and 25 patients received CMV-negative blood products plus IVIG. The incidence of CMV infection, CMV pneumonia, and idiopathic interstitial pneumonia was the same in each group. However, as reported in their previous trial, the authors noted a significant reduction in the incidence of grades 2–4 GVHD in the group receiving IVIG. The number and type of nonviral infections (bacterial and fungal), as well as overall survival, were similar in the two groups. The primary conclusion of this study was that high-dose IVIG reduces the incidence and severity of acute GVHD in allogeneic marrow transplant recipients (27).

In 1990 Sullivan and colleagues reported the largest controlled study to date on the use of IVIG for the prevention of infections and GVHD following allogeneic marrow transplantation (22). This trial was a randomized comparison of IVIG prophylaxis versus no treatment, and the primary study end points were acute GVHD, infection, interstitial pneumonia, and death. Patients randomized to the IVIG arm received Gamimune N at a dose of 500 mg/kg per dose, starting at day 7 prior to BMT, followed by weekly dosing through day +90 and monthly dosing through day +360. Data from the early phase of this study (through day +90) and the late phase of the study (days 90–360) have been reported separately (22,29). All CMV-seronegative marrow recipients received CMV-seronegative blood products. The study enrolled 369 evaluable patients. The primary findings from this study were as follows:

1. The overall incidence of CMV infection was equal in the two groups.
2. IVIG recipients had a significantly lower incidence of both Gram-negative sepsis and local bacterial infections.
3. The overall incidence of interstitial pneumonitis in CMV-seropositive recipients was significantly lower in IVIG recipients (13% versus 22%), although the incidence of CMV pneumonia between the two groups was not statistically significant. The decrease in interstitial pneumonia was only noted in adult patients (age >20).
4. The overall incidence of grades 2–4 acute GVHD was significantly lower in the IVIG group receiving HLA-compatible marrow (28% versus 43%, $p = 0.029$) and HLA-mismatched marrow (49% versus 71%, $p = 0.078$). Multivariate analysis of 325 evaluable recipients confirmed that the risk of acute GVHD was increased in the control group (relative risk = 1.63, $p = 0.0056$).
5. Overall survival was not impacted by the use of IVIG treatment. However, nonrelapse-related mortality was significantly reduced with IVIG therapy in adult recipients of HLA-compatible marrow (30% versus 46%, $p = 0.023$).

The results of the second part of this study—namely, the analysis of data from patients receiving monthly IVIG or no treatment from day +90 through day +360—were published in 1996 (29). Two hundred and fifty patients (123 IVIG, 127 controls) were evaluable. Between days 90 and 360 the incidence of bacteremia or septicemia per 100 patient-days of risk was the same in the two groups. The incidence of localized infection was slightly higher but not significantly so in the control group (0.44 versus 0.24; relative risk, 1.46; $p = 0.07$). IVIG administration did not impact on survival, on the incidence of bronchiolitis obliterans, or the incidence of death from chronic GVHD. Of potentially great importance was the observation that long-term IVIG administration may impact on long-term humoral immune system recovery. After discontinuation of IVIG treatment at day 360, it was noted that (a) serum IgG and IgA levels were significantly lower in the IVIG group compared with the control group at day 720 and (b) infections were less common in the control patients during the second year (0.12 versus 0.19; relative risk, 0.61; $p = 0.03$). The authors conclude that monthly administration of IVIG from days 90 to 360, in the absence of hypogammaglobulinemia, does not reduce late complications following allogeneic BMT and may impair humoral immune system recovery (29).

The use of IVIG as infection prophylaxis in allogeneic marrow transplant recipients was reported from Memorial Sloan Kettering Cancer Center in 1992 (30). Ninety-two allogeneic marrow transplant recipients (59 T-cell-depleted, 33 unmodified) were randomized to receive standardized lots of IVIG (Gammagard) or no immune globulin therapy. Patients were treated with 500 mg/kg every 2 weeks from day −7 through day +100, and then 250 mg/kg every 2 weeks from day +100 through day +180. IVIG did not alter overall or disease-free survival at either 1 or 3 years following transplant. The incidence of Gram-negative systemic infection was higher in the IVIG group than in the control group (26% versus 13%). IVIG did not decrease the incidence of CMV infection, CMV disease, or interstitial pneumonitis. However, IVIG recipients receiving unmodified marrow grafts had a significant reduction in the incidence of grade 3 or less acute GVHD (31.3% versus 64.7%, $p = 0.05$) (30).

Preliminary results from a large multicenter randomized double-blinded dose/response trial of IVIG for the prevention of infection and GVHD following allogeneic bone marrow transplantation were recently reported (31,32). Six hundred and twenty-seven recipients of an allogeneic marrow transplant were randomized to receive one of three dose levels of Venoglobulin-S on a weekly basis for 100 days and then monthly thereafter through 1 year following transplant. Dose levels were 100 mg/kg, 250 mg/kg, and 500 mg/kg. The primary end points of the study were the incidence of grade 2 or greater GVHD, nonrelapse mortality, and frequency and type of post-transplant infections. Patient characteristics—including age, underlying disease, type of transplant, HLA matching, CMV antibody status, GVHD prophylaxis regimen, type of transplant (related versus unrelated; unmanipulated versus T-depleted)—were similar in each dosage group. All patients were evaluated up to 12 months following transplant. The overall incidence of acute GVHD was similar for each dosage group (39% [100 mg/kg]; 43% [250 mg/kg]; 35% [500 mg/kg]; $p =$ not significant). The incidence of death from infection, sepsis, bacteremia, fungemia, CMV infection, CMV disease, interstitial pneumonia, and veno-occlusive disease was comparable and not significantly different for each dosage group. Overall survival was approximately 50% and was not statistically different across dosage groups. The preliminary conclusions from this large study are that the dose of IVIG did not appear to influence either the incidence of infectious complications, overall survival, or acute GVHD. Detailed subgroup analyses are currently still under way. The authors of this large study point out that if these data are confirmed after further subgroup analyses, they could have significant medical and economic ramifications for allogeneic transplant recipients, namely, that the widespread current use of IVIG for infection and GVHD prophylaxis may not be warranted (31,32).

The American Bone Marrow Transplant Group recently reported its large, multi-institutional study to determine whether high-dose intravenous immunoglobulin prevents severe infections during autologous bone marrow transplantation or equivalent high-dose myeloablative chemotherapy (33). Patients were randomized to either receive 500 mg/kg of IVIG once a week (Sandoglobulin) or receive no treatment, starting at the initiation of the preparative regimen and ending after the absolute neutrophil count recovered to ≥500 × 10⁹/L for 1 day. Primary end points for the study were the incidence of septicemia or other clinically proven infection, platelet use, and development of alloimmunity to platelet transfusion. Clinical infection, bacteremia, and fungemia occurred with similar frequency in each group. Death due to infection occurred in 4.9% of IVIG recipients and 2.3% of controls. Survival was higher in the control group, primarily because of a higher incidence of fatal veno-occlusive disease in IVIG recipients. The authors concluded that IVIG used in this manner in autologous BMT recipients and patients receiving high-dose myeloablative chemotherapy did not prevent infections and was associated with a higher incidence of fatal hepatic veno-occlusive disease (33).

Two meta-analyses looking at the efficacy of intravenous immunoglobulin in preventing complications after allogeneic marrow transplantation have now been published (34,35). Data from 12 previously published studies involving 1,282 patients were evaluated and synthesized. The authors concluded the following:

1. IVIG significantly reduces fatal CMV infection, CMV pneumonia, interstitial pneumonia, and overall post-transplant mortality.
2. IVIG reduces the incidence of acute GVHD.
3. IVIG is efficacious in preventing major complications of BMT in both CMV-negative and CMV-positive recipients (34,35).

The rationale for these studies is the plethora of contradictory information in the published literature about the therapeutic efficacy of IVIG in reducing CMV infection and disease, interstitial pneumonitis, GVHD, other infections, and mortality. This is in part due to variances in IVIG products used, treatment regimens, small numbers of study patients, study designs, patient eligibility, study end points, measurement techniques, and statistical analyses. Although these studies have concluded that IVIG has therapeutic efficacy, considerable uncertainty remains about the current indications for IVIG use in both allogeneic and autologous stem cell transplant recipients, particularly in the context of CMV prophylaxis. Numerous studies have now demonstrated that potent antiviral drugs such as ganciclovir are far more efficient than IVIG at suppressing CMV infection and preventing CMV disease (36–41). In addition, in response to well-controlled studies demonstrating positive immunomodulatory effects of IVIG (e.g., its effect on the incidence of GVHD), the use of IVIG for this indication has become the standard of care in many transplant units (22,25).

However, recent studies have begun to challenge this view (20,29–32). Until these issues are definitively resolved, the widespread use of IVIG in stem cell transplant recipients will remain empiric and controversial.

Passive Immunoprophylaxis and Treatment of Respiratory Syncytial Virus (RSV) Infections in Stem Cell Transplant Recipients

Passive administration of sera containing high titers of RSV-specific neutralizing antibodies has been shown to confer protection against infection in a cotton rat rodent model (42,43). In high-risk children the use of standard intravenous immunoglobulin at a dose of 500 mg/kg did not confer protection from subsequent RSV infection (44). Results of a multicenter study published in 1993 demonstrated that a hyperimmune RSV IVIG at a dose of 750 mg/kg once a month administered to children at high risk for RSV pneumonia protected against lower respiratory RSV disease (45). Monthly infusions at this dose level maintained the titer of RSV neutralizing antibodies at ≥1:250, a value considered to be protective to the lower respiratory tract. The RSV IVIG product (Respigam, Medimmune, Gaithersburg, MD) used in this study is now licensed for the prophylaxis of RSV infections in infants of less than 32 weeks gestation and infants less than 2 years of age at high risk for RSV disease (see Table 1).

RSV is a serious cause of pneumonitis in stem cell transplant recipients and carries a high mortality rate. RSV pneumonitis outbreaks have been reported from a number of transplant centers in the United States and Europe over the past 5 years (46–50). The mortality rate varies from 60% to 100%, dependent on the time prior to the institution of therapy. Two recent reports from Houston and Boston suggest that early treatment appears to have a beneficial effect on survival (49,51). In the series reported from the M. D. Anderson Cancer Center, 16 patients with RSV pneumonitis were treated with the combination of aerosolized ribavirin and IVIG containing high titers of RSV neutralizing antibodies (1:2,000 to 1:8,000). Therapy was with aerosolized ribavirin (20 mg/ml for 18 hours a day) plus IVIG (500 mg/kg every other day). Eight of the 16 patients survived (50%) (51). In this study initiation of therapy after the onset of respiratory failure was universally unsuccessful. This same group at M. D. Anderson studied the application of preemptive therapy with aerosolized ribavirin and IVIG to a total of 12 patients with upper respiratory RSV infection (52). In 10 of 12 patients, RSV remained confined to the upper respiratory tract and the patients did not progress to pneumonitis. The authors state that well-controlled prospective clinical trials designed to evaluate this preemptive therapy approach are warranted. DeVincenzo and colleagues report on the successful treatment of two BMT recipients with lower-tract RSV infection using aerosolized ribavirin and a single infusion of high-titer RSV immune globulin (Respigam, Medimmune) (49). Both patients received ribavirin at a dose of 6 g over 18 hours plus a single dose of RSV IVIG (1.5 g/kg). Both patients did not require mechanical ventilation and were discharged from the hospital within 2 weeks of treatment. Peak serum RSV neutralizing antibody titers obtained in these two patients were significantly higher than those achievable with standard IVIG. The beneficial effect of immune globulin on established RSV disease in animals is well established. Infusions of IVIG are capable of reducing the virus titer in lung tissue by a factor of 100 (53). RSV-IVIG has a five-fold greater *in vitro* RSV neutralizing activity compared with standard IVIG products and a tenfold increase in *in vivo* protective activity in the cotton rat RSV model (42). The reason high-titer RSV IVIG products are clinically efficacious is unclear. RSV infects surface epithelium in the respiratory tract, and the amount of neutralizing antibodies detectable at this site is only a tenth of that obtained in serum (42). Topical delivery of aerosolized antibody to the respiratory tract is an efficient way of clearing virus from the lung (54). This approach is currently being investigated in human clinical trials.

Passive Immunoprophylaxis of Varicella-Zoster Infection in Stem Cell Transplantation Recipients with Immune Globulin

Approximately 90% of adults have immunity to varicella-zoster virus (VZV), because most cases of primary varicella occur in children between the ages of 1 and 9 years. VZV infection is a frequent complication following both autologous and allogeneic stem cell transplantation and occurs either following reactivation of latent virus or, more uncommonly, after primary infection (55,56). Varicella-zoster infection in the stem cell transplant recipient results in primary disease (varicella or chickenpox) and recurrent disease (shingles). In the largest series reported to date, 18% of patients developed either primary or recurrent VZV infections within 3 years after BMT, the majority within the first 18 months. The projected incidence through 10 years following transplant was 52 ± 14%. Dermatomal zoster represented 62% of all infections, whereas 32% of patients had either central nervous system, disseminated, or visceral disease (pneumonia, hepatitis). All nondermatome-related VZV infection and VZV-associated death occurred within 10 months of transplantation (55). Risk factors for the development of recurrent VZV infection include age >10 years, radiation therapy in the preparative regimen, VZV seropositivity, severe GVHD, and use of immunosuppressive drugs, particularly post-transplant antithymocyte globulin (ATG) (55,56). The incidence and severity of VZV infections are similar in autologous and allogeneic stem cell transplant recipients (55,56).

Varicella is usually acquired by contact with persons infected with chickenpox, either by respiratory transmission or by direct contact. Varicella can also be acquired by direct contact with herpes zoster lesions.

Prevention of Disease with Varicella-Zoster Immune Globulin

Varicella-zoster immune globulin (VZIG) is produced by the American Red Cross (see Table 2). It is a 10% to 18% solution of the globulin fraction of human plasma and is packaged as single-dose vials, each containing 125 units of VZV antibody in a total volume of 2.5 ml or less.

1. Varicella-zoster seronegative children and adults who have received a stem cell transplant within the past 5 years should be given VZIG within 96 hours after close contact with a patient with either chickenpox or shingles. Close contact is defined as the following;
   a. Continuous household contact;
   b. Playmate contact (>1 hour of indoor play);
   c. Hospital contact in the same 2–4-bed room or adjacent beds in a large ward or prolonged face-to-face contact with an infectious staff member or patient.
2. VZIG is not recommended for the prevention of disease after exposure in varicella-zoster seropositive patients.

For maximum benefit, VZIG should be administered as soon as possible after presumed exposure and before 96 hours after exposure. Stem cell transplant recipients who are exposed again more than 3 weeks after a prior dose of VZIG. The drug is administered by deep intramuscular injection. Recommended dosage is one vial (125 units) per 10 kg of body weight.

Prophylaxis of Varicella-Zoster Infection in Autologous Transplant Recipients

The incidence and severity of varicella-zoster infection in autologous and allogeneic transplant recipients is similar (55). Recommendations for passive immunoprophylaxis with VZIG are the same for both autologous and allogeneic stem cell transplant recipients.

Immunoprophylaxis of Hepatitis B Virus Infection in Stem Cell and Solid Organ Transplant Recipients with Hepatitis B Immune Globulin

Hepatitis B virus (HBV) infection following either stem cell or solid organ transplantation can occur in the context of (a) transmission of HBV from a HBV-infected stem cell, organ, or blood product donor, or (b) reactivation of infection in a previously infected transplant recipient. Stem cell transplant recipients who are HBV surface antigen positive (HBsAg+) at the time of transplantation do not appear to have any additional liver complications or other nonhepatic sequelae in the post-transplant period (57). In contrast, stem cell transplant recipients who are HBV negative prior to transplant but receive marrow from a HBsAg+ donor are at increased risk for post-transplant severe liver disease (58). The presence of HBs antibodies in the recipient's serum at the time of transplant appears to be protective and may prevent severe liver damage (58).

Eighty percent of patients undergoing orthotopic liver transplantation as treatment for end-stage HBV-related liver disease become reinfected with HBV. However, immunoprophylaxis with hepatitis B immune globulin (HBIg) can not only reduce the rate of recurrence to 30% or less at 2 years following transplant, but also improve overall survival (59,60). These data have now been confirmed in further studies (61,62). Intravenous HBIG products are currently available only in Europe (60). All HBIG currently available in the United States is licensed for intramuscular administration only (see Table 2). However, these products are frequently administered intravenously, with the attendant risk of mercury toxicity from long-term use due to the infusion of thimerosol preservative (62). Future clinical products will likely be mercury-free. The dosage schedule and HBIG product have varied in published studies (59–62). HBIG has been administered intermittently to maintain a predetermined protective level of anti-HBs or has been given indefinitely on a regular monthly schedule. The fixed monthly schedule appears to be as effective as titer-based dosing (61,62).

There are currently no well-controlled randomized studies utilizing HBIG for prophylaxis of HBV infections following stem cell transplantation. However, recently published data from a retrospective study of transplant recipients in Italy receiving HBV-infected marrow suggest that the use of passive immunoprophylaxis or the presence of anti-HBs antibodies at the time of transplant appears to reduce the incidence and severity of post-transplant liver disease in these patients (58).

Immunoprophylaxis with CMV Hyperimmune Globulin or Standard IVIG to Prevent Cytomegalovirus and Other Infections Following Solid Organ Transplantation

In the United States approximately 10,000 kidneys, 1,600 hearts, and more than 2,000 livers are transplanted annually (8). Patients who undergo organ transplantation are highly susceptible to a number of infectious complications as a direct result of the high level of immune suppression required preventing graft rejection. Nosocomial infections predominate during the immediate post-transplant period (up to 30 days). Opportunistic viral, fungal, and bacterial infections are common during the later post-transplant period, especially during the first 6 months. Later, community-acquired infections tend to predominate. These include mycobacterial infections and fungal

pathogens. However, CMV infections remain the predominant and ubiquitous threat to solid organ transplant recipients. Symptomatic CMV infection occurs in 8% of kidney transplant recipients, 29% of liver recipients, 25% of heart recipients, and 39% of heart-lung recipients (63). The lack of cellular and humoral immunity in the recipient predisposes the patient to a high risk of CMV infection if the organ is derived from a seropositive donor. In addition, the use of post-transplant immune suppression with antithymocyte globulin or anti-T-cell monoclonal antibodies significantly increases the risk of CMV infection, particularly in CMV-seropositive recipients (64,65).

Management strategies for transplant patients at high risk of infections include prevention of exposure to infected blood products as well as prophylaxis and preemptive therapy with antiviral drugs such as ganciclovir. Prior to the wide availability and licensing of potent antiviral drugs, IVIG was extensively studied for the prophylaxis of CMV infection and disease as well as other infections in solid organ transplant recipients. Both standard IVIG products and CMV hyperimmune preparations have been used.

Use of Standard and CMV Hyperimmune IVIG Products for the Prevention of CMV and Other Infections in Solid Organ Transplant Recipients

Renal Transplantation

Randomized controlled trials in renal transplant recipients have conclusively demonstrated efficacy of IVIG products to prevent CMV infection and disease in some studies but not in others (66–72). Data from these studies are summarized in Table 5. Overall, the relative risk for the development of CMV infection and disease was reduced 29% in recipients receiving IVIG prophylaxis. In those studies where CMV-seronegative recipients received a seropositive kidney (D+, R−) the relative risk reduction was 45.6% in IVIG recipients when compared with those patients not receiving IVIG prophylaxis. However, caution is warranted when interpreting these combined data. Patients received markedly different IVIG regimens, and diagnostic criteria for defining CMV infection and disease varied widely. In addition, the total number of patients in each study was relatively small and patient characteristics were widely divergent. Nevertheless the use of IVIG appears to confer some protection against the development of CMV infection and disease, particularly in seronegative recipients receiving a seropositive organ.

The seminal study using CMV hyperimmune globulin (Cytogam, Medimmune) to prevent primary CMV infection in CMV-seronegative renal patients transplanted with kidney from a seropositive donor was published in 1987 by Snydman and colleagues (73). Fifty-nine CMV-seronegative patients received kidneys from seropositive donors and were randomized to receive CMV hyperim-

TABLE 5. *Clinical studies using either CMV-Ig or IVIG as prophylaxis for CMV and other infections following solid organ transplantation*

Study	Organ	Patients	Design	Product regimen	Symptomatic CMV infection/ disease	Outcome comments
Kasiske (66)	Kidney	Mixed	PP,SP,R,NPC	IVIG (Gamimune) 500 mg/kg, weekly for 12 weeks	IVIG 53% Control 77%	No effect on morbidity, organ rejection
Fehir (67)	Multiple organs*	Mixed	NPC,R,PP,SP	IVIG (Gammagard) 500 mg/kg, weekly × 4 months, bimonthly, × 8 months	IVIG 7% Control 6%	No efficacy reported; small number of patients for valid efficacy conclusions
Bailey (68)	Multiple organs*	D+ R–	R, PP	ACV with or without IVIG (Gamimune N), 300 mg/kg every 2 weeks × 10 weeks	IVIG + ACV = 80% ACV = 64%	Delay in onset of CMV disease in IVIG group (NS); No overt efficacy reported
Conti (69)	Kidney	D+ R–	R, PP, NPC	IVIG (Gammagard) 500 mg kg^{-1} week^{-1} ×2 wks, 250 mg kg week^{-1} ×5 wks versus GVC × 21 days	IVIG 22% GCV 21%	Both regimens equally effective compared with historical controls; GVC reported to be much cheaper than IVIG
Steinmuller (70)	Kidney	R+	R, NPC	IVIG (Sandoglobulin) 500 mg/kg q2 weeks ×3 doses 250 mg/kg q 2 weeks × 2 doses	IVIG 12%^{ss} Control 39%	CMV symptomatic disease significantly reduced in IVIG recipients; small number of patients
Fassbinder (72)	Kidney	Mixed	PP, SP, R	CMV-Ig (Cytotect) vs IVIG (Intraglobulin) 10 g iv, days 0, 18, 38, 58, 78	NR	Decreased severity of primary CMV disease in Cytotect group reported
Snydman (73)	Kidney	D+ R–	R, NPC	CMV-Ig (Cytogam) 150 mg/kg pre-tx; 100 mg/kg, weeks 2,4; 50 mg/kg, weeks 6, 8, 12, 16 vs no treatment	CMV-IgG = 21% No treatment = 60%	Significant reduction in CMV syndromes, fungal and parasitic disease; deceased mortality in CMV-IgG group
Cofer (74)	Liver	Mixed	PP, SP, R, PC	IVIG (Sandoglobulin) 500 mg/kg weekly to day 84 vs albumin control	IVIG 32% Control 20%	No overt benefit noted Lack of efficacy reported
Saliba (75)	Liver	D+ R– D– R–	PP	CMV-Ig 250 mg/kg, day 0-, 125 mg/kg every 10 days × 3 months versus no treatment	CMV-Ig = 27% Control = 86% (D+R– group)	Significant decrease in CMV symptomatic infection in D+ R– patients
Snydman (76)	Liver	Mixed	PP, SP	CMV-Ig 150 mg/kg pre-Tx and weeks 2, 4, 6, 8; 100 mg/kg, weeks 12, 16 vs placebo (1% albumin)	CMV-Ig 19% Placebo 31%	Reduction in symptomatic CMV infection (NS); no therapeutic effect noted in D+R– group
Snydman (77)	Liver	D+ R– R– treated with placebo	PP	Same regimen as Snydman (76)	CMV-Ig 14% Placebo 32%	Significant reduction in CMV disease in R– CMV Ig group

PP = Primary Prophylaxis; SP = Secondary Prophylaxis; R = randomized; NPC = not placebo controlled; NR = not reported; *= kidney, heart, heart-lung, liver, lung; ACV = Acyclovir; NS = not significant; SS = statistically significant.

mune globulin or no treatment. Patients received 150 mg/kg within 72 hours of transplantation; 100 mg/kg at weeks 2 and 4; and 50 mg/kg at weeks 6, 8, 12, and 16. Virologically confirmed CMV-associated syndromes were reduced by 60% in controls to 21% in the treatment group (p = <0.01). There was also a marked reduction in fungal and parasitic infections in the treatment group. CMV pneumonia was less frequent in the treatment group but was not statistically significant. Overall mor-

tality was also reduced in the treatment group (4% versus 14%). On the basis of these data Cytogam was licensed by the FDA for the primary prophylaxis of CMV infections in renal transplant recipients.

Liver Transplantation

Three randomized studies using either standard IVIG or CMV hyperimmune globulin have been reported in liver transplant recipients (74–76). Snydman and colleagues reported on 141 liver transplant recipients randomized to receive either Cytogam or placebo in a double-blind fashion (76). CMV immune globulin or placebo (1% albumin) were given at the same dosage and frequency as described in their earlier renal transplant study (see earlier) (73). CMV globulin reduced severe CMV-associated disease (multiorgan infection, pneumonia, or invasive fungal disease) from 26% to 12% (relative risk 0.39). CMV globulin was still protective in patients receiving T-cell antibodies. The overall rate of CMV disease of all types was reduced from 31% to 19% (relative risk, 0.56) in the CMV globulin group. The rates of CMV infection, graft survival, or patient survival were not influenced, and no effect on the D+ R− group was demonstrated, in contrast to the renal transplant study. However a reanalysis of the same data comparing CMV-seronegative recipients receiving CMV-Ig with seronegative recipients receiving placebo demonstrated prophylactic efficacy of CMV-Ig in the D+ R− group (77). The prophylactic efficacy of CMV-Ig in D+ R− patients was confirmed by a study conducted by Saliba and colleagues (75).

In summary, data from IVIG prophylaxis studies in solid organ transplant recipients suggest the following:

1. Renal transplant recipients appear to have the most benefit from the use of IVIG for primary CMV prophylaxis. This is most appreciated in the highest-risk group (i.e., D+ R− patients).
2. Therapeutic benefits are modified in the context of immunosuppressive drug use, particularly anti-T-cell antibodies.
3. The evidence to support the use of CMV hyperimmune globulin over standard IVIG products is marginal.
4. Most solid organ transplant centers now utilize alternate or additional methods of CMV prophylaxis (e.g., ganciclovir) in most patient groups (63).
5. Although the use of CMV hyperimmune globulin has been demonstrated to be cost-effective in D+ R− renal transplant recipients, CMV globulin is still more expensive than prophylactic or preemptive therapy with antiviral drugs (63,78).

CONCLUSION

The medical literature is replete with a plethora of contradictory information about the prophylactic and therapeutic efficacy of IVIG in both solid organ and stem cell transplant recipients. Despite a seemingly self-evident rationale for its use in the context of secondary hypogammaglobulinemia and post-transplant immunocompromise in stem cell transplant recipients, IVIG has not consistently been demonstrated to reduce CMV infection or disease, interstitial pneumonitis, GVHD, bacterial or fungal

infections, or overall post-transplant morbidity or mortality. Nevertheless, IVIG continues to be utilized as a standard of care in most stem cell transplant units worldwide. It is likely that the widespread use of IVIG in stem cell transplant recipients will continue, but until remaining efficacy issues are resolved one way or another by new clinical studies, its use in this patient population will remain controversial. It is more likely, however, that current medical economic pressures will force a rational reconsideration of the use of this expensive product prior to the publication of data from future well-designed, well-controlled, and adequately powered clinical trials. Similarly, the use of IVIG in solid organ transplant recipients is likely to decrease as more effective and cheaper pharmaceutical means of CMV prophylaxis are introduced.

REFERENCES

1. Janeway CA, Travers P. Janeway CA, Travers P, eds. *Immunobiology: the immune system in health and disease.* New York: Current Biology Ltd/Garland Publishing; 1994:5:28–29.
2. Lum LG. Recapitulation of immune ontogeny: a vital component for the success of bone marrow transplantation. In: Champlin R, ed. *Bone marrow transplantation.* Norwell, Ma: Kluwer Academic Publishers; 1990:27–54.
3. Witherspoon RP, Lum LG, Storb R. Immunologic reconstitution after human marrow grafting. *Semin Hematol* 1984;21:2–10.
4. Lum LG. The kinetics of immune reconstitution after human marrow transplantation. *Blood* 1987;69:369–380.
5. Parkman R. Immunological reconstitution following marrow transplantation. In: Forman SJ, Blume KG, Thomas ED, eds. *Bone marrow transplantation.* Cambridge, MA: Blackwell Scientific Publications; 1994: 504–512.
6. Storek J, Ferrara S, Ku N, Giorgi JV, Champlin RE, Saxon A. B cell reconstitution after human marrow transplantation: recapitulation of ontogeny? *Bone Marrow Transplant* 1993;12:387–398.
7. Medical Economics Data Inc. *1994 red book.* Montvale, NJ: Medical Economics Data; 1994.
8. University Hospital Consortium. *Technology assessment: intravenous immunoglobulin preparations.* Oak Brook, IL: University Hospital Consortium Services Corp.; 1995.
9. O'Reilly RJ, Keever CA, Small TN, Brochstein J. The use of HLA-non-identical T-cell-depleted marrow transplants for correction of severe combined immunodeficiency disease. *Immunodef Rev* 1989;1:273–309.
10. Fischer A, Landais P, Friedrich W. European experience of bone marrow transplantation for severe combined immunodeficiency. *Lancet* 1990;336:850–854.
11. O'Reilly RJ, Friedrich W, Small TN. Transplantation approaches for severe combined immunodeficiency diseases. In: Forman SJ, Blume KG, Thomas ED, eds. *Bone marrow transplantation.* Cambridge, MA: Blackwell Scientific Publications; 1994:849–873.
12. Ochs HD. Comparison of high-dose and low-dose intravenous immunoglobulin therapy in patients with primary immunodeficiency diseases. *Am J Med* 1984;76:78–82.
13. Liese JG. High versus low dose immunoglobulin therapy in the long term treatment of X-linked agammaglobulinemia. *Am J Dis Child* 1992;146:335–339.
14. Buckley RH, Schiff RI. The use of intravenous immune globulin in immunodeficiency diseases. *N Engl J Med* 1991;325:110–117.
15. Storek J, Saxon A. Reconstitution of B-cell immunity following bone marrow transplantation. *Bone Marrow Transplant* 1992;9:395–408.
16. Small TN, Keever CA, Weiner-Fedus S, Heller G, O'Reilly RJ, Flomenberg N. B-cell differentiation following autologous, conventional, or T-cell depleted bone marrow transplantation: a recapitulation of normal B-cell ontogeny. *Blood* 1990;76:1647–1656.
17. Meyers JD, Leszczynski J, Zaia JA, et al. Prevention of cytomegalovirus infection by cytomegalovirus immune globulin after marrow transplantation. *Ann Intern Med* 1983;98:442–446.

18. Winston DJ, Pollard RB, Ho WG, et al. Cytomegalovirus immune plasma in bone marrow transplant recipients. *Ann Intern Med* 1982;97:11–18.

19. Ringden O, Pihlstedt P, Volin L. Failure to prevent cytomegalovirus infection by cytomegalovirus hyperimmune plasma: a randomized trial by the Nordic Bone Marrow Transplant Group. *Bone Marrow Transplant* 1987;2:299–305.

20. Bowden RA, Fisher LD, Rogers K, Cays M, Meyers JD. Cytomegalovirus (CMV)-specific intravenous immunoglobulin for the prevention of primary CMV infection and disease after marrow transplant. *J Infect Dis* 1991;164:483–487.

21. Bowden RA, Sayers M, Flournoy N, et al. Cytomegalovirus immune globulin and seronegative blood products to prevent primary cytomegalovirus infection after marrow transplantation. *N Engl J Med* 1986;314:1006–1010.

22. Sullivan KM, Kopecky KJ, Jocom J, et al. Immunomodulatory and antimicrobial efficacy of intravenous immunoglobulin in bone marrow transplantation. *N Engl J Med* 1990;323:705–712.

23. Condie RM, O'Reilly RJ. Prevention of cytomegalovirus infection by prophylaxis with an intravenous, hyperimmune, native, unmodified cytomegalovirus globulin. Randomized trial in bone marrow transplant recipients. *Am J Med* 1984;March:134–141.

24. Kubanek B, Ernst J, Ostendorf P, Schfer U, Wolf H. Preliminary data of a controlled trial of intravenous hyperimmune globulin in the prevention of cytomegalovirus infection in bone marrow transplant recipients. *Transplant Proc* 1985;XVII:468–469.

25. Winston DJ, Ho WG, Lin C, et al. Intravenous immune globulin for prevention of cytomegalovirus infection and interstitial pneumonia after bone marrow transplantation. *Ann Intern Med* 1987;106:12–18.

26. Bowden RA, Fisher LD, Rogers K, Cays M, Meyers JD. Cytomegalovirus (CMV)-specific intravenous immunoglobulin for the prevention of primary CMV infection and disease after marrow transplant. *J Infect Dis* 1991;164:483–487.

27. Winston DJ, Ho WG, Bartoni K, Champlin RE. Intravenous immunoglobulin and CMV-seronegative blood products for prevention of CMV infection and disease in bone marrow transplant recipients. *Bone Marrow Transplant* 1993;12:283–288.

28. Bowden RA, Slichter SJ, Sayers MH, Mori M, Cays MJ, Meyers JD. Use of leukocyte-depleted platelets and cytomegalovirus-seronegative red blood cells for prevention of primary cytomegalovirus infection after marrow transplant. *Blood* 1991;78:246–250.

29. Sullivan KM, Storek J, Kopecky KJ, et al. A controlled trial of long-term administration of intravenous immunoglobulin to prevent late infection and chronic graft versus host disease after marrow transplantation: clinical outcome and effect on subsequent immune recovery. *Biol Blood Marrow Transplant* 1996;2:44–53.

30. Emanuel D, Taylor J, Brochstein J, et al. The use of intravenous immune globulin as prophylaxis for the infectious complications of allogeneic marrow transplantation. *Blood* 1992;80[Suppl. 1]:271a.

31. Winston DJ, Antin J, Wolff S, et al. Comparative efficacy of different doses of intravenous immunoglobulin for the prevention of graft versus host disease after bone marrow transplantation: results of a multi-center randomized double blind trial. *Blood* 1996;88:302a.

32. Wolff S, Winston DJ, Antin J, et al. Multi-center randomized double-blind dose response trial of IVIG for the prevention of infection after allogeneic bone marrow transplantation. *Blood* 1996;18:303a.

33. Wolff SN, Fay JW, Herzig RH, et al. High-dose weekly intravenous immunoglobulin to prevent infections in patients undergoing autologous bone marrow transplantation or severe myelosuppressive therapy. *Ann Intern Med* 1993;118:937–942.

34. Bass EB, Powe NR, Goodman SN, et al. Efficacy of immune globulin in preventing complications of bone marrow transplantation: a meta-analysis. *Bone Marrow Transplant* 1993;12:273–282.

35. Messori A, Rampazzo R, Scroccaro G, Martini N. Efficacy of hyperimmune anti-cytomegalovirus immunoglobulins for the prevention of cytomegalovirus infection in recipients of allogeneic bone marrow transplantation. A meta-analysis. *Bone Marrow Transplant* 1994;13:163–167.

36. Einsele H, Ehninger G, Steidle M, et al. Polymerase chain reaction to evaluate antiviral therapy for cytomegalovirus disease. *Lancet* 1991;338:1170–1172.

37. Schmidt GM, Horak DA, Niland JC, Duncan SR, Forman SJ, Zaia JA. A randomized, controlled trial of prophylactic ganciclovir for cytomegalovirus pulmonary infection in recipients of allogeneic bone marrow transplants. *N Engl J Med* 1991;324:1005–1011.

38. Goodrich JM, Bowden RA, Fisher L, Keller C, Schoch G, Meyers JD. Ganciclovir prophylaxis to prevent cytomegalovirus disease after allogeneic marrow transplant. *Ann Intern Med* 1993;118:173–178.

39. Goodrich JM, Mori M, Gleaves CA, et al. Early treatment with ganciclovir to prevent cytomegalovirus disease after allogeneic bone marrow transplantation. *N Engl J Med* 1991;325:1601–1607.

40. Forman SJ, Zaia JA. Treatment and prevention of cytomegalovirus pneumonia after bone marrow transplantation: where do we stand. *Blood* 1994;83:2392–2398.

41. Einsele H, Ehninger G, Hebart H, et al. Polymerase chain reaction monitoring reduces the incidence of cytomegalovirus disease and the duration and side effects of antiviral therapy after bone marrow transplantation. *Blood* 1995;86:2815–2820.

42. Siber GR, Leombruno D, Leszczynski J. Comparison of antibody concentrations and protective activity of respiratory syncytial virus immune globulin and conventional immune globulin. *J Infect Dis* 1994;169:1368–1373.

43. Walsh E, Schlesinger JJ, Brandriss MW. Protection from respiratory virus infection in cotton rats by passive transfer of monoclonal antibodies. *Infect Immunol* 1984;43:756–758.

44. Meissner HC, Fulton DR, Groothuis JR. Controlled trial to evaluate protection of high risk infants against respiratory syncytial virus disease by using standard intravenous immune globulin. *Antimicrob Agents Chemother* 1993;37:1655–1658.

45. Groothuis JR, Simoes EAF, Levin MJ. Prophylactic administration of respiratory syncytial virus immune globulin to high risk infants and young children. *N Engl J Med* 1993;329:1524–1530.

46. Couch RB, Englund JA, Whimbey E. Respiratory viral infections in immunocompetent and immunocompromised persons. *Am J Med* 1997;102:2–9.

47. Bowden RA. Respiratory virus infections after marrow transplantation: The Fred Hutchison Cancer Research Center Experience. *Am J Med* 1997;102:27–30.

48. Ljungman P. Respiratory Virus infections in bone marrow transplant recipients: the European perspective. *Am J Med* 1997;102:44–47.

49. DeVincenzo JP, Leombruno D, Soiffer RJ, Siber GR. Immunotherapy of respiratory syncytial virus pneumonia following bone marrow transplantation. *Bone Marrow Transplant* 1996;17:1051–1056.

50. Harrington RD, Hooten TM, Hackman RC. An outbreak of respiratory syncytial virus in a bone marrow transplant center. *J Infect Dis* 1992;165:987–993.

51. Whimbey E, Champlin RE, Englund JA. Combination therapy with aerosolized ribavirin and intravenous immunoglobulin for respiratory syncytial virus disease in adult bone marrow transplant recipients. *Bone Marrow Transplant* 1995;6:393–399.

52. Whimbey E, Englund JA, Couch RB. Community respiratory virus infections in immunocompromised patients with cancer. *Am J Med* 1997;102:10–18.

53. Prince GA, Hemming VB, Horswood RL, Channock RM. Immunoprophylaxis and immunotherapy of respiratory syncytial virus infection in the cotton rat. *Virus Res* 1985;3:193–206.

54. Prince GA, Hemming VG, Horswood RL. Effectiveness of topically administered neutralizing antibodies in experimental immunotherapy of respiratory syncytial virus in cotton rats. *J Virol* 1987;61:1851–1854.

55. Han CS, Miller WE, Haake RJ. Varicella zoster infection after bone marrow transplantation: incidence, risk factors and complications. *Bone Marrow Transplant* 1994;13:277–283.

56. Locksley RM, Flournoy N, Sullivan KM, Meyers JD. Infection with varicella-zoster virus after marrow transplantation. *J Infect Dis* 1985;152:1172–1181.

57. Reed EC, Myerson D, Corey L, Meyers JD. Allogeneic marrow transplantation in patients positive for hepatitis B surface antigen. *Blood* 1991;77:195–200.

58. Locasciulli A, Alberti A, Bandini G, et al. Allogeneic bone marrow transplantation from HBsAg+ donors: a multi-center study from Gruppo Italiano Trapianto di Midollo Osseo (GITMO). *Blood* 1995;86:3236–3240.

59. Samuel D, Muller R, Alexander G, et al. Liver transplantation in European patients with the hepatitis B surface antigen. *N Engl J Med* 1993;329:1842–1847.

60. Burbach GJ, Bienzle U, Neuhaus R, et al. Intravenous or intramuscular anti-HBs immunoglobulin for the prevention of hepatitis B re-infection after orthotopic liver transplantation. *Transplantation* 1997;63:478–480.

61. Terrault NA, Zhou S, Combs C, et al. Prophylaxis of liver transplant recipients using a fixed dose schedule of hepatitis B immunoglobulin. *Hepatology* 1996;24:1327–1333.

62. McGory RW, Ishitani MB, Oliveira WM, et al. Improved outcome of orthotopic liver transplantation for chronic hepatitis B cirrhosis with aggressive passive immunization. *Transplantation* 1996;61:1358–1364.

63. Patel R, Snydman DR, Rubin RH, et al. Cytomegalovirus prophylaxis in solid organ transplant recipients. *Transplantation* 1996;61:1279–1289.

64. Hibberd PL, Tolkoff-Rubin NE, Cosimi AB, et al. Symptomatic cytomegalovirus disease in the cytomegalovirus antibody seropositive renal transplant recipient treated with OKT3. *Transplantation* 1992;53:68–72.

65. Portela D, Patel R, Larson-keller JJ. OKT3 treatment for allograft rejection is a risk factor for CMV disease in liver transplantation. *J Infect Dis* 1995;171:1014.

66. Kasiske BL, Heim-Duthoy KL, Tortorice KL. Polyvalent immune globulin and cytomegalovirus infection after renal transplantation. *Arch Intern Med* 1989;149:2733.

67. Fehir KM, Decker WA, Samo T. Immune globulin (Gammagard) prophylaxis of CMV infections in patients undergoing organ transplantation and allogeneic bone marrow transplantation. *Transplant Proc* 1989;21:3107–3109.

68. Bailey TC, Ettinger NA, Storch GA. Failure of high-dose oral acyclovir with or without immune globulin to prevent primary cytomegalovirus disease in recipients of solid organ transplants. *Am J Med* 1993;95:273–278.

69. Conti DJ, Freed BM, Lempert N. Prophylactic immunoglobulin therapy improves the outcome of renal transplantation in recipients at risk for primary cytomegalovirus disease. *Transplant Proc* 1993;25:1421–1422.

70. Steinmuller DR, Novick AC, Streem SB, Graneto D, Swift C. Intravenous immunoglobulin infusions for the prophylaxis of secondary cytomegalovirus infection. *Transplantation* 1990;49:68–70.

71. Greger B, Vallbracht A, Kurth J. The clinical value of CMV prophylaxis by CMV hyperimmune serum in kidney transplant patients. *Transplant Proc* 1986;18:1387.

72. Fassbinder W, Ernst W, Hanke P. Cytomegalovirus infections after renal transplantation: effect of prophylactic hyperimmunoglobulin. *Transplant Proc* 1986;18:1387.

73. Snydman DR, Werner BG, Heinze-Lacey B, et al. Use of cytomegalovirus immune globulin to prevent cytomegalovirus disease in renal-transplant recipients. *N Engl J Med* 1987;317:1049–1054.

74. Cofer JB, Morris CA, Sutker WL. A randomized double blind study of the effect of prophylactic immune globulin on the incidence and severity of CMV infection in the liver transplant recipient. *Transplant Proc* 1991;23:1525.

75. Saliba F, Arulnaden JL, Gugenbeim J. CMV hyperimmune globulin after liver transplantation: a prospective randomized controlled study. *Transplant Proc* 1989;21:2260.

76. Snydman DR, Werner BG, Dougherty NN, et al. Cytomegalovirus immune globulin prophylaxis in liver transplantation: a randomized, double-blind, placebo-controlled trial. *Ann Intern Med* 1993;119:984–991.

77. Snydman DR, Werner BG, Dougherty NN. A further analysis of the use of cytomegalovirus immune globulin in orthotopic liver transplant patients at risk for primary infection. *Transplant Proc* 1994;26:23.

78. Tsevat J, Syndman DR, Pauker SG, Durand-Zaleski I, Werner BG, Levey AS. Which renal transplant patients should receive cytomegalovirus immune globulin? *Transplantation* 1991;52:259–265.

Subject Index